Clinical Ophthalmology

Clinical Ophthalmology

Edited by

Sir Stephen Miller KCVO MD FRCS
*Civil Consultant Emeritus (Ophthalmology)
Royal Navy; Consulting Ophthalmic
Surgeon, St George's Hospital, London;
King Edward VII Hospital for Officers,
London; the National Hospital, Queen
Square, London; Moorfields Eye Hospital,
London. Formerly Surgeon Oculist to
HM The Queen and to HM Household*

WRIGHT

London Boston Singapore
Sydney Toronto Wellington

Wright
is an imprint of Butterworth Scientific

All rights reserved. No part of this publication may be reproduced or transmitted in any form or by any means, including photocopying and recording, without the written permission of the copyright holder, application for which should be addressed to the Publishers, or in accordance with the provisions of the Copyright Act 1956 (as amended), or under the terms of any licence permitting limited copying issued by the Copyright Licensing Agency, 7 Ridgemount Street, London WC1E 7AE, England. Such written permission must also be obtained before any part of this publication is stored in a retrieval system of any nature.

Any person who does any unauthorized act in relation to this publication may be liable to criminal prosecution and civil claims for damages.

This book is sold subject to the Standard Conditions of Sale of Net Books and may not be re-sold in the UK below the net price given by the Publishers in their current price list.

First published 1987
Reprinted 1988
© **Butterworth & Co. (Publishers) Ltd, 1987**

British Library Cataloguing in Publication Data
Clinical ophthalmology
  1. Ophthalmology
  I. Miller, Stephen J. H.
  617.7   RE46

ISBN 0-7236-0754-0

Printed in Great Britain at
The Bath Press, Avon

Preface

On receiving an invitation from John Wright to edit a textbook on *Clinical Ophthalmology* I consulted some of my colleagues and together we came to the conclusion that the idea had great merit. There seems little doubt that candidates for higher diplomas often fail because of poor technique in writing answers to examination questions. Sometimes they fail because they are unaware of the particular interest of the examiner. This volume should eliminate some failures due to these aspects of inquisition for postgraduate diplomas and higher degrees.

There are two reasons for producing a new textbook in 1987. This is a time of rapid advances in technology, and these are affecting the whole of ophthalmology. It has been possible to invite contributors to this text who, in this decade, are at the peak of their form in ability, energy and experience.

Any editor who undertakes a task of this kind must expect some disappointment; nevertheless the main object of the written script – to bring into the daylight the personal and considered opinion of the super expert on the sub-specialty under discussion – has not been adversely affected.

In ophthalmology, as in medicine generally, the management of a clinical problem presents innumerable options, each with advantages and disadvantages. Although a list of options may help a candidate to answer an examination question it proves of limited value to the surgeon in the face of a crisis which demands an immediate decision.

The various chapters on the different aspects of the practice of ophthalmology declare the bias of surgeons and physicians, who know from experience what line of attack is likely to be successful. Their discussions are compressed and concentrated, eliminating discursive irrelevances, stressing always the important points in diagnosis and therapy. In *Clinical Ophthalmology* the basic principles and elementary techniques are taken for granted and are not described in detail; the subtle insights which separate the skilled from the pedestrian ophthalmologist are there for the taking.

This book fills a gap in the literature for postgraduates who are studying ophthalmology and for those who wish to keep in touch with modern developments.

My thanks are due to the authors who have taken so much trouble to write their chapters along the lines suggested to them by the Editor. It is also a pleasure to have the opportunity to say how helpful the staff of the publisher John Wright has been in piecing together this contribution to postgraduate education in ophthalmology.

S. M.

International Editorial Advisory Board

Professor Desmond B. Archer MB, BCh, FRCS, FRCS(Ed)
Department of Ophthalmology, Queen's Univerisity of Belfast

Professor A. C. Bird MD, FRCS
Professor of Clinical Ophthalmology, Moorfields Eye Hospital, London

Professor F. C. Blodi MD
Department of Ophthalmology, The University of Iowa

Professor Ian Constable
Professor of Ophthalmology, Department of Surgery, Royal Perth Hospital, Perth

Professor Gabriel Coscas
Clinique Ophthalmologique Universitaire de Créteil, Centre Hospitalier Intercommunal, Créteil

Professor Matthew D. Davis MD
Professor and Chairman, Department of Ophthalmology, University of Wisconsin–Madison Medical School

Professor August F. Deutman MD
Institute of Ophthalmology, Sint Radboud Hospital, Nigmegen, The Netherlands

Professor Morton F. Goldberg MD
Department of Ophthalmology, College of Medicine, University of Illinois at Chicago

Dr Arthur S. M. Lim
Chief, Department of Ophthalmology, National University Hospital, Singapore

Professor J. L. Van Selm MB, ChB(UCT) FACS, DOMS, RCP, RCS
Professor and Head of Department, Department of Ophthalmology, Medical School, Cape Town, South Africa

Contributors

Desmond B. Archer BAO, FRCS, FRCSEd
Professor of Ophthalmology, Queen's University of Belfast, Eye and Ear Clinic, Royal Victoria Hospital, Belfast
The Retina
   Macular Disease associated with Elevation of the Retina   223

M. A. Bedford MA, FRCS
Honorary Consultant Oncologist, Moorfields Eye Hospital, London
The Management of Ocular Tumours   352

Alan C. Bird MD, FRCS
Professor of Clinical Ophthalmology, Moorfields Eye Hospital, London
The Retina
   Retinal Receptor Dystrophies   199

R. J. Buckley MA, FRCS
Consultant Ophthalmologist and Director Contact Lens and Prosthesis Department, Moorfields Eye Hospital, London
Methods of Examination
   Specular Microscopy   61
The Cornea   129

G. J. Chader PhD
Laboratory of Vision Research, National Eye Institutes of Health, Bethesda, Maryland, USA
Physiology
   Biochemistry of the Eye   24

A. H. Chignell FRCS
Consultant Ophthalmologist, St Thomas's Hospital, London
The Retina
   Retinal Detachment Surgery   248

C. S. Cockram MB, BS, MRCP
Department of Medicine, Prince of Wales Hospital, Chinese University of Hong Kong
Systemic Diseases and the Eye
   Endocrine Disorders   553

J. R. O. Collin MA, FRCS
Consultant Ophthalmic Surgeon, Moorfields Eye Hospital, London
The Lids: Diseases and Treatment   379

P. I. Condon MCh, FRCS
Consultant Ophthalmic Surgeon, Regional Eye Department, Ardkeen Hospital, Waterford, Ireland
Systemic Diseases and the Eye
   Haematological Diseases   552

Robert J. Cooling FRCS, DO
Consultant Ophthalmic Surgeon, Moorfields Eye Hospital, London
Ocular Injuries   362

S. J. Crews FRCSEd
Consultant Ophthalmologist, Birmingham and Midland Eye Hospital and Dudley Road Hospital, Birmingham
Pharmacology and Toxicology   46

Françoise Cuendet
Hospital for Sick Children, Great Ormond Street, London and the National Institute of Child Health, London; Hopital de l'Enfance, Lausanne, Switzerland
Paediatric Ophthalmology   449

CONTRIBUTORS

T. R. Cullinan MSc, MD, MRCOG
Senior Lecturer in Environmental and Preventive Medicine, St Bartholomew's Hospital Medical College, University of London, and Department of Environmental and Preventive Medicine, St Leonard's Hospital, London
The Epidemiology of Blindness 571

A. M. Denman FRCP
Member of MRC Scientific Staff and Honorary Consultant Physician, Clinical Research Centre, and Northwick Park Hospital, Harrow, Middlesex
Immunology and the Eye
    Immunosuppression 505

C. J. Earl MD, FRCP
Consultant Neurologist, Middlesex Hospital, the National Hospital, Queen Square, London, and Moorfields Eye Hospital, London
The Visual Pathways
    Diseases of the Chiasm and Posterior Visual Pathways 346

W. Ernst
Department of Visual Science, Institute of Ophthalmology, University of London
Physiology
    Retinal Processing of Visual Information 1

Peter Fells MA, FRCS
Consultant Ophthalmologist, Moorfields Eye Hospital, London
Concomitant and Incomitant Squint
    Strabismus 412

T. J. ffytche FRCS
Consultant Ophthalmic Surgeon, St Thomas's Hospital, London, and Moorfields Eye Hospital, London
Methods of Examination
    Fluorescein Angiography 74

R. F. Fisher DSc, PhD, FRCS
Professor of Biophysical Ophthalmology, Institute of Ophthalmology, London, and St Mary's Hospital, London
The Lens
    Pathology of the Crystalline Lens 275

N. R. Galloway MD, FRCS
Consultant Ophthalmologist, Nottingham Eye Hospital
Methods of Examination
    Electrodiagnosis 97

J. S. Glaser
Professor, Departments of Ophthalmology and Neurological Surgery, Bascom Palmer Eye Institute, University of Miami School of Medicine, USA
The Visual Pathways
    Diseases of the Optic Nerve 321

A. M. Peter Hamilton FRCS
Consultant Ophthalmologist, Middlesex Hospital, London
The Retina
    Vascular Retinopathies: The Management of Diabetic Retinopathy 238
    Vascular Retinopathies: The Management of Diabetic Maculopathy 244

Roger A. Hitchings FRCS
Consultant Ophthalmologist, Glaucoma Unit, Moorfields Eye Hospital, London
Glaucoma 304

Lee M. Jampol MD
Professor and Chairman, Department of Ophthalmology, Northwestern University School of Medicine, Chicago, Illinois, USA
The Retina
    Inflammatory Diseases 186

Barrie Jay MA, MD, FRCS
Consultant Surgeon, Moorfields Eye Hospital, London; Dean, Institute of Ophthalmology, University of London
Hereditary Diseases 467

Jack J. Kanski FRCS
Consultant Ophthalmic Surgeon, Prince Charles Eye Unit, King Edward VII Hospital, Windsor, Berkshire; Northwick Park Hospital, Harrow, Middlesex
The Lens
    Cataract Surgery 282

C. M. Kemp BSc, PhD
Department of Visual Science, Institute of Ophthalmology, University of London
Physiology
    Retinal Processing of Visual Information 1

Colin M. Kirkness FRCS(Ed)
Lecturer, Department of Ophthalmology, Institute of Ophthalmology, London
The Lens
    Intraocular Lens Implantation 292

E. Kohner MD, FRCP
Consultant Physician in Medical Ophthalmology, Hammersmith Hospital, London, and Moorfields Eye Hospital, London
The Retina
    Vascular Retinopathies: The Management of Diabetic Retinopathy 238
    Vascular Retinopathies: The Management of Diabetic Maculopathy 244

P. K. Leaver FRCS
Consultant Ophthalmologist, Moorfields Eye Hospital, London
Methods of Examination
    Examination of the Ocular Fundus 70

T. J. K. Leonard MRCP, FRCS
Consultant Ophthalmologist, Charing Cross Hospital, London
Concomitant and Incomitant Squint
    The Ocular Motor System 425

Glyn Lloyd MA, DM, FRCR
Director of the Department of Radiology, Royal National Throat, Nose and Ear Hospital, and Consultant Radiologist, Moorfields Eye Hospital, London
Methods of Examination
    Radiology and the Orbit 87

A. G. A. Lyne FRCS
Consultant Ophthalmic Surgeon, Peterborough Hospital, and Scleritis Clinic, Moorfields Eye Hospital, London
Scleritis 147

David McLeod FRCS
Consultant Ophthalmic Surgeon, Moorfields Eye Hospital, London
The Vitreous and its Disorders 258

Amjad H. S. Rahi PhD, MD, FRCPath
Reader in Immunology, University of London, and Honorary Consultant Pathologist, Moorfields Eye Hospital, London
Immunology and the Eye
    Immunopathology 483

Marie Restori MSc
Senior Physicist, Moorfields Eye Hospital, London
Methods of Examination
    Ultrasonography of the Eye and Orbit 51

R. W. Ross Russell MA, MD, FRCP
Consultant Physician, Department of Neurology, St Thomas's Hospital, London; The National Hospital for Nervous Diseases, London; Moorfields Eye Hospital, London
Systemic Diseases and the Eye
    Carotid Artery Disease and Amaurosis Fugax 524

M. D. Sanders FRCP, FRCS
Consultant Ophthalmologist, National Hospital for Nervous Diseases, and St Thomas's Hospital, London
Concomitant and Incomitant Squint
    The Ocular Motor System 425

G. R. Serjeant MD, FRCP
MRC Laboratories (Jamaica), University of the West Indies, Kingston, Jamaica
Systemic Diseases and the Eye
    Haematological Diseases 552

Janet H. Silver MPhil, FBCO, FBIM
Principal Ophthalmic Optician, Moorfields Eye Hospital, London
The Management of Visual Disability 562

Redmond J. H. Smith MS, FRCS
Consultant Ophthalmic Surgeon, Western Ophthalmic Hospital, London, and St Mary's Hospital, London
Methods of Examination
    Gonioscopy 64

P. H. Sönksen MD, FRCP
Professor of Endocrinology, Department of Medicine, St Thomas's Hospital, London
Systemic Diseases and the Eye
    Endocrine Disorders 533

D. J. Spalton MRCP, FRCS
Consultant Ophthalmic Surgeon, St Thomas's Hospital, London
The Uveal Tract 162

Arthur D. McG. Steele FRCS, FRACO
Consultant Surgeon, Moorfields Eye Hospital, London
The Lens
   Intraocular Lens Implantation 292

David Taylor FRCS
Consultant Ophthalmologist, Hospital for Sick Children, Great Ormond Street, London; the Institute of Child Health, London; the National Hospital for Nervous Diseases, London
Paediatric Ophthalmology 449

S. M. Thompson FRCS, DObst
Senior Registrar, Birmingham and Midland Eye Hospital, Birmingham
Pharmacology and Toxicology 46

P. G. Watson FRCS
Consultant Ophthalmic Surgeon, Addenbrooke's Hospital, Cambridge; Honorary Consultant, Scleritis Clinic, Moorfields Eye Hospital, London
Scleritis 147

Richard A. N. Welham FRCS
Consultant Ophthalmic Surgeon, Moorfields Eye Hospital, London, and Royal Berkshire Hospital, Reading
The Lacrimal Drainage Apparatus 391

J. Williamson MD FRCS
Consultant Ophthalmologist, The Victoria Infirmary and Southern General Hospital, Glasgow
Systemic Diseases and the Eye
   Connective Tissue Disease 516

Peter Wright FRCS
Consultant Ophthalmic Surgeon, Moorfields Eye Hospital, London
External Diseases 107

Contents

Colour Plate Section   facing page 304

1 Physiology

    Retinal Processing of Visual Information   1
    W. Ernst and C. M. Kemp

    Biochemistry of the Eye   24
    G. Chader

2 Pharmacology and Toxicology   46
    S. J. Crews and S. M. Thompson

3 Methods of Examination

    Specular Microscopy   61
    R. J. Buckley

    Gonioscopy   64
    Redmond J. H. Smith

    Examination of the Ocular Fundus   70
    P. K. Leaver

    Fluorescein Angiography   74
    T. J. ffytche

    Ultrasonography of the Eye and Orbit   81
    Marie Restori

    Radiology and the Orbit   87
    Glyn Lloyd

    Electrodiagnosis   97
    N. R. Galloway

4 External Diseases   107
    Peter Wright

5 The Cornea   129
    R. J. Buckley

6 Scleritis   147
    P. G. Watson and A. G. A. Lyne

7 The Uveal Tract   162
    D. J. Spalton

8 The Retina

    Inflammatory Diseases   186
    Lee M. Jampol

    Retinal Receptor Dystrophies   199
    A. C. Bird

    Macular Disease associated with Elevation of the Retina   223
    Desmond B. Archer

    Vascular Retinopathies

        The Management of Diabetic Retinopathy   238
        E. Kohner and A. M. P. Hamilton

        The Management of Diabetic Maculopathy   244
        E. Kohner and A. M. P. Hamilton

    Retinal Detachment Surgery   248
    A. H. Chignell

9 The Vitreous and its Disorders   258
    David McLeod

10 The Lens

    Pathology of the Crystalline Lens   275
    R. F. Fisher

    Cataract Surgery   282
    Jack J. Kanski

    Intraocular Lens Implantation   292
    Arthur D. McG. Steele and Colin M. Kirkness

11 Glaucoma   304
    Roger A. Hitchings

12 The Visual Pathways

    Diseases of the Optic Nerve   321
    Joel S. Glaser

    Diseases of the Chiasm and Posterior Visual Pathways   346
    C. J. Earl

13 The Management of Ocular Tumours   352
    M. A. Bedford

14 Ocular Injuries — 362
Robert J. Cooling

15 The Lids: Diseases and Treatment — 379
J. R. O. Collin

16 The Lacrimal Drainage Apparatus — 391
Richard A. N. Welham

17 Concomitant and Incomitant Squint Strabismus — 412
Peter Fells

The Ocular Motor System — 425
M. D. Sanders and T. J. K. Leonard

18 Paediatric Ophthalmology — 449
Françoise Cuendet and David Taylor

19 Hereditary Diseases — 467
Barrie Jay

20 Immunology and the Eye
Immunopathology — 483
Amjad H. S. Rahi

Immunosuppression — 505
A. M. Denman

21 Systemic Diseases and the Eye
Connective Tissue Disease — 516
J. Williamson

Carotid Artery Disease and Amaurosis Fugax — 524
R. W. Ross Russell

Endocrine Disorders — 533
C. S. Cockram and P. H. Sönksen

Haematological Diseases — 552
P. I. Condon and G. R. Serjeant

22 The Management of Visual Disability — 562
Janet H. Silver

23 The Epidemiology of Blindness — 571
Tim Cullinan

Index — 579

Chapter 1

Physiology

Retinal Processing of Visual Information

W. Ernst and C. M. Kemp

THE ELECTRICAL SIGNAL FROM PHOTORECEPTORS

The electroretinogram (ERG) is the complex waveform of the voltage changes that can be recorded from the front of the eye when it is stimulated by a flash of light, and is a commonly used diagnostic aid in ophthalmology. The first wave of the ERG is known as the a-wave and its leading edge represents the onset of the electrical signal of photoreceptors.

What is the nature of this signal? To answer this question special techniques have to be used to isolate it from the components of the ERG which arise from other cells. One technique involves making local measurements of voltage in the region of the photoreceptors themselves in isolated animal retinae. This shows that in the dark there is an asymmetry between the plasma membrane in the receptor outer segment and the membrane elsewhere. Current flows into the outer segment from other parts of the receptor. The electrical circuit is completed inside the cell with current flowing through the junction between outer and inner segments. A small part of the extracellular dark current spreads to the front of the eye and the voltage associated with it contributes to the standing potential. Light suppresses some or all of the dark current depending on the intensity. Thus the signal of photoreceptors is a decrement of a dark current (*Fig.* 1).

To investigate the mechanisms involved more closely, individual receptors have been isolated either by pulling apart small fragments of retina or with the help of enzymes that digest the intercellular matrix. In some experiments the receptors are impaled with a microelectrode which can monitor the membrane voltage and can also be used to inject current into the cell; sometimes two intracellular electrodes are used, one for each function. In other

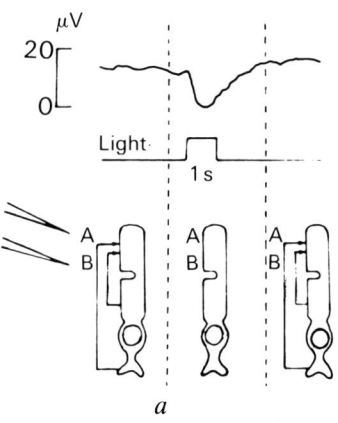
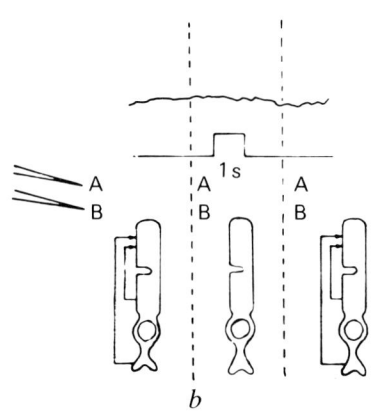

Fig. 1. Light eliminates the dark current of frog rods. In the experiment shown in (*a*), a pair of extracellular microelectrodes (A and B) has been introduced into the outer segment layer of an isolated frog retina viewed under a microscope. The top trace shows the voltage recorded between A and B as a function of time. The trace below indicates when a pulse of bright light is applied to the retina. That the voltage deflection caused by the light corresponds to the elimination of the dark current can be shown by withdrawing the electrode pair to a position outside the outer segments immediately after recording the trace in (*a*). The level of the trace now represents zero current flow between A and B (*b*), and this was the level of the peak of the light-induced deflection when the electrodes were still in the retina (*a*). The diagrams below the traces show what is happening to the current flow around a rod during the various phases of the experiment. More details can be found in Ernst W., Jagger W. S and Baumann C., *Nature* 1974; **248**, 253–5.

experiments a closely fitting micropipette is manoeuvred over the outer segment and the extracellular current flowing through the lumen is measured.

In a particularly elegant study the latter technique has been combined with intracellular recording. Examination of the way membrane current and membrane voltage are related shows that channels in the plasma membrane of the outer segment pass ions in the dark and are blocked by light. The term 'channel'

a rod, can close about 3–5 per cent of the total number of channels when having its peak effect. In the case of cones, the percentage, though about ten times smaller, is still relatively large, if one considers that only a single molecule of visual pigment among several million has absorbed light. Doubling the light intensity doubles the number of channels closed, hence halves the conductance of the plasma membrane, halves the current and doubles the hyperpolar-

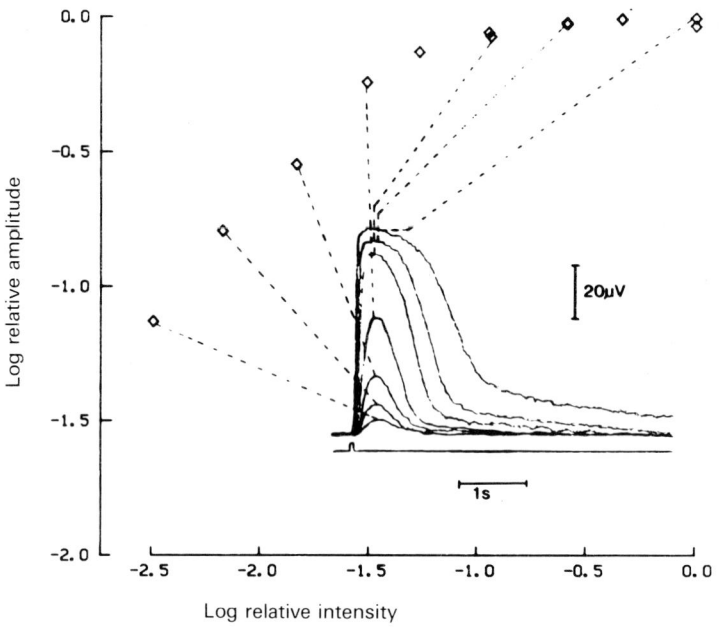

Fig. 2. Photoresponses recorded from baboon retinal rods and a double logarithmic plot showing relative amplitudes of the response peaks as a function of relative light intensity. A dark adapted, isolated, baboon retina was mounted as a membrane between the two compartments of a chamber containing an oxygenated, physiological saline at 37 °C (bicarbonate and Hepes buffer, pH 7·2; 1 mmol calcium ions). Included in the saline were 10 mmol sodium glutamate, which eliminates post-receptoral neuronal photoresponses, and 0·1 mg/ml D-600 (Knoll A. G., Ludwigshafen, W. Germany), which eliminates residual responses from Mueller cells. Light flashes of 40 ms duration (*see* trace below photoresponses) and of 502 nm wavelength, were shone on to the preparation through a window in the side of the chamber. The voltage across the retina was recorded via silver/silver chloride electrodes in electrical contact with the two compartments of the chamber, amplified (0–50 Hz bandpass), digitized and stored on a microcomputer. The responses to the dimmest flashes represent averages of several traces.

is loosely used to mean either a pore or a carrier mechanism. If the voltage across the membrane is measured with an intracellular microelectrode, a value in the region of 30–50 mV negative inside with respect to outside is obtained in the dark and the receptor hyperpolarizes on illumination. In the case of the rod outer segment, the light-sensitive channels account for almost all the conductance of the receptor plasma membrane. Sodium ions are the major current carriers across this conductance. Potassium ions carry most of the dark current across the plasma membrane in other regions. A sodium–potassium exchange pump prevents the concentration gradients for these ions from running down.

Light works in a graded manner. A very dim flash, which leads to no more than 1 photon absorbed by

ization. However, this linear relationship between response amplitude and light intensity has to break down as the number of channels that can be closed starts to run out. Eventually, practically all channels are closed and the response is said to be saturated; in the case of rods, typically a dark current of about 20–50 pA has been eliminated and the membrane has hyperpolarized to about −70 mV.

The relationship between peak response amplitude (A) and the light intensity (I) is approximately of the form:

$$A = I/(I + \text{constant}) \times A_{\max}$$

where $A_{\max}$ is the peak amplitude of a saturated response. *Fig.* 2 illustrates a series of responses to flashes of different intensity recorded as changes in extracellular voltages from baboon rods and the amplitude v. intensity function is shown alongside on a double logarithmic plot. When the value of the light intensity is small compared with the constant, the relationship simplifies to a proportionality between A and I. When the value of the light intensity is very large, the constant can be ignored and A equals its maximum value, A_{max}. When the values of intensity and constant are equal, A is half of A_{max}; the constant is therefore sometimes known as the semi-saturation constant.

The range of the electrical signal of a receptor is limited. The non-linearity in the relationship between amplitude and light intensity helps to expand the range of light intensities which can be signalled. From the point of view of discriminating relative intensity changes, a receptor operating in the non-linear region would be inefficient. Receptors, however, do have mechanisms enabling them to change the semi-saturation constant. In terms of the plot shown in *Fig.* 2, this would involve a shift of the curve to the right along the log intensity axis. Such mechanisms constitute part of the phenomenon of visual adaptation, which is the adjustment of sensitivity to light according to the prevailing conditions of illumination. They enable receptors to cope with large variations of light intensity.

The nature of the relationship between A and I – especially the efficacy of a single photon and the amplification this implies – points to an intermediate mechanism between the absorption of light and the closure of channels in the plasma membrane. An attractive explanation of the relationship is to assume that there is an internal transmitter mediating the flow of information from the visual pigment molecules to the ion channels of the plasma membrane; that the concentration of an internal transmitter varies in proportion to the photons absorbed; that the transmitter combines rapidly and reversibly with a limited number of sites on the plasma membrane; and that membrane conductance depends on the number of transmitter/site complexes. At low light levels the responses to light would then reflect the changes in the concentration of the internal transmitter, but as light intensity increased, the number of sites would become a limiting factor in shaping the responses and determining their amplitude. A_{max} would thus be a measure of the total number of light-controlled channels and the semi-saturation constant a measure of the extent of the change in internal transmitter per unit change of illumination.

Examination of the waveform of the responses to light, especially to dim light, provides further evidence for an intermediate mechanism between the visual pigment and the closure of the ion channels in the plasma membrane. For example, the rod responses of *Fig.* 2 were induced by flashes 40 ms long; yet for weak lights they took tens of milliseconds to develop and lasted more than a second. Such long delays are characteristic of both rods and cones, though cone responses are faster, especially in their decay. The mathematical descriptions of receptor waveforms at low light levels can be plausibly interpreted by assuming that there are three or more distinct steps in the build-up of the internal transmitter and one or more decay steps.

To summarize, the signal from a receptor is unlike one expected from a conventional neurone. Such a neurone signals by means of very brief depolarizations (spikes). The character of the waveform is invariant – the change either occurs or it does not (all-or-none) – and the information being signalled is contained in the number of spikes per unit time. By contrast, in a receptor the information is contained in the waveform of the slow hyperpolarizations, which are graded with light intensity and result from the closure of sodium ion channels in the plasma membrane of the outer segment. A study of these waveforms leads to the suggestion of a number of steps between the absorption of light and the closure of the channels. The mechanisms of transduction involved in these steps will now be examined.

RECEPTOR STRUCTURE

In considering transduction, it will be of value to recall the similarities and differences in the highly specialized structures of rods and cones. In each case the distal region of the cell consists of two segments connected by a narrow ciliary process. The outer segment in both rods and cones is responsible for capturing incident light and transducing it into an electrochemical signal, while the inner segment subserves the energetic and biosynthetic requirements of the cells.

The rod outer segment contains a large number of membranes arranged in an essentially parallel stack, so that these present the maximum surface area to light passing along the axis of the cell. Embedded within the membranes are the visual pigment protein molecules which absorb the light and trigger the process of receptor excitation. The membrane stack at the base of the outer segment is formed by invagination of the plasma membrane, and the pigment, which has been newly synthesized in the inner segment, is inserted into the membrane at this point. A short distance from the base, however, the membranes become pinched off to form closed, flattened vesicles or 'discs' separated from, and surrounded by, the plasma membrane. Like the discs, the plasma membrane contains rhodopsin, but since there are up to 2000 discs within the outer segment, only about 1 per cent of the pigment is located within the plasma membrane. Thus, almost all of the incident light which is absorbed by the outer segment will lead to photoactivation of visual pigment molecules in the discs. It follows that some method is required to transmit the information that a rhodopsin molecule in the disc membrane has absorbed a photon of light to the plasma membrane, where the permeability change then occurs. Hypotheses for this transduction mechanism will be described later.

Cone outer segments are generally both narrower and shorter than those of rods, but the major structural difference between the outer segments of the two cell types lies in the arrangement of the stacks of lamellae, which in the cone comprise a continuously folded single membrane virtually throughout the length of the outer segment. Thus, unlike those of the rod outer segment, almost all the membranes of the cone outer segment are in contact with the extracellular medium. In these receptors, therefore, there is no structural requirement for a messenger substance to signal the absorption of light, since the pigment molecules are themselves in the membrane that undergoes the permeability change. As we have seen, however, considerations based on the amplification of signals and delays in their processing show that cones, like rods, possess an elaborate transduction mechanism.

TECHNIQUES FOR INVESTIGATING VISUAL PIGMENTS

The visual pigments of rods and cones have until recently been characterized chiefly on the basis of their absorption spectra. Various spectrophotometric techniques have been used, each with its own merits and limitations. Early measurements were confined, for technical reasons, to extracts of the pigment solubilized with detergents. More recently, studies have been conducted on isolated, perfused retinae mounted inside the spectrophotometer: these have the virtue that the data obtained approximate more closely to those of the intact eye, but suffer from the drawback that they investigate the averaged behaviour of the pigments of a large number of cells and that any minority component is therefore swamped and remains undetected.

A variant, microspectrophotometry, has been used to examine the contents of individual photoreceptors on a specially adapted microscope. This otherwise powerful technique is limited by the rather noisy data (*see* p. 7) that are inevitably obtained when such small amounts of photosensitive pigment are studied by optical methods; it is impossible to use sufficient light to make high quality measurements, while avoiding bleaching substantial amounts of the pigment under investigation.

A further technique, fundus reflectometry, has been used to examine the visual pigments of living eyes non-invasively. As its name implies, the technique relies on measuring the light levels reflected from the fundus. By comparing these at a series of wavelengths for the fully light adapted eye (i.e., when all visual pigment has been bleached) with those obtained at the same wavelengths following full dark adaptation (when the retina contains its maximum complement of visual pigment), it is possible to construct difference spectra. If it is assumed that the only effect of changing the state of adaptation of the retina on fundal reflectivity is due to the presence or absence of the visual pigments, the difference spectra provide a measure of the pigment amounts and spectral characteristics. In practice, such an assumption has been found to be at least approximately justified, and the method has been used to examine the pigment levels and their distribution in the eyes of both normal humans and those with a variety of abnormalities, affecting primarily either cones (e.g. colour deficiencies) or rods (e.g. retinitis pigmentosa, stationary night blindness, vitamin A deficiency, fundus albipunctatus, Oguchi's disease). Very recently, instruments based on high sensitivity television cameras have been developed which enable the distributions of visual pigments to be mapped in relatively large areas of the retina simultaneously.

STRUCTURE OF THE RHODOPSIN MOLECULE

The visual pigment of rods, rhodopsin, is a membrane-bound glycoprotein, opsin, with a derivative of vitamin A, 11-*cis* retinal, attached as a prosthetic group. The full amino acid sequence of bovine opsin has recently been established and studies on the opsins of other species indicate that these are very similar in structure. Bovine opsin consists of 348 amino acids in a single polypeptide chain to which two carbohydrate side chains (comprising a total of some 11 sugars) are attached.

In addition to its insolubility, many other lines of evidence show that rhodopsin is integral to the disc membrane. For example, proteolysis of the molecule using digestive enzymes, such as papain, removes only part of the polypeptide. The molecule also projects from the membrane, however, both into the intradiscal space (where the N-terminal of the polypeptide and the oligosaccharide side chains are located) and into the cytoplasm. Since the C-terminal has been shown to be in the cytoplasm, it follows that the molecule spans the membrane (and thus could act in a gating fashion to release some small particle from the intradiscal space into the cytoplasm), and further that it spans it an odd number of times. Studies on the α-helical content and the distribution of the hydrophilic amino acids in the polypeptide chain have led to the suggestion that the molecule spans the membrane seven times (*Fig.* 3). Rhodopsin molecules are able to rotate and to move around the disc (but not to undergo 'tumbling'), so that they can interact with other molecules attached to the membrane. The viscosity of the membrane is, in fact, unusually low and reflects its composition, in which there is a high proportion of unsaturated fatty acids and a low cholesterol content.

Vertebrate rhodopsins, which are red, owe their colour to a broad absorbance band spanning the visible region. The spectra of the rhodopsins of almost all species show maximal light absorption close to 500 nm. The ability to absorb visible light results when the protein, which is colourless, combines with the pale yellow 11-*cis* retinal (*Fig.* 4). (In a few species, largely of amphibia and some freshwater fish, the chromophore that is bound to the protein is 11-*cis* didehydroretinal, derived from vitamin with opsin to form rhodopsin, was primarily the result of protonation, and there is now good evidence that this is the case. The site of attachment is fairly specifically tailored to accommodate the 11-*cis* isomer of retinal (although it does allow the formation of artificial pigments – isorhodopsins – with other *cis* forms

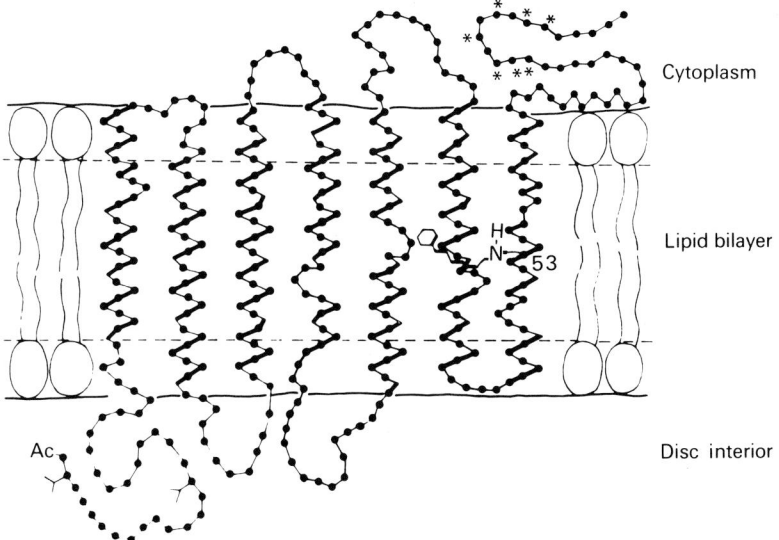

Fig. 3. The conformation of the bovine rhodopsin molecule in the rod disc membrane, which is a lipid bilayer. Each ● represents an amino acid. Also shown are the seven phosphorylation sites (*) near the C-terminal in the cytoplasm, the chromophore, 11-*cis* retinal, and the two oligosaccharides near the N-terminal inside the disc. (Derived from Hargrave P. A. *et al. Biophys. Struct. Mech.* 1983; **9**, 235–44.)

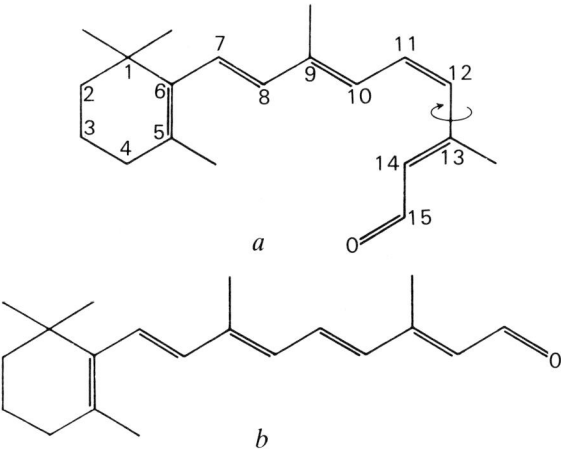

Fig. 4. *a,* The 11-*cis* isomer of retinal. The conformation shown is that which is found in the pure crystalline material. In rhodopsin the molecule may have undergone rotation around the 12–13 bond, as indicated by the arrow. *b,* all-*trans* retinal, the isomer produced by photolysis of rhodopsin.

A_2.) The retinal is attached to the ε-amino group of a lysine amino acid located 53 residues away from the C-terminal, by means of a covalent C–N Schiff base linkage. Schiff bases of retinal behave as indicator molecules, since protonation of the –N– atom causes their absorption spectra to shift to longer wavelengths. This property led to the assumption that the red shift, which occurs when retinal combines

which have a similar effective length). The site is buried within a hydrophobic region of the molecule, as indicated in *Fig.* 3.

RHODOPSIN BLEACHING

When rhodopsin absorbs light, it undergoes a long series of reactions, producing transient intermediates, each of which has different spectral properties. The reactions fall into two groups, the first of which is fast enough to be involved with the signalling processes of the rod, while the second is much too slow (*Fig.* 5). Only the initial reaction, in which rhodopsin is converted to bathorhodopsin, is dependent on light, and there is good evidence that during it the covalently bound 11-*cis* retinal is isomerized to the all-*trans* form (*Fig.* 4).

Bathorhodopsin is formed with very great rapidity (in about a million millionth of a second) and efficiency (about 70 per cent of all quanta absorbed by rhodopsin trigger the reaction). All the other reactions then proceed in both the dark and the light, and can only be prevented by reducing the temperature so that they become 'frozen'. The very rapid reactions (up to the formation of metarhodopsin I) appear to involve, primarily, minor alterations of the protein's internal structure, rather than any gross change to its exterior, such as might be expected if they were crucial for the transduction signal.

In contrast, the formation of metarhodopsin II is accompanied by major conformational changes, with the retinal binding site becoming exposed to the aqueous medium. The time scale of this reaction, which occurs in about a thousandth of a second, together with the major molecular changes it involves, have made it the favourite candidate for the initiation of the transduction process.

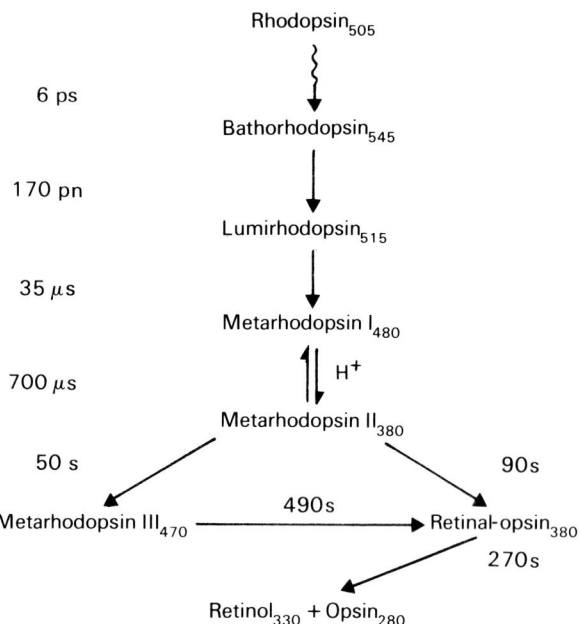

Fig. 5. The photolysis sequence of vertebrate rhodopsin in the intact, isolated retina, determined in conditions where a large fraction of the pigment is bleached. The wavelengths at which each of the intermediates absorb maximally are shown as subscripts and apply to the frog retina; reported values for other species vary slightly. The reaction half-lives are approximate. (Reproduced from Kemp C. M. (1984) *Biological Membranes,* **5,** 4–191, by permission of Academic Press, London).

It has been known for several years that, upon bleaching, rhodopsin becomes a substrate for a kinase enzyme which phosphorylates the protein at several sites close to the carboxyl terminal (*see Fig.* 3). This light-dependent activation is caused by changes in the conformation of rhodopsin itself: it has been shown that the kinase is potentially active in the dark adapted rod but is unable to phosphorylate unbleached pigment molecules. Although the rate at which the phosphorylation takes place was originally thought to be rather slow, there is now evidence that it is metarhodopsin II which is the specific product that acts as substrate for the kinase enzyme.

The decay reaction pathways of metarhodopsin II seem to depend upon the fraction of rhodopsin in the rod which has been bleached: when this is less than about 10 per cent (i.e., in conditions similar to those in which rods function), little or no metarhodopsin III is formed, and the reaction to retinal occurs rapidly. When greater fractions are bleached, a substantial proportion of metarhodopsin III is produced, which in turn decays to retinal. While the decay reactions of metarhodopsin II are too slow to be consistent with their playing a role in the onset of the transduction process, it has been suggested that they may be involved either in switching off the signal or in modifying the sensitivity of the rod.

The final, spectrally observable reaction in the bleaching sequence is the reduction of the all-*trans* retinal to the alcohol, retinol (vitamin A). This reaction is catalysed by a membrane-bound oxidoreductase enzyme within the outer segment.

RHODOPSIN REGENERATION

In order for rhodopsin to be regenerated so that the system is 'recharged', it is clearly necessary for the all-*trans* retinol to be both oxidized back to the aldehyde, and reisomerized to the 11-*cis* form. In retinae separated from the eyecup, these reactions do not occur and it has been established for many years that this is because of their dependence on the presence of the pigment epithelial cells which are normally adjacent to the photoreceptors. The nature of the interaction is still not fully clear: while it is known that the retinol formed as a result of bleaching is efficiently transferred to the pigment epithelium by specific retinoid transport proteins, no isomerase activity has been convincingly demonstrated within these cells. Very recently it has also been suggested that the glial cells may also be involved in the visual cycle, since immunochemical markers indicate that, like the pigment epithelium, these contain substantial quantities of a retinal-binding protein.

Just as the mechanisms underlying rhodopsin regeneration are still poorly understood, so too are the precise details of the time course of the process. Thus, although it has been claimed on the basis of fundus reflectometry data on humans that rhodopsin regeneration can be fitted by a single simple exponential curve, this has not appeared to be true for data obtained from other species (such as the cat), in which the measurements can be made with greater precision. What is clear is that rhodopsin regeneration in man is half complete by about 6 min following the extinction of a light bright enough to have bleached essentially all the pigment, and continues for about 25 min.

CONE PIGMENTS

While rhodopsin has been relatively well characterized, the cone pigments are much less fully documented, for several reasons. Chief amongst these have been the relative paucity of cones in almost all retinae (even in man they account for less than 10 per cent of the receptor population) and the instability of the pigments to *in vitro* treatments such as detergent solubilization, which rhodopsin readily survives. Measurement of their spectral properties in intact cones is also very difficult because of the small dimensions of the outer segments. Good quality spectra have recently been obtained for human cone pigments (*Fig.* 6), however, which indicate that the peak absorbance wavelengths of the 'blue-', 'green-' and 'red-'sensitive cones lie at about 435, 535 and 560 nm, respectively. The relative sizes of the populations of the three types of cells are not well established, though several lines of evidence indicate that blue-sensitive cones are much the least prevalent.

Human colour vision varies in sensitivity with wavelength in a manner which represents the summation of the spectral properties of the individual pigments, and is maximal at about 535 nm.

Although less universally established across species, it is generally assumed that the cone pigments are based on the covalent linkage of 11-*cis* retinal to proteins, the structures or conformations of which vary to account for the spectral variations of the pigments they form. (As in the case of rod pigments, there are some species in which the chromophoric group is based on the aldehyde derivative of vitamin A_2.) As yet the molecular details of the cone pigment proteins remain obscure.

CONE VISUAL CYCLE

Just as there is little information on the molecular properties of the cone pigments, so there are few data on the reactions of the visual cycle which they undergo. To date no convincing spectra for the intermediate products of bleaching have been described, though there is indirect evidence that such products exist. Because of the faster response characteristics of cone cells relative to that of rods, any intermediates occurring prior to, or giving rise to, transduction would be expected to be very short lived.

A major difference between the cone pigments and rhodopsin lies in their rates of regeneration following bleaching. In the human retina, cone pigment recovery following extensive bleaching is half complete in less than 2 min. It is also inferred from data on other species that the recovery of human cone pigments does not depend on the presence of the pigment epithelium, and can occur in the isolated receptor. This assumption appears to be borne out by microspectrophotometry, which has shown that cones obtained from light adapted human retinae contain substantial quantities of their pigment.

THE BIOCHEMISTRY OF TRANSDUCTION IN RODS

The characteristics of transduction in rods are well enough documented electrophysiologically that it is possible to define several criteria which must be met by any reaction scheme which is proposed to underly it. Thus, it must be able to account for the rapidity with which the permeability of the plasma membrane is modified following the absorption of light, the onset of which occurs within a tenth of a second. It must also account for the size of the change: given that absorption of a single photon leads to closure of at least 100 of the light modulated channels, a large amplification is required. The size and waveform of successive responses to absorptions of single photons do not vary, in contrast to what would be expected if they were the result of a simple diffusion limited process. Moreover, the time course of the rod's response is rather complex, with an S-shaped delay before its onset which shortens with increasingly intense light stimulation. This latency implies that a sequence of reactions is involved in the process, and is again evidence against a simple diffusion process. These delaying reactions do not have time courses that correspond to spectrally observable steps in the rhodopsin bleaching sequence.

Over the past decade or so, two basic models have been developed, one of which is centred on the

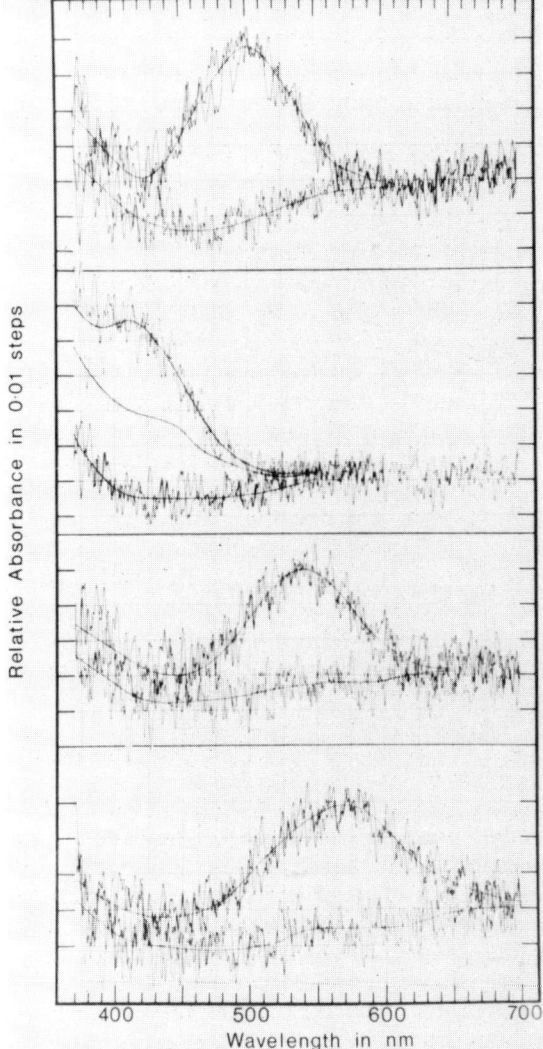

Fig. 6. The spectra of human visual pigments, obtained by microspectrophotometric measurements on individual photoreceptors. From top to botton the curves illustrate rhodopsin and the pigments of the blue-, green- and red-sensitive cones. (Reproduced from Bowmaker J. and Dartnall H. J. A. *J. Physiol (Lond.)*, 1980, **298**, 501–11.)

calcium ion, and the other on the cyclic nucleotide: 3′,5′-guanosine monophosphate (cGMP). Each of the schemes explains a section of the data, but equally each has problems; recently there has been a trend towards integrating elements of both into a combined model.

The calcium hypothesis is based on the fact that the disc membranes of the rod have a large amount of this ion associated with them, while the intracellular concentration of the free ion is four orders of magnitude lower. Calcium is known to be closely

series of well-documented reactions in the rod outer segment, which are initiated by light absorption by rhodopsin, and lead to changes in the intracellular concentration of cGMP. In the dark, the level of cGMP is over 50 μM, much higher than in most cells; light exposure of the cell causes this to drop substantially. As each rhodopsin molecule passes through its bleaching reaction sequence, it has been shown to trigger the exchange of GTP from the cytosol with bound GDP from many molecules of a protein also loosely bound to the disc membranes (*Fig.* 7). Thus

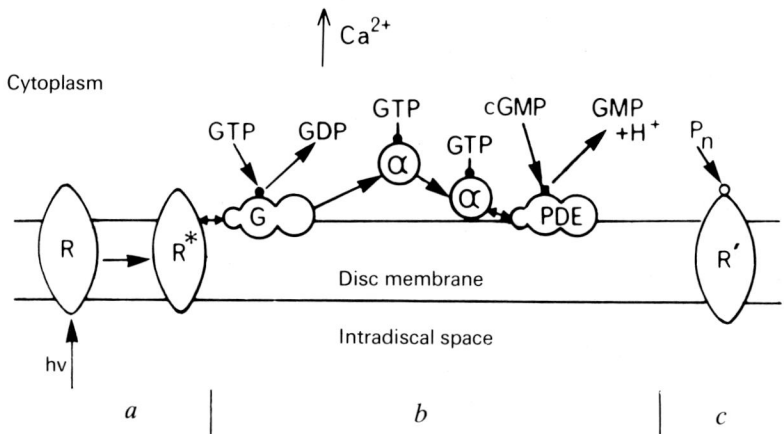

Fig. 7. The reactions triggered by rhodopsin bleaching which affect cGMP. Section (*a*) shows the light-induced conversion of rhodopsin (R) into the active form (R*) and the activation of the G-protein (G) which is trimeric and loosely bound to the disc membrane. Following the GTP/GDP exchange which occurs when the G-protein is active, the α subunit of the molecule dissociates from the membrane and subsequently interacts with and activates the trimeric cGMP phosphodiesterase (PDE) protein (section *b*). The phosphorylation of photolysed rhodopsin (R′) is shown in section (*c*). (Derived from Kemp C. M. *Biological Membranes*, 1984; **5**, 4–191, by permission of Academic Press, London.)

associated with changes in membrane properties so that the notion that it is released into the cytoplasm provides a plausible basis for the subsequent closure of the sodium ion channels in the plasma membrane. Moreover, electrophysiological experiments have shown that it is possible to mimic the effects of light and darkness on the output of the rod by manipulating the concentrations of calcium. The major problem of the model has been the difficulty of demonstrating that a release of calcium ions from the discs actually occurs following light exposure. Recent *in vitro* experiments, however, in which elaborate efforts have been made to ensure the tissue is kept metabolically active, do appear to establish that there is a substantial change in the extracellular concentration of the ion around the rod following light stimulation, implying that there is a mechanism for pumping out from the cell calcium which has been released from the discs.

Recent experiments, moreover, show a fall in intracellular calcium concentration with illumination. Also calcium buffering agents introduced into rods do not have the effects expected of them, if calcium ions were the internal messenger.

The major alternative hypothesis is based upon a

the absorption of a single photon leads to an amplified biochemical change in the outer segment. This GTP/GDP exchange protein (termed transducin, the G-protein, the gamma-protein or the 'helper' protein) is inactive when bound to GDP, but when replacement with GTP occurs, it in turn activates a second protein, the phosphodiesterase (PDE), which catalyses the conversion of cGMP to GMP.

There are therefore several stages of amplification in this overall reaction sequence, since the PDE is capable of hydrolysing large numbers of cGMP molecules. Even so, it has still been questioned whether the actual changes of cGMP which occur in intact rods following illumination are large enough to be compatible with this molecule's being the transduction messenger. While the reactions have been shown to be very fast in *in vitro* experiments, there are also doubts that they occur sufficiently rapidly in more physiological circumstances to account for the time scale over which transduction is initiated. Some of the problems disappear if it is assumed that the free cytoplasmic cGMP is only a part of the total normally measured.

There is evidence that changes in cGMP content within the rod cause changes to the plasma membrane consistent with its proposed role of internal messenger. Application of cGMP to the cytoplasmic side of excised patches of plasma membrane causes an increase in the membrane conductance. Experiments in which cGMP is applied to the inside of a truncated rod outer segment show that the cGMP conductance in the plasma membrane is suppressible by light, provided that GTP is present.

The picture has been further complicated by the demonstration that another light-dependent reaction in the outer segment results in the release of the sugar, inositol triphosphate, from the phospholipid, phosphotidyl inositol, which is a component of the disc membrane. Electrophysiological experiments have shown that modulating inositol triphosphate levels gives results consistent with its being the transmitter, at least in invertebrate photoreceptors.

RECEPTOR ADAPTATION

The limited extent over which receptors can vary the size of their electrical signals implies they would have a correspondingly limited operating range of illumination. However, this is supplemented by their ability to vary their sensitivity in order to follow changes in the prevailing light conditions. In light adaptation, the decrease in sensitivity which accompanies increased illumination occurs rapidly, and a new operating range is established within seconds.

By contrast, full dark adaptation in man can take nearly an hour, though in circumstances where the decrease in light levels is moderate, the necessary dark adaptation is completed within a minute or so. Dark adaptation of cones is more rapid than that of rods, as is evident from the familiar biphasic time course characteristic of human dark adaptation (*Fig.* 8, dashed curve). Thus, the increase in sensitivity, i.e. fall in threshold, which occurs during the first 3 or 4 min in darkness following intense light adaptation is due to the recovery of the cones, When this is complete, the sensitivity remains at a steady level for several minutes, while the rods are still less sensitive than the cones. After between 8 and 15 min in the dark, a new phase of dark adaptation begins as the rods become the more sensitive receptors and therefore determine the visual threshold.

As a result of the different absorption spectra of rhodopsin and the cone pigments, a shift in spectral sensitivity occurs (frequently termed the Purkinje shift), with blue light becoming relatively more effective than red in producing a response compared with the early phase. The extent to which the rod phase of adaptation appears to increase sensitivity over that of the cones therefore depends on the colour of the test stimulus used to monitor it. The retinal location and the size of the stimulus are also important. With a small spot of deep red light in the near peripheral visual field, no rod branch is apparent in the dark adaptation curve; the red sensitive cone pigment is always more sensitive than rhodopsin. Likewise, in the rod-free foveola no rod component is seen, no matter what the spectral composition of the stimulus. By contrast, in the mid and far periphery, where rods are numerous and cones are sparse, large spots, even if they are deep red, will always produce a rod component in the dark adaptation curve of a normal observer.

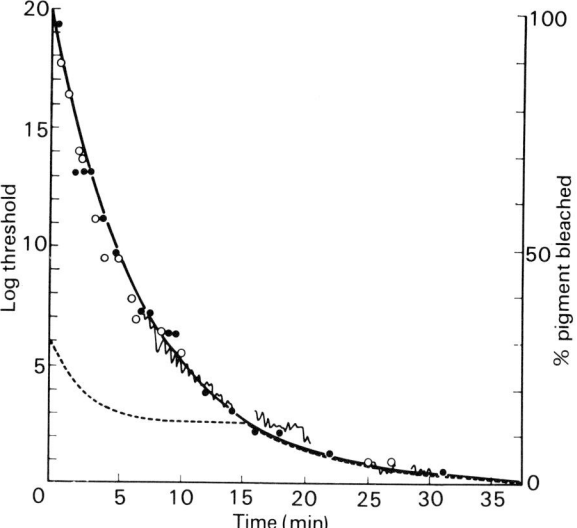

Fig. 8. Dark adaptation of an observer who has rod but no cone function (rod monochromat). the wavy trace is the course of the observer's dark adaptation after a full bleach over a range of about 6 log units (scale on left). The dashed line shows dark adaptation in normal observers, with thresholds determined by the cones for the first 15 min and then by rods for the remaining 25. The rod phase of the normal observer's curve coincides with the tail end of the rod monochromat's. The regeneration of rhodopsin (scale on right) follows a parallel time course in the monochromat (●) and normal observer (○). (Reproduced from Rushton W. A. H., *Handbook of Sensory Physiology* VII/I, 1972, pp. 364–94, by permission of Springer-Verlag, Berlin.)

The mechanisms which underlie dark adaptation are still unknown, but it is clear that a simple explanation based on the availability of visual pigment to absorb photons can be excluded. If this were the case, then when half the complement of pigment was bleached by the prevailing light, the probability of absorption of incident photons, and therefore the sensitivity of the receptor, would be expected to be approximately halved from the fully dark-adapted level. In fact, direct measurement has shown that such a degree of light adaptation is caused by a background light which causes only a very small fraction of the pigment to bleach. Further evidence that the availability of visual pigment does not limit the sensitivity of the receptor, when it is partially adapted, has been obtained from measurements of the levels of rhodopsin in human rods during dark adaptation (*Fig.* 8), since it is well established that their sensitivity is still depressed by a factor of about a thousand when 90 per cent of the visual pigment has regenerated.

A simple empirical relationship has been proposed, linking sensitivity to the visual cycle, i.e., the logarithm of the threshold elevation of the rod is proportional to the fraction of rhodopsin bleached. The data in *Fig.* 8 point to such a relationship. Further, the notion that recovery of sensitivity depends directly on the disappearance of bleached products is supported by the observation that in people with systemic vitamin A deficiency resulting in a reduced rate of scotopic dark adaptation (*Fig.* 9), rhodopsin regeneration is also slower than normal.

for why rhodopsin regeneration and recovery of sensitivity normally run in parallel but can be disassociated, a fact which implies a complex relationship. For example, it has been suggested that the presence of one or more of the intermediate products of rhodopsin bleaching causes substantial desensitization of the rod. The disappearance of the intermediates would influence both rhodopsin regeneration and sensitivity recovery. However, no single, spectrally

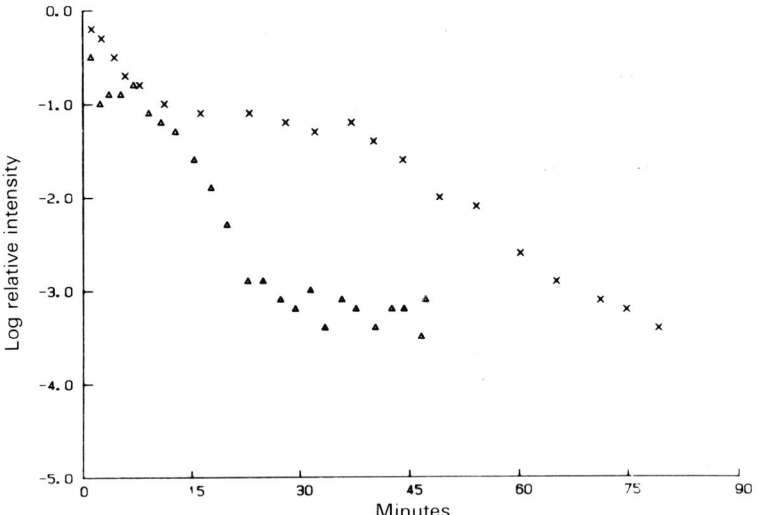

Fig. 9. Dark adaptation in vitamin A deficiency. A patient with primary biliary cirrhosis was given oral doses of vitamin A after initially showing no signs of rod function. Data were obtained 7 days after the treatment was started ($\triangle$) and the serum vitamin A level was 1 μmol l^{-1}. The progress of dark adaptation and the final rod threshold were within normal limits. Rhodopsin regeneration, measured by fundus reflectometry, was also normal. Subsequently the treatment was temporarily stopped: 15 days later the serum vitamin A level fell to 0·5 μmol l^{-1}. The second set of data (X) indicate an abnormally slow dark adaptation. Rhodopsin regeneration was also slowed. The data in both experiments are thresholds for detecting a small flashing spot of green light subtending 0·9° and presented at an eccentricity of 25° in the nasal visual field after a bright flash which bleaches extensive amounts of the visual pigment. (More details can be found in Walt R. P., Kemp C. M., Lyness L. *et al. Br. Med. J.* 1984; **288**, 1030–1.)

There are quantitative grounds, however, for questioning whether the relationship is truly a simple one. Clearly, in the extreme case when *all* the pigment has been bleached, the logarithmic relationship cannot hold, since it predicts a finite threshold elevation although the rod no longer has any rhodopsin to absorb incident light. Detailed study of the relationship in rods where relatively small fractions of pigment (less than 10 per cent) have been bleached likewise suggests that the relationship fails: the observed threshold elevation is larger than it would predict. Also in some observers the time constant for dark adaptation is nearly twice as long (11 min) as any reported value for the regeneration of rhodopsin (6 min). Finally, there are conditions, such as fundus albipunctatus disease, where there is a breakdown between rhodopsin regeneration, which occurs slowly, but is complete long before the recovery of sensitivity, which takes several hours to reach completion.

Several schemes have been proposed to account

identifiable intermediate qualifies for the role of desensitizing product. Both calcium and cGMP have also been involved in schemes explaining adaptation with the assumption that their levels are related to the visual cycle and are critical in regulating sensitivity. In yet another scheme, the phosphorylation of rhodopsin has been associated with rod light adaptation, and the subsequent dephosphorylation, which occurs *in vivo* with a time course similar to that of rhodopsin regeneration, has been proposed to underlie dark adaptation. For the moment, however, these proposals are all speculative and the relationship between sensitivity and the visual cycle is still obscure.

SYNAPTIC TRANSMISSION AND VOLTAGE-DEPENDENT MECHANISMS

The information that photons have been absorbed needs to be transmitted from receptors to the second-order neurones, the horizontal and bipolar cells. We have seen that light causes a hyperpolarization of the plasma membrane and this will include the membrane in the synaptic terminals of the receptor. If receptor synapses are like those of other neurones, calcium ions will enter them through channels which are controlled by the plasma membrane voltage; entry will be maximal when the membrane is relatively depolarized and will diminish with hyperpolarization; exocytosis of a chemical transmitter will be dependent on calcium entry. Thus, the effect of light, because it causes a membrane hyperpolarization, will be to reduce or stop the release of transmitter. Such a view accords with observations on how second-order neurones are affected by agents that normally block synapses, such as cobalt ions; their application is equivalent to bright light.

The mechanism just described requires a voltage-gated mechanism which passes calcium ions at the dark membrane potential but is deactivated by hyperpolarization. The existence of voltage-gated calcium channels outside the rod outer segment can be demonstrated by studying rods which have lost their outer segments. These are first superfused with a medium containing calcium ions and then one in which the calcium is replaced by cobalt. The cobalt ions block the calcium channels. For each medium the relationship between current and voltage is measured and the difference represents the properties of the calcium channels. (Steps are taken to block other voltage-gated channels, which would make the interpretation of the data more complicated.) It turns out that at the rod dark potential there is a constant small entry of calcium ions into the cell but that this is abolished by hyperpolarizations beyond about $-50\,\text{mV}$. Such a mechanism, if it exists at the rod synapses, could therefore be mediating the control of transmitter release by light-induced hyperpolarization.

The calcium mechanism is not the only set of voltage-gated channels in the rod. The existence of other mechanisms can be demonstrated by the technique of voltage clamping with intracellular microelectrodes: any small deviation from a given membrane potential is detected and counteracted by current injection. During illumination the changes in the injected current will therefore equal the changes in membrane current, but at a constant voltage, so that the voltage-gated mechanisms will not contribute. *Fig.* 10 (A) shows such current waveforms for various light intensities in an experiment on a salamander rod. By contrast, when there is no clamp and the experiment is repeated, the voltage waveforms of *Fig.* 10 (B) are obtained. In the second case the voltage-gated mechanisms are allowed to act and their effect is most marked for lights at the higher intensities which produce the greatest hyperpolarizations. Then the voltage waveform consists of a transient peak (sometimes called a 'nose'), followed by a plateau phase at a less negative level, followed in turn by recovery to the dark level. The explanation for this complexity is that, after a delay, the primary hyperpolarization activates, or 'gates', a secondary response which acts in the opposite direction; the observed waveform is a superposition of the two effects.

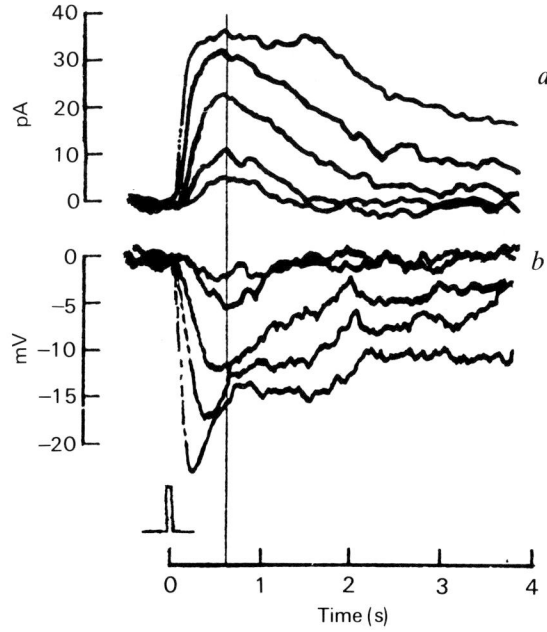

Fig. 10. Changes in the membrane current of an isolated salamander rod elicited by flashes of different intensities (A) are compared with the rod's normal voltage responses when the flash series was repeated (B). In A the membrane voltage was clamped at the dark level ($-47\,\text{mV}$). In B the responses were changes from this dark level. Traces for five intensities are superimposed. Response amplitude increases with flash intensity. Each intensity step represents a fourfold increase. The timing of a flash is indicated below the records. A vertical line has been drawn through the peak amplitudes of responses to dim flashes. (Reproduced from Bader C. R. Macleish P. R. and Schwartz E. A., *J. Physiol. (Lond.)* 1979; **296**, 1–26.)

The exact role of the voltage-gated mechanisms is still a matter of speculation: the calcium channels may directly control transmitter release; the other channels may play a regulatory part by bringing back the membrane voltage to levels at which further changes can be optimally signalled by the synapse; they may also help prevent instability of membrane voltage; they certainly shape the input to the synapse by emphasizing the onset of responses (the 'nose') and, as we shall see, they modify responses to spatial variations of light intensity. Their existence is a reminder that the traditional view of the receptor as a light transducer has to be complemented by recognizing its role as an active processor of information.

COUPLING BETWEEN RECEPTORS

The information processing carried out by receptors is emphasized by their electrical coupling to one another. This can be demonstrated by injecting current into one receptor and recording a voltage change in a neighbour and then injecting current into the neighbour and observing the voltage change in the first receptor. The passage of current survives the presence of extracellular cobalt ions, which block chemical synapses, and the effects can be quantitatively modelled by assuming an electrical network of receptors linked by passive resistances. Another way of showing coupling is to move a slit of light across the retina while recording from a single receptor. When the slit falls on distant receptors, a hyperpolarization is induced in the impaled cell and the effect is too large to be explained in terms of scattered light. *Fig.* 11 shows the result of such an experiment on a turtle cone. It leads to the idea of a receptive field. This is the property of a single neurone, in the present case a receptor. The receptive field of a cell is the area of retina whose stimulation influences the cell's responses.

The anatomical basis of inter-receptor coupling may be processes arising from the synaptic region, which make close contact with one another, or processes at the level of the inner limb. Inter-rod and inter-cone coupling has been demonstrated physiologically in a number of species and the anatomical basis for coupling appears to exist in primate retinae. Usually rods are coupled to other rods and cones of a particular type to similar cones, but in some cases cross-talk has been demonstrated.

Spatial resolution is downgraded by coupling: what then are its beneficial effects? To answer this question we need to introduce the idea of 'noise'. In the context of the visual neurones, the term is applied to events that produce changes in activity which look like those normally elicited by light but arise independently. For example, in receptors visual pigment molecules can bleach spontaneously: such bleaching events are not distinguishable from absorptions of photons. Another example might be fluctuations in the concentration of the receptor internal transmitter. The effect of coupling is that receptors will average their signals. Since the noise arising in one receptor is independent of the noise in another, averaging will tend to produce a flat baseline of activity against which the light-induced changes, which occur synchronously in the coupled receptors, can be more readily distinguished. However, for spots of light much smaller than the receptive field, coupling weakens the light-induced signal by dissipating it to the unstimulated receptors. Thus for the optimal effects of coupling in enhancing the signal to noise ratio, the number of rods coupled must be matched to the average size of the retinal image being detected.

How far hyperpolarization spreads from illuminated to unilluminated receptors depends on the relative values of the transmembrane and inter-receptor conductances. The presence of voltage-gated mechanisms complicates matters because their activation after a delay increases the transmembrane conductance. The initial phase of the light response propagates further than the phase after the mechanisms have become involved. Thus, the combination of coupling and voltage-gated mechanisms modifies the responses of receptors both in time and in space.

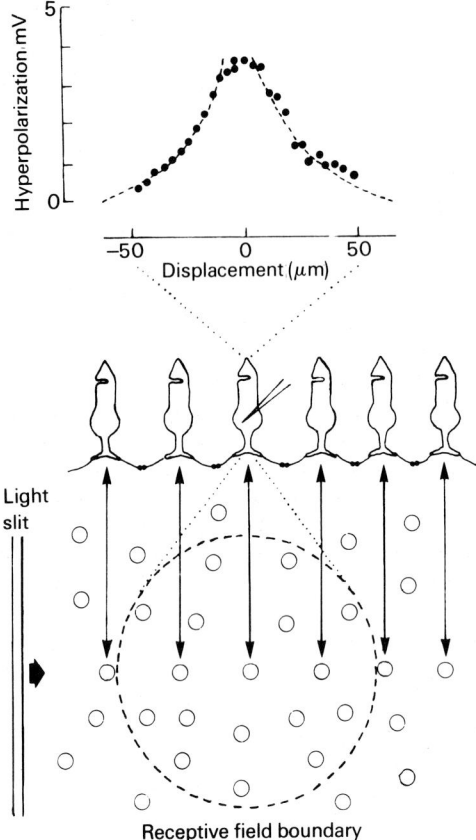

Fig. 11. Results of an experiment (*top*) providing evidence for coupling between cones in the turtle retina. (Adapted from Lamb T. D. and Simon E. J. (1976) *J. Physiol (Lond.)* **263**, 257–86.) A cone was impaled with a microelectrode and a slit was flashed at various positions on the retina. When the slit was centred over the impaled cone (0 μm displacement), a peak hyperpolarization of more than 3 mV was recorded. When the slit was displaced to either side, flashes elicited smaller hyperpolarizations, but these were still significant beyond the point where appreciable amounts of scattered light would fall on the impaled cone. *Middle:* the impaled cone and its neighbours along the axis of the slit displacement. The cones are shown linked to explain the spread of hyperpolarization. *Bottom:* a transverse view of the same (*see arrows*) and other cones. On the assumption of symmetry of connections, the dashed circle has been drawn to define the boundaries of the receptive field of the impaled cone.

PARALLEL FUNCTIONAL PATHWAYS IN THE RETINA

Before dealing with the detailed properties of each type of retinal neurone, it is helpful to take an overview of how information is passed through the retina. The turtle retina illustrates the main features of organization common to most vertebrate retinae and has the advantage that most of its cell types have been extensively studied. *Fig.* 12 shows a section through the retina and the responses to illumination of the neurones beyond the receptors. Generally, light falling anywhere in the receptive field of a receptor elicits a hyperpolarization. Beyond the receptors, however, it becomes common to find complex receptive fields owing to lateral interactions which can be both additive and subtractive. We shall therefore first consider what happens when small spots of light are centred on the receptive fields of the various neurones.

The bipolar cells can be divided into two functional types: those which hyperpolarize to the light, like the receptors, and those which do the opposite and depolarize. Both types produce sustained, graded responses. The hyperpolarizing bipolar cells synapse with ganglion cells in the outer part of the inner plexiform layer and cause these cells to hyperpolarize to light. The ganglion cells are the first neurones in the retina to transmit information by action potentials. Because such potentials are triggered by depolarization, in these cells spikes can be detected in the absence of illumination while, when light is shone, spike production is reduced or ceases. The depolarizing bipolars synapse with ganglion cells in the inner part of the inner plexiform layer and cause these cells to depolarize to light. Their spike production therefore occurs during illumination. Thus 'off' ganglion cells are 'switched off' by light and 'on' by dark, while the 'on' cells are 'switched on' by light and 'off' by dark. The 'off' and 'on' tags are also sometimes applied to the hyperpolarizing and depolarizing bipolar cells, respectively. From the level of the bipolar cells onward, the visual system has parallel 'on' and 'off' pathways. This may represent one solution to the restricted number of signalling levels available to a neurone; if there are two pathways for each part of the retinal image, one for signalling changes below the mean light level and the other for those above, the range of intensity changes that can be covered is doubled.

There are two main cell types which promote lateral interaction – horizontal cells in the outer plexiform layer and amacrine cells in the inner plexiform layer. The main response to light of horizontal cells is a graded hyperpolarization (*see Fig.* 13). They introduce a subtractive effect to the message transmitted to the bipolar cells (lateral inhibition). Thus an annulus of light in the receptive field of a bipolar cell may cause the cell to reverse its usual behaviour, so that a cell hyperpolarizing to small central spots of light will now depolarize, while a depolarizing bipolar cell will hyperpolarize.

This behaviour is carried forwards to the respective ganglion cells. The receptive fields of bipolar and ganglion cells are said to show centre–surround antagonism. Such antagonism means that a neurone will signal the difference between the local intensity at the field centre and the mean intensity across the field. Whereas the spatial pattern of receptor activity corresponds approximately to the variations of absolute intensity across the retina, the pattern seen in the bipolar cells and beyond is one of local deviations from mean intensities. Such a transformation increases the dynamic range of the neurones, allows an improvement in signal to noise ratio and eliminates redundancies in the intensity information, because relative changes rather than absolute values are signalled. It may also be the case that the transformation is a useful step towards higher level processing, for if we consider the whole array of bipolar cells or ganglion cells, then the maximum activity will be observed in those cells with receptive field centres in regions where intensity changes most

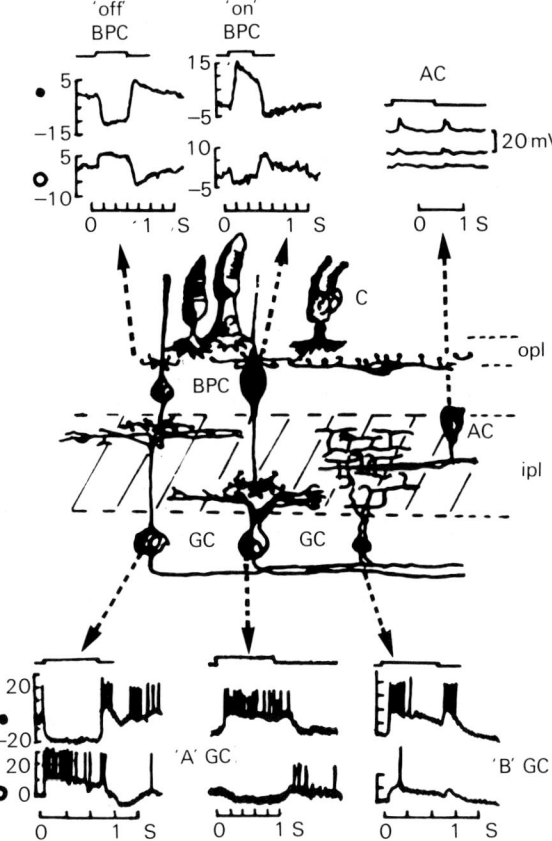

Fig. 12. Schematic drawing of the turtle retina, as seen in a radial section with representative responses of the various cell types excluding receptors. The labels 'opl' refer to the outer plexiform and 'ipl' to the inner plexiform layer. The label 'C' is associated with a cone, 'BPC' with two bipolar cells, 'AC' with an amacrine cell and 'GC' with three ganglion cells. The dashed arrows point to the responses obtained from these cells. For each cell the upper traces were obtained with a central spot and the lower ones with annular illumination. Stimulus duration is indicated above the records. The cells to the left-hand side belong to the 'off' pathway, depolarizing when a central spot goes off; the middle cells belong to the 'on' pathway, depolarizing when a central spot goes on. The behaviour of cells in both pathways reverses when annular illumination is used; responses are always sustained. The cells to the right-hand side depolarize both when the spot goes on and when it goes off. They do not show reversal of behaviour with annular illumination; responses die away after the onset or offset of stimulation. (Adapted from Marchiafava P. L., Weiler R. and Strettoi E. *The Physiology of Excitable Cells*, 1983, pp. 549–55, by permission of Alan R. Liss Inc, New York.)

sharply. Thus an edge of an object would be an effective stimulus and it may be that higher level processing, which has to produce the recognition of objects, is facilitated by having the intensity picture decomposed into 'edges' and 'blobs'. The existence of separate 'on' and 'off' pathways provides the means of signalling the direction of the intensity change.

The interposition of amacrine cells in the inner plexiform layer leads to a distinction between cells that respond in a sustained manner to illumination, such as all the ones we have considered so far, and those that respond only at the onset and/or offset of illumination, such as the amacrine cell illustrated in *Fig.* 12 and the 'B' type ganglion cell, which receives input from it. Thus, from the amacrine cell layer onwards there are parallel pathways of neurones with sustained (tonic) and transient (phasic) responses. The former pathway may be important in signalling luminance changes in the retinal picture, while the latter may provide the information necessary for such tasks as movement detection.

Horizontal Cells

The horizontal cell is the retinal interneurone which establishes centre–surround antagonism in the visual system. It does this by exerting a subtractive influence on the activity of cones. The turtle retina provides an intensively studied example of the mechanisms involved.

The existence of a negative feedback route from horizontal cells to cones is suggested by a comparison of the waveforms of the two types of cell when small and large spots of light are shone on the retina. The response of a cone to a large spot includes a prominent depolarizing inflection approximately coinciding with the peak of the horizontal cell hyperpolarization (*Fig.* 13); this is absent in the cone response to a small spot, which elicits only a small response from a horizontal cell. A more direct piece of evidence comes from injecting hyperpolarizing current into a horizontal cell and observing a depolarization in a neighbouring cone (*Fig.* 13*b*). Experiments with blocking agents suggest that a chemical synapse is involved. In the dark the cones release a transmitter which keeps the horizontal cells relatively depolarized and presumably leads to the release of their transmitter to the cones. This transmitter, however, has a hyperpolarizing action on the cone membrane, so that when light causes the reduction of release from both cones and horizontal cells, there is a tendency for the cones to depolarize. Thus the synapse from cones to horizontal cells is sign-preserving in terms of the polarity of the response to light (hyperpolarization leads to hyperpolarization), while the synapse from horizontal cells to cones is sign-inverting (hyperpolarization leads to depolarization).

Fig. 14 shows a diagram of a cone pedicle in the turtle retina. There are invaginations with a ridge of cone cytoplasm containing a synaptic ribbon and because of the presence of synaptic vesicles near these ribbons it is supposed that here the cone membrane is presynaptic to the horizontal cell processes that come into the invagination (proximal junction). Sometimes two cell processes are present on either side of the ridge to form a dyad; sometimes there is a third process at the base (possibly from a bipolar cell) to form a triad. Away from the proximal junctions are other specialized contacts between the cones and the horizontal cell processes (distal junctions), which may be the site of the feedback synapses, though the evidence is not clear on this point. There

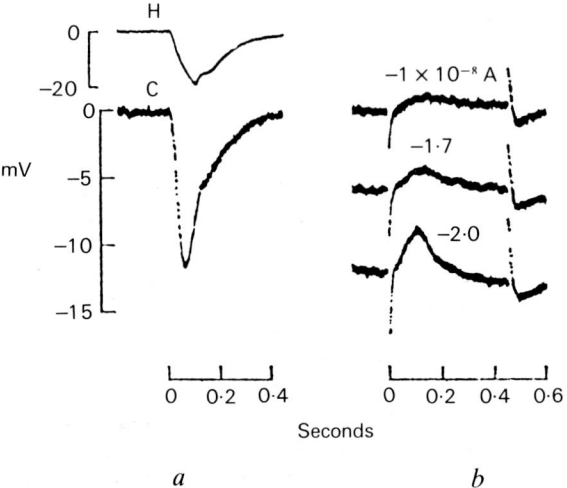

Fig. 13. *a*, Responses recorded simultaneously from a horizontal cell (H) and a cone (C) in a turtle eyecup to a flash of light occurring at time 0 and covering a large area. *b*, Responses of the cone are shown for three different steps of current injection into the horizontal cell. The artificial hyperpolarization of the horizontal cell mimics the effects of light on the feedback synapse in making the cone depolarize. (Taken from Baylor D. A., Fuortes M. G. F. and O'Bryan P. F. *J. Physiol. (Lond.)* 1971; **214**, 265–94.)

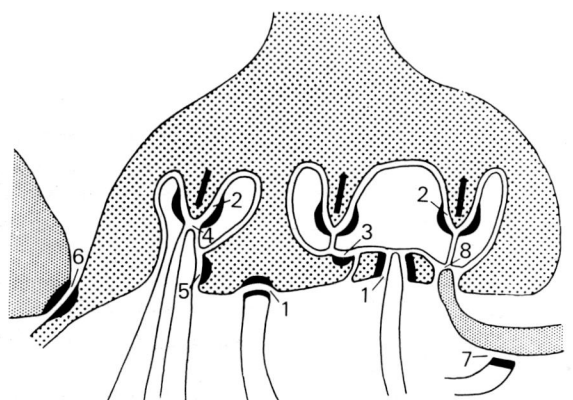

Fig. 14. Diagram of the specialized contacts of a cone pedicle in the turtle retina: (1) basal junctions; (2) proximal junctions of lateral processes (horizontal cell); (3) distal junction of a lateral process; (4) apical junction of a central process in a triad; (5) distal junction of a central process in a triad; (6) junction with an adjacent cone pedicle; (7) *en passant* junction of a basal process; (8) ending of a basal process. (Reproduced from Lasansky A. *Phil. Trans. R. Soc. Lond. (Biol.)* 1971; **262**, 365–81.)

are also basal junctions and gap junctions between adjacent cone pedicles.

What are the consequences for information processing of negative feedback? *Fig.* 13 shows that it accelerates the decay phase of the cone response: fast changes in the waveform are emphasized relative to slow ones. The feedback synapse also has spatial consequences, emphasizing boundaries of illumination in the pattern of cone activity. The hyperpolarization of a cone in the centre of an illuminated region will be 'damped' more by all the horizontal cells around than the hyperpolarization of a boundary cone, which will be affected only by those horizontal cells receiving input from the illuminated side of the boundary.

red. The hyperpolarization to green can be explained by a connection of the cell to green-sensitive cones. The depolarization, however, requires a more complex pathway. Red light falling on to red-sensitive cones causes them to hyperpolarize and hence the horizontal cells connected to these cones will also hyperpolarize. If these red-sensitive horizontal cells exert an inhibitory effect not only on the red-sensitive cones but also on the green-sensitive variety, the depolarizing influence of the red light will be communicated forwards to the green-sensitive horizontal cells.

The depolarizing influence, while always clear in the horizontal cells, is not always apparent in the green-sensitive cones. A way of demonstrating that

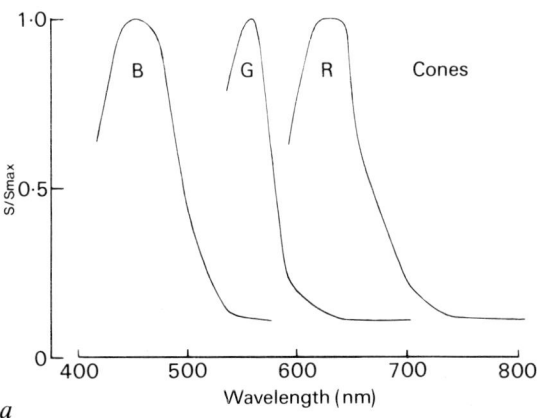
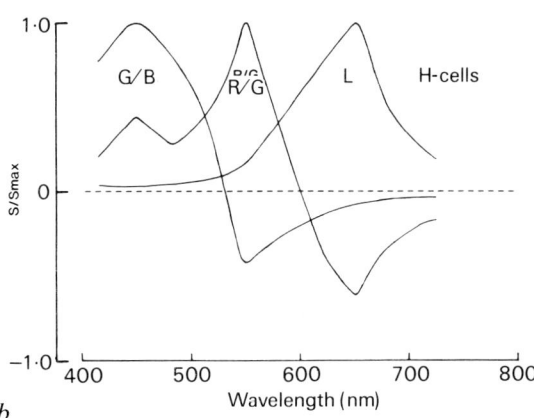

Fig. 15. *a*, Relative spectral sensitivity functions for three cone groups: blue-sensitive (B), green-sensitive (G) and red-sensitive (R). (Constructed from data given by Baylor D. A. and Hodgkin A. L., *J. Physiol. (Lond.)* 1973; **234**, 163–98.) Different cones of a given type showed considerable variability in their spectral sensitivities and recently have been further subdivided: the lines have been drawn to link mean values at various wavelengths. Regions where the presence of oil droplets markedly increased variability have been omitted. The spectral sensitivities of the turtle cones are more red-shifted than those of human ones (cf. *Fig.* 6) because the pigments have vitamin A_2, not A_1, as the chromophore. *b*, Similar spectral sensitivity functions for three horizontal cell types: blue-sensitive (G/B), green-sensitive (R/G), and red-sensitive (L). The presence of a subsidiary peak in the blue for the R/G function implies a direct input to these horizontal cells from the blue-sensitive cones. Positive values correspond to hyperpolarization and negative values to depolarization. (Redrawn with a linear abscissa from Fuortes M. G. F. and Simon E. J. *J. Physiol. (Lond.)* 1974; **240**, 177–98.)

The subtractive effects of horizontal cell activity extend not only to temporal and spatial processing, but influence the signalling of wavelength information. *Fig.* 15(*a*) shows the spectral sensitivities of responses recorded from three different groups of cone in the turtle retina. *Fig.* 15(*b*) shows the spectral sensitivities of responses from three different types of horizontal cell. For one type (red-sensitive cones and horizontal cells) the functions match well; for the other two the broad band cone functions have been transformed at the horizontal cell level to emphasize the wavelength changes; a wavelength change can even lead to a change in the polarity of the response (colour opponency).

To understand these transformations it is necessary to invoke subtractive effects between one colour system and another. Consider how a horizontal cell can hyperpolarize to green light and depolarize to

it does exist is to include strontium ions in the medium perfusing the turtle eyecup, since this promotes the production of large depolarizing spikes by the cone channels controlled by the horizontal cells. The strontium effect suggests that the channels controlled by the feedback transmitter pass calcium ions. *Fig.* 16 shows a strontium experiment with simultaneous recording from a green-sensitive cone and a horizontal cell. Red light produced depolarizing spikes in the cone and a depolarization in the horizontal cell with the 'cone' spikes apparent in the waveform. The main underlying pathways are illustrated in *Fig.* 16(*b*). A similar arrangement of connections will explain how change of wavelength will produce polarity inversion in the blue-sensitive horizontal cell.

The responses of horizontal cells are sometimes called S-potentials. Horizontal cells that hyperpolarize to most illumination, no matter what the

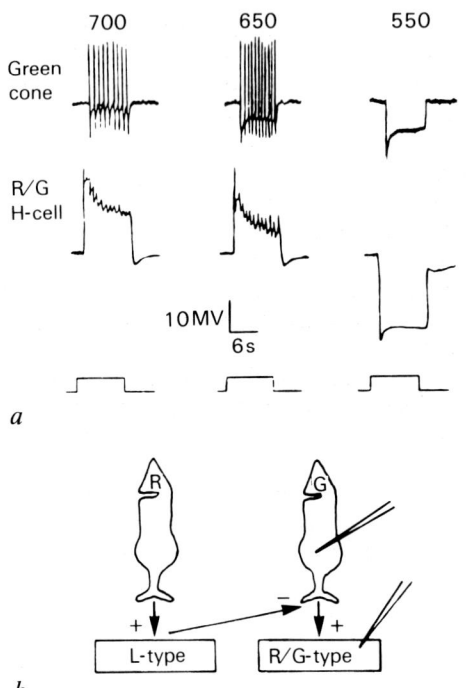

Fig. 16. *a*, The effect of steps of light of different wavelength on the responses of a green-sensitive cone (G) and a green-sensitive (R/G) horizontal cell in a turtle eyecup. The wavelengths are indicated above the voltage records and the occurrence of the stimuli are indicated below. Strontium ions are present in the eyecup perfusate to demonstrate the interaction of the red- and green-sensitive systems. Red lights (700 and 650 nm) cause a small sustained hyperpolarization in the G cone owing to absorption by the G pigment. However, the light is very effective in hyperpolarizing the red-sensitive (R) cones and the red-sensitive horizontal (L) cells. The latter produce the large depolarizing spikes in the G cone which ride on the sustained hyperpolarization. The spikes induce the depolarization seen in the R/G cell. By contrast, with green light (550 nm) there is reduced activity in the R system and the R/G cell reflects the hyperpolarization in the G cone resulting from absorption by the G pigment. Prominent depolarizing spikes are not usually seen in the voltage records of cones in a standard perfusate stimulated by light centred over the receptive field; they can be observed (i) with annular stimulation and an unmodified extracellular medium, (ii) with centred stimulation and a medium containing strontium ions, as described above, or barium ions, and (iii) with centred stimulation and a medium containing calcium ions at a higher than normal concentration. Current injection experiments (*see Fig.* 13) confirm that the cone spikes are the consequence of hyperpolarizing the membrane of L cells. (Taken from Piccolino M. and Newton J., *The S-Potential*, 1982, pp. 161–79 by permission of Alan R. Liss Inc, New York.) *b*, Diagram of the main pathways involved in the experiment. Plus signs indicate sign-preserving pathways, minus signs, sign-inverting ones.

wavelength, like the red-sensitive cells of the turtle, are called 'luminosity' or L cells. Those that hyperpolarize to some wavelengths and depolarize to others, like the green- and blue-sensitive cells, are called 'chromaticity' or C cells. A C cell that depolarizes to red and hyperpolarizes to green is called an R/G cell; one that depolarizes to green and hyperpolarizes to blue is called a G/B cell.

Some interesting facts emerge when the anatomical basis for horizontal cell receptive fields is examined. The functional fields are much larger than the dendritic fields of the neurones, even after the effects of cone coupling have been allowed for. The explanation lies in electrical coupling between horizontal cells. In the turtle retina there are two types of L cell, L1 cells generally having larger receptive fields than L2 cells. The L1 units turn out to be axon terminals linked together with no obvious cell bodies, while the L2 syncytium is formed from cell bodies in communication via gap junctions. Careful staining, however, reveals that terminals are linked to cell bodies via very thin, long axons. Yet L1 and L2 syncytia are functionally distinct, which implies that the axon does not conduct signals. Thus the functional and anatomical units do not correspond. A similar distinction has been found in the cat retina.

There is little evidence for feedback from horizontal cells to rods but rods do provide inputs to horizontal cells and therefore these cells may possibly mediate the influence of rod activity on cones. Psychophysical experiments show that such influences exist in human retina. In a conventional dark adaptation experiment an observer is asked to detect the presence of a flashing light and the threshold intensity for detection is measured. However, the experiment can be varied by asking the observer not just to detect the light but to detect whether the light appears to be flickering or not. If it is arranged that the flickering light can only be detected by cones (by making it deep red and flashing it at a rate too fast for rods to follow), then during cone dark adaptation the flicker detection thresholds fall, but once rod dark adaptation gets going, the thresholds start to rise and it is likely that the rise in these cone-determined thresholds is due to the gradual restoration of rod dark current during dark adaptation. There is some evidence that the effect is arising early in the retina and probably involves the horizontal cells.

BIPOLAR CELLS

Centre–surround antagonism in receptive fields first becomes a prominent feature of retinal neurones at the level of the bipolar cells, though a weak form of it can be detected in cones. *Fig.* 17 shows how the responses of the two types of bipolar cell change as a spot is swept over their receptive fields. *Fig.* 18 shows the pathways which may be involved. Typically, a bipolar cell will contact several receptors, except in special cases such as the primate fovea where there are one-to-one connections. The receptive field centre will be a little larger than the dendritic spread due to inter-receptor coupling. The effects of summation on spatial resolution are not as severe as might be thought from considering the properties of a single neurone. Spatial information can be retrieved by later processing, provided the ratio of bipolar cells to receptors remains high.

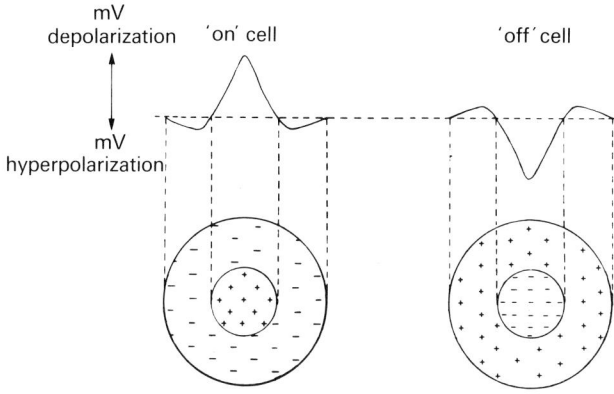

Fig. 17. Changes in membrane potential for an 'on' or centre-depolarizing bipolar cell (left) and an 'off' or centre-hyperpolarizing bipolar cell (right) when a spot or slit of light is moved across the equator of the cell's receptive field. The centre–surround organization of the field is shown below. Plus signs indicate regions giving a depolarizing response, minus signs, a hyperpolarizing one.

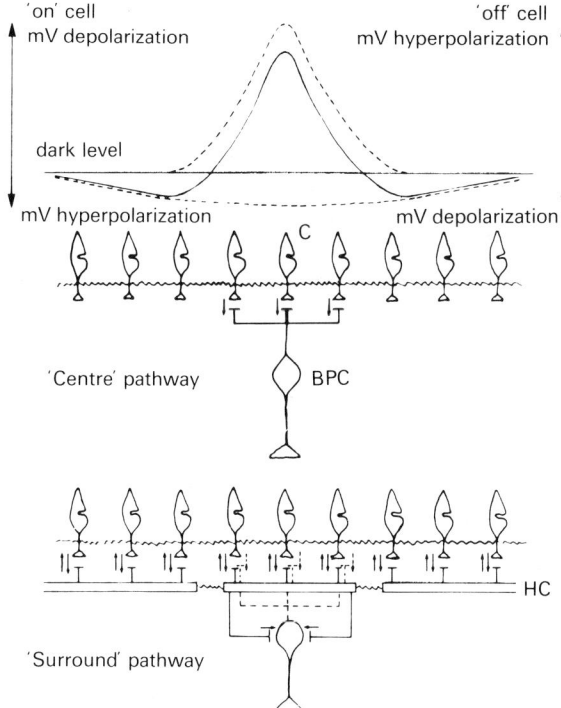

Fig. 18. Response profile of a cone-driven bipolar cell (*above*): up means depolarization for an 'on' cell and hyperpolarization for an 'off' cell. The dotted lines represent the centre and surround components which added together give the actual profile (solid line). The lower diagrams show the pathways which might be responsible for the profile. The centre component arises from the connection between cones and the bipolar cell. The surround component arises from two pathways: (1) cones to horizontal cells to bipolar cell; and (2) cones to horizontal cells to cones to bipolar cell.

The receptor to bipolar cell synapse leads to an amplification of signals. For example, in the dark adapted eye, photons absorbed in just a few of the rods connected to a rod-driven bipolar cell can lead to a large change in the membrane potential of that cell. Amplification is also seen in the synapses between cones and bipolar cells. Theoretical calculations show that the sign inversion which takes place in the signal between hyperpolarizing receptors and the depolarizing variety of bipolar cells is likely to achieve a higher level of amplification than sign preservation. All synapses interpose delays in the passage of information; a study of these delays shows that they are well matched to those already introduced at the receptor level; thus rod-driven synapses are slower than cone-driven ones, in keeping with the slower processing of information by the rod outer segments.

Some attention has been given to the nature of the conductance changes in bipolar cells induced by transmitters from the receptors. In the case of the hyperpolarizing bipolars, the transmitter released in the dark appears to increase the membrane conductance of the bipolar cell, probably to sodium ions. Hence light, by decreasing the transmitter and thereby decreasing the conductance, causes a hyperpolarization. In the case of some of the fish depolarizing bipolars, sign inversion is achieved in two ways: the rod transmitter decreases conductance to sodium ions while the cone transmitter increases the conductance to potassium or to chloride ions. In either case, a light-induced decrease of transmitter will cause a depolarization.

The pathways involved in the production of the surround are more complex than those of the centre and have still not been established with certainty, even in a well-studied retina such as that of the turtle. None the less, the scheme shown in *Fig.* 18 seems a plausible approximation for the cone system on the available evidence. The surround input is believed to be mediated chiefly through the horizontal cells acting via two routes; one through two synapses – horizontal cell to cone to bipolar cell; the other through one synapse – horizontal to bipolar cell. The electrical coupling of the horizontal cells will play an important part in defining the area and relative weight of the surround input.

We have already seen how various mechanisms such as the voltage-gated channels and the sign-inverting feedback synapse all tend to emphasize the onset and offset of light in the response waveforms. The centre–surround mechanism will also reinforce this effect because of the disparity in the delays of signals travelling in the two pathways owing to the different number of synapses that have to be crossed.

One of the possible roles we have attributed to centre–surround antagonism is the enhancement of the signal to noise ratio of the visual system. It can be shown that at low light levels, when this ratio will be small of necessity, the optimum strategy is for a neurone to have a large and weak surround, or not to have one at all. This seems to be the case for rod-driven bipolar cells responding to dim lights.

We have seen how colour opponency is introduced by horizontal cells. Such opponency can be found in some bipolar cells, though it is not universal. For example, in a study of 80 cone bipolar cells in the carp retina, the red-sensitive cones supplied the input to both the centre and surround of about half the cone-driven bipolar cells. In about one-third, single opponent fields were seen with the centre optimally sensitive to red and the surround to green. In about one-fifth the centre and the surround each showed opponency, with red central light eliciting hyperpolarization, green central light, depolarization, red peripheral light, depolarization, and green peripheral light, hyperpolarization. Another possibility is for opponency to exist in the centre of the field but be absent from the surround. Thus, in the turtle retina there are cells that hyperpolarize to green central spots of light, depolarize to red central spots and hyperpolarize to surrounds of any colour, i.e. there is centre–surround antagonism for some wavelength combinations and centre–surround synergism for others. The effect of colour opponency is to make the cells respond optimally to certain spatial combinations of colours.

The axons of the 'on' and 'off' bipolar cells terminate in different sublaminae of the inner plexiform layer. *Fig.* 12 shows that the 'off' cells terminate in the outer sublamina (sublamina A) and those of the 'on' cells in the inner sublamina (sublamina B).

PROCESSING IN THE INNER RETINA

To make sense of the properties of amacrine and ganglion cells, it is best to consider them together. The turtle retina makes a good starting point, because the classification of its ganglion cells is simple and has already been presented in outline. *Fig.* 12 shows there are two types: the A cells (including 'on' and 'off' varieties), which give sustained responses to illumination, and the B cells, which give transient responses. The properties of the A cells closely reflect those of the bipolar cells, with the 'off' ganglion cells synapsing in sublamina A of the inner plexiform layer where the terminals of the 'off' bipolar cells predominate, and the 'on' ganglion cells synapsing in sublamina B where the 'on' bipolar cells terminate. Type B cells, on the other hand, have new properties which are first encountered at the level of the amacrine cells. Their synapses are diffusely organized throughout the inner plexiform layer. Other distinguishing features between type A and type B cells are the larger size, the faster conduction and the higher firing rate of the former.

A way of testing for separate inputs to a cell is to polarize it with current injection to various levels and observe what happens to different aspects of the response. If one conductance is being controlled by the input, then the polarization will affect all aspects in a similar way; if more than one conductance is present, then the behaviour will differ according to the pattern of stimulation, e.g. surround responses will not be affected in the same way as centre ones. Such experiments support the view that each class of bipolar cell provides the main input to the corresponding class of type A ganglion cell.

By contrast, observations on type B cells show that they receive complex inputs, probably a mixture of direct contributions from the bipolar cells mixed with signals from the amacrine cells. There are at least three types of amacrine cell: those that respond with a sustained depolarization to light, those that respond with a sustained hyperpolarization and those that share transient properties with type B ganglion cells and respond to both onset and offset of illumination. The transient amacrine cells probably receive a depolarizing transmitter with a short-lasting action from both classes of bipolar cell. Thus their on-response would reflect the start of depolarization in the depolarizing bipolar responding to light going on and their off-response would reflect the start of depolarization in the hyperpolarizing bipolar cell responding to light going off. The contribution from both types of bipolar cell would lead to the disappearance of centre–surround antagonism. However, some differences remain between the effects of central and peripheral stimulation. Moreover, polarization experiments point to more than one conductance mechanism in these cells. The likely explanation is input from other amacrine cells, possibly of the sustained variety. The involvement of elaborate amacrine cell circuitry leads to a complexity in the properties of type B ganglion cells. For example, a proportion of them seem to be specialized for the detection of movement, responding optimally to a spot of light swept across them in a particular direction (the preferred direction), while remaining silent when the spot is moved in the opposite way (the null direction). This pattern probably results from the interaction of a depolarizing input from bipolar cells and hyperpolarizing one from amacrines, which arrives with a variable delay depending on which way and how fast the spot is moved. If the hyperpolarization is coincident with the depolarization, no response is detected, but if it follows it, the motion has an effect. Directionality is the consequence of an anisotropy of amacrine cell inputs: spots moved in the null direction may excite cells along a shorter pathway and therefore induce a shorter inhibitory delay than spots moved in the preferred direction.

In mammals the classification of ganglion cells is more complex. The cat has been the most intensively studied and, like the turtle, the various classes of cell have been designated either by letters or by brief descriptions of functional characteristics. The functional characteristics are those we have already encountered, such as whether responses are sustained or transient, whether firing rate is brisk or sluggish, what are the relative sizes of the cell bodies and what are the relative conduction velocities. Another important characteristic is whether a change in light in one part of the receptive field centre can be compensated by a change in the light in another part so that the cell does not respond, i.e. whether the cell behaves linearly in summing the activity of the inputs that make up its field centre. There are three main groups that emerge on these criteria. X cells have sustained responses, they fire briskly, their size and conduction velocity both lie in the middle of the respective ranges and they behave linearly. In many ways they resemble the A cells of the turtle. Y cells give transient responses, they fire briskly, they are the cells with the largest cell bodies and the fastest conduction velocities and they behave non-linearly. They have no exact parallel with the cells of the turtle, where the transient cells are sluggish, small and conduct slowly. Mammalian W cells probably represent the nearest parallel to the turtle B cells. They, however, include both sustained and transient neurones and some with concentric organization of their receptive fields and others that respond to stimuli of a particular type, such as local edges or movement in a particular direction. They fire sluggishly, have the smallest cell bodies and the slowest conduction velocities. Many of them show very non-linear and specialized behaviour. It is not clear whether W cells should be considered as a single class. Cutting across this X–Y–W classification there is the 'on' v. 'off' distinction. X and Y cells and some W cells show well-developed centre–surround antagonism.

The anatomical organization of the cone pathways in the cat looks similar to that seen in the turtle, with hyperpolarizing bipolar cells making contact with 'off' ganglion cells, both X and Y, in the outer part of the inner plexiform layer, sublamina A, and depolarizing bipolar cells with 'on' ganglion cells in the inner part, sublamina B. In each sublamina there are amacrine cells of a 'starburst' form which receive inputs from the local bipolar cells and other amacrine cells and contribute to the inputs of their local ganglion cells. It is thought that these amacrine cells modulate the response of the ganglion cells to information coming through the direct pathway from bipolar cells. Amacrine cells must also be responsible for the non-linearities seen in Y cells and for the fact that these cells can respond to stimulation presented remotely from the main centre–surround area of their receptive field.

The cat rod system differs from the picture given above in three respects: first, there appears to be only one type of bipolar cell, that is, one that hyperpolarizes to light; second, all information to the ganglion cells has to pass through amacrine cells; third, the rod bipolar cell terminates in sublamina B, not sublamina A. It seems that rod amacrine cells with postsynaptic (input) dendrites in B and presynaptic (output) dendrites in A, form part of the direct rod path to the 'off' ganglion cells. The route followed by rod signals to the 'on' ganglion cells is less clear but they may cross into the cone depolarizing bipolar

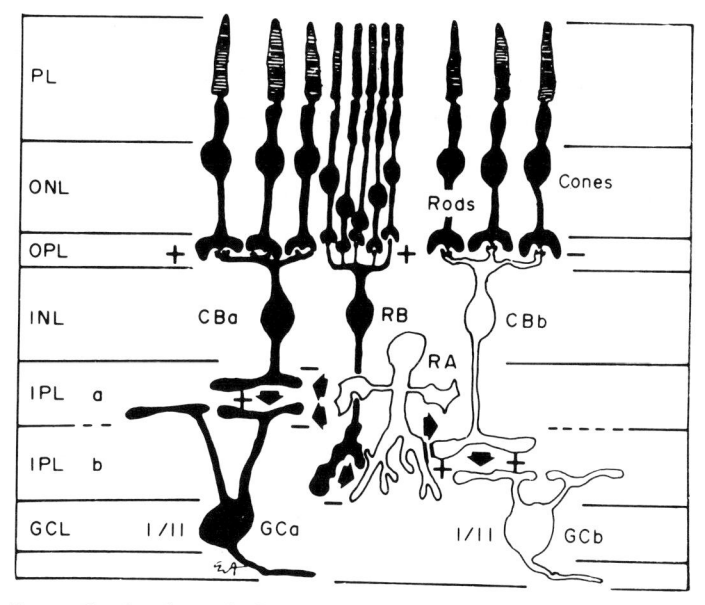

Fig. 19. Cone and rod pathways in the cat retina. Neurones giving hyperpolarizing responses to light are filled black; depolarizing neurones are not filled. In the outer plexiform layer (OPL) the same cones contact both type (a) cone bipolar cells (CBa) and type (b) bipolars (CBb) which have their synaptic terminals in different sublaminae of the inner plexiform layer (IPL). The bipolars contact ganglion cells of classes I and II. Rod bipolars (RB) give hyperpolarizing responses to light, thus apparently receiving excitatory synapses from rods in the OPL. Though the RB axon terminal is broadly stratified in sublamina (b), it contacts no ganglion cells (GC) directly. It synapses on the rod amacrine cell (RA) in sublamina (b). Since RA depolarizes to light, it must receive inhibitory synaptic input from RB. RA has chemical synaptic output to 'off' ganglion cells in sublamina (a); hence this synapse also has to be inhibitory (sign-inverting). The pathway from RA to 'on' ganglion cells is via large gap junctions (presumed electrotonic contacts) between it and type (b) cone bipolar terminals. (Reproduced from Famiglietti E. V. jun. *Vision Res*, 1983; **23**, 1265-79.)

cells via gap junctions in sublamina B, after which they are transmitted across the bipolar–ganglion cell synapse. In addition to the connection between rod bipolar and rod amacrine cells, the former contact another type of amacrine cell in what appears to be a reciprocal synapse involving the two-way flow of information. A process from the rod amacrine and one from this other amacrine type form a dyad arrangement with the bipolar cell. Some of the pathways described are illustrated in *Fig.* 19.

To add to the complexity of retinal processing, there is a class of neurone called the interplexiform cell which is postsynaptic in the inner plexiform layer and presynaptic to cells in the outer plexiform layer. The role of this centrifugal pathway is still obscure.

What are the functional roles of the X, Y and W parallel pathways? There is no consensus on this question as we have no clear idea of the higher processing carried out by the visual system and its information requirements. One suggestion is that Y cells detect some change in the pattern of illumination in the peripheral parts of the retina and carry a signal to the system controlling fixation so that eye movements bring the pattern on to the central retina where detailed analysis of the spatial information is performed by the X pathway. Certainly, X cells are concentrated in the central retina and their properties seem well suited to spatial analysis, while those of Y cells are suited to detection of peripheral changes. Another possibility is that the X system carries out the preliminary processing of information which will enable the brain to compute the existence of edges, their position and extent and the relative luminances on either side, while the Y system extracts information for movement detection. Yet another view of the X and Y systems is that the Y cells prepare the appropriate region of the cortex for the arrival of information down the slower X system, i.e., by decreasing the general tonic inhibition in a particular region of cortex corresponding to the retinal area where changes are taking place. The weakness of such speculations is that they assign no role to the W neurones, which form a large proportion of the ganglion cell population. For the moment, therefore, the exact reasons behind cell specialization and the segregation of information into parallel pathways remains a mystery.

THE ELECTRORETINOGRAM

We have already mentioned the electroretinogram in connection with the electrical signal of receptors. Extracellular current flows arise in the retina because conditions such as membrane permeability or local ion concentrations in or near one part of a retinal cell differ from conditions in another region of the cell. *Fig.* 20 shows how these currents spread to the front of the eye where they can be recorded as an electroretinogram. How much reaches the front will depend on the orientation of the cells generating the current and the relative resistances of the local and remote pathways. Cells that are organized along the radial axis of the eye and that span regions of high resistance will tend to make the most prominent contributions. Measurement of extracellular voltages and resistance across various parts of the retina and

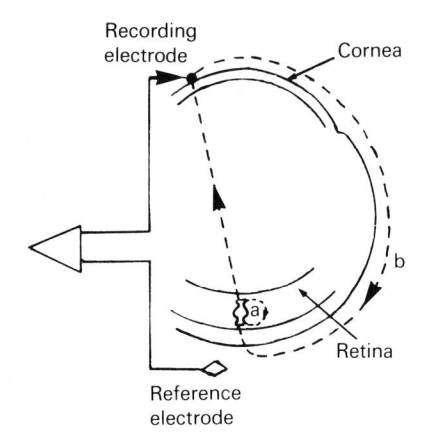

Fig. 20. Current flow (dashed line) from a retinal cell recorded with a corneal electrode.

across the pigment epithelium has localized the sources of the current flow to the receptors, to the Mueller cells, which span the retina from the receptor inner segments to the vitreous boundary, and to the pigment epithelium cells behind the receptors. Most of the electroretinogram is only indirectly related to signal processing by the retina.

The mechanism by which receptors produce their signal has already been considered. How do the Mueller cells respond to illumination? There is evidence that, like glia in other parts of the nervous system, they are sensitive to local changes in the concentration of extracellular potassium ions. In a region of a potassium increase the membrane of the Mueller cell will tend to depolarize, acting as a current sink, while in a region of a decrease it will tend to hyperpolarize, acting as a current source. *Fig.* 21 illustrates one model of what may happen to the level of potassium ions in different parts of the retina following illumination, and the current flows that ensue. The model assumes that the feet of Mueller cells forming the inner limiting membrane at the boundary between retina and vitreous have a particularly high permeability to potassium ions. This means that the feet will act as the current sources for the sinks created by local potassium increases or the current sinks for the sources created by local potassium depletion and there will be a current flow between the feet and the regions of potassium change. Three such regions are shown: in the vicinity of the receptors light causes a depletion (distal source), in the region of the outer plexiform layer light causes an increase (distal sink) and in the region of the inner plexiform layer light causes an increase (proximal sink). Each region generates a photocurrent which will be a component of the electroretinogram, though the two currents originating in the distal regions will be the most prominent because of the relatively long radial distance over which the current flows.

What causes the potassium changes? In the receptor, as we have seen, there is a dark current which, away from the outer segments, is carried across the plasma membrane by potassium ions. This outward, passive potassium flux is in balance with inward flux via a sodium/potassium exchange mechanism or 'pump' which exists to prevent the disappearance of the ionic gradients across the membranes. Light, by reducing the passive flux, creates a net inward movement and hence local depletion, probably in the region of the receptor inner limbs where the sodium 'pump' is presumed to be most active.

The mechanisms underlying the potassium increases are more obscure. In the outer plexiform layer the depolarizing bipolar cells are probably responsible for at least part of the effect, because treatments that selectively eliminate their responses but keep the hyperpolarizing cells functioning also abolish the b-wave component of the electroretinogram which arises from the distal source. The neurones involved in the proximal increase are not known. In primate retina the increase seems not to occur since no proximal sink has been found.

Fig. 22 shows how the various currents generated in the monkey fovea might add together to produce a local electroretinogram. Because of overlap of current sources and sinks, there is some uncertainty in the exact waveforms of the components. The receptor component is often referred to as the late receptor potential (LRP), or fast PIII, or distal PIII. The P terminology goes back to early work on the electroretinogram which showed that it could be disassociated into three underlying processes, i.e., PI, recorded as a positive-going wave at the cornea, very sensitive to anoxia; PII a positive-going wave, less

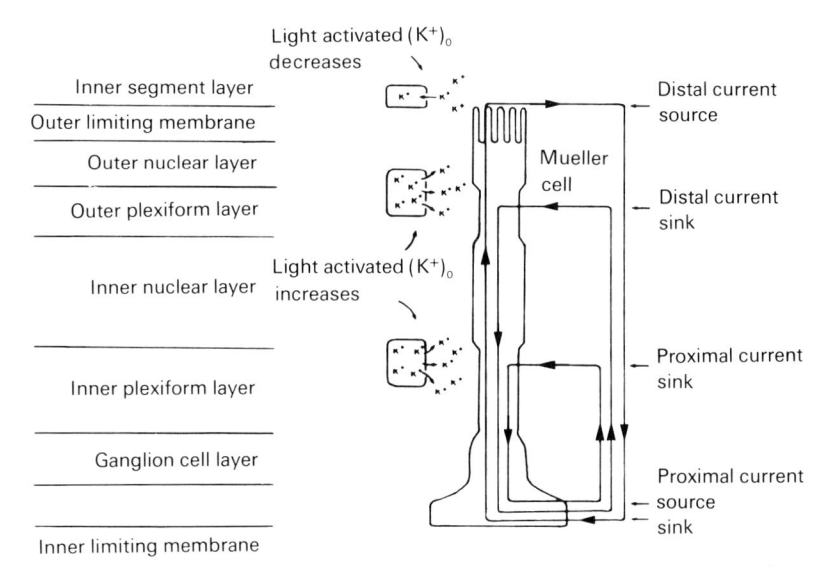

Fig. 21. Model for the generation of the electroretinogram. Local changes in extracellular potassium concentration are believed to occur in different retinal regions as a result of illumination. The sources and sinks of membrane current in the Mueller cell correspond to these regions and generate various components of current flow around the cell. (The model is based on data from frog retina and has been proposed by Newman E. A. and Odette L. L., *J. Neurophysiol.* 1984; **51**, 164–82.) There is still some dispute about the exact location of sources and sinks in the retinae of different species. For example, in primate retina there is no evidence of a proximal current sink, nor does current flow appear to be forced through the feet of the Mueller cells; rather there is a more extensive proximal region where current crosses the Mueller cell membrane to complete the circuit set up by changes in other regions.)

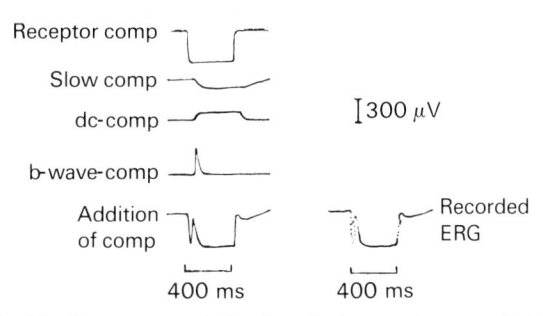

Fig. 22. Components of the foveal electroretinogram (ERG) obtained from a monkey eye with extracellular electrodes in the retina. On the left are shown the size and form of the components that would account for the observed ERG shown on the right. This local ERG is dominated by the receptor component and the b-wave component is relatively small; this differs from what is usually seen when the electroretinogram is recorded with corneal electrodes and wide field stimulation. (Redrawn from Valeton J. M. and Van Norren D., *Vision Res.* 1982; **22**, 381–91; the polarities of the components have been reversed to bring them into line with what is seen with corneal recording.)

sensitive to anoxia; and PIII a negative-going wave, least sensitive to anoxia. The slow component of *Fig.* 22 results from the distal current sink; it is also referred to as slow PIII. The dc and b-wave components both arise from the distal current source; they correspond to PII.

In an electroretinogram the addition of positive and negative components gives rise to waves. Thus, the leading edge of the receptor component produces the a-wave, while the presence of the b-wave component generates the b-wave. However, any wave in the electroretinogram should not be identified too closely with an underlying component, for though a single component may dominate in the production of a particular wave, other components contribute to the amplitude and form. It is important to remember this when considering the effects of various treatments on the electroretinogram. For example, it is clear from *Fig.* 22 that any change in the amplitude of the receptor component will also affect the amplitude of the b-wave and could also affect the timing of the b-wave peak.

The picture presented by *Fig.* 22 is still too simple, for we have yet to consider the contributions of the pigment epithelium cells (PI). Intracellular recordings of the voltage across the apical (receptor side) membrane, of the voltage across the basal (choroid side) membrane, together with extracellular measurements of the trans-epithelial voltage and of potassium changes in the space between receptors and the apical processes of the epithelial cells, have all been used to work out the electrical mechanisms of the pigment epithelium. *Fig.* 23 shows the three processes involved; light induces a hyperpolarization of the apical membrane, a delayed hyperpolarization of the basal membrane and a later, slower depolarization of the basal membrane. A potassium mechanism similar to the one which generates slow PIII of the Mueller cell will account for the apical hyperpolarization. The delayed basal hyperpolarization also appears to depend on potassium changes, though in a less direct way. The cause of the depolarization of the basal membrane, however, does not appear to depend on potassium changes in the retina and still requires explanation. Each of these processes contributes to the electroretinogram: the apical hyperpolarization together with its retinal counterpart, slow PIII, produces the c-wave; the delayed hyperpolarization contributes to a fast oscillation; the slow basal depolarization is solely responsible for the response called the light peak. The pigment epithelial components of the electroretinogram may appear very large because of the very large trans-epithelial resistance.

The light peak forms the basis of the electro-oculogram (EOG). The retina and pigment epithelium produce dark currents which give rise to an oriented standing potential across the eye. If electrodes are placed on either side of the eye and the dark adapted eye is repeatedly swivelled between a left and a right point, a change in the voltage between the electrodes is observed which is related to the standing potential. A similar measurement can be made for the light adapted eye and the ratio of the measurements reflects the size of the light peak seen in the dark adapted electroretinogram. The light peak turns out to be a very sensitive clinical indicator of retinal or pigment epithelial malfunction.

The form of the electroretinogram is very dependent on the pattern of stimulation. Frequently, the

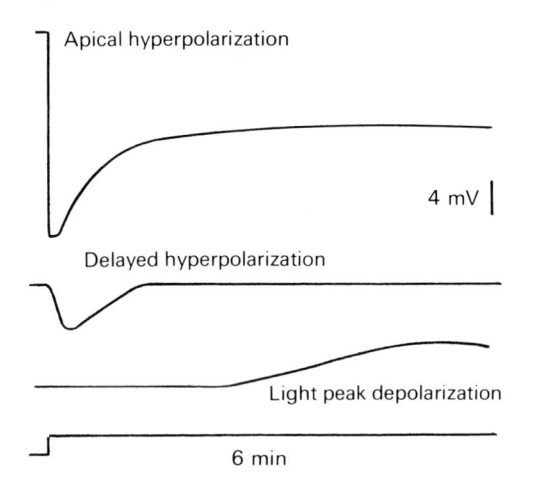

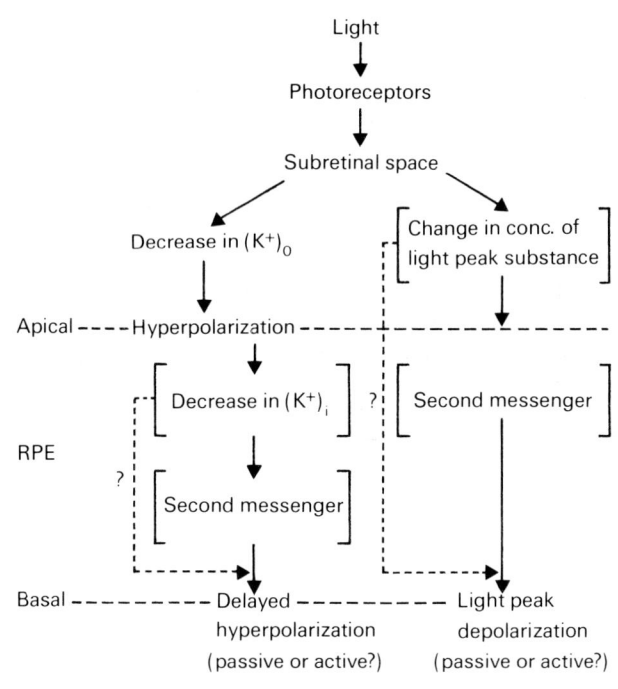

Fig. 23. The three components of the electrical response of a pigment epithelium cell to a step of light and the possible underlying mechanisms. Stages in brackets have yet to be demonstrated. Interrupted lines indicate alternative pathways. (From Steinberg R. H., Linsenmeier R. A. and Griff E. R. *Vision Res.* 1983; **23**, 1315–24.)

whole of the back of the eye is illuminated ('Ganzfeld' illumination); if only part of the eye is stimulated, the unstimulated regions act as a shunt pathway; less current reaches the front of the eye and the balance of contributions from the different components is altered. If coloured lights are used, separation of rod and cone components can be achieved, as illustrated in *Fig.* 24. Here stimulation by red light has produced cone a- and b-waves peaking at earlier times than the corresponding rod waves. Another type of stimulation often used is a chequer board pattern reversing in time. The response is called a 'pattern ERG' and there is some evidence that it reflects the output of the inner plexiform layer. It is clinically useful for studying conditions where a disturbance of the inner retina is suspected.

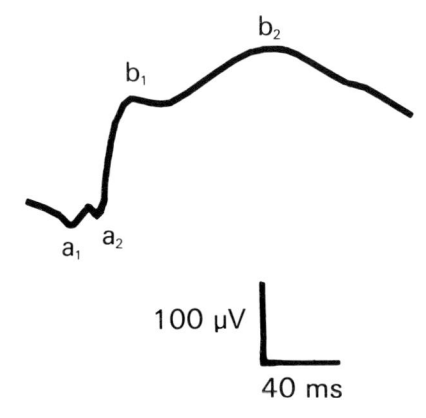

Fig. 24. A human electroretinogram elicited by a very short, bright red stroboscopic flash at the start of the record. The flash covers the whole eye (Ganzfeld stimulation). Separate cone (indicated by subscript 1) and rod (indicated by subscript 2) a- and b-waves are seen because the red light is very much more effective for cones than for rods and produces responses in the two systems with very disparate latencies.

One other form of electrical activity of the eye needs to be mentioned, and this is the early receptor potential (ERP) which, as its name implies, arises in the receptors as a very early response to light. Its origin lies in charge movements in the receptor plasma membranes associated with the bleaching of visual pigment molecules. Such movements produce brief flows of extracellular current around the receptors. To record a sizeable ERP a very large number of pigment molecules have to be bleached in a very short time, typically more than 10 per cent in less than 1 ms. The ERP is useful clinically for assessing the state of the visual pigments; in humans it is the cones which give the dominant contribution.

SUMMARY

At the level of the visual pigment molecules, information about the pattern of incoming light is in terms of numbers bleached. This is translated into the extent of receptor hyperpolarization by complex biochemical machinery in the outer segments. However, the translation is not exact; to cope with limited signalling range available, adaptive mechanisms are present which emphasize how the input departs from what has come in before. Receptors are not just transducers of light into chemical and electrical signals; they are active processors of information.

Throughout the retina mechanisms exist which emphasize intensity and wavelength changes in illumination both in time and across space. Voltage-gated mechanisms and negative feedback pathways provide examples of how changes in time are emphasized. The centre–surround organization, seen weakly at the receptor level and more strongly beyond, is an example of a mechanism for extracting spatial discontinuities; it also represents solutions to the problems of the limited range of neuronal signals, of information overload and of noise.

Parallel pathways are used for signalling different aspects of the stimulus to the brain and it seems probable that this arrangement serves several functions: one being to protect important features of the information from being degraded by noise and another being to combine the information into outputs convenient for computations in the brain. These will involve determining what patterns constitute surfaces of objects, what patterns correspond to shadows or textures, how surfaces are related to one another in a three-dimensional space and what movements are taking place. The computations in the retina thus can be thought of as part of the extraction and transformation of information required for these higher level activities. The retina must not be thought of as merely the transmitter of information to the brain but rather as the brain's forward extension.

Biochemistry of the Eye

G. Chader

The eye is a singular organ, consisting of several tissues integrated in function to facilitate the visual process. It contains a contrasting array of cell types from neural to epithelial to pigmented. It has perhaps the most metabolically active cell type in the body (the retinal photoreceptor cell) and the least active (the lens fibre cell). It demonstrates clinical entities that in some cases are systemic and in other cases are uniquely ocular; these can be studied in relation to visual pathology alone or to more generalized diseases affecting multiple cell types and tissues of the body.

Diseases that affect any tissue have underlying biochemical aetiologies. Thus, to understand, treat and cure a disease process, it is important to understand the normal biochemical functioning of the tissue in question and how, in the disease, the functioning goes awry.

CORNEA

As the first of the ocular tissues on which entering light impinges, the main functions of the cornea are (a) to remain clear and transparent, (b) to remain in proper conformation and curvature, since it affords the major refractive component of the eye, and (c) to provide a tough, flexible outer covering for the eye along with the sclera.

The sclera and conjunctiva constitute most of the outer surface of the eye and mainly consist of collagen fibres with lesser amounts of glycoproteins and proteoglycans. The sclera is an opaque tissue, due in part to its composition and the interweaving and cross-lamination of the large collagen fibrils, as compared to the cornea where collagen fibres and the spaces between them are smaller than one-half the wavelength of visible light.

Structure and Function

The cornea is an avascular structure composed of a thick layer of connective tissue, the stroma, encased anteriorly by the epithelial cell layer and posteriorly by a single cell layer, the endothelium. Two specialized membranes separate these layers: Bowman's membrane, composed mainly of type I and III collagens is found between the epithelium and stroma, Descemet's membrane; a specialized basement membrane composed mainly of type IV collagen, lies between the stroma and the endothelial cell layer.

Epithelium and Endothelium

The epithelium is a discrete cellular layer, normally five to six cells in thickness, covering the anterior surface of the cornea. As the outermost part of the cornea, the epithelium plays an important role in interacting with the external tear film and atmosphere as well as forming a barrier which prevents most foreign substances from entering the internal stroma. The epithelial cells are metabolically quite active, with mitotic activity prominent in the basal cell layer; this ultimately leads to cellular desquamation into the tear film. The rapid turnover in cells (every 7 days in some species) necessitates substantial protein and DNA synthesis and active transport processes in the cells for precursor uptake.

The endothelium is a single cell layer on the posterior corneal surface abutting the aqueous humour. In contrast to the epithelium, hyperplasia is not observed in the human endothelium; DNA synthesis is negligible in the mature cells. Rather, cell spreading appears to be the mechanism by which the endothelium responds to cell loss due to ageing or trauma. Fluid and ion transport, perhaps the most important function of the endothelium, will be discussed below.

Stroma

As with most connective tissues, the stroma is mainly acellular (90 per cent). The keratocytes present are tightly embedded in an extracellular matrix (ground substance). This matrix consists of highly ordered arrays of collagen fibres of uniform diameter lying parallel to the corneal surface. Proteoglycans and glycoproteins are found between the collagen fibres. A critical consideration in corneal transparency is the regular, parallel, repeating structure of the collagen fibrils and their relatively thin cross-section.

The term proteoglycan is now used for any macromolecule which consists of a protein core with carbohydrate side chains containing sulphate esters. The side chains attached to these proteoglycans are known as glycosaminoglycans (GAGs), a term that has largely replaced the term mucopolysaccharide. In general, a glycosaminoglycan is any higher molecular weight heteropolysaccharide unit containing serially repeating disaccharide amino-sugar residues (e.g. glucosamine or galactosamine) and a uronic acid, with the exception of keratan sulphate which has galactose in place of uronic acid. The term glycoprotein is reserved for a component that is mainly protein in nature but which contains smaller sized covalently bound sugar moieties in other than serially repeating array.

There are several distinct types of GAGs in most tissues. These include (a) the hyaluronic acids, which are unsulphated and may or may not be covalently linked to protein, and (b) several smaller sulphated types, including heparan sulphate, dermatan sulphate, chondroitin sulphate and keratan sulphate, which are normally protein-bound. The corneal stroma contains a chondroitin sulphate proteoglycan and a keratan sulphate proteoglycan. Proteoglycans are classified mainly by the type of sugar disaccharide present and the type of linkage that binds them to the core protein moieties. Chondroitin sulphates are mainly distinguished by their content of N-acetylgalactosamine and glucuronic acid; keratan sulphates predominantly contain N-acetylglucosamine and galactose (Fig. 1). The degree of sulphation can vary in these structures. Glycosaminoglycans demonstrate a relatively high degree of molecular weight polydispersity and chemical heterogeneity.

Keratan sulphates (KS) constitute well over half of the total GAG content of the cornea and can be divided into two main classes based on protein linkage. KS I, the type mainly localized in the cornea, is covalently bound to an asparagine residue through an alkalai-stable N-acetyl glucosamine linkage, while the skeletal (cartilage) type (KS II) exhibits an O-glycosidic linkage. The corneal keratan sulphates also differ from those in other tissues (e.g. cartilage) in their degree of sulphation and variable concentration of disaccharide. Sulphation appears to be cation-dependent with a Na^+K^+-ATPase involved in transport of sulphate into the cornea. Vitamin A and vitamin A deficiency appear to have no direct effect on the sulphation process. Sulphation increases dramatically at the time of corneal deturgescence in the chick embryo cornea, indicating that GAG sulphation may be intimately involved in corneal transparency.

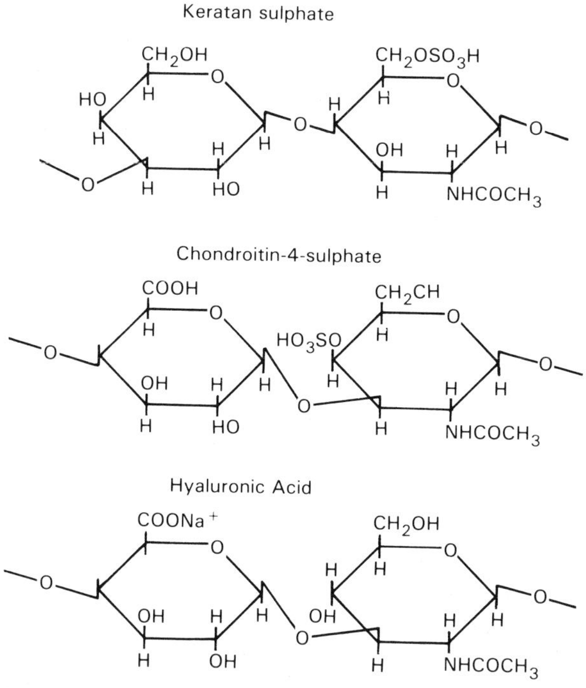

Well over 90 per cent of the stroma solid matter consists of protein; the greater part of this is collagen. Although several types of collagen have now been identified in the body, the type found in the cornea is type I collagen. It is similar to other collagens in that it has a typically high hydroxyproline content and also a high glycine content. It is highly glycosylated, possibly to aid in the orderly packing of collagen fibrils by promoting the proper interactions of collagen with glycoprotein. Proteoglycans may also play a role in fibril formation and arrangement. As pointed out above, the most unique feature of the corneal fibrillar system is its lamellar spatial arrangement and the small size of the individual fibrils (25–30 nm) as compared with other collagen types (>40 nm), as in the sclera. This small size is more typical of embryonic collagen. The distance between fibrillar arrays is less than that of the wavelength of light, thus minimizing light scatter. After corneal wounding, the collagen fibrils formed are of a larger size and are deposited in a less regular pattern; hence they interfere with transparency. Type III collagen is the type produced in stromal wound repair.

Corneal Metabolism

Nutrient Uptake

Since the cornea is avascular, nutrients must be obtained through diffusion from the tear film, from the limbal vessels or from the aqueous humour. The impermeability of the epithelium also limits entrance of most substances, particularly hydrophilic substances, into the cornea. An exception to this is oxygen, which can reach epithelial cells from the air dissolved in the tear film. A number of important metabolites, including vitamin A, are supplied to the cornea primarily through the limbal vessels. This is a selective process, however, and depends on the size and hydrophobicity of the substance in question.

Glucose Utilization

Glucose, the major energy source of the cornea, is supplied primarily from the aqueous humour through

Fig. 1. Repeating units commonly found in glycosaminoglycans.

the endothelium. It is passively transported through the corneal layers where it furnishes biosynthetic building blocks from its carbon skeleton as well as energy equivalents. Little glucose appears to enter the cornea through the epithelium; glucose is present in a several-fold lower concentration in the tear film than in the aqueous humour. The cornea is able to store glucose in the form of glycogen granules in both epithelium and endothelium.

Fig. 2 depicts the major modes of glucose utilization in the cornea. Besides direct use in polysaccharide synthesis, ATP is an end product of glucose metabolism through aerobic and anaerobic glycolysis. It has been estimated that 85 per cent of the total glucose in the cornea is utilized via aerobic glycolysis. Lactate, a major glycolytic product, is rapidly produced and is mainly removed by simple diffusion into the aqueous humour. Reducing equivalents as well as pentose sugars are produced through the pentose phosphate pathway (hexosemonophosphate shunt) in which glucose-6-phosphate is oxidized yielding pentoses and NADPH. It has been estimated that the pentose phosphate pathway accounts for 66, 66 and 37 per cent of the glucose oxidized in epithelium, stroma and endothelium respectively. The pentoses are especially important for use in DNA and RNA synthesis. Transaldoase and transketolase enzymes can also utilize the pentose phosphates to form triose phosphates and reform glucose. The shunt may serve another important role in the cornea, acting as an alternative energy pathway under conditions of metabolic stress. It is interesting that shunt activity increases considerably at the time of deturgescence in the embryonic cornea. The ability to utilize glucose by anaerobic glycolysis along with stored glycogen, allows for excellent tissue survival *in vitro* even in glucose-free medium.

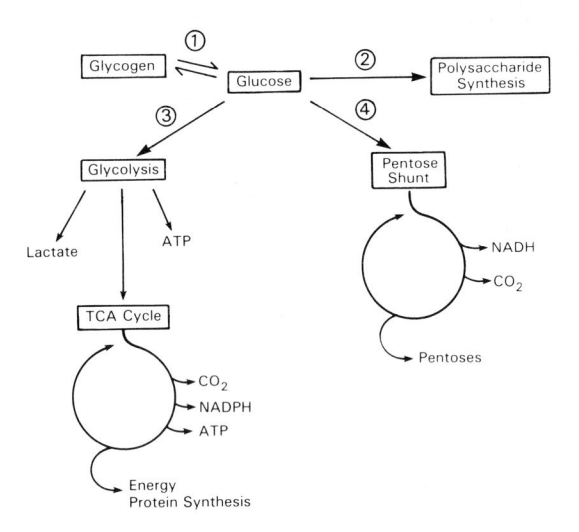

Fig. 2. Pathways by which glucose is (1) stored (2), utilized in glycoconjugate biosynthesis (3), utilized for energy production (4), utilized for reducing equivalents and pentose building blocks.

Keratocytes in the stroma appear to have a metabolic rate similar to that of epithelial cells and utilize glucose both aerobically and anaerobically. Most of the glucose in the endothelium appears to be metabolized through the Embden–Meyerhof pathway. The large number of mitochondria in endothelial cells suggests a high rate of aerobic glycolysis.

Adenosine and Glutathione

Besides glucose, two other low molecular weight compounds are of importance in corneal metabolism. Adenosine is known to spare and substitute for glucose in maintaining corneal integrity. Ribose, released by the hydrolysis of adenosine, can be used to synthesize glucose through a reversal of the pentose phosphate pathway and thus be a potent energy source.

Glutathione, a tripeptide composed of glycine, cystine and glutamic acid, is in high concentration in the cornea. The oxidized form (GSSG) is known to act in cells as a hydrogen acceptor and the reduced form (GSH), as a hydrogen donor. Although the role of glutathione in the cornea is yet unclear, it has a distinct stimulatory effect on the deturgescent mechanism. Total glutathione in the epithelium is high and comparable to that in retina; it is mainly found in the reduced form. In the endothelium, the level is approximately 50 per cent of that found in the epithelium, with GSSG accounting for about 60 per cent of the total (an unusually high percentage).

Normally, there is a balance between GSSG and GSH in corneal tissues, with a constant supply of NADPH produced by the pentose phosphate pathway necessary to maintain the reduced form. This balance suggests that GSSG/GSH may function as a redox system, protecting the cornea from free radical (peroxide) damage and protecting protein sulphydryl groups. Endothelial fluid transport is disrupted either when the total glutathione content is decreased by two-thirds or when the GSSG:GSH ratio is markedly altered.

Irrigating Solutions

Because of the need to maintain corneal integrity and function during surgery and under *in vitro* storage conditions prior to corneal transplantation, balanced salt solutions have been formulated which are generally based on the composition of aqueous humour. Most often used has been a glutathione–bicarbonate Ringer's solution (GBR), whose major ingredients are reduced glutathione, bicarbonate, glucose and adenosine. Because of rapid oxidation of GSH *in vitro*, GBR solutions are stable for only a matter of hours. To allow for a longer shelf-life, a newer solution has been devised, BSS Plus, which replaces the GSH with GSSG and deletes adenosine from the mixture. Control studies have shown that GSSG is similar to GSH in its ability to maintain endothelial function.

Perfusion of human corneal endothelium with BSS Plus allows for de-swelling at a rate of 24 μm/h.

Transport and Transparency

The small size and spatial arrangement of the collagen fibrils contribute to corneal transparency. Several years ago, it was proposed that a perfectly ordered long-range lattice structure of collagen fibres was present in the corneal matrix which allowed for destructive interference between scattered light waves and thus structural transparency. It is now known that only short-range order in collagen fibres is necessary (three to four fibres) to maintain transparency.

Besides the size and arrangement of collagen fibrils, the most important factor determining corneal transparency is fluid transport. The polyelectrolyte nature of the stromal matrix naturally attracts fluid; thus, the fluid must be actively pumped out of the cornea, keeping the cornea in a constant state of deturgescence. For this purpose, the epithelium and endothelium work in concert. The main function of the epithelium is to form an impermeable barrier to fluid influx from the tear film while the endothelial cells actively maintain corneal deturgescence. Epithelial cells do, however, actively transport sodium (Na^+) ions from the tear film into the stroma, utilizing a Na^+/K^+-ATPase pump. Concomitantly, chloride (Cl^-) is moved from the stroma into the epithelium and thence, by passive transport, into the tear film. Epinephrine and cyclic AMP enhance Cl^- transport and thus may be involved in maintaining corneal deturgescence. Cyclic AMP administration increases transparency in swollen corneae. The nucleotide stimulates Cl^- active transport in the epithelium, mediated at least in part, by β-adrenergic (catecholamines) stimulation of adenylate cyclase and possibly ascorbate inhibition of phosphodiesterase activities.

The predominant role of the endothelium in controlling fluid transport is due to several enzymic pump systems present in the endothelial cells which collectively regulate fluid and ionic transport across the cell layer. A Na^+/K^+-ATPase is present, which is several-fold more active than in epithelium. Ouabain, a specific ATPase inhibitor, blocks endothelial fluid transport. A bicarbonate-dependent ATPase has also been reported in endothelial cells; depletion of bicarbonate from incubation/perfusion medium induces swelling. The enzyme seems to be present in mitochondria and not on the plasma membrane; enzymic inhibition by thiocyanate is paralleled by inhibition of fluid transport. Carbonic anhydrase has also been implicated in the regulation of fluid transport since carbonic anhydrase inhibitors decrease the flow of fluid from stroma to aqueous humour. The enzyme has been localized almost exclusively in the corneal endothelium and, as in most tissues, produces bicarbonate (HCO_3^-) ions and hydrogen (H^+) ions. Besides these systems, a Na^+/H^+ pump has been postulated at the lateral plasma membrane surface. Passive ion movement also occurs in that K^+, Cl^- and HCO_3^- diffuse into the aqueous humour. In the contralateral direction, Na^+, Cl^- and HCO_3^- are passively moved from the aqueous into the cornea. Thus, a complex series of metabolically dependent and passive reactions occur in the endothelium and epithelium to maintain proper fluid/ionic balance and deturgescence in the cornea.

Corneal Disease

Several corneal disease entities are related to defects in biosynthesis, structure and function of corneal collagen and GAGs. In keratoconus, for example, altered biosynthesis, glycosylation and cross-linking of collagen have been reported as well as changes in GAG metabolism. A thickened Descemet's membrane is observed in Fuch's endothelial dystrophy with abnormal collagen fibril bundles. In corneal macular dystrophy, a defective conversion of a glycoprotein precursor to keratan sulphate has been uncovered. In endothelial corneal dystrophy, excess collagen is produced, resulting in a multilaminar structure posterior to Descemet's membrane. In Reis–Buckler's ring-shaped dystrophy, Bowman's membrane is replaced by short (8–10 nm) filaments, with subsequent disorganization of stromal collagen. The filaments may result from abnormal collagen biosynthesis or degradation.

Keratomalacia and generalized protein/calorie malnutrition have long been known to affect epithelial tissues. Effects are especially prominent in the cornea where xerophthalmia (drying) is an early manifestation with loss of goblet cells. Subsequent stages lead to keratinization, erosion, infection, perforation, etc. The biochemical basis of the disease lies in the dependence of epithelial cells on vitamin A for growth and development and, in the adult, for maintenance of differentiated function. It has been postulated that vitamin A is necessary for such maintenance, possibly through regulation of the biosynthesis of specific glycoproteins through the intermediate mannosyl retinyl phosphate (MRP). The synthesis of several high molecular weight corneal glycoconjugates is enhanced by retinoic acid, an active vitamin A metabolite; and thus retinoids may control the expression of the keratinizing phenotype.

Cyclic nucleotides may be involved in the pathology of corneal wound healing. Dibutyryl cyclic AMP inhibits the appearance of collagenous activity in ulcerated corneae *in vitro*. Similarly, an imbalance in the cyclic AMP/cyclic GMP ratio may be a problem in wound healing. Increasing cyclic GMP levels (carbachol) may help in this condition.

LENS

As with the cornea, the major function of the lens is to remain transparent and to furnish refractive power to the eye. Thus, the major interest in the lens pathologically is when either or both of these functions is disturbed, as in cataract. The lens is positioned in place by the zonular fibres, anchored to the ciliary body, and forms a barrier between the aqueous and vitreous humours. Also, as with the cornea, its position and function in the eye dictates much of its biochemical nature, both structurally and metabolically.

The lens is a truly unique tissue whose only close metabolic analogy is the red blood cell. It is of ectodermal origin and normally loses no cells during growth and maturation. Layers of cells are added to the original embryonic cells of the nucleus throughout life, as are rings on a tree, yielding a biological history of the tissue (albeit altered with age) from the centre to periphery.

Structure and Composition

The young adult lens is a pale yellow, soft, biconvex structure consisting of one main cell type, the fibre cell, and a single layer of epithelial cells on the anterior surface. It is surrounded by a strong, elastic typical basement membrane, the lens capsule. The fibres develop through maturation from the epithelial cells. These latter cells divide in the germinative zone near the lens equator. As they differentiate into mature, elongated fibres, they are pushed deeper into the lens interior. losing their nuclei in the process. Three distinct lenticular zones are thus formed: (1) the epithelial layer of dividing cells; (2) a cortex of differentiating, elongating cells; and (3) a central nuclear region of densely packed, mature fibre cells without nuclei and other cellular organelles. Thus, although the lens is a metabolically active tissue, there is a steep metabolic gradient from epithelial to cortical to nuclear fibre cell.

The components of the lens capsule are secreted by epithelial and cortical cells and are constantly if slowly renewed by these cells. The capsule itself is composed, in the main, of type IV collagen and GAGs (heparan sulphate). The collagen is heavily glycosylated. The GAGs probably help to determine the structural organization of the capsular matrix.

The lens has the highest protein concentration of any tissue – about 35 per cent of the total mass. About 90 per cent of all the proteins are the crystallins, a class of structural proteins specific to the lens. The term 'crystallin' generally is used to refer to lenticular water-soluble proteins, while 'albuminoid' is an older term which has been used in reference to water-insoluble proteins. The crystallins have been divided into three major families, α, β, and γ, based mainly on size and electrophoretic mobility. *Table* I gives some of the more important characteristics of the crystallins and MIP, the Main Intrinsic Protein of lens cell membranes. The crystallins have been highly conserved proteins during evolution, doubtlessly because of the need for lenticular transparency.

α-Crystallin is the largest crystallin type and is rather heterogeneous in nature. It consists of four basic subunits, two of which are direct gene products and two arise as post-translational modifications of the original polypeptides through deamidation. β-Crystallins are the most polydisperse in nature. They are usually found in β-pleated sheet and random coil structures, with the basic structure highly conserved during evolution. The γ-crystallins are quite small and do not aggregate. Structurally, they have a high degree of β-pleated sheet structure with a paucity of α-helices. The lenticular crystallin composition varies considerably from species to species and also varies with age. In the young human (10–19 years), the relative percentages of α-, β- and γ-crystallins are 37, 38 and 25 per cent respectively. By the eighth decade of life, however, the percentages are approximately 58, 34 and 9 per cent respectively.

The main intrinsic protein (MIP) has been studied as archetypical of insoluble membrane proteins and is specifically associated with the cellular gap junctions. It has a molecular weight of $2 \cdot 6 \times 10^4$ daltons but is processed to a molecular size of $2 \cdot 2 \times 10^4$ daltons during ageing. The highest concentration of the $2 \cdot 2 \times 10^4$ dalton species is in the lens nucleus, with little if any in the superficial cortical region. Other insoluble and membraneous proteins are present in the lens, with the percentage of such insoluble components (and higher molecular weight aggregates) increasing with age. There is no clear correlation, however, between formation of these entities and the development of lenticular opacities.

Table I. Properties of principal adult human lens proteins

Property	α-crystallin	β-crystallin	γ-crystallin	MIP
% of total (approx.)	55	35	10	>50 of membrane
Native form	Oligomer	Oligomer	Monomer	Insoluble
Mol. wt (daltons)	50–80×10^4	5–25×10^4	2×10^4	$\sim 2 \cdot 6 \times 10^4$
Subunits	4	Multiple	—	—
Subunit mol wt (daltons)	2×20^4	$2 \cdot 5$–$3 \cdot 5 \times 10^4$	—	—
Isoelectric point (pH)	$4 \cdot 8$–$5 \cdot 0$	$5 \cdot 7$–$7 \cdot 0$	$7 \cdot 1$–$8 \cdot 1$	—

Lens Metabolism

Glucose Utilization

As with the cornea, the lens is avascular and relies upon diffusion and active transport for its supply of metabolites and oxygen. Sugars, for example, enter by facilitated diffusion along a concentration gradient. Although all the pathways for glucose metabolism are present, it is probable that the lens depends on anaerobic glycolysis (i.e. >70 per cent of glucose goes to lactate) for energy equivalents since it lacks a blood supply and exhibits a low oxygen level. Glucose is essential for normal lens function and maintenance of transparency. A lens incubated under completely anoxic conditions but with sufficient glucose will remain clear for some time.

under normal circumstances (*Fig.* 3). The physiological function of this pathway in lens is still questionable. It may be that it utilizes the H^+ produced from glucose in the pentose phosphate pathway for subsequent energy production ('transhydrogenation').

Glutathione and Ascorbic Acid

These reducing substances are in particularly high concentration in the lens. Glutathione is present at $10 \,\mu mol/g$, a level higher than in any other tissue; over 90 per cent is found in the reduced (GSH) form. Although synthesis is high, enzymes hydrolysing this tripeptide have not been well studied in the lens. Ascorbate ($1 \,\mu mol/g$) does not appear to be synthesized in lens tissue, but rather enters from the

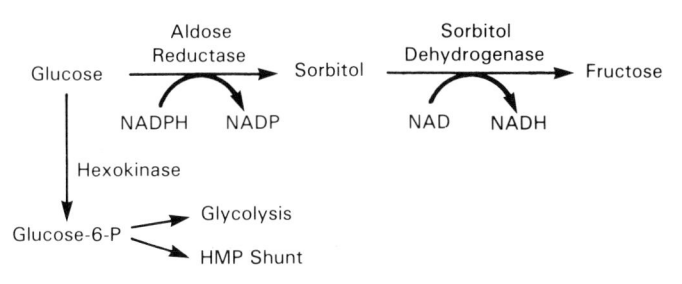

```
                    Aldose                    Sorbitol
                    Reductase                 Dehydrogenase
        Glucose  ────────────▶  Sorbitol  ────────────────▶  Fructose
                 NADPH  NADP              NAD   NADH
          │
          │ Hexokinase
          ▼
                    ▶ Glycolysis
        Glucose-6-P
                    ▶ HMP Shunt
```

Fig. 3. Competition for glucose between the sorbitol pathway and other metabolic pathways.

The enzyme hexokinase, which converts glucose to G-6-P, plays a particularly important role in lens metabolism due to its central role in sugar metabolism, its rate-limiting activity and its vulnerability to metabolic distress (e.g. hypoglycaemia). Hexokinase, through the production of G-6-P, also controls metabolism via the HMP shunt, a pathway which competes with the glycolytic pathway for G-6-P utilization. Thus, the first enzymes in these respective pathways (G-6-P dehydrogenase in the HMP shunt and phosphofructokinase in glycolysis) are also key enzymes in lenticular metabolic control. The HMP shunt is not usually very active in lens, utilizing less than 5 per cent of the total lens glucose supply. Other than in the epithelium, the lens cells would have little use for ribose, the major metabolic product of the shunt, although the reducing equivalents produced may be of importance.

The Sorbitol Pathway

The first hint of the importance of this pathway in lens metabolism came from the observation that polyols (sugar alcohols) were present in cataracts induced by high sugar concentrations. Thus, although of minor importance in most normal tissues, it assumes major importance in sugar and diabetic cataractogenesis as discussed below. In the lens, aldose reductase is quite sluggish, with the K_m for glucose estimated at 200 mM. It thus does not effectively compete with hexokinase for glucose and only a small fraction of the hexose is reduced to sorbitol

aqueous humour. The roles of these reducing agents in normal lens metabolism and in cataractogenesis remain controversial. They perhaps function in redox reactions, involving pyridine nucleotide and pentose phosphate metabolism. Certainly they could help protect lens proteins and their sulphydryls from oxidative damage by acting as free-radical scavengers.

Transport

As the lens is a unique encapsulated tissue, it appears to have developed a unique mode for maintenance of ionic homeostasis. This is known as the 'pump-leak' system, in which it is thought that an active cation pump (Na^+/K^+-dependent ATPase) exchanges potassium for sodium at the epithelium (Na^+ out, K^+ in) with sodium passively entering from the vitreous humour and potassium similarly leaving. Thus, the proper internal ionic balance is achieved (Na^+, 200 mM; K^+, 120 mM. An interesting corollary of this mechanism is that it assumes that lens cells do not individually regulate their ionic environment but rather act in concert. The entire lens thus effectively functions as a single cell. Many other substances are transported into the lens; free amino acids, for example, are concentrated to a high degree.

Transparency

Again, in analogy to the cornea, the lens remains clear due to both structural and biochemical factors.

Certainly, pump mechanisms, energy metabolism etc. all must operate adequately. Beyond this though, factors relating to the large size of the lens and its high cellular protein concentration must be overcome to insure that the lens is not opaque due to scattering of incident light. On a gross basis, lens fibres are indeed arranged in regular, repeating, ribbon-like arrays. On a molecular basis, it was proposed several years ago that lens proteins were arranged in 'paracrystallin' structures, well ordered over large distances. This is now known to have little to do with transparency, however, in that a generalized, higher-ordered lattice theory of transparency is not necessary to explain the phenomenon. Only short-range order appears necessary to fulfil all the theoretical and experimental requirements for transparency. It is interesting to note that *in vitro* experiments with lens protein solutions demonstrate that turbidity actually decreases in highly concentrated crystallin solutions due to short-range, ordered spatial configurations, as in dense liquids or glass.

Cataract Formation

Virtually any major insult to the lens, be it genetic, environmental, physical, metabolic or simple ageing, results in some form of opacification or loss of clarity. Although the aetiology of most cataracts must be generally considered to be multifactorial, several individual factors are known to contribute to the cataractogenic process.

Ageing

Alteration of shape for accommodative purposes is an important property of the human lens. With age, the lens soma 'hardens' and is less easily deformed; thus much of the accommodative ability of the lens is lost by the sixth decade of life. Physically and biochemically, age-related changes in lens proteins are numerous. Most prominent is the well-known conversion from soluble to insoluble form (up to 40 per cent in older lenses). These processes cannot be strictly correlated with senile cataract formation as mentioned before. Human cataracts contain more disulphide than in normal lens; thus it has been suggested that disulphide bonding of protein may result in insolubilization and opacification. Non-disulphide, covalent cross-linkage of crystallins is prominent in the lens nucleus as well and may also result in insolubilization. Since the lifetime turnover of crystallins is negligible, there is an age-dependent accumulation of D-aspartic acid in nuclear proteins due to racemization. As with cross-linking, this process may be related to the formation of aggregates and insoluble protein. Lens pigmentation increases as well as non-tryptophan fluorescence. These may be related to photo-oxidative damage as discussed below.

Photo-oxidation

A small percentage of ultraviolet light passes through the cornea and aqueous humour and may initiate photo-oxidative damage in the lens involving free or protein-bound tryptophan residues or other photosensitive elements. Such oxidation could result in fluorescent and pigmentary changes characteristic of ageing and cataractous lenses. It has been postulated that light activates an endogenous photosensitive agent (possibly a tryptophan or other amino acid oxidation product) in the presence of molecular oxygen to promote the ageing/cataractous processes. Activated ('singlet') oxygen is known to cause crystallin aggregation and pigmentary changes *in vitro*. Hydrogen peroxide (H_2O_2), another form of activated oxygen, may also be involved in these reactions.

Lipid peroxidation may also play a role in cataract formation. Fatty acid radicals can ultimately produce the compound malondialdehyde, a well-known cross-linking agent, which can attack enzymes and membrane components. Similarly, the generation of superoxide ($O_2^-\cdot$) and hydroxyl ($OH\cdot$) radicals has been postulated to be involved in cataract formation. The high concentration of glutathione (with ascorbic acid and vitamin E) and the presence of catalase and superoxide dismutase enzyme systems help to protect the lens from oxidative damage.

Sugar Cataracts

Strictly speaking, the term 'sugar cataract' only refers to the clinical entities seen in galactosaemia and juvenile diabetes, but it is used now in a somewhat broader context, e.g. adult diabetes. Excess sugar in the lens is converted by aldose reductase (*see Fig.* 3) to the corresponding sugar alcohol (glucose → sorbitol; galactose → dulcitol). This only occurs at unusually high levels of sugar in blood and aqueous (*see* discussion of the sorbitol pathway, above). The resultant alcohol is then unable to escape from the lens nor is it readily metabolized, and thus it accumulates within the cells making the cytoplasm markedly hypertonic. This induces a large movement of water into the lens, alteration of the Na^+/K^+ ratio, and concomitant swelling. The normal lenticular architecture is thus disrupted, leading to the formation of foci of interfibrillar and intracytoplasmic light scattering (i.e. water clefts and vacuoles), with resultant opacification. The many changes involved in the formation of sugar cataracts are depicted in *Fig.* 4.

It now appears that sugar cataracts (galactosaemic and diabetic) may be prevented and/or controlled in the not too distant future. In animal studies, inhibitors of the enzyme aldose reductase have been shown to delay and prevent cataract formation. Active agents have been fatty acids, tetramethylene glutaric acid, flavinoids and, more effectively, the synthetic compounds alrestatin and sorbinil.

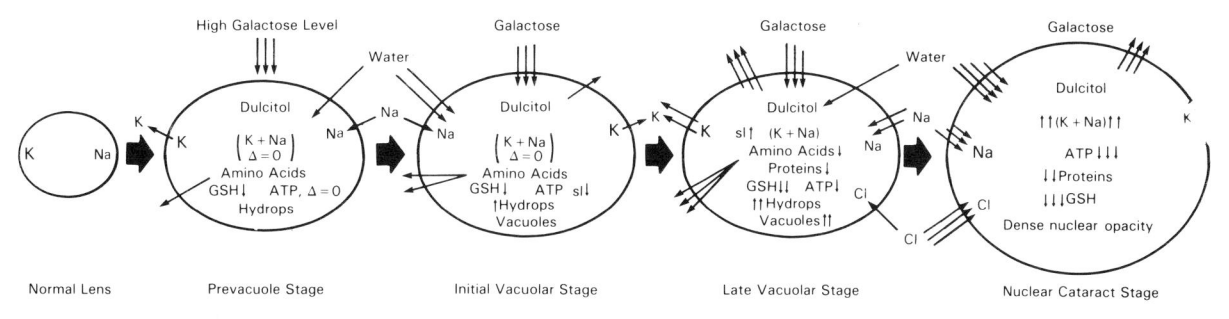

Fig. 4. Stages in sugar cataract formation. K: potassium; Na: sodium; GSH: glutathione; Cl: chloride; Δ = 0: no change in total K + Na; sl: slight change; arrows pointing up: increase; arrows pointing down: decrease. (Adapted from Kinoshita J., Kador P. and Datiles M. *JAMA* 1981; **246**, 257.)

Other Cataracts

For some time, posterior subcapsular cataracts have been known to be associated with long term steroid treatment. It is thought that the steroids may induce aberrant differentiation and migration of epithelial cells leading to the posterior opacification observed. It is known that typical glucocorticoid receptor proteins are present in the lens and that lens tissue can form glucuronide and sulphate conjugates of cortisol. Whether these processes are involved in cataract formation is yet unknown. Posterior subcapsular cataracts are also induced by ionizing radiation.

In addition, several nutritional cataract entities are known. Riboflavin-deficiency cataract, for example, may be related to inadequate functioning of the FAD-dependent glutathione reductase. Animal studies have indicated that suboptimal levels of vitamin E may compromise lens cell differentiation, leading to opacification. Lens opacities have also been reported in human subjects with hypocalcaemic tetany. An increased leakiness of membranes followed by hydration/swelling has been proposed as the cause of the hypocalcaemic effect.

Cataract Therapy

A number of agents have been reported to be useful in preventing or delaying cataractogenesis. In senile cataracts, nutritional supplements, including inorganic salts, sulphydryl and redox compounds and non-steroidal anti-inflammatory compounds have been used with controversial results. In radiation cataracts, antioxidants and free radical scavengers have been used to try to delay or prevent cataract formation. Undoubtedly the most potentially useful of these agents, the aldose reductase inhibitors used in sugar cataract control, have been discussed above.

OCULAR FLUIDS AND CILIARY BODY

This section deals with the tear film, aqueous humour and vitreous humour, together with aqueous production from the ciliary body. The primary function of each of these liquid or gel substances is to provide an optically clear passageway for light on its way to the retina. Other, more specialized functions, will be discussed more fully below.

Tear Film

Tears moisten and lubricate the anterior eye surface and allow for dissolved oxygen to enter the epithelial cells of the cornea. The tear film has a tripartite layered structure. The outermost layer is relatively hydrophobic and contains most of the lipids; these are secreted by the Meibomian glands. Below this is the aqueous layer, secreted by the main and accessory lacrimal glands. The bottom layer consists mainly of mucins secreted by the goblet cells of the conjunctiva.

Composition

The tear film is about 98 per cent water, the remaining 2 per cent being lipids, ions, proteins etc. The lipid composition is approximately 65 per cent cholesterol and wax esters, 15 per cent phospholipids, 4 per cent triglycerides, 2 per cent free fatty acids and 2 per cent free sterols. Vitamin A is also present in tears. A number of salts are dissolved in the water phase of the tear film, including sodium, potassium, chloride and bicarbonate. Many proteins are also present, notably immunoglobulins, interferons, complement, lysozyme, lactoferrin and a specific tear prealbumin (STP) which is synthesized in the lacrimal gland. Mucins are present, mainly in close juxtaposition to the corneal surface.

Function

The thin, hydrophobic surface layer of the tear film is thought to retard evaporation and to lubricate the motion of the lids over the cornea. The mucins act as a wetting agent, allowing for a stable interaction of the aqueous layer with the epithelial surface. In the aqueous layer, tear electrolytes act as osmotic regulators and physiological buffers, maintaining tear–corneal homeostasis. Besides these general functions, the individual components of the tear film fulfil specific functions. The immunoglobulins (IGG,

IgA, secretory IgA etc.) act in the immune defence system to protect the eye from microbial attack, as does complement. Lysozyme is another important lacrimal antimicrobial agent; interferon similarly protects against viruses.

Dysfunction

Dysfunction associated with the tear film most often is related to abnormal synthesis or secretion of one of the critical tear components (mucin, lipid etc.). Often this can be assessed by biochemical measurement of the components, e.g. lysosome or lactoferrin. Keratinization, associated with systemic vitamin A deficiency, results in decreased mucous secretion and tear film instability. Decreased amounts of antimicrobial agents will lead to infection and inflammation.

Aqueous Humour

The aqueous humour is a fluid secreted by the ciliary epithelium and is essentially a modified filtrate of blood serum. It contains no cellular components and only a small percentage (<1 per cent) of serum proteins, but has most of the small molecular weight electrolyte and nutrient constituents of serum. In addition, some constituents (e.g. ascorbate) are in much higher concentration than in serum, demonstrating the complexity of aqueous secretion.

Composition

Glucose is one of the most important of the aqueous humour constituents; it is usually found in slightly lower levels than in serum. Lactate, in contrast, is found at concentrations higher than in serum. Oxygen is present at a partial pressure of 55 mmHg. Most cations are present at serum levels but calcium is lower (~50 per cent). The cation balance is affected by the surrounding tissues; the lens, for example, secretes Na^+ into the aqueous; K^+, Cl^- and HCO_3^- are derived from the corneal endothelium. As might be expected, the major anions are chloride and bicarbonate. Organic constituents show a higher degree of variation from plasma levels due to tissue metabolism, active transport *v.* passive diffusion etc. Ascorbate and inositol are good examples of this since they are in much higher concentration in aqueous than in serum and are secreted by the ciliary epithelium by active transport. Some free amino acids are also found in high concentration in the aqueous, secreted in the main from the ciliary epithelium by an active process. Serum proteins are present in the aqueous but in very low amounts. They are mainly restricted to the smaller molecular weight proteins such as albumin; the α_1-acid glycoprotein (mol wt $4\cdot4 \times 10^4$) for example, is present in comparably much higher amounts than the immunoglobulins ($>15 \times 10^4$ mol wt). Insulin and the steroid hormones are also present and enter the aqueous humour by simple diffusion. Prostaglandins, however, appear to be actively released into the aqueous by the iris. Cyclic AMP has been detected in the aqueous at a level about the same as is found in serum.

Function

The aqueous humour provides a physiological bathing medium and nutrient source for the cornea, lens and other adjacent tissues as well as a repository for materials removed from these tissues. Its synthesis and secretion is in dynamic equilibrium; removal is through the outflow channels of the trabecular meshwork. As pointed out in the discussion of the cornea, aqueous oxygen and glucose are of critical importance to corneal function, fuelling the metabolic pumps of the endothelium such that deturgescence is maintained. The lens epithelium is similarly dependent on glucose, amino acids and dissolved oxygen in the aqueous. The extraordinarily high concentration of ascorbic acid (and relatively high glutathione) in aqueous humour may indicate a need for protection against oxidative damage to the tissues lining the anterior chamber.

Ciliary Body and Aqueous Humour Production

Both 'dialysis' (diffusion and ultrafiltration) and 'secretion' processes are important in aqueous production. There is a rapid exchange rate of water across the blood–aqueous barrier which enters passively into the chamber. Relatively little difference in osmolarity exists between the two fluid compartments. Most aqueous components are supplied through the ciliary body but contributions from corneal endothelium, iris and lens cannot be ignored.

Aqueous constituent secretion occurs from the ciliary processes. Tight junctions between the epithelial cells preclude movement of most large protein molecules from the ciliary stroma into the aqueous while allowing smaller, especially hydrophobic molecules to pass relatively freely. These cells exhibit high carbonic anhydrase and Na^+/K^+-ATPase activities necessary for normal aqueous constituent secretion (i.e. transport of Na^+, K^+, sugars, amino acids etc.). Inhibitors of Na^+/K^+-ATPase (e.g. vanadate, ouabain) and carbonic anhydrase (e.g. acetazolamide) inhibit aqueous production and lower the intraocular pressure (IOP).

Breakdown in the blood–aqueous barrier (osmotic agents, drugs, trauma etc.) can lead to both increased flow and altered composition of the aqueous humour. The aqueous then becomes much more like serum in its composition and is called 'secondary aqueous'.

IOP and Glaucoma

Intraocular pressure (IOP) can fluctuate considerably and is acutely affected by factors controlling production and outflow of aqueous humour. Pressure within ciliary process capillaries affects aqueous flow.

Vasoconstriction of efferent ciliary blood vessels favours increased aqueous flow; constriction of afferent vessels decreases ultrafiltration. β-Adrenergic-stimulated adenylate cyclase in the ciliary processes also mediates aqueous production. Outflow of aqueous is mainly by bulk flow through the trabecular meshwork and is dependent on differences between the IOP and episcleral venous pressure. The mucopolysaccharide material in the extracellular matrix of the trabecular meshwork may offer substantial resistance to aqueous outflow.

In glaucoma, the increased IOP is caused by increased resistance to outflow. In narrow angle glaucoma, physical blockage of the chamber angle by the iris increases IOP. In primary open angle glaucoma (POAG), the angle remains grossly normal but outflow resistance increases for reasons poorly understood. Many POAG patients demonstrate a marked increase of IOP when challenged over several weeks with topical or systemic glucocorticoids. Similarly, some people with normal eyes may develop steroid glaucoma after prolonged treatment with glucocorticoids. Abnormal sensitivity to steroids is a biochemical marker that may provide a clue to the trabecular derangement that causes glaucoma. Glucocorticoids have been demonstrated in the aqueous humour, albeit at a lower concentration than in serum. Differences have been found in the metabolism of cortisol by trabecular meshwork cells from normal and POAG patients grown *in vitro*. These differences are a one hundred-fold reduction in Δ^4-reductase activity and a four-fold reduction in 3-oxido-reductase activity. These enzyme defects are not observed in peripheral lymphocytes of POAG patients and thus may be of specific importance to glaucoma pathology.

Glaucoma treatment presently utilizes three categories of drug: carbonic anhydrase inhibitors (e.g. acetazolamide), which decrease aqueous formation: miotics (e.g. pilocarpine), which increase outflow through smooth muscle contraction; and adrenergics (e.g. adrenaline), which may affect both inflow and outflow. Timolol, a β-adrenergic blocking agent which reduces aqueous formation, has been found to be particularly useful in glaucoma therapy. The mechanism of action of these agents is yet unclear, especially since both α- and β-adrenergics are effective in lowering IOP; action, however, may be mediated by cyclic AMP, particularly in controlling outflow.

Vitreous Humour

The vitreous humour is a gel-like, avascular, specialized connective tissue that occupies most of the volume of the eye (up to 90 per cent in some species). It is attached to surrounding tissues, e.g. to ciliary body and to retina peripherally and at the optic disc. Its prime function is, again, transparency but it also interacts metabolically with its surrounding tissues and furnishes a viscoelastic component to the globe.

Composition and Structure

The major components of the vitreous are collagen and hyaluronic acid, with the collagen forming an interweaving network or superstructure for the hyaluronic acid and other components. A small number of hyalocytes are present in the vitreous and these synthesize and secrete matrix material.

Several collagen types are represented (types I to IV) and are produced by cells in the vitreous as well as by retinal glial elements. Depending on the ratios of collagen and hyaluronic acid, the vitreous body can be a gel or liquid. Hyaluronic acid (*see Fig. 1*) is a high molecular weight, unsulphated glycosaminoglycan (GAG) consisting of glucuronate and N-acetyl-glucosamine repeating units. Because of its large number of carboxyl groups, it acts as an acidic polyanion and is heavily hydrated. Soluble proteins present in the vitreous are low in concentration (<1 per cent) and are akin to those found in serum (e.g. albumin). Vitreous has a high ascorbate concentration. Most small molecules have an asymmetrical distribution in the vitreous due to differential production and/or utilization by the surrounding tissues.

Function

The natural resiliency of the globe is mainly due to the vitreous humour. Thus, it physically buffers the internal ocular organs from shock and trauma. It also acts as a nutrient and waste product reservoir for the surrounding tissues. Glucose is present at about half the concentration found in aqueous humour and is taken up and metabolized in retina and lens. Sodium and potassium are exchanged at the lens posterior surface: magnesium is secreted into the vitreous from the retina. Lactate and pyruvate diffuse from the retina into the posterior vitreous. There appears to be a generalized transretinal flow from the aqueous through the vitreous primarily due to powerful metabolic pumps located in the pigment epithelium. Radiolabelled compounds instilled intravitreally quickly reach the retinal outer segments and PE cells.

Vitreous Pathology

Both ageing and metabolic diseases can affect the vitreous body in composition and/or physical state. With age, the collagen network tends to collapse, forming small lakes of fluid in the matrix. Diabetes may change the collagen as well as the amino sugar content of the vitreous. Diabetes may also result in vitreal contraction of collagenous elements and detachment from the retina.

The hyaluronic acid polymer is relatively unstable and can easily depolymerize under a variety of pathological conditions, leading to a great decrease in viscosity. Depolymerization may occur due to action of: mammalian or bacterial hyaluronidases, ionizing radiation or catalytic reducing agents (organic or inorganic). It is interesting that a natural 'reducing' agent, ascorbate, is present in vitreous in high concentration; other such agents include cysteine, cuprous and ferrous ions. Vitreal changes related to hyaluronic acid metabolism can occur with injury both acutely, due to physical trauma and haemorrhage or, somewhat more chronically, due to the presence of a foreign object. Haemorrhage results in vitreal liquification and a decrease in hyaluronic acid content due to subunit depolymerization. Inflammation and clot formation is variable. The enzyme urokinase has been used experimentally to treat vitreal haemorrhage. Various foreign objects, usually present as a result of traumatic injury, also can lead to hyaluronic acid depolymerization and liquification. A foreign iron body (ferrous) leads to siderosis; copper implantation leads to chalcosis.

Intraocular Gels

The prevalence of vitrectomy and glaucoma surgery has led to great interest in the use of highly viscous hyaluronic acid solutions. Hyaluronic acid is a perfect natural gel which allows for both inert space filling and minimization of intraocular tissue adhesions.

THE RETINA–PIGMENT EPITHELIAL UNIT

The neuronal elements of the posterior segment should be considered as two functional units. First, the photoreceptor cells of the neural retina and their attendant pigment epithelial (PE) cells, whose respective major functions are the acceptance of the light signal (photoreceptor cell) and the metabolic and structural maintenance of the photoreceptor outer segments (PE cells). Secondly, the other neuronal cell types of the retina (bipolar, horizontal, amacrine and ganglion) function much as does the brain in signal processing and can be thought of as typical CNS elements. The major glial element of the retina, the Mueller cell, plays a role akin to that of the PE cell, i.e. affording structural and metabolic support to the retinal neurones. This section addresses the structural components and metabolism of the neural retina and the PE–choroid complex with special regard to the different structures and functions of the units described above.

Structure and Composition

The retina is a natural tissue slice, perfect for *in vitro* incubations. Within this 'slice', however, are several discrete layers which themselves are structurally and metabolically distinct. Primarily they are the photoreceptor–PE–choroid unit and the several nuclear and synaptic layers of the neural retina.

Photoreceptor Cell

Photoreceptor cells can be divided into two general types: rods and cones. Rod photoreceptors are long, cylindrical and mainly function in peripheral and in dim light vision. Cone photoreceptors are short, cone-shaped and function at higher light levels and in colour discrimination. For these purposes, four major types of light-sensitive visual pigments are present in vertebrate photoreceptors: rhodopsin (absorption max. 500 nm) is present in rods; red- (570 nm), blue- (400 nm) and green- (540 nm) sensitive pigments are found in cones.

Rhodopsin

The photoreceptor cell is a true neurone with a specialized organelle, the outer segment, which contains a number of unique structural proteins and enzymes. Most prominent of these is rhodopsin, the visual pigment, which comprises more than 80 per cent of the outer segment membrane protein. Rhodopsin is an insoluble, integral membrane glycoprotein of approximately 41 000 daltons having a protein core unit and two oligosaccharide chains consisting of mannose and N-acetylglucosamine linked to the protein through asparagine amino acid residues. It is thought to reside partially within the membrane bilayer as a transmembrane protein, spanning the bilayer in seven α-helical segments and having exposed C- and N-terminals extending into the cytoplasmic and intradiscal spaces, respectively (*Fig.* 5). It appears that about half of the rhodopsin molecule resides in the lipid bilayer, one-third on the cytoplasmic surface and the remainder on the intradiscal surface. It is known that light induces changes in rhodopsin conformation, e.g. at the C-terminus.

Rhodopsin is a conjugated protein having the ability to bind retinal as a prosthetic group in the dark, as will be discussed below. Retinal is bound in a covalent Schiff base linkage (C–N bond) to a lysine residue (position 53) within a hydrophobic region of the membrane (*Fig.* 5). The binding region is a sensitive area in rhodopsin's structure geared to communicate with the surface loops and easily change the external topography. The structure and/or function of rhodopsin can also be influenced in several other ways by co- or post-translational chemical modifications. Its α-amino terminus, for example, is blocked by N-acetylation, possibly protecting the protein from aminopeptidase proteolytic attack and prolonging its biological longevity. Rhodopsin can be phosphorylated in a light-dependent manner using ATP or GTP, a process catalysed by the enzyme rhodopsin kinase. Phosphorylation sites are at several serine and threonine residues clustered near the exposed C-terminus of the protein, leading to a strong negative charge in this region. The reaction is light-dependent in that light-induced conformational changes in rhodopsin rather than light-activation of the kinase enzyme *per se* triggers the reaction. Rhodopsin can also be acylated by long chain fatty acids (e.g. palmitate). This process may be involved in insertion of rhodopsin into nascent membranes at the outer segment base.

The outer segment contains several other unique protein constituents. A large (290 000 dalton) integral protein has been identified and localized only at the disc margins and disc incisures. Several peripherally bound proteins involved in cyclic nucleotide metabolism are known to be present and interact with rhodopsin. These will be discussed below.

precursor (e.g. ^{3}H-leucine) into newly formed discs and the subsequent apical movement, shedding and phagocytosis of the radiolabelled disc membranes. Light has a profound effect on the renewal process in that light and dark regulate both the rate of membrane addition to and loss from the outer segment. For example, there is a diurnal variation in amino acid incorporation into opsin in the inner segment. Moreover, disc shedding proceeds in a circadian

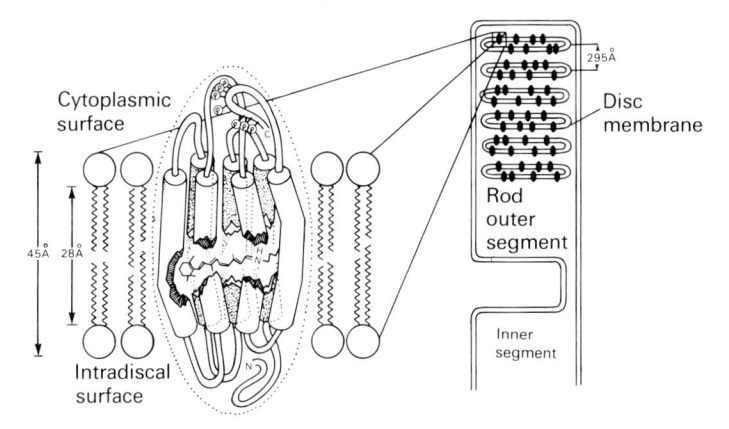

Fig. 5. Possible organization of rhodopsin into seven helical regions within the disc membrane lipid bilayer. Portions of three of the helical regions have been omitted to show schematically the orientation of 11-*cis* retinal within the membrane. (Adapted from Dratz E. and Hargrave P. *Trends Biochem. Sci.* 1983; **8**, 128.)

Lipids

The lipid components of the outer segment are also unusual in composition. They make up about 50 per cent of the outer segment mass. Of this, the phospholipids constitute the bulk (>80 per cent), with other lipids (e.g. cholesterol, free fatty acids etc.) the small remaining amount. A low cholesterol content allows for a relatively fluid, non-viscous membrane. Another factor ensuring high membrane fluidity is the extraordinarily high amount of long chain polyunsaturated fatty acids, especially docosahexaenoic acid, a 22-carbon atom fatty acid with six double bonds. The high membrane fluidity enables rhodopsin to move freely within the plane of the rod disc membrane and interact with other membrane constituents in coupled reactions. High levels of vitamin E, a potent antioxidant, are also present in outer segment membranes.

Renewal

Vertebrate rod photoreceptor cells continually renew their outer segments. The renewal process depends on (*a*) synthesis of new membrane components in the inner segment, (*b*) assembly of discs at the outer segment base; (*c*) displacement of discs towards the outer segment tip by new discs; and (*d*) disc shedding at the outer segment tip and phagocytosis of the shed packets by the pigment epithelium. This process can be demonstrated (*Fig.* 6) autoradiographically following the incorporation of a pulse of radiolabelled

manner in mammals, with a burst of shedding and phagocytosis occurring soon after the time of light onset. The process is not under pineal control but

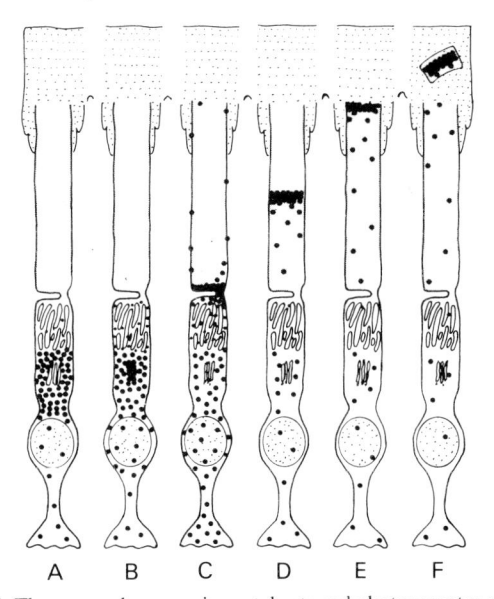

Fig. 6. The renewal process in vertebrate rod photoreceptor outer segments. A, After administration of pulse of radioactive amino acid or other membrane precursor, radioactivity (dark dots) accumulates in myoid region. B, Newly formed protein moves throughout cell and some is concentrated in Golgi apparatus for processing. C, Proteins migrate through cilium and are incorporated into newly formed membranes. D, New discs (non-radiolabelled) force the displacement of radiolabelled discs. E, Radiolabelled discs reach outer segment tip. F, Radiolabelled disc packets are shed and phagocytized by pigment epithelial cells.

is truly a light-entrained, circadian process since, once the animals are adapted to a particular light regime over a suitably long period of time, shedding will occur at the usual time even without the onset of light (i.e. continuous darkness). Melatonin, a tryptophan derivative synthesized in pineal and retina, has been postulated to be one of the signalling molecules in disc shedding. It is interesting to note that the retina contains the melatonin-synthesizing enzymes N-acetyltransferase (NAT) and hydroxyindole-O-methyl-transferase (HIOMT) and thus resembles the pineal in this respect.

Inner Segment

Connecting the outer segment to the inner segment is a modified cilium through which newly synthesized rhodopsin passes to be assembled into discs at the base of the outer segment. The cilium has a 9 + 0 arrangement of microtubules and is thought to be rich in the enzyme guanylate cyclase. The presence of calmodulin and actin indicates that calcium may regulate cytoskeletal interactions and membrane assembly in this region. The inner segment is perhaps the most metabolically active region of any cell known. It is packed with mitochondria, exhibits a most active Golgi apparatus where rhodopsin is processed and is the site of the electrophysiological pump mechanisms. The Na^+-K^+-ATPase used in maintaining the 'dark current' is present in the plasma membranes. The remaining portions of the cell are ordinary in nature, consisting of a parikaryon (nuclear zone) and a basal synaptic region.

Pigment Epithelium–Choroid

Posterior to the photoreceptor outer segments is a single cell layer of cuboidal, pigmented, neuroepithelial cells, the pigment epithelium (PE). This cell layer sits on a thin layer of connective tissue, Bruch's membrane, abutting a rich vascular network, the choroid, which acts as the major nutrient source for the retinal photoreceptors. PE cells are distinctly polarized into apical and basal surfaces morphologically and biochemically. Na^+/K^+-ATPase, for example, is present predominantly in the apical portion of the PE, at least in frogs. This enzymic pump mechanism is responsible for the vectorial transport of several ions including K^+, Na^+, Ca^{+2} and Cl^-. The terminal bars of the PE include a tight junction (zonula occludeus) which forms the basis of the blood–retinal barrier. This is analogous to the blood–brain barrier formed by the capillary endothelial cells. Thus the PE cell itself rather than the intercellular spaces forms the major route for nutrients and waste products to pass to and from the photoreceptors. The PE cell character is strikingly similar to the cuboidal cells of the brain choroid plexus.

Inner Retinal Neurones

These cells (bipolar, horizontal, amacrine, ganglion etc.) form alternating strata of nuclear and plexiform (synaptic) layers and begin the long series of steps in visual signal processing. Structurally, biochemically and functionally they are similar to brain neurones, having a cellular perikaryon containing the nucleus and most cytoplasmic elements and an array of axonal and/or dendritic processes. Neurotransmitter modulation of synaptic transmission is discussed below.

PE–Choroid Metabolism and Function

Being only a single cell layer and difficult to isolate, little is known about the general metabolism of PE cells. It does, however, perform some important, well-defined, biochemical and structural functions.

Support

The long PE cell microvillus processes lend mechanical support and orientation to the photoreceptor outer segments.

Pigment

The numerous pigment granules function to capture stray or damaging light. Melanosomes form as a result of the action of the enzyme tyrosinase within a premelanosome matrix. The enzyme oxidizes tyrosine to indole-5,6-quinone; the quinone then polymerizes on the matrix to form melanin. No tyrosinase activity is detected in mature melanosomes.

Transport/Barrier

The PE layer furnishes a major pump-transport system for the retina and the eye as a whole (transretinal flow). As fluid is pumped from the interphotoreceptor (subretinal) space into the choroid, adhesion of PE and retina is facilitated. Based on *in vitro* studies, it has been postulated that cyclic AMP may play a major role in controlling the fluid volume in the subretinal space. The tight junction elements are of critical importance in establishing the blood–brain barrier.

Nutrition

The PE layer acts as a 'feeder' layer for the retinal outer segments, supplying glucose, O_2 etc. and removing wastes.

Phagocytosis

PE cells phagocytize shed outer segment tips and degrade them into smaller components. For this purpose, the PE cell has an extremely active lysosomal system relative to other tissues. PE lysosomes are specialized in their content of hydrolytic enzymes for degradation of outer segment constituents such as rhodopsin. Active in this process are cathepsin D and phospholipase D as well as general acid proteases, lipases and glycosidases. Residual bodies form the end product of such action. Incomplete digestion, however, may lead to the formation of lipofuscin granules. These are highly fluorescent bodies which accumulate in cells with age. They are particularly numerous in the older PE cell, presumably due to the heavy demand placed on the phagolysosome system by the influx of shed outer segments, estimated to be 25–30 000/day in the rat.

Vitamin A

The PE cell acts as a storage depot for vitamin A for ultimate use in photoreceptor visual transduction. Storage is in the form of esters (e.g. palmitate).

RETINAL METABOLISM AND FUNCTION

General Metabolism

The retina as a whole has a high rate of metabolism; glucose utilization is along the glycolytic pathway with major usage through the tricarboxylic acid cycle. Thus, ATP is efficiently produced in most retinal layers. Lactic acid is produced in relatively large amounts, indicating active aerobic glycolysis. Oxygen is very important to the retina, which is particularly sensitive to anoxia. Retinal bleaching decreases oxygen uptake and ATP utilization, particularly in the photoreceptor cell where the decreased membrane permeability (sodium pump) and ATPase activity result in a lowered need for energy production by inner segment mitochondria. The pentose phosphate pathway is also present in retina, although its activity is low. Glucose, as well as being the major energy producing substrate, is used as a carbon source for the biosynthesis of many important other substances, e.g. glycoproteins and putative neurotransmitters such as glutamate, aspartate and γ-amino butyric acid (GABA). Glutamine, important in ammonia detoxification and as a biosynthetic donor of $-NH_2$ groups, is also derived from the glucose skeleton.

Taking advantage of the stratified nature of the retina, some of the most important information concerning intermediary retinal metabolism has been obtained using the microdissection and biochemical cycling/amplification techniques of Lowry and Passonneau. In this way, metabolite concentrations and enzyme levels can be determined in each retinal layer. As can be seen in *Fig*. 7, a glucose gradient extends through the retina from the choroid to the vitreous with an inverse gradient of lactate. Hexokinase, the enzyme which phosphorylates glucose as a first step in its metabolic utilization, is extremely active in the photoreceptor inner segments in the mitochondria-rich region and, to a lesser degree, in the synaptic layers of the inner retina. Phosphofructokinase, a key regulatory enzyme of glycolysis, and the other enzymes of glycolysis are present mainly in the inner retinal layers. Activity of these enzymes

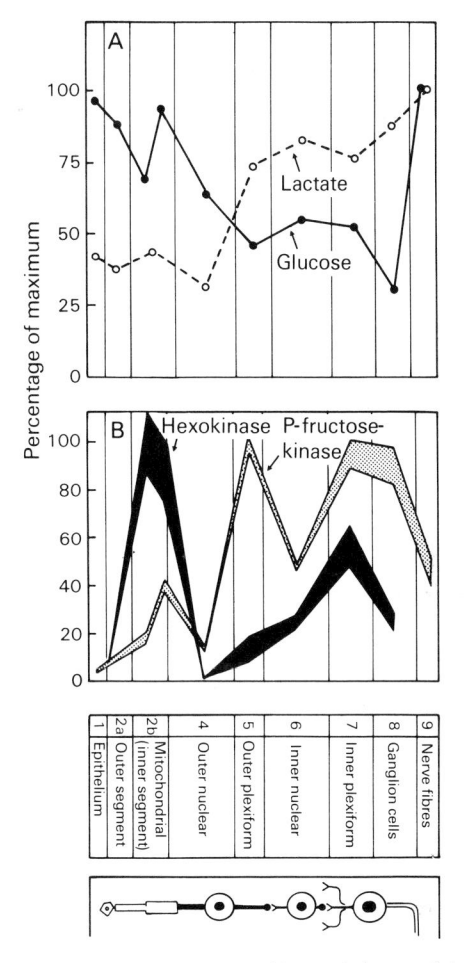

Fig. 7. A, Distribution of glucose and lactate in layers of the rabbit retina. *B*, Distribution of hexokinase and phosphofructokinase activities in layers of the monkey retina (*A*, Adapted from Matschinsky F. and McDougal D. *Prog. Clinicochem. Methods* 1968; **3**, 71. *B*, Adapted from Lowry O. In: Cohen M. and Snider R. (ed.) *Correlates of Neural Activity*, Harper, 1972, p. 178.

depends on retinal vascularity, e.g. higher in the relatively avascular rabbit retina and lower in the highly vascular monkey retina. These patterns therefore indicate (*a*) an exceptionally high rate of aerobic glycolysis in most retinae, (*b*) a gradient of metabolic activity utilizing glucose, O_2 etc., peaking in the photoreceptor inner segment, and (*c*) that metabolism in the inner retina is dependent on the degree of vascularization (i.e. O_2 supply) of these layers. In the photoreceptor cell, these results are compatible with the potentially large energy usage in maintaining the Na^+ current through Na^+/K^+-ATPase activity.

The Visual Cycle

In a broad sense, the visual cycle not only involves the rhodopsin bleaching events in the outer segment but the longer range movement of retinoid between retina and pigment epithelium (*Fig.* 8).

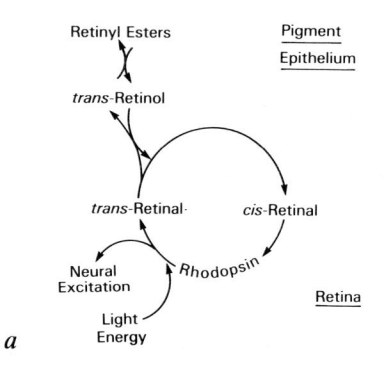

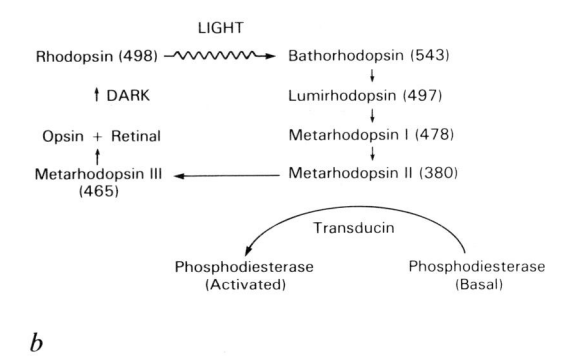

Fig. 8. *a,* Pathways of retinoid movement in the retina-PE unit. *b,* Intermediates in the visual cycle and coupling to phosphodiesterase activation. Absorption maxima are given in parenthesis for each intermediate.

Retinoid Movement

Vitamin A is supplied to the PE cell from the serum where it circulates bound to serum retinol-binding protein (RBP). Membrane receptors are present on the basal and lateral surfaces of the PE cell which recognize the RBP–retinol complex and effect the translocation of retinol into the cell. Within the cell, retinol is stored as retinyl esters prior to movement to the outer segment. The PE cell contains extremely high amounts of cellular retinol-binding protein (CRBP), a protein of yet unknown function but whose high affinity for retinol indicates that it may facilitate retinoid movement/function within the PE cell. The PE cell contains a second important protein, the cellular retinaldehyde-binding protein which specifically binds 11-*cis* retinoid isomers.

Movement of retinoid between PE cell and outer segment may be facilitated by a third protein, the interphotoreceptor retinoid-binding protein (IRBP). This is a protein unique to the eye, synthesized by the retina but secreted into the subretinal space (interphotoreceptor matrix). Its high concentration, specific location and affinity for retinoids makes this protein a prime candidate for an intercellular retinoid transport protein between retina and PE. Another method for returning retinoid to the PE cell is the process of outer segment shedding and phagocytosis.

In sum, PE stores of retinoid decrease in the dark; there is a flow of retinoid to the visual cell. The reverse occurs after strong bleaching; retinoid accumulates in the PE cell, while retinal decreases in the photoreceptor.

Rhodopsin Bleaching

In the outer segments 11-*cis* retinal is tightly bound to the protein opsin forming the visual protein, rhodopsin (*see Fig.* 8*b*). With light activation, the retinal is isomerized to the *trans*-configuration, initiating a series of changes in the opsin molecule which results in spectrally definable 'bleaching intermediates'. The reaction proceeds rapidly, with an approximate 1 ms time lapse between light stimulation and formation of metarhodopsin II. The conversion of metarhodopsin II to III occurs slowly; therefore it is probable that the step most important in visual transduction is the conversion from MI to MII. In regeneration, darkness allows for reformation of the Schiff base between 11-*cis* retinal and the lysine residue of opsin. The cycle is thus primed for acceptance of another visual signal.

In these reactions, retinoid must be altered chemically (aldehyde–alcohol conversions) and in configuration (*cis–trans* changes). A membrane-bound alcohol dehydrogenase is present in the visual cell and is involved in retinol dehydrogenation. The presence of a *cis–trans* isomerase enzyme has not been firmly established.

Cyclic Nucleotides

As in other neuronal tissues, the retina exhibits a high cyclic AMP level as well as high adenylate cyclase activity. The retina, however, demonstrates a uniquely high cyclic GMP level and guanylate cyclase activity with more than 90 per cent of the cyclic GMP present in the photoreceptor cells. Levels of cyclic GMP are high in dark adapted retinae; strong bleaching rapidly lowers the level. Moreover, a light-activated cyclic GMP metabolizing system has been found in the photoreceptor outer segment raising the possibility that cyclic GMP may function in the visual process as a link between rhodopsin bleaching and membrane conductance changes.

It appears that a complex series of events in the retina controls the concentration or metabolic flux of cyclic GMP through the activation of the enzyme phosphodiesterase (PDE). After bleaching, PDE activity is markedly increased. Activation is probably through the key rhodopsin intermediate, metarhodopsin II, and is mediated by the protein 'transducin' and the high energy compound GTP (*Table* II). In this process, rhodopsin structural changes allow for binding of transducin, an exchange of GDP for GTP on a specific site of the molecule and release of PDE from an inhibited state (i.e. activation). At present, GTP/GDP exchange on the transducin molecule is the only chemical reaction known to be directly catalysed by rhodopsin photolysis. This reaction results in a 'cascade' effect in that many cyclic GMP molecules are hydrolysed as a result of the capture of one photon of light in the outer segment. In an inactivation step, GTPase activity, intrinsic in the transducin molecule, hydrolyses the bound GTP to GDP, returning the PDE to basal activity. Finally, it has been suggested that rhodopsin phosphorylation acts as a 'turn-off' signal, returning rhodopsin back to a ground-state level.

Table II. Rhodopsin photolysis and phosphodiesterase activation: possible sequence

1	Light absorption	$R \xrightarrow{h\nu} R^* \text{ (MII)}$
2	GTP/GDP exchange	$T_{GDP} + GTP \xrightarrow{R^*} R^*\text{--}T_{GTP} + GDP$
3	PDE activation	$PDE + R^*\text{--}T_{GTP} \rightarrow R^*\text{--}T_{GTP}\text{--}PDE$
4	cGMP hydrolysis	$cGMP + HOH \xrightarrow{T_{GTP}\text{--}PDE} 5'\text{--}GMP + H^+$
5	PDE inactivation	$T_{GTP}\text{--}PDE \xrightarrow{GTPase} PDE + T_{GDP}$
6	R* inactivation	$R^* + ATP \xrightarrow{\text{Rhodopsin Kinase}} R\text{--}P + ADP$

Phototransduction

In dark-adapted vertebrate rods, a well-known 'dark current' flows (depolarization) owing to the movement of Na$^+$ ions out of the inner segment plasma membrane (pumped by Na$^+$/K$^+$-ATPase) and back into the outer segment. With light, the membrane becomes hyperpolarized due to the closure of the outer segment Na$^+$ channels and reduction of the ionic movement. One of the central questions in vision biochemistry concerns the nature of the coupling between rhodopsin photolysis and the membrane permeability changes. Since most of the outer segment rhodopsin is present in disc membranes physically separated from the plasma membrane ion channels, one or more low molecular weight soluble internal messengers must be present in the outer segment to couple these events. This messenger (or messengers) would then function to translate the photic stimulus into a chemical response at the plasma membrane level, and to amplify the response since the capture of only one photon can transiently decrease a rod's dark current by about 3 per cent.

Calcium has been postulated to be such a messenger. It is known to mimic many of the electrophysiological effects of light and to be present in the outer segment in high concentration. It has thus been suggested that, in the dark, Ca^{+2} is sequestered within the discs and that light stimulation releases the ion, allowing it to block Na$^+$ channels with resultant hyperpolarization. More recently, cyclic GMP has emerged as a strong candidate for the role of internal messenger (*Fig.* 9). It is in high concentration in rods (70 μmol/l) and mimics many of the effects of dark-adaptation. Intracellular injection of cyclic GMP, for example, causes membrane depolarization to the Na$^+$ equilibrium potential. Most strikingly, rhodopsin bleaching activates the enzyme phosphodiesterase (PDE), causing a sharp decrease in cyclic

POSSIBLE LIGHT EFFECT ON PHOTORECEPTOR

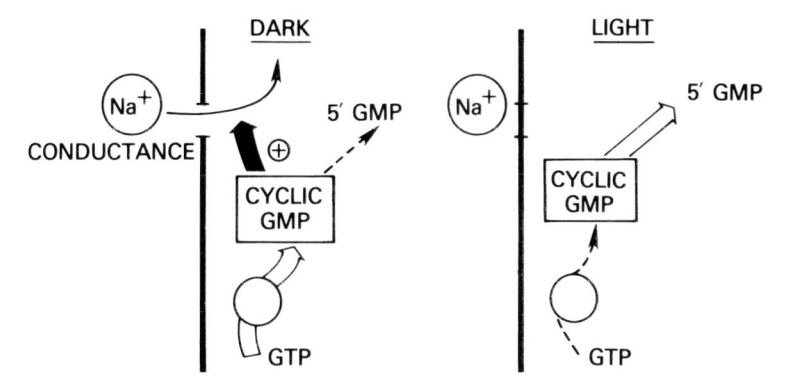

Fig. 9. Hypothetical effects of cyclic GMP in controlling membrane permeability in the rod outer segment. Left panel: In dark, the high cyclic GMP level could exert a positive effect on maintaining open sodium channels. Right panel: In light, phosphodiesterase is activated, cyclic GMP levels fall and sodium channels close.

GMP concentration. Only a small bleach results in the hydrolysis of many cyclic GMP molecules, yielding a high amplification of the photic signal.

As depicted in *Fig.* 9, cyclic GMP levels are high in the dark-adapted outer segment, since PDE activity is relatively low. Theoretically, then, this could allow for the maintenance of open sodium channels and flow of the 'dark current'. In light, PDE activity is stimulated; cyclic GMP levels drop leading to closing of the sodium channels and hyperpolarization. As yet, the coupling mechanism between the cyclic GMP metabolizing system and the membrane sodium channels has remained unexplored. Although the calcium and cyclic GMP theories are in apparent conflict, it is possible that both Ca^{+2} and cyclic GMP (as well as other, yet unknown, substances) act together in a chain of events involving membrane conductance changes including adaptation.

Retinal Neurochemistry

Along with the photoreceptor cell synapse, the inner retinal synapses function to (*a*) pass the photic stimulation on to the brain and (2) begin its processing into a coherent visual image. Surprisingly little is known about the specific neurotransmitters that function at the various synapses. Only for amacrine cells and a few other cells is there evidence for the presence and physiological function of particular transmitters. In part this is due to the wide variation in the occurrence and putative function of neurotransmitters and neuropeptides in different species. The following is a short description of several possible candidates for neurotransmitters in retinal synaptic transmission.

Monoamines

Adrenoreceptors are divided into α- and β-types based on agonist selectivity (α-type: adrenaline > noradrenaline > isoproterenol β-type: isoproterenol > adrenaline > noradrenaline ≫ dopamine). Highly specific antagonists are also useful in classification: phentolamine and propranolol for α- and β-types respectively. β-adrenergic receptors are closely linked to adenylate cyclase. Catecholamines are synthesized from tyrosine, starting with the enzyme tyrosine hydroxylase. Its enzymic activity is light-dependent in the retina and is probably modulated through cyclic AMP-dependent phosphorylation. Catecholamine action is terminated by (*a*) re-uptake into presynaptic terminals, (*b*) general diffusion or (*c*) enzymic degradation–monoamine oxidase (MAO) or catechol-O-methyl transferase (COMT). As demonstrated by fluorescence techniques, a minority of amacrine cells and some cells in the ganglion cell layer contain monoamine transmitters.

Dopamine interacts with two types of receptors in most neuronal tissues: D_1-receptors linked to adenylate cyclase and D_2-receptors which are cyclase-independent. In retina, most dopamine receptors seem to be of the D_1-type. Dopamine is present in certain retinal amacrine cells, in particular those that receive input and send their output to other amacrine cells. Pre-loaded ^3H-dopamine can be released from amacrine cells by light stimulation. Dopamine is also present in interplexiform cells in teleost fish retinae and some mammals, e.g. cebus monkey. An active dopamine-sensitive adenylate cyclase has been demonstrated in teleost horizontal cells. Since dopamine can transiently depolarize some horizontal cells, dopamine and its intracellular messenger, cyclic AMP, may modulate the light response at inner retinal synapses.

Serotonin (5-hydroxytryptamine, 5-HT) is another amine of probable use in the retina. It is formed from tryptophan in a series of steps beginning with the enzyme tryptophan hydroxylase. 5-HT appears to be present in an amacrine cell subset. Although indoleamine-accumulating neurones are well known in the retinae of several species and 5-HT is also present, tryptophan hydroxylase activity is quite low in the mammalian retina. This raises doubts as to the general role of 5-HT as a retinal transmitter, although its existence in the retinae of some species appears to be firmly established.

Acetylcholine

Cholinergic neurones are of two broad types: nicotinic and muscarinic. Nicotinic responses are elicited by acetylcholine (ACh) or nicotine, inhibited by α-bungarotoxin and curare, and are generally rapid excitatory responses. Muscarinic responses are elicited by ACh or muscarine, inhibited by atropine and are normally slower excitatory or inhibitory responses. ACh is synthesized from choline and acetyl CoA by the enzyme choline acetyltransferase; its action is terminated by acetylcholinesterase. Presynaptic cholinergic amacrine cells have been relatively well studied in the retina, affecting ganglion cell transmission. In turtle retinae, it has been postulated that cone photoreceptors are cholinergic.

GABA

γ-Aminobutyric acid (GABA) is an inhibitory transmitter in an amacrine cell subpopulation. It is primarily present in the inner synaptic layer although it may function as a neurotransmitter in horizontal cells of some species. GABA is synthesized from glutamate by the enzyme glutamic acid decarboxylase (GAD), which requires pyridoxal phosphate as a coenzyme. Inactivation by uptake systems and metabolism (e.g. GABA transaminase) takes place in both neurones and glia (Mueller cells) in some species. A well-defined role of GABA is to regulate the cellular influx of chloride ion, resulting in hyperpolarization (inhibition). It has also been suggested that GABA acts as a neuronal trophic factor during development. It seems likely that, in the CNS, GABA, benzodiazepine and chloride recognition sites are part of a single macromolecular complex.

Amino Acids

Aspartate, glutamate and glycine are putative neurotransmitters in the retina. As in most tissues, their synthesis and concentration in the retina are high due to their roles in energy metabolism and protein synthesis. Glutamate is synthesized from glutamine in nerve synapses by the enzyme glutaminase I. A glutamate/glutamine cycle has been proposed in neuronal tissue for glutamate inactivation. In this cycle, released glutamate may enter glial (Mueller) cells and be converted to glutamine which can then be released, taken up, reconverted to glutamate and returned to neuronal synaptic storage.

Aspartate and/or glutamate have been suggested as candidates for photoreceptor cell transmitters. They are present in significant amounts in photoreceptors and high affinity uptake systems for these substances are present in photoreceptor preparations. Aspartate aminotransferase, a marker enzyme for aspartate/glutamate, has been localized in cones and cone terminals in guinea-pig retinae. Horizontal cells are depolarized by aspartate and glutamate. Both aspartate and glutamate are also present in the ganglion cell layer in most species. D-aspartate, a marker analogue for glutamate and/or aspartate is accumulated by a small percentage (<10 per cent) of the ganglion cells of several species.

Glycine is a putative retinal neurotransmitter since: (*a*) it is in high concentration in the retina; (*b*) glycine receptors are present; (*c*) a high affinity uptake mechanism is present; and (*d*) there is a K^+- and a light-evoked release of glycine from the retina. In neural tissue, the major synthetic pathway for glycine may be from serine through the enzyme serine hydroxy-methyl transferase (SHMT). Serine inactivation at the synapse may be by re-uptake or by reconversion back to serine via SHMT.

Glycine is a fast-acting inhibitory transmitter in the CNS similar to GABA. In the retina, it is present in an amacrine cell subpopulation. Electrophysiologically, it inhibits target cells (e.g. horizontal, ganglion); it also affects the velocity specificity of ganglion cells. Strychnine, a glycine antagonist, blocks many of these effects; ^{3}H-strychnine binding is thought to indicate the presence of glycine receptors and is appreciable in retinal synaptosomal membranes.

Taurine

Taurine is the most abundant free amino acid in the retina; it is particularly high in the photoreceptor layer (50–80 mmol/l). This high concentration appears to be due to uptake from the plasma (through the pigment epithelium) rather than by synthesis in situ. A high affinity retinal uptake system has been demonstrated in photoreceptor cells as well as a light-stimulated release from retinae pre-loaded with radiolabelled taurine. Taurine-accumulating neurones are present in the cat retina and appear to be mainly a subpopulation of amacrine cells. The cat retina is particularly sensitive to taurine deficiency compared to other vertebrate retinae and quickly develops a photoreceptor degeneration when the animal is placed on a taurine-free diet.

The function of taurine in the retina is unclear. Its presence in inner retinal neurones may indicate a transmitter role acting as an inhibitory transmitter released by amacrine cells involved in the 'off' responses to light stimulation. In the photoreceptor layer, its extremely high concentration indicates its role is probably not in neurotransmission but rather as a regulator of ion fluxes (Na^+, K^+, Ca^{+2}). Taurine has been shown to enhance ATP-dependent Ca^{+2} uptake into frog rod outer segments.

Neuropeptides

Several peptides are known to be present in the retina. These may function as neuromodulators or neurotransmitters. Among those reported to date are met- and leu-enkephalins (ENK), vasoactive intestinal polypeptide (VIP), substance P, somatostatin, glucagon, neurotensin, luteinizing hormone–releasing hormone (LH–RH), and thyrotropin-releasing hormone (TRH). On the whole, these substances have been identified by their immunoreactivity. Due to variation in peptide structure from species to species and the problems inherent in immunological identification, the presence of most of these substances must yet be verified by more direct chemical and isolation techniques. The significance of TRH-like immunoreactivity, for example, is controversial in some species.

Different amacrine subpopulations demonstrate immunoreactivity towards enkephalin, somatostatin, glucagon and neurotensin. Substance P-like immunoreactivity is found in several amacrine types in the monkey retina and at least two in the chicken. Glucagon-like immunoreactivity in the chicken retina is also localized to amacrine cells, as is VIP and neurotensin. Thus, in vertebrates, the peptides are primarily associated with interneurones (amacrine cells). In invertebrates, however, this may not always be the case, since enkephalin-like immunoreactivity has been found in primary photoreceptors of the spiny lobster.

Little is known about the function of these peptides in the retina. Neurotensin and substance P have excitatory effects on ganglion cell activity; enkephalin amacrine cells may inhibit GABA amacrines, thus affecting the 'on-centre' ganglion cells. Biochemically, VIP has been shown to induce glycogenolysis in brain cortex and may play a similar role in the retina. It markedly increases cyclic AMP concentration in mixed retinal cell cultures and in the isolated carp horizontal cell. In the latter, it induces cell depolarization and a decrease in membrane resistance. Much work has yet to be done on the individual effects of these peptides and their possible interactions with the classical neurotransmitters.

Retinal Pathology

Diseases of the retina can be either of systemic origin (e.g. diabetes) or specific to the retina (e.g. hereditary retinal degeneration). The following are a few examples in which the biochemical aetiologies of the disease processes are of particular interest.

Uveoretinal Autoimmune Disease

Experimental allergic uveitis (EAU) is an autoimmune disease characterized by destruction of the retinal photoreceptors and general inflammation of the retina and uveal tract. The sensitizing agents are known to come from the visual cell layer and, in particular, a soluble retinal protein of about 50 000 mol wt has been implicated in the aetiology of the disease. This has been called the S-antigen (S = soluble) and, together with an insoluble rod outer segment protein (presumably rhodopsin), may be the major immunopathological agents in EAU. Although it has yet to be definitively proved, a good deal of evidence now indicates that the S-antigen could very well be the outer segment '48K protein'. IRBP has also recently been shown to produce EAU in test animals. The mechanism by which sensitization occurs, however, remains unknown.

Retrolental Fibroplasia (RLF)

From extensive studies, this condition is thought to be caused by elevated oxygen in premature infants. Pathology includes neovascularization, possibly due to aberrant spindle cell formation. Although the exact biochemical causes of RLF are unknown, it is probable that increased oxygen tension could lead to oxidative damage of sensitive retinal lipids and proteins in the rapidly growing and developing tissue. Clinically, vitamin E has been reported to have a somewhat protective effect.

Oxidation

In many cell types of the body, ageing results in the accumulation of autofluorescent, insoluble liproprotein pigment known as lipofuscin (ageing pigment). The older retinal pigment epithelial cell in particular contains a large amount of lipofuscin. PE cells exist in a high oxygen environment and ingest through phagocytosis a large amount of polyunsaturated fatty acids and other lipids that are highly susceptible to lipid peroxidation. This, as well as accumulation of partially hydrolysed membrane proteins (e.g. rhodopsin), can result in progressive accumulation of undigestible residual products in the PE cell. Animal models of the Chediak–Higashi syndrome, which is characterized by an abnormal cellular accumulation of unsaturated fatty acids, demonstrate greatly increased PE cell lipofuscin. Monkeys deficient in the antioxidant vitamin E exhibit a high lipofuscin content in PE cells of the macular region. In other animal studies, vitamin E deficiency or the lack of other antioxidants has also been found to result in disruption of outer segment membrane integrity and visual cell death presumably through lipid peroxidation. High light intensities or constant illumination are also known to result in outer segment damage. Although the mechanism is not clear, it is again likely that free radicals produced by lipid peroxidation play a role in the pathology. As in other ocular tissues, high levels of vitamin E and the enzyme superoxide dismutase, which reduces the superoxide radical to hydrogen peroxide, may help to protect the delicate outer segment membranes from oxidative damage.

Diabetic Retinopathy

Retinal complications of diabetes occur in proliferative and non-proliferative types. In non-proliferative retinopathy, microaneurysms form in the retinal capillary bed with exudates and haemorrhage. In the proliferative type, new vessels form along with the appearance of fibrous tissue. An early manifestation in the disease is the selective loss of retinal capillary mural cells prior to the appearance of microaneurysms while the other major cell type of the capillary lining, the endothelial cell, appears to be relatively unaffected. Since diabetes involves a general alteration in sugar metabolism, it has been suggested that excess sorbitol may accumulate in the retina somewhat analogous to the situation seen in the lens in sugar cataract formation. The enzyme responsible for sugar alcohol formation, aldose reductase, has been localized in the cytoplasm of mural cells from human retinal vessels. Moreover, aldose reductase has been implicated in the aetiology of a thickened basement membrane in the general vasculature of diabetics. In animal studies, thickening of retinal capillary basement membranes in galactose-fed rats was prevented by sorbinil, an aldose reductase inhibitor. It thus may be that aldose reductase-mediated sorbitol accumulation is basic to the pathological changes observed in mural cells in non-proliferative diabetic retinopathy.

Retinitis Pigmentosa

Retinitis pigmentosa (RP) is a family of diseases in man primarily affecting the retinal photoreceptor layer but ultimately leading to general retinal degeneration and blindness. In many RP types there is a distinct hereditary component. Recently, it has been shown that peripheral lymphocytes of RP patients are deficient in their ability to produce the lymphokine, γ-interferon. This finding affords a possible biochemical marker for at least some forms of RP and indicates that an altered immune response is one of the abnormalities associated with the disease. Otherwise, little is known about the biochemical aetiology in man but several excellent animal models are available for study.

RCS Rat

In this model, a layer of outer segment debris forms between the retina and PE in the early postnatal stages of retinal development. The primary defect has been pinpointed to an inability of the PE cells to phagocytize shed packets of outer segments. Biochemically, it has been found that affected PE cells have a lowered ability to esterify retinol leading to a small excess in free retinol. Free retinol is a known membranolytic agent and could adversely affect fragile outer segment membranes. It is not known, however, whether this mechanism is operative *in vivo*.

Mouse and Canine Dysplasias

The disease in the *rd* mouse, and in Irish Setter and Collie dogs, appears soon after birth, with rod outer segments degenerating even as they are elongating. This entity is then best defined as a dysplasia rather than a degeneration in that the outer segments never achieve a normal morphology before the pathology is observed. In these animals a defect in retinal phosphodiesterase (PDE) activity is observed prior to the pathological changes. The PDE deficiency leads to a large accumulation of cyclic GMP which, as with retinol in the RCS rat, could cause adverse effects. *In vitro* studies with normal human retinae indicate that, in fact, a large excess of cyclic GMP can lead to pathological changes in the photoreceptor cell layer.

It is hoped that the biochemical leads gleaned from the animal models will be of use in studying the defect in humans when such retinae become available for study.

Gyrate Atrophy

In contrast to human RP, it appears that the major biochemical defect in gyrate atrophy (GA) has been uncovered. GA is an inherited, autosomal recessive disease of the PE–choroid complex which generally results in ophthalmoscopically visible degenerative changes in the second or third decade of life as well as myopia, cataracts, night blindness and loss of peripheral vision. The enzyme ornithine aminotransferase (OAT) is deficient in cells of GA patients leading to markedly elevated serum ornithine levels. It is not clear, however, how the enzyme defect and/or hyperornithaemia cause the retinal degeneration. High ornithine levels are known to inhibit the enzyme arginine-glycine amidinotransferase, an important enzyme in creatine biosynthesis. It also is known that high ornithine concentrations inhibit protein synthesis in cultured chick embryonic PE cells. Vitreal injection of ornithine in monkeys has been shown to lead to marked oedema, specifically in the pigment epithelium. The effect was observed within 4 hours of injection and resulted in patches of PE cell death and secondary degeneration of the underlying photoreceptor cells.

It is known that the OAT enzyme uses vitamin B_6 (pyridoxine) as a cofactor; large doses of the vitamin have been administered to GA patients with a resultant lowering of serum ornithine in some (B_6-responsive) but not other (B_6-nonresponsive) patients. Restriction of dietary protein intake and foods high in arginine content have actually resulted in reversal of some of the effects of the disease as assessed electrophysiologically. There is good hope, therefore, for ultimate control of at least this one hereditary disease of retinal degeneration.

SELECTED REFERENCES

General

Anderson R. *Biochemistry of the Eye,* San Francisco, American Academy of Ophthalmology, 1983.
Davson H. *The Physiology of the Eye,* New York, Academic Press, 1972.
Graymore C. *Biochemistry of the Eye,* New York Academic Press, 1970.
Osborne N. and Chader G. *Progress in Retinal Research,* vol. 2, Oxford, Pergamon Press, 1983.
Records R. *Physiology of the Human Eye and Visual System,* Hagerstown Md, Harper and Row, 1979.
Zadunaisky J. and Davson H. *Current Topics in Eye Research,* vol. 1, New York, Academic Press, 1979.
Zinn K. and Marmor M. *The Retinal Pigment Epithelium,* Cambridge, Mass., Harvard University Press, 1979.

Cornea

Berman E. Proteoglycans of bovine corneal stroma. In: Balazas E (ed.) *Chemistry and Molecular Biology of the Intercellular Matrix,* vol. 2, New York, Academic Press, 1970, pp. 879–86.
Chakrabarti B. and Park J. Glycosaminoglycans: Structure and interaction. *CRC Crit. Rev. Biochem.* 1980; **8**, 225–313.
Dikstein S. and Maurice D. The metabolic basis to the fluid pump in the cornea. *J. Physiol. (Lond.)* 1972; **221**, 29–41.

Edelhauser H., Van Horn D. and Records R. Cornea and sclera. In: Records R. (ed.) *Physiology of the Human Eye and Visual System,* Hagerstown, Md, Harper and Row 1979, pp. 68–97.

Fischbarg J. and Lim J. J. Role of cations, anions and carbonic anhydrase in fluid transport across rabbit corneal endothelium. *J. Physiol. (Lond.)* 1974; **241,** 647–75.

Hart G. Corneal proteoglycans. In: McDevitt D. (ed.) *Cell Biology of the Eye,* New York, Academic Press, 1982, pp. 1–52.

Klintworth G. The cornea – Structure and macromolecules in health and disease. *Am. J. Pathol.* 1977; **89,** 718–808.

Langham M. *The Cornea.* Baltimore, Md. Johns Hopkins Press, 1969.

Maurice D. The structure and transparency of the cornea. *J. Physiol. (Lond.)* 1957; **136,** 263–86.

Maurice D. and Riley M. The cornea. In: Graymore C. (ed.) *Biochemistry of the Eye,* New York, Academic Press, 1970, pp. 1–104.

Riley M. Transport of ions and metabolites across the corneal endothelium. In: McDevitt D. (ed.) *Cell Biology of the Eye,* New York, Academic Press, 1982, pp. 53–95.

Rodrigues M. and Waring G. Anterior and posterior corneal dystrophies. In: Garner A. and Klintworth G. (ed.) *Pathobiology of Ocular Disease. A Dynamic Approach*, New York, Marcel Dekker, 1982, pp. 1152–65.

Lens

Bellows J. *Cataract and Abnormalities of the Lens.* New York, Grune and Stratton, 1975.

Bettelheim F. and Siew E. Biological-physical bases of lens transparency. In: McDevitt D. (ed.) *Cell Biology of the Eye,* New York, Academic Press, 1982.

Bloemendal H. The vertebrate eye lens. *Science* 1977; **197,** 127–38.

Bloemendal H. *Molecular and Cellular Biology of the Eye Lens.* New York, Wiley, 1981.

Delayne M. and Tardieu A. Short range order of crystallin proteins accounts for eye lens transparency. *Nature* 1983; **302,** 415–17.

Duncan G. *Mechanisms of Cataract Formation in the Human Lens.* London, Academic Press, 1981.

Kador P. Overview of the current attempts toward the medical treatment of cataract. *Ophthalmology* 1983; **90,** 352–62.

Kern H. Transport of organic solutes in the lens. In: Zadunaisky J. and Davson H. (ed.) *Current Topics in Eye Research,* vol. 1, New York, Academic Press, 1979, pp. 217–40.

Kinoshita J., Kador P. and Datiles M. Aldose reductase in diabetic cataracts. *JAMA* 1981: **246,** 257—61.

Kuck J. Metabolism of the lens. In: Graymore C. (ed.) *Biochemistry of the Eye,* London, Academic Press, 1970, pp. 261–318.

Paterson C. Crystalline lens. In: Records R. (ed.) *Physiology of the Human Eye and Visual System,* Hagerstown, Md, Harper and Row, 1975.

Spector A. The search for a solution to senile cataracts. *Invest. Ophthlmol. Vis. Res.* 1984; **25,** 130–46.

Zigler J. and Goosey J. Ageing of protein molecules: Lens crystallins as a model system. *Trends Biochem. Sci.* 1981, **6,** 1–4.

Ocular Fluids

Balazs E. *Chemistry and Molecular Biology of the Intercellular Matrix.* New York, Academic Press, 1970.

Bill A. Basic physiology of aqueous drainage. *Exp. Eye Res.* 1977; **25** (Suppl.), 291–304.

Bito L. The physiology and pathology of intraocular fluids. *Exp. Eye Res.* 1977; **25,** 273–89.

Bito L., Davson H. and Fenstermacher J. The ocular and cerebrospinal fluids. *Exp. Eye Res.* 1977; **25,** (Suppl.), 1–561.

Cole D. Comparative aspects of the intraocular fluids. In: Davson H. and Graham L. (ed.) *The Eye,* vol. 5. New York, Academic Press, 1974, pp. 71–161.

Cole D. Secretion of the aqueous humour *Exp. Eye Res.* 1977; (Suppl.), 161–76.

Doane M. Turnover and drainage of tears. *Ann. Ophthalmol.* 1984; **16,** 111–14.

Gloor B. The vitreous. In: Moses R. (ed.) *Adler's Physiology of the Eye,* 7th ed., St. Louis, Mosby, 1981.

Holley F. and Lemp M. Tear physiology and dry eyes. *Surv. Opthalmol.* 1977; **22,** 69–87.

Jordan A. and Baum J. Basic tear flow. *Ophthalmology* 1980; **87,** 920–30.

Mishima S. Clinical pharmacokinetics of the eye. *Invest. Opthalmol Vis. Sci.* 1981; **21,** 504–41.

Mishima S., Masuda K. and Tamura T. Drugs influencing aqueous humour formation and drainage. In: *Drug and Ocular Tissues.* Basle, Karger, 1977, pp. 128–287.

Moore J. and Tiffany J. Human ocular mucins: Origins and preliminary characterization. *Exp. Eye Res.* 1979; **29,** 291–391.

Nicolaides N., Kaitaranta J. and Rawdah T. Meibomian gland studies: Composition of steer and human lipids. *Invest. Ophthalmol. Vis. Sci.* 1981; **20,** 522–36.

Rapoport S. Sites and functions of the blood–aqueous and blood–vitreous barriers of the eye. In: Rapoport S. (ed.) *Blood–Brain Barrier.* In: *Physiology in Medicine.* New York, Raven Press, 1976, pp. 207–32.

Reddy V. Dynamics of transport systems in the eye. *Invest. Ophthalmol. Vis. Sci.* 1977; **18,** 1000–18.

Sears M. The Aqueous. In: Moses R. (ed.) *Adler's Physiology of the Eye,* 7th ed., St. Louis, Mosby, 1981, pp. 204–26.

Retina

Abrahamson E. and Ostroy S. Molecular processes in vision. Benchmark Papers in Biochemistry, vol. 3, Stroudsburg, Pa, Hutchinson Ross, 1981.

Berman E. Biochemistry of the retinal pigment epithelium. In: Zinn K. and Marmor M. (ed.) *The Retinal Pigment Epithelium*, Cambridge, Mass., Harvard University Press, 1979, pp. 83–102.

Bonting S. *Transmitters in the Visual Process*. Oxford, Pergamon Press, 1978.

Bridges C., Fong S.-L., Liou G. et al. Transport, utilization and metabolism of visual cycle retinoids in the retina and pigment epithelium. In: Osborne N. and Chader G. (ed.) *Progess in Retinal Research*, vol. 2, Oxford, Pergamon Press, 1983, pp. 137–62.

Chader G., Liu Y., Fletcher R. et al. Cyclic GMP phosphodiesterase and calmodulin in early-onset inherited retinal degenerations. In: Miller W. (ed.) *Current Topics in Membranes and Transport*, vol. 15, New York, Academic Press, 1981, pp. 133–56.

Davson H. *The Eye*, vol. 2B: *The Photobiology of Vision*, New York, Academic Press, 1977.

Dowling J. The chemistry of visual adaptation in the rat. *Nature* 1960; **188,** 114–18.

Hagins W. The visual process: Excitatory mechanisms in the primary photoreceptor cells. *Ann. Rev. Biophys. Bioeng.* 1972; **1,** 131–54.

Hargrave P. Rhodopsin chemistry, structure and topography. In: Osborne N. and Chader G. (ed.) *Progress in Retinal Research*, vol. 1, Oxford, Pergamon Press, pp. 1–52.

LaVail M. Analysis of neurological mutants in the inherited retinal degenerations. *Invest. Ophthalmol. Vis. Sci.* 1981; **21,** 638–57.

Lolley R. and Schmidt S. Metabolism of the vertebrate retina. In: Davson H. and Graham L. (ed.) *The Eye*, vol. 6, New York, Academic Press, 1974, pp. 343–78.

Miller W. Molecular mechanisms of photoreceptor transduction. In: Miller W. (ed.) *Current Topics in Membranes and Transport*, vol. 15, New York, Academic Press, 1981.

Miller W. Does cyclic GMP hydrolysis control visual transduction in rods? *Trends Pharmacol. Sci.* 1983; **4,** 509–11.

Rodieck R. *The Vertebrate Retina*, San Francisco, Freeman, 1973.

Shichi H. *Biochemistry of Vision*, New York, Academic Press, 1983.

Stein P., Rasenick M. and Bitensky M. Biochemistry of the cyclic nucleotide-related enzymes in rod photoreceptors. In: Osborne N. and Chader G. (ed.) *Progress in Retinal Research*, vol. 1, Oxford, Pergamon Press, 1982, pp. 227–44.

Wald G. Molecular basis of visual excitation. *Science* 1968; **162,** 220–39.

Watling K. Transmitter candidates in the retina. *Trends. Pharmacol. Sci.* 1981; **9,** 244–47.

Young R. Visual cells and the concept of renewal. *Invest. Ophthlmol. Vis. Sci.* 1967; **15,** 700–25.

Chapter 2

Pharmacology and Toxicology

S. J. Crews and S. M. Thompson

INTRODUCTION

No matter how active *in vitro*, a drug cannot work on the intact eye unless it reaches its receptors in adequate concentration. The bioavailability of drugs used in the eye depends on many factors.

Compliance

Many patients do not collect their prescribed drugs. Of those who do, many do not use the medication, or use it infrequently or incorrectly. Adequate and repeated explanation to the patient, as well as practical advice about dose timetables, helps to reduce 'non-compliance'.

Disposal

About 80 per cent of each eye drop drains immediately through the nasolacrimal canal. Normal tear volume is restored 2–3 minutes after instillation of drops. The purpose of viscous vehicles such as methyl cellulose and polyvinyl alcohol is theoretically to slow down this rapid drainage. As so much of a drop is lost so quickly, small drops of high concentration present more drug to the cornea than large drops of low concentration. In addition, dilution of the drop by tears occurs rapidly, particularly as the basal tear turnover rate of 16 per cent per minute can be trebled by the increased lacrimation caused by instilling an eye drop. Many eye drops do not contain buffers, so that the pH of the drop rapidly assumes that of tears, and irritation leading to increased lacrimation is reduced.

Drops larger than 50 µl cannot be accommodated by the cul de sac. For this reason, there should be an interval of 5–10 min between applying drops, if more than one type is being used.

Absorption

The main barrier to drug absorption through the cornea is the epithelium, which is lipophilic, and crossed readily by non-polar drugs. After entering the stroma, which is hydrophilic, passage of drugs through the endothelium into the anterior chamber is rapid. A drug is therefore best absorbed if its lipid–water partition coefficient makes it both lipid- and water-soluble. Thus the hemisuccinate or acetate ester forms of some corticosteroids are absorbed better than their more polar phosphate forms. In addition, free bases are more lipophilic than free ions, so the pH and dissociation constant (pKa) of the drug influence corneal absorption. Many ocular drugs are, however, unstable in the base form (atropine, pilocarpine, idoxuridine). They are stored in solutions of low pH, but not buffered, so that on instillation they rapidly approach the pH of tears (7·4), the concentration of free base rises and the absorption of the drug increases.

Pro-drugs are a recent development in the improvement of drug absorption through the cornea. A drug such as adrenaline is altered so that its derivative (dipivalyl epinephrine) is much more lipophilic, and therefore better absorbed. After absorption local esterases convert the pro-drug back to adrenaline.

Agents that reduce the surface tension increase corneal wetting and therefore present more drug for absorption. Some preservatives used in ocular solutions (such as benzalkonium chloride) also act as wetting agents.

Drug Vehicles

The main forms of drugs instilled into the eye are aqueous solutions, aqueous suspensions, ointments and ocular inserts. Each has a different influence in drug bioavailability. In solution the drug is totally dissolved and therefore available, but tissue contact time is short. In suspension, the drug is present as small particles kept suspended in an aqueous medium by a dispersing agent. Particles do not leave the eye as quickly as solutions, which increases the tissue contact time. However, the bottle must be shaken thoroughly before each use to ensure an adequate concentration of particles in each drop, and most patients do not shake the bottle at all. Ointments increase the bioavailability of a drug by increasing tissue contact time, and by preventing dilution and drainage of the active ingredient. However, they can be messy to use and blur the vision. Ocular inserts, which are placed in the upper or lower fornix for up to a week, allow a drug to be released at a continuous steady rate. This means that there is a constant therapeutic effect and fewer side effects.

A variety of inserts has been tried since the original 'lamellae' (gelatin impregnated wafers), were used 50 years ago. Some have employed water-soluble or erodable matrices but they have the disadvantage of a declining rate of release of drug coupled with a high initial dose and consequent enhanced drug side effects. Copolymer plastic inserts may be employed. The only one available commercially at the time of writing is Ocusert-pilo. A central drug-containing core is surrounded by flexible outer layers allowing a continuous delivery of pilocarpine in two strengths, pilo-20 releasing 20 μg/h and pilo-40, releasing twice this amount over approximately seven days with fewer side effects such as miosis or myopia. Despite many theoretical advantages, especially in disabled or poorly compliant patients, they have not achieved wide acceptance and are expensive. The development of drug inserts would seem to be logical when:

1. The drug's side effects are severe.
2. The mechanism of action suggests continuous drug presence (e.g. antiviral).
3. The drug half-life is short.
4. Repeated medication is unlikely (e.g. trachoma).

Soft contact lenses have also been used to deliver drugs. A 1 per cent pilocarpine presoaked hydrophilic lens applied in acute closed angle glaucoma was found to be as effective as pilocarpine 4 per cent drops. However, a presoaking time of 2 hours is necessary and prolonged high dose pilocarpine therapy is rarely needed for acute glaucoma. Soft lenses have also been used to deliver antibiotics and idoxuridine.

AUTONOMIC DRUGS

The anatomy of the autonomic supply to the eye and ocular adnexa is of importance in the understanding of drug action; lesions will affect their action and different drugs can be of help in neurological investigations. The effects of stimulating the parasympathetic or sympathetic system are shown in *Table* I.

Drugs are usually divided into four groups depending on whether they stimulate or antagonize the parasympathetic or sympathetic effector systems.

Cholinergic Drugs

These drugs can act either directly, similar to the peripheral or muscarinic action of acetylcholine, or indirectly, by blocking cholinesterase.

Acetylcholine

A quaternary ammonium compound, acetylcholine is the chemical transmitter at parasympathetic and sympathetic ganglia (inhibited by nicotine), neuromuscular synapses of skeletal muscle (inhibited by curare), CNS synapses and some post-ganglionic sympathetic endings. It is destroyed by cholinesterase, the unpleasant muscarinic actions can be abolished by atropine.

Used locally on the intact eye, acetylcholine is ineffective, but injection of a 1 per cent solution into the anterior chamber produces miosis lasting about

Table I. Main effects of stimulating the autonomic system

	Sympathetic	Receptor	*Parasympathetic*
Eye			
Radial muscle of iris	Contraction (mydriasis)	α	—
Sphincter muscle of iris			Contraction (miosis)
Ciliary muscle	Relaxation for far vision	β	Contraction for near vision
Lacrimal gland	—		Secretion
Heart	Increase in rate	$β_1$	Decrease in rate
	Increase in force of contraction		Decrease in force of contraction
Lung	Bronchodilatation	$β_2$	Bronchoconstriction
Arterioles			
Coronary	Constriction		dilatation
Skeletal muscle	or	$α_1β_2$	dilatation
Abdominal viscera	dilatation		—
Skin, mucosa, cerebral			dilatation
Stomach and intestine			
Mobility	Decrease	$αβ_2$	Increase
Sphincters	Contraction	α	Relaxation
Secretion	Inhibition		Stimulation
Liver	Glycogenolysis and gluconeogenesis	$αβ_2$	Glycogen synthesis
Urinary bladder			
Detrusor	Relaxation	β	Contraction
Sphincter	Contraction	α	Relaxation
Skin			
Sweat glands	Slight, localized secretion	α	Generalized secretion

10 min and is active even after retrobulbar anaesthesia. Side effects attributed to intracameral use include transient lens opacities, corneal oedema, retinal detachment, bradycardia and systemic hypotension.

Retrobulbar injections have been employed in retinal artery occlusion and quinine toxicity in an attempt to produce retinal and choroidal vasodilatation.

PREPARATIONS

Miochol (Cooper Vision), acetylcholine 1 per cent, mannitol 3 per cent.

Methacholine

Acetyl-β-methylcholine, Mecholyl, has been employed in 2·5 per cent solution, which produces miosis in 30 min in Adie's myotonic pupil or familial dysautonomia but not in the normal eye. Weak pilocarpine drops are now used more frequently in view of easier availability.

Carbachol

Carbachol produces a powerful miosis, similar to eserine in 3 per cent solution, with prolonged accommodative spasm. It has been used in chronic open angle glaucoma and by injection into the anterior chamber for operative miosis. Side effects tend to be more severe than pilocarpine, some of the toxicity to conjunctiva and corneal epithelium may be related to formulation.

PREPARATIONS

Isopto Carbachol (Alcon), carbachol 3 per cent, hypromellose 1 per cent.

Pilocarpine

Pilocarpine is an alkaloid obtained from a shrub of the pilocarpus species. It has muscarinic actions. It penetrates through the cornea producing a miosis in 10 min, with a peak at about 30 min lasting 6 h. The ciliary muscle contraction is of a shorter duration. There is wide individual and species variation. Variable intraocular pressure changes have been reported in normal human eyes. In one series a fall of 8 per cent was found in normal eyes whereas the fall in open angle glaucoma was 12–40 per cent. This fall is attributed to a widening of the trabecular spaces due to contraction of the long fibres of the ciliary muscle attached to the scleral spur. Certain viscous solutions (e.g. hypromellose, PVP) are added commercially to prolong the action of the drops. Vasodilatation occurs in the conjunctival vessels with increased aqueous flow in the aqueous veins. Intracameral injection may cause vasodilatation of iris vessels and hyphaema. Increased permeability is found in the blood aqueous barrier which may account for more postoperative uveitis in patients on miotic therapy. Ciliary spasm is greater in the young and is used in the treatment of accommodative squints, this spasm may be painful.

The commonest side effect is the decreased vision due to miosis and accommodative spasm, especially found in patients with central cataracts, and labelled 'The miotic life'. Follicular conjunctivitis is not uncommon, possibly related to the preservative; controversial toxic effects are lens opacities and retinal detachment. Systemic toxicity is only encountered after excessive use, such as intensive drop therapy which is never justifiable. The dangerous dose is 100 mg, which is contained in 5 ml of 2 per cent drops assuming 1 mg per drop. Mild toxicity is difficult to detect and may be more common than supposed. Symptoms include nausea, vomiting, salivation, sweating, bronchial spasm, hypertension and shock. Impure pilocarpine may contain jaborine, a stereoisomer, which has mydriatic and cycloplegic action. Mothers on topical therapy may give birth to infants with signs suggesting meningitis, i.e. restlessness, hypothermia and convulsions.

PREPARATIONS

Guttae pilocarpine hydrochloride 0·5 per cent, 1, 2, 3 and 4 per cent. Isopto Carpine (Alcon) contains hypromellose 0·5 per cent, Sno Pilo (Smith & Nephew) contains PVA. Slow release Ocusert (May & Baker) pilo 20, 20 µg/h for 1 week; pilo 40, 40 µg/h for 1 week. Pilocarpine nitrate minims (Smith & Nephew) 1, 2 and 4 per cent. Pilocarpine hydrochloride Opulets (Alcon) 1, 2 and 4 per cent.

Reversible Cholinesterase Inhibitors

Cholinesterase inhibitors can be divided into reversible, such as physostigmine, and irreversible, for example, phospholine. Because they act indirectly, they depend on an intact nerve supply and will not be effective after retrobulbar anaesthesia.

Physostigmine/Eserine

Originally obtained from the calabar bean, this drug was used as a poison in trials by ordeal. Systemically eserine, by inhibiting cholinesterase, frees acetylcholine to exert its muscarinic and nicotinic actions, the former can be blocked by atropine. Locally, physostigmine produces miosis in 10 min lasting about 4 h, though mild miosis may persist for several days. Ciliary spasm is variable and increases on voluntary accommodation, it can cause marked discomfort. Side effects are shown in *Table* II.

Physostigmine is rarely used nowadays, either on its own or combined with pilocarpine, but is sometimes employed to reverse mydriasis, a procedure not without risk.

Drops may turn pink or brown on storage due to formation of an oxidation product, rubreserine.

Table II. Side effects of anticholinesterase drops

Local:
  Epiphora
  Fibrillary twitching of lids
  Vasodilatation ... red eyes
  Miosis – lowers brightness and dark adaptation
        lowers VA if central cataract, visual field constricted
        pupillary pigment cysts – usually reversible
        increased IOP, especially if narrow angle
  Lens opacities, especially ecothiopate
  Ciliary spasm – variable myopia increased when reading or in bright light
  Pain in eye and head
  Iritis, posterior synechiae, retinal detachment
  Allergic reactions
Systemic (mainly irreversible anticholinesterases):
  GI – nausea, diarrhoea, abdominal cramps, salivation and intolerance to alcohol
  CNS – fatigue, muscular twitching, weakness, paraesthesia, insomnia, nightmares, drowsiness, convulsions, coma, asthma and pulmonary oedema
        abnormal reactions to relaxants
  CVS – hypo/hypertension, bradycardia and sweating

PREPARATIONS

Guttae physostigmine sulphate 0·25 and 0·5 per cent. Guttae physostigmine 0·25 per cent pilocarpine 2 and 4 per cent; physostigmine 0·5 per cent pilocarpine 4 per cent.

Neostigmine/Prostigmin

This agent has been employed locally as a weaker alternative to eserine in 3–5 per cent drops. Systemically 1–1·5 mg subcutaneously or intramuscularly is employed in diagnosis of myasthenia gravis combined with atropine 600 µg or as tablets 75–300 mg per day for treatment.

Edrophonium (Tensilon)

This has both anticholinesterase and direct action on the neuromuscular junctions. It is mainly employed in diagnosis of myasthenia gravis. The dose is 2 mg given initially intravenously and if no adverse reaction is encountered, a further 8 mg, which produces improvement to ptosis and diplopia in the next 5 min. It may be dangerous in asthmatics.

Irreversible

Cholinesterase Inhibitors

Demecarium (Tosmilen) consists of two neostigmine molecules used in 0·25–0·5 per cent drops. It produces a miosis which persists for 3–10 days and a reduction of intraocular pressure for 24 h and even up to 9 days. Side effects may be pronounced and are indicated in *Table* II.

PREPARATIONS

Demecarium bromide, Tosmilen (Sinclair) 0·25 per cent and 0·5 per cent drops.

Organophosphorous Compounds

These were developed as insecticides and war gases. They can have profound effects by depressing the cholinesterases in plasma, red cells and body tissues. Local ocular use can depress the cholinesterases in the body for up to 3 months after stopping therapy. The original preparation, dyflos, has been withdrawn and the only agent on the market is ecothiopate iodide (phospholine). Used as drops 0·03–0·25 per cent it produces a marked miosis which may last for 2–4 weeks, a ciliary spasm lasting 7 days, which increases on voluntary accommodation, and a fall in intraocular pressure maximal over 24 h. Drops are employed once or twice a day. Side effects locally and sytemically are indicated in *Table* II; the frequency and severity will be related to the strength of the drops used. The association of lens opacities (miotic cataract) is well established. These commence in the anterior subcapsular region after about one year's therapy, are mainly seen in the older age group but have been reported in children. These drops should not be employed in narrow angles as they may precipitate acute closed angle glaucoma. Systemically, anaesthetic complications have been reported with suxamethonium, where apnoea may be prolonged (*Table* II).

PREPARATIONS

Ecothiopate iodide (Ayerst) 0·03 per cent, 0·06 per cent, 0·125 per cent and 0·25 per cent once or twice a day.

Anticholinergic (Parasympatholytic) Drugs

The original alkaloids were obtained from plants of the order *Solanacea*. These medicaments inhibit the muscarinic action of acetylcholine by competition at the receptor site but vary in the effect on different parts of the body. In high dose they excite or depress the central nervous system in addition to blocking autonomic ganglia and skeletal neuromuscular junctions.

Atropine

This is the most powerful and prolonged of the group. The mydriasis can last for 12 days or more and the cycloplegia for 3 weeks, with frequent individual variation. Down's syndrome subjects are said to show an enhanced pupillary response. For maximal pupil dilatation atropine may be combined with phenylephrine. Subconjunctival injections are given as Mydricaine No. 1 or 2, a combination of atropine, procaine and adrenaline. Any rise of intraocular pressure is minimal in normal eyes but greater in open angle glaucoma and a marked rise can occur in narrow angles. This risk of precipitating acute angle closure glaucoma is present for all members of this group when used locally but least for tropicamide. The risk from systemic therapy is unlikely in premedication dose, but may occur with multiple drug therapy.

Systemic atropine helps to abolish the oculocardiac reflex. Systemic toxicity from topical use is seen especially in the very young and the old, a bottle of atropine 1 per cent could be lethal to a young child. These systemic side effects include dry mouth, red skin, tachycardia, raised body temperature, hallucinations, collapse and death. Prolonged local atropine medication quite frequently leads to contact allergy.

PREPARATIONS

Atropine sulphate eye drops 1 per cent. Isopto atropine (Alcon) 1 per cent hypromellose 0·5 per cent. Minims atropine sulphate (Smith & Nephew) 1 per cent. Opulets atropine sulphate (Alcon) 1 per cent. Mydricaine No. 1 atropine 0·5 mg, procaine 3·0 mg, adrenaline 1 in 1000, 0·06 ml in 0·3 ml. Mydricaine No. 2, twice these quantities in 0·3 ml.

Homatropine Hydrobromide

This is similar in action to atropine except that the duration is less. Mydriasis lasts only 24 h and cycloplegia 12–48 h.

PREPARATIONS

Homatropine hydrobromide eye drops 1 and 2 per cent; Minims Homatropine hydrobromide 2 per cent (Smith & Nephew).

Lachesine chloride

One per cent drops are used mainly when there is atropine allergy.

Hyoscine Hydrobomide

This is used little now but is another alternative to atropine, similar in duration of action to homatropine. CNS side effects are quite common.

PREPARATIONS

Eye drops 0·25 per cent.

Cyclopentolate (Mydrilate)

This is a popular short acting mydriatic in 0·5 and 1 per cent drops, producing mydriasis and partial cycloplegia in 20–30 min, lasting up to 24 h. It is relatively less effective in the dark iris. Being related to the hallucinogenic drugs, toxic symptoms have been reported of a temporary psychiatric nature in children, in whom 0·5 per cent drops are to be preferred.

PREPARATIONS

Mydrilate (WBP) cyclopentolate hydrochloride 0·5 per cent and 1 per cent. Minims cyclopentolate hydrochloride (Smith & Nephew), 0·5 per cent and 1 per cent drops in 15–30 min, lasting $\frac{1}{2}$ to 4 h. The cycloplegia may be too variable and brief for refraction.

Tropicamide (Mydriacyl)

The most rapid and shortest acting mydriasis and cycloplegia are produced by 0·5 per cent and 1 per cent drops in 15–30 min, lasting $\frac{1}{2}$ to 4 h. The cycloplegia may be too variable and brief for refraction.

PREPARATIONS

Minims Tropicamide (Smith & Nephew) 0·5 per cent and 1 per cent. Mydriacyl (Alcon) 0·5 per cent and 1 per cent.

Adrenergic Agents

The action of the various drugs has been elucidated but also made more complex by the identification of different receptor sites in the body, α and β, further subdivided into β_1 and β_2. In general, drugs are divided into adrenergic direct or indirect agents and blocking substances, however, it must be appreciated that few have only one action.

Adrenaline

This is normally produced in the adrenal medulla and chromaffin tissue and acts on α- and β-receptors. Instilled as weak drops into the eye (0·01–0·1 per cent), it produces vasoconstriction of conjuctival vessels (α-action). Weak solutions are injected in combination with local anaesthetic (e.g. lignocaine) and mydriatics (mydricaine) to prolong their action. A weak and variable mydriasis is seen with 0·1 per cent drops, which is more pronounced if the post-ganglionic sympathetic is sectioned and use is made of this in the diagnosis of Horner's syndrome. Similarly, a greater mydriasis may be found in acute pancreatitis and thyrotoxicosis (Loewi's test).

Stronger drops, i.e. 1 per cent, reduce the intraocular pressure, probably by both reducing aqueous secretion (β-effect) and increasing the outflow (α-effect). It is used twice daily and there may be a period of several weeks before the full effect is seen. This effect is enhanced and prolonged by guanethidine so that weaker concentrations down to 0·2 per cent are effective (*see below*), and is additive to pilocarpine and Diamox (acetazolamide). Because of its mydriatic action, it is contraindicated in closed angle glaucoma and may be dangerous in patients with narrow angles.

Side effects topically include a high rate of conjunctival hyperaemia and oedema with a follicular reaction of the conjunctiva; these reactions are claimed to be less with dipivefrin. Pigmentation of conjunctiva, cornea and soft contact lenses may be encountered after prolonged use (adrenochrome). Cystoid macular oedema is described mainly in aphakic patients, which is usually reversible but may take 6 months to improve. Systemic adverse reactions may occur with acute hypertensive crises or cardiac complications, usually in patients with pre-existing cardiovascular disease or interaction with monoamine oxidase inhibitors. Regional infiltration with accidental intravenous injection has caused death due to cerebral haemorrhage or ventricular fibrillation.

PREPARATIONS

Eppy (Smith & Nephew), adrenaline 1 per cent. Isopto Epinal (Alcon), adrenaline 0·5 per cent or 1 per cent; hypromellose 0·5 per cent. Simplene (Smith & Nephew), adrenaline 0·5 per cent or 1 per cent in a viscous vehicle. Epifrin (Allergan), adrenaline 1 per cent. Propine (Allergan), dipivefrin hydrochloride (0·1 per cent).

Phenylephrine

This is mainly an α-receptor stimulant. Weak strengths, e.g. 0·125 per cent, are incorporated in a number of solutions to whiten the eye; prolonged use, however, may induce conjunctival hyperaemia. A 10 per cent solution causes a variable mydriasis (less in dark irides) in about 30 min which lasts up to 4 h. Pigment cells are liberated into the anterior chamber. Some fall in intraocular pressure is encountered, except in narrow angles where an acute angle glaucoma can be precipitated. Combination of an anticholinergic agent and phenylephrine produces maximal pupil dilatation in uveitis or pupil block glaucoma, while it is used on its own for ophthalmoscopy without cycloplegia.

Widening of the palpebral aperture occurs in some individuals and can be used to treat Horner's syndrome. A reversible toxic keratopathy may be encountered in some individuals, rendering fundus viewing difficult, while tachyphylaxis is encountered on repeated administration. Systemic toxicity may be produced in elderly patients with cardiac disease, hypertension and those on monoamine oxidase inhibitors or tricyclic antidepressant drugs. A minim of 10 per cent phenylephrine contains approximately ten times the subcutaneous dose and therefore should not be injected subconjunctivally.

PREPARATIONS

Isopto Frin (Alcon), phenylephrine hydrochloride 0·12 per cent, hypromellose 0·5 per cent. Prefrin (Allergan) phenylephrine hydrochloride 0·12 per cent. Zincfrin (Alcon), phenylephrine hydrochloride 0·12 per cent, zinc sulphate 0·25 per cent. Phenylephrine eye drops, phenylephrine hydrochloride 10 per cent. Minims phenylephrine hydrochloride (Smith & Nephew) 10 per cent and 2·5 per cent.

Cocaine

In addition to its anaesthetic action, cocaine potentiates adrenaline and noradrenaline. Thus it acts indirectly and has no effect following sympathetic section. A 4 per cent solution will cause vasoconstriction and a variable mydriasis lasting up to 4 h, also widening of the palpebral aperture in a few individuals. A toxic keratopathy may complicate its use preoperatively, while closed angle glaucoma can occur. A combination with homatropine was in use for many years but is now little employed as cocaine is an addictive drug.

PREPARATIONS

Cocaine hydrochloride eye drops 4 per cent. Cocaine and homatropine eye drops, cocaine hydrochloride 2 per cent, homatropine hydrobromide 2 per cent.

Adrenergic Blocking Agents (Sympatholytic)

These are divided into those that block α- and β-receptors and those that impair the function of the nerve. Many of the agents have intrinsic adrenergic actions in addition, together with membrane stabilizing and local anaesthetic actions. The latter can complicate local administration.

α-Adrenergic Blocking Drugs

Thymoxamine

Thymoxamine 0·1 per cent or 0·2 per cent drops cause a miosis in 20–30 min lasting up to 2 h and are used to reverse the mydriasis induced by phenylephrine 10 per cent drops when repositioning of intraocular lenses is required. The 0·5 per cent drops cause a reduction in intraocular pressure and have been used in acute closed angle glaucoma.

Tolazine (Priscol)

This has been used subconjunctivally as a diagnostic test in glaucoma and by retrobulbar or intravenous injection in retinal artery occlusion.

β-Adrenergic Blocking Drugs

These agents inhibit catecholamines at β-receptor sites. They are similar structurally to β-adrenergic agents, e.g. isoprenaline. β-adrenergic effects are now subdivided into β_1 and β_2, β_1 being especially the cardiac effects, and β_2 bronchodilatation and vasodilatation in skeletal muscle (*see Table* I). The different blocking agents have various effects on β_1 and β_2 sites.

Although much experimental work has been done on the different agents, the main one on the market at the moment is timolol for topical ocular use; one of the main problems with the others has been tachyphylaxis, i.e. reduced action on repeated use.

Timolol

The 0·25 per cent and 0·5 per cent drops have been shown to reduce the intraocular pressure in chronic open angle and other forms of glaucoma lasting 12 h or more, and so are instilled twice daily. Timolol has the advantage over other antiglaucoma agents of not altering the size of the pupil or accommodation. Its effect seems additive to pilocarpine, adrenaline and acetazolamide. Tachyphylaxis appears relatively rare.

Ocular side effects are rare, but systemic adverse reactions such as bronchospasm and bradycardia are encountered and care must be exercised in patients with asthma and cardiac problems, especially heart block.

PREPARATIONS

Timoptol (Merck, Sharp & Dohme) eye drops, timolol maleate 0·25 per cent and 0·5 per cent.

Teoptic (Dispera) eye drops: carteolol hydrochloride 1 per cent and 2 per cent.

Other β-blocking agents used on clinical trials include: *Atenolol*, 4 per cent drops, reduced intraocular pressure but tachyphylaxis was common; *Pindolol*, 1 per cent drops, was also shown to reduce intraocular pressure in normal and glaucomatous eyes.

Adrenergic Neurone-blocking Agents

Guanethidine (Ismelin)

Five or ten per cent drops produce miosis and ptosis in 30 min, reaching maximum in 24 h with some reduction of intraocular pressure. It acts like a post-ganglionic sympathectomy, potentiating the action of direct adrenergic agents such as adrenaline or phenylephrine. As mentioned above (p. 50), the oculohypotensive action of adrenaline is enhanced and prolonged and therefore a variety of combinations are on the market for the treatment of glaucoma. Guanethidine 5 per cent drops alone are used in the treatment of dysthyroid eye disease, though intolerance is frequent.

PREPARATIONS

Ganda (Smith & Nephew) eye drops. 1 + 0·2, guanethidine monosulphate 1 per cent, adrenaline 0·2 per cent in viscous solution. 3 + 0·5, guanethidine monosulphate 3 per cent, adrenaline 0·5 per cent. 5 + 0·5, guanethidine monosulphate 5 per cent, adrenaline 0·5 per cent. 5 + 1, guanethidine monosulphate 5 per cent, adrenaline 1 per cent. Ismelin (Zyma) eye drops, guanethidine monosulphate 5 per cent.

Local Anaesthetics

These agents selectively block nerve conduction in smaller pain and sensory fibres and ideally are non-irritating with low systemic toxicity. They should act quickly and last as long as required for each type of operation. Adrenaline may be combined to prolong the action and hyaluronidase can spread the area when infiltration anaesthesia is employed.

Oxybuprocaine Hydrochloride (Benoxinate)

For applanation tonometry and minor surgery of short duration, 0·4 per cent drops are used.

PREPARATIONS

Minims Benoxinate oxybuprocaine hydrochloride 0·4 per cent (Smith & Nephew). Opulets Benoxinate oxybuprocaine hydrochloride 0·4 per cent (Alcon).

Amethocaine Hydrochloride

Used as 0·5 per cent and 1 per cent drops for short duration anaesthesia, but vasodilatation may be a drawback.

PREPARATIONS

Amethocaine hydrochloride eye drops 0·5 per cent and 1 per cent. Minims amethocaine hydrochloride (Smith & Nephew) 0·5 per cent and 1 per cent.

Proxymetacaine Hydrochloride (Proparacaine, Ophthaine)

The lack of stinging is of value with children.

PREPARATIONS

Ophthaine (Squibb) proxymetacaine hydrochloride eye drops 0·5 per cent.

Cocaine Hydrochloride

This is an alkaloid extracted from the shrub *Erythroxylum coca*. The first use of any local anaesthetic was in the eye in 1884, and this altered the whole pattern of ophthalmic surgery. Local drops 2–4 per cent give a prolonged anaesthesia for 10–20 min, accompanied by vasoconstriction and mydriasis (*see above*). As it forms a precipitate with iodine, cocaine has been employed in cauterization of dendritic ulcers. It is little used now except nasally for DCR operations in 5–20 per cent, in combination with adrenaline, which may be dangerous.

Lignocaine Hydrochloride

This is used as eye drops or by injection for infiltration anaesthesia.

When given by injection for regional anaesthesia, the duration of the nerve block is about 1½ h if combined with adrenaline. It is not advised to use stronger solutions than 1 per cent, though a variety of strengths are available: 0·5 per cent–2 per cent lignocaine with or without adrenaline 1 in 200 000 (500 μg/100 ml). The maximum dose is 200 mg of plain lignocaine or 500 mg if combined with adrenaline. The maximum dose of adrenaline is 500 μg. Toxic effects may occur at lower doses, especially if accidentally injected into a vein.

PREPARATIONS

Minims lignocaine and fluorescein (Smith & Nephew), lignocaine hydrochloride 4 per cent, fluorescein sodium 0·25 per cent.

Bupivacaine Hydrochloride (Marcain)

This can be used for regional anaesthesia where a prolonged action is required, up to 8 h. The disadvantage is its slow onset of action, up to 30 min. Consequently it is often given with lignocaine.

Solutions used are 0·25 per cent, 0·5 per cent and 0·75 per cent. The first two are available mixed with adrenaline 1 in 200 000. The maximum dose is 2 mg/kg in any 4 h period.

General Anaesthesia

This is being increasingly employed because of the complexity and duration of modern ophthalmic surgery. Control of the intraocular contents presents the main problem and pharmacological principles only will be described.

There are four components to be considered (Holloway, 1980):

1. Pressure from extraocular structures.
2. Aqueous volume.
3. Choroidal blood volume.
4. Vitreous volume.

Most anaesthetic agents reduce the intraocular pressure (IOP), with the exception of nitrous oxide. Intravenous thiopentone and halothane have been shown to reduce the IOP and the effect is proportional to the concentration of drug administered. The mechanism is not fully understood, but is suggested to be partially on the extraocular muscle tone and part centrally on the diencephalon, midbrain and hypothalamus. Ketamine intravenously has been used for monitoring ocular tension in buphthalmos as it was thought not to affect the pressure. However, small increases or a 25 per cent reduction have been reported in children. Non-depolarizing muscle relaxants such as tubocurarine block the transmitter actions of acetylcholine leading to ptosis, paralysis of extraocular muscle movements and a small drop in IOP due to reduction of muscle tone. The shorter acting non-depolarizing agents, such as pancuronium or alcuronium, do not alter the intraocular pressure.

Suxamethonium, a short acting depolarizing agent causes a rapid rise in IOP of 7–12 mm in 1–2 min, lasting about 5 min. It is probably safe in the intact eye, but may be dangerous in the opened eye, e.g. perforating injury, though simultaneous thiopentone administration will reduce this risk considerably. An alternative short acting non-depolarizing agent is fazadinium.

The extraocular muscles appear to be specifically resistant to the relaxant action of suxamethonium. Another remote risk with this drug is the prolonged apnoea, which may be encountered with patients on ecothiopate iodide drops. The suxamethonium induced rise in IOP may also be due to an increase in choroidal volume, as some rise still occurs after section of the extraocular muscles and canthotomy.

The choroidal blood volume may be reduced by lowering the systemic arterial pressure, providing the systolic pressure is lower than 90 mmHg. A marked fall in IOP usually occurs, which is greatest if the systolic pressure is reduced to 50–60 mmHg. Any cause which leads to an increase in the venous pressure will increase the choroidal volume and hence the IOP (e.g. a cough may raise the pressure to 40 mmHg). Increasing the P_{CO_2} will raise the IOP and lowering the P_{CO_2} will reduce the IOP. Increasing the P_{O_2} will lead to choroidal vasoconstriction and hence moderate hyperventilation will tend to reduce the IOP. Acetazolamide intravenously has been shown to increase the choroidal volume, which may lead to bulging of intraocular contents despite apparently low aqueous pressure.

Vitreous volume may be reduced by osmotic agents such as mannitol intravenously, commenced preoperatively, or an intravenous bolus of 50 per cent sucrose. The latter reduces the IOP in 5 min and can be given if the eye is tense during operation. Premedications are not used by all anaesthetists, but agents are chosen which avoid respiratory depression and nausea. Atropine is of help in abolishing the oculocardiac reflex.

OCULAR HYPOTENSIVE AGENTS

Carbonic Anhydrase Inhibitors

Acetazolamide

This is a sulphonamide derivative which reduces the intraocular pressure by inhibition of aqueous secretion. The bicarbonate in the aqueous is reduced and water secreted with it. This effect is independent of any diuretic action. A fall in IOP of 30–60 per cent occurs, lasting about 6–12 h after oral therapy. It is claimed that a more prolonged effect of 12–24 h may be obtained with sustained release capsules (sustets). A more rapid and certain action is produced with parenteral injection, intramuscular or intravenous. The pressure lowering effect of acetazolamide may be greater in advanced glaucoma than early glaucoma or normal eyes, as in the latter groups the drug is said to cause a reduced facility of outflow. The dose by mouth or injection is 250–500 mg initially followed by 250 mg every 6 h.

Prolonged acetazolamide medication depresses carbonic anhydrase activity throughout the body and this causes a high rate of side effects, especially in the elderly. By its action in the renal tubules it increases the excretion of bicarbonate, sodium and potassium resulting in a mild diuresis and a metabolic acidosis which may be fatal. Potassium supplements may be necessary for patients on high dose, long term therapy. Acetazolamide is contraindicated in renal and liver failure and also in patients with severe electrolyte imbalance. Side effects are malaise, anorexia, nausea, depression, anuria and bone-marrow depression may be rarely encountered. Transient myopia has been reported with this drug and other sulphonamides and diuretics.

PREPARATIONS

Acetazolamide tablets 250 mg. Diamox (Lederle), acetazolamide tablets 250 mg. Diamox Sustets, acetazolamide S/R capsules 500 mg. Sodium parenteral acetazolamide 500 mg vial.

Dichlorphenamide (Daranide)

Dichlorphenamide is an alternative carbonic anhydrase inhibitor. Unfortunately, most of the side effects of acetazolamide are likely to be encountered with this drug. The dose is 100–200 mg initially, then 100 mg every 12 h.

PREPARATIONS

Daranide (Merck, Sharp & Dohme), dichlorphenamide 50 mg.

Osmotic Agents

These agents are employed temporarily to withdraw fluid from the eye and thus reduce the intraocular pressure, especially in acute closed angle glaucoma. Their effect will depend on the rate of diffusion across the blood–aqueous barrier.

Mannitol

Mannitol is given by intravenous infusion over about 30 min as 10–20 per cent solution in total dose of 2 g/kg (50–200 g). It is contraindicated in congestive cardiac failure and pulmonary oedema. As a slow injection 40 ml of 20 per cent solution may be given over 2 min for a more immediate effect.

Urea

This is rarely used now as extravasation may cause tissue necrosis. The dose is 1–1·5 g/kg (40–80 g) intravenously 30 per cent urea solution in glucose infusion 5 or 10 per cent, given over about 45 min. It is contraindicated in renal and hepatic failure.

Glycerol

Glycerol is given orally as 1–1·5 g/kg of 50 per cent solution in saline. Lemon and soda can be added for taste as nausea may be caused. Care must be taken if general anaesthesia is to follow.

Local glycerol drops (20 per cent) have been employed to reduce corneal oedema temporarily to allow full ocular examination. They have also been used for prolonged therapy, as have hypertonic sodium chloride drops.

ANTI-MICROBIAL AGENTS

Antibiotics

Only the main antibiotics in use in ophthalmology are described here. For sensitivities *see Table* III. Recommended doses are available in standard handbooks of antibiotic therapy. Subconjunctival doses are given in *Table* IV.

Sulphonamides

Sulphonamides are rapidly absorbed from the gastrointestinal tract and are well distributed through all body compartments, including the eye.

Sulphacetamide is highly soluble and therefore used as drops (10–30 per cent).

Untoward effects are blood dyscrasias, crystalluria and hypersensitivity reactions including the Stevens–Johnson syndrome.

Penicillins

Benzyl penicillin (penicillin G) is given orally, as drops or subconjunctivally, intravenously or intramuscularly, and phenoxymethyl penicillin is given orally. They are still effective against many coccal infections, but most staphylococci produce a penicillinase (β-lactamase) which makes them resistant.

Methicillin is a penicillinase-resistant penicillin reserved for staphylococcal infections. It is given intravenously or intramuscularly and penetrates the inflamed eye. It can also be given subconjunctivally and into the vitreous.

Table III. Sensitivity to antibiotics of pathogenic bacteria more commonly encountered in ocular infections

Organism	Benzyl penicillin	Cloxacillin Methicillin	Ampicillin Amoxycillin	Carbenicillin	Cephaloridine	Erythromycin	Fusidate	Tetracycline	Chloramphenicol	Neomycin Framycetin	Gentamicin	Polymyxin	Sulphonamide
Staphylococcus aureus a	S	S	S	S	S(R)	SR	SR	SR	S(R)	SR	S	R	SR
Staphylococcus aureus b	R	S(R)	R	R	S(R)	SR	SR	SR	S(R)	SR	S	R	SR
Streptococcus pyogenes	S	S	S	S	S	S(R)	S	S(R)	S	R	R	R	SR
Streptococcus pneumoniae	S	S	S	S	S	S	S	SR	S	R	R	R	SR
Streptococcus faecalis	S(R)	R	SR	R	R	S	S	SR	S	R	R	R	SR
Neisseria gonorrhoea	S(R)	S(R)	S(R)	S(R)	S(R)	S	S	S	S	S	S	R	SR
Haemophilus influenzae	S	SR	S	S	S	S	S	S(R)	S	S	S	S	SR
Escherichia coli	R	R	SR	SR	SR	R	R	SR	SR	SR	S(R)	S	SR
Proteus spp.	R	R	SR	SR	SR	R	R	R	SR	SR	S(R)	R	SR
Pseudomonas aeruginosa	R	R	R	S(R)	R	R	R	R	R	SR	S(R)	S	R

S, sensitive; SR, both sensitive and resistant strains found; R, resistant; (R), resistant strains rare or resistance of moderate degree. *Staphylococcus aureus* B, B lactamase positive. A, B lactamase negative.

Table IV. Doses of subconjunctival antibiotics

Ampicillin	125 mg
Benzyl penicillin	500 000 u (300 mg)
Carbenicillin	100 mg
Cefuroxime	100 mg
Cephaloridine	50–100 mg
Chloramphenicol	100 mg
Cloxacillin	100 mg
Colistin	500 000 u
Flucloxacillin	100 mg
Framycetin	100–500 mg
Gentamicin	10–20 mg
Kanamycin	10–20 mg
Lincomycin	75–150 mg
Methicillin	500 mg
Neomycin	500 mg
Polymixin B	125 000–200 000 u
Spiramycin	10–20 mg
Streptomycin	250 mg
Ticarcillin	125 mg
Tobramycin	10–20 mg
Vancomycin	25 mg

Cloxacillin and flucloxacillin are also reserved for staphylococcal infections but are taken orally. Subconjunctival injection is not generally recommended.

Broad Spectrum Penicillins

Amoxycillin is better absorbed from the gastrointestinal tract but is otherwise similar to ampicillin, which can also be given periocularly.

The main use of carbenicillin and ticarcillin is against *Pseudomonas aeruginosa* and proteus strains resistant to ampicillin. Even more active against pseudomonas are azlocillin and piperacillin where parenteral administration is necessary. Ticarcillin can be given subconjunctivally, and carbenicillin subconjunctivally or into the vitreous.

UNTOWARD REACTIONS TO PENICILLIN

Hypersensitivity reactions are rash, fever, vasculitis and Stevens–Johnson syndrome. Toxic effects are rare, but include bone-marrow depression.

Cephalosporins

These are semi-synthetic antibiotics of similar structure to penicillin. Most are given parenterally and excreted by the kidney. They penetrate the inflamed eye.

The second generation drugs (such as cefuroxime, cephamandole and cefoxitin) are active against staphylococci, *Haemophilus influenzae* and enterobacteria.

Cefsulodin, a third generation cephalosporin, is active against *P. aeruginosa* but not staphylococci.

Ceporin and cefuroxime have been used subconjunctivally, and cephaloridine and cephazoline into the vitreous. In practice, there are usually other antibiotics with similar spectra available for use. Cephalosporins are useful in patients with penicillin sensitivity, although cross-sensitivity has been reported.

Aminoglycosides

Gentamicin and tobramycin are given parenterally. They penetrate the eye poorly, so are usually used periocularly, often for *P. aeruginosa* infection. Gentamicin can also be used intravitreously.

Untoward effects are ototoxicity and renal toxicity, directly related to plasma levels.

Neomycin and framycetin are used locally and subconjunctivally and have a wide spectrum. Untoward effects are skin hypersensitivity reactions, which occur in 4–8 per cent of patients using neomycin drops.

Tetracyclines

Tetracyline, oxytetracycline and chlortetracycline are slowly absorbed from the gastrointestinal tract and have short half-lives.

Minocycline and doxycycline are better absorbed and have longer half-lives, so need only be given twice and once a day, respectively. They are mainly used in the therapy of trachoma and other chlamydial conjunctivitis.

Chloramphenicol

This is employed locally in ophthalmic practice as a useful broad spectrum antibiotic. It can also be given subconjunctivally. Pseudomonas is resistant.

When used systemically bone-marrow suppression occurs once in 30 000 courses of therapy. A few cases of aplastic anaemia after using chloramphenicol drops have been reported.

Miscellaneous Antibiotics

Erythromycin is taken orally but does not penetrate the uninflamed eye. It is useful for patients hypersensitive to penicillin and in chlamydial infections in children.

Clindamycin is an oral drug with a similar antibacterial spectrum to erythromycin. Its chief interest is its action against *Toxoplasma gondii*, although it has not been widely used in human ocular toxoplasmosis.

The side effect of pseudomembranous colitis is uncommon.

Polymixin β is not absorbed from the gastrointestinal tract, and is used as eye drops or subconjunctivally. Proteus and some strains of pseudomonas are resistant.

Pyrimethamine is an anti-malarial drug used in the therapy of ocular toxoplasmosis in combination with a sulphonamide. It is given orally.

The side effect of megaloblastic anaemia is preventable if folinic acid is given concurrently.

ANTI-VIRAL AGENTS

These drugs are used locally in the eye. They are active against DNA viruses, especially herpes viruses, and in ophthalmology are used almost exclusively for herpes simplex type I infections.

Site of Action

All are effective against epithelial lesions. Acyclovir penetrates the stroma, producing therapeutic aqueous levels.

Toxicity

All can cause superficial punctate epitheliopathy, follicular conjunctivitis and allergic skin reactions. Punctal stenosis has been associated most often with idoxuridine, but has also been reported with other agents.

Idoxuridine (IDU)

IDU is a halogenated pyrimidine resembling the nucleic acid thymidine. After entry into the cell, the compound is phosphorylated and incorporated into both cellular and viral DNA. This results in faulty protein transcription, and damage to host and viral cells. It is available as 0·1 per cent drops (used hourly) and 0·5 per cent ointment (five times daily).

Vidarabine (Adenine Arabinoside)

This is an analogue of adenosine. After phosphorylation in the cell, it acts by inhibiting both viral and host DNA polymerase, preventing adequate synthesis of DNA. It is available as 3 per cent ointment (five times daily).

Trifluorothymidine (F_3T)

Like IDU, this is an analogue of thymidine. It is a potent inhibitor of thymidylate synthetase, which is necessary for DNA synthesis in mammalian and viral cells. The phosphorylated compound also acts like IDU by replacing deoxythymidine triphosphate in DNA, and causing faulty protein transcription.

It is used as 1 per cent drops.

Acyclovir (Acycloguanosine)

This is an analogue of guanine. In the infected cell it is phosphorylated by herpes-specific thymidine kinase. The resulting acycloguanosine triphosphate inhibits viral much more than host DNA polymerase. Acyclovir is therefore more virus-specific than the other antivirals and is less toxic to epithelial cells. It is available as 3 per cent ointment (five times daily).

ANTI-FUNGAL AGENTS

Although fungal infections of the eye are uncommon, they tend to be destructive unless treated by an appropriate anti-fungal agent for several weeks. Many fungi have been reported to cause ocular infection, but the most common ones are *Candida albicans*, *Aspergillus fumigatus* and *Fusarium solanii*.

The main anti-fungal agents and their sensitivities are shown in *Table* V. They may be divided into three families.

Polyene Antibiotics

Nystatin is fungistatic and fungicidal. It is used as 3·3 per cent eye ointment (100 000 u/ml), particularly for candida infections. It does not penetrate the cornea, and side effects are negligible.

Table V. Sensitivities of anti-fungal agents

Agent	Species
Nystatin	Candida
	Aspergillus
Amphotericin B	Candida
	Coccidioides
	Histoplasma
	Blastomyces
Pimaricin	Aspergillus
	Fusarium
Flucytosine	Candida
	Cryptococcus
Clotrimazole	Aspergillus
	Candida
	Rhizopus
Miconazole	Candida
	Penicillium
Econazole	Aspergillus
	Fusarium
	Penicillium
Ketoconazole	Candida
Thiabendazole	Fusarium
	Penicillium
	Phialophora
	Cladosporium

Amphotericin B is usually administered intravenously, and penetrates the aqueous but probably not the vitreous. It is toxic when used systemically: most patients develop impaired renal function and some develop anaemia, leucopenia or thrombocytopenia. It is occasionally used intravitreally or subconjunctivally (150–300 µg) where it may cause yellow discoloration of the conjunctiva.

Natamycin (Pimaricin) is active against the three main fungal organisms, and also many others, but does not penetrate deeper than the epithelium. It is used as a 5 per cent suspension or 1 per cent ointment.

Pyrimidine Anti-Fungal

Flucytosine (5-fluorocytosine) is taken orally, is not very toxic and penetrates to the anterior chamber. It is often used in combination with another anti-fungal agent because resistance can develop during treatment.

Side effects include bone-marrow depression, gastrointestinal symptoms and hepatomegaly.

Imidazole Antifungals

Clotrimazole has a broad anti-fungal spectrum. It is used as a 1 per cent solution in arachis oil.

Miconazole and econazole have broad spectra and low toxicity and miconazole is also active against many Gram-positive bacteria. Miconazole may be used orally or intravenously and topically as a 1 per cent solution in arachis oil. Econazole is used as a 1 per cent solution in arachis oil and is more effective than miconazole in infections by *Fusarium, Aspergillus* and *Penicillium* spp.

Ketoconazole is given orally and is particularly effective against *Candida* spp. It can cause hepatitis.

Thiabendazole is an anthelminthic agent which is active against some fungi. It is administered orally as tablets and topically as a 4 per cent suspension.

Ocular penetration of all the imidazole drugs in humans is unclear, although miconazole is known not to penetrate the rabbit eye. However, in practice these drugs seem to be effective against eye infections caused by sensitive fungi.

ANTI-INFLAMMATORY DRUGS

Non-Steroidal Prostaglandin Inhibitors

Following the demonstration of prostaglandins in the body and subsequently in the eye, it was shown that they are involved in the inflammatory process, especially in uveitis and also in traumatic miosis and secondary glaucoma.

Polyphloretin phosphate has been used locally as drops both in animals and in humans; it has a specific anti-prostaglandin action.

A number of drugs such as aspirin, phenylbutazone and indomethacin have been in use for many years for their anti-inflammatory action, which is in part due to inhibition of prostaglandin synthesis. Systemic administration has been shown to reduce the postoperative rise in intraocular pressure after cataract extraction. Pretreatment with topical indomethacin 0·5–1 per cent drops reduces the operative miosis and has been claimed to lower the incidence of cystoid macular oedema. Indomethacin has been employed systemically in episcleritis and scleritis. Oxyphenbutazone (Tanderil) is available as a 10 per cent ointment with or without chloramphenicol, and though it avoids some of the complications of corticosteroids such as viral replication or glaucoma, it is not widely used.

Antihistamines

The role of histamine in the induction of various allergic ocular disorders is still in doubt. Systemic antihistamines tend to produce sedation, which limits their usefulness for purely ocular conditions. The only topical anti-histamine available is antazoline.

PREPARATIONS

Otrivine–Antistin (Zyma) eye drops, antazoline sulphate 0·5 per cent, xylometazoline hydrochloride 0·05 per cent. Vasocon-A (Cooper Vision) eye drops, antazoline phosphate 0·5 per cent, naphazoline hydrochloride 0·05 per cent.

Sodium Cromoglycate

Mast cell stabilization by sodium cromoglycate drops is employed in vernal catarrh and other allergic disorders to reduce the itching and discomfort and avoid the complications of steroid therapy. The available preparations are Opticrom (Fisons) eye drops, sodium cromoglycate 2 per cent and eye ointment 4 per cent.

Corticosteroids (*Table* VI)

Following their identification, corticosteroids were found to be extremely useful in a wide variety of inflammatory ocular disorders, either topically, by subconjuctival injection, or systemically. They have been shown to act at numerous sites of the inflammatory process, both in the acute and chronic phases, often with seemingly opposite actions. In the acute phase they decrease capillary permeability and exudation. In the chronic, they inhibit fibroblastic activity and neovascularization. In general, topical administration will achieve a much higher dose than systemically to the anterior segment and is usually sufficient, whereas systemic administration is required for posterior segment affections and scleritis. The inflammatory suppression will be dependent on the dose and type of corticosteroid used.

The implications of this suppression must be carefully considered and the minimal dose used for long term therapy. Thus, postoperatively careful selection of the dose allows inflammation to be reduced without interfering with wound healing. For external lid affections use of a lotion or cream will avoid adverse reactions on the eye. Fluorometholone and clobetasone are claimed to penetrate less well into the eye and may be advantageous in conjunctival and superficial corneal conditions. Suppression of the inflammatory exudate in the eye with corticosteroids will also be accompanied by a reduction in beneficial substances such as antibodies, fibrinolytic factors and drugs. Similarly, steroids may delay the absorption of haemorrhage or lens matter.

Adverse Reactions

The side effects from systemic corticosteroid therapy are well dealt with in any standard textbook and must be carefully considered before therapy is commenced. Alternate day therapy may reduce the risk of adrenocortical insufficiency. In young children acute intracranial hypertension has been described due to reducing or stopping therapy, which may be fatal.

Posterior subcapsular lens opacities are associated with long term, high dose systemic therapy, rarely

Table VI. Topical corticosteroids available

Corticosteroid	Preparation	
Betamethasone sodium phosphate	Drops and ointment	Betnesol (Glaxo) 0·1%
	Drops and ointment	Betnesol-N (Glaxo) 0·1% + neomycin sulphate 0·5%
	Drops	Vistamethasone (Daniels) 0·1%
	Drops	Vistamethasone-N (Daniels) 0·1% + neomycin sulphate 0·5%
	Subconj.	Inj. betamethasone: 4 mg/ml
Clobetasone butyrate	Drops	Eumovate (Glaxo) 0·1%
	Drops	Eumovate-N (Glaxo) 0·1% + neomycin sulphate 0·5%
Dexamethasone	Drops	Maxidex (Alcon) 0·1%
	Drops and ointment	Maxitrol (Alcon) 0·1% + neomycin sulphate 0·35%, polymixin B sulphate 6000 i.u./ml or g
	Drops	Sofradex (Roussel) dexamethasone sodium metasulphobenzoate 0·05%, framycetin sulphate 0·5%, gramicidin 0·0005%
	Subconj.	Decadron (MSD) 4 mg/ml
		Oradexon (Organon), dose 2 mg
Fluorometholone	Suspension	FML (Allergan) 0·1%
	Suspension	FML (Allergan) 0·1% + neomycin 0·5%
Hydrocortisone acetate	Ointment	Chloromycetin hydrocortisone (P-D), chloramphenicol 1%, hydrocortisone acetate 0·5%
	Ointment	Cortucid (Nicholas) 0·5% + sulphacetamide sodium 10%
	Drops and ointment	Framycort (Fison) 0·5% + framycetin sulphate 0·5%
	Drops and ointment	Neo-Cortef (Upjohn) 1·5% + neomycin sulphate 0·5%
Prednisolone sodium phosphate	Drops	Minims prednisolone (S&N) 0·5%
	Drops	Predsol (Glaxo) 0·5%
	Drops	Predsol-N (Glaxo) 0·5% + neomycin sulphate 0·5%
Methyl prednisolone acetate	Subconj.	Depomedrone (Upjohn) inj. 40 mg/ml, dose 10–20 mg
Triamcinolone	Subconj.	Kenalog (Squibb) 40 mg/ml, dose 10–20 mg

from topical treatment. The risk is mainly from daily doses of 10–15 mg or more of prednisolone or equivalent for longer than one year. The mechanism is still obscure. Reducing the dose may prevent progression in early cases.

One of the main secondary effects from topical therapy is the aggravation of dendritic ulceration of the cornea to form an amoeboid ulcer. The other risk is steroid glaucoma, which is encountered more with the stronger topical agents, such as dexamethasone or betamethasone, less frequently with fluorometholone, clobetasone or dilute prednisolone (0·05 per cent). Numerous studies have shown that certain individuals are more susceptible and grades of steroid responders have been described. Patients with chronic simple glaucoma and their siblings are more likely to be steroid responders, as are myopes, diabetics without retinopathy and people with Krukenberg's spindle. The mechanism is still obscure, though increased resistance to outflow due to alteration in the mucopolysaccharide of the trabecular meshwork has been postulated.

ADVERSE DRUG REACTIONS

The more common adverse reactions encountered with topical medicaments either on the eye or systemically have already been mentioned, with the exception of allergy. Some systemic drugs that cause ocular adverse reactions will now be described.

Allergy

The lids and conjunctiva may be swollen dramatically in the generalized acute urticarial or angioneurotic oedema reaction to a wide variety of systemic drugs, penicillin being one of the commonest. An exudative conjunctivitis and keratopathy is encountered in the Stevens–Johnson syndrome which may be drug-induced, especially by the sulphonamide derivatives and tetracyclines. The eye condition may resolve without permanent damage or lead to dry eye, conjunctival shrinkage and corneal opacification.

Contact dermatitis due to topical drugs (dermatitis medicamentosa) is relatively common, atropine and neomycin being the most frequent causes. When antibiotics are combined with corticosteroids, the allergic reaction may be reduced sufficiently to obscure diagnosis. Preservatives in drops may be the cause and it is sometimes possible to change to a product with different preservative or use a preservative-free solution. Ointments are frequent sensitizers and one should avoid their long term use in atopic individuals.

Practolol Syndrome

Although this drug was withdrawn following the recognition of toxicity, patients still need treatment and the mechanism is still obscure. In severe cases the conjunctiva became keratinized and scarred, the cornea developed melting opacities and there were accompanying psoriatic skin eruptions, deafness, fibrinous peritonitis and pericarditis.

Phenothiazine Pigmentation

Patients on long term phenothiazine therapy may develop slate blue discoloration of the exposed skin and lids with gold brown pigmentation of the conjunctiva. Deposits may occur on the corneal endothelium and Descemet's membrane, also on the anterior lens epithelium. These ocular deposits rarely give rise to symptoms but do not disappear when the drug is stopped.

Corneal Deposits

Corneal deposits occur on the epithelium with a wide variety of drugs, especially the chloroquine compounds and amiodarone. In either case the deposits rarely cause symptoms and reverse on stopping therapy.

Pupil and Accommodation

Cycloplegia can be caused by a wide variety of systemic drugs which have an anticholinergic action. This may be distressing to the patient, especially if they are already mentally disturbed, or may lead to the prescription of unexpectedly strong presbyopic correction. The risk of closed angle glaucoma in susceptible patients from drugs with anticholinergic action, such as tricyclic antidepressants, is small.

Retina

Two groups of drugs concentrate in the pigment epithelium and choroid and may produce retinopathy, phenothiazines with a piperidine ring and chloroquine compounds. The only phenothiazine on the market with retinotoxic capabilities is thioridazine (Melleril) and the evidence is that there should be no danger provided the dose is kept below 800 mg/day. Retinal toxicity with high dose chloroquine compounds occurs in a proportion of patients who have received 250 mg or more a day for a period so that a total dose of 100 g has been exceeded. The fundal changes are first manifest at the maculae and may progress to a bull's eye appearance which is enhanced by fluorescein angiography. Central field defects may be detected early, as are colour vision defects and changes in the electro-oculogram and electroretinogram. The value of ocular monitoring is still controversial and it would seem preferable for the dose in all patients to be reduced before the total of 100 g is reached to 250 mg on alternate days or twice a week. There is very little excretion or detoxication of chloroquine compounds and they are retained in depots in the body for 5–10 years.

Toxic Amblyopia

Numerous drugs have been reported to cause occasional toxic optic neuropathy. The main one with clinical significance is ethambutol. This usually causes visual impairment of fairly sudden onset, recovery may take up to a year after stopping and some patients with permanent damage have been reported. The risk of toxicity is minimal providing the dose is kept to below 15 mg/kg and providing the renal function is good. With higher doses patients should be warned to report if any visual deterioration occurs. The visual evoked response may be helpful, especially in patients with communication problems.

Other Reactions

Acute toxicity is still seen in isolated patients taking quinine either from overdosage or those with idiosyncrasy. Some recovery of vision usually occurs despite residual constricted fields and optic atrophy. Acute intracranial hypertension with papilloedema has been described in children from vitamin A, nalidixic acid, tetracycline therapy or where corticosteroids have been stopped or reduced.

A number of drugs have been reported to cause diplopia or ocular palsies. Phenothiazines occasionally produce oculogyric crises. Some drugs cause abnormal or defective colour vision, especially digitalis, and this may be an early indication of overdosage.

ACKNOWLEDGEMENT

We thank Miss L. C. Dudley for checking the manuscript.

BIBLIOGRAPHY

Ellis P. P. *Ocular Therapeutics and Pharmacology*, 7th ed., St Louis, Mosby, 1985.
Goodman L. S. and Gilman A. *The Pharmacological Basis of Therapeutics*, 7th ed., London, Macmillan, 1985.
Havener W. H. *Ocular Pharmacology*, 5th ed., St Louis, Mosby, 1983.
Holloway K. B. Control of the eye during general anaesthesia for intraocular surgery. *Br. J. Anaesth.* 1980; **52,** 671.
Jones B. R. Principles in the management of oculomycosis (XXXI Edward Jackson Memorial Lecture). *Am. J. Ophthalmol.* 1975; **79,** 719–51.
Shell J. W. Pharmacokinetics of topically applied ophthalmic drugs. *Surv. Ophthalmol.* 1982; **26**(4), 207–18.

Chapter 3

Methods of Examination

Specular Microscopy
R. J. Buckley

Every artist is aware of specular (mirror-like) reflection by the cornea. The bright reflection of the principal light source at the air–tear interface immediately distinguishes the lustrous living eye from its dull lifeless counterpart. Invisible to the naked eye is a much dimmer reflection from the posterior corneal surface, at the endothelium–aqueous interface;* that reflection was first observed at the slit lamp by Vogt, and described by him in 1919.[1] Being interrupted by the cell boundaries and by other features, it carries an image of the endothelium, and thus allows observation of this monolayer.

VOGT'S METHOD

Examination of portions of the endothelium by Vogt's method is part of the routine assessment of the cornea at the slit lamp. A narrow, bright slit is aimed at the corneal epithelium and the area adjacent to this bright gleam, on the side opposite to the light source, is examined; the angle between incident and reflected rays should be 40–60°. Moving the microscope forwards less than 0·5 mm brings the endothelium into focus. High magnification should be used.

The method is limited by the curvature of the posterior cornea (which allows only a small area to be visualized), by eye movements and by the physical restrictions of the slit lamp, so that endothelial appearance is sampled, rather than comprehensively surveyed. Furthermore, the obliquity of the light reflexes distorts the image: the endothelium is not seen 'en face'.

NON-CONTACT SPECULAR MICROSCOPES

The so-called 'non-contact' clinical specular microscopes are essentially either high powered monocular photo-slit lamps (e.g. Nikon Endothelial Camera) or variants of the Brown macrocamera.[2] These instruments suffer the same disadvantages as the basic method of Vogt, enhanced by the greater magnification employed.

ACCESSORY OBJECTIVES

The epithelial (air–tear) reflex, which is about 95 times brighter than the endothelial (cornea–aqueous) reflex, is distracting. Partly to overcome this, and to provide more magnification, and to stabilize the eye, accessory objective lenses have been developed for use at the slit lamp.

That of Eisner is hand-held, being used in the manner of a gonioscope, and does not applanate the cornea. Buckley's objective is mounted in the tonometer in place of the normal prism, and does applanate the cornea.

CLINICAL SPECULAR MICROSCOPES

The clinical specular microscope is essentially Maurice's laboratory instrument of 1968.[3] He used a ×40 water-immersion objective with a saline-filled screw-on cap which applanated the cornea; the endothelium was thus held perpendicular to the axis of the microscope. The optics were longitudinally divided so that light travelled to the cornea through one half of the objective and was received at the ×10 eyepiece through the other half. The field of view was about 0·01 mm².

Using a horizontally mounted variant of this instrument, Sherrard in 1972[4] captured the first clinical endothelial specular photomicrograph (ESP).

Laing[5] and Bourne and Kaufman[6] described the first practical clinical instruments, which were liberated from the screw-on saline chamber by the use of the 'dipping cone' objective. In this objective the front component lens is prolonged forwards in the frustrum of a cone.

LARGE FIELD INSTRUMENTS

By 'optical tailoring' of the components of a laminated objective cone, and the routine use of a contact

---

* For angles of incidence near the normal, the percentage of the incident light reflected at the interface of two transparent media is given by:

$$R\% = \left[\frac{n_1 - n_2}{n_1 + n_2}\right]^2 \times 100$$

where n_1 and n_2 are the indices of refraction of the two media. For air–tears, this is 2·07 per cent; for cornea–aqueous, the precentage is 0·022. The refractive indices of air, tears, cornea and aqueous are taken as 1·0, 1·336, 1·376 and 1·336, respectively.

lens, an instrument was produced that could provide a field of view of up to 1 mm². This was the Pocklington (Keeler–Konan) instrument, as described by Sherrard and Buckley.[7]

Another approach was adopted by Koester,[8] in whose instrument, the PRO/Koester, a narrow slit of light oscillates rapidly, producing images which are reconstituted into a stationary large field (typically 0·65 mm²).

CLINICAL PRACTICE OF ESP

ESP is a clinical technique which is inoffensive to patients and easily mastered by the operator. The use of a thin plano high-water hydrogel contact lens renders local anaesthesia unnecessary in most cases. With the Pocklington instrument the lens, in addition to acting as part of the optical system, limits microsaccadic eye movements by friction, so providing a less mobile and more accurately focusable image at the observed magnification of ×130. Anteroposterior pulsations of the globe are absorbed by the flexibly mounted objective carriage.

POSTERIOR CORNEAL RINGS

When the human cornea is applanated, as by the flat-faced objective cone of the specular microscope, its posterior surface is thrown into a series of very shallow undulations. The sides of these wrinkles are tilted away from the perpendicular of the axis of the microscope, and so reflect light away from that axis; they are therefore seen as dark bands. The crests of the wrinkles are perpendicular and so appear bright. These 'posterior corneal rings' (PCRs), which are an applanation artefact, form in a pattern of concentric irregular horizontal ellipses, surrounding the axial region of the cornea. They may represent areas of 'tying' of the stromal lamellae, where their capacity to slip over each other is focally limited; perhaps they indicate the structure which holds the cornea in its normal complex aspheric shape.

Because the PCRs form in the same places at each examination, they may be thought of as a corneal 'fingerprint', unique to the individual; but more importantly, they supply a target for the relocation of specific areas of the endothelium and even individual cells.

PCRs are absent or vestigial in children and in certain abnormalities of the cornea such as keratoconus. They do not occur in the form seen in man in nonprimates, and the rabbit cornea, so often used as a model in research, seems not to wrinkle under any circumstances.

RELIEF MODE

A non-specular reflection, which allowed the pseudothree-dimensional observation of posterior corneal profile disturbances, was simultaneously described in 1981 by Hartmann[9] (as 'indirect specular microscopy') and by Sherrard and Buckley[10] (as 'the relief mode'). This seems to be a combination of marginal and indirect retroillumination from deeper structures (iris, fundus, lens, pseudophakos). Structures that disrupt the normally smooth posterior corneal surface can be observed alternately in direct and in indirect reflection, which greatly facilitates their interpretation.

ANALYSIS OF SPECULAR MICROGRAPHS

The development of the modern clinical instrument, with its field of view of 100 times the area of Maurice's original instrument, allowed a more realistic overview of significant portions of the posterior surface of the cornea, whose total area has been estimated as 147 mm² (*Fig.* 1).[11] Large disturbances, such as the PCRs, geographical dysplasia in the ICE syndrome, and surgical wounds, could be visualized and scanned (*Fig.* 2). The devastating effects of angle- and iris-supported lens implants could be fully appreciated. However, the sheer size of the field encouraged the tendency to count ever greater numbers of cells while

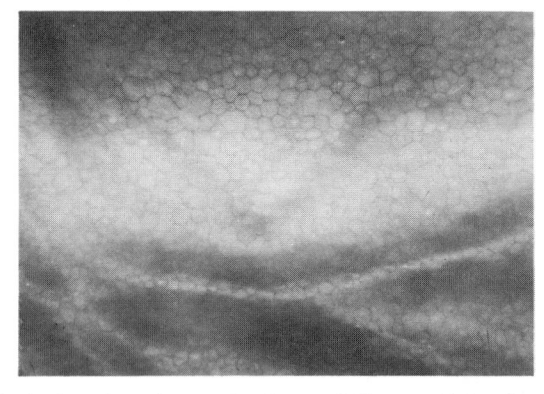

Fig. 1. Specular micrograph of normal 80-year-old female. The cells are irregularly enlarged. A portion of a posterior corneal ring is seen in the lower third of the field. (Magnification ×60).

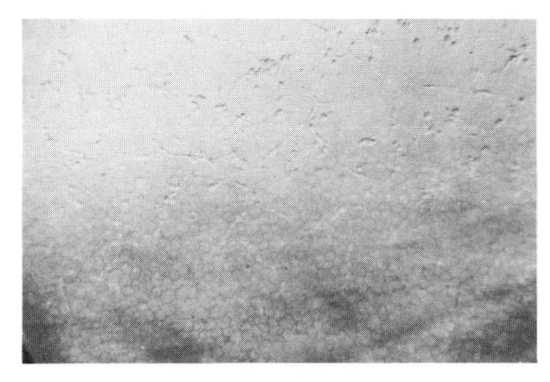

Fig. 2. Specular micrograph of 64-year-old patient with recurrent anterior uveitis following penetrating injury 3 years before. The cells are present in normal numbers. Many keratic precipitates are seen, with relief mode imaging in the upper third of the field. (Magnification ×60).

overlooking the characteristics of the cells themselves.

For a continuous cell monolayer, the regular hexagon is geometrically and thermodynamically the most stable polygon. The existence of unequal endothelial cell sizes, and cell shapes other than hexagons, was recognized and illustrated by Vogt. Waring[12] analysed individual cell areas and plotted histograms from which a 'coefficient of skewness' could be calculated. Increasing skewness correlated with advancing age, which absolute cell density did not. Heterogeneity of cell size has been termed 'polymegethism' and homogeneity, 'homomegethism'.[13]

Olsen,[14] in his study of cell population heterogeneity, concentrated on cell shape, and this approach was also adopted recently by Matsuda et al.[15] It appears that endothelial cells are capable of changing their shapes and areas in response to traumatic stimuli, presumably to make good defects in the monolayer caused by loss of individual cells. When this phase is over (a few weeks) there is a slower return to hexagonality. It is not known why some stressed endothelia, observed long after the insult, appear to have lost the potential to recover hexagonality.

An indication of the importance of cell morphometric analysis, in distinction from density measurement, is seen in the work of Schultz et al.[16] which demonstrates a reduced percentage of hexagonal cells in diabetes.

The application of automated image analysis to specular micrographic images is currently problematical and expensive. However, this is clearly a challenge that must be met if modern clinical specular microscopy is to advance as much in its second decade as it did in its first.

REFERENCES

1. Vogt A. *Klin. Monatsbl. Augenheilkd.* 1919; **63**, 233.
2. Brown N. A. P. *Br. J. Ophthalmol.* 1970; **54**, 697.
3. Maurice D. M. Cellular membrane activity in the corneal endothelium of the intact eye. *Experientia* 1968; **24**, 1094–5.
4. Sherrard E. S. 1972; Personal communication.
5. Laing R. A. et al. *In vivo* photomicrography of the corneal endothelium. *Arch. Ophthalmol.* 1975; **93**, 143–5.
6. Bourne W. M. and Kaufman H. E. Specular microscopy of human corneal endothelium in vivo. *Am. J. Ophthalmol.* 1976; **81**, 319–23.
7. Sherrard E. S. and Buckley R. J. Clinical specular microscopy of the corneal endothelium. *Trans. Ophthalmol. Soc. UK* 1981; **101**, 156–62.
8. Koester C. A scanning mirror microscope with optical sectioning characteristics: application in ophthalmology. *Appl. Optics* 1980; **19**, 1749.
9. Hartmann C. Die 'indirekte' Spiegelmikroskopie. *Ophthalmologica* 1981; **183**, 177–86.
10. Sherrard E. S. and Buckley R. J. The relief mode: a new application of the specular microscope. *Arch. Ophthalmol.* 1982; **100**, 296–300.
11. Bron A. J. and Brown N. A. P. Endothelium of the corneal graft. *Trans. Ophthalmol. Soc. UK* 1974; **94**, 863–73.
12. Waring G. D. et al. The corneal endothelium. *Ophthalmology* 1982; **89**, 531–90.
13. Rao G. N. et al. Endothelial cell morphology and corneal deturgescence. *Ann. Opthalmol.* 1978; **11**, 885–99.
14. Olsen T. Variations in endothelial morphology of normal corneas and after cataract extraction: a specular microscopic study. *Acta Ophthalmol.* 1979; **57**, 1014.
15. Matsuda M. et al. Serial alteration in endothelial cell shape and pattern after intra-ocular surgery. *Am. J. Ophthalmol.* 1984; **98**, 313–19.
16. Schultz R. O. et al. Corneal endothelial changes in Type I and Type II diabetes mellitus. *Am. J. Ophthalmol.* 1984; **98**, 401–10.

Gonioscopy

Redmond J. H. Smith

INTRODUCTION

The angle of the anterior chamber can only be seen easily with the aid of a gonioscopic contact lens. Troncoso[1] was the first to describe a practical system of gonioscopy by means of a self-illuminated hand-held microscope ('the gonioscope') and a contact lens. The system requires the patient to be recumbent and the gonioscope is usually suspended from the ceiling on a counter-balanced cord. This apparatus is not in use in the United Kingdom, where virtually all outpatient diagnostic gonioscopy is carried out at a slit lamp, whereas operating theatre gonioscopy is usually done with the operating microscope.

Optics

Owing to total internal reflection, a gonioscopic view is only obtainable in an average anterior chamber by a very oblique view, e.g. ray x in *Fig.* 1. (Ray y is totally internally reflected.) Either by artificially

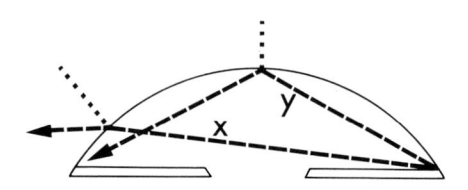

Fig. 1. Ray y is totally internally reflected at the corneal surface. Ray x escapes but only gives the chance of a very oblique view and only of a wide angle.

steepening the cornea by a steeply curved contact glass, e.g. Koeppe lens,[2] *Fig.* 2, or by redirecting a ray via a mirror incorporated in a contact lens, e.g. Goldmann lens,[3] *Fig.* 3, or an Allen Braley Thorpe lens, *Fig.* 4, a much more convenient view can be obtained. (Ray y now avoids total internal reflection.)

Types of Goniolens

A number of goniolenses have been designed either on the direct principle (as *Fig.* 2), to be used on the recumbent patient[2,4] and especially during goniotomy, or on the indirect principle (as *Figs.* 3, 4).[3,5–8]

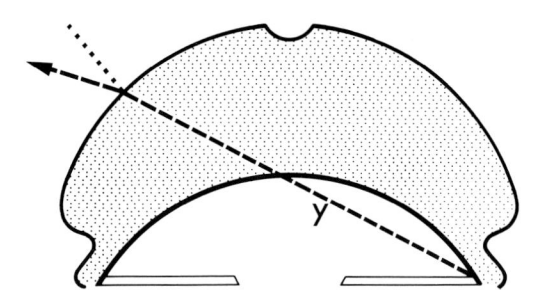

Fig. 2. Ray y now escapes from the cornea, also from the surface of the (Koeppe) lens as it is well clear of the critical angle. (Redrawn from Kolker A. E. and Hetherington J. jun. *Becker-Shaffer's Diagnosis and Therapy of the Glaucomas*, 5th ed. St Louis, Mo, Mosby, 1983.)

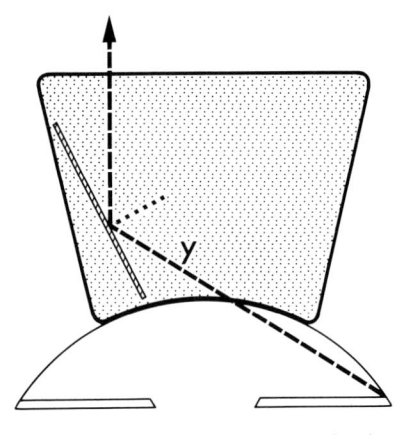

Fig. 3. The pathway of ray y in a Goldmann gonioprism. (Redrawn from Kolker and Hetherington.)

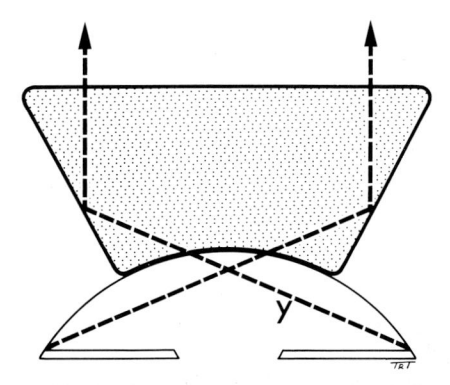

Fig. 4. The pathway of ray y in an Allen Braley Thorpe gonioprism. (Redrawn from Kolker and Hetherington.)

There are a number of variations possible; direct lenses can have a steep curve as already mentioned or a flat inclined face (*Plate Ia*).

Indirect lenses can have more than one mirror; there are, for example, single (*Fig. 5*) and double-mirror Goldmann lenses available (leaving aside the three-mirror lens which is principally for retinal work), and there are also four-mirror lenses available (*Fig. 6*).[6,7]

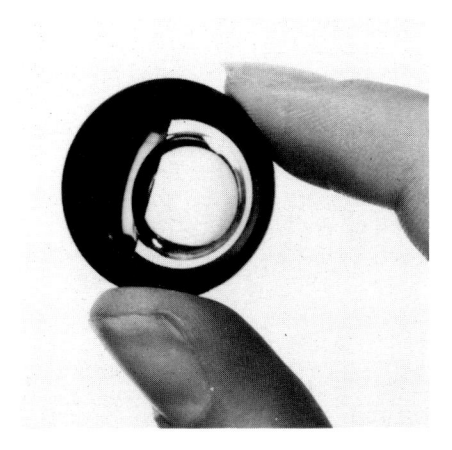

Fig. 5. The Goldmann single mirror lens.

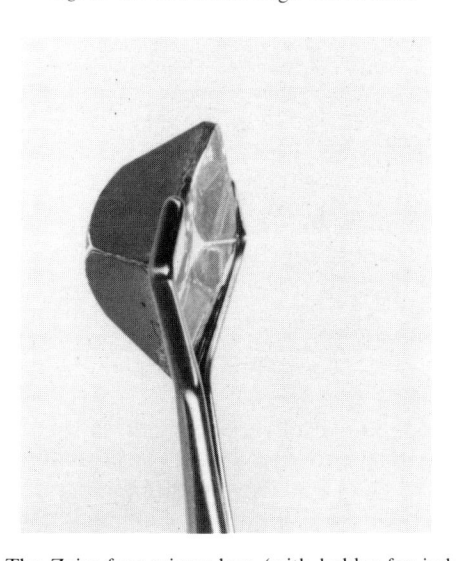

Fig. 6. The Zeiss four-mirror lens (with holder for indentation gonioscopy).

Indirect lenses, using total internal reflection instead of mirrors, have also been used, e.g. the lens of Allen and O'Brien[8] and the improved version of Allen Braley and Thorpe;[7] and an apparatus has been described for reversing the image in the gonioscopic mirror.[9] (It has even been pointed out that direct gonioscopy can be carried out without a lens if the medial canthal region is liberally flooded with saline.[10])

The radius of curvature of the corneal contact surface of the goniolens can be varied, for example in the Goldmann it is 7·4 mm, while in the Zeiss it is 7·7 mm and in the lens illustrated in *Plate Ia* it is 8·4 mm. Lenses with a steep curve tend to trap air bubbles unless skilfully inserted or internally irrigated, whereas low curve lenses avoid the bubbles but may produce corneal wrinkling.[11]

The diameter of the contact portion of the lens can vary and in some types, for example the Goldmann, the lens bears partly on the sclera at the limbus, whereas in others the bearing surface is only on the cornea.

Provision is made in some lenses, particularly direct lenses being used for surgery, for continuous irrigation via a channel built into the lens.[12] Another variation is to apply a vacuum to an internal channel, thus attaching the lens to the cornea by suction.[13]

Contact Fluid

Low curve lenses require no fluid as the tears suffice;[10,11] steep curve lenses can be inserted either with normal saline or with methyl cellulose in saline. (Methyl cellulose in water is not satisfactory as it causes corneal epithelial oedema.[14]) A recent report describes the use of KY jelly in goniolenses.[15]

CLINICAL APPLICATIONS

Normal Appearances of Angle Tissue

The gonioscopic view of the normal angle conventionally illustrated is usually that of the inferior angle by indirect gonioscopy, that is, with the mirror in the 12 o'clock position, as in *Fig. 7*. The structures seen from below upwards (in a wide angle) are as follows: the anterior surface of the iris (including the

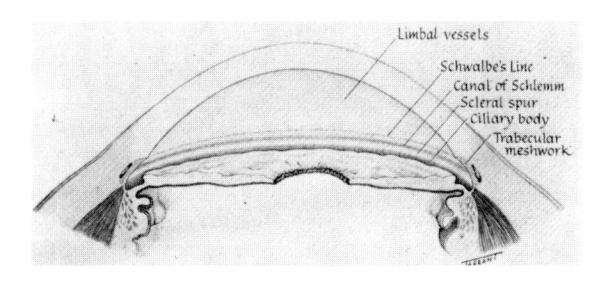

Fig. 7. Diagram of a typical angle with the principal structures marked.

pupillary edge only with a widely dilated pupil), the anterior aspect of the ciliary body, the scleral spur, the trabecular meshwork, including a darker band marking the canal of Schlemm, the line of Schwalbe at the anterior limit of the trabecular meshwork and finally the inner aspect of the cornea, through which limbal conjunctival vessels are usually seen.

The appearance of each structure is subject to a good deal of variation, mainly as a result of difference in pigmentation or partial, or sometimes almost total, obscuration by a brown or tan coloured spongy looking material called pectinate tissue. This is more commonly reduced to a patchy arrangement of strands of iris-coloured tissue extending from the base of the iris to the trabecular zone. These are called iris processes and they, or their more florid manifestation the pectinate tissue, become less and less obvious with advancing age. Thus, in patients in their sixties and seventies, iris processes are usually absent.

The appearance of the ciliary band is usually that of a non-homogeneous patchy texture, often somewhat paler than the iris and often showing coils of the major arterial circle as it runs circumferentially in the angle. In infant eyes it is common to see a series of darkish smudges in the ciliary region which appear to be dark segments of ciliary body showing through a relatively translucent iris base. These are almost invariably seen in buphthalmic eyes but are not known with certainty to be abnormal.

The scleral spur is a narrow pale band lying between the ciliary band and the trabecular meshwork. It may be partially obscured by some iridotrabecular pectinate tissue.

The trabecular meshwork is of a homogeneous light honey colour, little different from the cornea, but subject to a great deal of variability as to the amount of pigment deposited on it. When the meshwork is lightly or non-pigmented the canal of Schlemm can usually be seen as a shadowy band in the mid-trabecular zone, but if blood filling occurs, the canal appears as a red blush along the mid-trabecular zone. Where pigment is abundant in the meshwork it usually occupies approximately the same zone as Schlemm's canal, thus obscuring it. Pigmentation is often variable around the circumference.

In addition to this 'canal band', the meshwork may show some more erratically distributed particles of pigment, especially in the inferior zone. These give the impression of being mildly postpathological and may be seen in the angle in eyes with previous injury, uveitis or surgical operations.

Schwalbe's line marks the anterior limit of the trabecular meshwork and the periphery of Descemet's membrane. The line is usually a slightly wavering pencilled track delineated by fine black pigmentation, but occasionally it shows up as a sharp white line, presumably manifesting the edge of Descemet's membrane, which may be condensed into a slight ridge.

The chief variations in the appearances of the normal wide angle consist in variations in the amount of pectinate tissues (iris processes) and the degree of pigmentation of the trabecular meshwork. Racial coloration only applies in so far as the colour of the iris and pectinate tissues are concerned. The intrinsic pigmentation of the meshwork is unaffected by race: that is to say, an African eye may have a totally non-pigmented meshwork whereas a blue-eyed subject could have dense trabecular pigmentation.

Blood filling of Schlemm's canal can occur in an apparently random fashion during Goldmann gonioscopy in many normal eyes. The conditions that produce it are not exactly known, but are presumably concerned with various factors such as the pressure exerted on the episclera by the contact lens, the relative pressures in the canal and the episcleral veins, the pressure gradient across the trabecular meshwork and the pressure in the anterior chamber. There is a certain amount of evidence to suggest that blood filling occurs less easily in open-angle glaucoma than in normal eyes.[16,17]

Width of Angle

Variations in the depth of the anterior chamber and in the configuration of the peripheral part of the iris contribute to variations in the width of the angle.

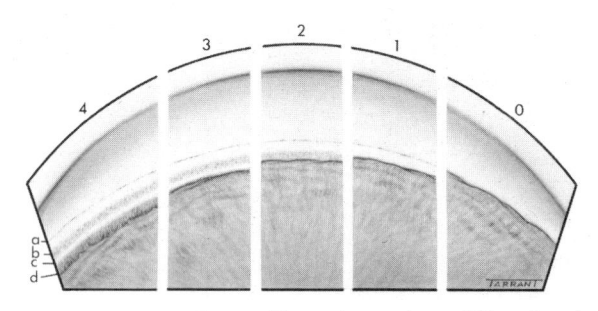

Fig. 8. Composite diagram illustrating various widths of angle. Note that in grade 0 none of the angle's features can be seen due to obscuration by the iris. At each grade, one item is revealed (a, Schwalbe's line; b, meshwork, including the Canal band; c, scleral spur; d, ciliary body band). Thus, in grade 4, all four principal structures are visible.

A so-called 'wide' angle is usually found where the configuration of the iris is flat, and the chamber is of a good depth, approaching 3 mm from posterior corneal surface to anterior lens capsule. A 'narrow' angle occurs where the anterior chamber approaches 2 mm in depth and where the iris, especially at its periphery, shows a well-marked anterior curvature (physiological iris bombé).

The appearance of a wide angle is such that all the structures mentioned previously can easily be seen, whereas in a narrow angle the base of the iris obscures them, only Schwalbe's line and part of the trabecular meshwork being visible. Between these two extremes, more or less of the angle structures can be seen, depending on the degree of obstruction of the view by the iris. Verbal descriptions such as 'wide', 'intermediate' and 'narrow' may be found in the literature.[18] Alternatively, some authors grade angles by a numerical system, a closed angle being designated 0, a narrow angle 1, up to the widest angle at grade 4.[19] *Fig.* 8 illustrates the grading from 0 to 4. (Note: one more landmark is seen at each grade.)

Furthermore, the width of the angle is not absolutely fixed, as small variations may occur with pupillary activity. Usually a moderate dilatation is accompanied by narrowing of the angle, although even this is by no means the same from eye to eye.

In a few angles, the configuration of the base of the iris is unusual, in that the major part of the surface is perfectly flat (plateau iris), while a sudden angulation occurs near the base giving a narrow angle in an eye with a relatively deep anterior chamber.

The width of the angle would be of only academic interest were it not for the fact that it could close if narrow enough. Many clinicians therefore grade angles in a functional way, e.g. closed, likely to close (very narrow), could easily close (narrow), could possibly close (medium narrow to medium), could not close (medium wide to wide).

Abnormalities of the Angle

Closure and Peripheral Anterior Synechiae

Primary closure, as in a narrow angle, is difficult to be sure of as the bulging anterior iris surface obscures the view of the recess. In other words, a very narrow angle may be virtually indistinguishable from a closed one. A slightly improved view may be obtained, especially when using a lens with a small corneal contact area such as a Zeiss four-mirror lens by pushing on the cornea, thus raising the pressure in the anterior chamber and reversing the physiological iris bombé, momentarily widening the angle (*Figs.* 6 and 9).[20] Switching the slit lamp on and off, thus producing movement of the iris, may also help in some doubtful cases of angle closure. (An extreme version of these measures to try to identify the openness of a very narrow angle is Chandler's manoeuvre, where the physiological iris bombé is reversed by paracentesis followed by refilling of the anterior chamber.[21])

Closures by peripheral anterior synechiae may be easy to distinguish, especially in an otherwise wide angle, when the adhesions of part or all of the base of the iris to the meshwork or even to the peripheral cornea can be seen. This type of closure is usually secondary to previous events – loss of the anterior chamber followed by subsequent reformation, persistent uveitis, rubeosis iridis and so on.

Congenital Anomalies

Primary congenital glaucoma is a hereditary condition with a typical gonioscopical appearance. The iris is usually flat and attached at its base to the trabecular meshwork, thus obscuring the scleral spur. The anterior surface of the iris appears hypoplastic and the alternating dark and pale patches mentioned previously are prominent.

There is reputed to be a faint grey membrane partially obscuring the view of the angle structures (Barkan's membrane),[22] and certainly if a goniotomy knife is drawn along just anterior to the iridotrabecular adhesions the iris does appear to drop back as though tethering by a membrane had been released. There is some doubt, however, about all these appearances as distinct from the normal in small infants.

Rieger's anomaly and the Axenfeld syndrome may be accompanied by gross deformity of the angle.[23] Large bridging adhesions sometimes occur, especially in Rieger's anomaly. Schwalbe's line may also look abnormally prominent.

In Axenfeld's syndrome the angle looks partially closed and the anterior leaf of the iris is extremely deficient, but in some cases the angle may look practically normal.

Neovascularization

In cases of prolonged retinal ischaemia following vascular accidents or diabetic retinopathy, neovascularization of the angle occurs crossing the scleral spur to ramify as fine capillary networks on the trabecular band (*Plate Ib*). There may be a number of such systems scattered randomly around the angle.[24] At this stage there is usually fine neovascularization present at the margin of the pupil.

The next stage in the gonioscopic picture is for the base of the iris to be drawn towards the meshwork, presumably due to contraction of fibrovascular tissue associated with the abnormal capillary system, and eventually anterior trabecular PAS (peripheral anterior synechiae) become firmly established.

It is usually possible to detect abnormal vascularization at the junction of the iris and trabecular tissue, and indeed in the latest stages free blood can be seen in the inferior angle (*Plate Id*). By this stage rubeosis of the iris has usually progressed to the stage of large

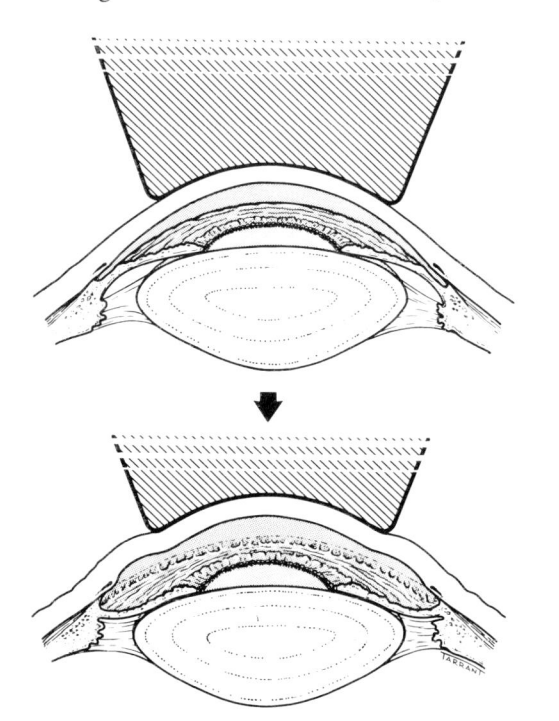

Fig. 9. 'Indentation' gonioscopy. The cornea is indented, the fluid displaced causes a reversal of the normal anterior curvature of the iris, thus momentarily widening the angle. (The increased volume in the posterior segment is accommodated by scleral distension.) (Redrawn from Kolker and Hetherington.)

confluent vascular channels linking the peripheral and peripupillary new vessel systems and ectropion uveae has also made its appearance. Intraocular pressure may begin to rise at any time following the first appearance of new vessels since the abnormal endothelial sheets which precede the vessels may be quite widespread but undetectable in the angle.

Heterochromic 'Cyclitis'

In Fuch's heterochromic cyclitis the angle is characteristic. There is a lack of pigment present, all the angle structures tending to have a 'washed out' appearance. At the base of the angle, however, mainly over the ciliary band, and to some extent over the scleral spur, are irregularly arranged fine capillaries.[25] The appearances are not unlike those seen in early rubeosis but the angle does not deteriorate to form peripheral anterior synechiae and bleeding does not occur spontaneously, but only if the eye is opened surgically.

Trauma

Following ocular contusion, especially where hyphaema or even iridodialysis have occurred, it is fairly common for secondary glaucoma of a persistent nature to come on later. This is thought to be due to damage to the meshwork at the time of injury and the gonioscopical appearances have been called 'traumatic angle recession'.

The angle is alleged to have a typical appearance, the chief characteristic being an apparent exaggeration of its width.[26,27] In the experience of the writer, however, such cases frequently show similar appearances in the other eye (which has suffered no damage). This suggests that the supposedly pathological appearance is simply a normal variant and the traumatic angle damage is actually too subtle to be visible by ordinary gonioscopy.

Traumatic cyclodialysis resulting in severe hypotension is occasionally seen. It can only be diagnosed by gonioscopy. The cleft between the scleral spur and the base of the iris allows a view directly into the suprachoroidal space and it may be possible to see one or more anterior ciliary vessels crossing the space from the scleral wall to the outer aspect of the ciliary body, a bizarre appearance.

Foreign bodies can also be found occasionally in the angle: in the case of glass this can be several years after an incident, its presence being unsuspected by the patient and the only symptom being recurrent attacks of corneal oedema.

Following perforating eye injuries, residual peripheral anterior synechiae may be found. These can vary considerably from virtually all the angle being closed to isolated 'PAS' (peripheral anterior synechiae).

Where synechiae are present, the iris can clearly be seen to be dragged forwards and its surface firmly adherent to the anterior part of the trabecular meshwork, or even further anteriorly to Schwalbe's line or to the cornea itself. In practice, the commonest event leading up to secondary angle closure is the 'flat chamber', which may occur after anterior segment surgery. In general terms, the longer the duration of flat chamber and the greater the amount of inflammation present, the more complete will be the angle closure.

In the early days of gonioscopy 'peripheral anterior synechiae' were much quoted as a possible cause of glaucoma, as though they were able to occur spontaneously. However, it is now known that virtually all peripheral anterior synechiae occur as the result of some prior event, such as injury or inflammation. There are two exceptions to this. Following primary angle closure glaucoma, peripheral synechiae may occur, as has been mentioned earlier, but they are far more likely to be extensive areas of complete closure than localized isolated synechiae. Spontaneous peripheral synechiae may also occur in progressive essential atrophy of the iris.[28] In this condition progressive angle closure occurs by a process of slowly progressive adhesion and cicatrization in the angle with marked shrinkage of the iris.

Inflammatory Changes in the Angle

In long standing uveitis patchy peripheral anterior synechiae may occur.[29] In some cases, however, especially in sarcoid uveitis where large pale keratic precipitates are found, the angle may show mounds of pallid inflammatory cells on the meshwork associated with secondary glaucoma. Occasionally such masses may be the only sign of the uveitis.

Pseudo-exfoliation of the Lens Capsule

The trabecular meshwork is usually, although not invariably, very heavily pigmented in pseudo-exfoliation. In addition, it may be possible to see flakes of the 'exfoliated' material.[30] These frequently stand up in a peculiarly prominent manner, suggesting one end might be impacted in the trabecular meshwork.

Pigmentary Glaucoma

In this condition, a remarkably dense band of pigmentation is present in the mid-trabecular band (*Plate Id*).[31-33] Pigment loss from the posterior iridic surface, pigment deposition on the posterior aspect of the cornea and pigment particles free in the aqueous humour are other signs of this condition.

Neoplasms

Gonioscopy may occasionally reveal a forward extension of a ciliary body melanoma and is useful to define the peripheral limits of any iris neoplasm.

REFERENCES

1. Troncoso M. U. *A treatise on gonioscopy*, Philadelphia, Davis, 1947.
2. Koeppe L. Über den derzeitigen stand der Glaukom forschung an der Gullstrandchen Nernstpaltampe sowie den weiteren Ausbau der Glaukom – Frühdiagnose vermittelst dieser Untersuchungs methode. *Z. Augenheilk*. 1918; **40,** 138–50.
3. Goldmann H. Zur technik der Spaltlampen mikroskopie. *Ophthalmologica*. 1938; **96,** 90–7
4. Lister A. Discussion on gonioscopy. *Proc. Roy. Soc. Med*. 1950; **43,** 1024–5.
5. Fertsch F. Van Beuningen's pyramid gonioscope. *Monatsschr. Fein. Mech. Optik*. 1952; **69,** 165–6.
6. van Beuningen E. G. A. Pyramid shaped gonioscope. *Klin. Monatsbl. Augenheilkd*. 1953; **122,** 172–8.
7. Allen L., Braley A. E. and Thorpe H. E. An improved gonioscopic contact prism. *Arch. Ophthalmol*. 1954; **51,** 451–5.
8. Allen L. and O'Brien C. S. (1945) Gonioscopy simplified by a contact prism. *Arch. Ophthalmol*. 1945; **34,** 413–14.
9. Heinzmann H. An additional apparatus for gonioscopy to be used with the Zeiss–Opton slit lamp. *Ber. deutsch. ophth. Gesellsh*. 1950; **56,** 128–31.
10. Cowen H. P. Pool gonioscopy. *Am. J. Ophthalmol*. 1957; **43,** 619.
11. Peczon J. D. Tears for gonioscopic fluid. *Am. J. Ophthalmol*. 1964; **57,** 838–40.
12. Grant W. M. and Chandler P. A. An arrangement for gonioscopy during surgery. *Arch. Ophthalmol. (Chicago)* 1954; **52,** 454–5.
13. Worst J. G. F. Gonioscopy with suction contacts lens. *Bull. Soc. Ophthalmol. Fr*. 1964; **64,** 909–20.
14. Smith R. J. H. and Watkins R. Corneal epithelial oedema. *Br. J. Ophthalmol*. 1978; **60,** 75.
15. Mehta H. K. A new use of KY jelly as a gonioscopy fluid. *Br. J. Ophthalmol*. 1984; **68,** 765–7.
16. Kronfeld P. C. Gonioscopic studies of Canal of Schlemm. *Am. J. Ophthalmol*. 1948; **31,** 1506–7.
17. Schirmer K. E. Gonioscopic assessment of blood in Schlemm's canal. *Arch. Ophthalmol*. 1971; **85,** 263–7.
18. Gorin G. and Posner A. *Slit Lamp Gonioscopy*, 3rd ed., Baltimore, Md. Williams & Wilkins, 1961.
19. Shaffer A. *Stereoscopic Manual of Gonioscopy*. London, Kimpton, 1962.
20. Forbes M. G. Gonioscopy with corneal indentation. *Arch. Ophthalmol*. 1966; **76,** 488–92.
21. Chandler P. A. and Simmons R. J. Anterior chamber deepening for gonioscopy at time of surgery. *Arch. Ophthalmol*. 1965; **74,** 177–90.
22. Barkan O. The pathogenesis of congenital glaucoma. Gonioscopic and anatomic observations of the angle of the anterior chamber in the normal eye and in congenital glaucoma. *Am. J. Ophthalmol*. 1955; **40,** 1–11.
23. Burian H. M., Braley A. E. and Allen L. External gonioscopic visibility of the ring of Schwalbe and the trabecular zone. *Trans Am. Ophthalmol. Soc*. 1954; **52,** 389–428.
24. Smith R. J. H. Thrombotic glaucoma: a clinico-pathological study. *Acta XVII Conc. Ophthalmol*. 1954; 1164–75.
25. Francescetti A. Heterochromic cyclitis (Fuchs' syndrome). *Am. J. Ophthalmol*. 1955; **39,** 50–8.
26. Alper M. G. Contusion angle deformity. *Arch Ophthalmol*. 1963; 455–67.
27. Roth A., Royer J., Gainet F. et al. Gonioscopic observation after ocular contusion. *Bull. Soc. Ophthalmol. Fr*. 1973; **73,** 323–30.
28. Hogan M. J. and Zimmerman L. E. *Ophthalmic Pathology*, Philadelphia, Saunders, 1962.
29. Smith R. J. H. *Clinical Glaucoma,* London, Cassel, 1965.
30. Dvorak T. G. Pseudo exfoliation of the lens capsule: Relation to 'true' exfoliation of the lens capsule as reported in the literature and role in the production of glaucoma capsulo-cuticulare. *Amer. J. Ophthalmol*. 1954; **37,** 1–12.
31. Sugar H. S. and Barbour F. A. Pigmentary glaucoma. *Am. J. Ophthalmol*. 1949; **32,** 90–2.
32. Malbran J. Pigmentary glaucoma and its relationships with congenital glaucoma. *Mod. Probl. Ophthalmol*. 1957; **1,** 132–46.
33. Perkins E. S. and Jay B. S. Pigmentary glaucoma. *Trans. Ophthalmol. Soc. UK*. 1960; **80,** 153–67.

Examination of the Ocular Fundus

P. K. Leaver

Examination of the ocular fundus in the intact eye was made possible with the introduction by Helmholtz in 1851 of his monocular direct ophthalmoscope.[1] Within a year, Ruete had described the indirect method[2] and in 1861 Giraud-Teulon designed the first binocular indirect instrument.[3] Nevertheless, it was to be more than 85 years before the advantages of stereopsis and the indirect optical principle were to be fully realized and developed for clinical use.[4] The introduction by Schepens of a head-mounted binocular indirect ophthalmoscope (*Fig.* 1)[4] and its skilful and painstaking use combined with

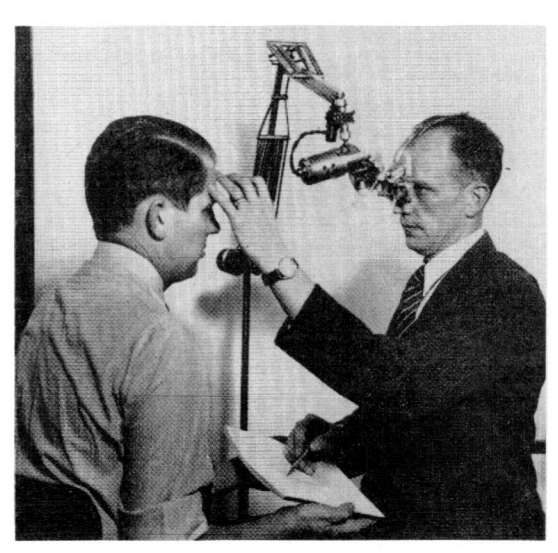

Fig. 1. Charles Schepens (1947) demonstrates his new head-mounted binocular indirect ophthalmoscope. (Reproduced by permission of the Editor of *Ophthalmology*, (formerly *Transactions of the American Academy of Ophthalmology and Otolaryngology*).

sceral depression,[5] in the management of retinal detachments was arguably the greatest advance made in fundus examination since that of Helmholtz 96 years earlier.

Methods of fundus examination are by no means limited to ophthalmoscopy and since the introduction of the slit lamp biomicroscope by Gullstrand in 1911[6] numerous workers have devised methods for using this instrument to examine the fundus. Koeppe in 1918 introduced a contact lens and later Goldmann designed the three-mirror lens which bears his name.[8] In 1923 Lemoine and Valois suggested the principle of using a high power concave pre-set lens[9] and this was later developed by Hruby.[10] Alternatively, a strong, convex pre-set lens can be employed, delivering a real, inverted image similar to that formed by the condensing lens in indirect ophthalmoscopy.[11, 12] More recently, this method has been modified and improved by Schlegel with the development of a contact lens for use with the slit lamp incorporating a very high power convex lens (*Fig.* 2).[13]

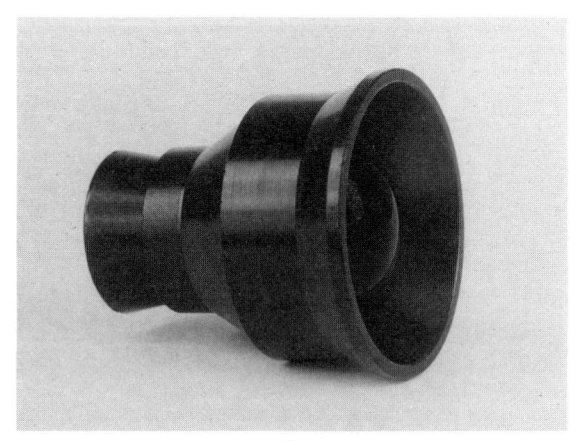

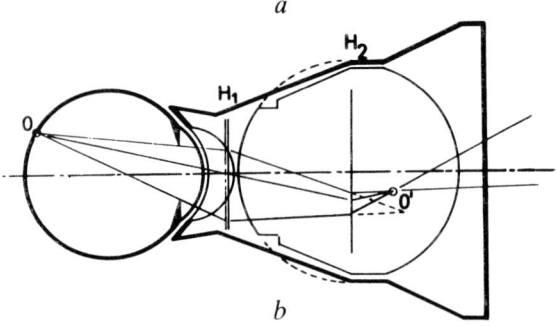

Fig. 2. *a*, The Rodenstock Panfundoscope contact lens devised by Professor Schlegel. *b*, Optical principles of the Panfundoscope lens.

DIRECT OPHTHALMOSCOPY

In general terms, because of its high magnification, small field and relatively low level of illumination, the direct ophthalmoscope is most useful for examining details at the posterior pole in eyes with clear optical media. However, the disadvantages of poor illumination have to a large extent been overcome by the introduction of more sophisticated power sources and halogen bulbs. Stronger light sources not only improve the visualization of fundus details with white light, but also facilitate the examination of blood vascular abnormalities and retinal pigment epithelial changes by the introduction of red-free or other filters. Although several attempts have been made to develop a binocular direct instrument, the results have not proved really satisfactory; but because the high degree of magnification offsets some of the disadvantages of monocularity, it remains a very useful instrument, particularly for examination of the posterior pole.

INDIRECT OPHTHALMOSCOPY

While monocular indirect ophthalmoscopy confers some advantages over the direct method, it was the development of a binocular indirect instrument with both the viewing system and light source mounted on a headband[4] which transformed the method of examining the peripheral fundus. It was no coincidence that Charles Schepens began to achieve dramatically better results in retinal detachment surgery using this instrument than had previously been possible,[5,14] as was readily appreciated by Lorimer Fison, who developed and popularized it in the United Kingdom. While the intensity of the light source is of great benefit in illuminating a large field, especially when the optical media are not clear, it is the freedom of movement and easily changed angle of view of the observer which facilitate examination of the peripheral fundus speedily and without difficulty.

The use of scleral indentation to complement binocular indirect ophthalmoscopy or slit lamp biomicroscopy with the three-mirror contact lens makes it possible to examine the entire ocular fundus, including the pars plana in an eye with a dilated pupil.[15] Furthermore, the introduction of the small pupil ophthalmoscope[16] and more recently the use of higher power aspheric lenses, make it possible to see the fundus even when the pupil is small or the optical pathway obstructed by lens opacities or lens/vitreous remnants.

SLIT LAMP BIOMICROSCOPY

Neutralization of the refractive power of the anterior corneal surface allows the slit lamp to be used to examine the ocular fundus. This can be achieved in a number of ways:
1. By placing on the cornea a contact lens with a flat anterior surface, a virtual upright magnified image of the posterior pole is obtained. Incorporating a system of angled mirrors in front of the plane surface then makes it possible to extend the field of view over the entire fundus, a method devised and developed by Goldmann.[7] Alternatively the image can be converted into a real inverted one by introducing a high power convex lens, as in the Rodenstock panfunduscopic lens (see Fig. 2b), a method which confers a very wide field of view.
2. Pre-set concave[10] or convex[11] lenses can be used, which achieve similar results without the need to touch the eye itself. Such lenses are particularly useful for examining the posterior pole in circumstances in which manipulation of the globe or lids is undesirable or where lack of patient compliance makes this impossible. Recent developments in the use of pre-set convex lenses with slit lamp microscopy[17,18] have advanced certain aspects of fundus photography, while some workers are using the Bayadi lens for clinical evaluation of diabetic retinopathy.[19]

CONDENSING LENSES

In recent years the quality of condensing lenses for use with the indirect ophthalmoscope has been greatly improved. Not only is a range of optical power (and hence of magnification, field and illumination) now available, but optical errors induced by the high refractive power of such lenses have been largely eliminated.

While it is easiest to use the lens with the highest power (+28 dioptres or more), and shortest focal length, and most difficult to use the lowest power lens (+14 dioptres or less), the +20 dioptre lens is perhaps most commonly chosen for general purposes.

In most instances there is little to be gained by using a lens of lower power than 20 dioptres because the small gain in magnification is outweighed by loss of field and difficulties in handling caused by the long focal length. The higher power lens, however, may be very useful, particularly in two instances:
1. Where the pupil is small and the optical pathway narrowed by opacities, the extreme intensity of the light will often permit an adequate view of the fundus.
2. In small children and other less cooperative patients the large field enables a rapid assessment of the fundus to be obtained.

SCLERAL INDENTATION

Scleral indentation or depression is a vital adjunct to examination of the peripheral fundus by binocular indirect ophthalmoscopy[5,14] and can also be used in association with the Goldmann three-mirror contact lens, a method introduced by Eisner.[20] The method was first described by Trantas in 1900, using his thumb nail through the tissues of the eyelid,[21] and is nowadays more commonly achieved by using the thimble depressor introduced by Schepens.[5] It is sometimes helpful to use depression directly on the surface of the globe rather than through the lids, especially over the region of the inner canthus where the latter may be difficult, and for this purpose a drop or two of local anaesthetic is necessary, while the same applies when using Eisner's funnel with the three-mirror contact lens.[20]

Indentation of the coats of the globe confers two advantages: first, peripheral structures can be moved centrally into the field of view, and secondly, movement of the depressor over the surface of the globe (or the globe over the depressor as the patient moves his eye) throws into relief structural relationships which may not be apparent when viewed in a two-dimensional manner, such as foci of lattice degeneration, flat retinal breaks or shallow retinal separations.[15]

Moveover it is not always appreciated that by gentle and painstaking manipulation of the thimble combined with voluntary movements of the eye, scleral indentation can be achieved as far back as the post-equatorial retina (*Fig. 3*).

In conclusion, detailed examination of the fundus can be accomplished by a number of different methods, each of which carries certain advantages and disadvantages. In most instances, examination with the binocular indirect ophthalmoscope should be the cornerstone of the procedure, complemented where necessary by one or more of the other methods discussed. While there is little in the peripheral fundus that cannot be detected using indirect ophthalmoscopy with scleral depression, even when the ocular media are not perfectly clear, the highly magnified stereoscopic view obtained by using slit lamp biomicroscopy is often valuable in establishing more precisely the nature of pathology thus detected. Moreover, when pathological changes are confined to the posterior pole and the media are clear, examination with the direct ophthalmoscope complemented by a simple fundus contact lens or pre-set lens may be more appropriate.

The use of the Eisner indentation funnel with the three-mirror contact lens requires special skills and demands a high degree of patient compliance, while high power convex lenses such as the Rodenstock Panfunduscope are probably more useful in the treatment than diagnosis of retinal disease.

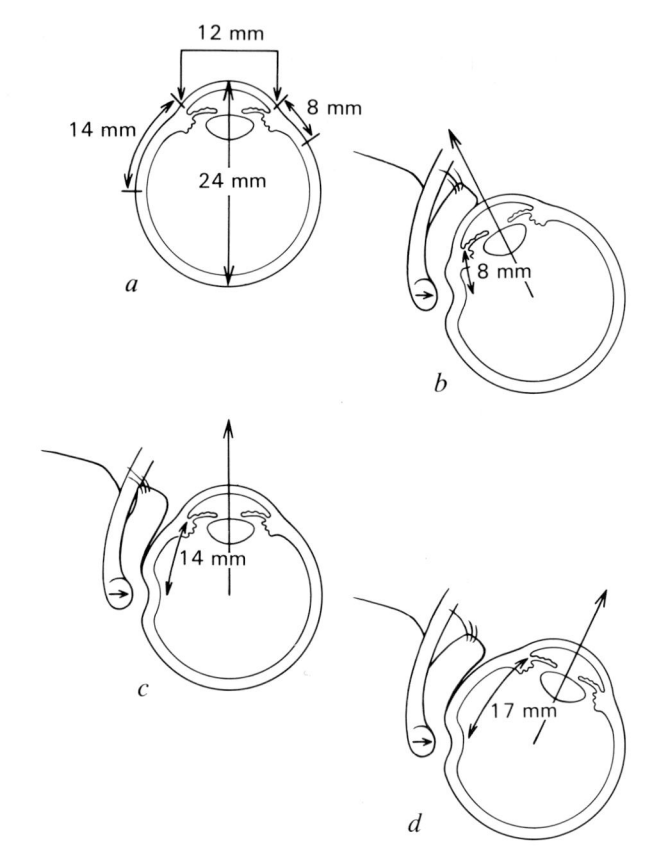

Fig. 3. Diagrams illustrating the extent of scleral indentation which can be achieved with the aid of the patient's eye movements. (Reproduced from Havener W. H. and Gloeckner S. L. *Atlas of Diagnostic Techniques and Treatment of Retinal Detachment* by permission of C. V. Mosby, St Louis.)

ACKNOWLEDGEMENTS

I am grateful to the Audio Visual Department, Moorfields Eye Hospital, for their help with the illustrations, and to Miss Heather Lucas for typing the manuscript.

REFERENCES

1. Helmholtz H. *Beschreibung eines Augenspiegels zur Untersuchung der Netzhaut in lebenden Auge.* Berlin, Forstner, 1851.
2. Ruete C. G. *Der Augenspiegel und das Optometer fur Practische Aerzte.* Gottingen, Dieterichschen Buchhandlung, 1852, pp. 1–27.
3. Giraud-Teulon. Ophthalmoscopie binoculaire on s'exercant par le concours des deux yeux associes. *Ann. Ocul.* 1861; **45**, 233–50.
4. Schepens C. L. A new ophthalmoscope demonstration. *Trans. Am. Acad. Ophthalmol. Otolaryngol.* 1947; **51**, 298–301.
5. Schepens C. L. Examination of the ora serrata region: Its clinical significance. *Acta XVI Int. Cong.* (London) 1950; **2**, 1384–93.
6. Gullstrand A. *Einfuhrung in die Methoden der Dioptrik des Auges der Menschen.* Leipzig, S. Hirzel. 1911.

7. Koeppe L. Die Mikroskopie des Lebenden Augenhinter Grundes mit Starken Vergroberungen un Fokalen Lichte der Gullstrandschen Nernstspaltlampe. *Albrecht von Graefe Arch. Ophthalmol.* 1918; **95**, 282–306.
8. Goldmann H. Zur Technik der Spaltlampenmikroskopie. *Ophthalmologica* 1938; **96**, 90.
9. Lemoine and Valois. Ophthalmoscopie microscopique du fond d'oeil vivant (sans verre de contact). *Bull. Soc. Franc. Ophthalmol.* 1923; **36**, 366.
10. Hruby K. Spaltlampenmikroskopie des Hinteren Augenabschnittes ohne Kontaktglas. *Klin. Monatsbl. Augenheilk.* 1942; **108**, 195–200.
11. El Bayadi G. New method of slit lamp micro-ophthalmoscopy. *Br. J. Ophthalmol.* 1953; **37**, 625–8.
12. Rosen E. Biomicroscopic examination of the fundus with a +55D lens. *Am. J. Ophthalmol.* 1959; **48**, 782–7.
13. Schlegel H. J. Ein einfache Weitwinkeloptik zur spaltlampenmikroskopischen Untersuchung des Augenhintergrundes (panfundoskop). *Documenta Ophthalmologica* 1969; **26**, 300–8.
14. Schepens C. L. Progress in detachment surgery. *Trans. Am. Acad. Ophthalmol.* 1951; **55**, 607–15.
15. Havener W. H. and Gloeckner S. L. *Atlas of Diagnostic Techniques and Treatment of Retinal Detachment.* St Louis, Mo, Mosby, 1967, pp. 22–35.
16. Hovland K. R., Elzeneiny I. H. and Schepens C. L. Clinical evaluation of the small pupil binocular indirect ophthalmoscope. *Arch. Ophthalmol.* 1969; **82**, 466–74.
17. Takahashi M. and Kajiura M. Fundus photography through the slit lamp microscope. *Jpn J. Clin. Ophthalmol.* 1975; **29**, 1319–23.
18. Kajiura M. Slit lamp photography of the fundus by use of aspherical convex preset lens. *Jpn J. Ophthalmol.* 1978; **22**, 214–28.
19. Blankenship G. Personal communication, 1984.
20. Eisner G. *Biomicroscopy of the Peripheral Fundus: An Atlas and Textbook.* Berlin, Springer, 1973, pp. 91–7.
21. Trantas. Moyens d'explorer a l'ophthalmoscope – et par translucidite – la partie anterieure du fond oculaire, le cercle ciliaire y compris. *Arch. Ophthalmol. (Paris).* 1900; **20**, 314–26.

Fluorescein Angiography

T. J. ffytche

INTRODUCTION

The development of fluorescein angiography in 1961 opened a new chapter in the history of ophthalmology, although few at the time could have predicted its eventual impact. For more than a hundred years observation of the retina, skilled as it was, had remained a static examination, limited in its understanding and burdened by the vagaries of individual interpretation. The new technique, described by Novotny and Alvis,[1] altered the picture absolutely and added a dynamic element to retinal diagnosis, stimulating interest and acting as a catalyst to parallel developments in therapy.

The basic principles of their original article have remained the same, only the instrumentation has been modified and become more sophisticated, and the past 20 years have improved the skill in interpretation and rationalized the indications and contraindications for the procedure.

PRINCIPLES OF FLUORESCEIN ANGIOGRAPHY

Fluorescein is an organic dye with a molecular weight of 376 and is produced commercially as its sodium salt. When injected intravenously it becomes extensively bound to serum albumin, but about 20 per cent circulates free in the plasma.

It is one of several chemical compounds exhibiting the property of fluorescence in that it absorbs light principally of one wavelength and emits it at a longer wavelength. Spectrofluorometric data on blood–fluorescein mixtures indicate that its maximum light absorption lies in the blue range of the spectrum at 490 nm, while the emitted wavelength, which gives the dye its fluorescence, is in the green–yellow range, between 520 and 530 nm.

In addition to its spectral characteristics, the property of sodium fluorescein most relevant to the ophthalmologist is its inability to cross two important barriers in the eye: *the retinal vascular endothelium and the retinal pigment epithelium*. It is the combination of these chemical and physiological properties that provides the basis for fluorescein angiography and its interpretation.

INSTRUMENTATION

There are many makes of fundus camera adapted for fluorescein angiography but their basic principles are the same, and choice depends on such factors as cost, reliability, availability of servicing and individual preference. The typical retinal camera photographs 30° of the fundus with a magnification of about ×2·5; wide angle cameras are available with fields of view up to 150°, but along with the increase in the area of retina photographed there is a concomitant reduction in magnification which affects visualization of finer details such as retinal capillaries and subretinal neovascular membranes – structures of great importance in the planning of therapy.

Cameras may also be adapted for angiography of the anterior segment and for ciné-angiography.

FILTERS

All instruments for fluorescein angiography incorporate a pair of matched optical filters. A blue *excitor* filter is placed over the light source so that emitted light can activate fluorescein as it circulates through the eye. A yellow–green *barrier* filter placed in front of the camera-back excludes non-fluorescent wavelengths and allows fluorescein together with a small amount of background detail to be recorded on black and white film.

Filter pairs vary within narrow limits but a popular combination is an excitor filter with peak transmission at 480 nm, together with a barrier filter with peak transmission in the region of 540 nm.

TECHNIQUE

Fluorescein angiography has established itself as a simple and safe outpatient examination in which an intravenous injection of the dye is given rapidly and its progress through the choroidal and retinal circulations recorded photographically, usually on black and white film.

Variations in the concentrations of fluorescein and the volume injected are used in different centres, but 5 ml of a 10 per cent solution or 2·5 ml of a 20 per cent solution are the most popular, although corresponding doses of 5 per cent and 25 per cent are also given. Dosage is reduced for small children. In some circumstances fluorescein may be given orally, in a dose between 1·25 and 2·5 g, although the quality of detail in the angiogram is often poor.

The standard angiogram is usually preceded by taking colour fundus photographs, often with stereoscopic pairs, and red-free pictures. A well-dilated pupil is helpful in producing good quality results, although it is possible to take reasonable photographs through pupils of medium or even small size.

The aim of the procedure is to deliver a rapid injection of the dye so that it retains its bolus form as it passes through the ocular circulation. The patient is positioned at the camera and a wide bore needle inserted into a large arm vein. Scalp vein infusion needles (No. 21) have proved very useful since they can be retained in the vein during the angiogram and allow the observer to inject and photograph without assistance.

Control photographs are first taken with both filters in position; they are important since they provide an indication of the efficiency of the filter combination and they allow background details to be contrasted with the fluorescence of the angiogram. They are also of value in detecting auto- and pseudofluorescence.

Following the control photographs, an injection of fluorescein is given rapidly and serial pictures at 1–1·5 s intervals are taken as the dye passes through the choroidal and retinal circulation. There is a variable delay between the time of the injection and the first appearance of the dye in the choroid. This arm-to-eye circulation time depends on systemic blood flow, being shortened in hyperdynamic circulations such as in the young, in anaemia and thyrotoxicosis. A prolonged arm-to-eye circulation time indicates a sluggish systemic blood flow and may be a feature of chronic chest disease or carotid artery stenosis, it may also indicate vagal slowing of the heart in response to the injection.

Under normal circumstances the dye enters the choroidal vessels between 8 and 12 s after injection. The duration of the passage of the fluorescein bolus through the eye depends on a number of variable factors which include the speed of injection and the state of the systemic and local circulation, but the first transit through the eye usually takes about 20 s.

Following serial photography of the passage of dye through the eye, late pictures can be taken 5 and 10 min after injection to record patterns of abnormal leakage.

SIDE EFFECTS

More than a million fluorescein angiograms have been performed in the past 20 years and their safety is proved by the very few reports of fatalities directly caused by the injection of fluorescein. The small size of the fluorescein molecule makes it unlikely to provoke an acute allergic reaction and anaphylaxis is exceptionally rare. Most deaths related to the procedure have occurred when there is underlying cardiovascular or cerebrovascular disease. Severe, but nonfatal complications have been reported in 0·4 per cent of angiograms and these include vasovagal attacks, bronchospasm, respiratory arrest, circulatory collapse, cardiac infarction, stroke and cardiac arrest. Although most centres do not perform a test dose on the grounds that fluorescein is non-antigenic and that true anaphylaxis is not dose-related, it is important that an emergency tray is available containing adrenaline, aminophylline and intravenous antihistamine preparations together with equipment for oxygen delivery and suction.

Minor side effects are fairly common and include nausea and vomiting, itching, rashes, sneezing and occasionally phlebitis at the site of injection, and if the injection is given extravascularly it will cause local pain. All patients should be warned that their urine will be discoloured for about a day and that their skin will take on a yellowish tinge for several hours.

Despite the known safety of the procedure, fluorescein angiography should never be undertaken unnecessarily and should be avoided in patients with cardiovascular and cerebrovascular disease and in those with a strong history of allergy or asthma. The procedure should probably also be avoided during pregnancy, although there is no evidence that it causes fetal abnormalities.

THE NORMAL ANGIOGRAM

The fluorescein angiogram may be divided arbitrarily into five phases: choroidal, arterial, arteriovenous, venous and late, each running into the other but each showing certain characteristics both in the normal and abnormal situation.

Choroidal Phase

Choroidal filling is patchy since the individual short posterior ciliary arteries show different filling times; but this mosaic effect is transient, lasting only a few seconds (*Fig.* 1) and a prolonged filling defect may indicate localized choroidal ischaemia. Visualization of the choroidal circulation is influenced by the density of the overlying pigment epithelium, with lightly pigmented fundi allowing much more of the choroidal fluorescence to be visible although the finer details are soon obscured by fluorescein passing through the overlying retinal vessels. The choriocapillaris is freely permeable to fluorescein and during the course of the angiogram the choroid becomes a lake of fluorescent blood prevented from spreading into the retina by the pigment epithelium. Defects in this barrier 'unmask' the choroidal fluorescence. In a significant proportion of eyes a cilioretinal artery may be present and since it is derived from the posterior ciliary circulation, it will also fill during the choroidal phase of the angiogram.

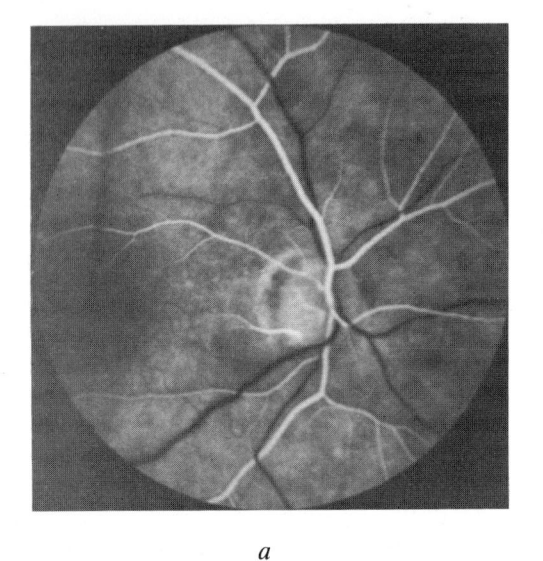

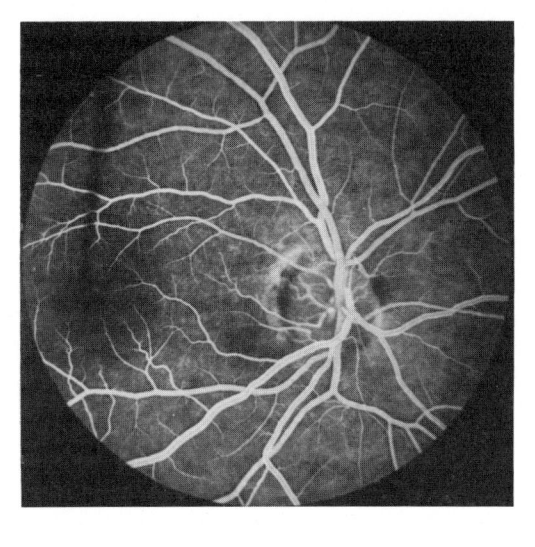

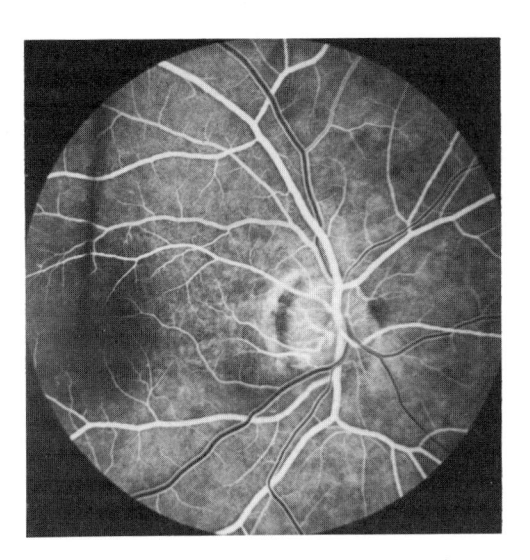

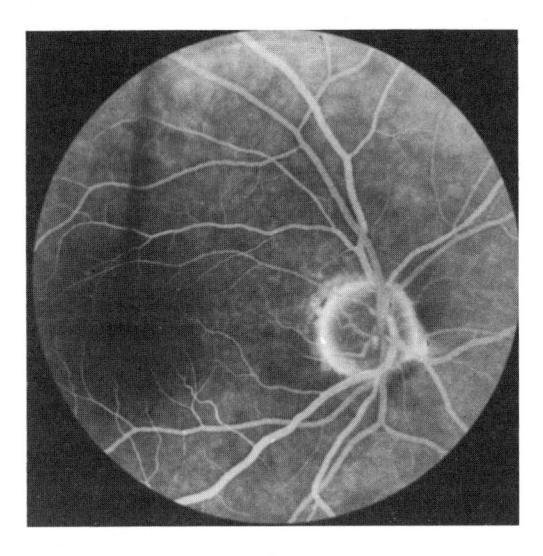

Fig. 1. *a*, Normal angiogram – arterial phase. *b*, Normal angiogram – early arteriovenous phase. *c*, Normal angiogram – arteriovenous phase. *d*, Normal angiogram – venous phase. *e*, Normal angiogram – late phase.

Arterial Phase

The retinal arteries begin to fill about 1·5 s after the commencement of the choroidal phase. The dye front of fluorescein can sometimes be recorded by ciné-angiography and its advancement along the retinal arteries plotted and the velocity measured. In the early stages of the arterial phase the contrast between the fluorescent arteries and the non-fluorescent veins is pronounced (*Fig.* 1*a*), but almost immediately venous and capillary filling commences and the transition into the arteriovenous phase is rapid.

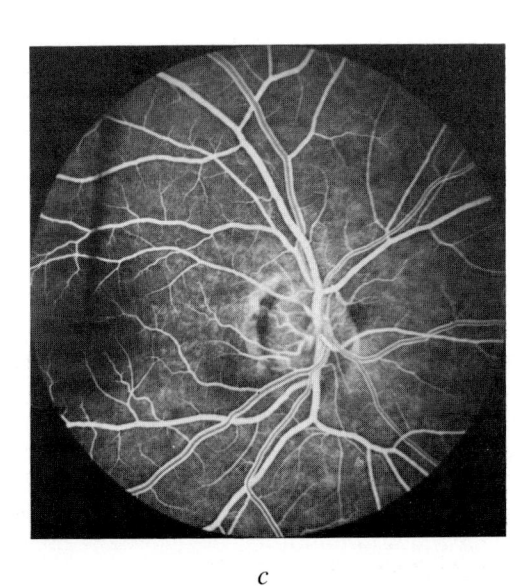

As the fluorescein passes through the retinal vessels the effectivity of the endothelial barrier becomes apparent. Under normal circumstances the dye does not traverse this barrier, which is formed by the tight junctions of the endothelial cells lining the retinal vessels, possibly aided by active sodium pump mechanisms within the cells themselves. Deficiencies of this barrier may result from a variety of causes and lead to leakage of fluorescein into the surrounding tissues to give the abnormal angiogram its characteristic appearance. Measurement of the diameter of the retinal vessels during angiography shows them to be about 10 per cent wider than on colour film. This is explained by the fact that the dye, which circulates in the plasma, fills the whole width of the vessel, whereas on colour photographs only the axial column of red cells is recorded, the peripheral plasma zone and vessel wall being normally transparent.

Arteriovenous Phase

As fluorescent blood enters the veins from the central areas of the fundus, it does not mix freely with the non-fluorescent blood returning from the periphery and laminar flow patterns are formed in the major veins near the disc (*Fig. 1b,c*). This feature characterizes the arteriovenous phase of the angiogram and at this stage the retinal capillaries show sufficient concentration of dye to enable them to be visualized. In normal conditions they are best seen against the dark background of the macular pigment, but in pathological conditions capillaries may be dilated and visible away from the central region (*see Fig. 4a*).

Venous Phase

As the arteries begin to empty the main volume of injected dye passes through the capillaries into the veins. The veins lose their laminar flow pattern as the non-fluorescent blood disappears from the lumen and their fluorescence equals that of the arteries in intensity (*Fig. 1d*). The capillaries in the macular region remain visible and in the normal angiogram no leakage occurs from any of the vessels.

Late Phase

As the dye leaves the eye there is a gradual decrease in the intensity of intravascular fluorescence, although recirculation produces visible fluorescence for several hours. The dye remains within the vessels although leakage from the iris and ciliary body produces fluorescence within the anterior chamber and vitreous, blurring the finer details of the posterior structures. Under normal conditions the optic disc may show a variable amount of fluorescence due to uptake of the dye by its glial components with a small amount of leakage at its margin, especially if there is a crescent of exposed choriocapillaris (*Fig. 1e*).

ABNORMAL FLUORESCENCE

The features of the fluorescein angiogram depend largely on the basic integrity of the two normal barriers to fluorescein leakage that exist in the fundus: the pigment epithelium and the retinal vascular endothelium. Disruption of either of these fundamental barriers gives rise to a variety of leakage patterns which by their distribution and rate of development give the abnormal angiogram its specific diagnostic value. The interpretation of fluorescein angiography relies as much on the appreciation of this dynamic evolution of fluorescein leakage as on the analysis of static patterns, and is greatly aided by stereoscopic visualization since leakage occurs at all levels of the retina and choroid.

In addition to fluorescein leakage, there are a number of other disturbances in the fundus which modify the appearance of the angiogram by increasing or reducing the intensity of fluorescein recorded by the camera. Abnormalities can therefore be divided into two broad groups: those causing hyperfluorescence and those causing hypofluorescence.

Hyperfluorescence

Autofluorescence

Certain lesions in the fundus have intrinsic fluorescence which is visible on control photographs. This property occurs in drusen of the optic disc and in astrocytic hamartoma.

Transmitted Fluorescence ('Window' Defect)

A breakdown in the pigment epithelium barrier allows normal choroidal fluorescence to become 'unmasked'. This fluorescence occurs early in the angiogram and decreases along with choroidal fluorescence in the later stages. It is observed in fundi with sparse pigmentation and in eyes with pigment epithelial degeneration or atrophy (*Fig. 2a,b*).

Active Leakage

This type of fluorescence is cumulative, its onset depending on its site of origin. Abnormal leakage may arise from disturbances of the *choroid*, either from local defects or elevation of the overlying pigment epithelium, such as central serous retinopathy (*Fig. 3a,b*) and pigment epithelial detachment, or from the presence of a subretinal neovascular membrane in disciform degeneration (*see Fig. 2a, b*), or in association with choroidal tumours. Leakage in these conditions commences early in the angiogram and increases in intensity, persisting long after the injection. The patterns are specific for the different lesions and are important both for diagnosis and for the planning of therapy. Late leakage following early hypofluorescence is a feature of conditions in which there is active inflammation of the choroid or swelling of the pigment epithelium. This appearance, known as 'reversed' fluorescence, is typical of choroiditis and placoid pigment epitheliopathy.

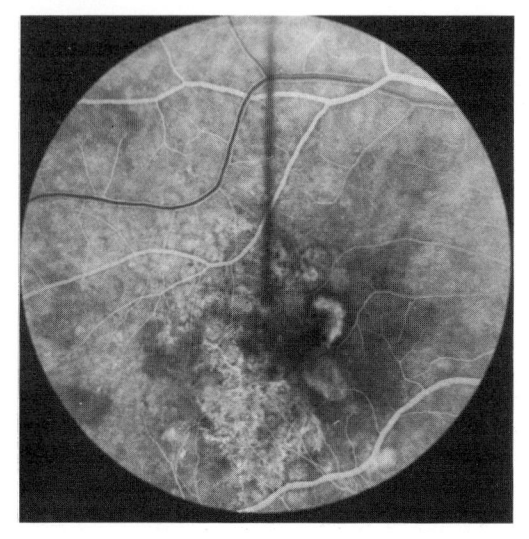

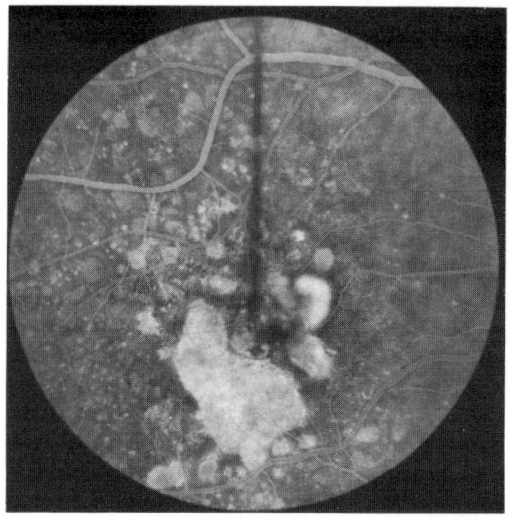

Fig. 2. a, Early arteriovenous phase in an eye with pigment epithelial degeneration and a subretinal neovascular membrane nasal to fixation. The 'window' defects in the degenerate pigment epithelium are observed together with the early fluorescence of the subretinal neovascular complex. *b*, Late phase showing active leakage from the subretinal new vessels. Scleral glow is seen in the large area of pigment epithelial degeneration.

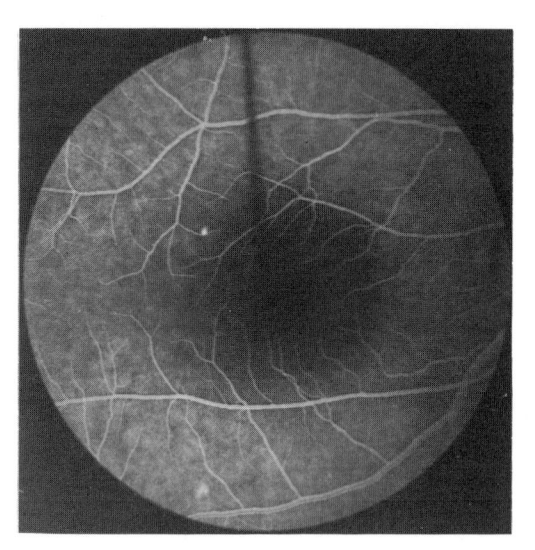

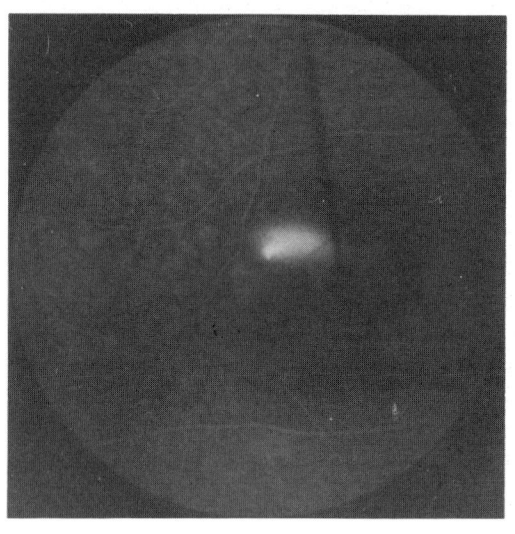

Fig. 3. a, Central serous retinopathy with a single focus of active leakage derived from the choriocapillaris. *b*, Late picture showing how active leakage continues to accumulate.

Active leakage may occur in the *retina* deriving from disturbances in the retinal vessels. Local leakage from retinal vessels is seen in hypoxia, inflammation or damage to the wall and in all new vessels (*Fig. 4a,b*). Retinal capillaries, particularly those on the optic disc and in the macular region, also leak fluorescein in conditions where oedema is present, and the fluid collects in extracellular tissue spaces to form the characteristic angiographic patterns of papilloedema and cystoid macular oedema (*Fig. 5*). Retinal leakage, whatever its cause, commences in the middle stages of the angiogram and accumulates slowly, except in the case of forward new vessels, which begin to fluoresce intensely early in the angiogram.

In conditions where late leakage patterns are diagnostic, oral fluorescein may be used since recording of the early features of the angiogram is unnecessary. This applies particularly to the demonstration of cystoid macular oedema and to new vessel leakage.

Pseudofluorescence

White surfaces in the fundus may reflect incident light and appear on the control photographs as fluorescent areas. This becomes increasingly evident in the late stages of the angiogram when fluorescein present in the aqueous and vitreous is activated by the blue light and the subsequent fluorescence is reflected off the white surfaces. Pseudofluorescence may be almost completely eliminated by correct matching of the filters but it occurs when there are opaque nerve fibres, plaques of exudate or with any flat white lesion.

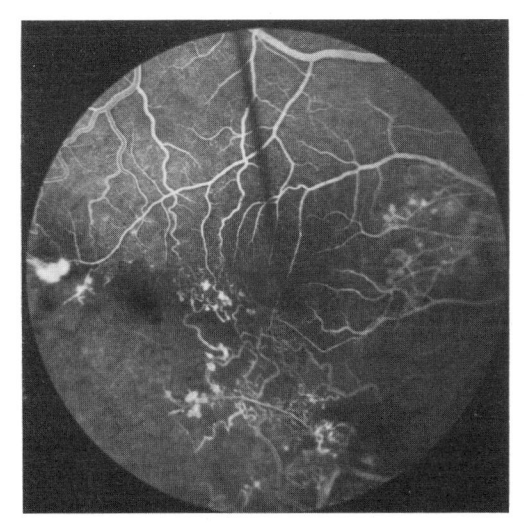

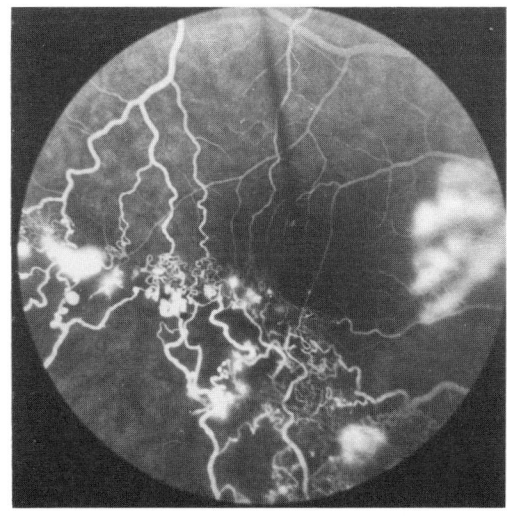

Fig. 4. *a*, Angiogram of branch vein occlusion showing an area of capillary non-perfusion with associated capillary abnormalities and new vessels arising from the disc. *b*, Later picture demonstrating active leakage from the retinal and disc new vessels.

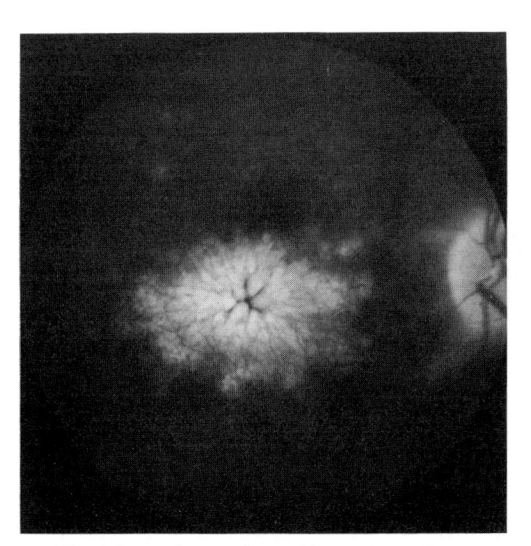

Fig. 5. Late picture of cystoid macular oedema.

Scleral Glow

The sclera normally takes up fluorescein in the same way as the skin. In the late stages of the angiogram those areas of the sclera at the posterior pole that are exposed or thinly covered by the pigment in the choroid and pigment epithelium will appear to glow (*Fig.* 2*b*). This feature also contributes to late fluorescence of optic disc tissues.

Hypofluorescence

Masking

Opaque material in the fundus will block fluorescence from tissues lying more posteriorly and the amount of masking depends on the density and degree of light absorption of the substance. Haemoglobin and pigment are the main masking agents in angiography but fluorescence may be obscured to a lesser extent by opaque nerve fibres, exudate and glial tissue.

Vascular Filling Defects

Areas of non-perfusion of the choroid, retina and optic disc show a decrease in the normal fluorescence and in diabetes and venous occlusion these areas may be extensive (*see Fig.* 4*a,b*). Their importance in the pathogenesis of new vessel formation, both in the retina and anterior segment, cannot be overstressed.

OTHER APPLICATIONS OF FLUORESCEIN ANGIOGRAPHY

Any blood vessel in the eye that is visible can be studied by fluorescein angiography, and cameras may be adapted to record changes in the normal and abnormal circulations of the iris, cornea and conjunctiva. Iris angiography is helpful in the demonstration of ischaemic and neovascular disturbances and is valuable in differentiating iris tumours. The results are, however, often difficult to interpret since leakage is a feature of normal iris vessels, particularly in the elderly. Abnormal corneal vessels may also be studied by anterior segment photography with the appropriate filters.

Ciné-fluorescein angiography has been used in the experimental situation to measure the velocity of blood through the retinal circulation and to calculate volume flow. The technique, however, does not lend itself easily to clinical studies and an accurate and safe method of measuring retinal blood flow in patients has yet to be developed.

The diffusion of fluorescein into the vitreous from the iris and ciliary body and retina may be measured in the normal and abnormal situation by the technique of vitreous fluorophotometry. This procedure involves the measurement of fluorescein concentrations in different regions of the vitreous by photometry and the plotting of a concentration curve. Variations in the shape of the concentration curves indicate changes in local capillary permeability, and subclinical fluorescein leakage from the retina may be detected early in pathological conditions such as diabetes.

CONCLUSION

Fluorescein angiography has had an enormous impact on the understanding of fundus disorders. This safe, simple and relatively inexpensive outpatient technique transformed ophthalmic diagnosis from an art into a science in the space of a few years. Many hitherto unrecognized fundus conditions were identified and well-established diseases were studied afresh. These advances would have been sterile were it not for the parallel developments in photocoagulation and medical therapy that have followed the increased knowledge created by angiography. It remains a most valuable investigation, contributing to the diagnosis of fundus disorders, to the planning and monitoring of therapy, and to the understanding of the clinicopathology of diseases of the choroid and retina.

REFERENCE

1. Novotny H. R. and Alvis D. L. A method of photographing fluorescence in circulating blood in the human retina. *Circulation* 1961; **24**, 82.

SUGGESTED READING

De Laey J. J. (ed.) *International Symposium on Fluorescein Angiography.* The Hague, Junk, 1976.
Hill D. W. Fluorescein angiography. In: Clifford Rose F. (ed.) *The Eye in General Medicine.* London, Chapman and Hall, 1983.
O'Connor P. R. Fundus photography and fluorescein angiography. In: Keeney A. H. (ed.) *Ocular Examination.* St Louis, Mo, Mosby, 1976.
Schatz H., Burton T. C., Yannuzzi L. A. et al. *Fundus Fluorescein Angiography: A Comprehensive Text and Atlas.* St Louis, Mo, Mosby, 1978.
Wise G. N., Dollery C. T. and Henkind P. *The Retinal Circulation.* New York, Harper and Row, 1971.
Yannuzzi L. A., Schatz H. and Gitter K. A. Interpretation of fluorescein angiograms. In: *The Macula.* Baltimore, Md, Williams and Wilkins, 1978.

Ultrasonography of the Eye and Orbit

Marie Restori

Ultrasonic 'pulse–echo' techniques are now used routinely in biometric studies, the assessment of eyes in which opacity prevents biomicroscopical examination and in the study of intraocular and orbital tumours. Ultrasonic pulses within the range of 5 MHz to 20 MHz are used, 10 MHz proving suitable for examination of most clinical conditions.

PULSE–ECHO TECHNIQUES

A large number of 'pulse–echo' techniques[1-6] have been used in ophthalmology. Only the A-scan and B-scan techniques are in routine use in most centres; at Moorfields Eye Hospital in London rapid B-scan and C-scan techniques are used in diagnosis.

A-scan Technique

Pulses of sound are sent from the transducer, if necessary via a couplant, into the eye; in the time interval between interrogating pulses of sound, echoes from eye structures are received by the same transducer and plotted as spikes on a cathode ray tube. The height of the spikes indicates echo amplitudes and the position of the spikes on the X-axis, the arrival time of the echoes at the transducer. The A-scan along a central axis of a normal eye is shown in *Fig. 1a*; the vitreous cavity is echo-free.

The nature of abnormalities giving rise to echoes is suggested by the amplitude, extent and movements of the echoes. A knowledge of the velocities of sound within the ocular tissue permits calculation of intraocular distances.[7] If the transducer is aligned such that the ultrasonic pulses travel along the optical or visual axis, high amplitude echoes will be received from the corneal, lenticular and vitreo-retinal boundaries and the axial length of the eye can be calculated. A large selection of A-scan equipment designed specifically for axial length measurement

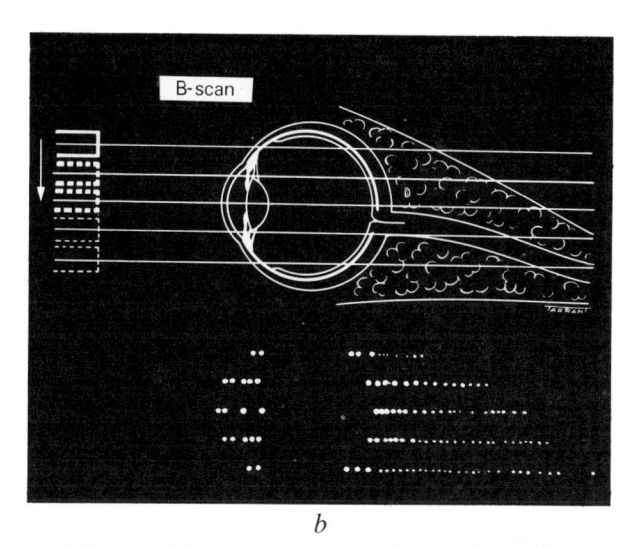

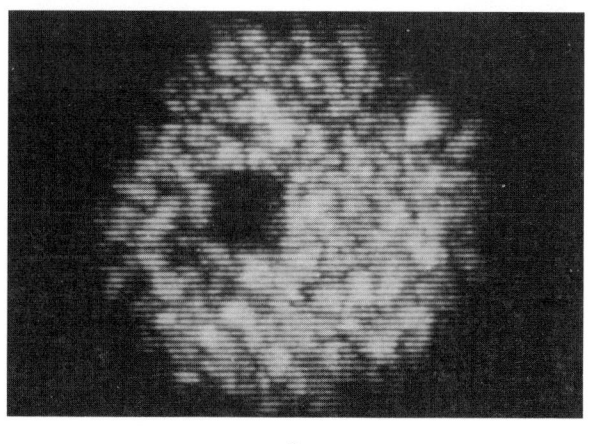

Fig. 1. a, A-scan technique. *b*, B-scan technique. *c*, C-scan section through orbital fat; optic nerve appears dark.

and formulae for calculation of intraocular lens implant power are available.[8]

B-Scan Technique

Coupling of the sound to the eye for the B-scan examination is generally to the closed eyelid via a gel, or if the anterior structures are of interest, to the open anaesthetized eye via a saline bath.

The transducer sends out interrogating pulses of sound and in the time interval between pulses echoes are received by the same transducer and plotted as spots, the brightness of the spot indicating the amplitude of an echo and its position the arrival time of the echo at the transducer. The transducer is moved to many positions across the eye and a series of brightness modulated spots are plotted to form a B-scan section, which is comparable to a histological section through the eye and orbit. Good grey-scale is required to enable echo amplitude to be judged from display brightness. The transducer can be moved in a straight line (*Fig.* 1*b*) or rocked through an angle to produce a linear or sector B-scan section respectively; both produce only partial outlines of the globe. A more complete outline of the globe (a compound B-scan) can be obtained by a combination of linear and sector tranducer movements. The transducer movement may be manual or mechanical; alternatively, transducers within an array may be fired in sequence electronically to simulate a moving transducer. Rapid or 'real-time' B-scanning permits two-dimensional dynamic studies of abnormalities during and following eye movements and may be vital in distinguishing abnormalities.[9]

B-scan sections are generally taken in the horizontal and vertical planes at regular intervals (usually every millimetre), with many directions of gaze.

Digital scan convertors may be used to digitize the information concerning the amplitudes and positions of echoes.

C-Scan Technique

The coronal plane of the eye and orbit is inaccessible to B-scan examination because the surrounding orbital bone proves a barrier to the sound. This plane

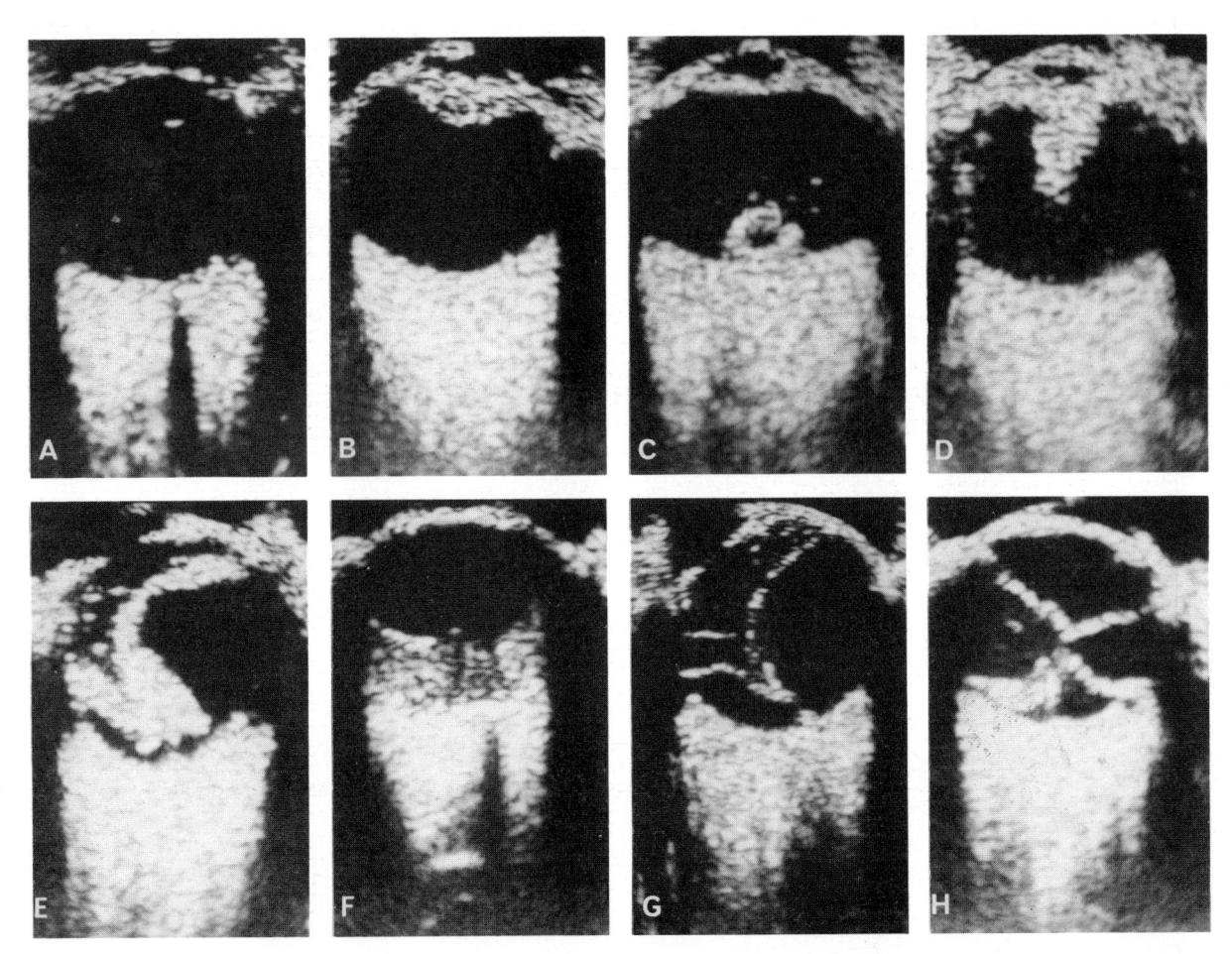

Fig. 2. Horizontal linear B-scan sections. *a*, Central section through normal eye and orbit. *b*, Cataract. *c*, Dislocated lens lying on retina; detached vitreous gel. *d*, Ruptured posterior lens capsule; lens material within vitreous. *e*, Detached collapsed vitreous gel; asteroid bodies within gel. *f*, Retrohyaloid haemorrhage. *g*, Deviated gaze; detached vitreous gel tethering to optic disc; intra-gel opacity. *h*, Fibrotic posterior hyaloid membrane inserting into posterior traction retinal detachment.

may be imaged, however, using a C-scan technique; this technique has been described in detail elsewhere.[4] The C-scan section presents a brightness modulated display of echoes from a certain depth and thickness of orbital tissue (*Fig. 1c*).

TISSUE CHARACTERIZATION

'Tissue characterization' techniques attempt to extract from ultrasonic signals those quantitative parameters which are intrinsic to the tissue itself and useful medically. Some techniques attempt to apply signal processing methods to obtain some quantitative measurement of the spatial arrangement of the scattering elements of tissue.[4] Others involve attempts at quantitative measurements of acoustical properties,[10] such as attenuation and velocity.

INTRAOCULAR DIAGNOSIS (RAPID B-SCAN)

The Lens

The normal lens (*Fig. 2a*) in linear B-scan section is internally acoustically clear; echoes arise from the central portions of the anterior and posterior lens boundaries. Cataracts may give rise to internal echoes (*Fig. 2b*) or the entire lens boundary may be outlined. If the normal posterior lenticular boundary echo is absent, the lens may be dislocated (*Fig. 2c*) or ruptured. Rupture of the posterior lens capsule (*Fig. 2d*) results in a series of echoes within the lens which extrude into the vitreous cavity.

The Vitreous

Vitreous opacities give rise to echoes of varying amplitudes within the normally acoustically clear vitreous cavity. In general, it is not possible to differentiate between opacities ultrasonically. Asteroid bodies (*Fig. 2e*) do, however, give rise to much higher amplitude echoes than haemorrhage or inflammatory cells.

Posterior Vitreous Detachment

Posterior vitreous detachment may be outlined by echoes arising from opacity confined to within the

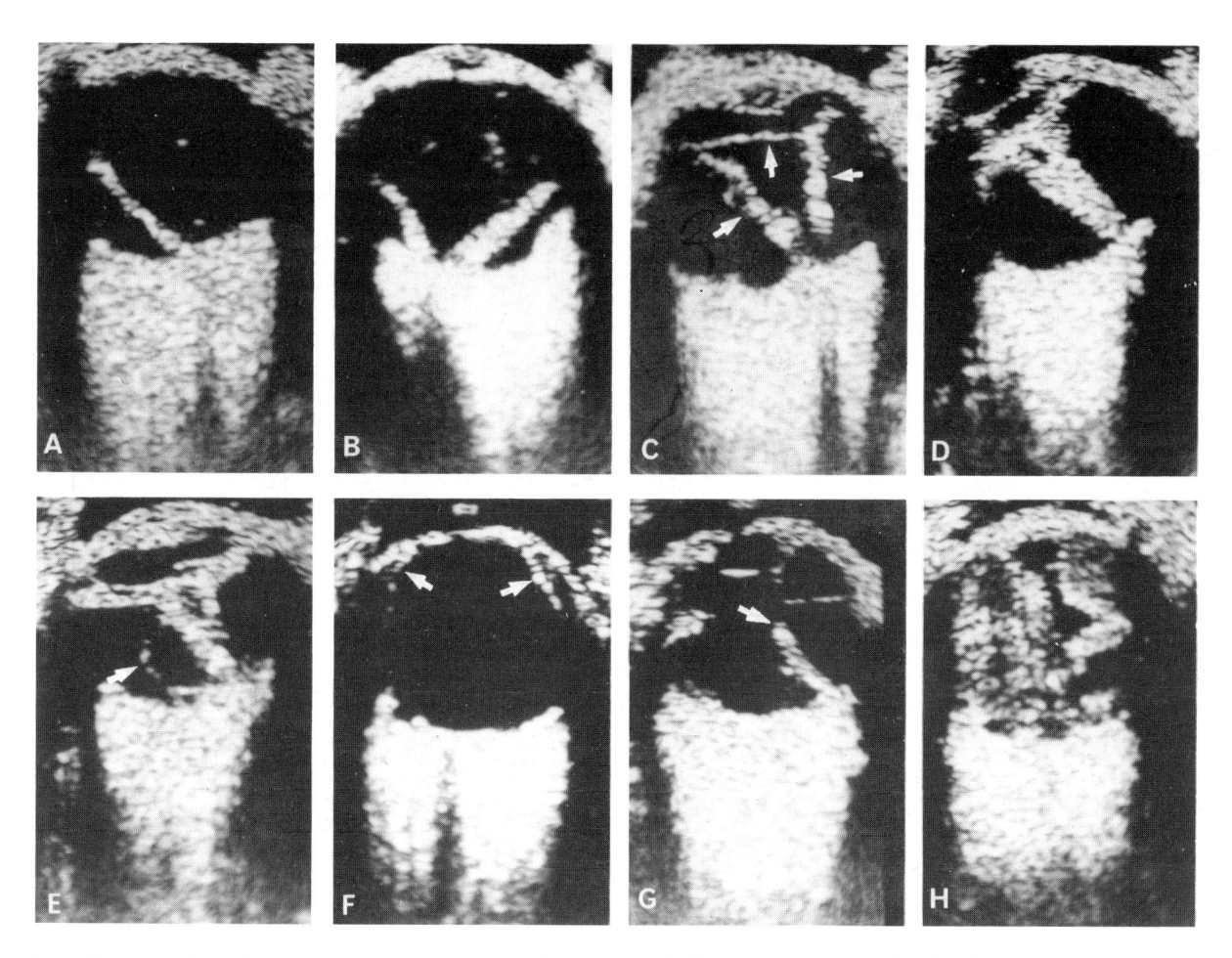

Fig. 3. Horizontal linear B-scan sections. *a*, Temporal retinal detachment. *b*, Total funnel-shaped retinal detachment; detached vitreous gel. *c*, Cataract; total retinal detachment; detached retracted vitreous gel ('triangle sign', arrows). *d*, Deviated gaze; total retinal detachment ('closed triangle'). *e*, Massive pre-retinal retraction; retinal 'cyst' (arrow). *f*, Shallow anterior annular choroidal detachment (arrows). *g*, Bullous nasal choroidal detachment with attachment to vortex vein (arrow). *h*, Suprachoroidal haemorrhage.

detached vitreous gel (*Fig. 2e*) or to the retrohyaloid space (*Fig. 2f*); the corporate mobility of such echoes on dynamic B-scan testing suggests the vitreous gel is detached. If both intra-gel and retrohyaloid opacity is present, the gel boundary can be recognized during dynamic studies. Alternatively (*Fig. 2g*), or additionally, a sheet of echoes along the gel boundary outlines the posterior vitreous detachment. Posterior vitreous detachment may be complete (*Fig. 2f*) or incomplete (*Fig. 3g*). Wide vitreo-retinal adhesions may indicate areas of epiretinal fibrosis and may be associated with traction retinal detachment[9] (*Fig. 2h*).

The Retina

Retinal detachments give rise to high amplitude echoes (*Fig. 3a*). A total rhegmatogenous retinal detachment is seen in central B-scan section as a bright line of echoes extending anteriorly to the ora serrata and tethering to the optic nerve head; a detached vitreous gel (*Fig. 3b*) is seen anterior to the detached retina. Typically a fresh retinal detachment gives rise to undulating movements on dynamic testing. The diagnosis of massive pre-retinal retraction is made when these undulations become damped or absent.[11] Often the 'triangle sign' (*Fig. 3c*), as described by Fuller et al.,[12] is present. Various configurations of triangle are possible depending on the degree of retraction of the vitreous gel and the angle between the retinal leaves at the level of the optic disc; the retinal leaves may be in apposition and a closed triangle (*Fig. 3d*) may be present. 'Cysts' may be seen on the anterior or posterior (*Fig. 3e*) aspects of the retina. The rigidity of the retina and the angle between the retinal leaves at the level of the optic disc give some indication of operability.

The Choroid

Shallow choroidal detachment (*Fig. 3f*) and bullous choroidal detachment are best demonstrated using saline bath coupling. Bullous choroidal detachments give rise to convex sheets of high amplitude echoes

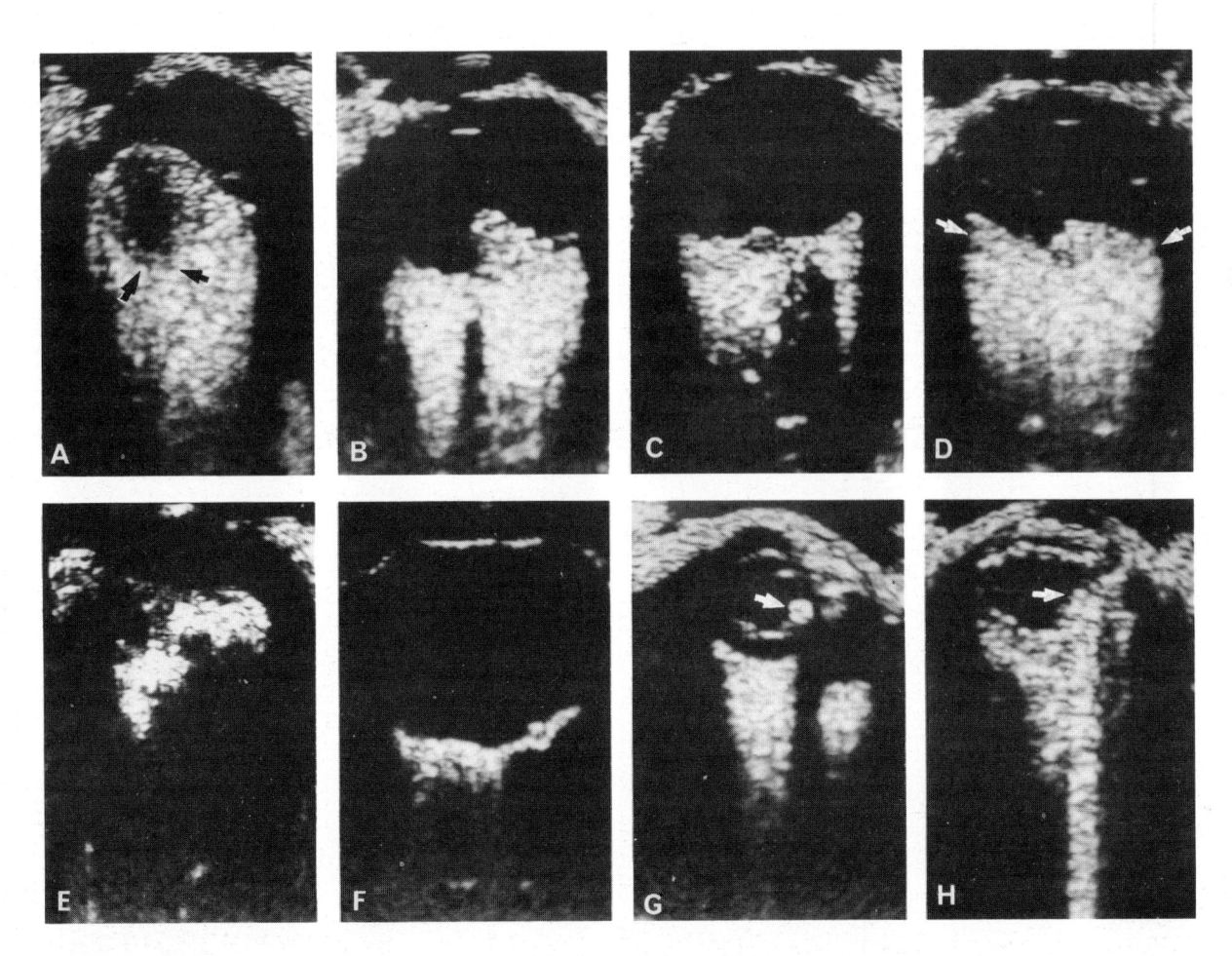

Fig. 4. Horizontal linear B-scan sections. *a,* Large malignant melanoma with posterior extraocular extension (arrows). *b,* Posterior 'collar-stud' malignant melanoma. *c,* Small malignant melanoma showing choroidal excavation. *d,* Large secondary deposit (arrows). *e,* Large retinoblastoma containing calcium. *f,* Choroidal osteoma; attenuation by calcium prevents visualization of orbital structures. *g,* Deviated gaze; phthisical eye with retinal detachment; foreign body (arrow) attenuating sound. *h,* Phthisical eye; foreign body (arrow) producing 'ringing'.

in B-scan section which extend anterior to the ora serrata; attachment to the vortex veins (*Fig.* 3g) may be detected. Suprachoroidal haemorrhage (*Fig.* 3h) may reduce the amplitude of the choroidal detachment echoes.

Intra-ocular Tumours

Tumours generally give rise to a group of well-defined echoes which appear on several adjacent B-scan sections and which can be made to adjoin the coats of the eye. On dynamic testing, tumours move as an integral part of the eye and show no after-movements. Macroscopic extraocular extension of a tumour (*Fig.* 4a) can be detected ultrasonically. Malignant melanomas[13] are usually rounded or 'collar-stud' in shape (*Fig.* 4b), with internal echoes of varying amplitudes; sometimes acoustically clear areas (*Fig.* 4a) are present internally. Choroidal excavation,[4] that is, replacement of normal strong choroidal echoes by tumour cell echoes of lower amplitude, may be seen in large or small (*Fig.* 4c) tumours. Secondary tumours are generally irregular in shape (*Fig.* 4d) and usually give rise to higher amplitude echoes than those from within malignant melanomas. Ultrasonically it may be difficult to differentiate between a gross disciform and a secondary deposit. The presence of calcium, which is both strongly reflecting and highly attenuating, may aid in the diagnosis of retinoblastoma (*Fig.* 4e) and choroidal osteoma (*Fig.* 4f).

It may be of value to follow the growth of tumours either prior to or during treatment; measurements may be taken to assess the maximum elevation and base diameter of a mass. A desk-top computer enables areas of tumour sections to be calculated and tumour volume to be computed.

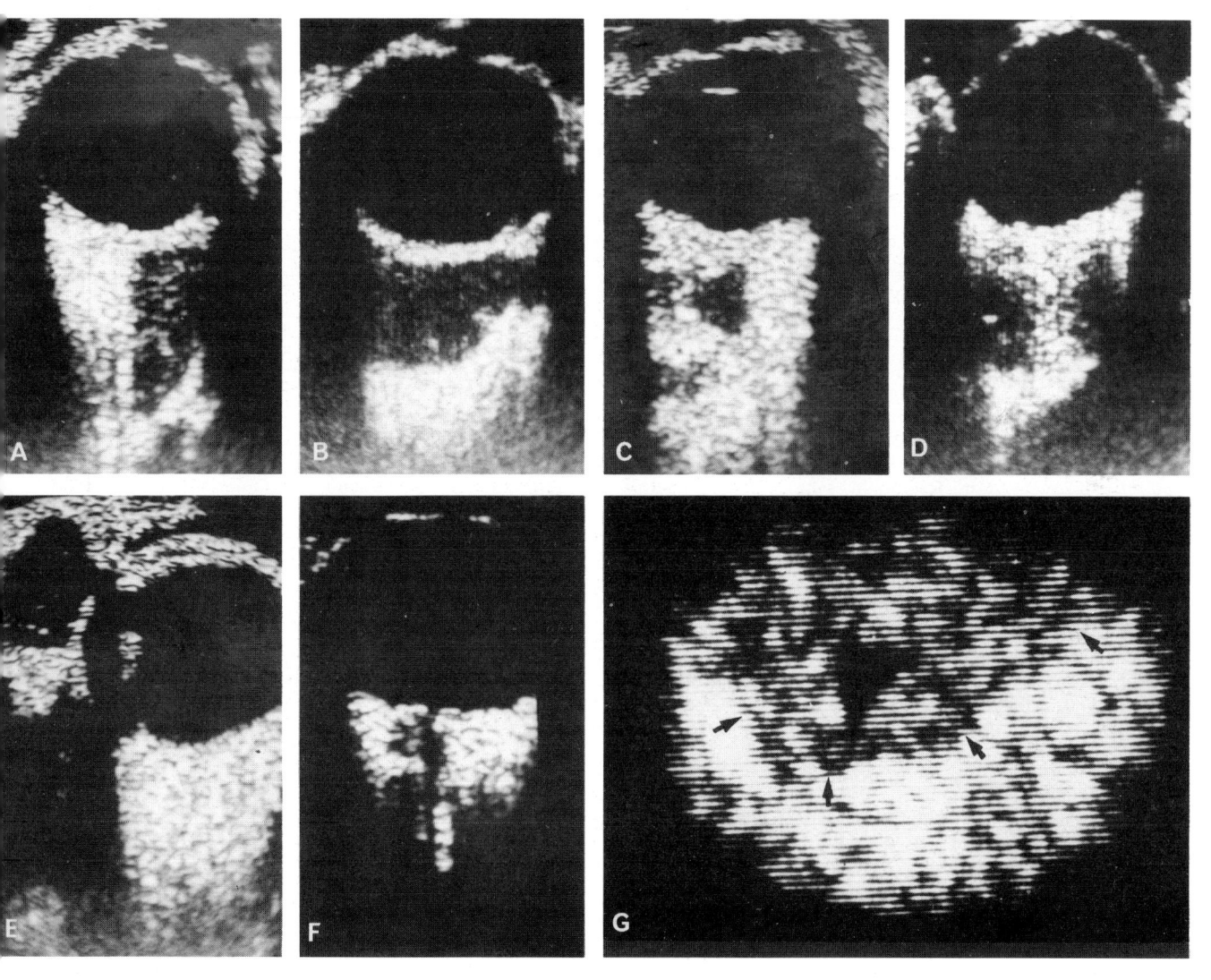

Fig. 5. Horizontal linear B-scan sections and C-scan section. *a*, Deviated gaze; cavernous haemangioma. *b*, Lymphoma directly behind the globe. *c*, Pseudotumour. *d*, Lymphocytic lesion of indeterminate nature. *e*, Lacrimal gland cyst. *f*, Optic nerve meningioma. *g*, Optic nerve meningioma (arrows); triangular atropic optic nerve.

ORBITAL DIAGNOSIS

X-ray computerized tomography has, to some extent, superseded the use of ultrasound in orbital diagnosis; it outlines lesions in relation to bone and shows the orbital apex and ocular muscles well. Ultrasound, however, is more useful in determining the exact nature of those lesions detected.

Ultrasonic diagnosis within the orbit is a pattern recognition process based on the location, shape (of both the anterior and posterior borders) of a mass, the distribution in both number and amplitudes of internal mass echoes, together with the attenuating properties of a lesion. Generally a particular type of tumour does not have a single pattern associated with it (an exception to this is the cavernous haemangioma, *Fig. 5a*), but several possible patterns. This is particularly so in the spectrum of conditions between lymphoma (*Fig. 5b*) and pseudotumour. Lymphomas may be echo-free internally or may contain echoes of varying amplitudes. Pseudotumours often produce a mottled appearance (*Fig. 5c*) to the orbital fat. Inflammatory signs,[3] such as fluid in Tenon's capsule and within the optic nerve sheath, may suggest the presence of pseudotumour. An overlap in the appearance between lymphoma and pseudotumour (*Fig. 5d*) may make ultrasonic differentiation difficult. Cystic lesions (*Fig. 5e*) are easy to demonstrate ultrasonically. Optic nerve lesions produce enlargement of the nerve shadow; many (*Fig. 5f*), but not all (*Fig. 5g*), are echo-free.

CONCLUSION

The A-scan technique is used for biometric studies and by many workers in diagnosis. The B-scan and C-scan techniques may be used in intraocular and orbital diagnosis; dynamic B-scan studies are essential in characterizing vitreo-retinal pathology. 'Tissue characterization' techniques hold promise of distinguishing abnormalities that are difficult to differentiate by other techniques.

ACKNOWLEDGEMENTS

The author would like to thank Alan Lacey for the photographic work, David McLeod for his helpful comments and Carol Clark for her secretarial assistance.

REFERENCES

1. Ossoinig K. Echography of the eye, orbit and periorbital region. In: Arger P. H. (ed.) *Orbital Roentgenology*. New York, Wiley, 1977.
2. Bronson N. R., Fisher Y. L., Pickering N. C. et al. *Ophthalmic Contact B-scan Ultrasonography for the Clinician*. Westport, Conn., Intercontinental Publications, 1976.
3. Coleman D. J., Lizzi F. L. and Jack R. L. *Ultrasonography of the Eye and Orbit*. Philadelphia, Lea and Febiger, 1977.
4. Restori M. and Wright J. E. C-scan ultrasonography in orbital diagnosis. *Br. J. Ophthalmol.* 1977; **61**, 735–40.
5. Restori M. Ultrasonic holography in ophthalmic diagnosis. *Br. J. Clin. Equip.* 1978; pp. 71–5.
6. Atkinson P. and Woodcock J. P. *Doppler Ultrasound and its Use in Clinical Measurement*. London, Academic Press, 1982.
7. Francois J. and Goes F. Ocular biometry. *Doc. Ophthalmol. Proc. Ser.* 1981; 29.
8. Hoffer K. J. Accuracy of ultrasound in intra-ocular lens calculation. *Arch. Ophthalmol.* 1981; **199**, 819–23.
9. McLeod D. and Restori M. Ultrasonic examination in severe diabetic eye disease. *Br. J. Ophthalmol.* 1979; **63**, 533–8.
10. Jones J. P. and Cole-Beuglet C. *In vivo* characterisation of several lesions in the eye using ultrasonic impediography. In: A. F. Metherell (ed.) *Acoustical Imaging*, vol. 8. London, Plenum Press, pp. 539–46.
11. Gregor Z., Restori M. and McLeod D. B-scan ultrasound in massive pre-retinal retraction. *Trans. Ophthal. Soc. UK* 1979; **99**, Pt 1.
12. Fuller D. G., Laqua H. and Machemer R. Ultrasonographic diagnosis in massive periretinal proliferation in eyes with opaque media (triangular retinal detachment). *Am. J. Ophthalmol.* 1977; pp. 460–4.
13. Sheilds J. A., McDonald P. R., Leonard B. C. et al. The diagnosis of uveal malignant melanomas in eyes with opaque media. *Am. J. Ophthalmol.* 1977; **84**, 375.

Radiology and the Orbit

Glyn Lloyd

METHODS OF INVESTIGATION

Investigation of the orbit is now based upon a combination of plain X-ray and computerized tomography. Other established techniques such as carotid angiography, orbital venography and ultrasonography are ancillary and not used routinely. Thus most patients with orbital disease can be managed without recourse to any invasive technique. The role of nuclear magnetic resonance (NMR) in orbital diagnosis is not yet fully established, but early studies suggest that in most conditions it can act as a substitute for CT scan and at the same time have certain advantages, especially in the diagnosis of vascular anomalies. However, since bone does not produce an NMR signal, this is a disadvantage in those conditions that cause bone changes in addition to soft tissue abnormality in the orbit. Paranasal sinus pathology, for instance, is likely to be better demonstrated by high resolution CT than NMR as at present developed.

Plain X-ray Changes

Alterations in the general radiographic density of the orbit are dependent upon a decrease or increase of the soft tissue contents; thus, in the presence of a space-occupying lesion causing proptosis, oedema of the soft tissues or chymosis, a decrease in orbital translucence is to be expected. Conversely, enophthalmos resulting from a decrease in the contents of the orbit, will produce a slight hypertranslucence. These changes in the soft tissue density of the orbit are of little practical diagnostic significance and simply reflect a change which is obvious clinically. Alterations in the size of the orbit are a common accompaniment of long standing orbital pathology. *Decrease* in size may occur after early enucleation of the eye before the orbit has reached adult size; it may also be seen in congenital microphthalmos and anophthalmos. *Enlargement* is normally the result of raised intraorbital pressure producing changes in the orbit analogous to those seen in the calvarium in raised intracranial pressure. Any growing tumour may produce these X-ray changes if sufficient time has elapsed, but the response of the orbit to a space-occupying lesion is more rapid in a child than an adult, and while orbital enlargement usually denotes a benign lesion of long standing, this rule is not applicable to children.

Invasion and erosion of the walls of the orbit may take the form of osseous destruction and is then usually due to a malignant primary or secondary neoplasm. Rarely it may be due to an infective process, such as tuberculosis. A local indentation of the orbital wall with clear-cut edges is characteristic of a benign tumour such as a dermoid cyst or epidermoid. Increased bone density or hyperostosis in the orbit may occur in a number of conditions, principally a pterional or sphenoid ridge meningioma, but it may also be due to osteoblastic metastases, fibrous dysplasia, Paget's disease and osteitis associated with chronic sinus infection.

Calcification within the soft tissues of the orbit is uncommon. Within the globe it may be present in the lens in senile cataract, and ossification may occur in the vitreous and choroid as a result of degenerative changes following injury or infection. Finely stippled calcification may be demonstrable in cases of retinoblastoma, and Taybi[1] has reported macroscopic global calcification in 14 of 22 children with retrolental fibroplasia. Calcinosis oculi has also been reported in hyperparathyroidism.

Calcification in the retro-orbital structures may be seen in meningioma of the optic nerve. This may take the shape of calcification within the sheath of the optic nerve (*Fig.* 1), or a finely stippled calcification may be present in the tumour mass, usually

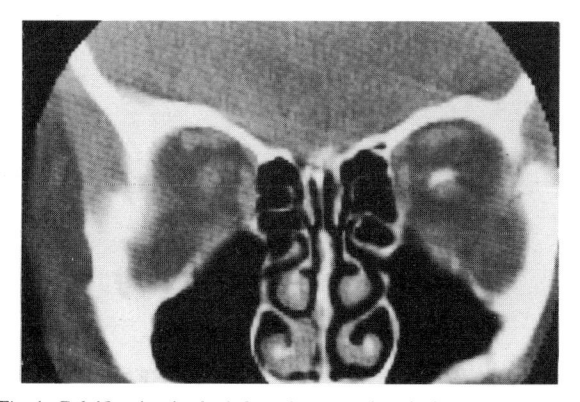

Fig. 1. Calcification in the left optic nerve sheath shown on coronal CT scan. This was a meningioma.

located towards the apex of the orbit. The identification of phleboliths in the orbit is an important observation in the differential diagnosis of patients presenting with proptosis and indicates the presence of abnormal veins in the orbit and a venous malformation (*Fig.* 2).

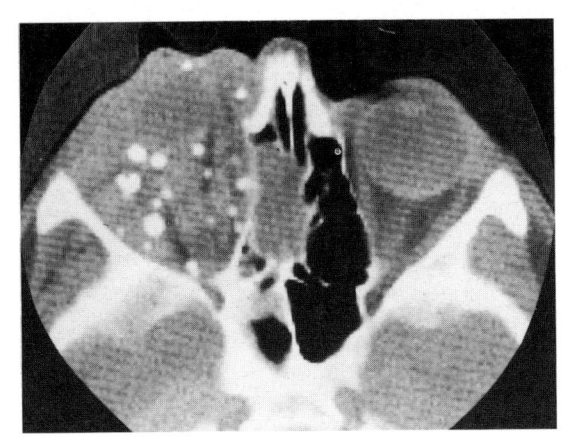

Fig. 2. Venous malformation shown on axial CT scan. Diffuse intra- and extraconal soft tissue mass with enlargement of the orbit and multiple phleboliths.

Computerized tomography

Plain X-ray of the skull and computerized tomography (CT) are now the dominant radiological investigations of the orbit, and the majority of patients presenting with exophthalmos can be totally evaluated by these techniques without further study.

Technique

The best apparatus for CT scanning of the orbit is a scanner that allows scans to be made in at least two planes. This means using an all-purpose scanner in which the scanning aperture is large enough to allow the head to be manipulated into the required positions to produce direct axial and coronal scans. Coronal sections should be obtained routinely, direct coronal scanning is necessary for adequate demonstration of orbital pathology. Reconstruction should be reserved for sagittal or oblique sections, which are not directly obtainable with most scanner designs. The attitude of the patient's head is important so that the best possible scanning plane can be obtained through the orbits. Satisfactory axial scans should include the globes and show the lens, optic nerve, lateral and medial rectus muscles on the same section. To do this, the position of the head should be adjusted so that the scanning plane forms an angle of 16–18° caudally from the orbito–meatal line. Optimum orbital scans will be obtained if the posterior clinoids are shown on scans that also include the optic nerves and clearly show the globes on both sides. For coronal scans the patient lies prone with the chin elevated. Alternatively, a similar position can be obtained by placing the patient supine with the head hyperextended.

Differential diagnosis of orbital mass lesions

There are three ways in which a differential diagnosis of orbital space-occupying lesions may be achieved:
1. By showing the site of origin of the lesion, for example the optic nerve.
2. By the shape and density of the lesion (CT morphology).
3. By consideration of the attenuation values before and after intravenous contrast injection.

Optic nerve tumours, whether gliomas or meningiomas, may be identified when the optic nerve is shown to be enlarged in both axial and coronal section. Further differentiation may be arrived at by consideration of the age of the patient: most optic nerve sheath meningiomas occur in the elderly and middle aged, whereas an optic nerve glioma is a disease of childhood and young adults. The presence of calcification in the tumour shown by CT indicates a meningioma; optic canal enlargement is the rule in gliomas and only seen in a minority of sheath meningioma.

Benign encapsulated tumours can be readily identified by their shape and even density. The commonest tumour in this group is a cavernous haemangioma *Fig.* 3. This gives a rounded contour, sometimes almost circular in outline, and is almost invariably intraconal in location. Another tumour that may be

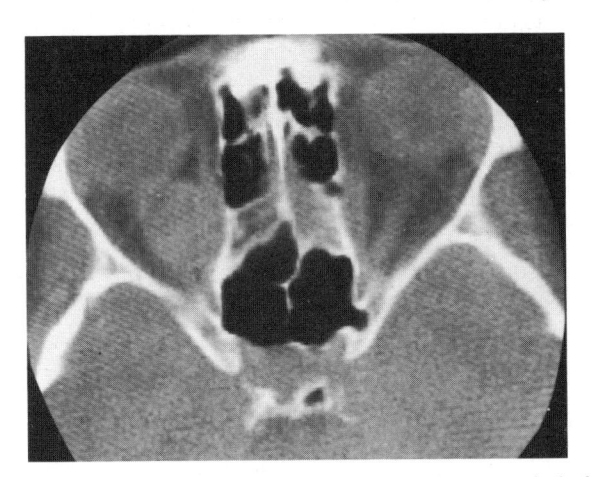

Fig. 3. Discrete rounded mass in the intraconal space typical of a cavernous haemangioma.

indistinguishable on CT from a cavernous haemangioma is a neurilemmoma; in general these are larger than the cavernous haemangiomas but it is usually not necessary to make a differentiation between the two tumours since the treatment is the same in either case; namely, excision by lateral orbitotomy. Another lesion that may present as a clearly defined rounded mass is an orbital varix.

When encapsulated tumours grow to a large size they may fill almost the whole of the intraconal space, but even the largest will invariably leave some translucence on the scan at the orbital apex, a point of differentiation from infiltrative processes in the muscle cone. The commonest of these is a granuloma or pseudotumour (*Fig.* 4). They may be distinguished from the clearly defined tumours described above by

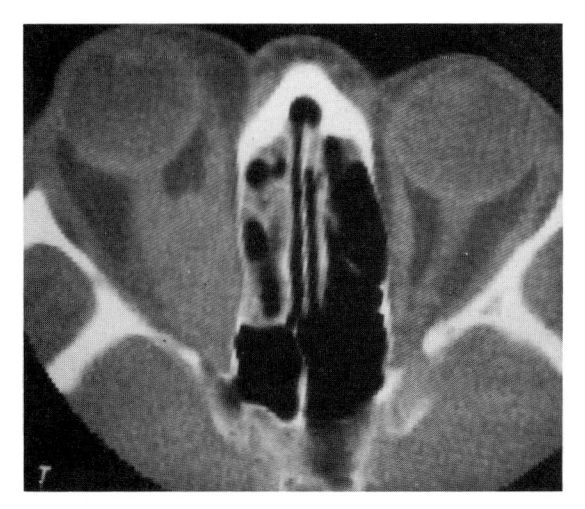

Fig. 4. Diffuse mass involving the intraconal space, optic nerve and medial rectus muscle. This was a non-specific inflammatory process or pseudotumour. Note the infection in the adjacent ethmoid cells.

their ill-defined edge and heterogeneous density, often involving the extraocular musculature. Other common lesions that may show an infiltrative process in the orbit are lymphomas and metastases. Although an absolute distinction between these lesions and the pseudotumour group is not always possible on CT, the characteristic distribution of the lesion in the orbit may suggest the diagnosis before biopsy (*see below*).

Contrast Medium

The injection of contrast medium for orbital CT scanning is no longer a routine procedure. If possible, post-contrast scans to show tissue enhancement are to be avoided since the injection of contrast converts what is essentially a non-invasive procedure into one which carries a similar morbidity and mortality to intravenous urography. The possibility of tissue recognition in the orbit by the behaviour of the attenuation values before and after contrast injection is severely limited, and since most patients with proved mass lesions will have either a biopsy or surgical excision of the lesion, contrast injection is seldom justified. Thus, for orbital scanning, contrast medium should be used to show up doubtful space-occupying lesions in better detail and when intracranial spread is suspected. If a clearly defined lesion is shown on the unenhanced scans, injection is usually unnecessary. One condition, however, can be diagnosed on the evidence of the attenuation values but without contrast enhancement: approximately two-thirds of dermoid cysts in the orbit show areas of negative attenuation due to the presence of fat or oil in the tumour (*Fig.* 5).

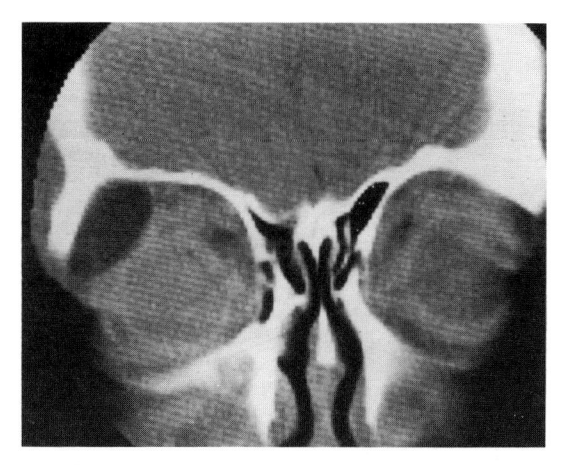

Fig. 5. Local area of low attenuation in the superolateral quadrant of the orbit due to a dermoid cyst.

Angiography of the Orbit

In addition to plain X-ray and CT scan, two angiographic methods of investigation of the orbit may be required in some patients.

Carotid Arteriography

CT scan has made carotid angiography unnecessary for the routine investigation of unilateral exophthalmos, and has taken over the role of angiography in the exclusion of intracranial lesions causing proptosis. This investigation should therefore only be carried out on selected patients, principally those with suspected vascular anomalies either in the orbit or middle fossa; for example, a dural arteriovenous malformation or infraclinoid aneurysm. In the orbit it should be remembered that approximately 25 per cent of space-occupying lesions may be classified as vascular anomalies and these are by their nature best demonstrated by angiography – by venography in the case of a venous malformation and by arteriography when there is an arteriovenous shunt. Arteriography may also be needed to define the blood supply to a vascular tumour in the orbit prior to surgery.

Technique

In a patient with proptosis, the essential requirement of arteriography is that it should combine an adequate study of the intracranial vessels with a detailed investigation of the orbit; and to do this some elaboration of normal technique is needed. For the injection of the contrast medium, straight needle puncture is not to be recommended because of the manipulation of the head required for the modified axial projection (*see below*). Displacement of the needle may result, with the inherent danger of an intramural injection.

Some form of catheterization or cannulation is therefore needed and also should provide a means of selective injection of both the internal and external carotid arteries.

For the angiogram series three projections are used. These are all magnified geometrically.
1. A standard lateral arteriogram series of the skull and a series of lateral macro-angiograms coned to the orbit.
2. An anteroposterior series.
3. A modified axial view to provide a plan view of the orbital vessels.[2]

Diagnosis

Orbital tumours may be shown by carotid angiography in three ways: by displacement of vessels; by the demonstration of a pathological circulation; and by deformation of the choroid crescent.

Orbital Phlebography

In the original technique the superior ophthalmic vein was filled from an injection into the angular vein either by cut down or by percutaneous puncture. This technique has now been superseded as the first approach to orbital venography by the method of frontal vein injection originally described by Vritsios.[3] In this method the injection of contrast is made into a frontal vein or main tributary. Immediately prior to injection a rubber band is placed around the forehead at the hairline, to prevent reflux of contrast medium over the scalp, and the facial veins also need to be occluded either by a compression bandage or by finger pressure applied by the patient. In some patients the most prominent forehead vein is the anterior temporal branch, and it can be used successfully to make the injection provided the temporal vein is occluded above the angle of the jaw by finger pressure. A 23-gauge scalp vein needle is normally used for the injection unless the veins are large enough to employ a 21-gauge needle, which will allow a more rapid injection.

Technique

The injection is made with 10–12 ml of 280 Conray or equivalent contrast medium. Films are taken after delivery of 5 ml and immediately prior to the end of the injection. A preliminary control film is also obtained for subtraction studies. Both orbital venous systems normally fill, provided sufficient contrast medium is used, and this is an advantage of the frontal vein approach since minor degrees of displacement of the veins on the abnormal side may be detected by comparison with the opposite, normal side. In over 90 per cent of patients frontal venography can be performed without anaesthesia and on an outpatient basis. In children, and in adults with difficult veins in whom venipuncture has failed initially, a general anaesthetic may be required.

Diagnosis

A tumour or other space-occupying lesion in the orbit may be demonstrated by venography in three ways: it may cause displacement of veins; it may obstruct the venous system in the orbit; or it may be revealed by the presence of a pathological venous circulation. These changes are often found in combination, but the type of change does indicate to a very great extent the likely pathology present; displacement is usually caused by a benign tumour; obstruction by an inflammatory or malignant process and pathological veins by a venous malformation.

DYSTHYROID EXOPHTHALMOS

The enlargement of the extraocular muscles which occurs in this condition may be clearly demonstrated by computerized tomography. In dysthyroid patients multiple rectus muscle enlargement is usually present, either bilaterally (most common) or unilaterally, sometimes accompanied by enlargement of the optic nerve. Single muscle enlargement may also occur in a minority of dysthyroid patients. The muscle enlargement tends to affect the belly of the muscle rather than its origin or insertion, and this may help in the differentiation from pseudotumour involving muscle. When this typical enlargement affects the medial recti it will produce a characteristic indentation on the medial orbital wall (*Fig.* 6). This will persist after regression of muscle enlargement and remains as evidence that the muscle has been enlarged in the past.

Brismar et al.,[4] have recorded a pitfall in the differential diagnosis of endocrine exophthalmos by computerized tomography. Owing to the enlarged rectus muscles in the apex of the orbit, simulated tumour

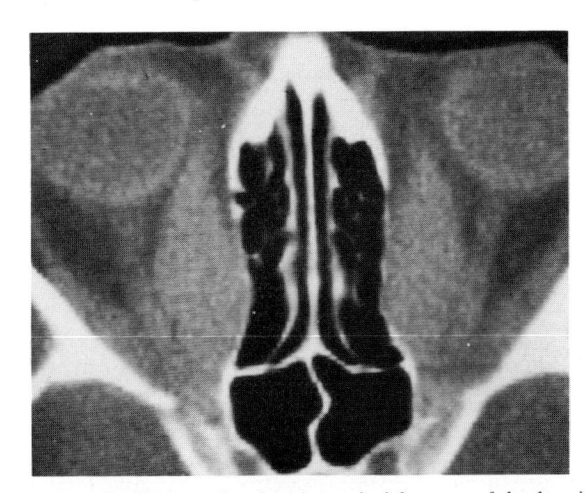

Fig. 6. Axial CT scan showing the typical features of dysthryoid disease. There is rectus muscle enlargement particularly affecting the medial recti, and indentation of the ethmoid labyrinth on both sides.

formation may be shown on the scan. This is explained by the tomographic section intersecting obliquely one of the enlarged muscles (usually the inferior rectus), thus producing a false tumour-like structure on the scan. The problem has been largely overcome by the routine use of coronal sections.

In some dysthyroid patients the fat content of the orbit may increase considerably and this may be the primary cause of the exophthalmos with little or no muscle enlargement. This gives a different CT appearance, with forward displacement of the eyeball, an increase in the intraconal space, and sometimes a characteristic angulation of the lateral rectus muscles at the point where they are held by the lateral check ligaments. Phlebography also gives a characteristic appearance in dysthyroid disease; the second part of the ophthalmic vein may be displaced downwards with an exaggerated upward concavity. This selective displacement of one part of the venous system is caused by the combined increased bulk of the levator palpebrae and superior rectus muscles lying immediately above this part of the superior ophthalmic vein.

UNILATERAL EXOPHTHALMOS

The causes of this condition can be divided for convenience of diagnosis into four main categories:
1. Dysthyroid disease (*see above*).
2. Intracranial lesions giving rise to unilateral proptosis.
3. Causes arising in the paranasal sinuses and nasopharynx.
4. Intraorbital space-occupying lesions.

In a small proportion of patients proptosis may be due to an intracranial lesion. A sphenoid ridge meningioma is the commonest intracranial lesion to cause unilateral exophthalmos. More frequently, the cause of the proptosis is to be found in the paranasal sinuses or nasopharynx, usually the result of a tumour, infection or mucocoele.

Intraorbital Space-occupying Lesions

Vascular Anomalies

Vascular anomalies in the orbit may be classified into ophthalmic artery aneurysms; arteriovenous malformations, haemangiomas; and orbital varices.

Ophthalmic Artery Aneurysm

Saccular aneurysms arising from the intraorbital course of the ophthalmic artery are extremely rare and there are fewer than six authentic cases in the literature.[5] The majority of ophthalmic artery aneurysms arise from the junction of the internal carotid and ophthalmic arteries and are designated carotid ophthalmic aneurysms.

Arteriovenous Malformation

The orbit is a relatively uncommon site for an arteriovenous malformation but because of the use of angiographic techniques the condition is being increasingly reported in the literature. The lesion may occur as a congenital anomaly or follow trauma to the anterior orbit.[6] Clinically the anomaly may present either as a pulsating exophthalmos, sometimes associated with an audible bruit, or as a simple proptosis. Carotid angiography is the essential investigation, both to show the nature of the lesion and its blood supply. Studies of the internal and external carotid vessels may be needed, since some of these malformations are fed in part from the external carotid artery.

Haemangioma

The orbital haemangiomas are divided into capillary and cavernous types. Capillary haemangioma is a lesion that occurs in infants and may give rise to unilateral proptosis. It is often associated with a superficial capillary naevus and may be demonstrated as a fine vascular network on carotid angiography or sometimes as a diffuse and extensive pathological circulation, in some patients fed from the external carotid.[6] Cavernous haemangioma, on the other hand, is a disease of adult patients, and some authors regard the condition as a more developed form of infantile capillary haemangioma. Orbital cavernous haemangioma is a benign encapsulated neoplasm or hamartoma which is typically found within the muscle cone and gives rise to an axial proptosis. The incidence of cavernous haemangioma is undoubtedly less than that normally reported. This is mostly because of the confusion in the literature between cavernous haemangioma and venous malformations in the orbit. The latter condition is more common than cavernous haemangioma and there is little doubt that many of the reported examples of cavernous haemangioma are in fact entirely venous and therefore should be classified with the venous malformations.

Diagnosis

The commonest change on plain X-ray is enlargement of the affected orbit. The cavernous haemangioma, being a slow-growing tumour, produces moderate degrees of orbital enlargement which can be demonstrated both by plain X-ray and by tomography. These tumours are well demonstrated prior to orbitotomy by CT scan, the lesion showing as a well demarcated tumour mass with even density values and a rounded margin. This investigation has made arteriographic studies unnecessary in most patients with this condition. Nevertheless, the most positive evidence of a cavernous haemangioma is often provided by arteriography. It may be possible to demonstrate 'venous pools' within the muscle cone in the capillary and venous phase of the examination, and these may be fed by contrast medium from the external carotid circulation.

Orbital varices

These may be primary or secondary.

CONGENITAL VENOUS MALFORMATION

A detailed description of this anomaly has been given by Lloyd et al.[7] and by Wright.[8] These patients usually give a history of proptosis dating from birth or early childhood and characteristically the proptosis is provoked or made worse by an increase of venous pressure in the head. Orbital varices may be accompanied by venous abnormalities elsewhere in the head and neck, particularly on the scalp of the affected side. Cases have also been recorded of associated venous malformations in other parts of the body and the condition may also be associated with the Klippel–Trenaunay–Weber syndrome.

DIAGNOSIS

The characteristic plain X-ray features which may be present in these patients are (a) enlargement of the orbit – this is often a gross enlargement since the venous anomaly is present from birth; (b) the presence of phleboliths in the orbit or in adjacent structures; (c) prominent vascular markings and venous 'lakes' in the frontal bone of the same side corresponding to the venous dilatations in the scalp.

By venography it is usually possible to identify two types of venous abnormality; either a local saccular dilatation of the veins in the orbit resembling a venous aneurysm, or a whole system of abnormal venous channels throughout the orbit.

To a large extent the CT morphology of venous malformations follows the venographic appearances. There may be a diffuse change often associated with phleboliths and affecting both the intraconal and extraconal space or they may present as a rounded mass intra- or extraconally. Intermediate forms also exist and a slightly irregular or lobulated intraconal mass may be very suggestive of a venous malformation. The clearly defined rounded varix in the muscle cone may present a problem in CT differential diagnosis, however, since it may be indistinguishable from the more common intraconal tumours such as a cavernous haemangioma or neurilemmoma. In this respect it is important to look for phleboliths. They occurred in 24 per cent of the varices in a series recorded by the author Lloyd[9] and were never seen in 45 histologically verified cavernous haemangiomas.

TRAUMATIC VARICES

Hanafee[10] has described venous lakes occurring in orbit after trauma originating from a tear of the superior ophthalmic vein at the superior orbital fissure and demonstrated by venography. In the author's experience it would seem likely that the most probable cause for so-called traumatic varices is the rupture of a pre-existing varix with extravasation into the muscle cone. This may occur spontaneously without trauma.

SECONDARY VARICES

The venous system in the orbit may dilate secondarily as a result of a caroticocavernous fistula or dural arteriovenous shunt in the middle fossa. Secondary dilatation of the ophthalmic veins may also be caused by an arteriovenous malformation, either in the middle or anterior fossa of the skull or to an intraorbital arteriovenous malformation. These lesions are best demonstrated by carotid arteriography.

Tumours of the Orbit

Orbital Meningioma

Meningioma in the orbit may occur as a primary tumour or it may be present as the secondary extension of a growth originating in the anterior or middle fossa of the skull.

PRIMARY INTRAORBITAL MENINGIOMA

These may be classified as extradural, arising within the orbit remote from the optic nerve, and sheath meningioma, arising from clusters of arachnoid cap cells found in the meningeal sheath covering the optic nerve.

The sheath meningiomas may be further subdivided into intracanalicular or foraminal tumours, and tumours arising from the retrobulbar part of the optic nerve. True intracanalicular tumours are, however, a great rarity and the majority of these so-called foraminal meningiomas are in fact extensions of intracranial tumours. The retrobulbar sheath meningiomas occur predominantly in middle-aged women. Characteristically they give little sign of their presence on plain X-rays, but may show minor variations in the size of the optic canal or calcification in the tumour. The radiological diagnosis is based upon the computed tomography findings. Visual deterioration in the middle-aged or elderly patient with obvious optic nerve enlargement on CT and minimal or no enlargement of the optic canal is characteristic of a sheath meningioma. Primary extradural meningiomas in the orbit usually present with proptosis before compressing the optic nerve. The majority of these show some plain X-ray evidence of their presence, such as localized or generalized orbital enlargement, hyperostosis of the orbital walls, or changes in the adjacent sinuses. In this group the tumour may be located inside or outside the rectus muscle cone and the CT changes are usually non-specific.

SECONDARY MENINGIOMA

These occur as an extension of a meningioma arising in the middle fossa of the skull or less commonly in the anterior fossa. Meningioma en plaque, affecting the greater and lesser wings of the sphenoid and taking origin in the region of the pterion, is the most common variety to affect the orbit secondarily (*Fig. 7*). In these patients the cause of the proptosis is the result of a hyperostosis on the lateral wall and roof

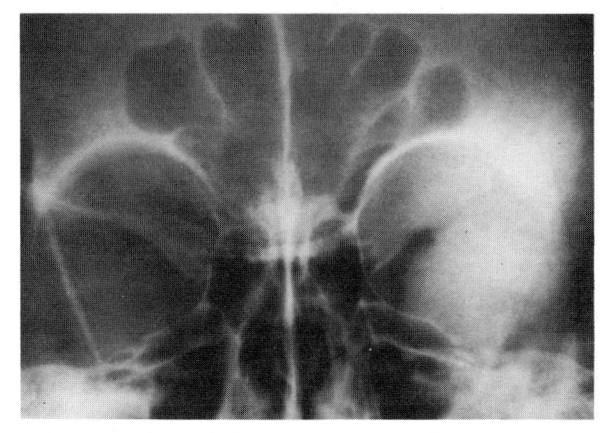

Fig. 7. Typical appearances of a pterional meningioma with hyperostosis on the greater and lesser wings of the sphenoid.

of the orbit, provoked by the meningioma affecting the inner surface of the greater wing of the sphenoid. The degree of hyperostosis and its extent is best assessed by tomography, particularly in the axial plane, and is often much more extensive than is suspected on plain X-ray.

Dermoids and Epidermoids

These tumours result from sequestration of the primitive ectoderm in the region of the orbit. Epidermoids occur when epidermal elements are solely concerned, and a dermoid when the deeper dermal layer is also involved.[11] Strict differentiation of the two types of tumour is to a large extent academic and many are of transitional type, but the dermoids are cystic and may contain oil, sebum, cholesterol and hair, while the epidermoids are solid tumours consisting of a mass of desquamated cells containing keratohyaline, encased in a capsule of well-differentiated stratified squamous epithelium. Both may arise in the diploe of the skull and bones of the orbit and in their growth expand both inner and outer tables, thus producing sharply demarcated bone defects on the radiographs, with well-defined and in some cases slightly sclerotic margins. They occur in characteristic locations in the orbit, more commonly in the superolateral quadrant, but they frequently occur in the medial part of the orbital roof, and sometimes in the greater wing of the sphenoid or lateral wall of the orbit, where they produce a very characteristic cyst-like appearance in the bone. Rarely, they may occur in the inferior part of the orbit.

Diagnosis

Dermoids may give a characteristic appearance on CT scan. The presence of oil or fat produces a localized area of low attenuation in the negative range of the Hounsfield scale (*see Fig.* 5). In the author's series this sign has been present in approximately two-thirds of surgically proved dermoids.

The superficially placed periorbital dermoids may also show minor X-ray changes. The most common locality for these tumours is the outer part of the upper eyelid and they may cause a shallow localized indentation on the orbital rim at its superolateral angle.

Neurofibromatosis

The changes in the orbit and adjacent parts of the skull which can occur in this condition are striking and characteristic. Typically, the orbit is enlarged, the sphenoid ridge elevated to the level of the orbital roof and there may be a large defect in the greater wing of the sphenoid forming the posterior boundary of the orbit producing an encephalocoele. This allows the cranial pulsation to be transmitted directly to the eye and orbital contents, thus producing a pulsating exophthalmos.

Diagnosis

The result of these changes is the so-called 'bare' orbit of neurofibromatosis seen on the postero-anterior radiograph.

Associated changes which may be present in the skull are (*a*) enlargement of the middle fossa, (*b*) enlargement of the optic canal due to the presence of an optic nerve glioma and (*c*) enlargement of the pituitary fossa.

Rhabdomyosarcoma

Rhabdomyosarcoma of the orbit, although a rare tumour in absolute terms, is nevertheless the most common cause of malignancy in the orbit of children, and the majority of these tumours occur in the first decade of life. Three histological types are recognized: embryonal rhabdomyosarcoma; differentiated rhabdomyosarcoma; and alveolar rhabdomyosarcoma, which is the most malignant variety with an invariably poor prognosis. Clinically, the condition presents with exophthalmos with rapid and even alarming progression[12] and this is often accompanied by a superficial swelling in the eyelids, canthi or fornices.

Diagnosis

Radiologically these tumours produce progressive enlargement of the orbit and later they may cause bone destruction with extension to extraorbital structures, including the temporal fossa and cranial cavity.

Enlargement of the orbit may be appreciated on plain X-ray. CT shows a bulky tumour, which usually enhances after injection of contrast medium, frequently occupies an anterior location in the orbit and may extend both intra- and extraconally, sometimes with involvement of the paranasal sinuses.

Lymphoma

Both benign and malignant lymphoma occur in the orbit. The so-called 'benign' lymphoma, however, is better termed benign reactive lymphocytic hyperplasia and should be classified as a variety of pseudotumour. However, the histopathology of these tumours gives no indication of the ultimate outcome: a tumour diagnosed benign may later disseminate and, conversely a histologically malignant tumour may not. Prolonged follow-up is in fact necessary to arrive at a diagnosis of benignity or malignancy. Separation of tumours into monoclonal and polyclonal cell types is also not a sure guide to prognosis; a substantial minority of polyclonal tumours disseminate, while well-differentiated monoclonal tumours do so rarely.[13]

Diagnosis

Lymphomas occur most frequently in the sixth and seventh decade and have an equal sex distribution. They tend to arise outside the muscle cone in the anterior orbit. On plain X-ray they seldom show any abnormality and on CT it is not always possible to distinguish a lymphoma in the orbit from other infiltrating processes, such as a pseudotumour or metastasis. However, some clue to the diagnosis may be derived from the location of the mass in the orbit. In a series of 46 histologically proved lymphomas, two-thirds were both anterior and extraconal in location. This gives rise to the characteristic pattern of these tumours: an anterior, palpable mass enveloping the globe in an elderly patient. Lymphomas arising in the orbit do not as a rule involve bone; only one of 46 patients showed bone erosion associated with the soft tissue mass.

Metastases

In contradistinction to the lymphomas, metastases commonly involve bone. On plain X-ray the typical appearance is that of an ill-defined osteolysis, often difficult to appreciate, but frequently accompanied by loss of the innominate line on the postero-anterior projection. Osteoplastic secondaries occur in the orbit, usually from a breast primary in women or prostate primary in men, and may be indistinguishable from the hyperostosis provoked by a sphenoidal meningioma. These changes can also be demonstrated on CT scan. In a series of 19 patients with proved metastases, 30 per cent showed bone destruction or sclerosis in addition to a soft tissue mass. Involvement of the extraocular muscle is also a feature of some metastases and a single rectus muscle may be involved without infiltration of other structures.

Lacrimal Gland Tumours

These may be benign pleomorphic adenomas; carcinomas, including adenocarcinoma, adenoid cystic carcinoma and undifferentiated types; or lymphomas. The prognosis of lacrimal gland tumours depends upon the histology and whether there is extension of the tumour outside the gland capsule. Benign mixed tumours, if completely removed with capsule intact, have a favourable prognosis, but in contrast the carcinomas, even after total exenteration of the orbit, result in a fatal outcome in almost all cases.

Diagnosis

Plain X-ray changes depend upon the histological type of tumour to some extent. In general the mixed cell type, of relatively slow growth and long duration, produces more obvious changes in the underlying lacrimal fossa. The most common sign is a local enlargement of the lacrimal fossa without bone invasion. This is seen in approximately 80 per cent of benign mixed tumours, but will also occur in some 50 per cent of carcinomas. Differentiation on plain X-ray is, therefore, not always possible. However, the diagnosis and pathological type may be suggested by a combination of conventional radiography and CT scan. X-ray signs of malignancy in lacrimal gland tumours include invasion and sclerosis of the adjacent bone of the lacrimal fossa, calcification in the tumour and extension of the mass outside the lacrimal gland area as demonstrated on CT scan. In addition to showing the size and extent of the tumour in the orbit, CT may demonstrate calcification, when not revealed by conventional techniques (*Fig.* 8). Early bone

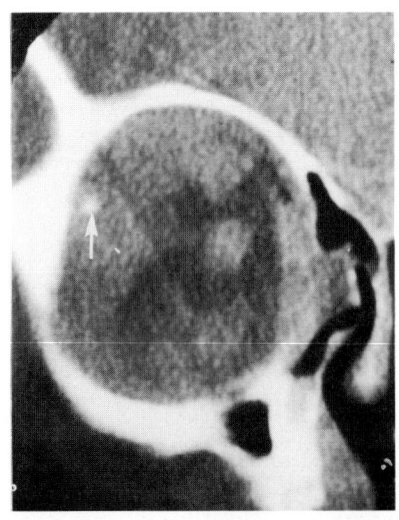

Fig. 8. Lacrimal gland carcinoma. There is a localized nidus of calcification (arrow) within the tumour mass. This was only demonstrated by CT scan.

erosion is also demonstrable at an early stage if high resolution CT is employed.[14]

Neoplastic involvement of the lacrimal gland may also be due to lymphoma. These tumours occur in an older age group than the epithelial tumours and on plain X-ray show minimal enlargement of the lacrimal fossa in approximately 50 per cent of patients, the rest showing no abnormality. The CT changes are also non-specific: either a simple enlargement of the lacrimal gland or a more widespread change as described above in the discussion of lymphoma.

Inflammatory Conditions in the Orbit

Acute Infection

Orbital cellulitis results from acute bacterial infection which in most patients is secondary to sinus infection, usually an ethmoiditis or maxillary antritis. A dental abscess may be the initial cause in some instances.

Diagnosis

In the author's series two-thirds of patients showed obvious sinus infection on plain X-ray, and very occasionally gas and a fluid level may be visible within the orbital soft tissues, indicating the presence of abscess formation. Computerized tomography will also show associated sinus infection with or without fluid levels in the sinuses. It is also useful to distinguish between pre-septal cellulitis, a less serious infection, and true orbital cellulitis, when the clinical diagnosis is in doubt.[15] In addition to the presence of sinus infection adjacent to the affected orbit, CT may show widening of the extraconal space between the ethmoids and the periorbita due to oedema or abscess formation. In addition, local rectus muscle enlargement due to extension of the inflammatory process may be demonstrated. It is important to localize abscess formation when it is present. Unequivocal evidence is provided when there is soft tissue gas with or without a fluid level. Ring enhancement after intravenous contrast will also suggest abscess formation.

Chronic Infection (Orbital and Retro-orbital Pseudotumours)

The name of pseudotumours has been given to a group of cases which are difficult to differentiate clinically from an orbital tumour but which on pathological investigation have proved to be of chronic inflammatory origin. Pseudotumours of the orbit present a difficult nosological problem as they are a spectrum of different conditions rather than a single entity. They occur throughout the orbit from the region of the lacrimal gland to the orbital apex and present very different signs and symptoms according to their position.

Diagnosis

Plain X-ray examination seldom shows any significant abnormality in the affected orbit, but some patients with pseudotumours show an associated clouding of the nasal sinuses due to infection or nasal polyposis. One other feature that may occur in the more posteriorly placed granulomas is an enlargement of the sphenoidal fissure. This has been observed in three patients and has been recorded by other authors.[16] In one instance it was associated with slight enlargement of the optic canal. On orbital venography, pseudotumours may produce a displacement of the venous system in the orbit, but the most characteristic venographic feature is a venous block, usually in the second or third part of the superior ophthalmic vein.[17] Positive evidence of an increased soft tissue density within the orbit may also be obtained by CT scan. Characteristically the changes are those of an infiltrative lesion, with an irregular ill-defined edge and variable density.

Analysis of a series of 61 patients with histologically proved pseudotumours showed that the lesions occurred with equal frequency in an anterior or posterior location in the orbit. Twenty-eight per cent were associated with enlargement of one or more rectus muscles and 16 per cent associated with sinus infection. In addition, one-third showed a diffuse mass in the orbital apex which is the characteristic location for these inflammatory processes. Although a similar appearance can be demonstrated in some patients with metastases or lymphomas, a mass filling the orbital apex with local muscle enlargement is very suggestive of this condition.

REFERENCES

1. Taybi H. Ocular calcification and retrolental fibroplasia. *Am. J. Roentgenol.* 1956; **76**, 583.
2. Lloyd G. A. S. A technique for the arteriography of the orbit. *Br. J. Radiol.* 1969; **42**, 252.
3. Vritsios A. Méthode de phlébographie des veins ophthalmiques, des veins de la face et des vaisseaux superfices du crâne. *Arch. Soc. Ophth. Grèce du nord* 1961; **12**, 223.
4. Brismar J., Davis K. R., Dallow R. L. et al. Unilateral endocrine exophthalmos: diagnostic problems in association with CT. *Neuroradiology* 1976; **12**, 21–24.
5. Henderson J. W. *Orbital Tumours*, Philadelphia, Saunders, 1973.
6. Dilenge D. Arteriography in angiomas of the orbit. *Radiology* 1974; **113**, 355.
7. Lloyd G. A. S., Wright J. E. and Morgan G. Venous malformations in the orbit. *Br. J. Ophthalmol.* 1971; **35**, 505.

8. Wright J. E. Orbital vascular anomalies. *Trans. Am. Acad. Ophth. Otol.* 1974; **78,** 606.
9. Lloyd G. A. S. Vascular anomalies in the orbit: CT and angiographic diagnosis. *Orbit* 1982; **1,** 45.
10. Hanafee W. N. Orbital venography. *Radiol. Clin. North Am.* 1972; **10,** 63.
11. Pfeiffer R. L. and Nicholl R. J. Dermoids and epidermoid tumours of the orbit. *Arch. Ophthalmol.* 1948; **40,** 639.
12. Jones I. S., Reese A. B. and Kraut J. Orbital rhabdomyosarcoma: an analysis of 62 cases. *Am. J. Ophthalmol.* 1966; **61,** 721.
13. Jacobiec F. 1983 Personal communication.
14. Lloyd G. A. S. Lacrimal gland tumours: the role of CT and conventional radiology. *Br. J. Radiol.* 1981; **54,** 1034.
15. Krohel G. B., Krauss H. R. and Winnick J. Orbital abscess. *Ophthalmology* 1982; **89,** 492.
16. Lombardi G. *Radiology in Neuro-ophthalmology* 1967; Baltimore, Williams and Wilkins.
17. Lloyd G. A. S. *Radiology of the Orbit*, Philadelphia, Saunders, 1975.

Electrodiagnosis

N. R. Galloway

All cells in the body exhibit bioelectrical potentials; that is, there is a difference in potential between the inside and the outside of the cell. This potential difference may be modified by some stimulus acting on the cell or by activity of the cell itself. The summed activity of groups of cells can often be recorded at a site remote from the source. We can, for example, place electrodes on the skin over the chest and record the electrical activity of the heart. When measuring the electrical activity produced by a sense organ it is necessary to stimulate the sense organ and measure the changes in relation to the stimulus. It has not been possible to measure spontaneous electrical activity which occurs during the act of seeing. By flashing a light or pattern in front of the eyes it is possible to detect and measure activity in the retina from electrodes placed on or near the eye, and in the occipital cortex from electrodes placed on the back of the scalp.

Such measurements have now become part of the clinical routine in many centres and it is becoming recognized that they can provide important information about the function of the visual pathway. The results of this type of test have the great advantage of being purely objective, but it must be borne in mind that they may be modified by 'disease' in the equipment as well as disease in the patient. To date the equipment for this type of test has been expensive and bulky and there has been a risk that the tests could become too divorced from the clinical scene, particularly if they are performed in isolation with no attendant medical staff.

The electrical changes produced by sensory stimulation are called 'evoked responses'. Strictly speaking there are three types of evoked response which are useful in the ophthalmic clinic. The electroretinogram (ERG) and the electro-oculogram (EOG) both arise from the eye itself, and the visually evoked potential, or VEP, arises from the occipital cortex and its neighbouring regions.

The size of these potentials is very small. The ERG and EOG may measure in the region of 0·5 mV (500 μV), the VEP is in the region of tens of μV. Our ability to measure smaller and smaller potentials with accuracy accounts for most of the clinical advances to date and there does not seem to be any limit to similar progress in the future.

THE ELECTRORETINOGRAM

There is a potential difference between the cornea and the posterior pole of the eye amounting to about 1 mV. This is known as the corneo-retinal potential and it was first described in the middle of the last century.[1] This potential is modified by the action of light and the resulting waveform is known to arise in the retina. The response to a brief flash of light is known as the electroretinogram, whereas the response to a prolonged light stimulus over many minutes is known as the electro-oculogram.

Method of Recording

The stimulus is an illuminated bowl which projects diffuse light into all parts of the fundus. The intensity of the light and the frequency and duration of flashes should be variable. In most clinics the pupils are dilated with a mydriatic and this certainly gives more controlled results in young normal subjects. In an elderly subject the pupil response to mydriatics may be variable, especially when the eye is diseased, and useful results can be obtained without resorting to mydriasis. The main electrode is often placed on the cornea itself in the form of a contact lens and the other electrode is positioned on the cheek. The contact lens electrode is beginning to be replaced by 'wick' electrodes in the conjunctival sac or skin electrodes on the eyelid. They give smaller responses than the contact lens.[2]

The minute responses obtained by any of these electrodes must be magnified before they are large enough to move the arm of a pen recorder and they are first fed through an amplification system. When very small responses are being recorded it is necessary to use an averaging computer which literally averages successive responses, giving one clear-cut response from a number of barely detectable ones.[3]

The Nature of the Response

A normal ERG is shown in *Fig.* 1. The important features of the waveform are the initial a-wave which is negative followed by the positive b-wave. The b-wave is disturbed by a ripple of three or four small wavelets known as the oscillatory potential. The time relationships and amplitudes should also be noted in *Fig.* 1. It is important to realize that the ERG is a mass response arising from large numbers of cells throughout the retina. The ERG as normally recorded may be unaffected by small areas of focal damage to the retina. The waveform shown in *Fig.* 1 is thought to be the sum of at least three different signals. These are firstly a slow negative wave arising from the inner segment of the receptors, and secondly a more rapid though slightly delayed positive wave arising from the Mueller cells. A third positive wave, which may be seen after the b-wave is thought to arise from the pigment epithelium. This part of the ERG is known as the c-wave and it is not usually recorded in the clinic by the methods at present in use.

Much work, both clinical and experimental, has been devoted to an investigation of the source of the ERG. Such investigations have involved the comparison of animals with predominantly rod retinae with those with cone retinae, the selective poisoning of different layers of the retina and the insertion of microelectrodes to different depths in the retina.[4] The wavelets on the b-wave appear to have a separate origin from the b-wave, and it has been suggested that they reflect feedback circuits in the inner retina.[5] The wavelets can be selectively abolished in animals by clamping the retinal circulation and a similar effect is seen in man after central retinal artery occlusion and in severe diabetic retinopathy.[6,7] One other component of the ERG can be demonstrated before the a-wave. This is called the early receptor potential (ERP). A very bright stimulus and special recording techniques are needed to produce it and its interest arises in the fact that it is thought to come from the outer segment of the receptors.

It is evident that the ERG arises from parts of the retina distal to the ganglion cells. Thus a normal ERG may be recorded from an eye with advanced optic atrophy provided that the outer layers of the retina are intact.

Factors Influencing the Response

The Stimulus

Fig. 2 shows how the waveform changes with intensity of the stimulus. As a brighter light is used, the a-wave continues to increase in size, whereas the b-wave reaches a maximum. The latency of the peaks shortens and the position of the wavelets on the b-wave changes. If a flickering light stimulus is used with a frequency of 30 Hz, then the resulting ERG is thought to arise mainly from the photopic neural mechanism since the response frequency of the scotopic neural mechanism does not exceed 20–25 Hz. At higher frequencies the ERG loses its characteristic waveform and becomes sinusoidal and eventually disappears as the electrical flicker fusion frequency is reached. Unfortunately, the use of a small focal stimulus does not elicit a localized ERG because light is scattered in the media, and for this reason a wide field is generally used in the clinic.[8] A recent attempt to produce a focal stimulus seems to have been more successful. In this technique a 4° white stimulus was projected through an ophthalmoscope.[9]

Over the past few years a considerable interest has arisen in the use of a patterned stimulus. If a recording is made while the patient is viewing a checker board of black and white squares which alternate successively and therefore give no overall luminance change, then a small response (about one μV) is obtained. Unlike the *flash* ERG, this response is often reduced on the side of the affected eye in patients with amblyopia and there is other evidence to suggest that it may arise in the ganglion cell layer.[10,11]

The Recording Equipment

Inadequately positioned electrodes or faulty connections can distort or abolish the response. To avoid

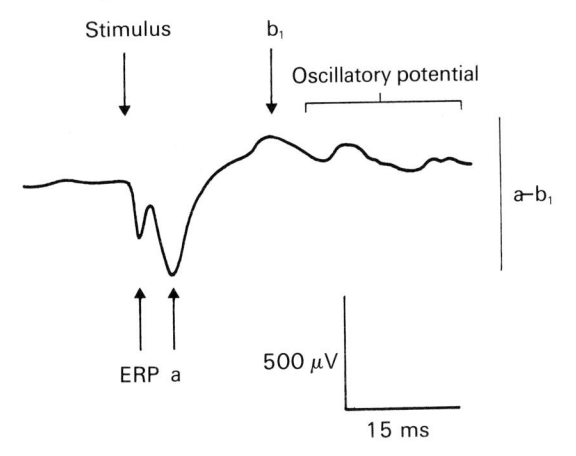

Fig. 1. A bright flash ERG showing the various components that can be recorded in the clinic. The ERP (Early Receptor Potential) is only seen with a bright flash. (*After* Galloway N.R. *Ophthalmic Electrodiagnosis.* London, Lloyd-Luke, 1981, p. 13.)

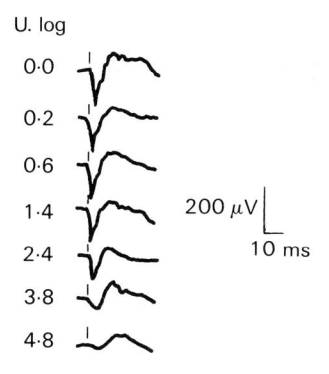

Fig. 2. The effect on the ERG of altering the strength of the light stimulus. Filters of increasing density have been placed in front of the flash from above downwards. The intensity of flash for the top trace is rather less than that for *Fig.* 1.

error every recording should be accompanied by an indication of the amplifier settings, and a calibration signal should be used.

Dark Adaptation

The ERG increases in size during dark adaptation. It also undergoes a change in waveform, the b-wave becoming slower and more rounded in the dark adapted state. These changes are thought to be due to the varying contribution of rod and cone components. Stimulation with red light under light adapted conditions favours the photopic ERG and stimulation with a subcone threshold blue light under dark adapted conditions favours the scotopic response.[12]

reduction in the amplitude of the ERG at an early stage in the disease process. The reduction in amplitude is out of proportion to the ophthalmoscopic changes and in some instances the ERG may be abnormal when the fundus appears normal. There is a relationship between the area of functioning retina and the ERG.[13] So far the ERG cannot indicate the prognosis or the inheritance pattern in an individual with retinitis pigmentosa, although studies of rod and cone responses have shown some promise[14-16] in this respect. An absent or very small ERG can therefore be useful confirmation of the diagnosis (*Fig.* 3*b*), but at present the test cannot be used to give a prognosis. In the case of children with suspected Leber's amaurosis, the ERG can play a more important primary

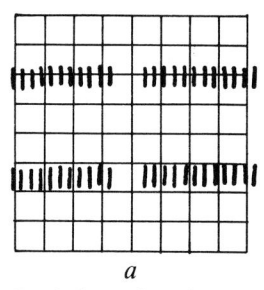

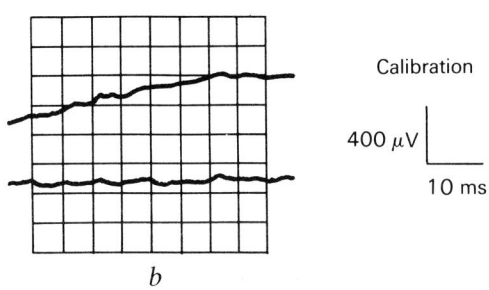

Fig. 3. Recordings from a patient with retinitis pigmentosa. *a*, A representation of the EOG. Each of the small vertical bars represents the size of the corneo-retinal potential. They have been recorded every minute. No change in potential is noted even though the lights are switched on at the point where there is a gap in the bars (q.v.). *b*, The lower trace shows the ERG with no response to light. (*After* Galloway N. R. *Ophthalmic Electrodiagnosis.* London, Lloyd-Luke, 1981, p. 91.)

Age and Sex

A small ERG can be elicited within hours of birth if a strong stimulus is used, but the ERG does not reach its adult value until the age of about 2 years. In adult life the size of the ERG gradually declines and it is slightly larger in women than in men.

The Effect of Disease on the Response

The ERG in response to a flash (but probably not to a pattern) arises from the receptors and bipolar cells in the retina. The ganglion cells may be damaged with associated optic atrophy and yet the ERG can be normal. Thus after optic nerve section the eye is blind with a normal ERG. The ERG in response to a flash is a mass response and focal areas of retinal damage such as senile macular degeneration may not be shown up by the ERG unless special stimuli are used. The ERG is therefore of most use in detecting diffuse retinal disease, either due to retinal dystrophy or the effect of drugs. A normal ERG can be recorded in the presence of dense opacities in the optical media and thus the value of the ERG is enhanced when the fundus is obscured in this way.

Inherited Retinal Degenerations

Patients with retinitis pigmentosa show a marked

diagnostic role and it should always be included in the examination under anaesthesia when the disease is suspected.

The ERG has also been used to detect female heterozygous carriers in families with sex linked recessive retinitis pigmentosa. Although the response to flicker and the size of the b-wave is affected in 50 per cent or more of these patients, the test is still not very successful in making the diagnosis in a given individual.

Other retinal degenerations have also been investigated by electroretinography; for example patients with choroideraemia and gyrate atrophy also show a disproportionate reduction of the response, as do patients with the progressive form of retinitis punctata albescens. Myopia is known to reduce the size of the ERG, a fact that needs to be considered when obtaining a series of 'normal' patients, and degenerative myopes may give very poor responses.

Diabetic Retinopathy

It has been known for some years that the oscillatory potential of the ERG is selectively abolished in patients with diabetic retinopathy (*Fig.* 4). The disappearance of these wavelets seems to reflect retinal ischaemia because a similar effect is seen in retinal vascular occlusion. The recording of the ERG in juvenile diabetics with a disease duration longer than 5 years has been shown to be valuable for the identification of those at risk for the development of proliferative retinopathy.[17]

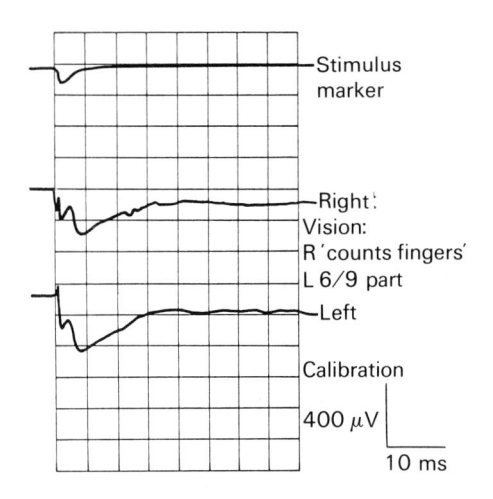

Fig. 4. The ERG in a patient with advanced diabetic retinopathy. Note that the ERG is a mass response and does not in any way reflect visual acuity. Note that the oscillatory wavelets are barely visible.

Retinal Detachment

When the retina becomes detached there is an immediate reduction in the size of the b-wave coincidental with the loss of vision. The amount of reduction of the b-wave depends on the extent of the detachment.[18,19] Apart from giving an indication of the extent of the detachment, the ERG may also give some guide to the surgical prognosis.[20] Examination of the fellow eye in detachment cases may also have some prognostic value.[19,21] Once the retina has been replaced surgically, the ERG also shows a gradual recovery, but this may lag behind the visual recovery. It is useful to perform electroretinography when a detachment is suspected behind a vitreous haemorrhage or when remnants of lens capsule obscure the view in a case of suspected aphakic detachment. It is important to remember that the ERG can be recorded even in the presence of dense opacities in the media, and providing that the stimulus is sufficiently bright, the response should be normal in the absence of disease.

Occlusive Vascular Disease of the Retina

When the retinal circulation is clamped experimentally in monkeys, the b-wave is reduced but the a-wave may increase in size. A more striking change is the disappearance of the oscillatory potential and this is seen both in monkeys after experimental occlusion of the retinal circulation and in man after occlusion of the central retinal artery.[7] Similar but less marked changes are seen in cases of central retinal vein occlusion (*Fig.* 5) and there is some promise that the ERG may help to predict those cases liable to develop neovascularization.

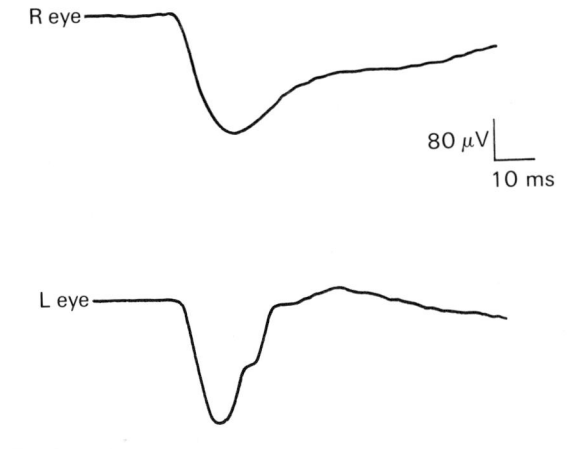

Fig. 5. ERG from each eye of a patient with a right central retinal vein occlusion.

The ERG and Injury to the Eye

The value of the ERG for the injured eye has been limited by lack of clinical data. The sparsity of such information may have been due to the difficulty in applying the test to a severely injured and painful eye. Many of the technical difficulties can now be overcome by replacing the traditional contact lens electrode by a cotton wick or gold/mylar one and obtaining the average of several responses. After blunt trauma or perforating wounds the ERG may initially be abolished. Within a few days this may recover, depending on the extent of the injury. In general it seems that when the response remains poor the prognosis is poor and such results may be useful when a view of the fundus is obscured.[22-24] Specific changes in the ERG in eyes suffering from siderosis bulbi were originally described by Karpe[25] and they have been confirmed by others. Karpe described the earliest changes in siderosis as 'negative plus', meaning a relative increase in the size of the a-wave. Subsequently the size of the b-wave diminishes giving a 'negative minus' type of response. Eventually the ERG becomes extinguished.

The ERG in Toxic and Deficiency States

Certain drugs; particularly those stored in the pigment epithelium, which are toxic to the eye, may cause alterations of the response, sometimes before there is any clinical evidence of toxicity. Chloroquine toxicity in particular may be detected in this way.[26,27] Many other drugs and poisons have been shown to produce abnormal electrical responses from the eye. These include quinine, lead, the phenothiazines, indomethacin and several others.

Indications for Electroretinography

These may be summarized as follows:
1. The confirmation or exclusion of the diagnosis of retinitis pigmentosa and related conditions.
2. The investigation of macular degeneration in children.
3. The investigation of vitreous haemorrhage.
4. The assessment of diabetic fundi, especially in the early stages of diabetic retinopathy when the media are opaque.
5. As a means of monitoring the possible toxicity of certain drugs.
6. In combination with the VEP to investigate unexplained poor vision.

THE ELECTRO-OCULOGRAM

If electrodes are placed on the skin of the medial and lateral canthi, electrical changes can be recorded when the eyes are moved from side to side. These electrical changes occur because the eye acts as a rotating dipole, as if it were a battery rotating in a conducting medium. When the eye is adducted the nasal electrode becomes more positive because the positive cornea moves towards it. The study of such changes is known as electro-oculography. Passive movements of the anaesthetized eye give the same response, demonstrating that muscle action potentials are not involved.

The recording of these changes has been widely used to monitor eye movements. The potential changes recorded can be shown to be proportional to the sine of the angle of deviation, but they are also influenced by any change in the size of the corneo-retinal potential. If the size of the eye movements is kept constant by asking the subject to move the eyes between two fixed points, then the recorded electrical changes become more closely related to the corneo-retinal potential.

The usual methods for recording the ERG are only suitable for measuring rapid responses and they become less accurate when attempting to measure slow long term changes of the corneo-retinal potential over minutes or hours. The technique of electro-oculography has been introduced into this field in order to allow the measurement of long term variations of the corneo-retinal potential in response to prolonged light stimuli.

If these electrical changes recorded from medial and lateral canthi are written out on paper as the eyes are moved from side to side, then each horizontal movement is represented by a saw-toothed deflection. When the eye movements are kept constant by using fixation lights and the patient is seated in a darkened room, the size of the saw-toothed deflections becomes smaller. If the lights are then switched on, the deflections increase in size over a period of about 7 minutes and then start to become smaller again even though the lights are still switched on. When the eyes are exposed to constant illumination after a period of darkness, the corneo-retinal potential shows slow rises and falls over a period of hours, taking the form of a damped oscillation. The measurement of the initial fall in the dark and subsequent rise in the light is the basis of a clinical test. A ratio is made of the lowest reading in the dark and the highest reading in the light. This ratio has become known as the Arden index. If the illumination of the retina during the period of light is kept at 20 000 scotopic trolands, the Arden index in normal subjects is between 2·5 and 3·0. The EOG is thought to arise from the pigment epithelium but its mode of production is not understood.

As a general rule those conditions which cause a reduction in the size of the b-wave of the ERG also produce a reduction in the value of the Arden index. For example, striking abnormalities are seen in the inherited retinal degenerations (*see Fig. 3a*), and the light rise is abolished by a total retinal detachment. An early reduction in the size of the light rise has been described in chloroquine retinopathy. The usual finding of parallel changes in the ERG and EOG probably reflects the generally diffuse nature of many forms of retinal pathology, but some exceptions are well recognized. For example, patients with vitelliform macular degeneration often show a striking reduction of the EOG in the presence of a normal ERG. From the practical point of view there are some situations where the EOG is simpler to perform than the ERG; for example, where no skilled assistance is available and where a contact lens or wick electrode cannot be tolerated, the EOG may be considered less upsetting to the patient. On the other hand, the EOG requires a cooperative patient because of the need for constant eye movements. When a patient is blind and cannot fix a light then the EOG is not easy to record with any accuracy. The electro-oculogram can now be fully automated and as such makes a useful back-up test for the electroretinogram.[20,28-30]

THE VISUALLY EVOKED POTENTIAL

The term visually evoked potential, or VEP, is currently used to refer to the electrical changes that can be recorded from the back of the scalp when the eyes are being stimulated by a flashing light or flashing pattern stimulus. In fact all the responses described in this chapter are 'visually evoked'. Electrical changes can also be evoked by other forms of sensory stimulus such as sounds, smells or stimulation of peripheral nerves. The changes evoked in the brain by visual stimuli were recorded in animals directly from the surface of the pia mater in the 1930s.[31] At that time it was realized that the alpha rhythm, seen on normal electroencephalographic traces, could be accentuated or 'driven' by exposing the eyes to a light flashing at the same frequency. When the eyes were exposed to flashes repeated at a frequency different from the alpha rhythm, then the electrical changes recorded from scalp electrodes became small and more or less lost against the normal spontaneous activity of the brain. The problem of detecting these small electrical responses was largely solved by the introduction of signal averaging. This ingenious technique, which involves the computer analysis of a large number of responses to consecutive flashes, allows the display of any waveform that is related to the stimulus, and eliminates unwanted background noise.

Method of Recording the VEP

The VEP is now measured routinely in many eye clinics throughout the world but its full clinical value is probably yet to be realized. Recording techniques are by no means standardized and the results from normal subjects vary considerably. Although some interesting facts about the response in disease have come to light, it is not often possible to make firm deductions about an individual case on the strength of the VEP alone. In order to record a VEP, four groups of equipment are needed. First a repeated visual stimulus is required. Second, electrical contact with the patient's scalp must be achieved by means of suitable electrodes. Third, electrical changes in these electrodes must be magnified by a suitable system of amplifiers. Fourth, an averaging computer and read out system is needed to display the information obtained.

The Stimulus

This may be presented as a diffuse flash of light or it may be a repeated pattern on a TV screen. The pattern is usually in the form of black and white chessboard squares whose size can be adjusted. Both these types of stimulus can also be varied in terms of luminance and frequency of presentation. It is important to distinguish between pattern reversal and pattern appearance because each may produce a very different response. In the case of pattern appearance a black and white checker board is presented in an on–off sequence, whereas with pattern reversal the luminance of the black and white squares is reversed alternately. It is also important to distinguish between a rapidly repeated stimulus and a slowly repeated stimulus. The rapidly repeated stimulus produces a sinusoidal type of response, referred to as the 'steady state' response. Stimuli repeated less than two or three times a second produce a characteristic waveform known as the 'transient' response.

The Electrodes

These must make good contact with the skin of the scalp, be electrically inert and have a low electrical resistance. Silver coated silver chloride electrodes are popular, a layer of electrode jelly being placed between electrode and scalp. Fitting the electrodes takes time and patience and is best performed by an experienced technician. The standard 'ten-twenty' system of electroencephalographers provides a useful variety of positions, although some prefer to state electrode positions as direct measurement from the inion. In practice, the choice of electrode position depends on the particular aspect of the VEP being investigated.

Amplification and Read Out

Each year improvements occur in the design and function of electronic equipment and one or two good systems designed specifically for the electrodiagnostic clinic are now available. It is useful to have a computerized protocol so that the technician has to give answers to questions and instructions which are printed on a video screen. In this way the type of stimulus is chosen and, when the recording is complete, the trace appears on the screen and is then printed out on paper together with all the details of stimulus parameters and calibration. At the same time a permanent record can be made on disc, the printed read out being kept in the patient's notes.[32]

The Normal VEP

The character of the normal VEP depends upon the type of stimulus being used and the position on the scalp from which it is being recorded (*Fig.* 6). It also varies greatly from one individual to another. In spite of this, reliable features, particularly of the transient response to a checker board stimulus, are beginning to be identified. In general three peaks are distinguishable: a positive peak at 70–100 ms, a negative peak at about 100–130 ms and a second positive peak at about 150–200 ms. This last positive peak is often prominent in pattern stimulus records and is especially sensitive to changes in contrast. The timing of these peaks depends on the exact nature of the stimulus and the position of the scalp electrodes. The response to a plain flash is smaller and less well defined and cannot easily be compared to a pattern response. Two important features of the normal VEP must now be considered.

1. Because of the relatively large macular representation on the occipital cortex, the response is mainly derived from the central few degrees of the retina. If the subject looks to the side of the stimulus there is a rapid fall off in size of response.

2. The nature of the response varies as the check size of a patterned stimulus is altered. In most subjects the transient response increases in amplitude as the checks become smaller, reaching a peak when the checks subtend about 15′ arc at the eye.[33] Although this can now be shown in trained normal subjects, it is not easy to demonstrate in the clinic with elderly patients.

We know therefore that the VEP bears some relationship to the visual acuity but some otherwise normal patients have very small responses. The recent interest in measuring vision by contrast sensitivity

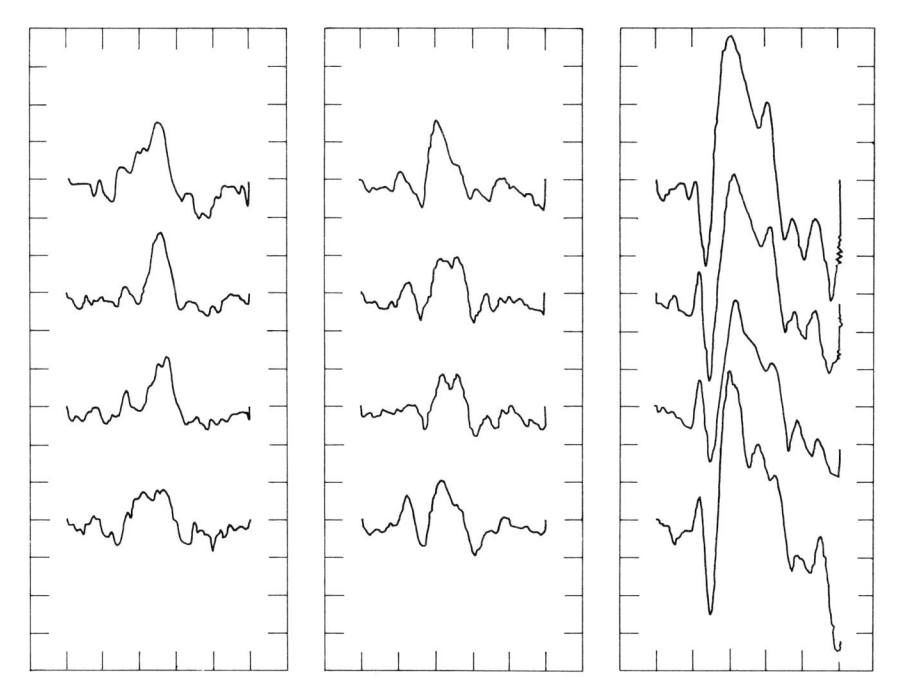

Fig. 6. The normal VEP. The traces are from three different subjects and were recorded from a single electrode immediately above the inion. Top trace, binocular; second, right eye; third, left eye; lower trace, repeat binocular. It can be seen that although the responses are typical for the individual, they vary considerably. These are responses to a pattern onset stimulus. Each vertical division represents 5 μV and each horizontal division 100 ms.

gratings has been accompanied by an interest in the response of the VEP to the same stimulus and here there may be a better correlation.[34,35] It seems likely that with better recording techniques and better means of obtaining the attention and proper fixation of the patient, the VEP will show more accurately the state of the central part of the visual field.

The VEP has also been used in attempts to make an objective assessment of refractive error,[36] but the method is no more accurate and is more expensive and cumbersome than other methods.

Factors Influencing the VEP

Age and Sex

The child's VEP is characteristically large and it has been shown that the amplitude reaches a peak in 5–8-year-olds. After a slight decline, a further increase occurs in the early 'teens and after this a gradual decline is seen over the years.[37,38] Sex differences in the responses are less evident, although in childhood males may have slightly larger responses whereas females have slightly larger responses in adult life.

Disease

RETROBULBAR NEURITIS

Abnormalities of the VEP in retrobulbar neuritis were described by Halliday in 1972.[39] It soon became apparent that careful measurement of the latency of the response was a good way of detecting previous attacks. Sometimes the VEP is the only remaining evidence of this. Because retrobulbar neuritis is often the first demyelinating episode of patients with disseminated sclerosis, the VEP can help to clinch the diagnosis when the next episode appears in some other part of the body. This delay in the response is not specifically seen in demyelinating disease and other possible causes of an altered response, such as amblyopia or macular disease, must be excluded.[39–41]

AMBLYOPIA OF DISUSE

The response to a patterned stimulus is abnormal from eyes with amblyopia, be it due to squint or anisometropia (*Fig.* 7). The response to a flash stimulus is usually normal from such eyes. Furthermore, when the amblyopic eye of a child is treated by occluding the other eye, the improvement in vision can be monitored by noting the corresponding improvement in the VEP. Subjective testing of visual acuity in children is not always easy and the VEP has unexploited possibilities in this field.[42–44]

HOMONYMOUS HEMIANOPIA

It has been shown that when a half field stimulus is used, a larger response may be obtained from electrodes placed over the *ipsilateral* hemisphere. That is to say the VEP is larger over the part of the occipital cortex which is not 'seeing' the stimulus. Such results are consistently found only if pattern reversal stimulation is used and the electrodes are placed in a transverse chain 5 cm above the inion and 5 cm apart. When half field stimuli are used in hemianopic patients the same paradoxical lateralization is evident, and furthermore it has been demonstrated in a patient who had undergone an occipital lobectomy. The rather surprising finding that a larger response is obtained over the inert hemisphere has been explained by the fact that the response originates from the medial and posteromedial surface of the cortex where neurones are transversely orientated. Whatever the explanation, the VEP promises to be a reliable test for hemianopia in children or elderly subjects.[45,46]

GLAUCOMA

Quite successful attempts have been made to relate VEP changes to loss of visual field in patients with glaucoma. A purely objective test for field changes could prove useful when the question of surgery may depend on deciding whether field loss has progressed. Using steady state VEPs to pattern reversal stimulation, clear cut alterations in phase and amplitude of the VEP have been demonstrated in patients with glaucomatous field defects. It must be remembered that the VEP reflects central rather than peripheral damage to the field and it may give erroneous responses when the field loss is mainly peripheral.[47,48] This explains why in some individual patients there seem to be discrepancies between the VEP and the amount of field loss.

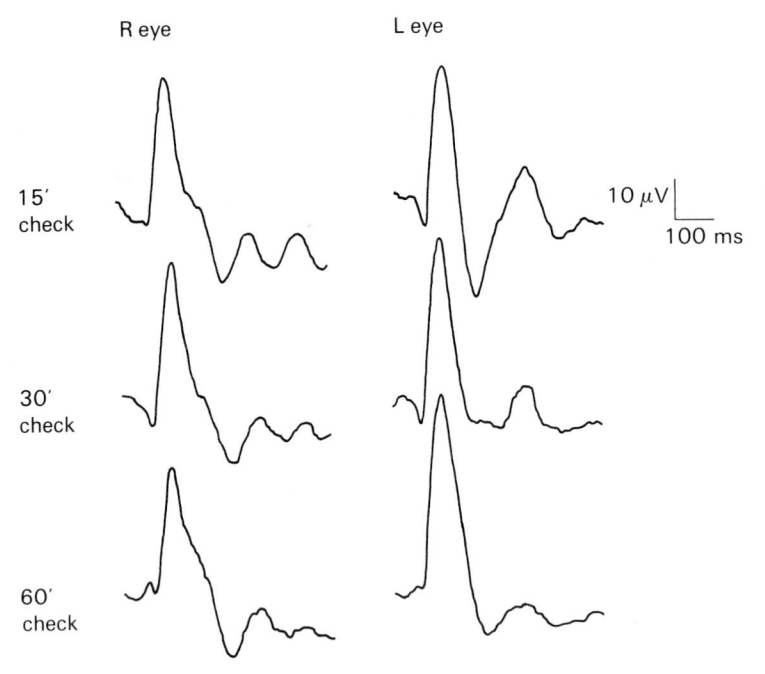

Fig. 7. The VEP recorded from each eye of a patient with right sided amblyopia in association with a squint. Note that the difference is most evident to the 15' check stimulus. Note also the late 'double hump' response.

HYSTERICAL AMBLYOPIA AND MALINGERING

There is no doubt that the VEP can be very useful in providing confirmatory evidence that the visual pathway is intact in these patients. The result can be affected if the patient deliberately defocuses or refuses to fix the centre of the stimulus pattern. A characteristic of hysterical responses seems to be large variations in the response from moment to moment. The first half of the test may produce an absent VEP and the second half a normal one.

Other Clinical Applications

It is possible to monitor the function of the optic nerve during orbital surgery by means of the VEP. The test has also been used alongside the ERG in order to help assess the prognosis before removing opaque media from the eye. The medicolegal value of the VEP has been stressed in post-traumatic cases. Visual disturbances following head injury are sometimes found in the absence of other clinical signs of residual injury and abnormal VEPs have been demonstrated in some of these patients.

Indications for Performing the VEP Test

These may be listed as follows:
1. The elucidation of unexplained visual loss.
2. The assessment of visual acuity in amblyopes.
3. The detection of *healed* retrobulbar neuritis.
4. The detection of hemianopia in difficult cases.

REFERENCES

1. Du Bois Reymond E. *Untersuchungen über thierische Elektricitat.* Berlin, Reimer, 1849, pp. 256–7.
2. Arden G. B., Carter R. M., Hogg C. et al. A gold foil electrode. Extending the horizons for clinical electroretinography. *Invest. Ophthalmol. Vis. Sci.* 1979; **18,** 421.
3. Van Lith G. Quantitative evaluation of the electroretinogram. *Ophthalmologica* 1981; **182,** 218–23.
4. Tomita T. and Yanagida T. Origins of the ERG waves. *Vis. Res.* 1981; **21,** 1703–7.
5. Wachtmeister L. Further studies of the chemical sensitivity of the oscillatory potentials of the electroretinogram (ERG). *Acta Ophthalmol.* 1980; **58,** 712–25.
6. Brown K. T. In: Straatsma B., Hull M., Alba R. et al. (ed.) *The Retina; Morphology, Function and Clinical Characteristics.* University of California Forum for Medical Science, University of California Press, 1969, pp. 319–68.
7. Stangos N., Rey P., Meyer J. et al. Averaged electroretinogram responses in normal human subjects and ophthalmological patients. In: Wirth A. (ed.) VIII Symposium of ISCERG. Pisa, Pacini, 1970; 277–304.
8. Armington J. C. In: *The Electroretinogram.* New York, Academic Press, 1974, p. 384.
9. Jacobson S. G., Sanberg M. A., Effron M. A. et al. Foveal cone electroretinograms in strabismic amblyopia. *Trans. Ophthalmol. Soc. UK* 1979; **99,** 353–6.
10. Arden G. B., Vaegan D. T., Hogg C. R. et al. Pattern ERGs are abnormal in many amblyopes. *Trans. Ophthalmol. Soc. UK* 1980; **100,** 453–60.
11. Seiple W. H. and Siegel I. M. Recording the pattern electroretinogram: a cautionary note. *Invest. Ophthalmol. Vis. Sci.* 1983; **24,** 766–99.
12. Adrian E. D. The electric response of the human eye. *J. Physiol. (Lond.)* 1945; **104,** 84.
13. Armington J. C., Gouras P., Tepas D. et al. Detection of the electroretinogram in retinitis pigmentosa. *Exp. Eye Res.* 1961; **1,** 74–80.
14. Arden G. B., Carter R. M., Hogg C. R. et al. Rod and cone activity in patients with dominantly inherited retinitis pigmentosa: comparisons between psychophysical and electroretinographic measurements. *Br. J. Ophthalmol.* 1983; **67,** 405–18.
15. Berson E. L., Gouras P., Gunkel R. D. et al. Rod and cone responses in x linked retinitis pigmentosa. *Arch. Ophthalmol.* 1979; **81,** 215–25.
16. Massof R. W. and Finklestein D. Rod sensitivity relative to cone sensitivity in RP. *Invest. Ophthalmol. Vis. Sci.* (ARVO abstracts), 1979; **18,** 263.
17. Larsen K. M., Larsen H. W. and Simonsen S. E. Oscillatory potential and nyctometry in insulin dependent diabetics. *Acta Ophthalmol.* 1980; **58,** 879–88.
18. Blach R. K. and Behrman J. The electrical activity of the eye in retinal detachment. *Trans. Ophthalmol. Soc. UK* 1967; **87,** 263.
19. Rendahl I. The clinical electroretinogram in detachment of the retina. *Acta Ophthalmol.*, 1961; **64,** 1–83.
20. Lobes L. A. The electro-oculogram in human retinal detachment. *Br. J. Ophthalmol.*, 1978; **62,** 223–6.
21. Tamai A. Electrophysiological studies on the fellow eyes of patients with idiopathic retinal detachment. II: Scotopic ERG findings. *Fol. Ophthalmol. Jpn.* 1977; **28,** 816–19.
22. Jayle G. E., Tassy A. F. and Ghnassia J. P. Intérêt pronostique de l'éléctrorétinogramme dans les traumatismes oculaires graves récents avec fond d'oeil invisible. *Bull. Soc. Ophthalmol. Fr. (Paris)* 1967; **67,** 685–90.
23. Gliem H., Moller D. E. and Kietzmann G. The prognostic value of ERG and EOG in blunt contusion of the globe. *Ophthalmologica (Basel)*, 1971; **163,** 411–17.
24. Crews S. J., Thompson C. R. S. and Harding G. P. A. The ERG and VEP in patients with severe eye injury. *Doc. Ophthalmol. Proc. Ser.* 1978; 15.
25. Karpe G. Early diagnosis of siderosis retinae for the use of electroretinography. *Doc. Ophthalmol. (Kbh)* 1948; Suppl. 100, pp. 1–66.
26. Arden G. B. and Fojas M. R. Electrophysiological abnormalities in pigmentary degenerations of the retina. *Arch. Ophthalmol.*, 1962; **68,** 369.
27. Kubota Y., Kubota S. and Asanigi I. The ERG of chlorquine in clinical retinopathy: The prognostic significance of abnormalities in the ERG. *Doc. Ophthalmol. Proc. Ser.* 1978; **15,** 95.
28. Arden G. B. and Kelsey J. H. Changes produced by light in the standing potential of the human eye. *J. Physiol. (Lond.)* 1962; **161,** 189–204.
29. Van Lith G. and Balik J. Variability of the electro-oculogram. *Acta Ophthalmol. (Kbh)*, 1970; **48,** 1091–6.
30. Galloway N. R. and Barber C. Automated electro-oculography. *Trans. Ophthalmol. Soc. UK* 1973; **93,** 269–75.
31. Fischer M. H. VEP from pia mater. I. Elektrobiologische Erscheinungen an der Hirnrinde. *Pflüg. Arch. Ges. Physiol. Mensch. Tiere* 1932; **230,** 160.
32. Billings R. J. Automatic detection, measurement and documentation of the visual evoked potential using a commercial microprocessor equipped averager. *Electroencephal. Clin. Neurophysiol.* 1981; **52,** 214–17.
33. Regan D. *Evoked Potentials.* London, Chapman and Hall, 1972, p. 109.
34. Parker D M., Salzen E. A. and Lishman J. R. Visual evoked response elicited by the onset and offset of sinusoidal gratings: latency, waveform and topographic characteristics. *Invest. Ophthalmol. Vis. Sci.* **22,** 675–80.
35. Riggs L. A. ERG, VER and psychophysics. *Doc. Ophthalmol. Proc. Ser.* 1977; **15,** 3–12.
36. Regan D. Rapid objective refraction using evoked brain potentials. *Invest. Ophthalmol.*, 1973; **12,** 669.
37. Dustman R. E., Schenkenberg T. and Beck, E. C. In: Rathe Kaner (ed.) *Developmental Psychophysiology of Mental Retardation.* Springfield, Ill., Thomas, 1976.

38. Sokol S., Moskowitz A. and Towle V. L. Age related changes in the latency of the visual evoked potential: Influence of check size. *Electroencephal. Clin. Neurophysiol.* 1981; **51,** 559–62.
39. Halliday A. M., McDonald W. I. and Mushin J. Evoked response in optic neuritis. *Lancet* 1972; **1,** 982.
40. Asselman P., Chadwick D. W. and Marsden C. Visual evoked responses in diagnosis and management of patients suspected of multiple sclerosis. *Brain* 1975; **98,** 261.
41. Lennerstrand G. Delayed visual evoked cortical potentials in retinal disease. *Acta Ophthalmol.* 1982; **60,** 497–504.
42. Arden G. B. and Bernard W. M. Effect of occlusion on the visually evoked response in amblyopia. *Trans. Ophthalmol. Soc. UK* 1979; **99,** 455–6.
43. Odom J. V., Hoyt C. S. and Marg E. Eye patching and visually evoked potential acuity in children four months to eight years old. *Am. J. Optom. Physiol. Optics* 1982; **59,** 706–17.
44. Sokol S. Pattern visual evoked potentials; their use in paediatric ophthalmology. *Intern. Ophthalmol. Clin.* 1980; **20,** 251–67.
45. Blumhardt L. D., Barrett G., Halliday A. M. et al. The asymmetrical visual evoked potential to pattern reversal in one half field and its significance for the analysis of visual field defects. *Br. J. Ophthalmol.*, 1977; **61,** 454–61.
46. Onofrj M., Bodis Wollner I. and Mylin L. Visual evoked potential diagnosis of field defects in patients with chiasmatic and retrochiasmatic lesions. *J. Neurol., Neurosurg., Psychiatr.* 1982; **45,** 294–302.
47. Cappin J. and Nissim S. VER in assessment of field defects in glaucoma. *Arch. Ophthalmol. (Chicago)* 1975; **93,** 9.
48. Ermers H. J. M., De Heer L. J. and Van Lith G. H. M. VECPs in patients with glaucoma. *Doc. Ophthalmol. Proc. Ser.*, 1974; 4 (XIth ISCERG Symposium), pp. 387–93.

Chapter 4

External Diseases

Peter Wright

DEFENCES OF THE OUTER EYE

The outer eye is a very good model of defence mechanisms, which can be broadly divided into two – physical protection and cellular and humoral protection. Physical protection is the gross and absolute protection offered by the lids, lashes, tears and epithelium of the cornea and conjunctiva.

Cellular and humoral protection is molecular and relative depending upon tear and tissue fluid constituents and cells present in the normal or inflamed conjunctiva.

Physical Protection

The lids play a major part in the protection of the outer eye, and loss of lids or impairment of their function leads to eventual loss of the eye by exposure and infection.

Effective lid function and closure requires:
- Normal lid height.
- Normal lid movement.
- Normal muscle tone.
- Normal blinking and reflex movements.
- Normal contour (even a small notch may be significant).

Functional shortening of the lids results from levator fibrosis and tarsal shrinkage in conditions such as trachoma, chemical burns and erythema multiforme, though many chronic inflammatory diseases can involve tarsus and levator.

The scarring process in the conjunctiva can also produce entropion with trichiasis and dry eyes and a combination of these increases the threat to the outer eye. Thus defects of lid closure, together with damage to the corneal epithelium from trichiasis and entropion with dry eyes, all combine to become a potent cause of potentially preventable blindness in hyperendemic trachoma in rural areas.

Tears and the precorneal tear film help maintain the normal conjunctival and corneal epithelial cells and the barrier that they offer. The fluid also serves a mechanical washing and diluting purpose. The mucoid components in the fluid act as a sticky trap for any particulate matter or debris which is then transferred by blinking into the mucus thread of the lower fornix and finally extruded into the inner canthus. Other tear constituents have more specific effects. These include the lipid, which has a spreading effect because of its surface activity and so stabilizes the tear film and conserves moisture. The mucus coats the epithelial surfaces, rendering them hydrophilic, and enables the complex precorneal tear film, which will be described later, to be formed and to remain stable. Lysozyme and non-lysozymal antibacterial factors are present with interferon to combat bacterial and viral infections. Antibodies may be naturally present in the tears or develop as part of the response of the outer eye to infection or antigenic challenge. Similarly a range of cells, including polymorphs, macrophages and lymphocytes, is seen and greatly increased in response to bacterial or viral stimuli. An intact layer of corneal and conjunctival epithelium is an important physical and functional barrier. The epithelium together with the tear constituents, including inflammatory cells, combine to produce the outermost line of defence.

The limbus is a specialized area of conjunctiva, having a greater number of multipotential cells and acting as an immunologically highly reactive site, comparable to a local lymph node.

Humoral Protection

This is provided by the four classic immunoglobulins found in tears and the periocular fluid.

1. IgG, the classic opsonizing, immobilizing, agglutinating, precipitating and complement fixing antibody, accounts for 80 per cent of all the antibody present in blood. Of the total IgG present in the body, 50 per cent is found in blood and 50 per cent in mucous membranes such as the conjunctiva.

2. IgM is a big molecule which protects intravascular spaces. It is normally only present in low concentration in tears but is often the first detectable antibody response, and in some infections may be the continued main response.

3. IgA is the protective antibody of mucous membranes generally, accounting for only 15 per cent of the total antibody in blood, but again 50 per cent is present in tissue, especially mucous membranes.

The ratio of IgG/IgA in tears is 1:5.

Secretory IgA (exocrine IgA) is a dimer, that is two molecules of IgA joined together by a non-immunoglobulin secretory piece. The production of the secretory piece and formation of the dimeric form occurs in the lacrimal gland. The dimeric form is more stable and resistant to digestion by acids and enzymes and so is important for the protection of the gut and mucous membranes generally from microbial infection.

4. IgE is normally only present in very small amounts in tears or blood. It is the 'reaginic' antibody of immediate hypersensitivity which, by fixing to basophils and mast cells, causes their degranulation with release of a great number of inflammatory mediators, including histamine, serotonin and the prostaglandin series.

Very high levels of IgE are characteristically found in tears and blood of patients with atopic disease and its conjunctival manifestations.

Different mechanisms of inflammation can occur in the conjunctival sac in response to widely varying stimuli.

Physical agents such as dust, sand or ice particles and radiations such as ultraviolet light produce a different response to chemical insults, whether simple chemicals or the complex radicals such as superoxides released by bacteria and inflammatory cells. Viruses and chlamydial agents again produce different patterns of reaction and repeated infection or concurrent bacterial infection may modify the response. Finally, immunogenic mechanisms may be primarily or secondarily involved in the inflammatory processes and may significantly influence the outcome. Recognition of these patterns of response is an important clinical aid to diagnosis and with practice it becomes possible not only to appreciate the obvious superficial hyperaemia, papillary or follicular changes in the conjunctiva, but also to observe and quantify the amount of cellular infiltration, vessel proliferation and fibrovascular activity present.

PATTERNS OF INFLAMMATORY RESPONSE IN THE CONJUNCTIVA

Hyperaemia of the conjunctiva is the first response and is seen with all types of irritation and inflammation. Passive hyperaemia also occurs most often in association with orbital and arteriovenous malformation. Change of blood flow within such a mass of abnormal blood vessels may produce sudden unilateral hyperaemia accounting for a red eye without any other signs of inflammation.

Oedema rapidly follows hyperaemia and varies greatly in amount depending on the type of inflammatory response, being greatest in IgE mediated hypersensitivity reactions. This is probably due to the type of mediators released and their effect on vascular endothelium. Haemorrhages may also occur as a result of the endothelial damage. Oedematous conjunctiva appears thicker and may bulge out between the lids (chemosis). It is, however, possible to see through the swollen conjunctiva and to observe the normal pattern of vessels within the conjunctiva and also in the tarsal conjunctiva, the deep, vertically running vessels lying on the surface of the tarsal plates.

Cellularity of the conjunctiva causes swelling and opalescence, which obscures first the deeper vessels and then the more superficial ones until finally only the surface pattern of the conjunctiva is recognizable, usually thrown up into an exaggerated variation of the normal. These superficial changes are the classic papillary and follicular responses which need to be carefully differentiated for diagnostic purposes. The normal conjunctiva contains fine vascular tufts which run vertically to the surface and become dilated and obvious in the early stages of inflammation. Following more prolonged irritation or inflammation, the vessel tufts become the central core of thickened polygonal tufts of tissue known as papillae. Variable degrees of cellular infiltration occur within these papillae and also, with time, hyalinization, to produce the typical chronic compound papilla seen in vernal conjunctivitis (*Plate* II*a*).

Follicles are clearer white or yellow aggregations of tissue found within the epithelium and having blood vessels around their periphery rather than centrally. Lymphoid tissue is absent from the conjunctiva at birth and rapidly develops within the first few weeks of life in response to exogenous antigenic stimuli (*Plate* II*b*). Thereafter resting nests of lymphoid cells remain within the normal conjunctiva but are quickly activated by any topical antigenic stimulus such as molluscum virus or drugs like eserine.

Finally, the fluid transudate within the tissue, with inflammatory cells and desquamated epithelial cells, combine to make the discharge that is the usual accompaniment of conjunctivitis and which, when examined as a conjunctival smear under the microscope, yields valuable clues to diagnosis.

LABORATORY AIDS TO DIAGNOSIS OF EXTERNAL EYE DISORDERS

Aids of value are bacterial culture, examination of discharge, conjunctival smears, scrapings and impressions, viral isolation and viral and chlamydial serology.

Bacterial cultures play little part in the management of the common type of bacterial conjunctivitis, which responds to topical antibiotic therapy in 48 h, but are essential in diagnosis and management of all cases of neonatal conjunctivitis, membranous conjunctivitis and suppurative keratitis. The latter, together with postoperative endophthalmitis, require first class microbiological investigation of special specimens taken by scrapings of the corneal lesions, anterior chamber and vitreous aspiration. Cultures from lid margins are essential in the long term management of the more severe forms of blepharitis, especially when associated with corneal or conjunctival hypersensitivity, since resistance of the organisms and development of contact dermatitis frequently occur and demand a change of therapy. Cultures taken with dry cotton tipped applicators yield few colonies or no growth, which is very rarely correct for any lid margin. Yield of organisms is greatly improved by moistening the swabs with tryptic digest broth or transport medium immediately before use. Other techniques such as alginate or Dacron swabs have no advantage over suitably moistened cotton tipped swabs. It is desirable whenever possible to avoid the use of topical anaesthetics when taking samples for culture since both the anaesthetic agents and the preservative in the drops can inhibit growth of susceptible organisms.

Conjunctival scrapings are really misnamed. The examination of the discharge from an inflamed eye may yield useful clues to the aetiology, and the clues are increased if some superficial conjunctival cells are included. These may be obtained by lightly rubbing the edge of a blunt platinum spatula against the everted anaesthetized palpebral conjunctiva. In some conditions cytology of specimens obtained from the fornix or from the limbus may be of value, as in trachoma and vernal disease respectively. Whatever the instrument used to obtain the sample, it should be blunt, and while moderate pressure may be needed to obtain a representative sample of cells, care should be taken to avoid any bleeding. This indicates excessive trauma to the conjunctiva and the red cells obscure other cellular detail in the final preparation. The material obtained on the scraper is smeared in a thin layer on a clean, degreased glass slide fixed in alcohol and stained with Geimsa's stain. For identification of bacteria or fungi Gram stain is preferable, and so for most cases at least two smears should be prepared. Cell types are noted and roughly quantified. Inclusions, if present, may be diagnostic (*Table I*).

Viral isolation is rarely helpful in establishing the diagnosis in unexplained conjunctivitis but may be of value if herpes is grown or not grown from corneal epithelial lesions resembling, but not typical of, dendritic figures. Facilities for chlamydial isolation are now often available at regional centres because of the increased incidence of chlamydial genital disorders. Isolates, however, are not easy to obtain from conjunctival swabs, especially later in the course of the disease, and serology of tears and blood are of more diagnostic help.

BLEPHARITIS AND BLEPHAROCONJUNCTIVITIS

Chronic low grade inflammation of the lid margin and appendages is one of the commonest problems in external eye disease. While it is not usually sight-threatening, the conjunctival and corneal complications can prove very painful and cause visual impairment.

Table I. Cytology

Cells	Differential diagnosis
Polymorphonuclear response	Bacterial Fungal Neonatal chlamydial Any severe membranous conjunctivitis
Mixed polymorph and lymphocytic response	Adult chlamydial infection
Lymphocytic response	Adenovirus Herpes simplex Epidemic haemorrhagic KC Molluscum 'Toxic' conjunctivitis from topical medication
Other diagnostic findings	*Diagnosis*
Mixed polymorph and lymphocyte response with plasma cells, Leber cells, giant cells and cytoplasmic inclusions	Established chlamydial infection
Eosinophils	Vernal disease Atopic KC Hay fever conjunctivitis Mucous membrane pemphigoid
Keratinized cells	Conjunctival epidermalization, dry eyes xerophthalmia, established mucous membrane pemphigoid

Seborrhoeic Blepharitis

This is the most obvious and least troublesome of the lid margin disorders. It is usually part of a generalized picture of seborrhoea (*Plate IIc*), with changes in skin folds and creases elsewhere and signs of scalp and eyebrow seborrhoea. The lids typically show waxy scaling of the margins with unsightly crusting, but few if any signs of inflammation of the lids or the conjunctiva. Attention to the seborrhoea elsewhere with simple cleansing of the lid margins with sodium bicarbonate lotion usually controls the problem. Secondary infection with staphylococci may increase the local irritation and redness and then a topical antibiotic ointment such as chloramphenicol 1 per cent at night is helpful. Such ointment should be applied sparingly to the lid margin and lash-bearing area only. There is no value to inserting the ointment into the conjunctival sac, which is invariably sterile in these cases, and the hydrophobic effect of the ointment base only serves to render more unstable the tear film which may already be compromised by the hydrophobic debris and epithelial squames.

Staphylococcal Blepharitis (Plate IId)

Chronic staphylococcal infection of the lid margin can involve either the anterior part of the lid margin, including the lash follicles, or the posterior part, including the meibomian glands.

Infection of the anterior part is usually with *S. epidermidis* or coagulase-negative strains. Erythema of the lid margin with crusting and exudate around the base of the lashes occurs with a very variable amount of irritation and few signs in the conjunctival sac. Sometimes coagulase-positive staphylococci are present and then localized ulceration occurs around the base of the lashes, each of which may then be located in a small collection of pus. This type of infection is prone to produce permanent scarring of the lid margin, persistent damage to the lash follicle and increased conjunctival and corneal signs.

Posterior lid margin disease involves the meibomian glands and is almost invariably associated with conjunctival and corneal signs. The clinical picture ranges from localized lid margin findings only to gross changes involving the skin of the lids and face, which comprise the typical features of acne rosacea. For the lesser changes in which lid margins, meibomian glands and conjunctiva or cornea only are involved without facial skin, the term 'ocular rosacea' has been used. This proves a helpful concept since treatment with oral low dose long term antibiotics as for acne rosacea is the only effective management.

In its milder forms, the changes seen are mainly a hyperaemia and telangiectasia of the skin of the intermarginal strip, which also becomes greasy or waxy in appearance. The meibomian gland openings become abnormal (*Plate* IIe) and the appearances vary between complete obliteration of the openings and exaggeration of the opening with a heaping up of the area and a central plug of white material. This is made up of keratinized epithelial cells and meibomian material which is probably abnormal in composition. Pressure on the lid over the tarsal glands produces either abnormal opaque cheesy material or nothing can be expressed. In the more advanced forms of the disorder multiple meibomian cysts develop and there is a loss of the sharp posterior lid margin, which becomes rounded. This is due to a quiet cicatricial change in the conjunctiva, producing a first or second degree entropion in which the lid margin is turned inward toward the surface of the globe so that the meibomian gland openings are dipped into the precorneal film and marginal meniscus or come directly into contact with the cornea and conjunctiva.

These mechanical changes in lid contour produce further disturbance of the outer eye by direct irritation and also by increasing the instability of the precorneal tear film. The pathological processes responsible for the changes are not fully understood, but it is suggested that the infection of the meibomian glands by staphylococci and other organisms producing bacterial lipases results in production of irritant and surface active compounds, including free fatty acids, which induce metaplasia of the lining epithelium of the meibomian glands, chronic irritation of the conjunctiva and disruption of the normal lipid layer of the tear film.

Phlyctenular Conjunctivitis

This condition occurs throughout the world and has historically been associated with poverty, malnutrition and tuberculosis. It presents as an ulcerated nodule in the conjunctiva associated with local hyperaemia and conjunctival cellularity, always in children, and more often girls than boys. It occurs in all climates but is said to be more common in spring and summer.

The clinical findings are distinctive and consist of a localized area of conjunctival hyperaemia in the centre of which develops a small white nodule (*Plate* II*f*). After a few days the centre of the lesion becomes necrotic and ulcerates through the conjunctiva, whereafter the lesion regresses leaving no trace. Phlyctens most often develop at the limbus but can occur anywhere in the bulbar conjunctiva and on the plica or caruncle. Phlyctenular keratitis is the comparable entity in the cornea, where marginal corneal nodules, infiltrates or ulcers may develop. Unlike the conjunctival lesions the corneal type is always followed by scarring and peripheral vascularization. Recurrences of the corneal lesions may occur at different points around the limbus, leading to a circumferential scarring and pannus, which if it extends to involve the central cornea may profoundly reduce vision. Conjunctival phlyctens give rise to few symptoms, but corneal lesions are very distressing, causing pain, lacrimation, blepharospasm and photophobia. Corneal or conjunctival lesions may develop in recurrent disease in the same patient, but not usually both together.

Swabs from the corneal and conjunctival lesions, even when ulcerated, show no bacteria and the condition is believed to be a hypersensitivity response of the type IV cell mediated immune kind. The lesions are therefore comparable to the bacterids of dermatology, in which skin nodules that do not contain bacteria develop but are an immune response to sensitization by an infection elsewhere, i.e. tuberculid in TB, monilid and trichophytid in monilidial and trichophyton infection. While tubercle was previously considered the commonest cause, staphylococcal lid disease is now thought to account for most cases. In some areas where parasitic worm infestations of the gut are common, phlyctenular disease may result from ocular challenge with antigen from ground-up ova in dust blowing into the eyes of patients with gut infestation and circulating antibodies to the parasite.

Sometimes the corneal phlyctens are indistinguishable from the corneal lesions of acne rosacea, further strengthening the concept of a spectrum of disease involving hypersensitivity to lid margin infection extending from simple blepharitis to florid acne rosacea.

Treatment of phlyctenular disease is with dilute topical steroid, which produces rapid resolution of symptoms and signs. Topical antibiotics play no part unless a purulent discharge suggests secondary bacterial infection. For patients with clinical signs of staphylococcal lid disease oral tetracycline or erythromycin may be indicated both to control the present attack and to prevent recurrences, particularly in corneal phlyctenulosis or the rosacea-like syndrome.

Staphylococcal Hypersensitivity

The concept of a hypersensitivity reaction to bacterial exotoxins, products of inflammation and disordered meibomian secretion is used to explain the conjunctival and corneal lesions which are seen in patients with active blepharitis. Swabs from the conjunctival sacs or corneal lesions in these cases are invariably sterile and there is no benefit from topical antibiotics but often subjective relief from topical steroids.

The findings, apart from the lid changes, are usually of a hyperaemic, cellular conjunctiva with a predominantly follicular response involving mainly the lower fornix. Conjunctival cytology reveals mainly lymphocytes and conjunctival cultures are sterile. Tryptic digest swabs from the lid margins are needed to establish the pattern of organisms present and will usually grow coagulase-negative staphylococci including *S. epidermidis*. This must be considered a pathogen in many ocular disorders, capable of causing suppurative keratitis and endophthalmitis and cannot be considered as a non-pathogenic commensal in many external diseases. Antibiotic sensitivity testing is essential because the *S. epidermidis* is often resistant to many antibiotics and previous prolonged topical therapy may have altered the sensitivity pattern. The cultures may also reveal unexpected mixed infections, including Gram-negative organisms.

Treatment of staphylococcal lid disease usually requires systemic therapy. Anterior lid margin changes may respond to topical therapy with antibiotic ointment alone, although some of these patients are staphylococcus carriers with evidence of staphylococcal folliculitis elsewhere and may require dermatological help and systemic treatment.

Gross meibomian abnormalities, such as cysts, need incision and curettage; local steroid injection has proved disappointing. The mainstay of treatment then is low dose oral antibiotics, usually tetracycline or oxytetracycline. For children prior to eruption of the permanent teeth, and in some adults with resistant organisms or lack of clinical response, oral erythromycin is indicated. Rarely a cephalosporin is required.

The normal dosage is 250 mg b.d. taken before food, avoiding milky drinks and antacids which may chelate or prevent absorption of the tetracyclines. The treatment needs to be continued for a minimum of 6 weeks, no effect usually being seen before 10 days. Treatment may be reduced to 250 mg daily for long term treatment, which may need to be indefinite if recurrences occur when treatment is stopped. For the conjunctival and corneal manifestations of staphylococcal hypersensitivity a topical steroid is helpful in bringing the condition more quickly under control. Provided the underlying lid margin disease is being treated, only dilute steroids are needed such as prednisolone 0·1 per cent o.d. or b.d., and can be discontinued within a few weeks while the oral treatment continues.

TOPICAL STEROID THERAPY

Topical steroids are widely used (and abused) in treatment of external eye disorders and serve a useful purpose in suppressing unwanted inflammation. Because of the risk of adverse reactions, such as steroid glaucoma viral and fungal enhancement and lens changes, it is desirable to use as little steroid as possible. Most of the inflammatory processes are very sensitive to steroids, which can be used in much weaker concentrations than normally employed. Steroid ointments are in general to be avoided because they provide large, long persisting, unquantified amounts of steroid and also apply high concentrations of steroid to the skin of the lid margin where adverse effects, including dermal atrophy and loss of pigmentation, may result.

The aim of treatment should be to use the minimum amount of topical steroid necessary and to taper the treatment as the inflammation improves. This is difficult using commercial, single strength preparations but is facilitated by use of a range of steroid drugs made up in semilog dilution series as shown in *Table* II. The starting point on the scale and frequency of instillation is based on a subjective assessment of the severity of inflammation (amount of

Table II. Moorfields series of semilog dilution of guttae prednisolone

Prednisolone 1%
Prednisolone 0·3%
Prednisolone 0·1%
Prednisolone 0·03%
Prednisolone 0·01%
Prednisolone 0·003%
Prednisolone 0·001%

hyperaemia, oedema, cellularity, etc.), and with reduction in any of these signs, the next weaker dilution is used until the treatment is discontinued. For long term treatment of disorders such as stromal keratitis it becomes easier to choose the exact level of treatment required at any time and to avoid most of the adverse reactions.

TEAR PRODUCTION AND DISORDERS OF THE PRECORNEAL FILM

Tears are produced by the main lacrimal gland and the accessory lacrimal tissue (known as the glands of Krause and Wolfring). A basic tear flow of 1–2 μl min^{-1} is normally produced and with reflex irritation or stimulation a flow many hundred times greater can be produced to dilute and wash away the irritant. The basic tear secretion is no longer thought to be the product of the accessory lacrimal tissue only and the whole mass of tissue is thought to respond as one unit to a varying stimulus from the outer eye and mediated by the parasympathetic nervous system alone. Sympathetic terminals are present in the lacrimal gland, but not associated with secretory acini, and no secretor motor function for them has been shown in man. Tears contain a number of proteins and other substances with more specific activity, forming part of the outer eye defences.

The tears flow from the lacrimal gland over the surface of the eye to be drained by the lacrimal puncta, and in doing so follow closely defined and limited pathways. The periocular fluid can be shown to exist in a number of functional subdivisions of static and moving tears when the movement of the fluid is revealed by introducing carbon particles or dyes into each area. The first of the functional subdivisions is in the upper and lower fornices and brought about by the close apposition of the lid margins above and below to the surface of the globe

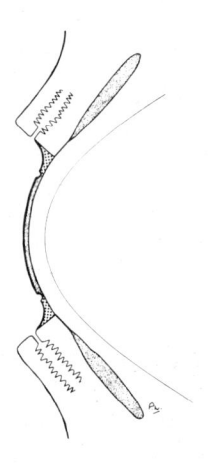

Fig. 1. Functional subdivision of the periocular fluid showing precorneal film, marginal meniscus and meniscus induced thinning.

(*Fig.* 1); the second comprises the marginal tear strip separated by the meniscus induced thinning from the third, the precorneal film (*Fig.* 2). During blinking all these areas are freely intermixed but immediately following a blink the tear fluid settles into these three areas and no further mixing occurs until the next blink. Tears from the lacrimal gland flow into the outer part of the upper fornix and then into the outer end of the upper marginal tear strip from whence they flow along the upper and lower marginal strips to drain into the upper and lower puncta. These marginal tear strips are roughly triangular in cross-section, with a concave meniscus on the anterior surface. This meniscus and the flow along the lid edge induces a linear thinning along the upper edge of the strip to define the central zone of tears, the precorneal film.

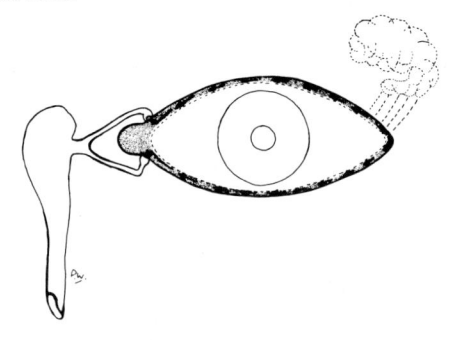

Fig. 2. Tear flow along upper and lower marginal strips.

Precorneal Film

This is a layer of fluid lying in front of the cornea and providing the optically perfect anterior surface for it. The film consists of a stable layer of fluid 5–8 μm thick which is laid down and renewed by every blink and which results from a unique series of physicochemical interactions between the corneal surface, mucous glycoproteins, fluid from the lacrimal gland and the meibomian secretion. The film is made up of three component parts: a deep mucous layer, a middle watery layer and a superficial lipid monolayer on the surface. Mucus, or more correctly a number of mucous glycoproteins, play an essential role in rendering the normal epithelial surface hydrophilic by lowering the surface tension below the critical point at which wetting can occur. The human corneal epithelium has on its surface very fine tufts and ridges known as microvilli and microplicae. The pattern of villi or plicae differs from species to species but is invariably present and can be seen on all corneal epithelial cells as they approach the surface. The individual microvilli are coated by a glycocalyx which is a product of the epithelial cell itself and this surface is then coated in turn by mucus derived from the goblet cells in the conjunctiva.

Goblet cells are present in all areas of the conjunctiva and in flat mount preparations have been shown in greatest density in the region of the plica semilunaris and in the lower nasal quadrant of the bulbar conjunctiva. They contain granules which histochemically have been shown to be sulphomucins and sialomucins comparable to those found in goblet cells of gut and bronchus. There also exists a non-goblet cell mucus system derived from the conjunctiva and also from the lacrimal gland. Within the superficial cells of the conjunctiva sub-surface membrane-bound vesicles can be shown with the same histochemical staining properties as goblet cells. An increase in these vesicles is said to occur in vernal conjunctivitis, contact lens induced papillary conjunctivitis and following sensory denervation. These changes may account for some of the apparent increase in mucus production seen with these disorders, but little is known about the factors controlling production and release of conjunctival or goblet cell mucus. The precise composition of ocular mucus and the ratio of sulphomucin to sialomucin have not been determined, but there is some evidence to suggest a shift towards sulphation following any chronic inflammation or irritation of the conjunctival sac. The possible effect of this change in composition of the mucus on viscosity and other physicochemical properties is not known.

The watery component of the tears is the product of the lacrimal gland and comprises a dilute solution of glycoprotein with other specific components already described. For the formation of the normal tear film this production of a watery glycoprotein solution is essential and resting tears can be shown to have a viscosity two to three times that of normal saline. The dissolved mucous glycoprotein comes from the lacrimal gland where histochemical and electron microscopic studies have shown individual acini to contain pure serous or mucous granules or a mixture of each. Again the factors influencing the release of these mucous glycoproteins into the tears are not known. Studies on the wetting properties of tears and tear substitutes have shown the potency of mucus to render the corneal epithelial surface water wettable, but this wettability is constantly threatened by the potential interaction of the surface lipid layer with the epithelium. It is suggested that the lipid normally covers the tear film, reducing evaporation, and contributes to the formation of the film after a blink by dragging some aqueous tears with it (Marangoni effect).

If the tear film thins, either by local evaporation of fluid or because of a surface elevation of the epithelium, surface lipid is able to come into contact with the cornea and renders the surface hydrophobic, producing the clinical picture known as break-up of the tear film. This is best demonstrated by instilling fluorescein into the tears and observing the precorneal film between blinks. Any surface irregularity will cause a constant recurring pattern of break up of the film revealed as dark areas in the green fluorescing film (*Plate* IIIa). With normal epithelium the break up seen is irregular and variable in onset. Break up time has been suggested as a measure of tear film stability and possibly an index of mucus production but has been shown to be unreliable and of no reproducibility. A non-invasive method employing a reflection of a circular grid pattern from the corneal surface, avoiding all drops or contact with the eyes, promises to give more consistent readings and may be a useful measure of tear film stability.

Tear film break up is probably the physiological stimulus to blinking, tear secretion and re-surfacing of the eye. In the presence of a persisting epithelial abnormality such recurring break up probably also plays a part in the subsequent pathology (as in Salzmann's nodular degeneration and metaplasia on pterygia).

Lipid Abnormalities

Lipid abnormalities or deficiencies are not well defined but irritable eyes with unstable precorneal film are seen as part of the picture of some forms of ectodermal dysplasia in which the lid margins are hypoplastic and the meibomian glands absent or malformed.

In blepharitis, especially that involving the posterior part of the lid with meibomitis, tear film instability is seen and thought to account for the epithelial keratitis across the lower part of the cornea seen in these patients. Excess mucus production probably rarely occurs but disordered mucus plays a part in several clinical entities.

DISORDERS OF MUCUS PRODUCTION

Mucus deficiency has been suggested as a cause of tear film instability and a reduction of goblet cell numbers has been shown in a wide range of disorders including chemical burns, trachoma, mucous membrane pemphigoid, most forms of cicatrizing conjunctivitis and keratoconjunctivitis sicca. Many of these disorders, however, are clinically associated with apparent excess of tenacious mucus and it is not known whether the mucus is altered in composition, simply less hydrated or altered in its physicochemical characteristics by changes in tear electrolytes and osmolarity.

Recent studies of the morphological characteristics of the epithelium and its associated glycocalyx have shifted the emphasis toward the corneal surface rather than the absorbed layer of mucus in interpretation of tear film instability problems.

Filamentary Keratitis

This is a disorder in which mucous strands attach to epithelial 'receptor' sites. The eyes may be wet or dry and the epithelial disturbance may be due to drying, as in keratoconjunctivitis sicca, disordered lid movements, as in involuntary blepharospasm, or to infection or other agents, as in adenovirus keratitis or the superficial punctate keratitis of Thygeson–Braily. In all these disorders the filament formation occurs generally over the surface of the cornea, stops at the limbus and never occurs on the conjunctiva, to which the mucous strands appear unable to attach.

In keratoconjunctivitis sicca the filaments tend to be present in the most exposed part of the interpalpebral area and are found mainly across the lower third of the cornea. In Theodore's superior limbic keratoconjunctivitis the filaments are found adjacent to the upper limbus and on the upper third of the cornea. The condition is poorly understood and consists of an intense papillary conjunctivitis affecting the upper fornix only, with redness of the upper bulbar conjunctiva, heaping up of the tissue at the upper limbus and filament formation on the upper part of the cornea in one-third of cases. The upper bulbar conjunctiva has been shown to be abnormal with disturbance of the normal microvillous pattern and squamous metaplasia. Thyroid dysfunction has been found in a proportion of cases but not all.

Treatment of filamentary keratitis is firstly the treatment of the underlying cause if possible, i.e. tear replacement for dry eyes, prevention of blepharospasm etc.; but since the filaments give considerable pain by traction on epithelial nerve endings, symptomatic treatment with acetylcysteine drops 10 or 20 per cent is often required. These drops sting, smell unpleasantly and are rather unstable. They dissolve excess mucus and give considerable relief of pain in many cases. If they do not do so, a suitable therapeutic soft contact lens may be tried, usually of medium to low water content, and will often give dramatic subjective relief by physically preventing mucus attachment to the cornea, though surface spoilation and mucus under the lens may preclude long term wear.

Superficial Mucous Plaques

These occur in dry eyes and also as part of the superficial keratitis seen in vernal disease. A coarse net-like arrangement of mucus occurs over the surface of the cornea and overlies an epithelial keratitis, (Plate IIIb). The mucus stains weakly with fluorescein but strongly with rose bengal, and is dissolved by quite weak acetylcysteine drops with improvement in signs and symptoms.

Vernal Plaques

Vernal plaques are uncommon oval-shaped lesions which develop on the upper part of the cornea as a late, chronic stage of uncontrolled vernal keratitis associated with active vernal disease (Plate IIIc).

The plaque appears to be an aggregation of mucus and fibrin forming an organized lamellar structure, which is histologically distinctive but does not give the histochemical staining reactions for mucous glycoproteins. Acetylcysteine has no effect on the plaque and treatment consists of vigorous treatment of the vernal conjunctivitis with topical steroids and sodium cromoglycate and careful surgical removal of the plaque by very superficial keratectomy. Intensive topical steroid therapy is continued until the epithelium is fully healed.

Ligneous Conjunctivitis (Plate IIId)

This rare disorder is most often seen in children but sometimes affects adults. It may follow acute conjunctivitis or surgical trauma to the conjunctiva, and results in dense membranous masses most commonly on the tarsal conjunctiva, sometimes involving all four lids and rarely the bulbar conjunctiva. Other mucous membranes, including genital and respiratory, may be the site of deposition of similar material. Removal of the membrane is always followed by recurrence. Pathological studies of the excised material have shown a characteristic histological picture of hyalinized connective tissue with much fibrin and inflammatory cells and mast cells. Treatment in the past has been unrewarding, but treatment with chromones, steroids and anti-fibrin agents following surgical removal has been of value.

FOLLICULAR CONJUNCTIVITIS (Table III)

Follicular hypertrophy of lymphoid tissue in the conjunctiva develops after birth and reaches its peak in preadolescent children. It is often referred to as folliculosis, implying enlargement without pathology,

Table III. Follicular conjunctivitis

Viruses	Herpes simplex
	Adenovirus
	Picornavirus
	Epstein–Barr virus
	Molluscum contagiosum
	Herpes zoster
	Influenza
	Newcastle virus
Chlamydia	Trachoma
	Paratrachoma
	Zoonoses – psittacosis
	– feline pneumonitis
	– cat scratch fever
Other infective agents	Actinomyces
	Vincent's organism
	Streptococci, Moraxella
Topical medication	Eserine, epinephrine (adrenaline), DFP, idoxuridine

and is comparable to the generalized lymphoid hyperplasia of the upper respiratory tract also seen at this age. While the latter may represent a response to chronic infection with a number of agents, including adenoviruses, no comparable causative agent has been found in the conjunctiva of these children. The follicles are usually present in the lower fornix and along the upper border of the tarsal conjunctiva towards the medial and lateral ends. Other signs of conjunctival inflammation such as hyperaemia and cellularity are conspicuously lacking and no treatment is indicated. Other enthusiastic attempts at treatment with topical antibiotics frequently add a toxic, allergic or irritative component which confuses the picture.

Acute Follicular Conjunctivitis (Plate IIIe)

This sudden inflammation of the conjunctival sac usually involves first one eye and then the other. It is sometimes associated with systemic features such as fever, malaise and regional adenopathy, and with a variable keratitis. The commonest causative agents are viruses, but not all viruses, common cold, measles, smallpox and vaccinia not doing so. Most typically a follicular response is seen in infections with adenoviruses, picorna viruses, herpes simplex and herpes zoster and chlamydia. Rarer causes include Newcastle disease, which is only seen in vets, laboratory staff and poultry workers.

Herpes Simplex Conjunctivitis

Herpes simplex virus infections are one of the most serious problems in external eye disease, mainly because of the corneal scarring that occurs, making herpetic disease and aphakic bullous keratopathy the commonest indications for penetrating keratoplasty in developed countries. The pattern of recurrent herpetic disease commonly seen is usually regarded as mainly a corneal problem and most conjunctival changes seen during long term treatment can be attributed to the unwanted effects of topical medication.

A follicular conjunctivitis is, however, always an accompaniment to a primary herpetic infection, especially involving the skin of the lids and face. Primary herpes infections (*Plate* III*f*) occur mainly in small children and in adolescents and young adults, and are thought to spread by kissing or other close personal contact. Ocular involvement usually follows development of lid margin vesicles but a conjunctival reaction alone can occur without any skin involvement. After an incubation period of 3–10 days an acute follicular conjunctivitis develops with a regional lymphadenopathy and variable mild constitutional symptoms of fever and malaise. Conjunctival ulceration and pseudomembranes may form, especially in small children, and conjunctival phlyctens may occur.

In about two-thirds of cases corneal involvement follows, taking the form of a coarse pleomorphic punctate epithelial keratitis without subepithelial involvement. These may resolve or persist with development of superficial stromal opacities or may progress to the formation of dendritic figures. These are always multiple unlike the single dendrites seen in recurrent herpetic disease (*Plate* IV*a*). The reason for this is not known. The follicular conjunctivitis alone does not require specific antiviral treatment, which is only indicated if corneal epithelial lesions are seen to develop, and the conjunctiva becomes normal without scarring in 2–3 weeks.

Corneal changes behave like recurrent herpetic disease and are slower to resolve. Herpes simplex virus infections of the eye are usually ascribed to type I virus and genital infections to type II. While this is generally true, neonatal ocular infections and others in adults can be shown to be due to type II and the ocular manifestations appear identical for the two subtypes. Because of the risk of enhancing herpetic infections, topical steroids are contraindicated in the treatment of follicular conjunctivitis, though sometimes used for symptomatic relief in the keratitis of adenovirus infections.

Adenovirus Infections

These viruses were originally called adenopharyngeal-conjunctival or APC viruses because they were isolated from adenoid tissue and from cases of acute upper respiratory infection in young adults. A number of subtypes of adenovirus have been distinguished serologically and the involvement of these various subtypes in upper respiratory tract (URT) or conjunctival disease can now be demonstrated by a rising titre of type-specific antibody. Types 1–7 have been associated with URT infections and types 1–27 with conjunctival disease. The clinical syndromes most commonly seen are pharyngoconjunctival fever (PCF), originally ascribed to type 3, and epidemic keratoconjunctivitis (EKC), originally described in type 8 infections. Recent outbreaks of EKC have involved other types, such as 12 and 22.

Pharyngoconjunctival Fever

The triad of clinical signs, fever, pharyngitis and follicular conjunctivitis, was recognized for many years before it was known to be caused by adenovirus. The onset is sudden, with an acute illness which is highly infectious and rapidly spreads through communities of children and young adults such as boarding schools or military personnel. All age groups may be affected. Transmission of the virus is by direct contact, droplet spray from coughing or on fingers and fomites such as towels and face cloths. Infection may also be acquired from swimming pools. The incubation period is about 5 days and following the development of conjunctivitis virus is shed from the conjunctival sac for roughly 2 weeks. It is this long period of virus shedding that accounts for the epidemics of infection that occur.

The constitutional symptoms vary and may be slight or severe, but the conjunctivitis is often the main complaint. One eye is often involved a few days before the other and the changes are more marked in the first affected eye. A watery discharge occurs and examination of a smear shows a lymphocytic response. The conjunctiva becomes hyperaemic, follicles develop, especially in the lower fornices, and preauricular and submaxillary adenopathy develops. The cornea is involved in a small proportion of cases with a fine epithelial keratitis which develops some discrete subepithelial opacity as the superficial lesions fade. The residual spots are usually few in number and the eyes are not usually irritable or photophobic once the acute phase has passed.

No treatment, including topical antivirals and steroids, appears to influence the course of the disease and usually a topical antibiotic drop such as chloramphenicol or neomycin only is prescribed to reduce the risk of secondary bacterial infection.

Epidemic Keratoconjunctivitis

This is a more severe, highly infectious keratoconjunctivitis, differing from PCF in the lack of fever and malaise and in the florid pseudomembrane formation and keratitis that occurs. The condition has been recognized for 100 years and was the 'superficial punctate keratitis' (SPK) first described by Fuchs. The infectious nature was rapidly recognized and epidemics were reported, the most famous of which involved many thousands of workers in the shipyards of the western coast of America during the Second World War (shipyard eye).

The condition mainly affects young adults and children may act as a clinically unaffected reservoir, helping its transmission. Outbreaks occur in the winter months and spread within families, schools or eye hospital outpatient departments. The incubation period after infection is about 8 days and virus is shed from the inflamed eye for 2–3 weeks. In the first phase a non-specific conjunctival hyperaemia and oedema develops, almost always in one eye only. The second eye may be involved after a few days, but is always less severely involved and may show keratitis without much conjunctival inflammation.

After a few days follicles develop in the upper and lower fornices and in severe infections a pseudomembrane forms on the conjunctival surface. Preauricular adenopathy develops at this time and is again usually asymmetrical. After 1 week the keratitis, which is the distinctive feature of the disorder, becomes apparent. The initial lesions are raised epithelial spots which rapidly develop a subepithelial and superficial stromal opacity beneath them (*Plate IVb*). The epithelial lesions have been shown to contain adenovirus and the subepithelial opacities are thought to represent an immune response to the presence of replicating virus in the epithelium as circulating antibodies to the infection develop. The epithelial lesions persist for 3 weeks, during which time considerable foreign-body-like discomfort is present and the subepithelial opacities persist for many months, certainly 3 months but up to 2 years has been reported. During this time variable impairment of vision and photophobia are usually present. The size and number of the spots of epithelial keratitis and the size of the subepithelial opacities varies with the subtype of adenovirus responsible for the infection.

Epidemic outbreaks in hospital outpatient departments may be caused by spread of the virus on instruments such as foreign body needles or tonometer heads, but by far the greater number of infections are transmitted by fingers to eye. Careful hand washing after examining all cases of potential adenovirus infection is the best preventive of epidemics. Washing of tonometer prisms under running water is preferable to pots of disinfectant but only properly sterilized instruments should be used with a separate slit lamp reserved for infected cases. Any medical person who develops an infection should not examine or treat patients for 3 weeks.

Atypical cases are often responsible for the start of an outbreak, for in addition to the asymptomatic upper respiratory infection of children already mentioned, mild adult cases may present without the telltale keratitis.

Treatment is largely symptomatic and supportive with cold applications and topical antibiotics to reduce the risk of secondary bacterial infection. Some claims have been made for the use of more potent antiviral agents such as tri-fluorothymidine and adenosine arabinoside, which may shorten the course of the disease but do not seem to influence the development of the subepithelial keratitis. Idoxuridine is completely ineffective.

For those patients with a large number of central stromal opacities causing disturbance of vision and photophobia, dilute steroid drops may be indicated and give symptomatic relief. Use of the dilution range previously described makes it possible to use the minimum amount of steroid necessary to relieve symptoms with least risk of adverse effects.

Picornavirus Infections

These viruses, so called because they are small (pico) RNA viruses, have recently been identified as the cause of outbreaks of atypical epidemic keratoconjunctivitis in which conjunctival haemorrhages develop and the keratitis is less striking and persistent than with adenovirus (*Plate IVc*).

Outbreaks of epidemic conjunctivitis with this agent have been reported in the Far East, Africa and England. The clinical picture differs from adenovirus infection in a number of ways. The incubation period is shorter, only 1–2 days, with an acute onset of painful conjunctivitis associated with subconjuctival haemorrhages (hence epidemic haemorrhagic conjunctivitis, EHC). The signs evolve rapidly over 6–12 hours with much lid swelling and chemosis, a watery discharge and usually a slight preauricular adenopathy. Upper respiratory symptoms or signs are uncommon. Few of the patients go on to develop a full follicular response in the conjunctiva, symptoms in the majority resolving within 1–2 weeks.

The keratitis consists of a fine epithelial disturbance, often with widespread intraepithelial microcystic change, but there is never any stromal involvement and the epithelial changes clear quickly, leaving no trace. The virus has proved difficult to isolate on normal cell lines in tissue culture, but when established in culture shows an enterovirus-like cytopathic effect. Neutralizing antibodies can be detected in the serum and a rising titre of antibody is the usual laboratory confirmation of infection. During outbreaks the clinical features and laboratory characteristics of the virus seem to change and it is not clear whether this is due to a change in the virus or whether different strains or subtypes of picornavirus may be involved. Although milder in severity and shorter in duration than adenovirus, EHC is very infectious and poses major potential problems of cross-infection under appropriate conditions.

Epstein–Barr Virus

This is the causative agent of infectious mononucleosis – glandular fever – which is a disease that takes many forms, one of which may predominantly affect the mucous membranes.

A mild conjunctivitis commonly occurs, is often unilateral and said to occur most often on the left side. The follicles that occur stand out as very white dots against an intensely injected conjunctiva. They may become confluent to produce an impressive white granulomatous mass, usually in the lower fornix, which together with the preauricular and submaxillary adenopathy, make up the condition known as Parinaud's oculoglandular syndrome (*Plate* IV*d*).

Keratitis does not occur and the conjunctival lesions resolve over a period of 2–3 weeks without any scarring.

Molluscum Contagiosum

This mildly infective skin lesion is due to a virus infection which causes hyperplasia of the epithelial cells, leading to the skin tumours having a fibrous capsule which divides into septa separating masses of the enlarged inclusion-containing epithelial cells. Molluscum lesions rarely occur directly on the conjunctiva but more often on skin around the eye (*Plate* IV*e*). This results in a follicular conjunctivitis mainly affecting the lower fornix, and a fine punctate epithelial keratitis which, if persistent, develops greyish subepithelial opacities and is associated with superficial vascularization. No virus has been identified in the conjunctival sac or in the corneal epithelial lesions and the ocular manifestations are attributed to toxic products from the virus or the infected epithelial cells.

Herpes Zoster

Ocular involvement by herpes zoster is well recognized but the conjunctival component is not usually an important one and swelling of the lids and periorbital tissues makes examination of the conjunctiva difficult. Sometimes the skin lesions are sparse and the keratoconjunctivitis may be the presenting feature. A follicular conjunctivitis with petechial haemorrhages and a preauricular adenopathy may occur. Sometimes more destructive changes are seen which progress to scarring and fibrosis. The diagnosis usually depends on the associated clinical features such as the skin rash and other signs of ocular involvement.

Chlamydia

Chlamydia agents have some of the features of viruses and some of bacteria and they cause trachoma, paratrachoma and lymphogranuloma venereum in man and a range of infections in animals including psittacosis, feline conjunctivitis and pneumonitis. Trachoma and paratrachoma are the most important ocular infections, and can be shown to be due to different subgroups of chlamydia which have been identified using micro-immunofluorescence techniques. Subgroups are lettered A–K, and groups A–D are associated with hyperendemic trachoma, while E–K are associated with paratrachoma, TRIC or oculogenital chlamydial disease.

Trachoma

Trachoma is a specific communicable ocular infection transmitted by direct eye to eye contact in overcrowded communities. Fingers, clothes and flies attracted to discharging eyes all serve to inoculate the causative agent. The condition has been known and recorded since earliest time. Records exist indicating that it was endemic in the Middle East over 2000 years BC and despite a vast amount of work relating to elucidation of cause, epidemiology, education, field work and large scale treatment, the condition remains one of the major causes of misery and preventable blindness in many parts of the world. The disease is essentially a follicular conjunctivitis with corneal complications in which subconjunctival inflammatory changes develop that progress to fibrosis, so that the final stages are complicated by all the changes of a cicatrizing conjunctivitis such as dry eye, entropion and trichiasis.

In the early stages, chlamydial conjunctival infections present with a mixed papillary and follicular response, the follicles being mainly in the fornices. Striking swelling of the tissues in the fornix occurs, the palpebral conjunctiva being tethered and less easily distended by inflammation.

The clinical picture varies in different parts of the world and this variability in appearance and in the eventual outcome may be associated with exogenous factors such as secondary bacterial infection, which increase the inflammatory response, and endogenous factors relating to the immune responses of the infected individual. An early fine epithelial keratitis develops and by the third week follicles are present and early pannus formation can be seen. The corneal signs tend to occur mainly in the upper part and limbal follicles develop at the upper limbus. The fibrovascular pannus progresses steadily towards the centre of the cornea and has active corneal infiltrates at its apex and within it. After some months the inflammation subsides, with necrosis and scarring of the follicles producing linear and stellate scars in the conjunctiva and the shallow pigmented depressions known as Herbert's pits at the limbus (*Plate* V*a*).

Severe scarring brings the major sight-threatening complications of lid deformity and dryness (*Plate Vb*).

Diagnosis is usually made on the clinical signs in a population known to be at risk of contracting the disease. Laboratory studies that help include conjunctival cytology, which reveals equal numbers of polymorphs and lymphocytes, with a few plasma cells, Leber cells and giant cells. The finding of cytoplasmic inclusions, iodine-positive, is diagnostic but only seen in 30 per cent of active cases. Isolation of chlamydia from conjunctival swabs requires specialized laboratory facilities, not widely available, and it only yields about 80 per cent positive results. Antibody studies on tears and blood are more helpful, being positive in almost 100 per cent of active cases. In trachoma high levels of antibody develop in tears and the protein subtype of the antibody changes as the infection progresses.

Treatment is now possible since chlamydia respond to a number of antibacterial substances, including sulphonamides and the tetracyclines, which are the mainstay of control of the disease.

Clinical response to oral medication may be slow, and although oral treatment over a 3–4 week period is effective, in mass treatment topical therapy is preferred, both to deal with hyperendemic trachoma and the seasonal epidemics of bacterial conjunctivitis and keratitis that occur in many of the affected communities.

The usual treatment regime is tetracycline ointment 1 per cent twice daily for 60 days, or intermittently for 5 days each month for 6 months.

Paratrachoma

Also known as oculogenital chlamydial disease or TRIC (trachoma resembling inclusion conjunctivitis), paratrachoma comprises an oculogenital infection with chlamydial agent acquired during sexual intercourse. Other names such as adult inclusion conjunctivitis are not appropriate, since the patient will often have evidence of chlamydial infection elsewhere. Neonatal inclusion conjunctivitis due to chlamydia occurs as a result of ocular contamination through the infected birth canal, but even these infants may show evidence of genital infection or respiratory infection, with a pneumonia-like syndrome.

In adults TRIC presents as an acute follicular conjunctivitis after a short incubation period of 3–4 days. Although one eye may be affected first, both are usually equally affected and show symmetrical signs later. Preauricular adenopathy, when present, is slight and painless. Initially the follicular response is greatest in the lower fornix but later the follicles increase in number in the upper fornix and along the upper border of the tarsal conjunctiva (*Plate Vc*). At this stage the inflammation may begin to resolve, but in most patients with ocular and genital infection the condition runs a chronic course, with development of keratitis and pannus. The corneal changes consist of a fine punctate epithelial keratitis (PEK), first seen in the upper part of the cornea, which progresses to a coarser PEK associated with subepithelial opacities forming EKC-like lesions. Epithelial changes may come and go for many months before pannus is seen, developing superiorly at first. Bulbar follicles, including follicles on the plica and caruncle, develop in the chronic stage of the disease. Diagnosis is made on the history of ocular and genital symptoms and signs together with the typical conjunctival cytology previously described. Micro-immunofluorescent studies of the antibodies in tears and blood are of the greatest help in confirming the diagnosis. The class of antibody present again helps to confirm the stage of the infection and the presence of high titre of antibody in blood strongly suggests genital and pelvic infection also.

Treatment of this group of patients involves close cooperation between ophthalmologist and genitourinary physicians, for although eye-to-eye transmission of the infecting agent can occur, the usual transmission is venereal, and examination, treatment and follow-up of all sexual contacts as well as the patient are required. Failure to do so means re-infection and chronic disease which can on occasion become sight-threatening with florid pannus and pronounced cicatrizing change like classic trachoma.

The usual treatment is with oral tetracyclines given in a full dose for a maximum of 3 weeks, after which cytology, serology and isolation studies from the eye and genital tract should be repeated. Topical therapy alone has no value and is not additive in effect but only irritant. Viable chlamydial organisms cannot usually be found in the conjunctival sac 48 hours after commencement of systemic treatment alone.

Neonatal Inclusion Conjunctivitis

Ophthalmia neonatorum is now an uncommon disease which is more often due to staphylococcal infection rather than the gonococcus. However, infections with *Neisseria gonorrhoeae* and mixed infections do occur and must be carefully excluded. Conjunctival smears and repeated bacterial cultures are mandatory in all cases of ophthalmia neonatorum. Neonatal inclusion disease always presents at 1 week or later. This late onset does not rule out bacterial causes, for although gonococcal conjunctivitis usually presents within 1–3 days, pneumococcal infections may present at 1 week and streptococcal infections still later, at 8–14 days.

The infant presents with an acute mucopurulent discharge and the conjunctiva appears hyperaemic and swollen. A papillary pattern becomes evident but follicles do not develop unless the disease persists for many weeks. Untreated, the condition may resolve spontaneously, when conjunctival scarring usually remains but rarely causes problems of lid position.

Diagnosis is confirmed by conjunctival cytology, isolation of the agent from conjunctival discharge and by serology of the baby and both parents. The latter will almost invariably be found to have serum antibodies to chlamydia of the oculogenital subtypes, confirming long standing genital infection which requires expert investigation and treatment. Early treatment of the infected baby is desirable and systemic therapy with oral erythromycin may have some advantages because of the risk of extension of the infection to the respiratory tract, causing neonatal pneumonia.

Topical therapy with tetracycline ointment or erythromycin is also effective, and is usually continued for 3 weeks.

Chlamydial Zoonoses

The chlamydial agents normally responsible for animal disease may on occasion be transmitted by direct ocular inoculation to the owner of the pet, or laboratory workers. Parrots, budgerigars and cats are the usual animal vectors and the conjunctivitis caused by the psittacosis or feline pneumonitis agent is usually a mild, self-limiting follicular reaction without keratitis or pannus. Treatment is with oral tetracycline but not sulphonamides, to which this subgroup of chlamydia is resistant.

Other Infective Agents

A number of other agents are recorded as causing follicular responses, but most, such as streptococci, moraxella infections or mixed infection with Vincent's organism, are rare. More frequently seen is the mucopurulent discharge accompanying actinomycotic infections of the canaliculi (streptothrix). Such an infection, especially of the upper canaliculus, may not be obvious and can be associated with a florid conjunctivitis with follicular component. An epithelial keratitis may also develop. Treatment consists of removal of the bulk of the cheesy material from the infected canaliculus and repeated syringeing of the lacrimal passages with concentrated penicillin solution.

Drops and 'Toxic' Follicular Changes

A number of topical eye medications can, after prolonged administration, give rise to a follicular conjunctival hypertrophy. The number of substances causing such a reaction is vast, but typically it occurs with alkaloids, antivirals such as IDU and a number of antiglaucoma preparations including eserine, DFP and adrenaline drops. The follicles mainly develop in the lower fornices, but bulbar follicles are common and a ring of limbal lymphoid tissue may develop, sometimes described as limbitis (*Plate* V*d*). The corneal epithelium is almost always abnormal with a widespread coarse epithelial keratitis in which many opaque 'sick' epithelial cells may be seen. Sometimes these become heaped up into a vortex pattern or tongues of abnormal thick epithelium containing microcysts may extend in from the limbus towards the centre of the cornea. More prolonged application may result in conjunctival metaplasia and appearance of keratin on the conjunctival surface. Swelling of the mucous membrane in the lacrimal system occurs and canalicular stenosis or obstruction may develop. When the causative agent is stopped the conjunctival signs regress over some weeks, but the corneal signs may take over a year to clear and may persist indefinitely. Conjunctival scarring frequently follows this type of toxic response. The nature of the reaction is not clearly understood, hence the term 'toxic'. It is almost certainly not a type I hypersensitivity phenomenon and the skin irritation typical of type IV contact dermatitis is absent.

A true allergic response is always papillary, as in atopic conjunctivitis or hay fever conjunctivitis, and never follicular. The follicles are thought to be due to antigenic stimulation caused by breakdown products of the medication, possibly combined with proteins. It is suggested in the older literature that this type of follicular reaction occurred more often in the past and became less frequent when purer, more stable topical preparations with preservatives became available.

Papillary Conjunctivitis (*Table* IV)

This is the term given to the formation of vascular papillae within the conjunctiva, usually as a chronic

Table IV. Papillary conjunctivitis

Allergic disorders	Hay fever conjunctivitis
	Atopic conjunctivitis
	Vernal disease
Chronic irritation	Keratoconjunctivitis sicca
	Contact lenses
	Prostheses
	Nylon suture ends
Topical medication	Atropine sensitivity and other contact dermatitis with conjunctivitis
	Drop and ointment vehicles
	Preservatives

response and most typically seen in chronic allergic disease of the outer eye. Papillae consist of tufts of vessels growing vertically from the deeper conjunctival vessels so that they are seen on the surface of the conjunctiva as fine red dots. Around the central vascular core there develops an infiltration with lymphocytes, plasma cells and often eosinophils. With persistence of the inflammation there is increasing organization of the papillae seen as hyperplasia of the overlying epithelium, hyalinization of the superficial stroma and formation of deep crypts containing many goblet cells between the individual papillae.

This produces a fine polygonal mosaic-like pattern which reaches its most florid form in the giant compound hypertrophic papillae or cobblestones of vernal disease. Papillae are distinguished from follicles by the presence of a central tuft of vessels, their shape and colour. Old, hyalinized papillae may appear avascular and white like follicles, but usually retain the polygonal shape. The papillary reaction is really only visible on the tarsal conjunctiva and so is not well seen in the lower fornix, where only a narrow strip of tarsal conjunctiva is present, but is typically seen on the broader upper tarsal conjunctiva.

Acute Atopic Conjunctivitis (Hay Fever Conjunctivitis)

This is probably the only true type I immediate hypersensitivity response seen in the outer eye. Typically these are patients known to have recurrent seasonal ocular and upper respiratory symptoms precipitated by pollens, often showing other evidence of atopy. The reaction may be very acute, with hyperaemia overshadowed by massive oedema and chemosis. Prolonged, less acute attacks give rise to a papillary conjunctival response with hyperaemia, less oedema but a copious watery discharge in which numerous eosinophils are found. The ocular features are seen at their most florid following conjunctival challenge tests in sensitized individuals. In the fully developed hay fever syndrome reflex hyperaemia and irritation of the eyes from the inflamed upper respiratory mucosa occurs and treatment is required for both areas to give adequate relief of ocular symptoms and signs. Other exogenous antigens including animal products such as hair, dander, wool and feathers, can cause a similar reaction. Skin tests to suspected allergens are usually positive and helpful in diagnosis and management of this group of patients.

Chronic Atopic Conjunctivitis

This is a chronic papillary response associated with very troublesome subjective symptoms, particularly intense itching and burning sensations and photophobia if keratitis supervenes.

In contrast to these dramatic complaints, the objective findings are often apparently slight, consisting of a diffuse papillary change in which the mucosa appears rather pale and milky. The papillae are small and very uniform in size. Bulbar conjunctival changes are limited to hyperaemia and very little oedema or chemosis occurs. Symptoms are made worse by external irritants such as cigarette smoke or hot dry atmospheres and by rubbing the eyes.

Diagnosis is made on the clinical signs and a history of other personal or family atopic disease, though no atopic history will be obtained in at least half the cases. Conjunctival cytology usually reveals numerous eosinophils and examination of blood and tears shows raised levels of IgE. A raised level of IgE can be considered diagnostic but the test may have to be repeated on a number of occasions before a positive result is obtained. This group of patients, with symptoms often greatly in excess of signs and poor response to most conventional medication, are easily dismissed as neurotic.

In those patients with extensive atopic eczema, especially if involving the skin of the eyelids, the picture can become considerably complicated by secondary bacterial infection of the lid margins with staphylococci. In very chronic cases it may be difficult to separate the signs due to atopy from those caused by bacterial hypersensitivity, and treatment of both may be required. A small proportion of patients with atopic eczema, usually young men, go on to develop a very troublesome keratitis with development of thick opaque epithelium containing microcysts (Hogan's syndrome). Superficial vascularization may follow and considerable photophobia and visual impairment results. The condition responds badly to all topical therapy. Keratoconus is the other corneal condition complicating all allergic conjunctivitis.

Vernal Disease

This is a chronic, recurrent keratoconjunctivitis of children and young adults, often showing seasonal exacerbation, in which characteristic cobblestone papillae develop in the upper tarsal conjunctiva together with limbal changes including limbal follicles. The disease occurs world wide but may take slightly different forms, the palpebral form (*Plate* V*e*) being most common in the West, while the bulbar form occurs more frequently in the Middle East and West Indies (*Plate* V*f*). In general it appears more troublesome in warmer climes but is always a disease of youth, rarely persisting after the age of 25 years.

The onset is unusual before the age of 5 years, boys are affected more often than girls and the condition burns out spontaneously after 5–10 years. Remissions lasting as long as 2–3 years can occur. Exacerbations generally occur in spring and summer in the northern hemisphere (hence 'vernal' conjunctivitis) and in autumn and winter in the southern, but recurrences of active disease may occur at other warm periods during the year. The disease is rarely active in the cold months. Roughly one-third of patients have a personal history of atopic disease either eczema or asthma, and another third have a history of atopic disease in a first degree relative. The remaining third have no history of atopy whatever.

The main presenting features are itching, redness and a mucoid discharge. Ptosis, often asymmetrical, may also occur as a result of the increased mass of the upper lid. The itching or irritation is intense and always parallels the activity of the disease. The discharge is both watery and tenacious. Epiphora is always seen, but in addition the patients describe strings of tenacious mucoid material which accumulate in the fornices, especially when the disease is active, cause increased irritation and can be pulled out as thick ropy strands. Increased numbers of goblet cells and of epithelial sub-surface mucous vesicles can be shown histologically. It is not known whether the mucous glycoproteins secreted are changed in type or whether the physiochemical properties are altered by admixture with protein and cellular debris to produce the abnormal viscosity. Vernal conjunctivitis occurs in two forms, palpebral and bulbar, either separately or together, and either may occur in exacerbations in one individual. The palpebral form affects only the upper tarsal conjunctiva and the appearances of the more easily examined lower fornix are usually normal. Careful examination of the upper fornix by eversion of the upper lid is essential for the diagnosis and follow up assessment of therapeutic response, requiring special skills on the part of the ophthalmologist to obtain cooperation in these unhappy children.

The appearance of the upper tarsal conjunctiva is diagnostic, with flat topped papillae, which with age become hyalinized and white, so that they have some resemblance to follicles. Palpebral follicles never occur in vernal disease alone and are always evidence of additional infection, typically with trachoma in the Middle East. Sometimes the hypertrophic process may be very marked, producing long finger-like masses of tissue which despite their appearance do not cause mechanical damage to the cornea (*Plate VIa*). Keratitis only occurs with active conjunctival inflammation and never occurs from even the most vicious-looking compound papillae that are not inflamed. The fibrovascular core and hyaline material persist in the papillary excrescences and judgement of the degree of activity depends on the recognition of signs of inflammation, i.e. redness, swelling, oedema, cellularity of the conjunctiva and amount of discharge (*Plate VIb*). Actively swollen papillae are tightly packed together and become separated and distinct as the inflammation is controlled so that they appear more striking and threatening. Inactive papillae of this type, however, are never associated with keratitis and mechanical removal by surgery, diathermy or cryotherapy is never indicated.

The limbal form of the disease develops as a widening swelling and opacification of the limbus, initially superiorly but also in other areas, forming in some cases a complete ring of perilimbal tissue (*Plate VIc*). Within this swollen limbal zone discrete limbal nodules or vegetations may develop. These are papillary, having a central vascular core unlike the true bulbar follicles seen with viral infection and drug reactions. White chalky spots within cyst-like formations occur (Trantas' dots) and consist of eosinophil debris. Clear cyst-like spaces or ocelli are also seen. Superficial vascularization develops deep to persistent limbal changes and may be complicated later by secondary lipid infiltration of the cornea. Limbal vernal is not usually associated with discharge and causes fewer symptoms. The most troublesome symptoms are caused by the keratitis which develops with severe uncontrolled active palpebral disease and which poses the main threat to vision in this condition.

The first sign of corneal involvement is the appearance of greyish spots in the superficial epithelium, especially in the upper third of the cornea. These spots gradually spread and extend to form a diffuse grey mass of superficial epithelial cells and mucus which may cover the entire cornea. Shedding of this layer produces the typical vernal erosion or ulcer which is oval, lying horizontally across the upper third of the cornea. The epithelium around the edge becomes thickened and opaque and the base of the erosion becomes covered by aggregated mucus, protein and cellular debris which eventually form a dense, firmly adherent mass known as a vernal plaque. The erosions are very indolent, healing slowly if the conjunctival inflammation is not controlled and considerable vascularization may ensue. Vernal plaque persists indefinitely once the epithelium grows back over it, though sometimes portions of the plaque break up and extrude through the epithelium.

Treatment of all forms of allergic eye disease is difficult and prolonged. The underlying pathological process appears to be the release of a wide range of inflammatory mediators from conjunctival mast cells and basophils. These are caused to degranulate and release their products by type I, IgE mediated mechanisms or by other less clearly defined routes. These may involve mechanical factors and other immunological processes. For those allergic phenomena such as acute atopic conjunctivitis, when a single specific antigen is recognized on clinical grounds or by skin tests, desensitizing or hyposensitizing treatment is usually helpful. In chronic atopic disease such treatment may help other atopic manifestations but does not usually influence the conjunctivitis. In vernal disease it is useless.

Antihistamines are disappointing both topically and systemically mainly because they offer a pharmacological answer to only one of the many potential mediators involved. Topical antihistamines give no lasting benefit and are potent contact sensitizers with prolonged use. Newer antihistamine-like compounds affecting mast cells and basophils have proved disappointing and newer specific H_1 and H_2 blockers have not been systematically studied in the conjunctiva.

The mainstays of treatment remain topical steroids and disodium cromoglycate (DSCG). DSCG was shown nearly 20 years ago to be a potent inhibitor of IgE mediated mechanisms, stabilizing mast cells and preventing their degranulation by favourably influencing the calcium gating of those cells. It has subsequently become an established form of treatment in allergic asthma and rhinitis and to some extent in gastrointestinal disease. In these disorders it appears to have a high degree of effectivity and a unique lack of adverse effects. Its effectivity as a topical ophthalmic preparation is less clear, though careful controlled studies have shown its value. Drops of DSCG have tended to sting and compliance with usage tends to be poor. For useful therapy the drops must be instilled four times daily. Newer formulations offer prospects of greater comfort and less frequent application. Its principal value seems to be as a steroid sparing agent, enabling lesser concentrations of steroid to be employed as adjunctive therapy. Thus in vernal disease only the mildest forms of the disease can be controlled by DSCG alone, probably less than 20 per cent of cases. Treatment with steroids is usually dramatically successful but needs to be prolonged because of the nature of the disease and complications of steroid therapy are frequently seen in this group of patients. Once again the availability of a suitable range of dilutions of steroid makes possible the desirable level of treatment for each stage of activity of the disease.

Vernal keratitis requires special mention since the keratitis is difficult to control and potentially sight-threatening. The development of keratitis always indicates active uncontrolled palpebral disease and it is a great mistake to reduce treatment such as topical steroid because of the appearance of corneal epithelial changes. Other corneal pathology, including herpes, can rarely complicate vernal but should still have characteristic features. The development of typical vernal keratitis is a signal to increase the topical steroid therapy and not reduce it. Vernal erosions and early plaque formation may be helped by dilute acetylcysteine drops in addition to steroid and DSCG in full dosage. Established vernal plaque requires surgical excision by superficial keratectomy after the conjunctival inflammation has been controlled.

Limbal vernal is usually easier to control than the palpebral form and often responds to DSCG alone or to short courses of dilute steroid. The development of steroid glaucoma should always be watched for and the children should be encouraged to expect applanation tonometry at every visit. It usually proves easy to do once the cooperation of the child and parent has been obtained. Steroid glaucoma is a real problem in treatment of external eye diseases with topical steroid and probably affects 10 per cent of cases. It can usually be managed by reducing the strength of the steroid or changing to one of the steroids with reduced potential to raise the intraocular pressure, such as clobetasone or fluormethalone. Unfortunately, these are often insufficient to control severe inflammation and it may rarely be necessary to combine potent topical steroid with antiglaucoma medication such as oral acetazolamide. Subsequent treatment with dilute steroids may then be possible without significant rise in intraocular pressure.

Keratoconjunctivitis Sicca

Primarily a deficiency of the lacrimal gland secretion, keratoconjunctivitis sicca (KCS) can be compounded by disorders of mucus production and other factors such as lid position and function which normally contribute to the lubrication of the outer eye and formation of the normal precorneal film, previously described.

Rarely tear deficiency may be congenital (alacrimia). Babies who do not cry are not suffering from alacrimia. The even rarer condition of Riley–Day syndrome (familia dysautonomia) presents with recurrent or persistent corneal epithelial ulceration in the presence of defective tear secretion and absent corneal and conjunctival sensation. Corneal opacification, perforation and endophthalmitis can rapidly supervene and the visual prognosis for these children is extremely bad. Dry eyes in childhood are otherwise associated with a good prognosis, provided secondary factors such as infection and disorders of lid position do not complicate the picture.

Most frequently dry eyes present in adults, women more often than men. Impairment of tear flow can follow surgical extirpation of the lacrimal gland, intentional or accidental, damage to its nerve supply, or damage to the lacrimal ductules by ill advised dissection in the region of the palpebral lobe of the lacrimal gland during ptosis or other orbital surgery or as the result of a cicatrizing conjunctivitis. Any of the foregoing can lead to a unilateral problem; spontaneous dry eye is usually a bilateral symmetrical disorder due to an autoimmune destruction of the lacrimal gland tissue. Although classically associated with rheumatoid arthritis and a dry mouth in the triad of Sjögren's syndrome, it is most often associated with other systemic immune disorders and systemic diseases such as lupus erythematosus and scleroderma in its various forms.

Only 14 per cent of patients with rheumatoid arthritis have dry eyes and this is not usually severe, although other ocular complications of rheumatoid disease such as corneal melting and guttering and scleral disease may be much more troublesome and visually disabling.

Symptoms from dry eyes are non-specific and result in the condition being overdiagnosed (usually on the basis of an inadequate history and a badly performed Schirmer's test). The usual complaints are of a hot, burning or gritty sensation made worse by cigarette smoke, sun, wind or central heating. Examination of the eye at the slit lamp reveals a reduced volume of tears in the marginal tear strip and an abnormal thinned precorneal tear film containing an excess of mucus and debris (*Plate VId*). These two findings are the most useful diagnostic indicators of a dry eye state and are doubly significant if the patient is subsequently shown to have any keratitis, which would have been expected to increase the reflex lacrimation. Instillation of rose bengal drops stains the dry epithelium of the cornea and conjunctiva to give a dramatic picture of interpalpebral staining in a severe case (*see Plate* III*b*). Lesser degrees of staining occur and are more difficult to interpret. Mucus strands and filaments also stain strongly. Unfortunately rose bengal stings and irritates dry eyes badly, probably because of the loss of the buffering capacity of the normal tears. This stinging, however, provides another useful test of lacrimal gland function since one can watch at the slit lamp the rate of wash out of the dye from the conjunctival sac. Lissamine green has been proposed as an alternative dye but gives weak staining and has not proved popular (*Plate VIe*). Fluorescein is of no use for, although the conjunctiva takes up the dye the fluorescence cannot be made out against the white sclera. Rose bengal staining, if obscured by intense conjunctival hyperaemia, can be made more obvious by viewing in the red free filtered (green) light of the slit lamp which makes the stained areas fluoresce bright blue.

A widespread epithelial keratitis maximal in the lower part of the cornea and usually absent from the part covered by the upper lid occurs and may be complicated by the mucus deposition previously described.

The diagnosis is made on the clinical findings and no simple, reliable test of tear production exists which can be said absolutely to confirm the diagnosis. Schirmer's test is a crude, unquantifiable and unpredictable test which has been shown to have no reproducibility on repeated testing. It must be remembered that in careful repeated studies even normal individuals have been shown to give an apparently pathological reading of less than 5 mm wetting on one occasion. A single test must therefore never be regarded as diagnostic but at best as a confirmation of the general clinical impression from slit lamp examination of normal or grossly reduced tear production. More specialized studies of tear constituents, such as lysozyme estimations, give more consistent results and are of value but not widely available. The older technique of lysozyme estimation using plates coated with micrococcus lysodikteus and measuring zones of inhibition around samples is being superseded by enzyme-linked immunosorbent assay systems (ELISA) which are increasingly used for other measurements. It may therefore be easier to obtain diagnostic measurements of tear constituents in the future.

Treatment of dry eyes consists primarily in rehydration, either by conserving the limited volume of tears produced or supplementing them with artificial tears. Excess mucus usually proves less troublesome once adequate hydration has been achieved but persistent filaments may require 10 or 20 per cent acetylcysteine drops.

Punctal occlusion to conserve the few tears produced is often of dramatic benefit. It is desirable to carry out a preliminary temporary occlusion of the upper and lower canaliculi with gelatine rods to exclude the possibility of overflow epiphora. Unfortunately gelatine rods cannot be obtained commercially but must be locally produced by drawing out threads of gelatine from a hot viscous solution on glass or plastic rods. The pliable threads are air dried to produce stiff rods which can be cut up and stored indefinitely.

Gelatine occlusion is not done to demonstrate improvement, which often takes some weeks after occlusion, but to ensure epiphora will not occur. The gelatine dissolves in a matter of days and to obtain permanent occlusion of the puncta the terminal lining of the canaliculus is destroyed with the electric cautery heated to black heat. It is usually desirable to occlude both upper and lower canaliculi since the upper can easily drain a very significant amount of tear fluid and regular examination of the puncta at the slit lamp is desirable, especially if increase in symptoms unexpectedly occurs. A tiny pinhole opening only may be present but drain an important volume of tears. Repeated attempts at occlusion are required in some patients.

Artificial tear supplementation remains the most important form of therapy and a wide range of drops has been evolved. In general an artificial tear drop has been shown to give best subjective relief if slightly alkaline with an optimal pH around 8·5. Viscosity and hydrophilic qualities are conferred by the incorporation of hydroxypropylmethyl cellulose and commercial polymers have been produced of unknown composition and uncertain value but designed to reproduce the physicochemical characteristics of mucus. Recent work has focused attention on the hyperosmolarity of the periocular fluid in dry eye states and the possible role of osmolarity in the causation of the epithelial changes seen. Some commercial hypotonic tear supplements have been produced but are probably not sufficiently hypo-osmolar to restore normality to the dry eye and none has been evaluated in a controlled clinical trial.

Other forms of treatment, such as constant infusion apparatus to deliver fluid continuously to the eye, have been suggested and much ingenuity devoted to the propulsion systems. Unfortunately the main problem is still the delivery of the fluid to the eye and the polythene tubing employed is easily displaced from the inner or outer canthi and easily blocked if fluid other than saline or water is used. Infection of the reservoir is also a major threat to these compromised eyes.

Stimulation of tear production is not a realistic form of treatment in most patients because oral parasympathomimetic drugs produce unacceptable gastrointestinal side effects and in most there simply is not sufficient remaining functional lacrimal gland tissue to give a useful response.

Conjunctival inserts have been suggested as treatment using the principle of an osmotic pump to transfer fluid from the conjunctival blood vessels into the tear film by raising tear osmolarity. These have had very limited clinical trial and would seem to be contraindicated on theoretical grounds if hyperosmolarity of the tear fluid does play any part in the development of the epithelial changes seen in KCS.

Methyl cellulose inserts have been produced, designed as small hard pellets of dry methyl cellulose which slowly dissolve over the day to produce a constant layer of 'mucoid' material over the surface of the eye (*Plate* VI*f*). Only three clinical trials of these devices have been reported and subjective acceptance has in general been poor, due to worsening of vision from irregular thickening of the precorneal film, irritation by the pellet and spontaneous extrusion. Patients with profound reduction of tear flow, associated irregular corneal surface and poor vision seem to tolerate the devices better than those with lesser pathology in whom the abnormal precorneal film and bulky marginal tear strip produce unacceptable visual disturbance.

Sudden unexpected worsening of symptoms in a patient with previously well controlled KCS occurs from time to time and is due to secondary infection or toxicity (usually from preservatives). Patients with KCS tolerate blepharitis badly and appropriate treatment of staphylococcal lid margin disease is necessary at all times. Toxicity from preservatives is often difficult to detect at onset but the steady worsening of symptoms despite increased use of artificial tears and burning rather than relief when the drops are instilled suggest the possibility. Confirmation comes from the appearance of signs of toxicity in the corneal and conjunctival epithelium where a widespread coarse epitheliopathy develops over the surface of the cornea with thick grey epithelium sometimes developing a vortex pattern. Rose bengal usually shows widespread staining of the conjunctiva, including that on the surface of the globe and in the fornix outside the interpalpebral zone where normally it would be protected by the lids from drying. Use of an alternative drop with a different preservative or preservative-free solutions solves the problem. Punctal occlusion, if not previously carried out, is of great help in this situation by reducing or abolishing the need for frequent drops.

CONTACT LENS INDUCED PAPILLARY CONJUNCTIVITIS
(Giant Papillary Conjunctivitis, GPC)

This is the contact lens 'look-alike' of vernal conjunctivitis. Histologically the appearances of the two conditions are almost indistinguishable but the clinical features differ significantly. The condition was originally described in wearers of soft contact lenses but is also seen in association with hard contact lenses, prostheses and mechanical trauma from protruding nylon suture ends. There is no increased frequency of personal or family history of atopic disease in patients with GPC compared to controls.

The typical patient with contact lens induced GPC has worn the lenses successfully for a long period, usually in excess of a year, and gradually develops slight itching, mucoid discharge and reduced tolerance of the lens which no longer centres properly but tends to be drawn up by blinking. The eye usually remains white and the lower fornix shows only minimal papillary changes if any, so that the cause of the problem may not be detected for some time if the upper lid is not everted during routine follow-up examination. The changes in the upper palpebral conjunctiva are striking with the formation of a number of discrete giant cobblestone-like compound hypertrophic papillae, similar to those seen in vernal disease (*Plate* VII*a*). The cobblestones are usually relatively few in number but with increasingly severe and chronic disease extend downwards over the surface of the tarsal plate towards the lid margin. They also become very hyalinized and are then known as 'white heads' by contact lens practitioners.

The aetiology of the condition remains obscure. The initial hypothesis was an allergic response triggered by proteinaceous deposits on the anterior surface of the lens, but since identical GPC occurs in wearers of hard contact lenses, with prosthesis and suture ends of inert material, it seems likely that mechanical factors play a major role. The exciting material does not need to be foreign since GPC has been personally observed in a patient in whom the keratin on the surface of a limbal keratin plaque formed a pointed excrescence which came into contact with the under surface of the upper lid to produce a typical response.

Treatment is removal of the offending cause. After cessation of contact lens wear the papillae resolve over a period of months. When the disease is active the tops of the papillae are said to stain with fluorescein but this is lost as the papillae resolve. Finally, only stellate white subepithelial lesions remain and may further resolve with time. Refitting with a new lens of the same material and physical parameters does not give lasting relief but refitting with a thinner lens of different material with good edge contours is usually satisfactory, although repeated episodes of GPC can occur in response to different materials. Although the condition does resolve spontaneously, it has been suggested that DSCG may relieve symptoms sooner and enhance the rate of resolution of the changes enabling refitting to be carried out more quickly. Steroids appear to offer no benefit in this disorder.

Treatment of the prosthesis-related cases is more difficult and repolishing or replacement of the prosthesis with the same material may not be curative. A glass prosthesis sometimes solves the problem but is difficult to obtain and fragile. Sometimes the only course is to use DSCG to ameliorate the symptoms and observe the changes. The whole process does seem to have a natural history and will often appear to 'burn out' in a couple of years.

Suture-related cases resolve rapidly if the exposed end is removed or cut flush with the surface of the globe. Only stiff suture ends such as nylon or Prolene seem to cause the problem, which does not occur with flexible or soft material such as virgin silk, further suggesting a mechanical effect.

Contact Dermatoconjunctivitis

A type IV hypersensitivity response to prolonged contact with a wide range of chemicals and drugs, this is a well-recognized dermatological phenomenon (*Plate* VII*b*). Topical ophthalmic medication can produce such a reaction in the skin around the lids and atropine is probably the commonest cause, with antibiotics, especially penicillin and aminoglycosides such as neomycin, soframycin and gentamicin. The list of potential causes would be vast but the clinical syndrome is very distinctive, with a weeping eczematous reaction in the skin involving all areas with which the medication comes into contact so that the cheek and even the ear may be involved if tears carry the diluted allergen to these parts. Lesser skin involvement presents as a dry, shiny, reddened appearance with altered wrinkling of the skin. The conjunctiva is hyperaemic with a generalized papillary response affecting the lower fornix more than the upper. Keratitis rarely occurs. Itching of the whole periorbital area is intense and distressing. Conjunctival cytology shows a lymphocytic response with masses of eosinophils. This pattern of true contact sensitivity gives a high incidence of positive skin tests to the allergen and is to be contrasted with the 'toxic' follicular response to topical medication previously described.

Sometimes the conjunctival changes persist after withdrawal of the offending agent and substitution of an alternative compound. In these cases a sensitivity to the vehicle, especially ointment base, and more rarely to the preservative in the drops can be shown.

Treatment consists of elimination of the causative medication, which may not be easy to determine if more than one topical preparation is being used. A steroid cream gives relief of skin itching and a water-soluble cream preparation is preferred to avoid the risk of continued sensitivity to a common ointment base.

CICATRIZING CONJUNCTIVITIS (*Table* V)

Many types of conjunctival inflammation resolve without any scarring. Purulent conjunctivitis, even when recurrent, leaves no scars. Other inflammations, including all types of membranous conjunctivitis, are associated with residual fibrotic change which may be focal, linear or in diffuse sheets. Chemical and thermal burns produce a variable amount of damage to conjunctiva and deeper tissues with subsequent fibrosis. A number of disorders which involve skin and mucous membrane changes are associated with the most progressive and disagreeable conjunctival scarring that occurs and are major causes of pain and blindness. Finally, some types of topical therapy can produce a chronic inflammation which proceeds to cicatrization.

Table V. Cicatrizing conjunctivitis

Infection	Membranous conjunctivitis, i.e. severe adenovirus
Trauma	Chemical burns
	Thermal burns
Oculocutaneous disorders	Mucous membrane pemphigoid
	Linear IgA disease
	Dermatitis herpetiformis
	Erythema multiforme
	Toxic epidermal necrolysis
Chronic inflammation	Topical medication
	Chronic atopic conjunctivitis

The reason why some types of inflammation are followed by fibrosis is not known, but in general the inflammatory process tends to involve the submucosa and the epithelium with an intense cellular reaction in all layers. The final activation and proliferation of the fibroblasts is probably under the control of mediators such as leukotrienes. The lack of understanding of the fundamental mechanisms involved makes the treatment of this group of disorders all the more difficult.

Membranous Conjunctivitis

If trachoma is the infection producing most conjunctival scarring world wide, then membranous conjunctivitis of all types is the second. Bacterial causes of membranous conjunctivitis such as diphtheria are now rare and the commonest infective agent involved is adenovirus.

Following a severe adenovirus infection quite considerable amounts of scarring may remain (*Plate* VII*c*), with localized symblepharon formation resulting in pockets of conjunctiva in the fornices. Fortunately the fibrosis does not usually involve the palpebral conjunctiva or tarsus close to the lid margin, so entropion rarely ensues. If it does, lid everting surgery can safely be carried out without fear of recrudescence or enhancement of the previous fibrotic process.

Chemical Burns

This is a complicated subject, and the final outcome for the various parts of the eye and adnexa depend on a number of factors, mainly the nature of the chemical and the length of time it remains in contact with the tissue. The main problems following chemical burns involve the cornea and are discussed in Chapter 14, but significant conjunctival scarring always occurs and the resulting disorder of tear production and disturbance of lid position and function require meticulous attention, especially if corneal surgery is planned in these cases.

Oculocutaneous Disorders

This portmanteau term is used to cover a group of disorders involving skin and mucous membranes, having different aetiologies, not always clearly understood, but generally involving immune mechanisms. While the final appearance of most of these disorders may appear superficially similar, there are important underlying differences which influence management. In particular, it is essential to distinguish between those conditions in which relentlessly progressive cicatrization occurs, influenced to a limited extent only by treatment and always made worse by surgery, and the others where an acute process resolves completely to produce a static fibrous scar which is eminently treatable by surgery.

Mucous Membrane Pemphigoid

This is the most unpleasant of the chronic relentlessly progressive cicatrizing disorders, having some resemblance to the bullous skin eruption pemphigoid. All mucous membranes can be involved in a small proportion of cases of cutaneous pemphigoid, but in mucous membrane pemphigoid the skin lesions are few or absent. Although the patient may present with initial involvement of only one mucosal surface, others are almost always involved during the course of the disease. The ocular changes have in the past been described as 'ocular pemphigus', a bad term which should not be used. Pemphigus is a skin disorder in which intra-epidermal blistering occurs as the result of antibody mediated damage to the intercellular attachments. Ocular involvement in pemphigus is not common and when it does occur the conjunctiva becomes intensely hyperaemic with occasional blistering. The changes in the conjunctiva are strictly intra-epithelial and always resolve without scarring, and these alone are ocular pemphigus.

Pemphigoid was so named because of its resemblance to pemphigus (meaning blister) but was later differentiated on histological grounds from pemphigus. Unlike the intra-epithelial changes of pemphigus, those in pemphigoid involve the dermo–epidermal junction, where an antibody directed against basement membrane determinants causes inflammation and separation to produce thick-walled subepidermal skin blisters. The antibody in pemphigus is usually present in serum in high titre and can be demonstrated in tissue. The pemphigoid antibody is never present in such high titres and may be absent in cases of mucous membrane disease only. The antibody can, however, be demonstrated by direct immunofluorescence in tissue biopsied from active skin or mucous membrane lesions.

The relationship between bullous pemphigoid of the skin and cicatricial mucous membrane pemphigoid is not clear, but the antibody directed against basement membrane zone determinants appears to be common to the two disorders and cutaneous pemphigoid can be localized with severe scarring, usually on the scalp.

Ocular involvement in cicatricial mucous membrane pemphigoid may present in several ways. Often the onset is insidious with non-specific conjunctival redness, discharge and irritation, involving one or both eyes, but acute conjunctival lesions with ulceration may occur (*Plate* VII*d*). Blisters are rarely seen on the conjunctiva or cornea, but chronic epithelial erosions are a common feature of the later stages. The sequel to the chronic conjunctival inflammation is the development of subconjunctival fibrous tissue causing shallowing of the fornices, entropion and mechanical limitation of movement of the globe. Early involvement of the conjunctiva in the canthal region occurs (*Plate* VII*e*) and loss of the normal architecture in the inner canthal region with flattening or obliteration of the normal conjunctival folds, plica and caruncle is an important early diagnostic sign. The cornea is not affected in the earliest stages and lack of visual impairment accounts for the late diagnosis of many cases. Eventually an epithelial keratitis develops with peripheral corneal vascularization which extends centrally and may be accompanied by stromal infiltrates and a thick fleshy pannus around the whole limbus (*Plate* VII*f*). Involvement of lacrimal ductules in the outer part of the upper fornix finally results in a dry eye with further conjunctival metaplasia and keratinization.

The combination of dryness, abnormal lid closure, entropion and trichiasis results in further damage to the ocular surface and may be complicated by infection, leading to perforation and loss of the globe.

The diagnosis of cicatricial mucous membrane pemphigoid is not easy to make in the early stages of the disease and laboratory investigations are not helpful. Biopsy of the fornix conjunctiva is contraindicated because of the risk of increased activity and scarring, although biopsy of bulbar conjunctiva seems safer. Biopsy of buccal mucosal lesions when present is of greatest value, allowing direct immunofluorescence to detect antibody at the basement membrane zone and so confirm the diagnosis.

Treatment is difficult and no single therapeutic regime predictably controls the disease, which has a variable natural history. Some patients have a relentlessly progressing course, others may have spontaneous remission for a period of months or years and then show reactivation. Acute ulcerative lesions of the conjunctiva respond to intensive topical steroids but topical therapy is of very little value apart from rehydration with artificial tear drops if dryness develops. Oral steroids are disappointing and fail to control the disease even in high dosage. Immunosuppression with oral cytotoxic drugs such as azathioprine or cyclophosphamide seems to offer greater hope of arrest of the disease but side effects of all these drugs are a major problem, especially in older patients.

Surgical treatment of this group of patients is particularly unrewarding, since further fibrosis and scarring follows all attempts to divide adhesions or implant mucous membrane, and probably the only worthwhile procedures are those for dealing with trichiasis, electrolysis or cryotherapy. The poor results from surgical treatment in pemphigoid are in sharp contrast to the excellent results obtained in dealing with the ocular complications of erythema multiforme and Stevens–Johnson syndrome.

Linear IgA Disease

So called because a linear deposition of IgA is seen at the dermo–epidermal junction in lesional skin and mucous membrane, the condition may represent one form of pemphigoid but does seem to have a high incidence of mucous membrane involvement. Patients presenting with buccal mucous membrane lesions due to IgA disease have been shown to have a high incidence of conjunctival involvement, often asymptomatic (*Plate* VIII*a*).

Dermatitis Herpetiformis

This is rarely associated with mucous membrane inflammation and scarring. The typical itchy skin rash, diagnostic finding of IgA antibody in a papillary distribution in skin and rapid response to sulphones, all make for speedy diagnosis and early treatment. This may partly account for the lack of conjunctival cicatrization in most patients with papillary DH. Sulphones such as dapsone have also been used to treat pemphigoid, though it has not been established whether the classic type with IgG basement membrane zone antibody or the linear IgA variant is more likely to respond.

Erythema Multiforme

This is an acute disease in which skin lesions, papules and blisters develop with inflammation of mucous membranes. The condition varies and is not always a severe systemic illness but may present with only minor skin lesions and more troublesome conjunctival or oral manifestations. Ocular involvement is usually equated with the Stevens–Johnson syndrome, which is better defined as erythema multiforme with involvement of at least two mucosal surfaces. Children and young adults are most often affected and although the aetiology is not known, a number of infective agents, including herpes simplex virus and mycoplasma pneumoniae, and drugs of many types especially antibiotics, have been implicated.

The onset of the illness occurs with a prodromal period of several days during which fever, general debility and upper respiratory symptoms develop. Drugs administered during this period may be unfairly blamed for the subsequent rash and other features of the illness. During the prodromal period and before the skin rash develops, conjunctival hyperaemia with mucoid discharge occurs (*Plate* VIII*b*). The systemic and cutaneous manifestations have been shown to be due to localized vasculitis and progression of the changes in the conjunctiva results in localized infarction with the formation of necrotic membranes (*Plate* VIII*c*). Healing takes place with fibrosis, resulting in focal static scarring.

Topical and systemic steroids control the vasculitis in the earliest phases but are of no value later once conjunctival infarction has occurred. Conjunctival adhesions may develop, but are always soft and lack the dense fibrous subconjunctival component seen in mucous membrane pemphigoid (*Plate* VIII*d*). Unless widespread scarring or localized changes in the upper fornix damage the lacrimal ductules, the eyes are not dry but more often wet with epiphora caused by mucosal scarring occluding the lacrimal drainage system. Acute secondary bacterial infection with corneal ulceration and endophthalmitis may cause visual loss in the early phase of the illness but later complications may also occur due to disorders of lid position and movement, abnormalities of lashes and keratin formation on the palpebral and bulbar conjunctiva (*Plate* VIII*e*). In sharp contrast to pemphigoid, these changes in erythema multiforme are always amenable to surgical treatment and early recognition and correction avoids much preventable damage to the outer eye.

Entropion of the upper lid is dealt with by a lid everting operation such as Trabut's procedure combined with recession of the posterior lamella to reduce the risk of exposure. Lashes are treated by cryotherapy and cicatricial bands of conjunctiva can be divided, readjusted by Z-plasty, or other mucous membrane can be implanted.

Toxic Epidermal Necrolysis (TEN)

TEN occurs in two forms, that affecting young children, known as the Ritten type, and that affecting adults, known as Lyell's syndrome. Ritten type TEN is caused by exotoxins of a particular staphylococcus, while Lyell's syndrome is very like erythema multiforme in its ocular manifestations. Varying degrees of conjunctival scarring, entropion and lash problems may ensue and respond well to surgical treatment after the acute illness has passed.

Chronic Inflammation

Chronic inflammation may produce cicatrization and this is most commonly seen after prolonged administration of topical drugs for chronic glaucoma. Many compounds have been implicated, including DFP, phospholine iodide, eserine and epinephrine (adrenaline). Preservatives in eye drops can also be responsible. This type of conjunctival cicatrization is sometimes known as pseudopemphigoid (*Plate* VIII*f*). It is not known whether the topical drug induces immunological changes of true pemphigoid, but bullous pemphigoid of skin has been reported following use of topical fluorouracil. After the topical agent is discontinued, the inflammation and surface metaplasia usually disappear but the fibrous tissue persists and surgical treatment for lid and lash disorders may be required. A few patients with pseudopemphigoid show exacerbation or progression just like cicatricial mucous membrane pemphigoid and it seems possible that a persistent immunological abnormality has been triggered by the topical therapy.

FURTHER READING

The dry eye. (Cambridge Ophthalmology Symposium). *Trans. Ophthalmol. Soc. UK* 1985; **104,** 351–498.
Duke-Elder W. S. *System of Ophthalmology,* vol. VIII. St Louis, Mo. Mosby, 1965.
O'Connor G. Richard (ed.) *Immunologic Diseases of the Mucous Membrane.* New York, Masson, 1980.
Wilson L. A. *External Diseases of the Eye.* London, Harper & Row, 1979.

Chapter 5

The Cornea

R. J. Buckley

THE NORMAL CORNEA

Introduction

The cornea is a round convex area in the fibrous envelope of the eye. Though its collagen fibres are continuous with those of the opaque sclera, it is transparent. Collagen makes up 71 per cent of its dry weight (but only 16 per cent of its wet weight, as the normal cornea is 78 per cent water). Its refractive index is usually taken as 1·376.

Dimensions

The anterior periphery of the cornea forms an ellipse with a horizontal diameter of 11·7 mm (normal range: 11·0–12·5 mm) and a vertical diameter of 0·9 mm less. The posterior surface is circular with a diameter of 11·7 mm (normal range not established).

Shape

A central zone of the cornea, forming a horizontal ellipse of approximately 5 mm × 3 mm, is usually almost spherical. Away from this zone the curve of the cornea is increasingly flatter, more so nasally than temporally and more above than below. Adult corneae are usually slightly toric. Usually the steeper meridian is within 15° either side of vertical ('with the rule astigmatism'). Astigmatism is regular when the axes of different curvature are mutually at a right-angle. Tight sutures at or near the periphery of the cornea (e.g. cataract section, graft–host interface) produce a central steepening, and not a flattening, which at first thought might seem more likely.

Power

The central zone of the cornea supports the most powerful refracting surface of the eye, which is the air–tear film interface. Its radius of curvature is 7·8 mm (normal range: 6·75–9·25 mm). The power of this surface is 48 dioptres, which is four-fifths of the total refractive power of the eye (60 dioptres).*

Thickness

The central thickness of the cornea is 0·52 mm (normal range 0·50–0·54 mm); this is most often measured optically using a pachometer attachment on the slit lamp (such as the Haag Streit Depth Measuring Attachment No. 1 on the Haag Streit 900). It can also be measured ultrasonically, using a probe applied to the corneal surface (examples: Jedmed Pachysonic, Storz Corneo-Scan). A contact objective, such as that of the contact specular microscope, may also be used: the distance between the points at which the superficial epithelium and the endothelium are in focus is measured, and a 'real and apparent depth' correction is applied. Away from the central area the cornea gradually thickens, so that it is perhaps 0·65 mm at its periphery.

Histology

The human cornea is described as having five layers, as set out in *Table* I.

Table I. Approximate actual and percentage thicknesses of the layers of the normal adult cornea

Layer	Thickness (μm)	% thickness
Epithelium	50	10
Bowman's layer (BL)	10	2
Stroma	440	84
Descemet's membrane (DM)	15	3
Endothelium	5	1
Total	520	100

---

* The power of a spherical surface, radius r, between two media of refractive indices n and n_1, is given by the formula $[(n_1 - n)/r]$. The actual interface under discussion is that between air and the tear film, but the tear layer forms what is virtually a curved plano lens on the corneal surface, and so the power calculation can omit this layer. If n_1, (cornea) is taken as 1·376, n (air) is 1·0, and r is 0·0078 m, i.e. 7·8 mm

$$\frac{n_1 - n}{r} = \frac{1 \cdot 376 - 1 \cdot 0}{0 \cdot 0078} = 48 \cdot 2 \text{ dioptres}$$

The total power of the cornea must take into account the small negative power of its posterior surface, radius 7·3 mm. Here, n_1, (cornea) is 1·376, n (aqueous) is 1·336 and r is −0·0073 m:

$$\frac{n_1 - n}{r} = \frac{1 \cdot 376 - 1 \cdot 336}{-0 \cdot 0073} = -5 \cdot 5 \text{ dioptres}$$

The total power of the cornea, in these examples, is $48 \cdot 2 - 5 \cdot 5 = 42 \cdot 7$ dioptres.

Stroma

The stroma consists of collagen fibrils, regularly arranged and of uniform diameter, which lie in approximately 200 bundles (lamellae) parallel to the corneal plane. They are embedded in a hydrated matrix of proteoglycans (molecules with a protein core and glycosaminoglycan side chains). This matrix is said to exert a 'swelling pressure' which draws water into itself. The stroma is populated by keratocytes, lying in and between the collagen lamellae, which have long slender branching and communicating processes. Neither these cells nor the other cells present in the stroma (see Table II) are fixed, but are able to move through the tissue in response to a number of stimuli.

the tear film. The flat surface cells are united by desmosomes which totally surround the circumference of each cell: these are known as zonulae occludentes or 'tight junctions'. The tight junctions render the epithelium impermeable to water, electrolytes, nutrients, metabolites and most micro-organisms. The tears do not, therefore, 'nourish' the cornea, but they do transmit the gases which pass between the environment and the eye surface.

Descemet's Membrane (DM)

The stroma is bounded posteriorly by Descemet's membrane, which is the basement membrane secreted by the most posterior cell layer, the endothe-

Table II. The components of the normal cornea

Layer	Main cell type	Other cells present	Collagen
Epithelium	Epithelial (basal wing, surface cells)	Melanocytes, polymorphs, dendrites of neurones, Langerhans cells (at periphery)	Type IV (basement membrane)
BL	None	None	Fine random fibres
Stroma	Keratocyte (Stromacyte)	Histiocytes, plasma cells, mast cells, polymorphs, lymphocytes	200 lamellae, types I (mainly), III, IV
DM	None	None	Fine random fibres. Mainly type IV
Endothelium	Endothelial cells	Lymphocytes	None

Bowman's Layer (BL)

The stroma is bounded anteriorly by a condensation of collagen, containing no cells, known as Bowman's layer (it is not a membrane). This layer is mechanically very resistant, but if breached is not regenerated. The basement membrane of the epithelium lies on its anterior surface.

Bowman's layer acts as though it restrains the cornea anteriorly; thus stromal swelling takes place in a posterior direction. Epithelial swelling is in an anterior direction.

Epithelium

The epithelium consists of a basement membrane, attached by hemidesmosomes to a layer of basal cells, two or three layers of wing-shaped cells, and two layers of superficial cells. Basal cells, as they mature into wing cells and then surface cells, become flattened but not keratinized. The potential for keratinization is present, as is seen in conditions such as vitamin A deficiency. Epithelial turnover time is roughly 7 days. If a part of the basement membrane is denuded by trauma, surrounding cells spread within hours to fill the defect.

The surface of the epithelium, which is smooth on light microscopy, is actually peaked and ridged into microvilli and microplicae 0·5 μm high. These excrescences interact with and stabilize the basal layer of

lium. Descemet's membrane increases in thickness through life, from 2 μm at birth to 20 μm in old age. It consists of collagen amorphously arranged, and glycoproteins which include fibronectin. It is very resistant to trauma and to pathological processes. A 'Descemetocoele' can sometimes maintain the integrity of the eyeball for long after the epithelium and stroma have been lost. When split, Descemet's membrane behaves as if it were elastic, and retracts and rolls inwards (i.e. towards the stroma) on itself.

Endothelium

The endothelium is possibly derived from neuroectoderm (rather than mesoderm, which forms the keratocytes of the stroma, or surface ectoderm, which forms the epithelium). At birth there are 300 000–400 000 endothelial cells per cornea, giving a density of around 3000/mm². Viewed from the posterior surface, the cells of this monolayer are polygonal (mostly hexagonal) and they are about 20 μm across. Their thickness is 5 μm. Under normal circumstances, the endothelial cells are not regenerated and thus age with the individual. There is a gradual loss of cells, and loss of the homogeneity of size and shape of the survivors, throughout life.

The functional reserve of the endothelium is considerable. There is no established relationship between cell density and function, but it is likely that up to 80 per cent of the cells may be lost before corneal decompensation becomes inevitable. The cells of a depopulated endothelial layer appear larger than normal in the two-dimensional view afforded by specular reflection, but they may not be actually enlarged. Their volume probably remains constant as they spread out, and so they become progressively thinner.

The endothelial cells contain organelles characteristic of cells engaged in active transport and protein synthesis. At the posterior intercellular borders there are maculae occludentes (focal tight junctions) separated by 3 nm-wide gaps. As a result, the endothelium presents only a partial barrier to the passage of small molecules. Furthermore, larger molecules, and small particles, can pass by endothelial pinocytosis.

Transparency, Hydration and Thickness

All these qualities are interlinked. The lattice theory of Maurice proposes that the relationship of the spacing of the collagen fibrils (30–60 nm) to the wavelength of visible light (400–700 nm) causes the destructive interference of light scattered in every direction other than that of the incident beam. If this spacing is altered, transparency decreases.

The hydration of the cornea is normally 78 per cent. It is kept at this level by a balance of factors, the most important of which are the swelling pressure of the stromal matrix (60 mmHg) which tends to pull water into the stroma, the pump function of the endothelium, which tends to draw it out of the cornea into the anterior chamber, and the partial barrier of the endothelial maculae occludentes, which impedes movement in either direction.

If the barrier function is compromised, for example by perfusion of the anterior chamber by a solution low in calcium ions, or one outside the tolerated range (6·8–8·2) of pH, the leakage of water into the cornea will exceed the capacity of the pump, and corneal oedema will result.

The consequence is identical if, with the barrier intact, the pump fails. Any disturbance of endothelial metabolism can reduce pump activity. Examples familiar to the corneal physiologist are lowered temperature and perfusion of the anterior chamber with ouabain (which inhibits ATPase).

When either the endothelial barrier or the metabolic pump fails, water enters the stroma, drawn in by the swelling pressure and pushed in by the intraocular pressure. This raises corneal hydration above 78 per cent, increasing thickness (central thickness >0·52 mm), and reducing transparency. This water is trapped within the cornea by the tight junctions of the superficial epithelium (though *artificial* dehydration of the eye surface does reduce corneal hydration) and must leave by the posterior surface when endothelial function is restored. Chronic endothelial failure, for example in Fuchs's dystrophy, results in permanent corneal oedema with sub- and intraepithelial cyst formation (i.e. bullous keratopathy) and eventually in loss of epithelial integrity.

Metabolism

The function of the swelling pressure/intraocular pressure and endothelial pump balance, impeded by a leaky barrier, is to allow nutrients to reach the avascular cornea from the aqueous, and metabolites to leave. Glucose, amino acids and lipids diffuse, or are actively transported, across the endothelium, and the water which accompanies them is pumped back into the anterior chamber.

The most actively metabolizing layers of the cornea are the epithelium and the endothelium; their levels of activity are probably similar. The epithelium, being ten times thicker than the endothelium, requires a proportionately larger supply of metabolic substrates.

Like other tissues, the epithelium can metabolize glucose both aerobically and anaerobically. An intermediate product of both pathways is lactic acid, which in the presence of oxygen is further oxidized to carbon dioxide and water. Under anaerobic conditions, however, lactic acid accumulates. Epithelial lactic acid diffuses into the stroma, raising the osmolarity of the hydrated proteoglycan matrix, and causing water to be drawn in from the aqueous. The conditions that produce hypoxia (e.g. an occlusive contact lens), by encouraging anaerobic metabolism and the accumulation of lactic acid, thus produce increased stromal hydration, with consequent increase in thickness and decrease in transparency.

Oxygen and Carbon Dioxide

Table III shows that, in theory, the corneal epithelium is not normally exposed to a Po_2 of less than 55 mmHg. Experiments suggest that its requirement is only 15–25 mmHg. The overnight swelling of the cornea (normally 3–5 per cent) is therefore probably not associated with the reduced oxygen supply, but rather with the reduction of tear osmolarity during sleep, and perhaps also with the reduction of pH (from 7·3 to 7·1) and with the increase of temperature (about 2 °C) which occur on eye closure.

When the eye is open, a steep oxygen gradient (155 mmHg to 55 mmHg) exists across the thickness of the cornea. When the eye is closed, this gradient is abolished. The Po_2 at the endothelium is unaffected by eye closure because it is maintained by the aqueous.

A gradient (trace to 55 mmHg), in the opposite direction, exists for carbon dioxide when the eye is open. This gradient also is abolished on eye closure.

The carbon dioxide leaving the cornea of the open eye amounts to 21 mm^3 cm^{-2} h^{-1}, while oxygen enters at only 5 mm^3 cm^{-2} h^{-1}. This excess of carbon dioxide

Table III. The partial pressures of oxygen and carbon dioxide at three levels in the cornea in open and closed eye conditions

		Source of O_2	P_{O_2} (mmHg)	P_{CO_2} (mmHg)
Epith	Open eye	Air	155*	(Trace)
	Closed eye	Tarsal vessels	55	55
Mid stroma	Open eye	Air	95	25
	Closed eye	Tarsal vessels	44	55
Endo	Open eye	Aqueous	55	55
	Closed eye	Aqueous	55	55

* At sea level.

is not generated solely by corneal metabolism, but also from the other ocular structures with which the aqueous comes into contact.

Corneal Metabolism and Contact Lenses

Every contact lens affects corneal metabolism, no matter how briefly it is worn. *Table* IV suggests the very different conditions imposed by lenses of different types and materials.

The least physiologically compatible lens type is the flush fitting scleral of polymethylmethacrylate (PMMA), which is now seldom used. The corneal oxygen supply is contained solely within the drop of normal saline inserted with the lens, and there is no tear exchange. Not surprisingly, this lens could be worn only for an hour or two before epithelial oedema became gross, with the onset of haloes and the blurring of vision. Persistent wearing of occlusive lenses produces rapid corneal vascularization in response to the induced hypoxia.

Corneal lenses move freely on the eye surface during blinking, exchanging 10–20 per cent of the subjacent tear layer per blink. Oxygenated tears are thereby brought in contact with the cornea. It will be apparent that the fit of corneal lenses (which determines the position and mobility on the eye) is directly related to their ability to deliver oxygen to the cornea. Gas permeable corneal lenses, which are dimensionally similar to PMMA corneal lenses, permit the passage of atmospheric oxygen through their substance, in addition to providing tear pumping action.

Hydrogel lenses, which are usually of 'semi-scleral' size, cling to the eye and have no significant tear pumping properties. Their oxygen permeability is linearly related to the water content of the material. A range of materials, of water content 38–79 per cent, is available. Oxygen transmission depends also on lens thickness; a thin low water content lens may transmit as much oxygen as a thick high water content lens. Lens thickness is dictated by optical power and by the strength of the material. These are some of the factors that are borne in mind when choosing a lens for a particular eye. Lens trial is the final test, as corneae are quite individual in their responses to lens-induced hypoxia.

Silicone rubber is in many respects the ideal contact lens material. It has a higher refractive index than many hydrogels, is very tough and is very permeable to gases. Unfortunately its surface is naturally hydrophobic and has to be specially treated to allow adequate wetting.

Table IV. Some properties of various contact lenses

	Flush (sealed) scleral (PMMA)	Fenestrated or slotted scleral (PMMA)	Corneal PMMA	Corneal gas permeable	Hydrogel	Silicone rubber
Route of O_2 to cornea	Static tear pool under lens	Tear pool exchanged by air bubble pump on blinking	Tear pump (10–20% exchange per blink)	(a) tear pump (b) from air through lens	From air through lens	(a) from air through lens (b) tear pump
Permeability to gases	Impermeable	Impermeable	Impermeable	Fairly to very permeable, depending on material and thickness	Fairly to very permeable, depending on water content and thickness	Very permeable
Typical diameter	20–23 mm (oval)	20–23 mm (oval)	8–10 mm	8–10 mm	12·5–14·5 mm	10·5–12·5 mm
Refractive index	1·49	1·49	1·49	1·47 (CAB)	38% 1·435 60% 1·415 75% 1·379	1·435

Extended Wear of Contact Lenses

The oxygen environment of the daily wear lens is the air, which at sea level gives a Po_2 of 155 mmHg (falling with altitude to about 50 mmHg at the summit of Everest). When a contact lens is worn during sleep, the oxygen tension at its anterior surface is 55 mmHg. A hydrogel lens which transmits sufficient oxygen to the cornea when the eye is open may not do so in the relatively hypoxic condition of lid closure. Extended (day and night) wear of hydrogel lenses results in overnight corneal swelling which is greater than normal. The cornea may not, in fact, resume its normal thickness after a day of wakefulness. Chronic oedema may well be a factor in the predisposition to corneal infection which is the most serious drawback of this mode of optical correction.

The Limbal Vessels

At the extreme periphery, the cornea derives its gaseous and metabolic requirements from the limbal vessels. However, the major bulk of the cornea should be considered to be avascular.

CONGENITAL ABNORMALITIES

Congenital abnormalities of the cornea are rare. They can occur in isolation, but are more usually associated with other ocular defects.

Abnormalities of Size: Enlargement

The horizontal diameter of the cornea at birth is 10 mm. The adult dimension of 11·7 mm is reached in about 2 years.

Megalocornea

Megalocornea is considered to be present if the cornea is found to be of adult size at birth, or 13·0 mm or greater (in horizontal diameter) after the age of 2 years.

In *simple megalocornea*, which is very rare indeed, the large corneae are clear and of normal thickness and central curvature, and there are no associated ocular abnormalities or systemic disorders.

The cornea is exactly similar in *anterior magalophthalmos*, but the iris and angle are also abnormal, and there may be systemic defects. Patients with this X-linked recessive condition tend to develop glaucoma and early cataract. Both complications usually respond to conventional treatment.

Much commoner than either of the two foregoing conditions is *buphthalmos* (ox-eye), in which the coats of the eye are stretched, and the corneal diameter thus usually increased, by infantile glaucoma. Buphthalmos is progressive: it may begin as early as late fetal life, is usually apparent before the end of the first year after birth, and ceases by the age of 3 years. Sixty per cent of patients are male; some 65 per cent of cases are bilateral, though often asymmetrical; and some 85 per cent of cases are sporadic, the remainder showing autosomal recessive transmission.

The cornea shows splits in Descemet's membrane (Haab's striae) and enlarged endothelial cells, and is often thickened by oedema. Decompensation is not uncommon, either in infancy or in later life. Presumably this is due either to the failure of the endothelium to clothe the splits in DM, or to endothelial depopulation with consequential loss of barrier function and pumping ability.

The anterior chamber angle is abnormal, and glaucoma is present, which produces retinal nerve fibre damage as in adult forms of glaucoma. Goniotomy or other forms of glaucoma surgery can arrest the glaucoma and the corneal enlargement.

The cornea usually appears to be enlarged in *keratoglobus* but its diameter is often normal; the appearance is largely attributable to excessive protrusion, which is due to abnormal thinness. The condition is bilateral. It has autosomal recessive transmission. There is an association with thin blue sclerae (which may lead to its diagnosis soon after birth), joint hypermobility syndrome and the Ehlers–Danlos group of syndromes.

Because of the thinness, steepness and lack of rigidity of the cornea, it is prone to spontaneous rupture of Descemet's membrane, with the production of hydrops corneae as in keratoconus. The entire cornea is quite liable to rupture if traumatized; the same is true for the sclera if this is also thin.

Abnormalities of Size: Reduced

Microcornea

In nanophthalmos (dwarf eye) the eye is normal except that all its dimensions are reduced. The term microphthalmos implies a small abnormal eye. Microcornea occurs, by definition, in both conditions, rarely as an isolated abnormality, and in association with congenital anomalies of the anterior segment.

Microcornea exists if the horizontal diameter, at birth, is less than 10 mm. Measurement may be difficult if the limbus is 'scleralized' and thus difficult to locate. The cornea is usually fairly flat, which produces a hyperopic refractive error unless associated with a short axial length. Even if the cornea is clear and the remainder of the eye is normal, the eye is usually amblyopic.

Treatment of microcornea is confined to correction of the refractive error, if this results in improved vision, and treatment of the glaucoma which often supervenes. The blemish of unilateral microphthalmos can often be concealed by a painted scleral contact lens ('cosmetic shell').

Abnormalities of Transparency

Waring proposes, as a mnemonic for the differential diagnosis of neonatal cloudy cornea, the acronym STUMPED (Sclerocornea, Tears in DM, Ulcer, Metabolic, Posterior corneal defect, Endothelial dystrophy, Dermoid).

Sclerocornea

The peripheral cornea is white and vascularized, resembling the sclera with which it blends. The centre of the cornea is more or less transparent in the various forms of the condition. Sclerocornea occurs as an isolated abnormality but is more usually associated with anterior chamber cleavage syndrome (Rieger's syndrome, Peters's anomaly).

Tears in DM

When the pressure on a neonatal cornea exceeds a certain limit, Descemet's membrane ruptures. It tears in linear or curvilinear fashion, and the edges roll inwards (i.e. towards the stroma) on themselves. Endothelial function is massively disturbed in the region of the tear and localized corneal oedema results. This is resolved when endothelial migration over the edges of the tear re-establishes the continuity of the monolayer. Then it is possible to see the tear as a broad parallel-sided band with brightly reflecting edges (Haab's stria). Specular microscopy often shows a reduced endothelial cell density within the band and indeed the total endothelial population of the cornea may be depleted. The decompensation of such corneae in later life is well known.

Pressure from within (glaucoma) or on the outside of the globe (e.g. forceps birth trauma) can cause DM splits. They do not usually occur after the second year of life, except in association with another corneal disease (most commonly keratoconus).

Ulcer

Congenital herpes simplex keratitis, which is very rare, can occur either locally or as a feature of systemic infection.

Bacterial ophthalmia neonatorum was a common cause of neonatal blindness until silver nitrate prophylaxis was proposed by Credé in 1884 (2·5 per cent aqueous solution; stronger than 1·0 per cent solution now rarely used).

Neither the herpes simplex virus nor the gonococcus are impeded by the epithelial barrier of the cornea: they can pass directly through the cell membranes.

Metabolic

Metabolic causes of corneal opacity are not usually seen at birth, but during the first few years of life. They are all rare; for this reason, they are merely listed here.

Mucopolysaccharidoses
  IH (Hurler)
  IS (Scheie)
  IIIB (Sanfilippo)
  VIA ⎫
  VIB ⎭ (Maroteaux–Lamy)

Mucolipidoses
  I
  II
  III
  IV
  GM_1 gangliosidosis I (generalized gangliosidosis)

Lipid diseases
  Angiokeratoma (Fabry)
  α-lipoprotein deficiency (Tangier)
  Crystalline dystrophy (Schnyder)

Protein disorders
  Infantile cystinosis (Fanconi)
  Tyrosinosis
  Oculocerebrorenal syndrome (Lowe)

Posterior Corneal Defects

These defects may occur separately, or in association with other manifestations of mesenchymal dysgenesis of the anterior segment (anterior chamber cleavage syndrome). They are best categorized by the 'step-ladder classification' devised by Waring (*Table* V).

Posterior Keratoconus

The posterior corneal depression is usually sharply circumscribed. Earlier ophthalmologists referred to this condition as 'keratoconus posticus circumscripta'. The associated stromal opacity may be minimal or even absent, and the defect may present as a cause of amblyopia or refractive error. The refractive indices of the cornea (1·376) and of the aqueous (1·336), being similar, abnormalities of the posterior corneal profile do not greatly affect the total refractive power of the eye. The endothelium is functional and oedema is rarely seen.

Only if the posterior excavation of the cornea is extensive and deep does ectasia result, when keratometry will probably indicate irregular astigmatism. This ectasia is not analogous to that of the usual form of keratoconus, when ectasia occurs early in the disease process and is related both to corneal thinning and to an abnormality of stromal collagen.

Endothelial dystrophy

Congenital hereditary stromal dystrophy, congenital hereditary endothelial dystrophy, posterior polymorphous dystrophy: all may produce corneal opacity

Table V. Mesenchymal dysgenesis of the anterior ocular segment: stepladder classification

Posterior keratoconus	Peters' anomaly*†			Posterior embryotoxon	Axenfeld's anomaly*	Rieger's syndrome*	Irido-gonio-dys-genesis*	Anterior chamber cleavage syndrome*
Posterior corneal depression	Posterior corneal defect and opacity	Posterior corneal defect and opacity Iris adhesions to opacity margin	Posterior corneal defect and opacity Iris adhesions to opacity margin Lens apposition to opacity					Posterior corneal defect and opacity Iris adhesions to opacity margin Lens apposition to opacity
				Prominent Schwalbe's ring	Prominent Schwalbe's ring Iris strands to Schwalbe's ring	Prominent Schwalbe's ring Iris strands to Schwalbe's ring Hypoplastic anterior iris stroma	Iris strands to Schwalbe's ring Hypoplastic anterior iris stroma	Prominent Schwalbe's ring Iris strands to Schwalbe's ring Hypoplastic anterior iris stroma

* May have developed glaucoma.
† Von Hippel's internal corneal ulcer, if inflammatory.
From Waring G. O., Rodrigues, M. M. and Laibson, P. R. Anterior chamber cleavage syndrome. A stepladder classification. *Surv. Ophthalmol.* 1975; **20,** 3. Used with permision of the Survey of Ophthalmology.

at birth. They are further mentioned in the section on dystrophies.

Dermoid

A dermoid of the cornea may be difficult to differentiate from the opaque vascularized cornea which is sometimes seen as part of Peters's anomaly. An ultrasound examination may demonstrate the normality of the remainder of the anterior segment, and a biopsy might show a variety of tissues, such as hair follicles, skin glands and fat. Usually the whole thickness of the cornea is not involved and a lamellar keratoplasty may produce a clear cornea.

CORNEAL OPACIFICATION

Since transparency is the normal state of the cornea, almost any process which upsets its anatomy or physiology results in opacification of some degree. The common causes of loss of transparency of a previously normal cornea are: oedema; drying; deposition; cellular infiltration; vascularization; scarring.

Oedema

As previously discussed, the water content of the cornea is normally exactly regulated. If either of its limiting membranes is disturbed, this equilibrium is upset. Hydration, thickness and transparency are directly interrelated.

Epithelium

Minor trauma to the epithelium (e.g. corneal foreign body, contact lens abrasion) produces a slight stromal oedema immediately beneath the lesion, which disappears when epithelial continuity is restored. This could be explained on the basis that the epithelium has a barrier function, so that a breach allows tears to enter the stroma; this is probably the case, but it is possible that, in addition, the epithelium has a water pumping activity similar to, but much less important than, that of the endothelium. Hypoxia (e.g. contact lens occlusion, abnormal atmosphere) produces corneal oedema by the accumulation in the epithelium and stroma of epithelial metabolites.

Endothelium

Any disturbance of the endothelium rapidly produces corneal oedema. Typical causes, each with the same end result, are given, with some examples.

Anatomical

Intraocular surgery with depletion of cells.
Rupture of DM (trauma, keratoconus, buphthalmos).

Rapid rise of IOP, reinforcing swelling pressure (surgery, acute glaucoma).

Functional

Aqueous changes (anterior uveitis, anterior segment ischaemia).

Infection (herpes simplex virus, mumps virus).

Immune reaction (cytotoxic T-lymphocytes in graft rejection).

Chemical damage (moderate alkali injury).

Post mortem (aqueous stagnation).

Eye banking (refrigeration slows metabolic pump).

Local damage to the endothelium, such as that adjacent to a surgical incision, or that caused by spontaneous rupture of Descemet's membrane (hydrops corneae), is repaired by the sliding of adjacent cells until the defect is closed. In the case of spontaneous rupture, these cells then secrete a new DM in the bared area. From the appearance of hydrops to its resolution usually takes 4–6 weeks.

Assessment

Assessment of corneal oedema depends upon its approximate degree. When oedema is mild, transparency is hardly affected (and certainly cannot be measured clinically). The appropriate measurement here is of corneal thickness. A central reading of greater than 0·54 mm in a previously normal cornea should be taken as evidence of oedema. The pachometer is the ideal instrument with which to follow changes of corneal thickness and thus to document the progress of a treated graft rejection or resolving postoperative oedema. Above 0·65 mm, readings become increasingly difficult, as the posterior cornea becomes wrinkled and the end point is difficult to ascertain.

Vision

Stromal oedema does not usually affect vision until the epithelium becomes oedematous also. The bullae of epithelial oedema cause the appearance of rainbow haloes around white lights. When these bullae become large or coalescent they have a more significant effect on vision, and in addition, when they rupture they cause pain.

Drying

Local drying of the cornea, in eyes with normal tear function, can occur if the spreading of the tear film is interrupted. Conjunctival elevations, for example following horizontal rectus surgery for squint, frequently produce saucer-shaped depressions (dellens). The cornea may be reduced to one-half of its normal thickness, or less, and be locally opaque, but there is no permanent disturbance of any layer and rehydration cures the condition.

The tear film and its continuity are crucial in the maintenance of corneal transparency. It is important to remember that a cornea can be dry in the presence of copious tears, if they are not wetting it, or if the normal lid action is absent (examples: exposure keratitis, and beside or beneath an anhydrous contact lens). In order for aqueous tears to form a film, a mucin layer must cover the hydrophobic epithelial surface, which in turn must be able to retain this layer. Conjunctival goblet cell disease results in mucin abnormality or deficiency (examples: Stevens–Johnson syndrome, avitaminosis A, ocular pemphigoid). The surface microanatomy of the epithelial layer normally features structures which interact with the mucin layer but is abnormal in certain conditions (for example, in sensory innervation deficiency).

Deposition

A variety of substances, both organic and inorganic, can be deposited in the corneal tissues with resulting loss of corneal transparency.

Calcium

Band keratopathy is discussed in the section on degenerations. Localized or generalized calcium deposition, occurring at the level of Bowman's layer, can follow any chronic inflammation. It is often seen in association with superficial stromal neovascularization. Calcific degeneration of all levels of the cornea is seen in phthisis bulbi and following severe chemical injury.

Silver

The historical use of silver nitrate solution in the prophylaxis of ophthalmia neonatorum has already been mentioned. Where this practice is continued it probably represents no hazard to the cornea. Unfortunately, that ancient remedy the silver nitrate stick ('lunar caustic'), which should probably be confined to museums of ocular therapeutics, is still found in eye clinics in some parts of the world. It is employed in chronic conditions of the external eye, the exact diagnosis of which, one suspects, sometimes eludes its champions.

Silver deposition in the cornea, if not iatrogenic, can also result from chronic exposure to silver compounds used in industrial processes. However it is topically applied, silver is deposited in the deepest layers of the stroma, where it produces an even bluish-grey discoloration (argyrosis corneae).

Iron

A ferrous foreign body on the cornea is a common minor injury. In that warm, damp environment the metal begins at once to oxidize. Rust stains the epithelium and, if Bowman's layer is breached, the superficial stroma also. The foreign body and the surrounding necrotic corneal tissue will fall away naturally, but less residual staining probably results if they are removed, using an aseptic technique which is followed by antibiotic prophylaxis.

An iron-containing pigment is commonly seen in the normal cornea in the Hudson–Stähli line. This deposition, which occurs at the level of the basal epithelial cells, is seen in the form of a roughly horizontal brown line at the junction of the upper two-thirds and the lower third of the cornea; it does not extend to the limbus. Similar lines are sometimes seen in association with corneal and limbal irregularities, such as drainage blebs and radial keratotomy scars. An iron line surrounding the base of the cone in keratoconus is known as Fleischer's ring. These lines probably mark boundaries of differential tear movement or tear pooling; the iron is probably derived from the tears.

In siderosis due to a retained intraocular ferrous foreign body, the stroma becomes diffusely brown-stained.

Copper

In hepatolenticular degeneration (Wilson's disease) a copper compound is deposited at the level of Descemet's membrane in a ring separated from the limbus by a clear interval. It is usually of a bluish or brownish colour, and it fades away when the systemic disease is treated.

Copper has been used since the earliest times (e.g. Ebers papyrus 1500 BC) in the treatment of trachoma and other chronic conditions of the external eye, often in the form of a stick or crystal of the sulphate ('blue stone'). Its main effect seems to have been a mild corrosion of the conjunctiva, resulting eventually in fibrosis which may well have curtailed other inflammations; the fibrosis, however, would lead to cicatrization and loss of conjunctival goblet cells, with consequential drying and corneal opacification. Topically applied copper is not usually deposited in the cornea, but this may occur in chalcosis following the retention of a copper-containing intraocular foreign body.

Mercury

Mercury, and some other heavy metals, is deposited in the posterior cornea when present at abnormally high levels in the body fluids. Such depositions are usually seen in workers in industry who are exposed to these metals or to their salts. Clinically, mercury deposition closely resembles argyrosis corneae.

Melanin

The normal Negro limbus is pigmented by melanocytes. In chronic conditions involving the limbus or the corneal epithelium, such as trachoma or vernal keratoconjunctivitis, this pigment may spread over the corneal surface. It is related that 'black cornea' is a presenting complaint in vernal disease in parts of Africa.

Melanin is rarely seen clinically in the cornea of the eye of white races, but histological evidence shows that melanocytes can be found in the epithelium and at other levels of the normal cornea.

Blood

Blood staining of the cornea occurs: in long-standing hyphaema; rarely, as an extension of a large subconjunctival haemorrhage; if abnormal corneal vessels bleed into the stroma.

Immune rings

A Wessely ring sometimes surrounds an area of antigenic activity in the cornea. It is made up of neutrophils attached at the site of antigen–antibody complex deposition. The antigen, from the centre of the ring, might consist for example of microbial protein, while the antibody diffuses in from the limbus. Such reactions occur commonly and repeatedly in other tissues but they are uniquely prolonged and visible in the cornea, because of its avascularity and transparency.

Lipid

Lipid deposition usually results from corneal neovascularization, and so is most often seen in relation to abnormal vessels. If these approach the visual axis there is a possibility that lipid will affect vision. The majority of patients with such deposition have no systemic lipid abnormality.

The arcus juvenalis seen in vernal disease is related to vascular activity in the limbus and peripheral cornea at the superior pole (and, rarely, at the inferior pole). This is a disease of childhood. Young patients (<30 years) with arcus who show no evidence of ocular disease should be investigated for disorders of fat metabolism.

Plaque

Corneal plaque is the rare consequence of chronic epithelial erosion or failure. In vernal disease a round or horizontally oval greyish-white plaque may be deposited in an area of epithelial macroerosion, usually in the upper third of the cornea. It consists of cellular debris, fibrin and mucus. Plaque perpetuates the failure to re-epithelize which caused it, and resists medical therapy; surgical excision (by superficial keratectomy) produces better results.

Plaque also occurs in chronic cases of herpes zoster keratitis, herpes simplex keratitis and, occasionally, in keratoconjunctivitis sicca.

Cornea Verticillata

In cornea verticillata (vortex dystrophy) metabolites or drugs are deposited in the epithelium in a pattern resembling a mare's tail, a spiral galaxy or a maelstrom. It is most commonly seen in patients on systemic treatment with phenothiazines, chloroquine, indomethacin and amiodarone. In these cases it is the drug or a metabolic derivative which is deposited. As a rule, neither symptoms nor permanent damage results. In Fabry's disease the deposition is sphingolipid (trihexose ceramide).

The rare *separate* entity of cornea verticillata, once described, is now thought to be a manifestation of Fabry's disease.

Abrasion and Erosion

Disturbance of the superficial epithelial cells is a common sign of a variety of insults to the corneal surface.

Mechanical

Simple slight abrasion of the cornea by contact with objects in the environment of the cornea (fingers, clothing, contact lenses etc.) results in disturbance of the superficial epithelium. More forceful abrasion will disturb the basal layer and its basement membrane also. These injuries are painful but heal rapidly, usually without the complications of infection or scarring. Initial healing is by spread of adjacent epithelial cells; the rate of epithelial mitosis then increases. During healing the cornea is protected by increased tearing, an overproduction of mucus which clothes the epithelial defects, and ptosis or blepharospasm. If most of the corneal epithelium is lost, conjunctival epithelium spreads centrally to cover the bare area. This epithelium differs in its surface characteristics from corneal epithelium, but it differentiates to the corneal type in days or weeks. Until then its transparency and tear-retaining characteristics are abnormal.

Mechanical damage to the epithelium is facilitated if it or its basement membrane are abnormal. The hypoxia caused by contact lens occlusion and the chronic oedema resulting from endothelial failure are examples of processes that increase epithelial fragility. Recurrent erosion and diabetic epithelial breakdown are attributable to abnormalities at the desmosomal level.

A mechanical keratitis sometimes results from environmental factors. Particles reach the conjunctival sac in various industrial processes and can cause an irritative keratoconjunctivitis. Man-made mineral fibres used in the insulation of buildings, for example, rockwool, are particularly prone to produce such a condition.

Radiation

A variety of electromagnetic radiations causes cellular damage to the cornea. The most familiar example is photophthalmia caused by ultraviolet light (especially of wavelength 250–315 nm). This is seen as snow blindness, arc eye and following exposure to UVB sun lamps. Following a latent period of some hours, the epithelium breaks down in punctate fashion in the exposed area. Healing occurs by spread and mitosis of surrounding cells.

Chemical and Toxic

Acids and alkalis cause epithelial erosion. The penetration of acids is arrested by the coagulation of protein which they produce, but alkalis penetrate rapidly. For this reason the alkali injury is the more serious. Ammonia, lime and caustic soda or potash burns can destroy all the living cells of the cornea. A severe alkali burn, however, can initially produce a white eye with a clear cornea. The whiteness of the sclera and conjunctiva is caused by infarction of blood vessels, and the dead yet clear cornea does not at first imbibe water as its proteoglycan matrix has been denatured and the swelling pressure thereby eliminated.

A tremendous variety of substances, organic and inorganic, particulate and in aerosol, gaseous and liquid, are toxic to the corneal surface if exposure is sufficiently prolonged and concentrated. To produce damage to the cornea, such substances must first contaminate and/or disrupt the tear film. Many topical drugs and their preservatives are toxic, especially when applied to an eye which is not in a normal state of health.

Cellular infiltration

Infiltration of the corneal tissues by inflammatory cells occurs in a wide variety of conditions, and must inevitably result in local or generalized, temporary or permanent, partial or complete, loss of transparency.

Viruses

Adenovirus

Adenovirus keratitis is usually seen in association with the follicular conjunctivitis of epidemic keratoconjunctivitis (EKC), with types 8 and 19 most often implicated. This acute condition, usually not associated with respiratory symptoms, presents as unilateral or asymmetrically bilateral keratoconjunctivitis with preauricular lymphadenopathy. The keratitis is at first diffuse but around the seventh day it becomes coarse and punctate. Virus particles have been demonstrated by electronmicroscopy of these lesions. About a week later, cellular infiltration by polymorphs appears beneath some of the epithelial lesions (subepithelial keratitis). This may persist for from 3 months to 2 years; it disappears on topical treatment with steroid, but can reappear when treatment is stopped. This infiltration marks an immune response to the presence of virus in the epithelium.

Adenovirus also causes pharyngoconjunctival fever (PCF), and here type 3 is the commonest cause. A pharyngitis and fever accompany the conjunctivitis, but the cornea is not usually involved.

Herpes Simplex

Herpes virus hominis can cause, in non-immune individuals, a keratoconjunctivitis similar to that produced by the adenovirus, but vesicles on the lid skin and small ulcers of the lid margins are often present and assist in the diagnosis.

In a previously exposed host (up to 90 per cent of the adult population), the corneal manifestations of herpes simplex infection are usually unilateral and predominate over the conjunctival signs. The virus, normally latent within the trigeminal ganglion, reaches the cornea via the Vth nerve. Recurrent keratitis often occurs at times of immunological change, such as systemic illness, immunosuppressive treatment, or systemic steroid therapy.

The early recurrences usually produce morphologically characteristic epithelial manifestations (dendritic, amoeboid or punctate keratitis), but later stromal and endothelial involvement becomes apparent, often in association with anterior uveitis. Several immunological mechanisms are implicated, both humoral and cell mediated, and as it is the inflammatory response to these which causes most of the corneal damage, it is logical to use anti-inflammatory as well as anti-viral drugs in the therapy of the disease.

Steroids inhibit chemotaxis and polymorph lysosome disruption, and possibly damage sensitized lymphocytes; they may also inhibit the local production of antibody. Their use in herpes simplex keratitis must, however, be supervised by an experienced practitioner who can observe, interpret and act on the signs of such complications as the enhancement of viral replication in the epithelium, secondary infection by bacteria or fungi, steroid glaucoma and cataract and the rebound phenomenon which follows the abrupt withdrawal of steroids.

Antimetabolic drugs which damage viral DNA include idoxuridine (IDU) and adenine arabinoside (Ara-A), which have poor penetration and are used particularly in epithelial disease, and trifluorothymidine (F_3T), acycloguanosine (acyclovir) and bromovinyldeoxyuridine (BVDU), which have better penetration and are used in stromal disease and in keratouveitis. Acyclovir and BVDU are more specific for virus than for host cells, and are therefore less toxic to the corneal tissue than are the other antivirals mentioned.

Herpes Zoster

The varicella virus, which causes chickenpox and herpes zoster, produces ocular and periocular disease when, like the herpes simplex virus, it colonizes the trigeminal ganglion. About 40 per cent of patients with herpes zoster ophthalmicus (HZO) have corneal disease at some stage of their illness. Acutely, a fine punctate epithelial keratitis or a dendritic ulcer (from which virus particles can be isolated) is sometimes seen. (The raised 'pseudo-dendrites' which also occur are adherent mucus and can be wiped off the corneal surface.) These early features may be accompanied or followed much later by a disciform keratitis which resembles that of herpes simplex and which is probably caused by a similar immunopathological process. Corneal sensation is always reduced after herpetic keratitis of either type, but more so in zoster than in simplex. As a result, neurotrophic disease (epithelial breakdown, trophic ulceration, stromal melting) is a relatively common manifestation of zoster keratitis.

Treatment of HZO is with topical steroid preparations plus antibiotic for the prophylaxis or treatment of bacterial secondary infection. Antivirals (IDU, Ara-A, and especially oral BVDU) have been shown to be effective in herpes zoster, but their role in treatment of the keratitis remains to be established.

Paramyxoviruses

The measles virus causes a punctate epithelial keratitis which requires no treatment; however, in association with malnutrition, a severe ulcerative keratitis, perhaps with corneal perforation, can result.

The mumps virus can rarely cause a dacryoadenitis with associated follicular conjunctivitis and superficial keratitis. More rarely still, it causes a unilateral endothelial keratitis which results in pancorneal oedema. When this clears (in days or weeks) a profound endothelial disturbance and depletion is seen.

Chlamydiae

Chlamydiae contain both DNA and RNA but are obligate intracellular parasites. The species *Chlamydia trachomatis* includes the agents of trachoma, inclusion conjunctivitis and lymphogranuloma venereum.

Corneal scarring due to trachoma is a major world cause of blindness. Though there may be diffuse punctate epithelial and subepithelial keratitis in the early stages, the cornea is more significantly involved when affected by vascularization and infiltration (pannus) extending from the upper limbus. This process results in fibrosis, which may cause visual loss, but the most important route to corneal blindness is via tear depletion, entropion and trichiasis caused by the chronic conjunctival disease.

Inclusion conjunctivitis (TRIC), an oculogenital disease, resembles the early stage of trachoma, but resolves without scarring, pannus or tear deficiency. Epithelial keratitis, followed by subepithelial keratitis resembling that of EKC, disappears on treatment with specific agents.

Both early trachoma and inclusion conjunctivitis respond to oral treatment with sulphonamides and tetracyclines. Where trachoma is hyperendemic, bacterial infection is usually an important complication, and topical treatment is then more relevant, though the organism is not necessarily eradicated.

Bacteria

The cornea is surrounded by bacteria: they are always present on the lid margins and often on the conjunctival surfaces; but bacterial keratitis is rare in the normal cornea. Where corneal resistance is lowered, bacterial infection becomes common. Causes of lowered resistance include acute or chronic epithelial loss (e.g. simple abrasion, vernal keratitis), previous corneal infection (e.g. herpes simplex keratitis), hypoxia (e.g. contact lens occlusion), impaired sensation (e.g. HZO, leprosy), exposure (e.g. lid defect, VII paralysis), dry eye (e.g. Sjögren's syndrome) and systemic illness (e.g. disseminated malignant disease, immunosuppression).

When bacterial infection occurs, the outcome depends on the organism, its toxins and its enzymes; the position on the cornea; the response of the host tissues; and the therapy given. Some infections (e.g. staphylococcus, moraxella, haemophilus, klebsiella, nocardia, *Escherichia coli*) are characteristically less progressive than others (e.g. streptococcus, pseudomonas, clostridium). The latter group possess proteases including collagenase which facilitate spread through the cornea. Some members of both groups elaborate toxins which damage cells (acting on membranes, or on protein synthesis) or neutrophils. The bacterial products are frequently antigenic, with the result that the immune response of the host forms a significant part of the clinical picture.

Staphylococcus, pseudomonas, *Streptococcus pneumoniae* and moraxella are the commonest causes of bacterial central corneal ulceration. Staphylococcus, haemophilus and moraxella account for most peripheral infections.

Bacterial keratitis causes blurred vision, pain, photophobia, red eye, sticky discharge and swollen lids. The accompanying conjunctivitis is usually non-specific. An anterior uveitis is usually present; pneumococcal keratitis frequently produces a hypopyon. The identity of the organism may be suspected from the clinical appearance and from a knowledge of the history, but it should always be investigated bacteriologically. Ideally, treatment is begun only after corneal scrapings have been Gram-stained and inoculated on to culture media. Unless significant numbers of a single organism are found in the Gram-stained smear, a combination of two antibiotics, rather than a single antibiotic, is recommended. Typical combinations are methicillin–gentamicin and cefuroxime–ticarcillin. These drugs should be given subconjunctivally and then every $\frac{1}{2}$–1 hour in drop form. When the culture and sensitivity results are available, the therapy can be modified as necessary.

Fungi

Fungal keratitis is commoner in tropical and subtropical regions than in temperate climates. Many different fungi have been known to cause keratitis, but the commonest are *Fusarium solani*, *Aspergillus* spp. and *Candida albicans*. Most of these organisms are ubiquitous and only become corneal pathogens when the cornea is injured or diseased.

Fungal keratitis often takes the form of a stromal keratitis with overlying epithelial ulceration; the edge of the infiltrate is feathery and there may be satellite lesions and/or immune rings. The appearances are not wholly specific, however, and investigation is required to prove the diagnosis. Corneal scrapes are examined in Gram-stained and Giemsa-stained smears, and are inoculated into media such as Sabouraud agar, brain–heart infusion and thioglycollate broth.

Antifungal agents used in mycotic keratitis include the polyenes (e.g. amphotericin B, nystatin, natamycin), the imidazoles (e.g. clotrimazole, econazole, ketoconazole, miconazole) and 5-fluorocytosine. A polyene and/or an imidazole are effective against filamentous fungi such as fusarium and aspergillus. An imidazole and 5-fluorocytosine are recommended for candida infections.

Steroid preparations enhance fungal keratitis in the stage of active infection and should not be used. They may be used, with great caution, at a late stage with the objective of reducing associated stromal infiltration or anterior uveitis.

Protozoa

Amoebic keratitis is very rare, despite the ubiquity of the organisms. Occasionally an outdoor injury will result in an indolent corneal lesion with stromal infiltration and recurrent epithelial breakdown, from which only acanthamoeba can be isolated. Treatment is with topical Brolene (propamidine) and steroid, and must be prolonged to ensure immobilization by encystment of the organisms. The residual scarring will usually necessitate penetrating keratoplasy.

Interstitial Keratitis

Interstitial inflammation of the cornea occurs in congenital syphilis, acquired syphilis, tuberculosis, sarcoidosis, leprosy, onchocerciasis, Wegener's granulomatosis and in Cogan's syndrome. In each case an immunological mechanism is postulated.

The stroma becomes oedematous, and then infiltrated. Vision is much affected; photophobia and pain (due to concomitant uveitis) may be severe. Blood vessels migrate into the deep stroma, producing the naked eye appearance of 'salmon patch'. The condition resolves spontaneously, leaving diffuse scarring which tends gradually to clear, and 'ghost vessels'. The vision improves, and may be compatible with a normal lifestyle, but endothelial damage may result in later corneal decompensation.

Cogan's syndrome links non-leutic interstitial keratitis, vestibulo-auditory symptoms and systemic occlusive vascular disease. This rare condition also shows a strong association with systemic vasculitis.

Non-infective Hepatitis

Superior limbic keratoconjunctivitis (of Theodore), superficial punctate keratitis (of Thygeson) and nummular keratitis (of Dimmer) are conditions in which no infective agent has been convincingly demonstrated.

In *Thygeson's superficial punctate keratitis* multiple discrete white or greyish dots appear in the epithelium with the production of discomfort or foreign body sensation and photophobia. The lesions are slightly raised and stain with fluorescein. They fade away and are replaced by new lesions, and the clinical course of the condition is relapsing, with a duration of 2–4 years. A slow virus aetiology has been proposed but not substantiated.

All the currently used treatments (topical antivirals, topical steroids and therapeutic hydrogel contact lenses) have shown success in managing the symptoms and signs, if not in limiting the course of the disease.

Vascularization

Vascularization of the cornea is always abnormal. The extension of blood vessels into the stroma is always preceded by cellular infiltration, with or without oedema, whether of infective, toxic, hypoxic or immune aetiology. Familiar clinical examples are trachoma, contact lens related hypoxia or irritation, and corneal graft neovascularization.

Whatever the neovascular stimulus, the initial dilatation of limbal capillaries and venules results in the leakage into the corneal tissues (usually the stroma) of leucocytes and serum proteins. The vascular endothelium proliferates and migrates, possibly in response to a factor released by polymorphs. Prostaglandins too have a role in neovascularization. A proteinase inhibitor which has been demonstrated in cornea, cartilage and other tissues can be shown experimentally to inhibit the process; presumably some such system protects the avascularity of the normal cornea.

A mild degree of pannus does not threaten vision, but some clinical types of neovascularization can progress to the central cornea, where they cause visual loss. Examples are seen in herpes simplex stromal keratitis, interstitial keratitis, atopic keratoconjunctivitis and following chemical, thermal or mechanical injury. Fibrous tissue and lipid deposition, following in the wake of the vessels, further decrease transparency.

Anterior segment fluorescein angiography, by revealing leaking new vessels, can give an indication of areas that are proliferating. If the neovascular stimulus can be removed, vessel growth usually ceases. If lipid deposition still continues, and poses a threat to vision, laser photocoagulation may succeed in closing the vessels. The same technique can be used in an attempt to create an avascular bed in preparation for keratoplasty.

Scarring

Clean wounds of the cornea heal by avascular scarring. A surgical wound, such as a corneal cataract section or a refractive keratoplasty incision, initiates epithelial sliding within 6 h and cover is usually complete within 24–48 h. At this time polymorphs are removing cellular debris. By day 3 or 4, the epithelial wound plug begins to regress and the adjacent stromal keratocytes are lined up along the wound margins, secreting collagen (especially type II) and glycosaminoglycans (especially keratan sulphate). Fibroblasts invade the wound by the end of the first week. Collagen deposition continues, and cellular infiltrate regresses, so that by 2 months the wound is strong and devoid of inflammatory cells. It is found that wound strength continues to increase for many months.

The new collagen fibrils are of large diameter and are not organized in a regular lattice as are the fibrils in normal cornea. The wound, though avascular, is therefore opaque. It is observed clinically that this opacification fades slowly over several years.

Scarring, if accompanied by neovascularization, results in the deposition of more fibrous tissue than accompanies the avascular process. Such a response is seen after some chemical injuries (e.g. exposure to mustard gas), after infections (e.g. herpes simplex stromal disease, bacterial suppurative keratitis) and after penetrating injuries, when the new vessels may extend from the iris as well as from the limbus.

DEGENERATION

Age-Related

Vogt's Limbus Girdle

Vogt's limbus girdle is frequently seen in middle-aged and elderly people. It appears in the interpalpebral zone both nasally and temporally, and there may or may not be a clear interval between it and the limbus. The opacity is at the level of Bowman's layer and is of no clinical significance, but it must be differentiated from early deposits due to hypercalcaemia.

Arcus Senilis

Arcus senilis occurs in nearly all late middle-aged and elderly people. A clear zone is present between it and the limbus. The deposition, which occurs at all levels of the stroma, is of lipid. An arcus present in early adult life may be a manifestation of hyperlipidaemia. In a later age group, but below the age of 60 years, it may indicate a raised serum cholesterol.

Pathological

Band Keratopathy

Band keratopathy (band-shaped degeneration) is seen in hypercalcaemia and as a sequel to almost any severe ocular disease, especially uveitis of childhood. Calcium is deposited in the superficial stroma, in Bowman's layer and in the deep layers of the epithelium. The distribution in the interpalpebral zone, with a clear interval between the ends of the band and the limbus, is characteristic.

If band keratopathy obscures useful vision it can be removed by superficial keratectomy or lamellar keratoplasty, or chemically with the chelating agent disodium edatate.

Salzmann's Nodular Degeneration

Salzmann's nodular degeneration is rare but can follow a variety of chronic corneal inflammations, especially rosacea keratitis and trachoma. The hyaline deposits are associated with areas of destruction of Bowman's layer and of the subjacent stroma. Clinically the bluish-white elevations may cause recurrent discomfort, due to epithelial loss from their surfaces, and visual loss if they impinge on the central zone. The condition can be treated by lamellar keratoplasty, but similar changes may develop in the graft if the corneal environment (which presumably contributed to the original disease) cannot be improved.

Terrien's Marginal Degeneration

Terrien's marginal degeneration is a rare bilateral condition which chiefly affects males in early middle age. The pathogenesis is unknown. Vascularizing peripheral infiltration is followed by stromal thinning and the appearance of a gutter just within the limbus. Before this is clinically obvious, keratometry may show a marked corneal astigmatism, which is responsible for the visual deterioration characteristic of this condition. If the gutter becomes ectatic, or if it perforates, a freehand peripheral keratoplasty may be required.

Pellucid Marginal Degeneration

This condition is discussed in the section on ectasia (p. 146).

Mooren's ulcer

Mooren's is a chronic marginal ulcer which begins as peripheral stromal infiltration and proceeds to epithelial loss and stromal melting. The lesion extends around the cornea, and usually resolves when it has encompassed the periphery, but in some cases it extends centrally, destroying the entire cornea. The condition runs a course of many months and often demoralizes through the pain it causes.

Mooren's ulcer has some of the hallmarks of an immunopathological disease. Immunoglobulin has been found bound to corneal epithelium, and autoantibodies to epithelium are sometimes found in the serum (though this finding is not specific for this condition).

Treatment is on the whole unsatisfactory. Current practice includes the use of therapeutic contact lenses, topical steroid, topical collagenase inhibitors, systemic immunosuppression, conjunctival excision and sclerokeratoplasty.

Climatic Droplet Keratopathy

Climatic droplet keratopathy (Labrador keratopathy, spheroidal degeneration) is related to ageing and/or corneal disease, and/or climatic conditions. It is most often seen in people who spend much time out of doors, especially in hostile climates. Small 'droplets' accumulate at the level of Bowman's layer, beginning in the peripheral interpalpebral zone and spreading centrally. In marked cases, vision is affected.

Vitamin A Deficiency

Corneal xerosis and keratomalacia are rare in the West but are common where diet is deficient in vitamin A and protein. Xerosis presents as a rough, keratinized, non-wetting corneal surface. The tears may be normal in composition and quantity. Treatment with vitamin A supplements reverses the process and the corneal surface is restored to normality.

Ulceration and keratomalacia are more severe manifestations of vitamin A deficiency. Stromal melting follows epithelial loss and in the extreme form, keratomalacia, which is seen in starving young children, the melting process is very rapid. Vitamin A appears to have a role in the reduction of collagenase production by damaged corneal tissue, and this process may be accelerated in its absence.

If the stromal melting has not resulted in perforation, immediate treatment with large doses of vitamin A may halt the process.

DYSTROPHY

Corneal dystrophies are inherited disorders (autosomal dominant with variable expression, except macular dystrophy, which is autosomal recessive). There is no associated systemic abnormality, except a possible disorder of fat metabolism in central crystalline dystrophy (Schnyder). Age of onset is within the first two decades of life but later for two of the commonest dystrophies, epithelial basement membrane dystrophy (Cogan) and late hereditary endothelial dystrophy (Fuchs). One layer of the cornea is primarily abnormal, but others are usually secondarily involved (the exception is macular dystrophy, which affects both the stroma and the endothelium primarily). Dystrophy is usually bilateral, though often asymmetrical. The process is usually confined to the central cornea, but in some types it extends to the limbus. Usually the primary defect does not greatly affect vision; however, the secondary consequences, such as epithelial oedema, sub-epithelial fibrosis, stromal oedema and vascularization, often do.

Most corneal dystrophies are very rare. *Table* VI summarizes some of their distinguishing features.

Anterior membrane

The commonest epithelial dystrophy is epithelial basement membrane dystrophy.

Epithelial Basement Membrane Dystrophy

Also known as map-dot-fingerprint dystrophy and Cogan's dystrophy, this is a true dystrophy but it is often confused with traumatic recurrent epithelial erosion. It is likely that half or more of patients with recurrent erosion have the dystrophy. The history of trauma that is often elicited may be misleading or may simply indicate unusual epithelial fragility. The finding of symptomless changes in the epithelium of the other cornea will confirm the diagnosis.

The condition occurs in working-age adults. Most cases are asymptomatic, and are observed by chance. However, when recurrent erosion occurs, the pain is usually severe and disabling. Large sheets of loose epithelium should be detached. Lubricating drops by day and ointment by night may reduce friction on the epithelium, as may padding for 1–2 days. A thin plano high water content hydrogel contact lens may give symptomatic relief, but logically this treatment should be continued (with changes of the lens as necessary) for 2–3 months. The condition remits spontaneously after an interval of a few months to a few years, but can recur.

Stroma

Much has been written about the stromal dystrophies, despite their rarity. The abnormal substance appears either within the keratocytes (e.g. macular and fleck dystrophies) or between the collagen fibrils (e.g. granular, lattice and central crystalline dystrophies). The substance may be a normal product present in excess (e.g. glycosaminoglycans in macular and fleck dystrophies) or a product not normally found in the cornea (e.g. 'hyaline' in granular dystrophy, amyloid in lattice dystrophy and cholesterol in central crystalline dystrophy).

Posterior membrane

Descemet's membrane is secreted by the endothelial cell and accumulates throughout life. If the cell is abnormal or is in some way stressed, it can produce excess or abnormal collagen. Abnormal cells become depleted in numbers more rapidly than normal cells, with loss of barrier and pump functions, and the early onset of stromal and later epithelial oedema.

Late Hereditary Endothelial Dystrophy (Fuchs's Dystrophy)

Small numbers of guttata are frequently seen on slit lamp specular microscopy of the easily observed (i.e. central) regions of the corneae of middle-aged and elderly people. It is not clear whether the progression to Fuchs's dystrophy is inevitable, given time, or indeed to what extent this true dystrophy resembles normal age-related endothelial degeneration. Dystrophic patients with accumulating, enlarging and coalescing guttata remain asymptomatic until easily measurable stromal oedema results. The vision is not much affected, and comfort not at all, until epithelial oedema supervenes. Because Fuchs's dystrophy is fairly common, the graft patient may receive a donor cornea destined to manifest the same condition, which event may then be interpreted as 'recurrence in the graft'.

Posterior Polymorphous Dystrophy (of Schlichting)

This is another common dystrophy, which may remain asymptomatic indefinitely. It is often found by chance by ophthalmologists and opticians at routine eye examinations and refractions. There are three main appearances, which may occur separately or together, and be asymmetrical between the two corneae. These are vesicles, curvilinear lines and geographical lesions, all seen at the level of Descemet's membrane. These appearances are caused by the focally thickened deposition of abnormal collagen by the endothelial cells on the posterior surface of the membrane. They may be present in normal endothelial numbers, or depleted. The individual lesions of posterior polymorphous dystrophy have been observed by endothelial specular photomicrography (ESP) to persist unaltered for some years.

ECTASIA

Keratoconus

Keratoconus is sometimes dominantly or recessively transmitted, but it is usually sporadic. There are associations with other ocular conditions (e.g. ectopia lentis, congenital cataract, aniridia, retinitis pigmentosa) and with systemic conditions (e.g.

Table VI. Outline characteristics of some corneal dystrophies

Name	Other name	Layer	Other layers involved	Heredity	Age at onset	Progression	Laterality
Epith. basement membrane dystrophy	Map-dot-fingerprint; Cogan	Epith.	None	Auto. dom.	Any: usually after 30 yr	Self-limiting	Bilateral
Juvenile epith. dystrophy	Meesman	Epith.	None	Auto. dom.	<1yr	Progressive to middle age	Bilateral
Ring-shaped dystrophy	Reis-Bücklers	BL	Epith. ant. stroma	Auto. dom.	Childhood	Progressive to early middle age	Bilateral
Granular dystrophy	Groenouw I	Stroma (pan-)	BL	Auto. dom.	<10yr	Slowly progressive	Bilateral
Lattice dystrophy	None	Stroma (esp. ant.)	Epith., BL	Auto. dom.	<20yr	Slowly progressive	Bilateral (sometimes unilateral)
Macular dystrophy	Groenouw II	Stroma (pan-)	Epith., BL, DM, endo.	Auto. rec.	<10yr	Progressive	Bilateral
Central crystalline dystrophy	Schnyder	Stroma (ant.)	BL	Auto. dom.	<1yr	Slowly progressive	Bilateral
Fleck dystrophy	Speckled dystrophy (Francois)	Stroma (pan-)	None	Auto. dom.	? Congenital	Non-progressive	Bilateral (sometimes unilateral)
Central cloudy dystrophy	Francois	Stroma (esp. post.)	None	Auto. dom.	? Congenital	Non-progressive	Bilateral
Congen. hereditary stromal dystrophy	None	Stroma (pan-)	None	Auto. dom.	Congenital	Non-progressive	Bilateral
Late hereditary endo. dystrophy	Fuchs	Endo.	DM, stroma; Bl, epith.	Auto. dom. (F:M = 4:1)	Middle age; rarely, in 1st–3rd decade	Progressive	Bilateral, asymmetrical
Posterior polymorph. dystrophy	Schlicting	Endo.	DM, stroma BL, epith	Auto. dom.	Congenital	Non-progressive or slowly progressive	Bilateral, asymmetrical
Congen. hereditary endo. dystrophy	None	Endo.	DM, stroma BL, epith.	Auto. dom.; Auto. rec.	<2yr; Congenital	Slowly progressive; Non-progressive	Bilateral

atopy, Ehlers–Danlos syndromes, Down's syndrome, Marfan's syndrome). For these reasons it should probably not be considered to be a corneal dystrophy.

The basic abnormality is of corneal collagen, which results in thinning and subsequent ectasia of the central area (not necessarily centred on the geometrical axis). Bowman's layer becomes fragmented and scarred in the region of the cone. Fine vertical striae in Descemet's membrane at the centre of the cone, seen in bright specular reflection at the slit lamp, clearly visible corneal nerves, and an iron ring (Fleischer's ring) often forming an inferiorly displaced, horizontal ellipse at the level of the basal epithelial cells, are classic signs. Episodes of hydrops corneae occur if Descemet's membrane splits spontaneously.

Keratoconus is always bilateral, though usually asymmetrical; it occurs more frequently in males than in females; its first clinical manifestation, increasing myopic astigmatism, usually appears in the second decade of life. Localized changes of thickness precede the ectasia, but these do not cause symptoms. The condition is progressive, usually for 5–10 years. However, only a small proportion of cases come to keratoplasty.

Position in cornea	Effect on vision	Other symptoms	Histopathology	Histo. stain	Management	Recurrence in graft
Usually central	Transient; slight or moderate	Pain of RE	Maps: intraepith. BM Dots: intraepith. cysts. F'prints. intraepith. BM & fibrillary material	—	MRE; LK if very severe	No
General	Transient, slight	Often nil; sometimes pain of RE	Intracyto-plasmic vacuoles containing fibrillary material	—	Usually nil; rarely SK, LK, PK	Yes
Central	Slight at first; increasing	Pain of RE to early middle age	Sub-epithelial microcysts	—	MRE; SK; LK; PK	Yes
Central	Slight at first; moderate after early middle age	Pain or RE (uncommon)	Rods & filaments of 'hyaline' (non-collagenous protein)	Masson trichrome: red	PK in early middle age	Yes
Central	Slight to moderate at first; severe in middle age	Pain of RE	Aligned fibrils of amyloid	Congo red (red & green dichroism); also birefringent	MRE; PK in middle age	Yes
General	Moderate to severe	None	Excess GAG (? keratan sulphate I) in keratocytes	Alcian blue; colloidal Fe	PK in early middle age	Yes
Central	Slight	None (dense arcus)	Cholesterol crystals; neutral fat droplets	Schultz (cholesterol blue-green)	Screen for metabolism abnormality, sometimes PK	Yes
General	None	None	Excess GAG in keratocytes; lipid vacuoles	Alcian blue; colloidal Fe (for GAG)	None	—
Central	None	None	?	?	None	—
Central	Severe	Nystagmus	Abnormal collagen lamellae	—	Early PK	No
Central: later general	None at first, progressive later	Pain of BK in later stages	Endo. atrophic; abnormal collagen post. to DM	Collagen layer PAS +ve	None at first; later manage BK; finally PK	No
General	None if non-progressive; moderate to severe if progressive	None if non-progressive; pain of BK in later stages if progressive	Endothelium epithelioid; abnormal collagen post. to DM	Collagen layer PAS +ve	None if non-progressive; possibly PK if prog.	No
General	Severe	— Nystagmus	Endo. atrophic; abnormal collagen post. to DM	—	Sometimes early PK	Yes

BK, bullous keratopathy; BL, Bowman's layer; DM, Descemet's membrane; GAG, glycosaminoglycan; LK, lamellar keratoplasty; MRE, management of recurrent erosion; PK, penetrating keratoplasty; RE, recurrent erosion; SK, superficial keratectomy.

Initially, spectacles may adequately correct the refractive error. As the astigmatism becomes higher or irregular, corneal contact lenses become necessary. The fit of the lenses must be reviewed at regular intervals during the stage of progression. When corneal lenses become too uncomfortable or too unstable to be serviceable, scleral lenses may be successful. These are hand made in PMMA from moulds of the eyes and are pierced by fenestrations or slots, or channelled on their back surfaces, to provide good tear exchange on eye movement and blinking. Contact lenses neither accelerate nor arrest the progression of keratoconus.

When lens wearing time becomes too short, or when the corrected vision drops to 6/18 or below because of scarring of Bowman's layer, keratoplasty should be offered. Penetrating keratoplasty is traditional, and should replace at least the areas delineated by Fleischer's ring, but a lamellar procedure can also be considered. In the absence of deep scars following episodes of hydrops, the posterior stromal lamellae, Descemet's membrane and the endothelium can be retained, and a thick donor lamella applied. Endothelial rejection does not occur after such a procedure. The dissection of the host stroma is time-consuming and difficult.

Pellucid Marginal Degeneration

This is a non-hereditary, non-inflammatory corneal thinning disorder. It occurs inferiorly in the peripheral cornea, being separated from the limbus by 1–2 mm. There is high, irregular astigmatism of the cornea above the affected area, but here there is no thinning or scarring, and there is no iron line. Hydrops sometimes occurs. Histology shows irregularity and patchy loss of Bowman's layer.

The condition is very rare. It appears in the 20–40 years age group and affects the sexes equally. Management requires contact lenses (probably scleral lenses) and if these are not practicable or tolerable a large corneal graft is indicated. Inferiorly, the graft has to be very close to the limbus, which enhances the likelihood of subsequent vascularization and rejection.

FURTHER READING

Buckley R. J. *The Cornea*. Spalton D. J., Hitchings R. J. and Hunter P. A. (ed.) *Slide Atlas of Ophthalmology*, vol. 6. London, Gower, 1983.
Duane T. D. (ed.) *Clinical Ophthalmology*, vol. IV. Philadelphia, Harper and Row, 1982.
Duke-Elder S. (ed.) *System of Ophthalmology*, vol. VIII. London, Henry Kimpton, 1965.
Leibowitz H. M. (ed.) *Corneal Disorders: Clinical Diagnosis and Management*. Philadelphia, Saunders, 1984.
Smolin G. and Thoft R. A. (ed.) *The Cornea*. Boston, Mass., Little, Brown, 1983.
Waring G. O., Rodrigues M. M. and Laibson P. R. Corneal dystrophies, parts I and II. *Surv. Ophthalmol.* 1978; **23**, 71–122, 147–68.

Chapter 6

Scleritis

P. G. Watson and A. G. A. Lyne

Scleritis is an inflammatory disease of the sclera which may cause visual impairment and even loss of the eye if inadequately treated. Episcleritis, on the other hand, is a benign inflammation of the episclera, not resulting in permanent damage to the eye and not associated with systemic disease to any significant extent. It is therefore of paramount importance that the ophthalmologist distinguishes between these two conditions and treats them accordingly.

While it is true that some patients are not easily categorized, especially in the early stages, in the majority of cases distinction can be made and revision of the diagnosis should not often be necessary.

Careful attention to the following features will help to effect an accurate diagnosis.

DISTINGUISHING FEATURES

Pain

Pain may be severe in scleritis, so severe in fact that a patient may ask for removal of a seeing eye. It is deep and boring in character, often preventing sleep or waking the patient early in the morning. The pain, which is situated behind the affected eye and spreads to the forehead, jaw, face and temple, tends to be continuous rather than intermittent. It is only partly relieved by analgesics such as aspirin or paracetamol but is relieved immediately by adequate treatment of the scleritis.

Episcleritis causes discomfort rather than pain, usually described as a burning sensation, feeling of a foreign body, itching or irritation. It is, however, never so severe as to cause loss of sleep or prevent working. Indeed, the patient may be unaware of anything wrong unless an observer tells him he has a red eye.

Vascular Pattern

Because of the superficial situation of the dilated vessels in episcleritis, the redness is more akin to the bright red appearance of conjunctivitis than the deep purple congestion of scleritis which, although much more widespread, resembles the colour changes seen in uveitis.

The vessels overlying the sclera are in three layers (*Figs.* 1, 2).

1. The superficial conjunctival plexus is derived from the terminal branches of the superior tarsal

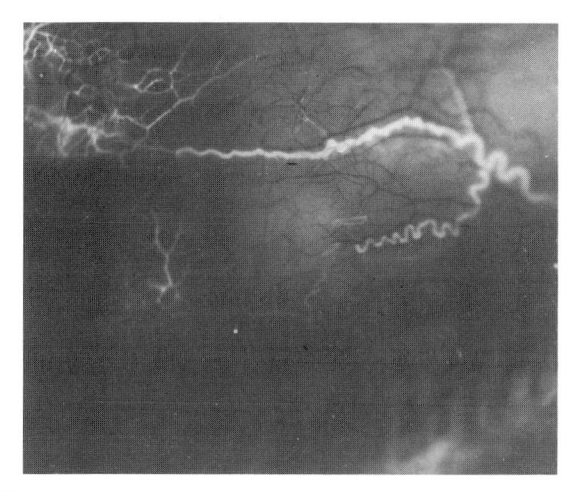

Fig. 1. Normal anterior segment fluorescein angiogram, 62-year-old male, 18·6 s. Early arterial phase. Dye has appeared simultaneously in the limbal perforating vessels and the main large perforating artery.

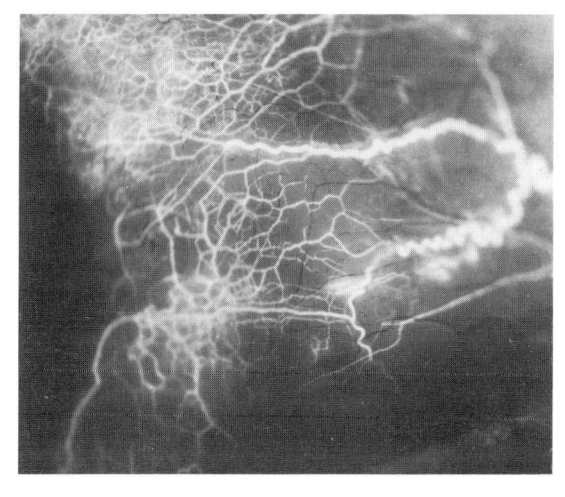

Fig. 2. Normal anterior segment fluorescein angiogram, 62-year-old male, 25·4 s. Mid venous phase. The larger veins are now full. Leakage is occurring from the capillary bed at the limbus. The conjunctival vessels are beginning to fill. In this angiogram they did not fill completely until 34 s.

arcade and anastamoses with the limbal marginal plexus of vessels.

2. The superficial episcleral vessels, which have a radial distribution, are those which lie in the deep layers of Tenon's capsule and are derived from perforating vessels, probably derived from the long posterior ciliary vessels with some contribution from the anterior ciliary vessels overlying the muscles. The perforating arteries penetrate the sclera from within and immediately give off branches to supply the limbal marginal arcade before passing backwards towards the rectus muscles and giving branches to both layers of episcleral tissue (*Fig.* 1).

3. The deep episcleral vessels which lie directly on the sclera form a network over it and are derived from the same source as the superficial plexus. The elevation of these vessels by a swelling of the sclera is most easily seen in nodular disease but can also be evaluated by observation of the margin of an area of diffuse scleritis or episcleritis. The vessels are best seen in the red-free light of the slit lamp when they show up as dark against the green background. It must be remembered that an area of scleritis always has an overlying congestion and sometimes infiltration of the episclera, but the reverse is not the case. If the congestion is very severe it is sometimes helpful to contract the superficial vessels with 10 per cent phenylephrine to reveal the state of the underlying vasculature.

Anterior segment angiography produces a recordable picture of the dynamics of the vascular response and can be extremely helpful in diagnosis and in deciding the type of treatment to be used in both episcleral and scleral disease.[1]

Corneal Changes

Although episcleritis may cause corneal oedema if it occurs adjacent to the limbus (even to the extent of leaving permanent changes), the corneal changes in this condition are minimal.

Scleritis is accompanied by corneal changes of one type or another in about 30 per cent of cases.

Even when the scleritis has been resolved, with or without treatment, the type and distribution of the corneal changes may give an indication of the scleritis which preceded them. A more detailed description of the corneal changes will be found under the appropriate section later in this chapter.

Uveitis

Uveitis is only seen in episcleritis when the reaction is so intense that the whole ocular vasculature is affected. The presence of a uveitis is strongly suggestive of scleral involvement, particularly when the inflammation overlies the ciliary body.

Although uveitis accompanies scleritis in approximately 30 per cent of cases, it rather surprisingly perhaps is not more common in necrotizing than other types of scleritis. When it does occur, however, the prognosis is worse and the condition much more difficult to treat. Uveitis is a sinister sign.

Scleral Translucency

While in certain patients with a very severe necrotizing scleritis and in scleromalacia perforans, scleral tissue is indeed lost, the sclera is not necessarily destroyed but may become more transparent. It is more accurate to speak of scleral translucency than of scleral thinning, which has been the commonly used term in the literature, since there is not always actual thinning present. The colour change is caused by reorientation of the collagen fibrils following inflammation and has the appearance of a dark area of sclera through which the underlying choroid can be seen. During the acute episode it is not easy to see, but even then it can usually be detected provided that the patient is *examined in daylight* and with care. True scleral translucency is a very important sign to look for when trying to establish the differential diagnosis, since it is rarely seen in any other condition apart from scleritis.

One other appearance that might be confused with this condition is racial pigmentation or benign congenital melanosis of the sclera, which, on superficial examination, is similar. Careful examination upon the slit lamp will show the typical deposits of pigment subconjunctivally which have a more violaceous colour than scleral disease, the eye is not inflamed and there will usually be a difference in colour of the two irides.

Senile elastosis or scleral hyaline plaque is a common appearance, consisting of areas of scleral translucency in the interpalpebral area in front of the insertion of the recti muscles. As its name implies, it is usually seen in the elderly and the sclera is not reduced in thickness, although it may be transparent. These changes are not as marked as those seen after scleritis and are never associated with any inflammation.

Corneal Sensitivity

Necrotizing scleritis is associated with quite profound loss of sensitivity. Resolution of the disease process is accompanied by recovery in sensitivity. The commonly used instrument of Cochet and Bonnet is capable of giving a reproducible result provided that allowance is made for the limits of the device and too much importance is not attached to small differences in filament length.[2]

NOMENCLATURE

There has been considerable confusion in the literature with regard to the nomenclature of scleral disease.[3] In particular, the terms episcleritis and scleritis have been confused, which accounts, for example, for the difference in the incidence recorded for these two conditions in association with such systemic diseases as rheumatoid arthritis.

Other terms, such as episcleritis periodica fugax, episcleritis multinodularis, brawny scleritis, deep scleritis, annular scleritis, gelatinous scleritis, massive granuloma of the sclera, malignant scleritis, progressive sclerokeratitis, have all been used. It is suggested that such descriptive terms are best avoided and that the terminology set out in *Table I* be adopted. The diagnosis can be made by clinical observation and has the virtue of simplicity and reproducibility. Since it is based not only upon the site of the inflammatory process but also has regard to the activity of the disease, it can be used as a basis for treatment.

Table I. Classification of episcleritis and scleritis

Episcleritis	
Simple	High flow
	Normal vasculature
Nodular	High flow
	Normal vasculature
	Local rapid leakage
Scleritis	
Diffuse	Slow flow
	Abnormal vasculature
Nodular	Slow flow
	Abnormal vasculature
	Deep local leakage
Necrotizing	
With inflammation	Slow flow
	Venular shut down
	Vaso-obliteration
	Re-routing of blood
Without inflammation (Scleromalacia perforans)	Absent flow
	Arteriolar occlusion
	Large bypass vessels

Necrotizing scleritis and scleromalacia perforans, although the most serious forms of scleritis, are fortunately the least common and account for 12 per cent of all cases.

They are the only form of scleral inflammation in which there is loss of scleral tissue, which can be extremely rapid. Because of this, and because there are often important systemic associations with these varieties of scleritis, early investigations and vigorous treatment is mandatory.

EPISCLERITIS

By definition, the term episcleritis means an inflammatory process occurring in the episclera. It is therefore necessary to examine a little more closely what is meant by the episclera.

The episclera is the thin, dense vascularized layer of connective tissue overlying the sclera and situated beneath Tenon's capsule.

It contains bundles of collagen, which are continuous with those of the sclera, and contains the same vessels as those which perforate the sclera. Some elastic fibres are present as well as some unmyelinated nerve fibres. The episclera blends with the subconjunctival tissues and Tenon's capsule a few millimetres behind the limbus and becomes very thin posterior to the equator of the eye.

Episcleritis is a benign recurrent inflammation of the episclera, involving the overlying Tenon's capsule but not the underlying sclera. It tends to run a limited course of between 10 days and 3 weeks and will resolve spontaneously. The diagnosis should be reconsidered if any one attack lasts longer than 3 weeks. Its incidence is difficult to determine because the majority of cases are probably treated by the patient's own general practitioner or at the local ophthalmic department without referral to the more specialized centres where records of incidence are compiled. However, there is no doubt that it is a much more common condition than scleritis, being twice as common in women than men.

The usual course of events is that the eye becomes quite quickly inflamed with a feeling described as gritty, burning and hot or as a feeling of a foreign body. It is quite commonly present upon waking and may not be accompanied by any discomfort at all, the patient only being aware of it on looking in the mirror because an observer has pointed it out. The discomfort is always related to the eye and never to the face, head or periorbital region.

Recurrence is common and attacks tend to come in bouts. Although patients will often relate the onset of an attack to minor trauma or some other episode which they consider relevant, these occurrences are rarely found to have any true significance. There does seem to be a seasonal element involved with many patients, a spring or summer association being the commonest finding but there is no significant association with atopic disease. There is, however, a definite association with gout.

The nodular form of the disease (*Plate IXa*) tends to resolve more slowly than the diffuse, even with treatment, and the symptoms tend to be rather more severe. Apart from this, there is little difference in behaviour of the two forms of episcleritis. Neither form of the condition has any significant systemic implications, apart from a few patients who in the early stages of connective tissue disease develop a recurrent episcleral inflammation. They do not appear, however, to develop scleritis later.

Recurrent attacks occurring over several years produce no serious damage to sclera or cornea, although minor degrees of scleral translucency and corneal infiltration may occasionally occur if the recurrences are always at the same site.

Episcleritis is to some degree a diagnosis of exclusion and the other causes of redness of the anterior segment of the globe must be considered and excluded before the diagnosis is made. Although the eyes may sometimes water, no true discharge occurs in episcleritis, although the lids may be stuck upon waking by a slight serous discharge or excess tears. There are no associated papillary or follicular changes as might be expected in a bacterial or viral conjunctivitis. Anterior uveitis, as judged by flare and cells in the anterior chamber, is, as has already been stated, rare in episcleritis and only seen in very acute inflammation.

Other conditions that may occasionally be confused are a foreign body lodged in the bulbar conjunctiva or punctum, which can cause a nodular swelling, and an inflamed pinguecula may sometimes cause confusion with episcleritis. They can always be distinguished by observation on the slit lamp. Pingueculae are situated in the conjunctiva in the interpalpebral area. They may have lipid deposits within them and sometimes become eroded on the surface and stain with fluorescein.

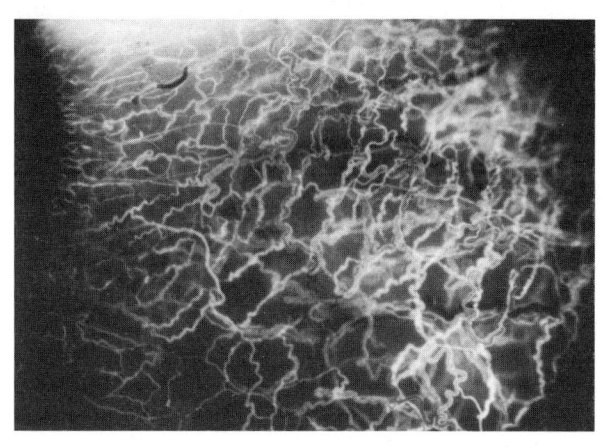

Fig. 3. Simple episcleritis. Anterior segment fluorescein angiogram, 16 s. Within 3 s of the appearance of the dye in the circulation the whole of the vascular bed is filled. The vessels, however, although leaky, are otherwise entirely normal.

Examination

The episclera will be seen to be acutely inflamed with dilated vessels, either diffusely or in a nodular distribution. The flow in these vessels is very fast (*Fig.* 3). This can be confirmed by anterior segment angiography.

In diffuse episcleritis, although the whole of the eye is often involved to some extent, the maximum inflammation is confined to one or two quadrants. The interpalpebral area is more commonly affected than those areas covered by the lids. Marked episcleral and conjunctival oedema caused by massive vascular leakage may be present, in some cases so much so that the conjunctiva and episclera may protrude between the lids. A nodule may be tender, but not to the same degree as occurs in scleritis, nor is the pain referred outside the eye. However, photophobia and temporary myopia due to ciliary spasm may caused acute distress and disablement. Patients with episcleritis are often self-conscious about their appearance, which is often thought to resemble that of an alcoholic hangover, and understandably this causes concern, especially in young women. Even though it is known that this is a benign condition, it does merit our attention. Anybody who has suffered a red eye, and had it pointed out to him by every person he meets, will understand the reason why treatment is sought.

Corneal Changes

Corneal changes are rarely seen in episcleritis. A lesion adjacent to the limbus may cause localized corneal oedema and a small resulting nebula.

Dellen are quite often seen in association with episcleritis if the limbus is swollen to any extent. This lesion, in which the superficial epithelium and some of the stroma of the cornea adjacent to a limbal swelling becomes thin, has been thought to be due to desiccation of the area because the lid is prevented from being in contact with it. However, desiccation is rarely seen but rather a pool of stagnant tear fluid is more often present in the facet, which will resolve if the limbal swelling is eliminated. The only consequence may be slight superficial vascularization of the cornea. The deeper stromal opacities which occur as a result of scleritis are not seen in episcleritis.

Aetiology

The cause of episcleritis is rarely found. Because of its seasonal incidence, it has been suggested that episcleritis is a type 1 hypersensitivity reaction, but intensive further investigations have not borne this out. Contact with external agents may certainly cause the onset of an attack, but this is exceptional.

In a series conducted at the Scleritis Clinic at Moorfields Eye Hospital, London, it was found that 11 per cent of patients with episcleritis had raised uric acid levels and 7 per cent had clinical gout,[4] so this condition must always be looked for. Patients with rosacea and psoriases often develop a localized episcleritis during the course of the disease.

Although it has often been stated in the past that episcleritis is associated with the connective tissue disorders, rheumatoid arthritis, tuberculosis, syphilis and other granulomas such as sarcoidosis, we have found this so rarely that unless there are clinical manifestations of the diseases, or the disease is intractable, we no longer investigate this group of patients extensively for these diseases.

Treatment

Although the disease will resolve spontaneously given time, most patients will request treatment in an attempt to speed up the process. They should, however, be actively discouraged from using medication unless the condition is exceptionally severe.

Local steroids render the eye more comfortable and have been shown to resolve the episcleritis a few days earlier in most cases but for treatment to be effective the patient must instill drops at at least hourly intervals as soon as any trouble is detected because the steroids are acting by stabilizing the vascular endothelium and preventing the release of vasoactive amines and polymorph breakdown. If an attack is allowed to develop, it will pursue its full course whatever further treatment is given. The patient is told to put the drops in every 2 hours until his symptoms improve, closing his eye after instillation for at least 30 s in order to allow the preparation to be absorbed rather than disappearing down the nasolachrymal duct. The frequency of medication can then be reduced to 4 hourly until the redness has resolved and gradually tailed off over a period of 3–4 days.

As with all frequent steroid medication the patient must be monitored for raised intraocular pressure and if this should occur it is advisable either to stop all steroid medication or to change to a preparation that is less readily absorbed into the anterior chamber and thus less likely to raise the tension, such as clobetasone or fluorometholone.

Cold compresses applied to the closed lids may afford symptomatic relief if the inflammation is severe. Other local preparations, such as Oc. Tanderil, are effective if steroids need to be avoided but many patients do not like using ointments and some complain of burning after a few days' use. Failure to respond to local therapy may sometimes occur and in these cases it may be necessary to use systemic non-steroidal preparations.

Flubiprofen (Froben) has been shown to be the most effective of the non-steroidal anti-inflammatory agents. This should be started with a dosage of 300 mg daily and reducing to half this level when control is achieved. Indomethacin 25 mg three times a day is also very effective if the response is poor to Froben.

If no response occurs to the above measures, the diagnosis should be seriously reconsidered since the likeliest possibility is that the patient is suffering from scleritis rather than episcleritis.

SCLERITIS

It must be emphasized that scleritis is not a common condition and in one series constituted only 0·08 per cent of all new referrals to an ophthalmic department.[5] The average ophthalmologist will only see a handful of cases in his career unless he happens to work in a specialized unit, and it is partly for this reason that much difficulty is experienced in treating these unfortunate patients. Early effective treatment can abort the disease process before extensive damage to the eye has occurred but so often patients present with eyes which are the subject of severe scleral destruction, complicated by glaucoma and visual loss, which is irreversible because of inadequate treatment over a period of years.

Anterior Diffuse Scleritis

This is the commonest form of scleritis, more so in women than men and showing peak incidence in the 40–70 years age group. It is uncommon in the very young and very old and is bilateral in 45 per cent of cases.

The onset is typically more gradual than episcleritis but if the patient has had previous attacks he will be aware of it at a stage before anything definite can be seen, and he will usually be right.

Pain varies from moderate to severe, so severe in fact that the patient is unable to sleep and is typically wakened by it in the early hours of the morning.

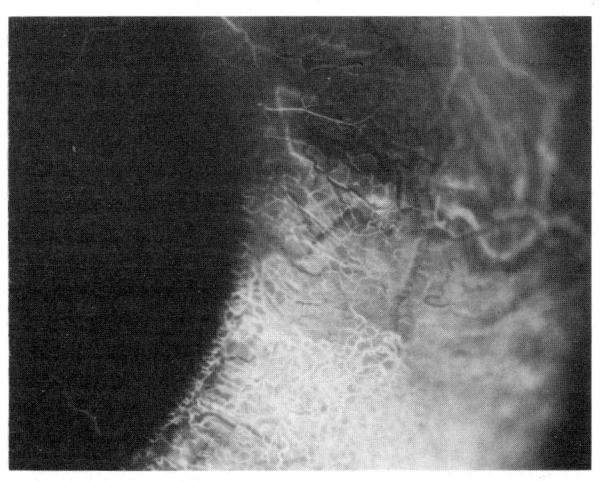

Fig. 4. Diffuse anterior scleritis. Anterior segment fluorescein angiogram, late venous phase, 24 s. One area of the superficial episcleral vasculature has remained unperfused even though this is at the site of maximum vascular congestion and the vessels appeared dilated (*see* Plate IX*b*).

It is situated in the eye and radiates from it in the distribution of the ophthalmic division of the trigeminal nerve, commonly to the jaw and temple. Photophobia may also be severe with epiphora but there is no other discharge. Blurred vision may be due to the complications of the disease or may simply be due to the photophobia and reluctance to open the eye.

Upon examination redness of the anterior segment will be seen in one or more quadrants. The colour of the inflamed eye, which is best examined in daylight, varies from salmon pink to purple, quite unlike the bright redness of episcleritis.

Anterior segment fluorescein angiography is a valuable investigation in this condition. Two types of response are found. The first, found in those patients with early diffuse disease, have a rapid flow pattern identical to that seen in episcleritis (*Fig.* 3). These patients, if treated, will respond rapidly and will not progress. The second pattern is one of intermittent venular closure (*Fig.* 4, Plate IX*b*). If untreated, these patients will show rapid progression of disease. Early treatment will allow the vessels to become reperfused, but if treatment is delayed, then this vascular closure becomes permanent (*Fig.* 5) and part of the episcleral network can only become reperfused by the formation of new vessels (*Plate* IXc). It is at the stage of irreversible vascular closure that necrotizing scleritis occurs because of the intense cellular activity which results from the vasculitis. This causes proteoglycan changes and alteration of the fibrocytes in the sclera and eventual collagen destructive changes. This destruction of tissue in turn leads to an autoimmune response in which there is an influx of cells of the lymphocytic series and further progressive destruction of the connective tissue.[6]

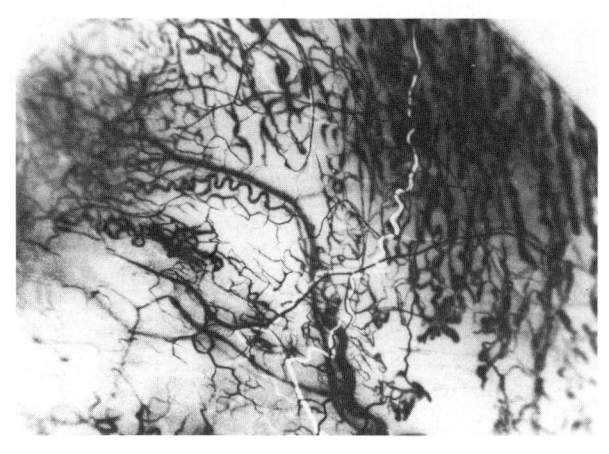

Fig. 5. Early necrotizing scleritis. Subtraction fluorescein angiogram, late venous phase. Even at this late phase there are areas of total non-perfusion. The large vessel running from 12 o'clock does not carry blood at any stage in the angiogram.

It may be possible, also on inspection in daylight, to see areas of scleral translucency which are the result of previous attacks of scleritis.

Although both sclera and cornea are composed of collagen fibres, they are opaque and transparent respectively, because of difference in fibre size, arrangement and the nature of the proteoglycan ground substance. In the cornea the collagen fibres are of the same diameter and are arranged in parallel bundles crossing at right-angles to one another whereas those of the sclera are irregular in size and are arranged in a meshwork. Severe scleral inflammation results in many cases in rearrangement of collagen fibrils or replacement of the collagen by fibrous connective tissue and a change in the constitution of the ground substance, which causes the sclera to become translucent, allowing the choroid to be seen through it. Ultrasonography shows that although there may be actual thinning of the sclera, this is not necessarily so.

Recurrence of scleritis often occurs at the edge of such a translucent lesion and the recurrence in turn may result in further scleral translucency so that the disease process extends in a circumferential manner around the globe a few millimetres behind the limbus.

Scleritis occurs initially most often between the 10 and 2 o'clock positions. It is therefore important always to raise the upper lid in cases of suspected scleritis.

Although progression may occur from above around both sides of the anterior segment, it is more common to see active recurrence on only one side of an area of scleral translucency. Separate foci can arise at any point but progression is almost always circumferential and rarely does the inflammation extend into the area of the limbus or back towards the equator.

If treatment is inadequate or unsuccessful in arresting the progression of the scleritis around the globe so that an area of translucency and possibly thinning encircles the cornea, severe visual loss, uveitis and glaucoma are the rule. An eye which has reached this state is virtually a lost eye, and every effort must be made to prevent this from occurring. The cause of visual loss in these patients appears to be somewhat similar to those in whom anterior segment necrosis has occurred, in that there is uveitis, glaucoma followed by phthisis and secondary retinal changes. Cataract formation can occur rapidly.

Nodular Scleritis

This type of scleritis is rather less common than the diffuse variety. The distinction between it and nodular episcleritis is made primarily by observation that all the vessel layers are displaced forwards by the underlying scleral swelling whereas in nodular episcleritis the deep episcleral vasculature can be seen lying on flat sclera. The nodule, which is a localized area of swollen sclera, can occur at any point on the globe but is usually situated a few millimetres behind the limbus, similar to the initial diffuse lesion, and in the interpalpebral area. The nodule is extremely tender, immobile and surrounded by dilated episcleral vessels.

The disease pattern follows the same course as the diffuse scleritis, in that the nodule tends to heal, leaving behind it an area of translucent sclera which may be the site of further recurrences. Slow outward progression of the disease occurs unless treated. The nodules should never be biopsied, even though they look tempting. Not only is the histology never helpful, but they almost always contain soft pultaceous material which, if allowed to escape, leaves a bare area of sclera. If they are treated medically, however, this material forms a matrix on which collagen is deposited and no residual deposit persists.

Necrotizing Scleritis

All scleritis is necrotizing to some extent but it is the acuteness and severity of the process seen in some patients which merits the term 'necrotizing'. Although the scleritis seems to be similar initially, its course, instead of occupying a period of months or years, is compressed into days or weeks. In addition, certain significant features are seen which occur only in necrotizing scleritis.

Generalized systemic disease is found in about 40 per cent of patients with scleritis but this proportion rises to 60 per cent or more of those with necrotizing disease. These patients often have the more severe types of connective tissue disease; indeed 30 per cent of these patients with necrotizing scleritis die within 5 years unless the systemic disease is vigorously treated. The importance of early diagnosis of this type of scleritis can be readily appreciated because, quite apart from the systemic implications of the disorder, ocular destruction will rapidly ensue. The majority of eyes lost from scleritis are lost because of inadequately treated necrotizing disease.

Although necrotizing disease can occur in a patient with severe long standing diffuse scleritis, the majority of them describe an acute onset to their disease which develops over a period of a few days, rarely of more than a week or two. The pain is often very severe indeed, so much so that the patient is unable to open his or her eye or to sleep, and profuse watering often accompanies the pain and photophobia.

All the features of diffuse and nodular scleritis may be seen in necrotizing disease but in a more acute form. There are also signs that may occur at some stage in the disease and are of importance from the diagnostic and prognostic point of view.

Avascular Areas

An area of vascular shutdown may be present in the middle of an inflamed area of sclera (*Plate* IXc). The area may be small initially, requiring examination on the slit lamp or fluorescein angiography to distinguish it, but it may be macroscopic and visible by the naked eye. The fluorescein angiographic appearance in necrotizing scleritis is characteristic. There is always an element of vascular closure, usually on the venous side of the circulation, at or adjacent to the area of maximum inflammation (*Plate* IXb, *Figs*. 4, 5). The vascular pattern is so distorted that it is difficult or impossible to distinguish between the normal vasculature and newly formed or bypass vessels (*Plate* IXb,c, *Figs*. 4 and 5). Those vessels, which are carrying blood, may show patchy early leakage and there is often deep early and late staining of the affected sclera from vessels deep to the site of inflammation. As the disease progresses, large areas become completely non-perfused.

The appearance of these areas of avascularity implies that the disease process is very active and that the eye needs immediate intensive treatment, or if the eye is already being treated, that treatment is inappropriate or inadequate.

If left without treatment, this avascular area may go on either to scleral lysis or sequestrum formation.

Scleral Lysis

In some patients with necrotizing scleritis an area of sclera can be seen simply to be dissolving away, leaving a few fibres at the base of the lesion, which cover the choroid beneath. This is probably the result of arteriolar occlusion adjacent to and within an area of severe and active scleritis (*Plate* IXd). The area, which is usually a few millimetres in diameter, will be found to contain a white sticky substance – all that remains of the sclera. The area immediately adjacent to the slough is always acutely inflamed. Although these areas appear to be in imminent danger of perforation, they rarely do so unless the eye has been subject to trauma or glaucoma. With treatment a slough may heal and should never be removed otherwise the eye will be left permanently with an area of scleral tissue loss.

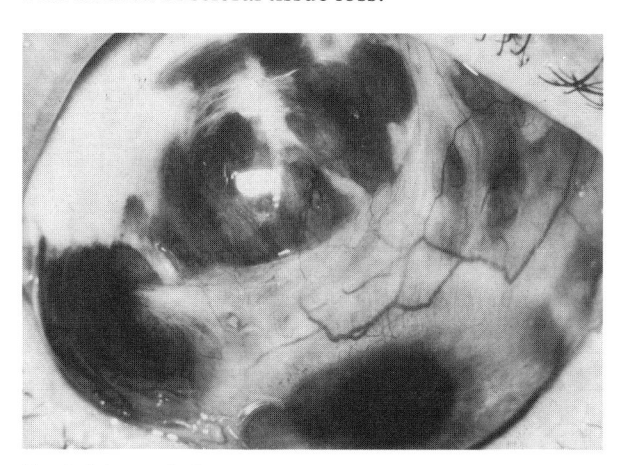

Fig. 6. Scleromalacia perforans. Total sequestration and removal of the sclera. This lesion has remained unchanged for 15 years and needs no treatment. Staphyloma formation will not occur unless the intraocular pressure becomes high.

Scleromalacia Perforans

This is a specific condition found almost exclusively in elderly female patients with long standing rheumatoid arthritis in which the arteriolar supply becomes obliterated.[7] An area of sclera becomes yellow in colour and then often, together with the overlying episclera and conjunctiva, completely separates from normal sclera (*Fig*. 6). This sequestrum of sclera becomes dead white in colour and will eventually absorb, leaving behind it a large punched out area of very thin sclera with choroid visible at its base. Again, actual perforation is rare and these lesions can be safely left.

Corneal Changes in Scleritis

Scleritis can be associated with corneal changes in approximately 30 per cent of patients. Most are of no importance, but occasionally the changes can be so severe that active steps have to be taken to prevent serious complications.

Marginal Guttering

Although marginal guttering is usually related to an area of active scleritis, it can occur in a separate part of the eye. Fluorescein angiography reveals a total vascular shut down *in advance* of the active guttering lesion, new vessels closing in behind as the lesion heals. Only in acute necrotizing sclerokeratitis are both sclera and cornea affected together.

The gutter, which can occupy large segments of the cornea, consists of a loss of corneal epithelium and stroma which can extend down to Descemet's membrane. Although a descemetocoele can occur, perforation is rare and conservative management is indicated unless actual leakage of aqueous occurs. These gutters are often surprisingly painless and the patient may be unaware that anything is amiss. Even perforation can occur, become blocked by iris and thus heal without much in the way of symptoms except for mild redness which is often mistakenly treated as a conjunctivitis with antibiotic drops.

Deposition of lipid is often seen on the corneal side of the gutter when this has been present for any length of time.

Peripheral Corneal Thinning

Peripheral corneal thinning sometimes occurs in patients who have active scleral disease and in whom the marginal plexus is particularly involved. In these patients the gutter is shallow and heals with partial opacity and superficial vascularization in part or all of the corneal circumference. If the area is localized to one quadrant, then the globe may expand in this axis. In another form the thinning is so uniform that at first sight the patient seems to be wearing a microcorneal contact lens so that it is sometimes known as 'contact lens cornea'. This particular lesion is usually seen with long standing rheumatoid arthritis.[8] Peripheral corneal thinning is also seen in association with dellen formation when there is an intense localized limbal oedema.

In acute diffuse anterior scleritis and in some patients with acute necrotizing scleritis an 'immune ring' can be seen spreading out in a centrifugal manner from an area of limbitis. Prompt treatment with steroids locally usually causes such a lesion to regress rapidly without any corneal destruction, but if left, an area of opaque cornea remains. This condition is most commonly (but not exclusively) seen following a severe attack of herpes zoster ophthalmicus.

Acute Necrotizing Sclerokeratitis

This term has been applied to a very acute form of necrotizing scleritis accompanied by an acute keratitis. The appearance is of a very rapid onset of acute anterior scleritis with a deep gutter which transgresses the limbus (*Plate* IX*e,f*). This change is characteristic of patients suffering from polyarteritis nodosa, or Wegener's granulomatosis. Corneal perforation is quite liable to occur if the scleral disease is not controlled.

Sclerosing Keratitis

This lesion consists of a change in the deep layers of the cornea such that they become opaque, resembling fibres, and take on a glistening appearance which resembles candy floss. Although this appearance is sometimes seen after chemical burns, it is unusual to find it except after scleritis. This type of keratitis is not heavily vascularized as a rule and is not typical of any particular type of scleritis.

Nummular Keratitis

Nummular opacities, frequently adjacent to Descemet's membrane, are occasionally found in association with scleritis in young patients but the appearance is uncommon and does not seem to have any particular aetiological associations.

Uveitis

Uveitis is surprisingly uncommon (only about 30 per cent of all patients with scleritis show any evidence of uveitis) but if it is observed, it is a sinister sign. Rather surprisingly, the severity of the inflammatory element of the scleritis does not correlate with the occurrence of uveitis, for example, all of the patients seen with scleromalacia perforans showed evidence of uveitis whereas only 40 per cent of the patients with necrotizing disease had signs of it. Uveitis only seems to occur when the vasculitis affects the vessels of the ciliary body and the scleritis has extended backwards towards the equator. Patients with sclerouveitis are notoriously difficult to treat and many have multiple complications.

Glaucoma

Open angle glaucoma is slightly more common in scleritis patients than it is in the general population. An already damaged trabecular meshwork will be further compromised by the scleral inflammation so that a potential glaucoma is converted into a manifest one.

If the diffuse scleritis is associated with a limbitis, then the intraocular pressure will rise markedly, resembling an attack of closed angle glaucoma. Gonioscopy will reveal that the angle is open in these patients and the glaucoma will resolve if the scleritis is treated. If these patients should be operated upon it will be found that the scleral tissue is swollen and oedematous, blocking the trabecular meshwork. This mechanism of glaucoma has been proved histologically.[9]

Closed angle glaucoma can occur as a primary closed angle attack distinguished from the acute open angle variety above only by gonioscopy. PAS formation is very unusual but can result in a form of chronic angle closure glaucoma.

Steroid induced rise in intraocular pressure is often seen in patients receiving frequent dosages of local steroid for episcleritis. It is, however, no more common in scleritis than in the general population.

Posterior Scleritis

This type of scleritis can be more difficult to diagnose than any other form because of the varied ways in which it can present. If the inflammatory changes in the posterior segment are associated with an anterior scleritis, the diagnosis is made easier, but if the inflammation is confined to the posterior segment it can be very difficult. In fact, in a review of enucleated eyes of those with a *primary histological* diagnosis of posterior scleritis, 40 per cent had not had the diagnosis made correctly before the eye was removed.[10]

One of the difficulties is that posterior scleritis is *apparently* very rare. Scleritis itself is an uncommon condition and, even allowing for considerable under-diagnosis, posterior scleritis constitutes only 6 per cent of the scleritis patients. It is therefore not a condition that automatically springs to mind when signs of a posterior disorder are seen.

As posterior scleritis is an inflammation involving the sclera behind the equator, the signs and symptoms are therefore not only those that would be expected from such an inflammation but also includes the associated inflammation of adjacent structures.

Pain

This can be quite severe in posterior scleritis but usually not as severe as that which accompanies anterior scleritis and certainly not as severe as that which occurs in necrotizing disease. Pain in scleritis appears to be more severe the more anterior in the globe the inflammatory disease is situated.

Reduction in Visual Acuity

Some change in visual acuity is universal in posterior scleritis, varying from slight blurring of vision to an almost complete loss. This is commonly due to the haziness of the vitreous, which is almost always present to some degree but may also be the result of retinal changes, particularly macular oedema and oedema or granulomatous involvement of the optic nerve. Central retinal vein occlusions can occur at this stage. Diagnosis can be extremely difficult because of the hazy vitreous.

Fundus Changes

Some degree of exudative detachment is present in about half the cases of posterior scleritis. The inflammatory change in the sclera extends to involve the choroid and manifests itself as an exudative retinal detachment or uveal effusion. *The diagnosis of posterior scleritis should be considered in all patients with exudative or other retinal detachments where no hole can be found.*

A localized granuloma of the sclera may be seen as a mass in the fundus which can be mistaken for a malignant melanoma and in the past some of these eyes have been enucleated because of this. Careful examination together with fluorescein angiography can help to avoid this error. The fluorescein angiographic appearances are those of a very early choroidal leakage with rapid leakage into the suprachoroidal or subretinal space. The current management of malignant melanoma does not always include immediate enucleation, so that a course of treatment can be given which will allow resolution of the secondary detachment and clarification of the diagnosis. Resolution of the detachment will usually occur readily, with the appropriate treatment leaving a mottled pigmentary change of the corresponding sector of the fundus. Resolution may be quite slow in the older patients in particular, taking several months to completely clear.

Ultrasonography with the appropriate probe and high resolution CT scanning will confirm that there is often quite considerable thickening of the sclera, at times to two or three times its normal thickness. This can be seen in all histological specimens.

Macular Oedema

This is the commonest cause of decreased visual acuity in all types of scleritis, particularly when the scleritis is associated with uveitis and involves several quadrants of the globe. It is particularly likely to occur in posterior scleritis and may be accompanied by optic disc oedema.

The cystoid macular oedema is of the same type seen in all types of uveitis and particularly those chronic forms of the disease and is as resistant to treatment. Although treatment of the scleritis often results in improvement of visual acuity, residual macular scarring and fibrosis may remain, leaving a permanent central scotoma.

Proptosis

Some degree of proptosis is seen in half the cases of posterior scleritis. This proptosis may be associated with limitation of eye movements and lid retraction of the lower lid upon attempted elevation and is a result of an extension of the granulomatous process into the extraocular tissues. A patient presenting with a combination of any of these symptoms and signs, i.e. pain, lowered visual acuity, exudative detachment, choroidal effusion, macular oedema, proptosis, limitation of extraocular movement or lid retraction, should be considered to have posterior scleritis, unless proved otherwise.

The diagnosis can be confirmed by ultrasonography, fluorescein angiography and resolution with treatment by systemic steroids.

Posterior scleritis does not have any clear association with connective tissue disease or other systemic disease. However, when such association does occur, it tends to be with the more acute forms of connective tissue disease such as polyarteritis nodosa, vasculitis or polychondritis.

HISTOLOGY

Biopsy of episcleral and scleral nodules is very rarely of value and should only be undertaken if there is no other possible way to establish a diagnosis. Large nodules containing necrotic material will fibrose if treated but if incised the material is lost and an area of scleral dehiscence remains. Biopsies that have been done usually showed little beyond necrotic collagen and a mixture of cells, lymphocytes, macrophages, plasma cells and fibroblasts.

Such histological material as is available, therefore, has been obtained from eyes that have been enucleated and are the result of necrotizing scleritis rather than any other form of the disease. The reason for removal has been intractable pain, secondary glaucoma often as a result of central retinal vein occlusion, uveitis, perforation of a scleral area of thinning, corneal ulcer, or a misdiagnosis of melanoma.

The basic lesion of such cases is a granuloma which consists of a central area of necrosis showing fibrinoid necrosis and loss of fibrocytes from the sclera (*Fig.* 7). Surrounding this area of necrosis is a region of new vessel formation with the vessels derived from neighbouring episcleral and choroidal vessels. The new vessels are cuffed with lymphocytes and often show medial necrosis. Further away from the necrotic centre is an area of cellular infiltration which consists of lymphocytes, plasma cells, macrophages and giant cells. Fibroblasts are present and the collagen fibres show a splaying of their fibrils. If the changes are anterior and near enough to the cornea, similar changes may be seen in the collagen fibres of the cornea.

The light microscopical characteristics of scleritis may be thought of therefore as fibrinoid necrosis, cellular infiltration with a variety of cells (but not usually polymorphs), vasculitis and fibrin deposition. Electron microscopy reveals that the first changes occur in apparently normal tissue away from the necrotic area and first affect the proteoglycan covering of the collagen fibrils, together with activation of the scleral fibrocytes. As the lesion is approached, the activity becomes more intense and the changes extend to the collagen itself, which unravels, splays and splits (*Fig.* 8). It is uncertain whether the fibrocytic activation is the result of cellular invasion of the sclera or the cause of it, or the extent to which the vascular proliferation is the result of extraneous inflammatory responses.

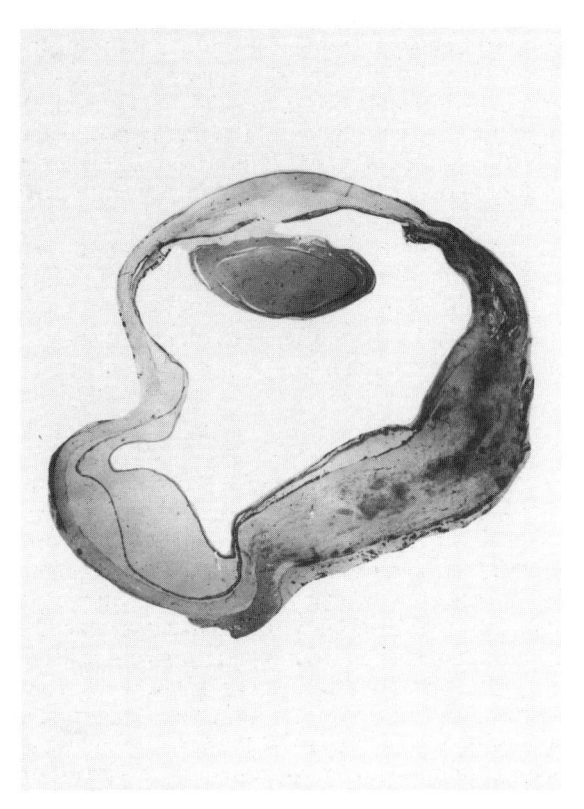

Fig. 7. Anterior and posterior scleritis. An eye removed because of intractable pain and loss of vision. The diagnosis of scleritis was not made before the eye was removed. The patient presented with loss of vision, a very red painful eye and uveitis. A cataract obscured the fundus view. The thickened sclera is the result of a necrotizing granuloma which involves both the anterior and posterior sclera and has given rise to an exudative detachment.

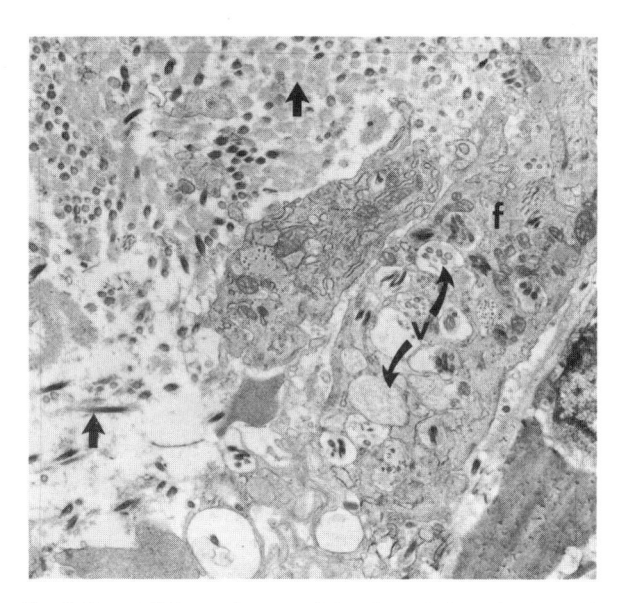

Fig. 8. Intracellular and extracellular degradation of collagen in an area of scleral destruction. An active fibroblastic cell (f) shows numerous intracellular vacuoles (v) containing collagen fibrils in various stages of breakdown. In the adjacent matrix, swelling and unravelling of collagen fibrils is evident (vertical arrows). ($\times 7425$.)

PATHOGENESIS

Although the exact sequence of events which leads to and causes persistence of scleral destruction is not yet fully understood, a great deal is known of the events which lead up to it and, in consequence, how this ultimate disaster can be avoided.

The cytological changes within excised eyes have been extensively studied.[11–13] The changes in the sclera are of a chronic granulomatous disorder characterized by fibrinoid necrosis, destruction of collagen together with cellular infiltration with polymorphonuclear leucocytes, plasma cells, lymphocytes and macrophages. The granuloma is surrounded by multinucleate epithelioid giant cells and old and new vessels, some of which are thrombosed showing the characteristics of a vasculitis.

Vasculitis

The changes associated with this vasculitis can be detected by fluorescein angiography of the anterior segment of the eye. In the earliest stages of the inflammatory response the flow in the vessels is rapid but if the inflammation persists then the flow is reduced, first in one small area, but later this becomes generalized (*Figs.* 4, 5). If the inflammation is suppressed in the early stages these vessels can open up again but if there is any prolongation of the response the vessels become thrombosed and occluded and abnormal bypass channels form (*Plate* IXc). Once the inflammatory response is brought under control new vessels then invade this area. If the disease is allowed to progress then the sclera, overlying episclera and sometimes conjunctiva begin to necrose (*Plate* Xa,b), the disease progressing outwards from the central area (*Plate* IXd). If arteriolar occlusion occurs, as in some systemic vasculitises or in the vasculitis of rheumatoid arthritis, areas of infarcted sclera can occur without any inflammatory response (scleromalacia perforans) (*see Fig.* 6).

Granulomatous Changes

The changes in a scleral granuloma extend far beyond the site of the apparent destructive change. The first changes that can be detected are in the mucopolysaccharides of the sclera, remote from the lesion. As the granuloma is approached, the fibres are pushed further apart by mucoid oedema and the collagen fibrils first bulge, then separate and finally unravel. The only cellular change in this region is an apparent increase in the number and activity of the fibrocytes. Within the granuloma, however, the cellular component increases dramatically, the region being infiltrated by plasma cells, lymphocytes and macrophages, some of which aggregate to form giant cells. There is fibrinoid necrosis and the fibrocytes are degenerate or disappear altogether. In this region there are tufts of new vessels which have their origin in the episcleral or choroidal vasculature. Both the new and old vessels show medial necrosis, mucopolysaccharide deposition and occasional thrombosis. Many have fibrin deposited in and around them.

Granulomatous changes of this type suggest that the lesions are immunologically induced either from locally produced antigens (type IV delayed hypersensitivity reaction) or from circulating immune complexes which have for some reason precipitated within the eye and initiated an immune response (type III reaction).[14] They also indicate that there is both an extracellular and a cellular component to the condition, the extracellular component being that which is responsible in the first instance for activating the scleral fibrocytes and for the damage to the proteoglycan matrix and binding site on the collagen fibril. This damage would appear to arise from substances diffusing from activated cells remote from the exact site of damage.

In type III reactions the vascular response is the result of antigen–antibody conjugation at sites in the vessel wall. These complexes are precipitated in the venule wall and activate complement inciting an acute inflammatory response.

Polymorphonuclear leucocytes are probably essential to the development of such inflammatory responses; they can be activated within the circulation by a variety of stimuli including complement (particularly C_5A), or as a response to immune complexes outside the vessels. They marginate and adhere to the endothelial cells, or at gaps where endothelial cells have contracted apart. Endothelial cell damage and consequent vascular permeability is produced by prolonged contact with marginated neutrophils and monocytes, probably by superoxide discharge and lysosomal enzyme release from these cells. The leucocytes then migrate across the endothelium to the extravascular tissue which may be the site of the noxious stimulus. A complex series of reactions can then occur within the vessel, in the vessel wall and outside. Multiple mediators such as adenine nucleotides, kinins, leucotrienes, prostaglandins and platelet activating factor are released, which dilate or contract the vessel wall depending on their concentration and the type of vessel involved.

These changes would account for the vascular changes seen on fluorescein angiography and for the association with many other systemic disorders in which immune complex deposition is known to occur.

Association with Other Disorders

If immune complex deposition were the only mechanism through which scleritis evolved it might be expected that immune complexes would be found in the vessel walls of all patients with this disease. Indeed if the patient is known to have a systemic vasculitis, such as periarteritis nodosa, Wegener's granulomatosis or the severe vasculitis of rheumatoid arthritis, then immune complexes can indeed sometimes be demonstrated in the vessel wall. However, prolonged searches in many patients with scleritis have shown either nothing or only immunoglobulins but not immune complexes, which implies that immune complex deposition is not the only mechanism by which vascular damage can occur.

It is not possible to diagnose the type of connective tissue disease likely to be present from the characteristics of the scleritis but it does seem that those patients with scleromalacia perforans and 'contact lens cornea' are likely to have rheumatoid arthritis of many years' standing, while those displaying the

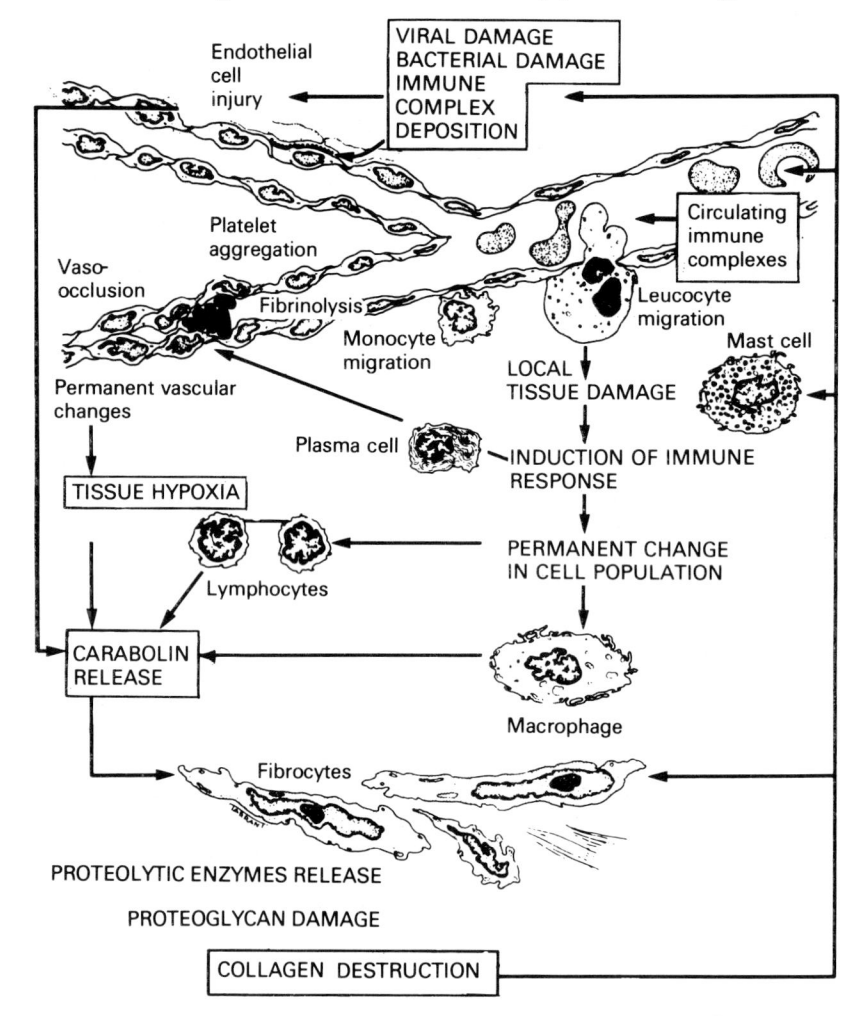

Fig. 9. A possible scheme for the induction and persistence of scleral disease.
(Reproduced from 'The nature and treatment of scleral disease', *Trans. Ophthal. Soc. UK.* Vol. 102, p. 279 (1982)).

Nevertheless, scleritis is associated with connective tissue disease in approximately 40 per cent of cases and investigation must therefore be directed to the detection of this group of conditions.

Rheumatoid arthritis is the commonest of the connective tissue diseases and there is therefore a definite association between scleritis and rheumatoid disease. To look at it the other way round, the incidence of scleritis in rheumatoid arthritis has varied between 0·15 and 0·67 per cent depending on the series studied, the only exception to this being the series of Jayson and Jones[15] in which an incidence of 6·3 per cent was found. A high proportion of such scleritis patients with rheumatoid arthritis showed seropositive erosive arthritis with vasculitis and had a high mortality.

so-called acute necrotizing sclerokeratitis are likely to have one of the acute connective tissue diseases.

Other Precipitating Causes

It has been noticed that scleritis frequently follows a local insult to the eye, whether this be the trauma of any ocular operation, cataract extraction or lensectomy, iridectomy or trabeculectomy (*see Fig.* 7).[16] It also follows chronic infections, as with an infected retinal detachment plomb, or infection with herpes zoster ophthalmicus. In all these situations there is an interval of 10 days to several months between the initiating trauma and the subsequent scleritis, which starts at the site of the original injury, spreading circumferentially from it. It was found that there was no particular surgical procedure that gave rise to scleritis more than any other and no particular suture used. The characteristic of these patients was that either the normal inflammatory response following surgery failed to resolve and the eye went into a state of necrotizing scleritis or alternatively, after a period of quiescence which could last up to a year, recurrence of inflammation occurred at the site of the previous surgical trauma. In the case of patients who had undergone cataract extraction the inflammation occurred at the corneoscleral junction.

It would appear, therefore, that the initial scleral inflammation can come about in several ways (Fig. 9). An episode in the eye which may be of a trivial nature, e.g. a mild infection, induces an inflammatory response which results in a local immune response which, if it is allowed to persist, gives rise to tissue damage, and will result in the development of autoimmunization. Usually the antigen is eliminated and the response subsides, but should the vessel remain permanently altered, circulating immune complexes may be precipitated in its wall giving rise to the local reaction. Although detectable vascular changes can be seen on fluorescein angiography in the eyes of patients with known immune complex disorders and those who have a systemic vasculitis, no inflammation will be seen in the eyes of these patients unless the ocular vessels are or have previously been damaged. We have also shown by fluorescein angiography that scleral destructive changes do not occur without a preliminary diminution of the blood supply. It would seem, therefore, that the target for the abnormal and persistent immune response is the endothelial cells of the microvasculature and that the pathological process can be precipitated by trauma whether it be mechanical or biological. If the insult is severe enough then vascular closure will result, hypoxia of the tissue occurs and the chain of catabolic destruction is initiated.

INVESTIGATION OF SCLERITIS

It follows from the previous discussion that there are two separate but interrelated causes of the sceral inflammation. The first is the local insult, which can give rise to an autoimmune response, and the second is the presence of a systemic disorder, which can give rise to a vasculitis that can affect the periscleral vasculature.

The most potent external source of local stimulation is herpes zoster although other viral or bacterial infections have been known to cause the response and these particularly chronic staphylococcal infections, syphilis, tuberculosis and gout should be sought and treated, as this may be sufficient to inhibit the inflammatory response.

Herpes Zoster

This condition, when the ophthalmic division of the trigeminal nerve is involved, gives rise to scleral or episcleral complications in about 6 per cent of cases.

There appear to be three separate patterns as a result of scleral or episcleral involvement in herpes zoster ophthalmicus:

(a) there may be a transient episcleritis in the vesicular stage which clears spontaneously;

(b) other patients may develop a nodular scleritis or episcleritis which clears spontaneously between the tenth to fourteenth day after the start of the disease;

(c) a few patients develop a necrotizing scleritis in the recovery stage at the site previously involved by an episcleritis early in the disease, which may relapse but remains confined to the same site.

Treatment of (a) should be by locally applied antiviral agents and steroid drops, on the assumption that it is viral in origin; (b) should be treated with local steroids and (c) with systemic steroids.

General Investigations

Because of the known association with other connective tissue disease and immune complex disorders, inquiry should be made of stiffness in the limbs or back, morning stiffness, joint swelling, skin rashes, numbness and tingling in the limbs, ulceration of mucous membranes.

Laboratory tests should include a full blood count and ESR, serum uric acid, specific tests for syphilis and an immunological survey which should include rheumatoid factors, antinuclear factor, immunofluorescence studies and immune complexes by the polyethylene glycol method. The advantage of this method is that a percentage of circulating pathological immune complexes are measured. If they are present in high concentrations these can be used to monitor the dosage of treatment required to keep the disease under control. Indeed, because scleritis is an 'end organ' disorder, the treatment depends not so much on the diagnosed disease as on the local manifestations of this disorder. The systemic disease only becomes of importance when this is known to produce a systemic vasculitis or circulating immune complexes can be demonstrated.

TREATMENT OF SCLERITIS AND EPISCLERITIS

The body has developed highly complex systems to produce and maintain the inflammatory reaction because it is essential to mount a rapid and vigorous response locally from small beginnings and from a large variety of different stimuli. This means that the response to a particular stimulus will not activate all the available mechanisms. If these defence mechanisms are overcome, then disease results and investigation is directed towards detecting which is the predominant system involved. Because there are different activators and inhibitors for each part of the response, treatment is directed at restoring this relationship to normal. The vascular abnormalities that accompany scleral inflammation are now amenable to investigation, particularly with fluorescein angiography. Because these are at the root of the pathological changes and indicate the severity of the disorder, the type of treatment selected now depends largely on what is seen on the angiogram.

In those patients with simple episcleritis in whom the vasculature is normal and the inflammatory response confined to vasodilatation and exudation (possibly due to mast cell activation) then the process will be self-limiting so that either no treatment or at most local medication with steroid or other anti-inflammatory drops will suffice. The one possible exception to this is gout, in which the mechanism is due to phagocytic vacuole disruption and should therefore be treated by uricosuric therapy, supplementing this as need be by local steroid therapy.

Treatment of those patients with nodular episcleritis, diffuse and nodular scleritis in whom the vascular tree is open (*Fig. 3, Plate* IXa) but in whom the response is prolonged, will always be successful with the non-steroidal anti-inflammatory agents. At present no satisfactory local preparation is available but as most of these patients also have a systemic vascular instability they are probably better treated systemically.

The situation alters immediately large sections of the vascular tree become shut down (*Figs. 4, 5, Plate* IXc). Specific therapy for such conditions as syphilis is given if indicated; otherwise a short course of one of the systemic non-steroidal anti-inflammatory agents such as indomethacin 100 mg daily or Froben 300 mg daily is started. If there is an immediate improvement in *both* the clinical condition and the vascular flow pattern, then these are continued at a much reduced dosage (this can be assessed using the red-free light of the slit lamp). If, however, after 1 week the clinical condition or the vascular flow is not improved, then a short, very intensive course of high dose steroid is given. The usual routine is 80 mg for 1 day reducing by 10 mg steps to 20 mg over 7 days and then, depending on the response, withdrawing the drug completely over the next 2 weeks or continuing on a maintenance dose of between 7 and 12·5 mg daily. It should be possible to withdraw the steroids completely within 1 month. This can be achieved either by alternate day therapy or 1 mg reductions. While long term maintenance therapy is often unnecessary, if it is required it is highly individual and must be determined for each person. It may sometimes be necessary to add a non-steroidal anti-inflammatory agent to reduce the systemic steroid dosage to an acceptable level.

Local steroid therapy is ineffective on its own but may sometimes be valuable as an adjunct to other systemic therapy in order to reduce the dosage required. It has, however, no place in the long term treatment as it has been responsible for many of the complications seen. Subconjunctival steroids are not only ineffective but also contraindicated because the trauma (and possibly some component of the injected drug) can induce a destructive scleritis.

Patients with destructive scleral disease need to be assessed in far greater detail. It appears only to be necessary to break the vicious cycle of inflammation for therapy to succeed. The cycle can be broken either at the site of local tissue destruction and antibody production, or at the level of the vascular endothelium or in certain instances at the central site of lymphocyte production. Sometimes a single course of therapy may be sufficient to achieve this, although more usually some continuing suppressive therapy is required until healing has occurred. It is particularly important, therefore, to identify those patients with immune complex disease and those with systemic immunologically induced disorders. The majority of patients with necrotizing scleritis in which there is a large inflammatory element affecting particularly the venules respond to a short oral course of high dose steroid therapy. There remain a few who do not.

Those who have conditions in which the whole of the immune system is involved, e.g. Wegener's granulomatosis, need treatment aimed at the suppression of the production of the lymphocytes. This is best achieved by the primary use of immunosuppressive drugs, such as cyclophosphamide together with steroid (*Plate* IXf). Others in whom the inflammatory response is excessive will respond best to chlorambucil and steroid and yet others who have a systemic vasculitis or only circulating immune complex disease will need only steroid.

To avoid the terrible complications of long term, high dosage steroid therapy and to block all the available receptor sites, pulse therapy has been introduced for the very severe disease and for those who are unable to tolerate oral steroid (*Plate* IXa,b). The patient is admitted to hospital and a single dose of methyl prednisolone of as much as 1 g is given intravenously over a period of a few hours. Depending on the response, the dose is repeated at weekly intervals for up to 4 weeks. No other therapy is given in between other than a low maintenance dose of steroid (e.g. 7·5 mg/d) or drugs that had been known to keep the condition quiescent between attacks.

In those patients with extremely high circulating immune complexes (80–100 per cent PEG) and in certain others who are resistant to other forms of medication, cyclophosphamide 500 mg is given as a bolus and repeated at intervals. Because of the dangers of cystitis, the patient must be fully hydrated and an intravenous infusion of fluid administered for 24 h after the injection to ensure a good diuresis.

A very low maintenance level (as low as 50 mg a week on some patients) can then often be achieved. These massive dosage regimes are not without risk and may have to be repeated at intervals. They must, therefore, be reserved for the very severe intractable disease and administered by a physician conversant with their use. However, given the correct indications, the results can be dramatic and sight saving and can often result in a permanent cure of an otherwise intractable condition. It is probably true to say that no patient should ever have reached the point where this form of treatment is necessary had they been adequately observed and treated at the onset of the disorder.

Scleritis is a medically treatable disease and surgery for excision and replacement of damaged sclera is rarely necessary and must be reserved for those patients in whom it is almost certain that the source of the inflammation is autoimmune, e.g. following a localized infective initiating process which has given rise to a primary or a self-perpetuating ulcer. Excision of the damaged tissue removes the source of the antigen but should never be undertaken in the presence of untreated active disease.

Many of the major difficulties in diagnosis arise from posterior scleritis, largely because the vascular network of the sclera of the posterior segment cannot be seen. It has to be assumed that the granuloma causing posterior scleritis has a similar course to those seen in the anterior segment and should be treated in the same way. In practice this is successful and although most patients require systemic steroid therapy to control the disease, some recover using non-steroid anti-inflammatory agents alone.

True scleromalacia perforans, which is due to infarction of the arteriolar supply of a section of the anterior segment, can only be treated in the very earliest stages of the disease before sequestration occurs. This change can always be detected clinically by a yellow discoloration of the sclera. Once resorption starts, treatment is not only ineffective but also meddlesome. Unfortunately the patients rarely have any symptoms and only present when the disease is far advanced. It is unusual therefore to have to treat scleromalacia perforans unless there are secondary complications.

Scleritis, however severe, is almost always treatable but it is essential to investigate the condition completely so that toxic drugs are not given to those who do not need them and effective therapy is given to those who do.

REFERENCES

1. Watson P. G. and Bovey E. Anterior segment fluorescein angiography in the diagnosis of scleral inflammation. *Ophthalmology* 1985; **92**, 1–11.
2. Lyne A. G. A. Corneal sensitivity in scleritis and episcleritis. *Br. J. Ophthalmol.* 1977; **61**, 650–4.
3. Watson P. G. and Hazleman B. L. *The Sclera and Systemic Disorders.* London, Saunders, 1976, pp. 91, 130, 142.
4. Watson P. G. and Hayreh S. S. Scleritis and episcleritis. *Br. J. Ophthalmol.* 1976; **60**, 163–91.
5. McGavin D. D. M., Williamson J., Forrester J. V. et al. Episcleritis and scleritis. A study of their clinical manifestations and association with rheumatoid arthritis. *Br. J. Ophthalmol.* 1976; **60**, 192–226.
6. Watson P. G. The nature and treatment of scleral inflammation (Doyne Memorial Lecture). *Trans. Ophthalmol. Soc. UK* 1982; **102**, 257–81.
7. Van der Hoeve J. Scleromalacia perforans. *Arch. Ophthalmol.* 1934; **11**, 111–18.
8. Lyne A. G. A. Contact lens cornea in rheumatoid arthritis. *Br. J. Ophthalmol.* 1970; **54**, 410–15.
9. Wilhelmus K. R., Grierson I. and Watson P. G. Histopathologic and clinical associations of scleritis and glaucoma. *Am. J. Ophthalmol.* 1981; **91**, 697–705.
10. Fraundfelder F. T. and Watson P. G. Evaluation of eyes enucleated for scleritis. *Br. J. Ophthalmol.* 1976; **60**, 227–30.
11. Kostenitsch J. Über einen Fall von Skleritis; pathologische anatomische Untersuchung. *Arch. Augenheilk.* 1894; **28**, 27–35.
12. Parsons J. H. *Pathology of the Eye*, vol. 1. London, Hodder and Stoughton, 1904.
13. Francois J. Ocular manifestations in collagenoses. *Adv. Ophthalmol.* 1970; **23**, 1–54.
14. Lachmann P. and Peters J. *Clinical Aspects of Immunology*, 4th ed. Oxford, Blackwell, 1982.
15. Jayson M. I. and Jones D. E. Scleritis and rheumatoid arthritis. *Ann. Rheumat. Dis.* 1971; **30**, 343–7.
16. Lyne A. G. A. and Lloyd Jones D. Necrotizing scleritis and after ocular surgery. *Trans. Ophthalmol. Soc. UK* 1979; **99**, 146–9.

Chapter 7

The Uveal Tract

D. J. Spalton

The uveal tract consists of the iris, ciliary body and choroid lying in continuity. It is derived from both neuroectoderm and mesoderm; neuroectoderm forms the muscles of the iris and ciliary body and the pigmented epithelium of the ciliary body; mesoderm forms the uveal stroma. Melanocytes from the neural crest are scattered throughout the tract and produce the characteristic pigmentation of the iris and fundus seen on ophthalmoscopy. Apart from the specialized muscular function of the iris and ciliary body the uveal tract is concerned with the nutrition of the eye both by the secretion of aqueous humour and the maintenance of the outer retina from the choriocapillaris. The vascular supply of the tract is derived from the anterior and posterior ciliary circulations from the ophthalmic artery. The rate of blood flow is exceptionally high, venous blood returning by the vortex veins to the orbital veins.

CONGENITAL ANOMALIES OF THE UVEAL TRACT

The fetal fissure of the optic vesicle closes at 7–8 weeks of fetal life to form the optic cup. This process begins centrally in the fissure and spreads anteriorly and posteriorly, in the inferomedial meridian. Defects in the closure mechanism will produce a coloboma. These may vary in size and shape from the gross to the trivial but are always characterized by their inferomedial axis. They may involve the iris, ciliary body, choroid or optic disc.

Coloboma

Chorioretinal colobomas are characterized by hypoplasia or absence of the choroid in the inferomedial axis. Mild degrees of colobomatous change can be seen as thinning of the retinal pigment epithelium and choroidal pigmentation and in many patients there is associated asymmetrical hypoplasia or tilting of the optic disc as well. More severe degrees are seen as the absence of the choroid leading to atrophy of the overlying retina so that the underlying sclera is viewed as a white, often staphylomatous, expanse. Sometimes a coloboma of the retina will be separated by an island of normal retina from a peripheral coloboma or the optic disc. Visual acuity will be affected if macular fibres are involved. Colobomas of the iris and ciliary body usually show absence of the lens zonule too, sometimes producing an indentation in the equator of the lens.

Aniridia

This can be inherited either in a dominant or sporadic manner. The condition is bilateral and is associated with nystagmus, corneal opacities and photophobia.

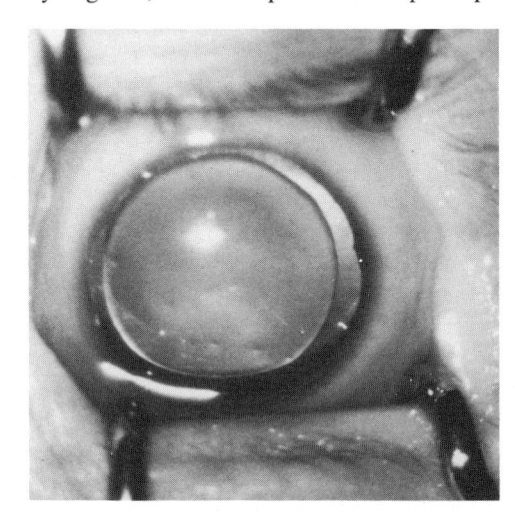

Fig. 1. Bilateral aniridia in a baby with the sporadic pattern of disease. A vestigial frill of iris root can be seen.

A vestigial frill of iris root can normally be seen on gonioscopy, which frequently forms peripheral anterior synechiae to occlude the angle and produce an intractable glaucoma which is difficult to control and is the most serious consequence of the condition. Sporadic cases have a high incidence of an associated nephroblastoma (Wilm's tumour) and this must be excluded by intravenous pyelography or ultrasound in all affected children (*Fig.* 1).

UVEITIS

Despite a great deal of experimental research the immunology of uveitis is still largely not understood. Many animal models have been developed but none of these uveitides is completely identical to the human disease: none of them shows the typical relapsing course of the human disease and while the current experiments with retinal 'S' antigen produce a syndrome similar to sympathetic ophthalmitis, the experimental disease still shows fundamental clinical and pathological differences.

The production of a uveitis requires an initiating event, perpetuation of the inflammatory response, followed by resolution of the inflammation and quiescence or relapse. O'Connor[1] has emphasized the role of tissue damage as an initiating event in uveitis, which can occur through trauma, infection or immunological injury. A simple illustration of this is the corneal abrasion which is sometimes associated with a mild anterior uveitis. In this situation it can be shown experimentally that retrograde (antidromic) impulses in the sensory corneal axon cause release of inflammatory mediators from the iris into the anterior chamber to produce a mild anterior uveitis. A mechanism such as this may help to account for the mild uveitis which sometimes accompanies a viral keratitis and which resolves on healing, but whilst a uveitis is a common feature of traumatic or surgical abrasion of the cornea, these patients do not suffer from recurrent inflammation, indicating other factors are involved.

Circulating immune complexes may have a role in this initiation and recurrence of uveitis. If aggregations of antigen and antibody are formed in the blood and deposited in the uveal vessels with binding of complement, an Arthus type of inflammatory reaction may be initiated and perpetuated. Both pathological and experimental work shows that this is a possibility but searches for circulating immune complexes in anterior or posterior uveitis have been inconclusive[2,3] and furthermore, uveitis is uncommon in diseases such as glomerulonephritis which have been shown to have this aetiology. However, a few rare diseases (such as serum sickness) do manifest a uveitis and factors such as the size and shape of the immune complexes, the presence of damaged uveal blood vessels, the type of immunoglobulins involved and their means of detection may be important. The alternative explanation has been put forward that their presence may be only an epiphenomenon or even beneficial to the patient, indicating recognition and removal of an offending antigen.[4]

The eye has a number of unique factors which affect its immune response. There is a dual blood supply from the retinal and choroidal systems and the absence of a lymphatic drainage means that an intraocular antigen must pass through the blood–ocular barrier to the blood to the site of immunological recognition. Following this central recognition and processing of the antigen, immunocompetent cells are formed which find their way back to the eye by the blood. Little is known about the precise cells and their location involved in this process of central recognition but it appears that both T and B lymphocytes are involved and that the situation may be further complicated by cooperation between these two cell types, as well as the various T cell subsets, so that the type of lymphocytic reaction can change during the course of the disease.[5] A factor that may modify the immune response is the avascularity of the ocular tissues, which retards removal of antigen leaving a reservoir which perpetuates the inflammatory response. When immunocompetent cells return to the eye they are deposited within the uveal vasculature and remain there as immunocompetent memory cells, even after the inflammation has resolved. From experimental work it appears that not all these cells are specific for the initiating antigen alone, but that other lymphocytes which react to other antigens in the host's immunological repertoire are also deposited at the same time.[6] After the attack resolves and the initiating antigen is removed, these cells remain, converting the uveal tract into an accessory lymph node with a diverse range of memory cells that can be potentially reactivated at a future date by stimulation with a range of appropriate antigens, a feature that might help to explain the nonspecific recurrence of uveitic attacks.

Genetic and racial factors and sex also influence the development of uveitis. The association of certain patterns of HLA antigens with various uveitic syndromes such as acute anterior uveitis, Behçet's disease and the Vogt–Koyanagi–Harada syndrome are well known, as is the great racial variation of incidence of different uveitic diseases. Sex plays a smaller role but some diseases, such as acute anterior uveitis with ankylosing spondylitis or Reiter's disease, are more common in males, while chronic anterior uveitis with Still's disease is more common in females.

Classification of Uveitis

Uveitis is a generic term given to an inflammatory process within the uveal tract. This inflammation may affect all or part of the uveal tract, but since the iris, ciliary body and choroid lie in continuity with each other, it is not surprising that a focus of severe inflammation in one region may spill over to affect the adjacent area. Thus a severe iritis may be accompanied by a cellular infiltration of the anterior vitreous from an inflamed ciliary body ('iridocyclitis') or a choroiditis by anterior uveitis. Uveitis may be due to a 'primary' immunological disease within the eye or be a secondary but important feature of ocular trauma or infection. There is no one classification or description of the disease that is entirely satisfactory or which can be applied to all types of uveitis and the clinical categorization of uveitis relies on a combination of clinical signs, anatomical findings and pathological processes where these are understood.

Endogenous uveitis has been used to describe inflammation of the uvea produced by an inflammation from a source within the body, usually gaining access to the eye by the blood stream, whereas an exogenous uveitis is preceded by perforation of the globe. Either type can be divided into infectious or non-infectious types but usage of these terms is becoming redundant as the understanding of immunology blurs their distinction. It is, however, useful in the clinical sense to think of uveitis as primary (idiopathic) or secondary (associated with some known factor whether it be traumatic, infective or immunological). Pathologically non-suppurative inflammation can be divided into acute (polymorphonuclear leucocyte infiltration), chronic non-granulomatous (lymphocytic and plasma cell infiltration) or chronic granulomatous (epithelioid cell infiltration). The latter two categories of this pathological classification can be alluded to by the clinical findings in the eye; 'granulomatous' uveitis produces typical large white 'mutton fat' keratic precipitates (KP), iris nodules (Koeppé or Busacca nodules) or stromal infiltration, and a diagnosis of granulomatous uveitis has been used to indicate that one of the 'granulomatous types' of disease, such as sarcoid, tuberculosis or syphilis, may be the underlying aetiology. Such clinical findings have limited implications. It can sometimes be difficult to decide whether or not the KP have a granulomatous appearance and some diseases, such as sarcoid, may be present in either a granulomatous or non-granulomatous manner, and in many cases of clinically granulomatous uveitis no evidence of any granulomatous disease is found. The appearance of the KP probably alludes more to such factors as antigen–antibody ratios than to the clinical cause of the disease.

A useful clinical distinction is whether the inflammation is acute or chronic. Acute anterior uveitis is associated with photophobia, pain and redness, which reflects the severity of anterior chamber involvement and usually has a relatively short clinical course which resolves over a few weeks, whereas these features are absent in chronic disease. Some diseases start, however, with an acute presentation and then become chronic, whereas others will have acute episodes within a chronic course.

These acknowledged difficulties in the classification of uveitis have led to an attempt at international definitions. The International Uveitis Study Group has proposed the following terms, classifying the disease anatomically.

1. Anterior uveitis to include inflammation extending posteriorly as far as the pars plicata. This term includes iritis, iridocyclitis, anterior cyclitis.
2. Intermediate uveitis – a rather poor name for inflammation of the pars plana and peripheral retina to include terms such as pars planitis, peripheral uveitis, peripheral retinitis etc.
3. Posterior uveitis is located behind the posterior hyaloid face and may be focal, multifocal or diffuse.
4. Panuveitis, implying involvement of the whole uveal tract.

Isolated macular oedema may be a manifestation of anterior or intermediate uveitis. Other suggested but more controversial criteria are the onset, which may be classified as sudden or insidious; the duration, classified as short if of less than 3 months'; grades of activity, classified as none, mild or severe; and the pattern, single or repeated. Perhaps the most useful information in the clinical management of a patient is to determine the anatomical localization of the inflammation as this will help to predict the clinical signs, natural history of the disease and its likely visual consequences, and to describe the patient as completely as possible, i.e. 'a 55-year-old woman with a chronic anterior uveitis and secondary glaucoma and a mild acute relapse, presenting initially with herpes zoster ophthalmicus 9 months previously'.

In other patients a uveitis may be secondary to another disease such as keratitis, scleritis or retinal vasculitis. This distinction is made on the site of the primary inflammatory reaction which is not always easy to know: in both posterior uveitis and retinal vasculitis there may be infiltration and leakage from retinal vessels and the distinction is made by comparison of the degree of retinal vascular involvement shown by infiltration, haemorrhage and occlusion to posterior uveitis.

Clinical Presentation of Uveitis

The presentation of uveitis depends on the severity of inflammation, the site within the eye and its rapidity of onset, and the sequelae on the severity, site and duration of the inflammation.

Acute anterior uveitis (AAU) is one of the causes of a red, painful eye. Patients usually present with a short history of a few days of pain and photophobia and, as with any inflamed eye, there may be a watery discharge which can be confused with a conjunctivitis. Pain from uveitis can usually be distinguished from that due to conjunctivitis, as in the former the pain has a deep, aching or boring character behind or around the eye, whereas conjunctivitis produces a gritty foreign body sensation. The pain from uveitis originates in the iris and ciliary body and is eased by paralysis of these muscles with atropine. Photophobia is often a prominent symptom. The conjunctival hyperaemia that is seen with acute anterior uveitis typically has a circumlimbal or ciliary distribution, whereas that from conjunctivitis produces a diffuse reaction. This hyperaemia is caused by the anastamosis of the conjunctival and ciliary circulations in the circumlimbal region with overspill of intraocular inflammation producing the hyperaemia. While the distinction of ciliary or conjunctival hyperaemia is useful, a severe anterior uveitis may produce such an intense hyperaemia that the whole conjunctiva becomes inflamed and this distinction cannot be made.

Visual acuity in AAU is affected only if the inflammation within the anterior chamber is sufficient to obscure the media and patients with mild uveitis will not usually complain of blurred vision. With a less acute or more indolent anterior uveitis there is correspondingly less pain and redness of the eye, the symptoms and intraocular signs remaining the same, although less marked. The most extreme example of this is seen in the chronic anterior uveitis of childhood associated with Still's disease, in which there is a complete absence of pain or redness of the eye and the affected child presents with visual loss from band keratopathy, glaucoma or cataract in a totally white eye.

Commonly posterior uveitis does not produce a red eye unless there is overspill of inflammation into the anterior chamber or a panuveitis. Patients usually present with floaters from vitreous debris or blurred vision from vitreous haze or cellular infiltration of the vitreous gel, or macular oedema; occasionally an intense chorioretinitis involves the macula or the overlying retinal nerve fibre layer to produce a noticeable field defect. Vitreous cellular infiltration is the equivalent of cells in the aqueous humour, but because of the more restricted circulation they are often localized to the area of inflammation, for example over the pars plana with intermediate uveitis, the optic disc with a papillitis or a focus overlying toxoplasmic chorioretinitis. Vitreous cellular infiltration can persist for a prolonged time and in chronic cases there is often some opacification of the gel by cell debris and proteinaceous fluid which obscure vision, although this is rarely severe enough to justify removal by vitrectomy.

The classic signs of inflammation within the anterior chamber are keratic precipitates (KP), flare, cells and posterior synechiae. With inflammation of the ocular blood vessels the blood–ocular barrier breaks down, causing leakage of leucocytes and protein into the ocular media. Leucocytes ('cells') can be seen within the aqueous humour by an intense narrow slit lamp beam and appear as spots similar to dust in a sunbeam (*Fig.* 2). The increased exudation of protein produces a 'flare' within the aqueous humour which defines the slit beam in a similar way to a car headlight cutting into a foggy night (*Fig.* 3). Cells circulate within the anterior chamber by convection currents to become deposited on the corneal endothelium, frequently in the inferior quadrant where they are seen as KP (*Fig.* 4). The presence of cells correlates with the degree of inflammation within the eye, appearing and disappearing accordingly. Severe inflammation, however, can produce permanent damage of the blood–ocular barrier and a flare may persist indefinitely as evidence of this, even after the uveitis has resolved. Really severe inflammation within the anterior chamber can lead to leakage of fibrinogen, the largest of all plasma proteins, to produce a fibrin clot within the aqueous ('plastic uveitis') or such gross leucocyte exudation that a hypopyon is formed by the precipitation of the leucocytes.

Posterior synechiae are adhesions between the pupil margin and anterior lens capsule, which may

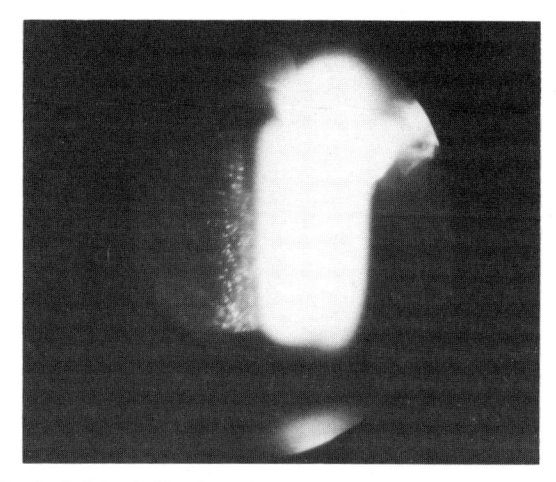

Fig. 2. Cellular infiltration of vitreous can be seen in an aphakic patient with severe posterior uveitis.

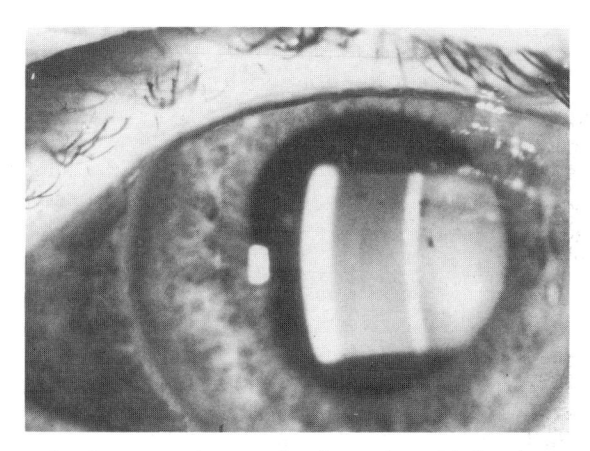

Fig. 3. A heavy proteinaceous flare in a patient with chronic anterior uveitis. Patches of pigmentation can be seen on the anterior lens surface where posterior synechiae have been ruptured by mydriasis.

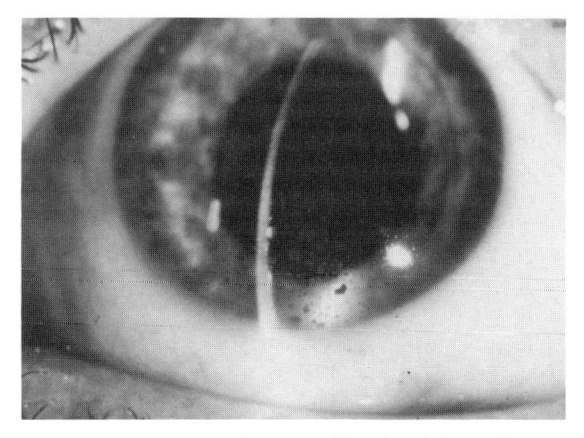

Fig. 4. Granulomatous KP in an eye with a chronic 'granulomatous' uveitis are seen on the inferior quadrant of the corneal endothelium and have a large, globular, mutton fat appearance. Note the whiteness of the eye.

progress to seclude the pupil, preventing dilatation and leading to the formation of iris bombé from the restriction of aqueous humour circulation. A cyclitic membrane which also occludes the pupil often occurs at the same time. Their prevention by mydriasis is one of the cornerstones of the treatment of uveitis. Accumulation of cells can sometimes be seen on the iris itself. These are known as Koeppé nodules when they appear on the pupillary margin or Busacca nodules when they are seen on the anterior stromal surface of the iris; both types of cellular accumulation are considered to be signs of granulomatous uveitis. They disappear without trace on successful control of the inflammation, although Koeppé nodules may lead to the formation of posterior synechiae if untreated. Discrete swellings within the iris stroma are occasionally seen in 'granulomatous' disease. Vasculitic disease of the radial iris blood vessels can produce sectorial iris atrophy with pupillary spiralling and loss of the iris pigment epithelium, most easily seen as iris transillumination when observing the red reflex. Such iris damage is a particularly common finding in anterior uveitis associated with herpes zoster.

A useful bedside diagnostic test that has been recently described for an anterior uveitis is the painful consensual pupillary light reflex.[7] In a unilateral case of anterior uveitis a bright light will produce a painful, direct and consensual pupillary light reflex in the affected eye. This is only seen in the presence of intraocular inflammation and thereby helps to exclude the other causes of a painful red eye.

With posterior uveitis the cellular infiltration is limited to the vitreous cavity. Accumulations of cells are seen scattered within the gel or as larger accumulations attached to a vitreous membrane or detached posterior hyaloid face. When this cellular debris is sited near the retina the patient notices floaters produced by shadows cast on the retina as the debris crosses the visual axis. In almost all cases of posterior uveitis fluorescein angiography shows leakage from the retinal vessels, particularly the veins. Further evidence of retinal vascular involvement can be seen as whitish fluffy infiltration around the retinal vessels, retinal haemorrhages or vascular occlusion occasionally leading to capillary closure and neovascularization. A retinal arteritis is rare. Macular oedema may be seen with anterior uveitis but is more commonly a feature of posterior uveitis.

Visual Loss in Uveitis

An attack of acute anterior uveitis rarely produces any ocular morbidity but prolonged inflammation, particularly with posterior uveitis or chronic anterior uveitis, is associated with visual loss from cataract, glaucoma or retinal damage, either as a result of post-inflammatory destruction, macular oedema or vascular occlusion and subsequent neovascularization. Visual loss from band keratopathy sometimes occurs in chronically inflamed eyes and this is a well-recognized feature of the chronic anterior uveitis associated with Still's disease; corneal decompensation from endothelial cell damage is usually restricted to severely diseased eyes.

Some degree of cataract formation is frequently apparent in most patients after about 2 years of chronic inflammation. The earliest changes occur in the posterior subcapsular zone and are seen initially as a polychromatic lustre which progresses to a localized posterior subcapsular opacity and eventually to maturity with progressive visual loss. The aetiology of these lens changes and the reason for their location is not understood, but the possibilities include derangement of lens metabolism from the primary immunopathology or changes in the permeability of the lens capsule or cellular membrane of the lens fibres leading to secondary metabolic changes. Phospholipases are released from lysozymes and mast cells during inflammation and have the potential to damage the phospholipid structure of the lens capsule, increasing its permeability which would disrupt metabolism in the lens and allow access to the sequestered antigens.[8] Similar morphological cataractous changes are seen as a result of topical or systemic steroid therapy and in many patients this is a contributing factor, although, of course, either condition occurs in isolation. This side effect of steroid therapy does not influence its usage as the risks of uncontrolled intraocular inflammation to vision are greater. Miosis and posterior synechiae enhance the effects of lens opacities by restricting pupillary diameter.

Cataract surgery in uveitis calls for careful clinical judgement as there are risks of exacerbating both the uveitis and producing postoperative glaucoma. It is of the greatest importance to control the intraocular inflammation and intraocular pressure as completely as possible prior to surgery and the results are better if the uveitis has 'burnt out'. Surgical techniques lie between intracapsular or extracapsular surgery or lensectomy, with or without concomitant vitrectomy. A sector iridectomy is often required to ensure a reasonable postoperative pupillary aperture. The type of surgical procedure is dictated by experience and the clinical circumstances, for example, patients with Fuch's heterochromic cyclitis do well with intracapsular extraction whereas children with Still's disease seem to do better with a lensectomy and vitrectomy procedure. Sometimes cataract surgery has a beneficial effect on a uveitic eye, producing a quieter eye postoperatively that is easier to manage. Intraocular lens implantation is contraindicated in all uveitic eyes, with the possible exception of Fuchs' heterochromic cyclitis.

Glaucoma in uveitis occurs by both open or closed angle mechanisms. Open angle glaucoma can be caused in the acute episode by clogging of the trabecular meshwork with inflammatory debris or an associated inflammatory trabeculitis and in some patients prolonged anterior uveitis leads to open angle glaucoma from trabecular destruction or 'sclerosis'. Topical steroid therapy will produce open angle glaucoma in genetically susceptible individuals and this may complicate the management of a uveitic eye. Closed angle glaucoma may result from formation of peripheral anterior synechiae occluding the angle, or pupillary seclusion by circumferential posterior synechiae or an inflammatory cyclitic membrane producing iris bombé and secondary angle closure. Neovascularization of iris with secondary angle closure is an occasional, but devastating complication of severe uveitis. Treatment is based on adequate suppression of inflammation, mydriasis and medication to restrict aqueous humour formation. Severe and prolonged intraocular inflammation can result in ocular hypotony from destruction of the ciliary body.

Retinal damage can result from direct retinal destruction as part of the primary inflammatory process such as a retinochoroiditis due to toxoplasmosis, for example, or secondary to involvement of the retinal pigment epithelium as in the Voght–Koyanagi–Harada syndrome. The most common cause of visual loss from uveitis, however, is macular oedema. This is a common finding in the presence of posterior uveitis, but the susceptibility of individual patients varies enormously. Some patients develop marked severe cystoid macular oedema with even mild inflammation; others seem to be able to tolerate much more severe inflammation without macular damage. Occasionally cystoid macular oedema is seen with an anterior uveitis, although careful examination will always show some degree of vitreous infiltration, but most commonly macular oedema occurs with primary inflammation in the posterior segment. Visual acuity correlates poorly with macular oedema and some patients maintain reasonable acuity despite marked macular changes. Mild degrees of macular oedema can only be diagnosed by careful stereoscopic biomicroscopy or fluorescein angiography but a prolonged photostress test is a useful clinical adjunct. Mild degrees of macular oedema disappear on resolution of the inflammation, with consequent visual recovery. More severe oedema may resolve without visual improvement due to permanent macular damage but a few of these patients will show some visual recovery several months to years later if the eye remains quiet, presumably due to the recovery of outer retinal metabolism. Steroids are by far the most effective drug in treating macular oedema, although other anti-inflammatory drugs can play some part. Photocoagulation is not beneficial and is contraindicated.

Lipid exudation into the retina is comparatively uncommon with inflammatory eye disease when compared to other vascular retinopathies. An occlusive retinal vascular disease is a feature in some patients, particularly those with Behçet's disease, sarcoidosis or Eales's disease. These diseases tend to produce a phlebitis more commonly than an arteritis with the sequelae of visual loss from branch retinal vein occlusion and retinal ischaemia with the subsequent risks of neovascularization, vitreous haemorrhage and retinal traction detachment.

Treatment of Uveitis

The absorption of topical drugs by an inflamed eye with damaged blood–ocular barriers is totally different from that of a non-inflamed eye and this must be clearly recognized when choosing ocular therapeutic agents as a substantial amount of experimental work on ocular pharmacology has been carried out on quiet eyes and is not directly relevant to patient management.

Steroids and mydriatics are the cornerstones of treatment of uveitis. Mydriasis prevents the formation of posterior synechiae and relieves pain by reducing spasm of the iris and ciliary muscles. Atropine is the most effective topical mydriatic drug, producing intense and prolonged pupillary dilatation. It is usually given as 1 per cent or 2 per cent drops once or twice a day; ointment can be used but the associated greasiness is less pleasant for the patient.

At the initiation of treatment local heat to the affected eye potentiates the therapeutic effect and is comforting. Atropine will sometimes produce a localized allergic dermatitis and in children the drops may be absorbed in sufficient quantity to produce systemic side effects of dryness, flushing and tachycardia; in children atropine ointment is easier to administer and less likely to produce systemic absorption. Patients with mild anterior uveitis find that the image degradation from mydriasis and loss of accommodation can be inconvenient and a less potent and shorter-acting mydriatic, such as cyclopentolate, homatropine or tropicamide, is indicated for such patients and for those with skin allergy to atropine. They can be administered once or twice a day and are particularly useful if given at night just to keep the pupil mobile. Subconjunctival mydriatics are of great use in breaking down established posterior synechiae or relieving pupillary block and iris bombé.

Steroids can be given topically, periocularly or systemically. Topical steroids are very effective in the control of anterior uveitis and of less use with posterior segment inflammation. Dexamethasone, betamethasone and prednisolone are used in descending order of potency. Systemic absorption with adrenal suppression is not seen as a clinical problem with topical medications but important localized side effects are induction of glaucoma, cataract or exacerbation of herpes simplex keratitis. Steroid-induced glaucoma is seen in genetically susceptible individuals and takes several weeks of topical treatment to appear, and in view of this intraocular pressure must be monitored in all patients on topical steroid therapy. It is often difficult in a patient to separate the other types of open angle glaucoma seen with uveitis from steroid induced glaucoma and susceptibility to steroids should always be considered in the assessment of the clinical situation. Steroid-induced glaucoma seems to be related to potency of the topical steroid and the frequency of its administration. Clobetasone and fluoromethalone have been introduced as they are associated with a lower tendency to steroid-induced glaucoma. They do, however, appear to be less potent in their action within the eye and this may explain their reduced effect on the intraocular pressure. Steroid-induced cataracts are only seen after 1–2 years of local therapy and begin as a polychromatic lustre in the posterior subcapsular zone and progress to a posterior subcapsular opacity which cannot be differentiated from that due to the uveitic disease process itself.

Steroids by periocular injection are of great value in the management of severe anterior or posterior uveitis and its prevention following surgery. High intraocular levels can be produced for several days from a single subconjunctival injection of 4 mg betamethasone without significant systemic effects. Depot preparations of steroids are available, but while these produce prolonged therapeutic action, they have the drawback of uncertain therapeutic levels and create problems at the site of injection where the medication itself may produce a chronic red inflammatory plaque. Detailed techniques have been described to ensure that the steroid injection is given into various potential anatomical spaces, such as the subconjunctival or sub-Tenon's space. It seems naïve, however, to presume that these fascial planes will also prove to be pharmacological barriers, as the drug may spread laterally in the tissues as well as vertically through them. Probably the only worthwhile distinction to make is between subconjunctival or deeper retrobulbar injection, where the orbital tissues will retain the drug in the proximity of a posterior inflammatory focus. Retrobulbar injections are, of course, contraindicated where the orbital tension is already increased as there is the potential risk of producing optic nerve compression. Subconjunctival injections will leak out through the conjunctiva into the conjunctival sac to penetrate the eye through the cornea as well as the sclera. They are usually given after topical anaesthesia and can be administered at the same time, although in different sites, as mydriatics or antibiotics and the injection can be repeated within a few days, depending on the tolerance of the patient.

Uncomplicated anterior uveitis can virtually always be managed by topical medication. This is, however, very much less effective in the management of posterior segment disease where periocular or systemic treatment is required if the inflammation is of any great severity. Systemic steroids carry the well-known side effects of adrenal suppression and Cushingoid effects. They must be used with care and to carry out particular therapeutic aims. Patients with mild posterior uveitis, normal vision and no macular oedema should be encouraged to tolerate the vitreous floaters and mild photophobia without recourse to systemic steroids as the side effects of treatment can outweigh the therapeutic advantages. Systemic steroids are especially useful in the management of vitreous inflammation and macular oedema and are by far the most effective drug in this situation. The dosage is monitored by the therapeutic response of the patient and the side effects, induction of diabetes, weight gain and exacerbation of systemic hypertension being particularly important. Macular oedema responds unpredictably to systemic steroids; some patients respond well, others partially and some not at all.

While prostaglandins may have a role as mediators of intraocular inflammation, prostaglandin inhibitors such as indomethacin have not been shown to have any therapeutic place in the treatment of uveitis. Some authorities believe, though, that they may be of use in preventing post surgical inflammation.

In patients with severe posterior uveitis or retinal vasculitis uncontrolled by steroids, either because of Cushingoid effects or inadequate therapeutic response, cytotoxic drugs have a role in increasing the therapeutic effect or allowing reduction of steroid dosage to tolerable levels. The main drugs used in the treatment of uveitis are azathiaprine, chlorambucil or colchicine. Cyclophosphamide is rarely used. Clinical experience shows that these agents are undoubtedly effective, especially in controlling retinal vasculitis such as in Behçet's disease where their effect is sight saving, though no controlled clinical trials have been performed. Azathiaprine, when used in combination with systemic steroids, is particularly useful in allowing the dosage of steroid to be reduced to acceptable levels. All these drugs carry the well-known hazards of immunosuppression; bone marrow suppression, possible induction of lymphoma, secondary infection, chromosome damage and potential sterility, so that they must be used with caution and careful monitoring of the ocular response to allow minimum doses to be used and with the co-operation of a physician to monitor their side effects. Other drugs such as levamisole have been used in selected cases, but evidence of their benefit is anecdotal.

Recently considerable interest has been shown in the usage of cyclosporin A in the treatment of severe posterior uveitis. This drug, developed for use in transplant patients, has the ability to interfere with the maturation of T cells by interfering with the production of interleucline II, without producing generalized immunosuppression. Initial reports of its use in uveitis have been encouraging, but these studies have been uncontrolled. The drug is extremely expensive and has serious toxic side effects so that its future role has still to be fully assessed. It produces renal toxicity, systemic hypertension, gingival hyperplasia and hirsutism in women. A pronounced ocular inflammatory rebound on withdrawing the drug can be devastating. Nevertheless, it appears to be effective, particularly in Behçet's disease, and is an indication of the way that the future pharmacology of uveitis will move from 'blanket' immunosuppression into more precise and specific immunotherapy, paralleled by a better understanding of the basic immunopathology.

SPECIFIC TYPES OF UVEITIS

Acute Anterior Uveitis

There are numerous diseases associated with acute anterior uveitis (AAU), but in the absence of other clinical evidence the most common associations in Caucasians are sarcoidosis, Reiter's syndrome and ankylosing spondylitis. These diseases, however, only account for about 5 per cent of the total number of cases. Other entities that present as anterior uveitis are Fuch's heterochromic cyclitis, panuveitis or 'overspill' anterior uveitis from primary posterior segment, corneal or scleral disease and herpes simplex or zoster which are usually diagnosed from the history and findings of associated corneal and cutaneous disease. The routine investigation of a new patient is dictated by the clinical history and findings and can usually be restricted, in the absence of other clinical indications, to screening by X-rays of the chest and sacroiliac joints and a blood count sedimentation rate. Both tuberculosis and syphilis are rare causes of uveitis these days, but it is important not to forget them and to search for them where indicated, otherwise more detailed or sophisticated investigations should be reserved for the unusual or atypical case.

The acute attack of AAU usually starts over a few days and experienced patients can predict a relapse in the earliest stages. Uniocular disease is more common than bilateral, but the other eye may be the one to be affected in subsequent recurrences. The severity of the attack is indicated by the clinical symptoms and signs. Very severe attacks may produce a fibrin clot in the anterior chamber, which is sometimes known as 'plastic' uveitis; a hypopyon is, however, rare in acute anterior uveitis without an associated systemic disease such as Behçet's disease. The posterior segment should be examined under mydriasis in all patients. A mild cellular reaction in the anterior vitreous gel is not uncommon. These patients are sometimes termed as having an iridocyclitis. Otherwise, retinal examination should be normal, although some cystoid macular oedema can occasionally be found.

Prompt treatment of acute anterior uveitis (AAU) with topical atropine and steroids produces relief, the atropine preventing the formation of posterior synechiae and relaxing the painful ciliary spasm. An uncomplicated attack of AAU can be expected to resolve over 4–6 weeks on treatment with a very low risk of visual morbidity and patients can almost invariably be controlled by topical or subconjunctival steroids without recourse to systemic therapy.

Reiter's disease is the triad of non-specific urethritis or bacillary dysentery, arthritis and ocular involvement, either as a mucopurulent conjunctivitis or anterior uveitis. Patients are usually HLA B27 positive and typically young males. The urogenital form of the disease seems to be associated with chlamydial infection and about 2 per cent of males attending VD clinics with non-gonococcal urethritis develop Reiter's disease. The dysenteric form follows shigella, salmonella or yersinia infection. Patients develop acute arthritis and eye signs 1–4 weeks later. The arthritis is usually limited to large joints, particularly the knees, and the sacroiliac joints. Keratoderma blennorrhagicum of the palms and soles of the hands and feet and circinate balanitis may occur. A few patients progress to a chronic arthritis and other complications such as plantar and Achilles tendon fasciitis, and aortic incompetence. Rheumatoid factor is negative and in the majority the disease is a self-limiting acute illness (ref 75).

Approximately 20 per cent of patients with ankylosing spondylitis will suffer an attack of anterior uveitis, which may be the presenting sign of the disease, and patients may suffer 6–8 attacks of AAU before the disease remits in later life. Ankylosing spondylitis is seen predominantly in young males and has usually presented by the age of 50. The sacroiliac joints are the first to be affected. The disease initially affects the site of attachment of tendons or ligaments or joint capsule, to be followed by ossification. In the spine this can eventually lead to ossification of the intervertebral discs and a rigid 'bamboo' spine. The hip joints can be severely affected. Other manifestations are aortitis in a minority of patients with long standing disease, and respiratory difficulties from restricted chest movement. Patients require referral to a rheumatologist for systemic anti-inflammatory treatment and advice on maintaining their spinal mobility by active exercise. Ocular inflammation from sarcoidosis is discussed below.

Definite evidence of the importance of genetic factors in AAU was established in 1973[9] when the high association of the HLA B27 tissue antigen with the disease was demonstrated. About 50 per cent of patients with AAU will be positive for B27, whereas the incidence in a control population is in the region of 10 per cent. AAU has an incidence of about 12 per 100 000 in a Caucasian population per year, whereas in the HLA B27 population the incidence is 1 in 1300 a year.[10] There is no major difference in acute anterior uveitis between patients with B27 and those without except that B27 positive patients tend to have more severe ocular inflammation. Other unknown or environmental factors must be important: not all B27 positive people develop uveitis or the other B27 associated arthritides (e.g. ankylosing spondylitis or Reiter's disease). Conversely, a patient may develop ankylosing spondylitis in association with B27 and may or may not ever suffer an attack of uveitis.

There are three ways in which the mechanism of the HLA B27 association with AAU might be explained. Molecular mimicry might exist between a pathogen and the B27 antigen which might allow the pathogen to gain entrance to the body without elimination. Alternatively, the HLA antigen might act as a binding site for the pathogen or might act purely as a genetic marker for some unknown associated gene which controls the immune response; this latter hypothesis would explain the existence of the disease in B27 negative patients. HLA B27 is represented on cells throughout the body and the particular susceptibility of the anterior uveal tract is unexplained, but some suggestions have been made. *Klebsiella pneumonia* is a common bowel inhabitant and there is some research which suggests that bowel growth of this bacteria might be related to the initiation or relapse of AAU, and the theories of molecular mimicry and antigen binding have been supported to some extent by the finding of immunological cross-reactivity of some strains of *Klebsiella pneumonia* and HLA B27 lymphocytes. It has been suggested that exacerbations of acute anterior uveitis could be related to the finding of positive bowel cultures of klebsiella;[11,12] furthermore, lymphocytes from B27 positive patients are lysed by an extract from klebsiella.[13] The bacteria is, however, a ubiquitous organism in the human bowel and the relevance of these findings awaits carefully controlled studies.

No other immunological or serological marker apart from HLA B27 has been identified in patients with AAU. Studies of autoantibodies, immunoglobulin fractions or T cell subsets show no significant difference from control populations. An initial report of an association of an α_1 antitrypsin phenotype with AAU has not been confirmed by other studies.[76]

Chronic Anterior Uveitis with Still's Disease

About 10 per cent of cases of arthritis in children are indistinguishable from adult rheumatoid arthritis or ankylosing spondylitis, but in the other 90 per cent the disease differs both clinically and pathologically. Juvenile chronic arthritis (or Still's disease) can be divided into three main subtypes by the presentation and pattern of joint disease. The systemic type presents in children of 1–5 years of age with fever, skin rash, lymphadenopathy and hepatosplenomegaly; ocular involvement is rare. The polyarthritic type is seen most frequently in girls. Systemic symptoms are not prominent, but there is either an acute or insidious onset of symmetrical arthritis of the small joints of the hands, feet or neck. The arthritis is persistent and crippling, but ocular involvement is uncommon and this is almost always restricted to the pauciarticular type, which is the most common form. Both sexes are equally involved with arthritis limited to less than five joints, and these are usually large joints such as the knee, ankle or elbow.

The pauciarticular type can be divided into early (less than 8 years of age) or late onset and chronic iridocyclitis is most commonly seen in girls with the early onset form. The arthritis is rarely disabling but some children with the late type eventually progress to ankylosing spondylitis. Typically rheumatoid factor is negative in all types and ocular involvement strongly correlates with the presence of anti-nuclear antibodies (ANA).

In a series of 160 patients with juvenile arthritis and uveitis, 95 per cent had a pauciarticular type of disease and 82 per cent were ANA positive.[14] There is no correlation with HLA A and B antigens, but HLA DR5 appears to be associated with an increased risk of ocular involvement.

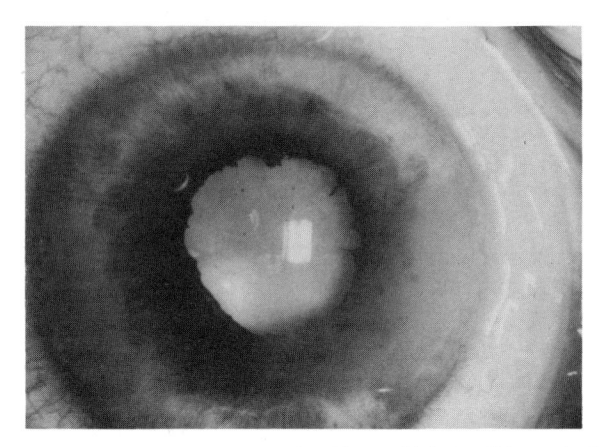

Fig. 5. Still's disease. The eye is white and iris detail is masked by an early band keratopathy. Full mydriasis is prevented by posterior synechiae to a cataractous lens. (Patient of Mr J. Kanski.)

Affected children usually present with visual loss and chronic anterior uveitis and occasionally the uveitis may precede the joint symptoms by up to 2 years. The uveitis may be found at presentation and usually develops within a year of onset of the arthritis, but it is essential that all children with the pauciarticular form, and particularly those with positive antinuclear antibodies, are kept under ophthalmic supervision. Development of uveitis after 5 years of joint disease is unusual.

Typically the disease is bilateral and the eye is completely white and painless. Unless the iridocyclitis is picked up by routine examination, children present with visual loss from band keratopathy, glaucoma, cataract or macular oedema (*Fig.* 5). Pathology shows[15] that there is an intense inflammation of the iris and ciliary body with plasmacytes secreting IgM and IgG antibodies, and it is likely the other features of the ocular disease are secondary to this iridocyclitis.

The treatment of the chronic anterior uveitis is difficult. Most cases are controlled by topical or systemic steroids, but in a few, cytotoxic therapy may be needed.[16] The band keratopathy is treated in the usual way, by scraping and washing with sodium versenate. If cataract surgery is required, conventional surgery seems to do badly and it appears that a lensectomy through the limbus or pars plana with partial or total vitrectomy is the treatment of choice, but there is a high incidence of visual loss from cystoid macular oedema. Secondary glaucoma is a devastating complication that responds poorly to standard medical or surgical therapy.

It is important to remember that sarcoidosis in children can present in an almost identical way to Still's disease, both in the ocular and systemic manifestations.

Fuch's Heterochromic Cyclitis

This is a distinctive type of uveitis that is quite different in its natural history from any other and which tends to be under-diagnosed because of the subtlety of its physical signs. Patients present with insidious visual loss or blurring from the corneal KP, cataract or glaucoma. Virtually all patients develop a cataract and about 50 per cent develop glaucoma with time, which is due to a fine neovascularization of the angle. Paracentesis ruptures these vessels producing a hyphema and this, too, has been considered a diagnostic sign.

Affected eyes are usually white, although mild injection can be seen. The diagnosis is made on the findings of a white eye with typical small spidery KP spread over the whole posterior corneal surface. These differ from normal KP by their lack of a smooth globular appearance and their diffuse distribution in contrast to the normal localization of KP to the inferior cornea. The cellular reaction and flare in the anterior chamber is usually mild and another distinctive feature is the absence of formation of posterior synechiae. The pathognomic features are, however, in the iris. The iris of the affected eye is relatively depigmented, appearing paler or bluer than the fellow eye, this colour change can be subtle and is best observed by examining both eyes in natural daylight. The stromal surface of the iris, too, has a fluffy moth-eaten appearance and with prolonged disease marked stromal atrophy can occur. Fluorescein angiography demonstrates ischaemic changes in the iris vasculature. A cataract appears in the posterior subcapsular zone in most patients and frequently progresses to maturity over a period of years. Sometimes a cellular infiltrate can be found in the anterior vitreous and some patients have been noticed to have pigmented spots of chorioretinitis or low grade periphlebitis in the peripheral retina.

Most commonly the disease is unilateral but bilateral cases do occur. They are more difficult to diagnose as both irides become depigmented and the diagnostic heterochromia is lost. Depigmentation is relative and in Negro eyes the iris still retains its brown colour. In these difficult cases the clue to the diagnosis lies in the appearance of the KP and the texture of the stromal surface of the iris. Thus heterochromic cyclitis differs from other types of chronic anterior uveitis by the appearance of the KP, iris heterochromia with atrophy and superficial stromal changes, absence of posterior synechiae and the late incidence of cataract and glaucoma.

Treatment of the inflammatory reaction appears to make no impact on the natural history of the disease. In the absence of pain or posterior synechiae there is no need for mydriasis and topical steroids merely hasten the development of cataract and complicate the management of the glaucoma. Affected eyes respond well to intra- or extracapsular cataract surgery or trabeculectomy.[17]

The aetiology is completely unknown. The disease appears in males or females and can be first diagnosed from childhood to old age; occasional familial cases occur. The heterochromia has suggested a dysfunction of autoimmune innervation by analogy to the heterochromia seen with congenital Horner's syndrome but pupillary size is unaffected in heterochromic cyclitis and no other clinical or pharmacological evidence of sympathetic paralysis has been found. There are few pathological studies on affected eyes but changes in number and size of the melanocytes and the melanosomes have been demonstrated on electron microscopy[18] together with neuronal atrophy. Immune complexes are found in the aqueous humour in a large percentage of patients[19] and O'Connor has postulated that the disease might be due to some type of localized occlusive vasculitis,[20] though a recent electron microscope study suggests that the primary immunological reaction may be towards iris melanocytes.[77]

Herpes Zoster

The ophthalmic division of the Vth cranial nerve is particularly susceptible to involvement with herpes zoster. Following a previous infection with chickenpox, the virus lies latent in the dorsal root ganglia of the spinal cord to be reactivated at a later date passing down the nerve to become manifest in its cutaneous sensory distribution. Attacks of herpes zoster (shingles) can be precipitated by malaise, immunosuppression or malignant disease, although most patients have no underlying disease. Recurrent attacks or multiple cutaneous nerve involvement are exceptionally rare.

Herpes zoster ophthalmicus is frequently preceded by pain in the area of distribution of the first division of the trigeminal nerve, which can be severe, to be followed by cutaneous erythema and vesicles a few days later. Ocular involvement is said to be more common if the nasociliary branch of the trigeminal nerve is involved, as this has an intraocular distribution, but this is not invariable. The cutaneous vesicles are anaesthetic, they appear together in a crop with erythema, oedema and a toxic reaction and are sometimes followed by secondary infection. The rash lasts for 10–14 days and heals by scabbing. The patient usually feels very ill and debilitated. Post-herpetic neuralgia in the cutaneous distribution of the affected nerve occurs to some extent in most patients but in a few is a permanent and disabling complication. Ocular involvement tends to be more common and severe with severe cutaneous involvement but this is not always the case and the eye can be affected with mild cases and vice versa.

Some degree of conjunctivitis is extremely common and in the first few days pseudodendrites may be seen on the corneal epithelium with or without stromal keratitis. An anterior uveitis is found within a few days in the affected eye in about 40 per cent of patients[21] and can persist for up to 2 years. The initial presentation is usually of a subacute anterior uveitis frequently with some degree of corneal anaesthesia and the presence of a stromal keratitis, but anterior uveitis is seen in the absence of this. Apart from an occasional optic neuritis, involvement of the posterior segment is very rare.

A particular feature of herpes zoster uveitis is the high incidence of iris changes that are seen. Areas of pigment epithelial loss are easily seen by iris retro-illumination and sectorial iris atrophy has been found in up to 25 per cent of patients.[22] Pathological material shows the underlying process in the eye varies from patient to patient and can be a vasculitis with ischaemia, a chronic neuritis or arteritis or direct virus infiltration of the structure involved.[23]

During the course of the illness the uveitis tends to become chronic, with acute exacerbations. Glaucoma may be a management problem and intraocular pressure must be monitored. Other occasional ocular findings, apart from the corneal disease and uveitis, are ocular motor palsies, scleritis and late cataract.[23] Optic neuritis is a rare but well-documented association and a contralateral hemiplegia is occasionally seen from vasculitis of the internal carotid artery due to contiguous spread of inflammation within the cavernous sinus. Evidence of an inflammatory reaction in the CSF may be found during the acute illness.

The conventional treatment of herpes zoster anterior uveitis has been to use topical steroids and atropine which often has to be continued for 1–2 years. It has been suggested, however, that treatment with acyclovir orally in the acute vesicular stage of the rash reduces the risks of subsequent ocular complications and that a mild uveitis is best treated with topical acyclovir rather than steroids as the inflammation resolves more rapidly, with fewer recurrences.[24] These observations await confirmation.

There is some evidence that herpes virus infection, either herpes zoster or simplex, may play a part in the aetiology of the acute retinal necrosis syndrome[25,26] (see Chapter 8, p 187).

Herpes Simplex

An anterior uveitis is a common accompaniment of herpes simplex keratitis and in these cases where there is a typical history of corneal ulceration with vascularization and scarring and corneal anaesthesia there is no difficulty in diagnosis. Iris involvement and glaucoma are common, but whether this is due to viral invasion or an immune hypersensitivity is not clear.

Occasionally herpes simplex also appears to be able to produce anterior uveitis in the absence of a history of corneal disease or signs of corneal scarring. This is difficult to diagnose and the frequency of isolated uveitis is unknown but the virus has been isolated from the anterior chamber in a number of cases. Systemic acyclovir would be a logical addition to standard therapy where this was found to be the case.

Herpes simplex has also been shown to produce a chorioretinitis in the neonate, infection being contracted through the skin during birth. Infected infants usually have disseminated disease and encephalitis.

Toxoplasmosis

Toxoplasmosis is one of the few uveitic syndromes that can usually be diagnosed from the morphology of the fundus lesion. The reservoir for *Toxoplasma gondii* is in the cat and in man the parasite has a predilection for neural tissue. Infection is usually caused by transplacental infection of the fetus from a primary infection of a non-immunized mother. In the worst cases the fetus is severely affected with intracranial infection producing mental retardation, epilepsy, hydrocephalus, characteristic intracranial calcification and retinochoroiditis. More commonly the ocular lesions are the only manifestation of congenital infection. Circumscribed chorioretinal scars are seen in the posterior pole of one or both eyes. These are usually densely pigmented with areas of atrophy and well-defined edges and vary from one-quarter to about 3–4 disc diameters in size; they may be isolated or several may be seen in the same eye (*Fig.* 6). Acuity is affected if the macula or its fibres are involved but otherwise the scars produce an arcuate field defect of which the patient is usually unaware. These quiescent lesions are signs of previous retinochoroiditis and need no active treatment.

Further disability from the disease is caused by the reactivation of retinochoroiditis at these sites. This usually occurs in or adjacent to a previous congenital scar and is seen as a white exudative area with overlying vitreous cellular infiltration, sometimes there is considerable exudative retinal periphlebitis and peri-arteritis associated with active disease. Toxoplasmosis does not appear to be associated with posterior or anterior uveitis in the absence of focal retinal lesions but occasionally an area of focal white retinochoroiditis occurs in the absence of apparent previous retinal scarring and this is presumed to be due to reactivation at the site in the retina of a previous subclinical lesion. Reactivation can occur at any site and a common place is adjacent to the optic disc. This characteristic lesion was known as 'Jensen's juxta-papillary choroiditis' and in the older literature was ascribed to a tubercular origin; toxoplasmosis is now recognized to be the most common course.

Acquired toxoplasmosis in the non-immunized adult can be associated with a febrile illness, lymphadenopathy and hepatosplenomegaly, and serological testing of the adult population indicates a high incidence of previous toxoplasmic infection, most of which must be due to subclinical disease. Retinal involvement with acquired toxoplasmosis is very rare but has been proved to occur.[27]

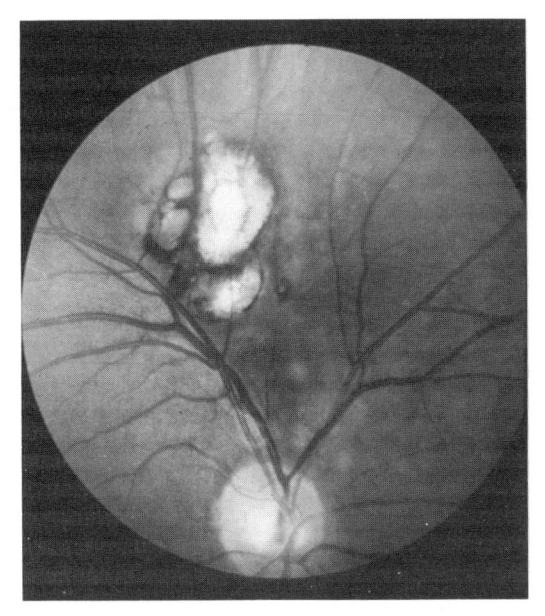

Fig. 6. Quiescent toxoplasmic chorioretinitis. Loss of the overlying retinal nerve fibre layer, which is seen as a dark groove, produced a corresponding inferior nasal arcuate field defect.

The diagnosis of toxoplasmic eye disease is made on the findings of characteristic fundus lesions and positive serology indicating previous toxoplasmic infection. The toxoplasma dye test is specific and accurate but results of serological titres do not correspond to the reactivation or level of activity of ocular disease. Thus low serological titres are compatible with active retinochoroiditis and there is a documented case where titres of 1:1 were found in the serum and yet histological examination of the eye confirmed the presence of toxoplasma gondii.[28] Thus any level of positivity in the serum demonstrates that the patient has been exposed to toxoplasmosis in the past. Further information may be gained in the future by looking for the presence of IgM antibodies, indicating recent infection or by measuring titres in the aqueous or vitreous humour although this will rarely be required in clinical practice.[29] In a prospective study of the incidence of congenital toxoplasmosis in non-immunized mothers there was a serum dye test conversion rate of 1 per cent during pregnancy. Of these pregnancies, 80 per cent produced children with ocular lesions and of these affected children 40 per cent had visual loss attributable to the toxoplasmosis,[30] although no child lost vision in both eyes. It is also of interest that in this long term study no child developed evidence of CNS disease.

Recently work with toxoplasmosis in animal models has clarified the pathophysiology of the disease.[31] Invasion of retinal cells by the organism results in intracellular multiplication until the cell ruptures to infect adjacent cells. T lymphocytes and macrophages are attracted to the lesion and in an immunologically competent host these destroy the parasite.[32] In later phases B cells infiltrate the lesion and the rising levels of local antibody may produce a hostile environment for the parasite which then becomes encysted[33] and which may remain dormant for many years. During this time host immunity falls and if spontaneous rupture then occurs the cycle of reinfection can be established. It seems likely therefore that the retinal damage that is produced with reactivation of a lesion is due to direct retinal invasion by the parasite and secondary retinal destruction from the associated inflammatory response.

Toxoplasma gondii is sensitive to sulphas (sulphadiazine) and pyrimethazine but early trials of treatment with these drugs did not seem to confer any advantages. The disease usually runs a self-limiting course, resolving over a period of months with further retinal scarring, depending on the degree of reactivity in the original lesion. Some authorities suggest that if the optic disc or macula is threatened systemic steroids are indicated to reduce the destructive inflammatory response. While this is often helpful, a few cases do deteriorate while on steroids and some untreated patients develop a severe endophthalmitis. *Toxoplasma gondii* is sensitive to clindamycin and it would appear that treatment for 3–4 weeks with this drug alone or in combination with sulphadiazine is more effective in limiting retinal damage and speeding recovery.[34] It could be hoped too that such treatment would kill the parasite and reduce the risk of cyst formation and, therefore, further future recurrences. No therapy appears to destroy the organism once encysted.

Toxocara

Toxocara canis is a nematode which has a life cycle dependent on the dog. The larva matures in the intestine, producing eggs which are deposited with the faeces and which remain viable in the soil for several years; 10–30 per cent of soil samples from American parks are contaminated with the ova. Reingestion by the dog is followed by release of larva from the eggs, migration from the gut throughout the body (second stage) and the cycle is completed by pulmonary infestation, larvae being coughed up and swallowed to mature in the gut (third stage). Transplacental spread of larvae occurs and puppies are the most common reservoir and source of human infection.

In humans, *Toxocara canis* produces either a systemic illness (visceral larva migrans) or ocular disease. Both are uncommon. Visceral larva migrans is seen in young children, usually of 1–4 years of age, who present with a systemic illness, fever, eosinophilia and hepatosplenomegaly. Ocular involvement is very uncommon with this illness, but this is seen in older children (4–8 years of age) who usually do not have a history of systemic disease.

Ocular disease is unilateral. In the eye the larva produces either preretinal or subretinal granulomas which lie at the posterior pole or periphery. Posterior uveitis is usually low grade although some patients develop a chronic endophthalmitis.[35–38] Vision is lost from direct macular involvement with the granuloma, retinal traction or posterior uveitis. The inflammation has been attributed to death of the larva and release of soluble antigens from the cuticle,[39] but recent work with a primate model of the disease led to alternative and interesting conclusions.[40] These authors developed a model of infection by injection of the larva into the vitreous cavity. They were able to show that there is a variable inflammatory response to the larvae, the eye always forming less granulomas than the number of injected larvae. Live larvae could be demonstrated in the retina without inflammatory reactions and some granulomas were shown to contain no larva or fragments of them. Their results were consistent with live freely mobile larvae, able to produce a tissue reaction in one area and leave this area to produce another reaction elsewhere. Hence their concept is of inflammation produced by living larvae rather than dead (which has important therapeutic consequences) and is analogous to the recent experimental work on toxoplasmosic retinitis. They were also able to demonstrate evidence of both vascular spread and transtissue migration of the larvae, some making their way along the optic nerve to the brain. The larva has a diameter of 18–21 μm and can become trapped in vessels of that size by haematogenous spread.

Diagnosis of toxocara infestation is made by an Elisa test (enzyme-linked immunosorbent assay) which can be performed on the serum or aqueous or vitreous humours. Serum tests have to be interpreted with caution as a significant number of the normal population have positive titres and these may not correlate with ocular findings. A case has been reported of a 4-year-old child presenting with leucocoria, a low Elisa titre of 1:4, in whom a typical larva was found on histological examination of the eye.[41] Elisa testing of aqueous humour is useful in confirming a doubtful diagnosis of toxocara. The most serious differential diagnosis of leucocoria, other than toxocara, in this age group is retinoblastoma and the potential risk of seeding a retinoblastoma from paracentesis must be borne in mind.

Most cases of ocular toxocariasis settle to leave an inactive granuloma in a quiet eye. Systemic steroids have been advocated for chronic endophthalmitis. Anthelmintic drugs do not appear to be as helpful, but there has been recent interest in the role of pars plana vitrectomy in cases with chronic endophthalmitis or visual loss from retinal traction.[42,43]

Syphilis

Syphilis was once considered to be a common cause of uveitis but since the Second World War the incidence has declined and the disease is now comparatively rare. In recent years, however, an increase has been seen again, particularly in the homosexual population, and the disease must always be borne in mind because of its potentially serious complications if left untreated. The decline in incidence has been due to routine screening programmes in pregnancy, random use of antibiotics and more precise serological tests with careful interpretation to exclude false positive reactions. There has also been a suggestion that the treponema is becoming less virulent with primary infections, and although cardiovascular and neurological complications are still seen, gummas have become exceptionally rare.

The description of syphilis and its general manifestations by Csonka[44] in the *Oxford Textbook of Medicine* is comprehensive and the reader is referred to this chapter for a full description of the systemic effects of the disease. Ocular disease is seen with early and late congenital syphilis and secondary syphilis; optic atrophy and pupillary abnormalities are features of late neurological disease.

Congenital syphilis is now rare. The fetus is infected from the mother at any stage of pregnancy but fetal lesions only develop after the fourth month and treatment prior to this time prevents the disease in the infant. The severity of the disease depends on how recently the mother became infected and the degree of treponaemia. The risks are greatest with recent infection but are still present 4 years after the secondary stage in the mother. A normal child may be born between two infected children and this can be accounted for by transient phases of treponaemia or reinfection of the mother. Infected children can present with fulminant congenital syphilis at birth or signs of early secondary syphilis. A diffuse chorioretinitis can occur at this stage but this is rarely seen in the active phases by an ophthalmologist and the diagnosis is made later in life by the appearance of the fundus, together with the history and serology.

The retinal changes are characteristically bilateral and produce late diffuse patchy atrophy and hypertrophy of the retinal pigment epithelium, sometimes known as the pepper and salt fundus. The fundus appearances vary widely and can simulate retinitis pigmentosa with optic atrophy and retinal vascular attenuation. The differential diagnosis is usually easy to make, by the association of other stigmata of congenital infection such as nerve deafness, nasal and dental deformities and interstitial keratitis. Visual function is normally very much better than would be expected with a similar degree of fundus change from retinitis pigmentosa.

Late congenital syphilis develops in an apparently normal child in the 5–30 age group. The ophthalmic hallmark is active interstitial keratitis and iritis, chorioretinitis appears to be less common at this stage. In these patients the development of cardiovascular disease is said to be rare while neurological complications occur in about 15 per cent of patients. Ophthalmologists, however, see burnt out interstitial keratitis quite commonly in elderly patients who have never had specific antibiotic therapy and yet have relatively little evidence, if any, of neurological complications.

Syphilitic uveitis is seen as a feature of acquired secondary syphilis either accompanying the skin rash or independently, preceding or succeeding it. It is particularly important to think of the diagnosis in an atypical or indolent anterior uveitis, especially in homosexuals or those patients with a military, naval or travelling background. Syphilis also produces changes in the posterior segment in the secondary stages which can vary widely. There is usually a mild cellular reaction in the vitreous and optic nerve involvement, such as papillitis or ischaemic anterior optic neuropathy, is common. Frequently there are areas of discrete palish yellow lesions at the level of the retinal pigment epithelium and serous retinal detachment with subretinal fluid in the posterior pole. Syphilitic uveitis readily responds to treatment with penicillin and systemic steroids.

All patients should have a neurological and CSF examination and sexual contacts should be traced and treated.

There are a number of serological tests that must be used to make a conclusive diagnosis. The VDRL test is a reaginic antibody test. This is used as a screening test, becoming positive early in the disease, and the titre can be used to monitor the success of treatment or reinfection. The TPHA test is a highly specific haemagglutination test using inactive fragments of *Treponema pallidum* which can be used for routine screening. The FTA–ABS is an indirect fluorescent antibody test using dead *Treponema pallidum* which is made very specific by absorption of other antigens with Reiter treponemes. It becomes positive early in the disease and remains positive after successful treatment. The activity of infection can be assessed by looking for IgM (active disease) or IgG (inactive or previous infection) antibodies.

In recent years it was thought that spirochaetes could survive in the anterior chamber of the eye after apparently successful treatment, but these findings have been largely discounted as artefactual or due to other non-pathogenic spirochaetes.

Tuberculosis
Ocular involvement with tuberculosis occurs as a result of direct infection of the uveal tract or as an immunological reaction to the infection elsewhere in the body.

Choroidal tubercles are a feature of miliary TB. The acute lesions are subretinal, slightly elevated yellowish lesions about one-quarter of a disc diameter in size. During the early phase of fluorescein angiography they are hypfluorescent, but they leak diffusely in the later stages. They are not often seen by the ophthalmologist at this stage as the patient is usually moribund and in the healed phase the chorioretinal scarring might be confused with that from other causes such as toxoplasmosis or syphilis.

Hypersensitivity to TB has a special place in the history of uveitis and its causes. At one time syphilis and TB were thought to be responsible for a substantial number of cases of uveitis, but over the years TB has become a much less recognized association. This is due both to the decreased prevalence of TB in the Western World, a better appreciation of the role of skin testing with PPD and a more critical appraisal of the natural history of the disease and treatment. TB is, however, associated with either granulomatous or non-granulomatous chronic iridocyclitis or occasionally a retinal vasculitis in some cases. Schlaegel[45] has popularized the concept of testing patients with chronic iridocyclitis by a Mantoux test and giving those with a strong reaction a 'therapeutic trial' of a 3-month course of isoniazid. Some patient's eyes undoubtedly improve and these patients are then assumed to have a tuberculous uveitis and given formal chemotherapy. There are, however, both practical and theoretical problems with this approach, which cannot be applied to the British population where the vast majority have already been vaccinated with BCG and will therefore have a positive Mantoux test. There is also a possible risk that short courses of treatment with only one chemotherapeutic agent might lead to the development of a resistant bacteria with potentially grave implications for the treatment of the patient and a risk to the community in general.

Peripheral neovascular retinopathy (Eales's disease) is especially common in India and it is possible that some racial or genetic hypersensitivity to TB exists to account for this. We have seen a florid retinal vasculitis progressing to retinal neovascularization in Indian or Arab patients who have had pulmonary tuberculosis confirmed by sputum culture of the bacilli. In the late phases these patients have an identical appearance to 'Eales's disease' and it is possible that in other patients the neovascular retinopathy may be the end result of a previous inflammatory retinal vasculitis caused by some type of immunological hypersensitivity to tuberculin in a genetically predisposed population.

Intermediate Uveitis
This disease occurs in children and young adults and the diagnosis is made on the clinical findings. The name is synonymous with pars planitis, peripheral

uveitis, chronic cyclitis or other pseudonyms and recently 'intermediate uveitis' has become the approved term in an attempt to standardize uveitis terminology.

Patients present with an insidious onset of floaters from vitreous debris or blurred vision from macular oedema. The disease is usually bilateral but often asymmetrical and in some patients unilateral. The eye is white with quiet anterior chambers or a few cells and flare, though a few patients have a more marked anterior uveitis. The vitreous gel shows a cellular infiltrate. Posterior vitreous detachment is common and with severe inflammations cellular aggregations may be seen on the retrohyaloid face. In some patients accumulation of cells known as 'snowballs' are seen in the inferior vitreous gel and others have 'a snowbank' of white cellular exudate overlying the inferior pars plana. There may be low grade vascular sheathing of the peripheral retinal veins or small pigmented scars in the peripheral retina and there may be mild swelling of the optic disc consistent with a posterior uveitis. The clinical picture varies from patient to patient and often is relatively static in each patient over the course of the disease: snowbanks do not seem to fluctuate much in the short term.

The aetiology of the disease and the origin of the cells in the vitreous is unknown but it would seem likely that they come from either the retinal vessels or through the pars plana and settle by gravity in the inferior fundus. No pathology of the acute case is available but histological examination of late cases shows that the snowbank consists of astroglial cells,[46] although this is probably different in the acute stage. The vitreous infiltrate obtained at vitrectomy has been studied in a few cases and conflicting results have been found. Kaplan[5] found the cells to be mainly B cells with a sparsity of T lymphocytes; Green et al. reported the findings in seven eyes with long standing disease removed at enucleation and in two vitrectomy specimens.[46] They found the snowbank to be composed of collapsed vitreous collagen and astrocytes. Their patients showed vitritis, optic disc oedema and retinal phlebitis, but in contrast the uveal tract was not inflamed and both vitrectomy specimens showed granulomatous inflammation of the vitreous. These findings, they suggest, are consistent with a vitreoretinal inflammation, rather than a uveitis.

Most patients have a good visual prognosis, the disease burning out over a number of years. Visual loss in the minority is from macular oedema, haziness of the vitreous gel or cataracts with long standing disease and occasionally from vitreous haemorrhage or retinal detachment. A few patients develop neovascularization in the snowbank or elsewhere in the fundus.[47] Topical steroids do not help the posterior uveitis but are useful in controlling overspill inflammation in the anterior chamber. Macular oedema may respond to subconjunctival or systemic steroids but in many patients remains refractory. Cytotoxic drugs are also of little benefit. If there is no macular oedema and the vitreous haze is not of such severity to cause visual disability the patient does not need systemic steroid treatment. Cryotherapy to the inferior snowbank has been reported to be helpful in amelioration of the inflammation and vitrectomy appears to have a beneficial effect on carefully selected patients.

A few patients are found to have either sarcoidosis or multiple sclerosis as an underlying aetiology.

Retinal Vasculitis

The differentiation of retinal vasculitis from posterior uveitis, i.e. retinal blood vessel inflammation from choroidal inflammation, can be difficult. Retinal periphlebitis is very much more common than periarteritis. Retinal vasculitis is recognized clinically by perivascular sheathing, usually around a retinal vein, which can be demonstrated angiographically by leakage of fluorescein – sometimes progressing to occlusion of the vessel, and associated retinal haemorrhages. There is, however, an invariable accompanying vitreous cellular infiltrate and the clinical differentiation from posterior uveitis depends on the predominance of retinal vascular signs to posterior uveitis. In contrast, virtually all patients with a posterior uveitis show retinal vascular leakage angiographically and in some instances, such as intermediate uveitis, a low grade retinal peripheral periphlebitis is a common finding. Thus there can be a spectrum of inflammatory signs from a distinctive primary retinal vasculitis (e.g. sarcoidosis or Behçet's disease) to a primary uveal inflammation. The situation is further complicated as conditions such as toxoplasmic retinochoroiditis often show considerable 'secondary' retinal vasculitis in their acute stages.

In some conditions both retinal and uveal mechanisms undoubtedly play a part and these well-recognized clinical contrasts might in the future be explained by analogy with the experimental work on retinal S antigen where the disease can be modulated from vasculitis to uveitis by changing the experimental dosage of antigen or the animal model. It may be, therefore, that a vasculitis or uveitis reflects the site of the immunopathology to a similar antigen rather than a totally different disease process. Such a concept would explain why a single disease such as sarcoidosis can affect the eye in so many different ways.

Eales's disease is the name given to the group of idiopathic retinal vasculitides where other recognized causes have been excluded. It is a heterogeneous group of disorders, usually presenting in young adults either in the inflammatory stage or later, as the effects of a neovascular retinopathy, when the inflammation has burnt out. Other causes such as haematological (e.g. Sickle cell disease), metabolic (diabetes), or circulatory disorders (slow flow retinopathy) must be excluded. Central retinal vein occlusion in young adults frequently is associated with a mild vitreous cellular infiltration and has been termed a benign vasculitis by some authors. These patients, however, in the author's experience, rarely have any other signs of local or systemic inflammatory disease and are much more likely to have a vascular or haematological cause of their ocular problem.

Behçet's disease

The classic signs of this disease are the triad of oral ulceration, genital ulceration and uveitis, but the disease has a multisystem spectrum and skin changes, arthritis, venous thrombosis, bowel and neurological involvement can be found.[48] The condition was first described in Turkey and is more common in people of Middle Eastern or Japanese origin (in Japan it is the cause of 20 per cent of cases of uveitis), although it is being increasingly well recognized in the Western world, where the signs are frequently less florid. It usually affects adults in young to middle age and is slightly more common in men than women.

Oral ulceration occurs in 99 per cent of patients and often precedes involvement of other systems by several years. Patients suffer bouts of painful aphthous ulceration which cannot be differentiated either clinically or pathologically from the common aphthous ulcer. Genital ulceration is less common (79 per cent) and can occur anywhere on the genitalia, the symptoms are more noticeable in men.

Cutaneous involvement (90 per cent) is seen as erythema nodosum on the legs, but more commonly as pustules, similar to a staphylococcal lesion and also usually on the lower limbs. A curious sign demonstrated by a few patients is dermatographia – light friction on the skin leads to formation of a wheal within a few minutes: some patients show a rapid inflammatory response to skin puncture (e.g. venepuncture).

Arthritis is common, usually quite mild and tending to affect the large joints such as the knee. Venous occlusions are a common feature and can affect small or large vessels, producing for example deep venous thrombosis in the legs, superficial thrombophlebitis or occlusion of the inferior vena cava so that the venous return from the lower body comes through the cutaneous veins in the abdominal wall producing the characteristic 'caput Medusa' appearance. Gastrointestinal involvement is uncommon but patients do tend to become folate deficient from a vasculitis of the bowel. Neurological signs occur in about 10–15 per cent of patients. The most typical pattern is of a mild to moderate relapsing and remitting illness affecting the brainstem or spinal cord which can be difficult to differentiate from multiple sclerosis. Benign intracranial hypertension is seen in a few patients.

Ocular involvement varies in severity from patient to patient but is seen in 75 per cent of patients and is the most serious feature of the disease. Anterior uveitis is the most widely recognized feature but involvement of the posterior segment is almost universal and is responsible for the blinding complications. Patients present with posterior or panuveitis. Hypopyon formation is a noticeable feature of the anterior uveitis in some patients, which tends to occur repeatedly throughout the illness and, in contrast to HLA B27 anterior uveitis, often appears in a relatively white eye. The posterior uveitis is severe and diffuse. Macular oedema is a common cause of visual loss but the disease is distinguished from other causes of posterior uveitis by the retinal features, which can be so characteristic as to suggest the systemic diagnosis. In the acute phase superficial patches of retinal infiltration are seen. These vary in size from one-quarter to 1 or 2 disc diameters. They usually occur as creamy white polymorpholeucocytic infiltrates in the superficial layers of viable retina that are not directly related to large retinal vessels, either in the posterior pole or equatorial areas. These lesions evolve and resolve over a period of several weeks, leaving apparently normal retina, without retinal pigment epithelial (RPE) scarring. Branch vein occlusion is common and in the presence of posterior uveitis should suggest the diagnosis of Behçet's disease. It is frequently followed by capillary closure and the devastating complications of neovascularization, vitreous haemorrhage, or retinal detachment. Progressive retinal destruction is seen with time and in the terminal stages the fundus appearance is of optic atrophy, gross attenuation of retinal arteries and veins with comparatively little RPE change.

If the ocular complications are untreated, the visual prognosis is not good, most patients becoming blind within 3–4 years of the onset. Men are said to have a worse visual prognosis than women. Systemic steroids are helpful in controlling the inflammation but most patients require cytotoxic therapy as well. Azathioprine, chlorambucil or colchicine appear to be the drugs of choice. Careful management of the steroid and cytotoxic therapy improves the visual prognosis,[49] although the side effects of treatment can be severe. More recently cyclosporin A has been used successfully in the management of Behçet's disease and appears to offer great future potential.

The diagnosis is made on the clinical features. No laboratory test is helpful, though in the acute relapse the ESR may be raised with a leucocytosis. The aetiology is thought to be due to a viral infection of a genetically susceptible individual. Ocular involvement is associated with the HLA B5 antigen and in particular the BW51 subtype. Patients with this tissue type have a ×6 relative risk factor.[50] The racial distribution of this antigen and the disease has been attributed to the spread of the antigen by the nomadic tribes along the old silk routes. No virus has been identified consistently in the oral or cutaneous lesions but there is indirect evidence that herpes simplex virus may play a role.[51] High levels of circulating immune complexes are also found in the serum of patients[52] and probably play some part in the pathogenesis.

Sarcoidosis

This is a multisystem disorder characterized by the production of non-caseating granulomas of unknown aetiology. Virtually any tissue or organ can be involved and although well-recognized patterns of involvement are seen, the disease is a great mimic of other diseases so that it must be considered as part of the differential diagnosis in many diverse clinical situations. The patient's symptoms and signs depend on the organs involved, the quantity of granulomatous tissue and its site within the organ and its activity. The disease occurs from childhood to old age, and there are geographical and racial variations in its incidence, being more common in females and American blacks and in some areas of the USA. The aetiology is unknown, but speculation suggests some type of infective cause or agent, or combination of these in genetically predisposed people. The most common manifestations are in the lung, skin, eyes, reticuloendothelial system, bones and joints. The true incidence of most types of involvement is unknown as in a large majority of patients involvement of any one particular system is subclinical and therefore depends on the degree and enthusiasm of investigation.

Pulmonary disease is the most common manifestation and yet in a substantial number of patients is entirely subclinical, being diagnosed, for example, on routine chest X-ray. Involvement of the lung is often used to classify and stage the disease. On the radiological appearances sarcoidosis can be divided into bilateral hilar lymphadenopathy (BHL), and lung infiltration or lung infiltration alone. These patterns tend to correlate with the prognosis or progression of disease from acute lymphadenopathy to chronicity and fibrosis, but must not imply the assumption of a necessary temporal sequence. Many patients present with an acute syndrome of BHL, erythema nodosum and arthritis and in a large percentage of patients this is a self-limiting disease which resolves without treatment within 3 years.

Ocular involvement occurs in about 25 per cent of patients and is seen as either infiltration of the ocular adnexa, intraocular inflammation or infiltration of the retrobulbar visual pathways.[53] Most ocular disease presents in the early phases of acute systemic sarcoidosis and new ocular manifestations become less common 2 years after the onset or in the chronic stages of the disease.

Involvement of the adnexa is most frequently seen as cutaneous infiltration of the lids, conjunctiva or lacrimal glands. Circumscribed and discrete granulomas within the orbit are very rare, as is myositis of the external ocular muscles.[54] The most common pattern of orbital involvement is an orbital apex syndrome from infiltration of the orbital apex by granuloma.

Lacrimal gland involvement is probably more common than is recognized. With acute disease the gland can be bilaterally infiltrated and enlarged and palpated through the skin, although in this form it is usually asymptomatic. Biopsy of the gland can be performed to confirm the diagnosis but if necessary this should be performed through the skin rather than the conjunctiva as this can damage the lacrimal ductules and potentially cause later tear deficiency. Gallium scanning shows lacrimal uptake in up to 75 per cent of patients with acute sarcoidosis and in most of these patients the gland is not palpable. Lacrimal infiltration may also occur with salivary gland infiltration (Mikulicz's syndrome) or uveoparotid fever (Heerfordt's syndrome). Dry eyes are unusual in the acute phases, presumably because the accessory glands maintain tear secretion, but a few patients develop dryness with the chronic fibrotic stages of the conjunctival disease.

Cutaneous involvement can be seen as discrete skin tumours, lupus pernio or sometimes as pearly 'millet seed' granulomas along the lid margin. Cutaneous involvement provides an opportunity to obtain a biopsy. Conjunctival involvement more commonly affects the inferior fornix where it produces a chronic follicular type of change. Biopsy of apparently normal conjunctiva, however, shows histological changes in some patients and 'blind conjunctival biopsy' has been advocated as a useful test in patients where the diagnosis of sarcoidosis is in doubt.[55]

Sarcoidosis produces either an anterior or posterior uveitis. Anterior uveitis is usually a feature of the acute BHL–erythema nodosum stage of the disease and most patients will have a uveitis of sufficient activity and severity to produce symptoms, but a chronic anterior uveitis of the type seen with Still's disease can rarely occur. The anterior uveitis may be acute or chronic, granulomatous or non-granulomatous. Most patients will have bilateral disease, but unilateral or asymmetrical involvement is well recognized. An anterior uveitis with granulomatous KP, Busacca or Koeppé nodules on the iris or stromal infiltration should suggest that sarcoidosis is considered in the differential diagnosis of the patient. Involvement of the angle of the anterior chamber by granulomas on the trabecular meshwork has been said to be common and diagnostic of sarcoidosis.[56] This is seen on gonioscopy as discrete white granulomas on the trabecular meshwork and all patients with sarcoid uveitis should have a gonioscopy. Glaucoma may be present in these patients but frequently intraocular pressure is normal. The granuloma may resolve completely with treatment or leave patches of peripheral anterior synechiae and a chronic secondary angle closure glaucoma.

Posterior uveitis may occur in the absence of anterior uveitis. It is responsible for most of the visual morbidity and may take a variety of patterns similar to pars planitis, bird shot retinochoroidopathy, retinal vasculitis or localized infiltration of the choroid or optic disc.[57,58] The classic description is of retinal vasculitis. This typically involves the small equatorial retinal veins and in its most marked form is seen as a focal fluffy white perivascular cuffing (candle wax dripping) which can progress to venous occlusion, peripheral closure and neovascularization (in our own series[57] this was the most common cause of visual morbidity). Small vessel involvement is reflected by a retinopathy of retinal haemorrhages and cotton wool spots but most patients show some signs of larger retinal venous disease as well. Involvement of the central retinal vein or retinal arteries is uncommon. Some degree of vitreous infiltration is always found on careful examination of patients with retinal vasculitis but the degree of vascular involvement can be difficult to identify and in these patients fluorescein angiography is of great help in demonstrating focal phlebitis. A few patients with posterior uveitis develop retinal or optic disc neovascularization in the absence of areas of capillary closure and this is presumably due to an angioblastic effect of the vitreous inflammation, these patients often respond well to steroids with regression of the neovascular tissue.

Optic disc swelling can be a common feature of any posterior uveitis and with sarcoidosis can be due to local tissue oedema, local infiltration by granulomatous tissue in the disc or papilloedema from neurosarcoid with raised intracranial pressure. In most patients it is a reflection of the posterior uveitis and resolves with this but sarcoidosis is an important differential diagnosis of bilateral or unilateral optic disc swelling of unknown aetiology. All such patients require careful examination of the vitreous for cells which will at least provide evidence of an inflammatory aetiology.

Choroidal involvement is relatively uncommon, although discrete granulomas can occur at the level of the retinal pigment epithelium[59] or choroid[60] and several of our own patients have had a similar fundus appearance to bird shot retinochoroidopathy.

Although most cases of sarcoidosis have a self-limiting and resolving pattern the disease can take a chronic progressive course with long term bodily and ocular morbidity, and in view of the wide differential diagnosis of its protean manifestations, it is important to make an accurate diagnosis and to confirm this histologically, where possible. The chest X-ray will be abnormal in about 75 per cent of cases but whether or not radiological changes are present, bronchoscopy with bronchial or transbronchial biopsy will produce positive histology in the majority of cases of early sarcoidosis and this is the primary investigation of choice. Bronchial lavage also demonstrates a lymphocytosis with excess of T helper lymphocytes in contrast to the peripheral blood where there is a relative paucity of these cells. The Kveim test involves the intradermal injection of an extract of sarcoid spleen and biopsy of the injection site about 6 weeks later. The test gives similar results to bronchoscopy and biopsy, being positive in about 75 per cent of patients with acute sarcoid and 30–40 per cent with chronic disease. It does, however, suffer from the defects of being prolonged and cumbersome as well as requiring good tissue extract and expert pathological interpretation. It is influenced by concurrent steroid therapy and is occasionally positive with other granulomatous disease (e.g. Crohn's disease) and therefore the Kveim test is becoming superseded. A number of other tests that help to provide circumstantial diagnostic information are available. Sarcoid granulomas contain activated macrophages which take up radioactive gallium and this can be a useful, though expensive, technique of demonstrating the localization of sarcoid tissue. Sarcoid granulomas produce angiotensin-converting enzyme, and the finding of increased serum levels of this enzyme is useful evidence, but this enzyme can be raised with other granulomatous diseases and is occasionally negative in active sarcoidosis and therefore the results are not diagnostic. Instead it provides circumstantial evidence of the diagnosis and is useful in the follow-up of patients as an index of amount of active granuloma, falling with treatment and rising with relapse. Other useful tests are cutaneous anergy to tuberculin, increased levels of serum lysozyme, hypercalcaemia and increases in plasma proteins which reflect the increased B cell activity seen in many patients. Circulating immune complexes are often found in patients with the acute BHL–erythema nodosum stage of sarcoidosis.

Sympathetic Ophthalmitis

Sympathetic ophthalmitis (SO) is exceptionally rare. It has been estimated that there are on average only about 10 new cases a year in the USA. The typical clinical course of events is of a perforating injury to one eye which is followed after a latent period by a granulomatous panuveitis in the fellow (sympathizing) eye. The patient presents with redness, photophobia, pain, lacrimation and blurred vision in this eye with a panuveitis leading to visual loss from glaucoma, cataract and retinal destruction.

It is doubtful whether sympathetic ophthalmitis occurs in the absence of a penetrating injury. In those cases where this is not apparent, serial sections invariably reveal subclinical perforation of the globe. The disease is seen from childhood to old age, there is no sex preponderance and race does not seem influential, indicating that the degree of uveal pigment is probably not important.[61] In about 90 per cent of cases there has been either traumatic (50 per cent) or surgical perforation of the globe and in most cases uveal tissue can be found incarcerated in the wound, microscopically if not macroscopically. Sympathetic ophthalmitis is occasionally seen in association with perforation of corneal ulcers or malignant melanoma with invasion of the sclera. Most traumatic cases involve perforation of the anterior segment with damage to the lens and ciliary body. The incidence following routine uncomplicated intraocular surgery is exceptionally low and it has been suggested that it has further decreased with microsurgery and better wound closure. However, vitrectomy techniques have made possible attempts to salvage severely injured eyes that would previously have been enucleated and there have been a few reports in recent years of sympathetic ophthalmitis following vitrectomy in these cases.

The latent interval between perforation and inflammation of the sympathizing eye is very variable. Frequently the exciting eye never completely settles down after injury but SO can be seen to follow a completely quiet white eye. About 65 per cent of cases present within 2 weeks to 3 months of the original injury and the majority have occurred within 2 years. There are, however, well reported cases occurring many years after the initial trauma,[62] but sometimes these severely injured exciting eyes have had a more recent event.

Clinically sympathetic ophthalmitis must be distinguished from phacoallergic uveitis due to lens trauma. This distinction is made on the finding of choroidal involvement with sympathetic ophthalmitis and the absence of this in phacoallergic uveitis, which is cured by removal of the lens. A breech in the lens capsule with associated pathological signs of phacoallergy is seen as an additional feature in 25–40 per cent of cases of sympathetic ophthalmitis.

Early enucleation of the exciting eye within 2 weeks of the onset of symptoms in the fellow eye has a beneficial effect on the outcome. After this time no therapeutic effect is seen from enucleation, although it does allow the diagnosis to be confirmed histologically. Occasionally the exciting eye may have useful vision and sometimes it may eventually have better vision than the sympathizing eye so that careful clinical judgement is essential prior to enucleating an eye with visual potential. The final visual acuity correlates with the severity of inflammation in the exciting eye. Prior to the advent of steroids visual loss was the final outcome in most patients but now steroid treatment results in a final visual acuity better than 6/36 in about 90 per cent of patients. Sympathizing eyes tolerate cataract or glaucoma surgery reasonably well providing the inflammation has been controlled before surgery.

The diagnosis is made on clinicopathological grounds as the pathological findings are not completely diagnostic. Most reports have been made on the pathology of the exciting eye; there have been naturally few examinations of the sympathizing eye but these would seem to indicate that the changes are the same in each eye. The characteristic findings are of a diffuse granulomatous uveitis of the whole uveal tract, without necrosis and sparing the choriocapillaris. The cellular infiltrate is basically lymphocytic and epithelioid with sparse plasma cells; eosinophils are prominent especially in early cases (prior steroid treatment may influence the choroidal cellular infiltrate). The epithelioid cells in the choroid phagocytose uveal pigment. Dalen–Fuchs' nodules are a characteristic but not a pathognomic finding and are found in about 50 per cent of patients. These focal accumulations of the retinal pigment epithelium are seen most commonly in the equatorial retina and consist of RPE cells, transformed RPE cells, epithelioid cells and sparse lymphocytes.[63,64] The retina is not involved by sympathetic ophthalmitis but involvement of the sclera by the inflammation along the uveal emissary veins is common and probably accounts for the failure of evisceration to prevent SO, in contrast to enucleation.

A case of sympathetic ophthalmia following vitreous surgery has recently been studied in detail with electron microscopy and monoclonal antibody techniques.[64] The choroidal infiltrate was found to be composed of predominantly T lymphocytes of the suppressor/cytotoxic category and only 5 per cent of cells were B lymphocytes. The epithelioid cells in the choroid showed antigenic determinants suggesting that they were bone-marrow derived monocytes. The Dalen–Fuchs' nodules were found to be composed of a mixture of histiocytes and RPE cells with small numbers of T cytotoxic/suppressor cells. The authors speculate that the immunopathology is a T cell delayed hypersensitivity mechanism directed at surface antigens shared by photoreceptors, RPE cells and choroidal melanocytes, all of which have a common neuroectodermal origin.

The immunopathology of the disease has fascinated ophthalmologists since it was first described. There are two basic theories surrounding the aetiology which are that the disease is caused by some type infection, presumably viral, or an autoimmune process. Despite numerous attempts, no infective agent has ever been consistently identified. Many experiments have been carried out in an attempt to produce the disease by immunization with uveal extracts or melanin and these have failed except to show that melanin is very unlikely to be the primary causative antigen. Many early experiments were difficult to interpret due to the use of impure and mixed antigens or those obtained from a different species, and carefully performed studies indicate that purified uveal homogenates do not consistently produce an experimental uveitis that is clinically or pathologically acceptable as SO.

There is at present great interest in the role of retinal S antigen in the aetiology of sympathetic uveitis. This antigen, derived as a soluble protein from the outer segments of the photoreceptors and probably identifiable as rhodopsin kinase, will produce a bilateral granulomatous uveitis in experimental animals when injected subcutaneously with adjuvant. While this model has some features in common with sympathetic ophthalmitis it does have some defects. These are that the pathological appearances of the experimental disease are dosage-, species- and adjuvant-dependent, that most clinical sympathetic uveitis results from a penetrating wound of the anterior segment without retinal involvement and hence no release of S antigen, and that the pathological pattern of the human disease does not correlate with the extent and severity of the original injury. Furthermore, the presence of retinal S antigen can be found in the normal population without ocular disease and is also an incidental finding in other patients with specific types of uveitis as, for example, with toxoplasmic retinochoroiditis. Some of these problems may be explained by the method of sensitization to S antigen which appears to be important. Rao and Wong have shown that intravitreal injection of S antigen fails to produce uveitis in the fellow eye while subconjunctival injection of the same amount of antigen does.[65] This suggests that the absence of lymphatics in the choroid allows the antigen to be removed by the blood without sensitization whereas the subconjunctival route, in analogy to a perforating injury, leads to drainage to the regional lymph nodes and a different type of immune response. Other retinal proteins such as interreceptor binding protein and opsin have recently been shown to have uveitogenic properties, and studies with these various proteins have led to the development of important animal models of ocular inflammatory disease. It is, however, impossible to say at this time how these antigens relate to human disease.

Lens-Induced Uveitis

This condition is sometimes known as phacoallergic uveitis or phacouveitis and must not be confused with phacolytic glaucoma where an intense macrophage response is seen in the presence of a hypermature cataract with an intact but leaky lens capsule and a secondary open angle glaucoma. Patients with lens-induced uveitis present with a unilateral red eye with clinical signs of a granulomatous anterior uveitis, usually a few weeks after rupture of the lens capsule. Breeching of the lens capsule is an obligatory clinicopathological diagnostic requirement.

Pathology shows a zonal granulomatous reaction around the break in the lens capsule or the lens remnants. Polymorpholeucocytes are found adjacent to lens; these are surrounded by macrophages and giant cells and outside these lie lymphocytes. Lens-induced uveitis is seen in association with sympathetic ophthalmitis in about 25 per cent of cases and this has led to suggestions that there are some similarities in the aetiology. It has been speculated that a breech in the lens capsule allows access of the sequestered lens antigens to the immune system. The disease is very rare, particularly when considered in terms of the numbers of potential patients who have had extracapsular cataract surgery, many of whom will have small amounts of residual lens matter remaining; possibly denaturation of lens proteins may have some role in the aetiology. Clinically the disease can be distinguished from sympathetic ophthalmitis by demonstrating absence of choroidal thickening by ultrasonography and by its cure with removal of the lens remnants where this is technically possible.

AIDS

The acquired immune deficiency syndrome was first recognized in promiscuous American homosexuals in the early 1980s when outbreaks of *Pneumocystis carinii* pneumonia, Kaposi's sarcoma and other opportunistic infections occurred in the homosexual population of California and New York. With the identification of the clinical syndrome, it became immediately apparent that patients suffered a severe and widespread defect of cellular immunity with cutaneous anergy, lymphopenia, depletion of T helper cells and an increased ratio of T suppressor to helper cells. In 1984, Gallo and colleagues identified the virus HTLV-III as the cause of the syndrome.[66] Transmission of the disease is through sexual or haematogenous contact and the disease has now reached epidemic proportions in homosexuals, drug addicts and haemophiliacs, although it appears to have been endemic in Central Africa in the heterosexual population for many years. The incubation period appears to be from a few months to 2 years but only a minority of infected persons appear to develop the clinical disease of AIDS.

Patients are susceptible to a limited range of viral, bacterial and fungal infections such as herpes zoster and simplex, mycobacteria, *Pneumocystis carinii*, toxoplasma, candidiasis, cryptococci, cytomegalo virus infections as well as Kaposi's sarcoma. Some patients develop a dementia during the illness due to HTLV-III viral encephalopathy. Persistent generalized lymphadenopathy affecting lymph nodes in more than one extra-inguinal site for over 3 months in the absence of any other cause occurs in some patients. Patients develop fatigue, weight loss, malaise and fever and once the disease is clinically manifest the outcome appears to be fatal.

Ocular complications of AIDS are well recognized. The HTLV-III virus can be identified in tears and corneal tissue which has marked implications for sterilization of ophthalmic equipment or corneal transplantation. So far, however, there is no evidence of infection through tear secretions and the chances of infection by this route appear to be low. Kaposi sarcoma lesions can be seen in the conjunctiva. Herpes zoster ophthalmicus has become a well recognized feature.

A retinopathy is a frequent occurrence at some stage in the illness. Patients may develop cottonwool spots which do not differ in any way from those seen in other conditions. Histological examination has failed so far to show evidence of viral infection in these lesions and it has been postulated that they are microinfarcts from high levels of circulating immune complexes. Cottonwool spots appear to be a poor prognostic sign both for further ocular problems[67] and for the life expectancy of patients.[68] Cytomegalovirus retinitis is the most common ocular infection although other ocular infections such as herpes simplex retinitis, toxoplasmosis, cryptococcus and *Mycobacterium avium intracellulare* have been reported. In a study of autopsy eyes from 75 patients with AIDS, Holland found cottonwool spots in 65 per cent of the eyes, no micro-organisms or viral particles could be found in these lesions. Cytomegaloviral retinitis was the only common infection found – 28 per cent of the cases had a cytomegalo virus retinopathy. They hypothesized that the retinal microvascular changes predisposed to cytomegalovirus infection by allowing access of viral particles to the retina during viraemia.[69]

Treatment of cytomegaloviral infection with AIDS is unsatisfactory. The infection responds to dihydroxy propoxymethylguanine (DHPG), but the retinopathy relapses after treatment with further retinal destruction. Maintenance chemotherapy has been used to prevent relapse but the logistics of arranging daily treatment are often insurmountable and the efficiency is unproven.

Ocular Histoplasmosis

This disease is recognized in the USA and other parts of the world where infection with histoplasma capsulation is endemic.[70] This spore is not found in Britain but an identical fundus disease occurs which is known by the poor name of 'presumed ocular histoplasmosis syndrome' (POHS). The aetiology of the British cases is unknown and no treatment appears to be effective. The features of the condition are peripapillary choroidal atrophy and focal spots of RPE atrophy in the posterior pole or equatorial retina. The vitreous gel is completely quiet.

The importance of the disease is that patients lose central vision in early middle age from disciform macular degeneration. Much experimental work on the disease has been done[71] which basically demonstrates an initial phase of fungaemia with focal depositions of the spore in the choroid and low grade choroidal inflammation and subsequent damage to the overlying retinal pigment epithelium (RPE). In other areas the RPE remains normal but new fundus lesions appear with time in these eyes and these are presumed to be due to non-specific reactivation of old choroidal foci. Paramacular lesions cause a high risk of later disciform degeneration and, if this develops, some patients have lesions amenable to laser photocoagulation.

Uveitis with Neurological Disease

Neurological symptoms with inflammatory eye disease are seen with neurosarcoidosis, Behçet's disease, the VKH syndrome, Whipple's disease and multiple sclerosis (MS) as well as with the recognized bacterial, parasitic and viral infections that affect the nervous system.

Rucker first described peripheral periphlebitis in the eyes of MS patients with 'snow balls' in the vitreous overlying the retina.[72] Further studies have confirmed that this is a relatively common finding which occurs in about 10 per cent of patients, probably being underdiagnosed as the peripheral retina is not frequently carefully examined by neurologists. Pars planitis and granulomatous iridocyclitis are also found in a few patients[73] with MS. Characteristically, the retinal periphlebitis is peripheral, low grade and asymptomatic with a mild cellular reaction in the vitreous; vascular occlusion and obliteration are not seen.

In a recent study[74] lymphocytic or granulomatous retinal periphlebitis was found in the eyes of 4 out of 47 patients with known MS on pathological examination. The retinal lesions are granulomatous in comparison to the non-granulomatous lesions seen around venules in MS brains, and areas of retinitis without associated vascular lesions were found, indicating that the inflammatory response in the eye may not solely be restricted to vascular tissue. Peripheral retinal vascular lesions were found to correlate with optic nerve pathology in the same eyes, although this was not an invariable association. The clinical significance of these retinal changes in MS is unknown, but affected patients are said to have a greater incidence of chronic progressive MS than those without. It has been suggested that the retinal and CNS lesions may have a common immunological aetiology: both are perivenous inflammatory infiltrates and the fact that there is no myelin in the human retina leads to speculation that the ocular and CNS changes might represent a primary phlebitic process which leads to demyelination in the brain.

Uveitis with Bowel Disease

Various types of inflammatory eye disease have been reported with a variety of bowel diseases; the dysenteric form of Reiter's disease has already been mentioned. Ocular complications of ulcerative colitis appear to be extremely uncommon and in some reports it is possible that ulcerative colitis and Crohn's disease have been confused, with the ocular disease being wrongly attributed. Crohn's disease is associated with a wide range of ocular manifestations and it has been estimated that up to 10 per cent of patients will have some eye manifestation.[75] Episcleritis is the most common sign, scleritis is less common and a destructive subepithelial keratitis has been described which has preceded overt abdominal disease and led to the diagnosis of the bowel disease being made. Both iridocyclitis and choroiditis can occur and the inflammatory signs fluctuate with the activity of bowel disease and clear up with its surgical excision. Whipple's disease is an exceptionally rare bowel disease due to infiltration by an unknown bacterial species. Neurological involvement is not uncommon and papillitis or choroiditis can occur either in conjunction or isolation to this. Ocular disease clears up when the bowel disease is treated with the appropriate broad spectrum antibiotic.[76]

The parasite *Giardia lamblia* has been found in the faeces of a few patients with retinal arteritis and iridocyclitis[77] which has been unresponsive to steroid treatment, but has improved on treatment with antiparasitic drugs.

THE PIGMENT EPITHELIOPATHIES

This is a group of diseases where the major clinical and pathological changes are thought to occur at the level of the retinal pigment epithelium (RPE). Krill's disease is a rare finding of a faint pigmentary stippling of the RPE in the posterior pole, usually found coincidentally. It is thought to be due to a viral pigment epitheliitis. Acute multifocal placoid pigment epitheliopathy, geographic choroiditis and bird shot choroidopathy are described in Chapter 8.

American patients with the disease have some American Indian ancestry. The disease has seasonal peaks of incidence in the spring and autumn.

The clinical picture is of an acute bilateral granulomatous panuveitis in the 20–50 years age range, sometimes preceded by a few days of prodromal illness with nausea, headache, orbital pain and meningism. In some patients the uveitis is less marked and serous retinal detachment and RPE changes predominate. Serous retinal detachments or pigment epithelial detachments are common in the acute phase and a spotty yellowish disturbance of the RPE can often be seen in the posterior pole. Fluorescein angiography shows a pattern similar, though more diffuse to acute multifocal placoid pigment epitheliopathy, with early masking of the choroidal pattern and late staining of the RPE. Patients respond to systemic steroids and the disease has a better visual prognosis than sympathetic ophthalmitis, usually subsiding over a period of months, although relapses

Fig. 7. Poliosis of the eye lashes (*a*) and vitiligo (*b*) in a 17-year-old Arab boy with the VKH syndrome.

Vogt–Koyanagi–Harada Syndrome

VKH syndrome is a rare disease in the West but represents about 8 per cent of cases of endogenous uveitis in Japan. This racial incidence is related to tissue type antigens HLA BW54, DWa, DR4 and MT3. BW54 and DWa are specific Japanese antigens and MT3 carries a 74·5 per cent increase in relative risk.[78] It has been suggested that non-oriental patients frequently have some oriental ancestry and this appears to be borne out by the fact that many

can occur. There are many clinical and pathological similarities to sympathetic ophthalmitis, except that involvement of the choriocapillaris is seen pathologically in the VKH syndrome while this is relatively spared in sympathetic ophthalmitis.

In the acute stages patient may have dysacousia, which is usually mild, meningism and a lymphocyte pleocytosis of the CSF. In the recovery phases vitiligo and poliosis (white eye lashes, brows or patches of hair) can be found as well as localized areas of alopecia (*Fig.* 7).

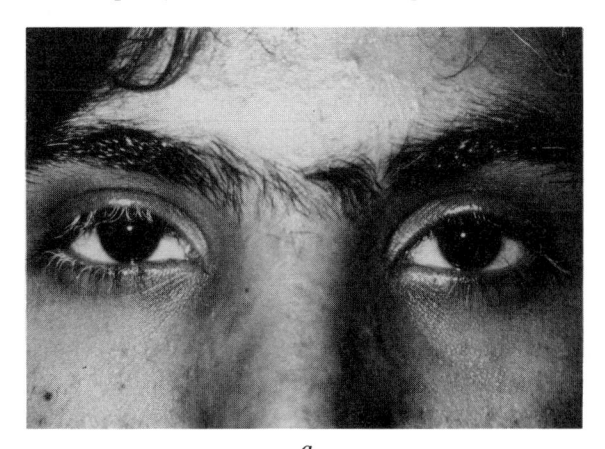

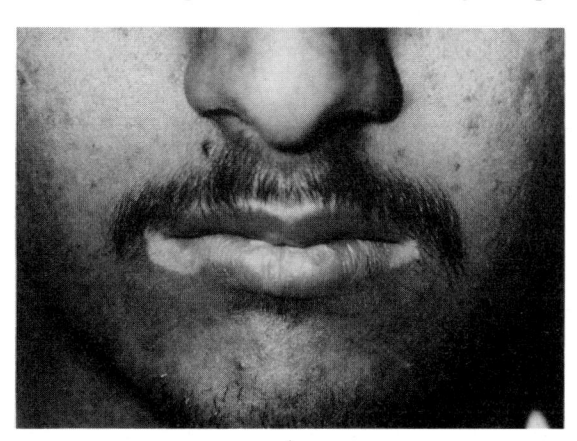

REFERENCES

1. O'Connor G. R. Factors related to the initiation and recurrence of uveitis. *Am. J. Ophthalmol.* 1983; **96**, 577–99.
2. Char D. H., Stein P., Masi R. et al. Immune complexes in uveitis. *Am. J. Ophthalmol.* 1979; **87**, 678–81.
3. Dernouchamps J. P. and Michiels J. Circulating antigen antibody complexes in the aqueous humour. In: Silverstein A. M. and O'Connor G. R. (ed.) *Immunology and Immunopathy of the Eye*. New York, Masson, 1979.
4. Dumonde D. C., Kasp E., Graham E. et al. Anti-retinal autoimmunity and circulating immune complexes in patients with retinal vasculitis. *Lancet* 1982; **2**, 787–92.
5. Kaplan H. J., Aarberg T. M. and Keller R. H. Recurrent clinical uveitis. Cell surface markers on vitreous lymphocytes. *Arch. Ophthalmol.* 1982; **100**, 585–7.

6. Shimada K. and Silverstein A. M. Induction of booster antibody formation without specific antigenic drive. *Cell. Immunol.* 1975; **18**, 484–8.
7. Au Y. and Henkind P. Pain illicited by consensual pupillary reflex. A diagnostic test for acute iritis. *Lancet* 1981; **2**, 1254–5.
8. Secchi A. G., Fregona I. and D'Ermo F. Lysophosphatidyl choline in the aqueous humour during ocular inflammation. *Br. J. Ophthalmol.* 1979; **63**, 768–70.
9. Brewerton D. A., Caffrey M., Nicholls A. et al. Acute anterior uveitis in HLA 27. *Lancet* 1973; **2**, 994–6.
10. Perkins E. S. Hereditary and congenital factors in inflammation of the uveal tract. *Trans. Ophthalmol. Soc. UK* 1981; **101**, 304–7.
11. Ebringer R., Cawdell D. and Ebringer A. *Klebsiella pneumoniae* and acute anterior uveitis in ankylosing spondylitis. *Br. Med. J.* 1979; **1**, 383.
12. Willshaw H. E. Acute anterior uveitis and *Klebsiella aerogenes*: A casual relationship? *Br. J. Ophthalmol.* 1981; **65**, 796–7.
13. Druery C., Bashire H., Geczy A. F. Search for klebsiella cell wall components cross-reactive with lymphocytes on B27. *Hum. Immunol.* 1980; **1**, 151–60.
14. Kanski J. J. Clinical and immunological study of anterior uveitis in juvenile chronic polyarthritis. *Trans. Ophthalmol. Soc. UK* 1976; **96**, 123–30.
15. Merriam J. C., Chylack L. T. and Albert D. M. Early onset pauciarticular juvenile rheumatoid arthritis – a histopathological study. *Arch. Ophthalmol.* 1983; **101**, 1085–92.
16. Kanski J. J. Care of children with anterior uveitis. *Trans. Ophthalmol. Soc. UK* 1981; **101**, 387–90.
17. Liesegang T. J. Clinical features and prognosis in Fuch's uveitis syndrome. *Arch. Ophthalmol.* 1982; **100**, 1622–6.
18. Melamed S., Lahav M., Sanbank U. et al. Fuch's heterochromic cyclitis: an EM study of the iris. *Invest. Ophthalmol. Vis. Sci.* 1978; **17**, 1193.
19. Dernouchamps J. P. Thesis, Universite Catholique de Louvain, 1981.
20. O'Connor G. R. Fuch's heterochromic cyclitis (Doyne Lecture). *Trans. Ophthalmol. Soc. UK* 1985; **104**, 219–31.
21. Womack L. W. and Liesegang T. J. Complications of herpes zoster ophthalmicus. *Arch. Ophthalmol.* 1983; **101**, 42–5.
22. Marsh R. J., Easty D. L. and Jones B. R. Iritis and iris atrophy in herpes zoster ophthalmicus. *Am. J. Ophthalmol.* 1974; **78**, 255–61.
23. Hedges T. R. and Albert D. M. The progression of the ocular abnormalities of herpes zoster, histopathological observations in 9 cases. *Ophthalmology* 1982; **89**, 165–77.
24. Magill J., Chapman C. and Masangam M. Acyclovir therapy in herpes zoster infection: a practical guide. *Trans. Ophthalmol. Soc. UK* 1983; **103**, 111–14.
25. Fisher J. P., Lewis M. L., Blumenkranz M. et al. The acute retinal necrosis syndrome: part I and II. *Ophthalmology* 1982; **89**, 1309–16.
26. Topilow H. W., Nussbaum J. J. and Freeman M. et al. Bilateral acute retinal necrosis. *Arch. Ophthalmol.* 1982; **100**, 1901–8.
27. Akstein R. B., Wilson L. A. and Teutsch S. M. Acquired toxoplasmosis. *Ophthalmology* 1982; **89**, 1299–1302.
28. Zscheile F. P. Recurrent toxoplasmic retinitis with weakly positive methylene blue dye test. *Arch. Ophthalmol.* 1964; **71**, 645–8.
29. Rollins D. F., Tabbara K. F., O'Connor G. R. Detection of toxoplasma antigen and antibody in ocular fluids in experimental ocular toxoplasmosis. *Arch. Ophthalmol.* 1983; **101**, 455–7.
30. Loewer-Sieger D. H., Rothova A., Koppe J. G. et al. Congenital toxoplasmosis – a prospective study based on 1821 pregnant women. *Uveitis Update. Proceedings of the 1st International Symposium on Uveitis, Helsinki 1984.* Saari K. M. (ed.) Amsterdam, Excerpta Medica, pp. 203–7.
31. Culbertson W. W., Tabbara K. F. and O'Connor G. R. Experimental ocular toxoplasmosis in primates. *Arch. Ophthalmol.* 1982; **100**, 321–3.
32. Shirahata T., Shimizu K. and Suzuki N. Effects of immune cryptocyte products and serum antibody on the multiplication of toxoplasma in immune peritoneal macrophages. *Parasitenk* 1976; **49**, 11.
33. Shimada K., O'Connor G. R. and Yoneda C. Cyst formation by toxoplasma gondii. *Arch. Ophthalmol.* 1974; **92**, 496–500.
34. Tabbara K. F. and O'Connor G. R. Treatment of ocular toxoplasmosis with clindamycin and sulphathiazine. *Ophthalmology* 1980; **87**, 129–34.
35. Ashton N. Larval granulomatosis of the retina due to toxocara. *Br. J. Ophthalmol.* 1960; **44**, 129–48.
36. Duguid I. M. Chronic endophthalmitis due to toxocara. *Br. J. Ophthalmol.* 1961; **45**, 705–17.
37. Duguid I. M. Features of ocular infestation by toxocara. *Br. J. Ophthalmol.* 1961; **45**, 789–96.
38. Hogan M. J., Kimura S. J. and Spencer W. H. Visceral larval migrans and peripheral retinitis. *JAMA* 1965; **194**, 1345–7.
39. Byers B. and Kimura S. Uveitis after death of larva in vitreous cavity. *Am. J. Ophthalmol.* 1974; **77**, 63–6.
40. Watzke R. C., Oaks J. A. and Folk J. C. *Toxocara canis* infection of the eye, correlation of clinical observations with developing pathology in the primate model. *Arch. Ophthalmol.* 1984; **102**, 282–91.
41. Seare S. S., Moaged K. and Albert D. M. Ocular toxocarasis presenting as leucocoria in a patient with low Elisa titres. *Ophthalmology* 1981; **88**, 1302–6.
42. Belmont J. B., Irvine A., Benson W. et al. Vitrectomy in ocular toxocarasis. *Arch. Ophthalmol.* 1982; **100**, 1912–15.
43. Hagler W. S., Pollard Z. F., Jarrett W. H. et al. Results of surgery for ocular *Toxocara canis*. *Ophthalmology* 1981; **88**, 1081–6.

44. Csonka G. W. Syphilis. In: Weatherall D. J., Ledingham J. G. G. and Wanell D. A. (ed.) *Oxford Textbook of Medicine*, vol. 1, ch. 5. Oxford, OUP, 1983.
45. Schlaegel T. F. Bacterial and protozoal uveitis. *Trans. Ophthalmol. Soc. UK* 1981; **101**, 312–16.
46. Green W. R., Kincaid M. C., Michels R. G. et al. Pars planitis. *Trans. Ophthalmol. Soc. UK* 1981; **101**, 361–7.
47. Felder K. S. and Brockhurst R. J. Neovascular fundus abnormalities in peripheral uveitis. *Arch. Ophthalmol.* 1982; **100**, 750–4.
48. Editorial. Behçet's disease. *Japn. J. Ophthalmol.* 1974; **18**, 291–4.
49. Mamo J. G. Treatment of Behçet's disease with chlorambucil. A follow-up report. *Arch. Ophthalmol.* 1976; **94**, 580.
50. Ohno S., Ohguchi M., Hirose S. et al. Close association of HLA BW51 with Behçet's disease. *Arch. Ophthalmol.* 1982; **100**, 1455–8.
51. Eglin R. P., Lehner T. and Subak Sharpe J. H. Detection of RNA complementary to herpes simplex virus in mononuclear cells from patients with Behçet's syndrome and recurrent oral ulcers. *Lancet* 1982; **2**, 1356–60.
52. Lehner T. and Barnes C. G. (ed.) *Behçet's Syndrome*. London, Academic Press, 1979.
53. Karma A. Ophthalmic changes in sarcoidosis. *Acta Ophthalmol.* 1979; Suppl. 141.
54. Stannard K. and Spalton D. J. Sarcoidosis with infiltration of the external ocular muscles – case report. *Br. J. Ophthalmol.* 1985; **69**, 563–6.
55. Nichols C. W., Eagle R. C., Yanoff M. et al. Conjunctival biopsy as an aid in the evaluation of the patient with suspected sarcoidosis. *Ophthalmology* 1980; **87**, 287–91.
56. Iwata K., Nanba K., Sobuc U. et al. Ocular sarcoidosis, evaluation of findings. *Ann. NY Acad. Sci.* 1976; **278**, 445–54.
57. Spalton D. J. and Sanders M. D. Fundus changes in histologically confirmed sarcoidosis. *Br. J. Ophthalmol.* 1981; **65**, 348–58.
58. Obenauf C. D., Shaw H. E., Sydnor C. F. et al. Sarcoidosis and its ophthalmic manifestations. *Am. J. Ophthalmol.* 1978; **86**, 648–55.
59. Gass J. D. M. and Olson C. L. Sarcoidosis with optic nerve and retinal involvement. *Arch. Ophthalmol.* 1976; **94**, 945–50.
60. Marcus D. F., Bovino J. A. and Burton J. C. Sarcoid granuloma of the choroid. *Ophthalmology* 1982; **89**, 1326–30.
61. Lubin J. R., Albert D. M. and Weinstein M. 65 years of sympathetic ophthalmia. A clinicopathological review of 105 cases (1913–1978). *Ophthalmology* 1980; **87**, 109–21.
62. Kinyoun J. L., Bensinger R. E. and Chuang E. L. 30 year history of sympathetic ophthalmia. *Ophthalmology* 1983; **90**, 59–65.
63. Font R. L., Fine B. S., Messner E. et al. Light and electron-microscopic study of Dalen Fuch's nodules in sympathetic ophthalmia. *Ophthalmology* 1982; **89**, 66–75.
64. Jakobiec F. A., Marboe C. C., Knowles D. M. et al. Human sympathetic ophthalmia: An analysis of the inflammatory infiltrate by hybridoma-monoclonal antibodies, immunochemistry, and correlative electron microscopy. *Ophthalmology* 1983; **90**, 76–95.
65. Rao N. A. and Wong V. G. Aetiology of sympathetic ophthalmitis. *Trans. Ophthalmol. Soc. UK* 1981; **101**, 357–60.
66. Gallo R. C. et al. Frequent detection and isolation of cytopathic retro-virus (HTLV-3) from patients with AIDS and at risk of AIDS. *Science* 1984; **224**, 500.
67. Pepose J. et al. Acquired Immune Deficiency Syndrome: Pathogenic mechanisms of ocular disease. *Ophthalmology* 1985; **92**, 472–84.
68. Humphry R. C., Weber J. N. and Marsh R. J. The ophthalmic findings of a group of ambulatory patients infected by Human T Cell Lymphotrophic virus type III: a prospective study. *Br. J. Ophthalmol* 1986; in press.
69. Holland G. N. et al. Ocular disease in Acquired Immune Deficiency Syndrome: clinicopathological correlations. *Proceedings 4th International Symposium of the Immunology and Immunopathology of the Eye*. 1986, in press.
70. Feman S. A., Podgorski S. F. and Penn M. K. Blindness from presumed ocular histoplasmosis in Tennessee. *Ophthalmology* 1982; **89**, 1295–8.
71. Smith R. E. Studies of the presumed ocular histoplasma syndrome. *Trans. Ophthalmol. Soc. UK* 1981; **101**, 326–34.
72. Rucker C. W. Sheathing of retinal veins in multiple sclerosis. *JAMA* 1945; **127**, 970–3.
73. Chester G. H., Blach R. K. and Cleary P. E. Inflammation in the region of the vitreous base. *Trans. Ophthalmol. Soc. UK* 1976; **96**, 151–7.
74. Arnold A C., Pepose J. S., Hepler R. S. et al. Retinal periphlebitis and retinitis in multiple sclerosis. *Ophthalmology* 1984; **91**, 255–62.
75. Knox D. L., Schachnak A. P. and Mustonen E. Primary, secondary and coincidental ocular complications of Crohn's disease. *Ophthalmology* 1984; **91**, 163–73.
76. Avila M. P., Jalkh A. E., Feldman E. et al. Manifestations of Whipple's disease in the posterior segment of the eye. *Arch. Ophthalmol.* 1984; **102**, 384–90.
77. Knox D. L. and King J. Retinal arteritis, iridocyclitis and giardiasis. *Ophthalmology* 1982; **89**, 1303–8.
78. Ohno S. Vogt–Koganagi–Harada's disease and sympathetic ophthalamia. *Uveitis Update. Proceedings of 1st International Symposium on Uveitis, Helsinki, 1984*. Saari K. M. (ed.) Amsterdam, Excerpta Medica, pp. 401–5.
79. Lee D. A., Barker S. M., Daniel W. P. et al. The clinical diagnosis of Reiter's syndrome. *Ophthalmology* 1986; **93**, 350–6.
80. Fearnley I. R., Spalton D. J. et al. α_1-Antitrypsin phenotypes in acute anterior uveitis. *Br. J. Ophthalmol.* 1986, in press.

Chapter 8

The Retina

Inflammatory Diseases
Lee M. Jampol

DISEASES OF UNKNOWN AETIOLOGY
Serpiginous (Geographic) Choroiditis

Serpiginous choroiditis[1-4] is a chronic recurring disease usually seen in young to middle-aged patients (30–70 years old) who present with visual loss. underlying choroidal vessels and frequently pigmentary clumping (*Figs.* 1, 2). Patients may present with recurrences in either eye and the majority of cases show multiple episodes. Subretinal neovascularization may be seen.[4] With involvement of the macula, permanent central visual loss is seen. Amsler grid

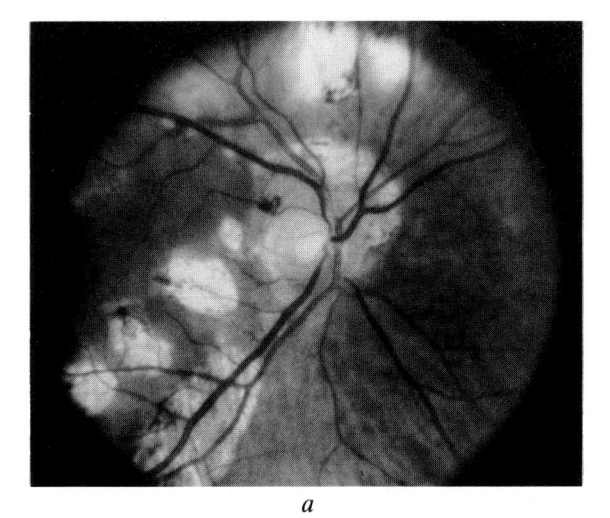

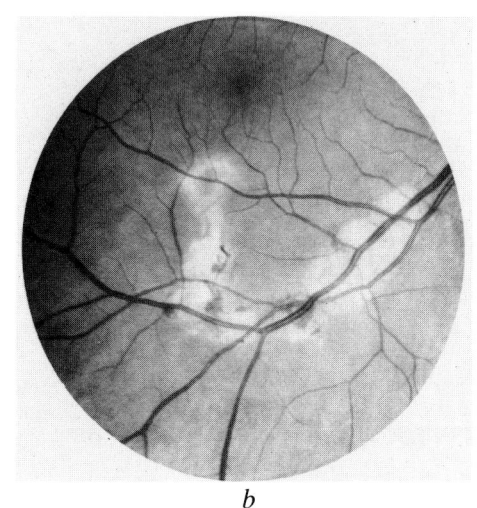

Fig. 1. Serpiginous choroiditis: multiple healed foci of inactive disease are seen near disc (*a*); *b*, choroiditis tracking toward fovea. Several years later, fovea became involved.

Although only one eye usually demonstrates central visual loss initially, there is often evidence of previous activity in both eyes. The clinical findings include the presence of vitreous cells and occasionally anterior chamber reaction. The fundus acutely shows white 'oedematous' appearing lesions, apparently at the level of the retinal pigment epithelium and choroid. The lesions are usually seen in the peripapillary area, but may be present in the macula or other areas of the posterior pole or even the periphery. Recurrences usually spread away from the disc in a serpentine fashion. These recurrences usually are located adjacent to areas of previous activity that had 'healed'.

Fluorescein angiography during the acute phase shows early blockage of fluorescence with marked late staining of the lesions. Activity of the lesions lasts for several weeks with the gradual development of atrophy of the retinal pigment epithelium and

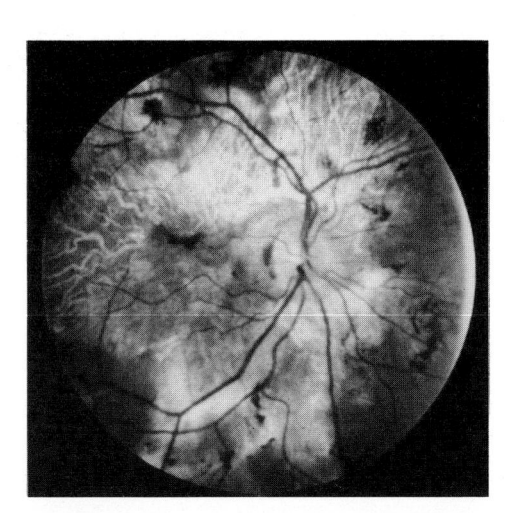

Fig. 2. Another patient demonstrates advanced 'end stage' serpiginous choroiditis.

testing reveals dense scotomas corresponding to areas of active or healed choroiditis.

The aetiology of this disease remains unknown. A tuberculous aetiology has been suggested by some studies. No evidence of active tuberculosis has been documented in the cases that we have seen.[4] Systemic evaluations in these patients have been unrewarding.

Therapy in these patients is difficult. Some patients appear to respond to systemic corticosteroids but the effect on the ultimate visual outcome is uncertain.

The differential diagnosis includes primarily acute posterior multifocal placoid pigment epitheliopathy (APMPPE). In patients with APMPPE, the lesions resolve more rapidly with less atrophy of the retinal pigment epithelium and choroid. The lesions usually have a simultaneous onset bilaterally and recurrences are rare. Patients with serpiginous choroiditis have recurrent episodes, with activity present at different times in different eyes. Unlike serpiginous choroiditis, visual recovery is the rule in APMPPE.

Birdshot (Vitiliginous) Chorioretinopathy

This disease, of unknown cause, usually presents in older individuals with complaints of gradual loss of central vision or floaters.[5-8] The patients may also complain of nyctalopia. Visual acuity may vary from 20/20 to 20/100. There is evidence of a chronic intraocular process characterized by vitreal cells and debris. The patient shows multiple grey, white or yellow areas present at the level of the deep retina or retinal pigment epithelium, with the lesions scattered throughout the posterior pole (*Fig.* 3). Involvement may be unilateral or bilateral. The patients may also show evidence of retinal vascular dilatation and leakage, cystoid macular oedema and optic disc oedema. Some patients also demonstrate mild anterior segment inflammation with some fine keratic precipitates (KP). Some observers have described arteriolar narrowing and vascular sheathing in the fundus.

There are no pars plana exudates so the process can be distinguished from pars planitis.

Birdshot chorioretinopathy has a chronic course with visual loss usually related to macular oedema rather than the vitreal reaction. With time, the acute RPE lesions become more atrophic, and multiple depigmented spots may be seen.

An association of birdshot chorioretinopathy with HLA A29 has been reported.[7,8] In addition, *in vitro* studies of lymphocytes of these patients demonstrate a response to retinal S-antigen (an antigen isolated from outer segments of photoreceptors).[7] There is thus evidence of an autoimmune process. A possible association with vitiliginous patches of the skin has been reported.[6] Electroretinography in these patients often demonstrates decreased photopic and scotopic b-waves, although the scotopic response is usually more severely impaired.[8] Some of the patients may demonstrate moderate elevation of final rod thresholds on dark adaptation testing.

Therapy of birdshot chorioretinopathy is unsatisfactory. There may be a mild ameliorating effect from systemic or periocular corticosteroids but usually these are of limited value. The final visual outcome may be limited by the macular changes.

Acute Retinal Necrosis Syndrome (ARN)

ARN is a recently recognized entity, probably first reported in the ophthalmic literature by Urayama,[9] as Kirisawa's uveitis. Patients present with unilateral or bilateral uveitis in association with necrotizing retinitis.[9-12] Often the anterior chamber reaction is noted, first with marked flare, cells, keratic precipitates, posterior synechiae and vitritis. Subsequently a necrotizing retinitis becomes apparent in one or both eyes. There is often marked vascular sheathing, vascular occlusion and retinal infarction and haemorrhages (*Fig.* 4).

The retinitis is often first seen in the peripheral

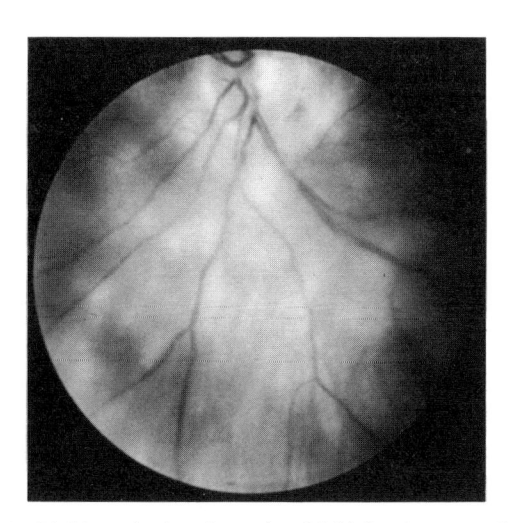

Fig. 3. Birdshot chorioretinopathy. Multiple almost confluent yellow–white lesions at level of deep retina or RPE.

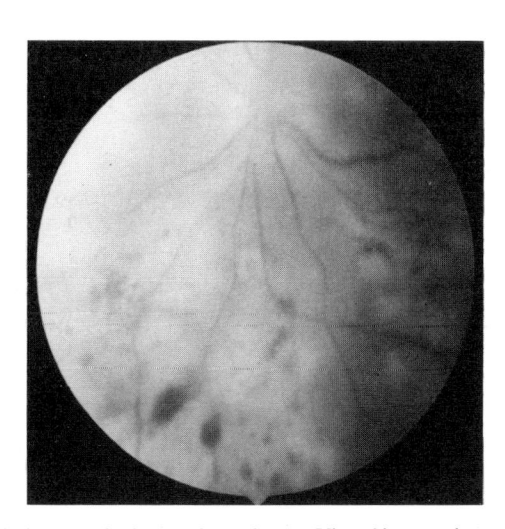

Fig. 4. Acute retinal necrosis syndrome. Vitreal haze and necrotizing retinitis with vasculitis and haemorrhages are seen.

fundus, although occasionally the changes are seen in the posterior pole. Whitening of the retina and the retinal pigment epithelium is noted and in some patients there appears to be choroidal involvement. Serous elevation of the retina may be seen. A posterior progression of the retinitis is usually noted. If the retinitis involves the macula, central visual acuity is destroyed. More commonly, healing of the retinitis occurs with the development of mottled pigmentation and scarring. With healing of the disease, however, vitreoretinal traction develops and results in tractional or more commonly rhegmatogenous retinal detachment in up to two-thirds to three-quarters of the cases. This retinal detachment is difficult to repair with standard buckling surgery or vitrectomy and often results in loss of vision in the eye.

development of retinal detachment, the possibility of prophylactic buckling or vitrectomy has been raised. The value of this therapy awaits further definitive clinical studies.

The Multiple Evanescent White Dot Syndrome (MEWDS)

This recently described syndrome[15] is a cause of unilateral, or rarely bilateral, visual loss in young patients (usually female). The patient often presents with visual loss. A granularity to the foveal area may be noted as well as the presence of multiple small 100–200 μm white dots present at the level of the pigment epithelium or deep retina (*Fig.* 5). These are most concentrated in the perimacular area and

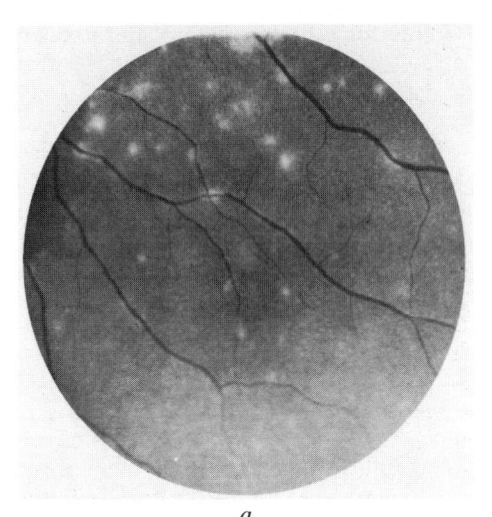

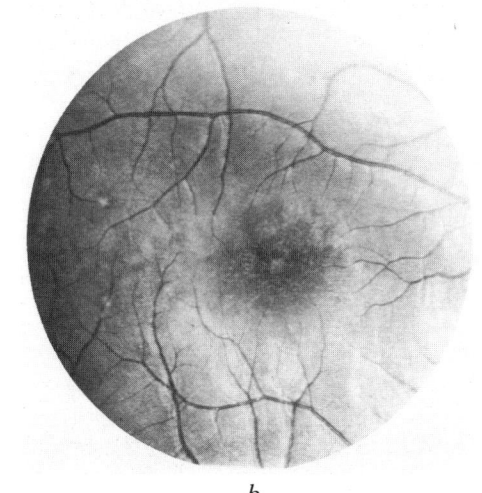

Fig. 5. Multiple evanescent white dot syndrome (MEWDS). *a*, Characteristic white dots; *b*, granular pathognomonic appearance of fovea.

The similarity of the retinitis of ARN to viral retinitis (cytomegalovirus or herpes simplex) has suggested involvement of a virus. In one case, a herpes virus was isolated from the eye, though it was not completely identified.[11,12] A possible association with herpes zoster ophthalmicus has been noted.[13] Herpes zoster has now been identified in two eyes with ARN. Serologic evidence of herpes virus infection has also not been demonstrated systemically, but recent measurements of intraocular antibody levels do implicate herpes zoster and perhaps other herpes viruses.

The differential diagnosis of acute retinal necrosis syndrome includes viral retinitis, toxoplasmosis (which usually is more localized) and Behçet's disease (*see below*).

Therapy of acute retinal necrosis syndrome is presently unsatisfactory. Antiviral agents, especially acyclovir, are being tested. Anticoagulation has also been used because of the frequent occurrence of retinal vascular occlusion. Aspirin has also been suggested as a possible therapy to prevent vascular occlusion.[14] In view of the high rate of subsequent

gradually become less prominent as the equator is approached. The patients may show signs of ocular inflammation with vitreal cells, retinal vascular sheathing and optic disc oedema. Fluorescein angiography often reveals evidence of leakage from disc capillaries, retinal vessels and perhaps at the level of retinal pigment epithelium. Acutely the electroretinogram and the early receptor potential are diminished. Over a several week period, healing is seen with a return of the central vision to normal or near normal levels. A dramatic improvement in the electroretinogram and early receptor potential has also been documented. The aetiology of this disease is uncertain. Systemic evaluations in these patients have been unrewarding.

In view of the excellent visual prognosis, no therapy is indicated. No response to steroids has been noted in these patients.

Behçet's Disease

Behçet's disease is a systemic disease with ocular manifestations.[16-18] The patients often present with aphthous ulcers, which may involve the mouth (stomatitis) or the other mucous membranes (e.g. genital ulcers). Dermatitis may be present and the patient may show arthritis, thrombophlebitis, or meningoencephalitis. Ocular involvement may cause blindness, while meningoencephalitis may cause neurological disability or even death. The disease is more common in men than in women and is usually seen in young adults. It is much more common in Middle Eastern and Far Eastern ethnic groups than Caucasians. An association with HLA B5 has been reported.

Behçet's disease will frequently present as an iritis, which in its classic form shows a hypopyon. With topical and systemic corticosteroid therapy now available, the incidence of these hypopyons has markedly decreased. Usually the iritis is bilateral and nongranulomatous. In addition, vitreal cells may be seen as well as evidence of disc oedema, retinal vasculitis (which may involve either the arterioles, the veins or both) and macular oedema. Cotton wool spots, vascular occlusions, ischaemia of the retina, and retinal haemorrhages may be seen. Visual loss in these eyes is often related to retinal vascular occlusion, macular oedema or disc involvement. Anterior segment complications (iritis) may also cause visual loss.

Therapy of the ocular disease has included topical, periocular and systemic corticosteroids. In cases where no response to steroids is seen, immunosuppressive drugs, particularly chlorambucil, have been utilized.

Diffuse Unilateral Subacute Neuroretinitis (DUSN)

DUSN, initially called the unilateral wipe-out syndrome, is often observed in young patients.[19] Patients in the acute phase present with unilateral vitreous cells, mild anterior chamber reaction, papillitis, and sometimes white spots of the retina. Recent work has suggested that this syndrome is related to the presence of an intraocular nematode, which may be one of at least two different species. This nematode is apparently not *Toxocara canis*. The worm may be visualized intraocularly in some cases. Toxins liberated by the parasite result in progressive visual loss, optic atrophy, arteriolar narrowing and pigmentary changes in the fundus. Patients may initially present at this stage, often unaware of the onset of visual loss. The presence of the unilateral optic atrophy, arteriolar narrowing and bone spicule pigmentation, may suggest either unilateral retinitis pigmentosa or a previous choroidal infarction. The worm is usually not demonstrable at this time. Possible therapies during the acute phase include photocoagulation of the worm or surgical removal of the worm. Experience with these modalities at present is limited.

Acute Macular Neuroretinopathy

This entity, initially described in 1975 by Bos and Deutmann, is a disease of young adults, mostly women, which may be unilateral or bilateral.[20,21] The patients sometimes have a history of a preceding viral illness. There is often a complaint of decreased vision, although the central visual acuity may be normal. The patients demonstrate multiple paracentral scotomas. This is associated with petal-shaped or multiple round lesions in parafoveal area which are a darker red than the surrounding areas. The lesions appear to be present in the deep retina or retinal pigment epithelium. Fluorescein angiography is usually normal, although there may be very slight hyperfluorescence in the areas of involvement. Electroretinography has been normal. These patients have prolonged loss of vision but there may be a gradual improvement. The paracentral scotomas may disappear. The retinal lesions may become less apparent with time, although permanent damage to the retina may be visualized.

Acute Retinal Pigment Epitheliitis

This entity[22,23] was first described in 1972 by Alex Krill. It is usually seen in young adults and is characterized by an acute loss of vision which may be minimal or down to the level of 20/100. It may be unilateral or bilateral. There is a normal anterior segment but the posterior pole demonstrated discrete clusters of small brown or greyish spots (usually two to four spots) in the involved macula. There maybe a yellow or white halo around each of these spots. Fluorescein angiography during the acute stage shows central hypofluorescence with a surrounding halo which is normal or slightly hyperfluorescent. Electroretinography and visual evoked responses are normal. The electro-oculogram has been subnormal in a few cases. The lesions usually evolve over a 6–12 week period. The central visual acuity usually returns to normal. The lesions become darker or fade and the lighter areas surrounding the darker spots may remain or fade.

The aetiology of this disease is unknown. It may represent a viral syndrome. No therapy is indicated in view of the good visual outcome.

Acute Posterior Multifocal Placoid Pigment Epitheliopathy (APMPPE)

This disease,[24,25] first described by Donald Gass in 1968, is often preceded by a prodromal influenza-like illness. It is usually seen in adolescents and young adults, both males and females. Both eyes are usually affected, although occasional unilateral cases are seen. The patients may show mild iritis or episcleritis and the vitreous may contain cells. Disc oedema may be seen. The classic feature of disease, however, is the presence of multiple cream-coloured placoid lesions, which may be somewhat geographic in configuration, scattered in the posterior pole (*Fig.* 6). Fluorescein angiography initially shows hypofluorescence (*Fig.* 6) with late staining of the lesion. During the acute phase, the patient may have meningeal signs and elevation of cerebrospinal fluid protein with pleocytosis.[26] Electroretinography and electro-oculography are normal.

The placoid lesions in APMPPE rapidly evolve, usually in 7–10 days, with the development of mild pigmentation. Unlike serpiginous choroiditis, the underlying choroid survives intact (without atrophy).

cases, rubeosis iridis, cataract and secondary glaucoma have been reported.

Cases initially thought to be Eales's disease have subsequently been shown to represent sickle cell retinopathy, talc retinopathy and other entities responsible for peripheral retinal neovascularization.[28] However, there does appear to be a group of patients, especially in Third World nations, and

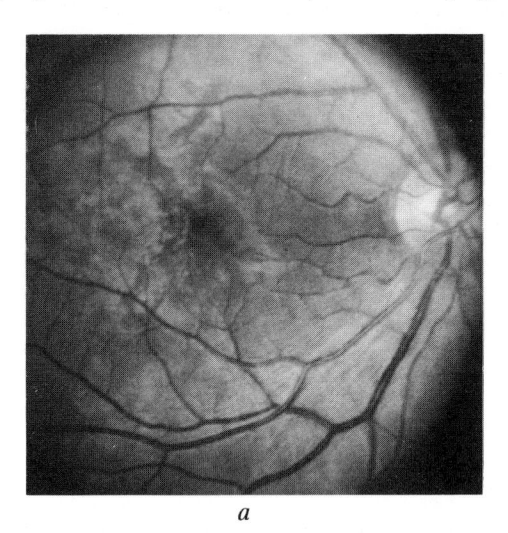

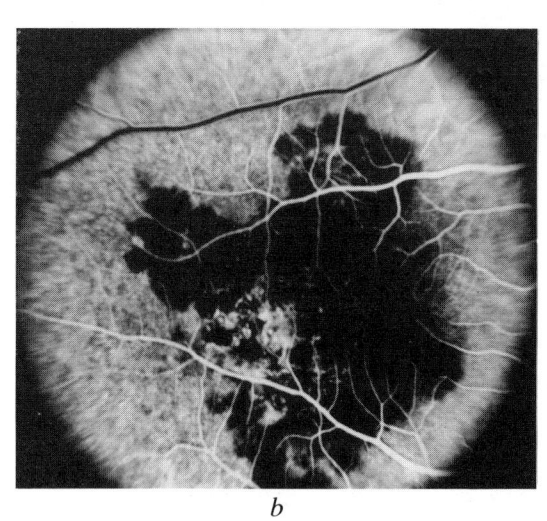

Fig. 6. Acute posterior multifocal placoid pigment epitheliopathy. *a*, Subacute lesion; *b*, fluorescein angiogram shows blockage or non-perfusion of choroidal circulation.

The visual recovery is slower than the resolution of the ophthalmoscopic appearance and may take up to 6 months. In most cases, however, central visual acuity does recover. Unlike serpiginous choroiditis, recurrences in this disease are rare, although they have been occasionally noted. In the rare unilateral cases, the second eye may become involved several weeks or months following the first eye. In these cases, the diagnosis of serpiginous choroiditis must be considered.

This disease is thought to represent either a pigment epithelial inflammatory disease (viral?) or choroidal ischaemia due to choroidal vasculitis. A controversy has existed as to whether the hypofluorescence seen on the angiogram acutely represents choroidal non-perfusion[27] or simply blockage by opaque retinal pigment epithelium. This controversy has still not been resolved.

Eales's Disease

In 1882, Henry Eales described the association of retinal haemorrhage with epistaxis and constipation. The term Eales's disease is presently applied to a variety of peripheral retinal vaso-occlusive processes of unknown aetiology.[28–30] These patients will often shown signs of an idiopathic retinal vasculitis with peripheral capillary non-perfusion. There is vascular sheathing and there may be peripheral retinal neovascularization, which can cause vitreous haemorrhage and rhegmatogenous retinal detachment. In severe

especially among young males, where the development of bilateral peripheral retinal vaso-obliteration with peripheral retinal neovascularization is seen. Systemic disease is usually not found in these patients, although an association with a positive tuberculin skin test has been suggested. In a few cases, active tuberculosis is present. One must separate from the Eales's disease category patients with other causes of peripheral retinal vaso-obliteration, including sarcoidosis, acquired diseases of connective tissue, and many others.[28]

Therapy of Eales's disease includes the use of corticosteroids and, in cases with retinal neovascularization, direct or scatter type photocoagulation. Since what is presently called Eales's diseases may well represent a wastebasket category for a wide variety of diseases associated with peripheral retinal neovascularization, the efficacy of these therapies undoubtedly depends upon the underlying causes of the retinal vascular obliteration.

INFECTIOUS DISEASES OF THE RETINA

Parasitic Infestations

Toxocariasis

Toxocara infestation of the eye is a disease caused by a round worm, *Toxocara canis*.[31] *T. canis* is an intestinal parasite present in dogs, especially puppies. Human infestation occurs by accidental ingestion of infective ova. It is frequently due to association with puppies or contact with dirt or soil contaminated by dog faeces. Once the ova are ingested, they penetrate the bowel wall and then pass via the blood stream to multiple organs throughout the body. If there is widespread systemic involvement, a syndrome called visceral larval migrans is present. This is characterized by fever, hepatomegaly and eosinophilia. These patients usually do not have ocular involvement.

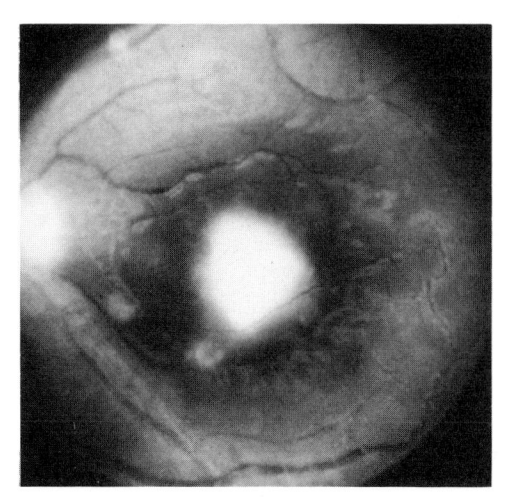

Fig. 7. Acute Toxocara granuloma in macular area.

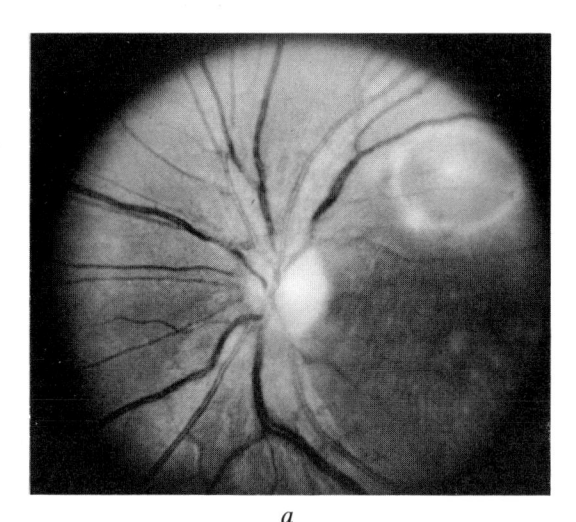

test) for toxocara. Paracentesis or vitreous aspiration demonstrating many eosinophils also supports the diagnosis.

Therapy consists of the use of systemic and periocular corticosteroids to suppress the inflammation in the active phases of the disease. Usually the granuloma eventually becomes inactive. Rare cases may require surgical intervention. Anthelmintic drugs have not been proved to benefit the ocular disease.

Cysticercosis

Ocular involvement can occur secondary to the presence of a cysticercus organism.[32,33] *Cysticercus cellulosae* is the encysted larval form of the tapeworm, usually the pork tapeworm, *Taenia solium*. In areas of the world *T. solium* is common. Cysts occur in the human as a result of accidental ingestion of ova.

Cysticercus may be found in the lids, ocular adnexa, or in the vitreous or subretinal space (*Fig. 8*). Therapy consists of surgical removal of the encysted organism. Medical therapy with praziquantel does not seem to be of value for intraocular cysticercus.[38]

Toxoplasmosis

Toxoplasma gondii is an obligate intracellular protozoal organism, which is the most common cause of

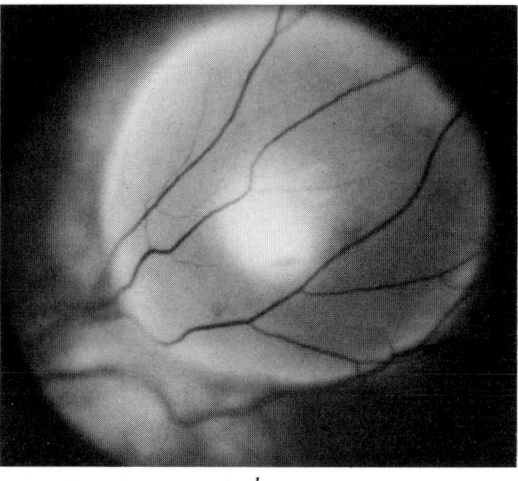

a *b*

Fig. 8. Cysticercus cellulosae. a, Parasite is visible superior to macula in subretinal space. *b,* Several months later lesion has grown dramatically in size.

Three distinct presentations of ocular involvement have been described. Occasionally this disease can present as a unilateral endophthalmitis. A localized posterior pole granuloma can also be seen (*Fig. 7*) and can cause preretinal or subretinal fibrosis and traction. Traction retinal detachment may occur. Also peripheral inflammatory masses may be present causing peripheral vitreoretinal traction.

The diagnosis of ocular toxocariasis can be made by the presence of one of these three clinical syndromes, usually in a young patient, and a positive (1:8) titre enzyme linked immunosorbent assay (Elisa

infectious retinitis. In most cases, infection of the retina appears to represent reactivation of congenital infection.[34] Congenital toxoplasmosis occurs when the mother is infected by the organism for the first time during pregnancy. Infection can be due to exposure to cat faeces, unpasteurized milk, or eating undercooked meat. Acute infection by toxoplasmosis may be asymptomatic or can result in a flu-like syndrome or sometimes 'infectious mononucleosis'. Lymphadenopathy, fever and malaise may be seen. Pneumonitis, myocarditis and meningoencephalitis are much rarer findings. Each year in the United

States, more than 3000 infants are born with congenital toxoplasmosis. Findings include chorioretinitis (*Fig.* 9), hydrocephalus, intracerebral calcification and convulsions. Retinitis can be seen with congenital or rarely acquired toxoplasmosis.

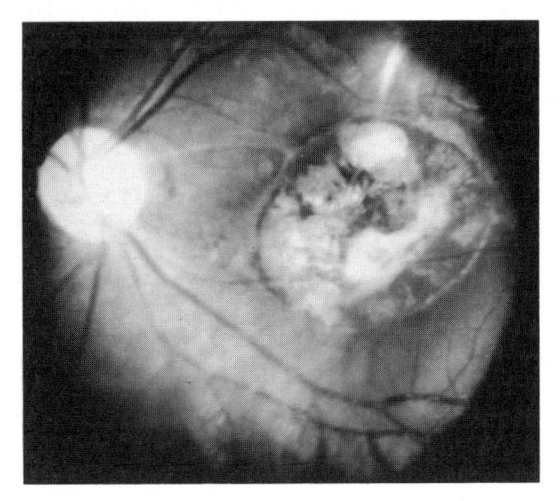

Fig. 9. Congenital toxoplasmosis. Large inactive chorioretinal scar with overlying vitreal organization.

The acute lesion of toxoplasmic retinitis is a yellow or white fluffy area in the periphery or posterior pole (*Fig.* 10). There is usually mild non-granulomatous anterior uveitis, and marked vitreous cellular reaction. There is often a variable sheathing of the retinal veins or arterioles adjacent to the area of retinitis.

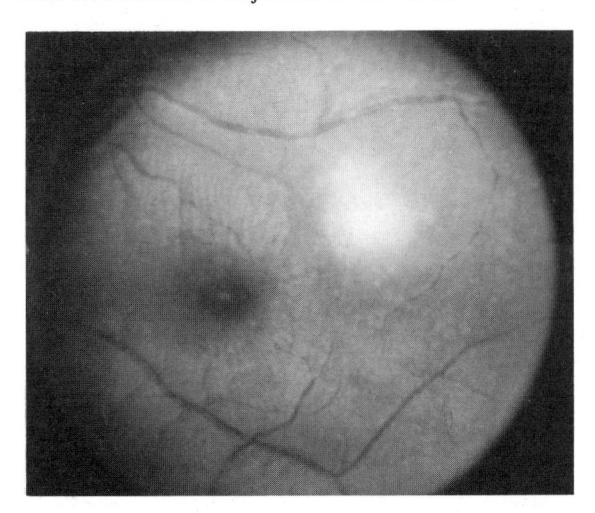

Fig. 10. Active toxoplasmic retinitis. Adjacent retinal vascular sheathing is apparent.

The inflammation may involve primarily the optic disc, the peripapillary area, the macular area, or anywhere in the fundus. Although the clinical appearance is usually the key to the diagnosis of toxoplasmosis, a Sabin–Feldman dye titre or a fluorescent antibody test can be confirmatory. Any positive titre in association with a consistent clinical picture is sufficient grounds to make the diagnosis.

If the retinitis is not threatening the macular area or disc, management includes only watching the patient. If the disc or macula is involved or threatened, therapy includes the use of sulphonamides, Daraprim with the concurrent use of leukovorin (sulpha) to protect the patient's bonemarrow, and the use of systemic corticosteroids to minimize destruction of ocular tissues. Periocular steroids are contraindicated as the high level of steroids attained suppresses the immune response to the organism. Recently clindamycin has also been utilized systemically or periocularly in severe cases. The risk of pseudomembranous colitis as a complication of clindamycin must be kept in mind.

Our usual starting doses for therapy include triple sulpha, 2 g as a loading dose and 1 g four times a day; Daraprim 100–150 mg as a loading dose and 25–50 mg a day for 4–6 weeks. The patient's white blood cell count and platelet count should be checked weekly. Leukovorin (folinic acid) 10 mg twice a week, should be added to protect the bone-marrow. Clindamycin 300 mg q.i.d. may be used. Spiramycin has been utilized as a secondary drug for toxoplasmosis, although its value for ocular toxoplasmosis is uncertain.

In severe cases attempts have been made to destroy the organism using laser photocoagulation or cryopexy. The value of these modalities remains uncertain.

Viral Infections

Rubella

If a pregnant woman becomes infected with the rubella virus for the first time, especially during the first trimester of pregnancy, congenital rubella infection may occur. Rubella in these pregnant women may result in abortion and stillbirth and if the baby survives, there may be heart disease including patent ductus arteriosus, pulmonary stenosis or ventricular septal defect. In addition, mental retardation and genitourinary abnormalities may be present.

The ocular manifestations of congenital rubella include the presence of microphthalmia, hyperopia, glaucoma, iris hypoplasia (with poor dilatation of the pupil), cataract and iridocyclitis. The changes are often bilateral, but may be asymmetric. Retinal involvement[35] may occur in utero; the retinitis is inactive by the time the baby is born. A salt and pepper appearance of the fundus with fine white dots and black clumps of pigment is seen (*Fig.* 11). Areas of retinal pigment epithelial atrophy and irregularity are present. The choroidal vasculature is normal. Despite the widespread pigmentary changes in the fundus, electroretinography is usually normal.

Retinal involvement in this disease usually does not result in impaired central vision, although the late development of subretinal neovascularization has been reported.[36]

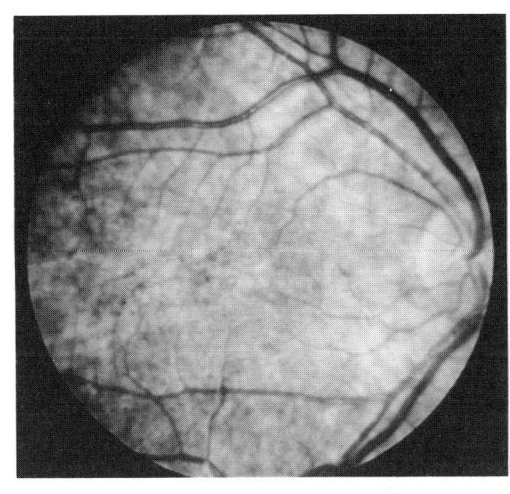

Fig. 11. Salt and pepper retinopathy of rubella.

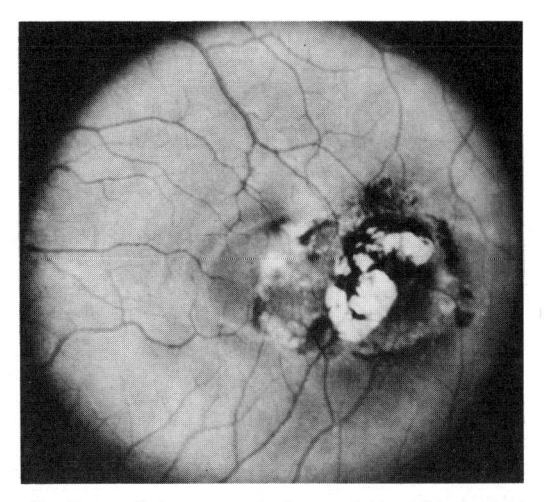

Fig. 12. Congenital cytomegalovirus retinitis. Macular lesion is apparent.

Measles Virus

Infection with measles virus may involve the retina in two clinical settings. During acute measles infection in an immunosuppressed patient, retinitis has been described.[37] During the 'slow viral' infection caused by measles virus, subacute sclerosing panencephalitis (SSPE), about half the cases show posterior pole chorioretinitis, which may be the presenting sign of the disease.[38,39] SSPE is usually seen in children who had previously had measles infections before the age of 2. Then at approximately 7 years of age, they show personality changes, inappropriate behaviour, intellectual deterioration, myoclonic jerks, seizures, paralysis and progressive dementia. Examination of the fundus may reveal low-grade active retinitis, usually in the macular area. This may be mistaken for macular degeneration, toxoplasmosis or cytomegalovirus. Usually there is minimal vitreous cellular infiltration.

Cytomegalovirus

Cytomegalovirus is a herpes virus which, like the other herpes viruses, contains DNA. Infection by this virus is characterized by the development of enormous cells with intranuclear and intracytoplasmic inclusions. About 80 per cent of the population is infected by the age of 13. The infection may be asymptomatic or may present as a respiratory infection, gastrointestinal upset or a mononucleosis-like syndrome. Congenital infections and infections in immunodebilitated patients are much more severe.

Congenital cytomegalovirus infection may result from an intrauterine or a birth canal infection. About 1 per cent of neonates are infected. The symptoms vary from none to the presence of prematurity, fever, failure to thrive, thrombocytopenia, anaemia, pneumonitis, gastroenteritis, hepatitis, splenomegaly, microcephaly and evidence of cerebral calcification. Congenital infection may be complicated by the presence of a necrotizing retinitis that closely resembles toxoplasmosis. Macular chorioretinal scars may result in loss of central vision (*Fig.* 12). Other ocular manifestations of congenital CMV infection include microphthalmos, cataract, uveitis and optic nerve hypoplasia.

Cytomegalovirus retinitis in adults is almost invariably seen in immunosuppressed or immunodebilitated patients.[40,41] It is uncertain if this represents a primary infection or more likely a reactivation of a previously acquired infection. It is frequently seen in patients with renal or heart transplants and patients with leukaemia or lymphoma. Recently CMV has also been commonly noted in patients with AIDS (acquired immunodeficiency syndrome). Manifestations of acquired cytomegalovirus infection include pneumonitis, gastrointestinal ulcers, skin ulcers, rash, hepatitis, anaemia, myocarditis, mononucleosis syndrome, neuropathy and necrotizing retinitis.

During the acute phase, the necrotizing retinitis usually presents in the mid-peripheral retina with a series of small whitish opacifications that may be present at the level of retinal pigment epithelium or the retina (*Fig.* 13). With time, these whitish lesions grow

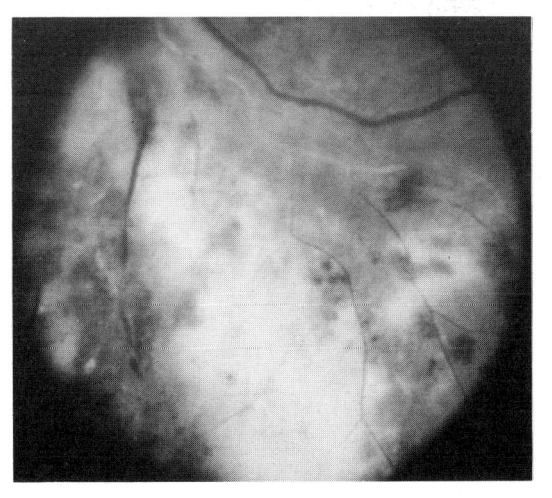

Fig. 13. Cytomegalovirus retinitis in renal allograft recipient. Classic necrotizing retinitis with vascular sheathing and haemorrhages.

in size and become confluent. Adjacent retinal vascular sheathing is common and may involve arterioles or veins (*Fig.* 14). Retinal vascular occlusion occurs with resulting retinal ischaemia or intraretinal haemorrhages. With time, the retinitis heals with mottling of the retinal pigment epithelium. The inner

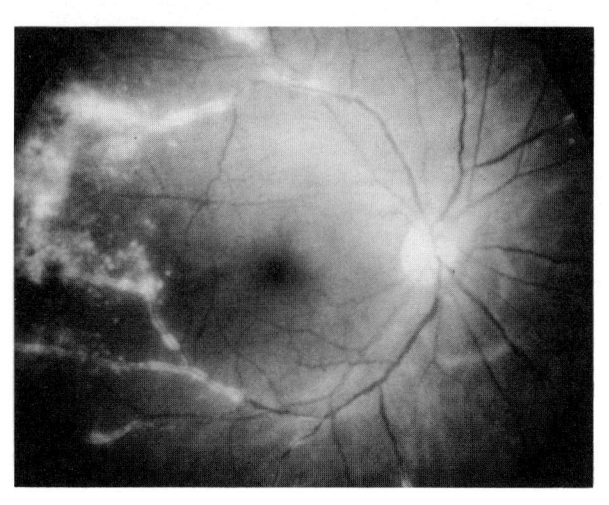

Fig. 14. Prominent posterior vascular sheathing in patient with CMV retinitis.

layers of the retina may be relatively spared. The vascular sheathing gradually disappears. The diagnosis of cytomegalovirus retinitis is confirmed by positive viral cultures of the urine, buffy-coat of the blood or ideally the vitreous or retina. Examination of cells in the retina and in other tissues may reveal the typical inclusions and giant cells. Electron microscopy may show the virus; changes in viral serologic titres can also help to document cytomegalovirus infection.

Unfortunately no drug treatment for cytomegalovirus retinitis is of proved value. A decrease in immunosuppressive drugs appears to help. Antiviral drugs like adenine arabinoside and acyclovir have been tried but without proved efficacy. As a result, the morbidity and mortality of CMV infection is high in these immunodebilitated patients. Recent studies have suggested that DHPG (dihydroxypropoxymethylguanine), a compound related to acyclovir, may be of benefit in patients with CMV infections, including retinitis.

Herpes Simplex

Herpes simplex retinitis[42] may be seen in three clinical settings:
1. Newborns with congenital disseminated herpes simplex infection.
2. Adults with herpes encephalitis.
3. Immunodebilitated patients with systemic herpes simplex infection.

The retinitis has been shown to be a direct viral infection of the retina. The retina and pigment epithelium are involved. Vasculitis and necrotizing retinitis similar to cytomegalovirus infection may be seen (*Fig.* 15). Retinal detachment is a frequent sequela. Antiviral drugs like acyclovir and a decrease in immunosuppressive drugs may be of some value in these patients.

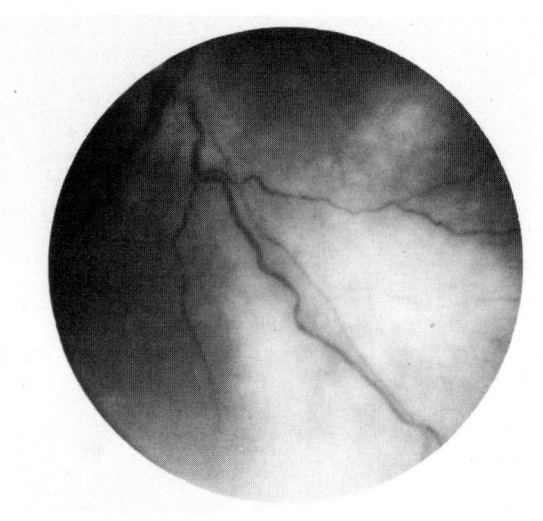

Fig. 15. Necrotizing herpes simplex retinitis in immunosuppressed renal allograft recipient with disseminated herpes simplex.

Herpes Zoster

Herpes zoster may also produce a necrotizing retinitis.[43] This manifestation is rare compared to the other ocular manifestations of zoster, which include skin vesicles, corneal involvement, cranial nerve or optic nerve involvement and iridocyclitis.

Syphilis

Ocular involvement by syphilis can occur in association with congenital infection or it can be seen with secondary or early latent syphilis. In patients with congenital syphilis, the retina may show a salt and pepper pattern of bone spicular pigmentation (*Fig.* 16). Widespread retinal involvement by these pigmentary changes can produce 'pseudoretinitis pigmentosa'. Patients with secondary or early latent syphilis may show papillitis, retinal vasculitis, retinal oedema or a diffuse chorioretinitis characterized by the presence of marked anterior chamber reaction, vitreous cells and a necrotizing retinitis.[44]

The diagnosis of syphilitic retinitis is made by the combination of a suggestive clinical picture with a positive FTA-ABS or TP-MH test. The use of a screening test such as the VDRL is not adequate to exclude ocular syphilis.

Intraocular Fungal Infections

Candida Retinitis

The commonest cause of fungal retinitis is Candida. This may be related to exogenous infection following

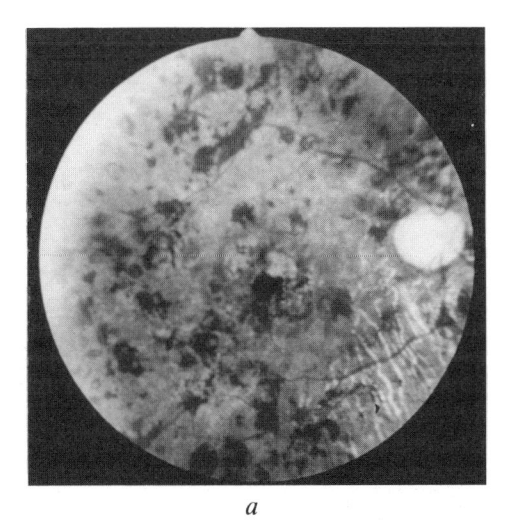

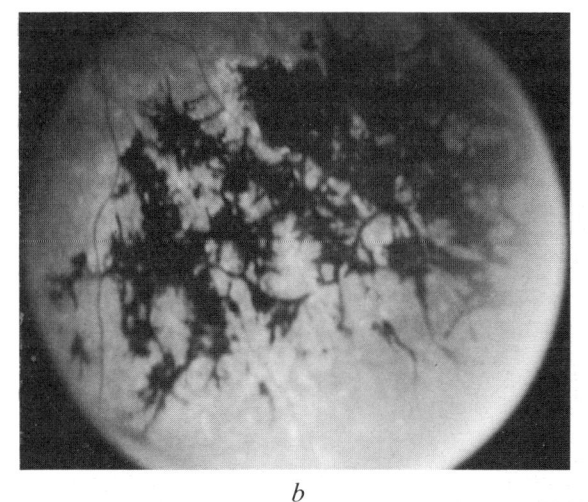

Fig. 16. Inactive syphilitis retinitis (congenital lues). *a,* Posterior pole; *b,* extensive bone spicule pigmentation in periphery.

surgery or trauma to the eye. More commonly, it is associated with haematogenous spread of Candida in an immunosuppressed or debilitated patient.[45,46] Predisposing factors for the haematogenous spread of Candida to the eye include the use of antibiotics, previous surgery (especially gastrointestinal tract surgery), intravenous infusions or drug abuse, use of systemic corticosteroids or other immunosuppressive agents, the presence of malignancy, diabetes or liver disease including alcoholism. We have commonly seen Candida retinitis in drug addicts, leukaemics, or renal transplant recipients.

Candida retinitis often initially presents as a white, fluffy vitreal infiltrate overlying a small focus of chorioretinitis (*Fig.* 17). Multiple lesions may be seen in each eye. With time the lesions grow and then eventually organize. Traction may be exerted on the underlying disc and macula or other areas of the retina. Left untreated, a diffuse endophthalmitis may develop. Usually however, the lesions heal or the patients die. Therapy of Candida retinitis includes the use of systemic amphotericin B, in some cases in combination with fluorocytosine. In debilitated patients, death is a frequent outcome of systemic involvement. In some patients drug therapy has resulted in the clearing of the infection. Vitrectomy may be of some value in treating Candida endophthalmitis.

Aspergillus Endophthalmitis

Aspergillus, especially *A. fumigatus,* can be a cause of a severe ocular infection in immunodebilitated patients.[47,48] A diffuse endophthalmitis develops with destruction of the eye. This is often a manifestation of systemic involvement. The organism shows a predisposition to invade blood vessels, similar to the behaviour of the phycomycetes. Ischaemia of the eye, including the appearance of central retinal artery occlusion, may be a presenting sign.

Phycomycetes

Direct intraocular infection by the phycomycetes is very rare. However, in patients with orbitosinocerebral infection with the phycomycetes, involvement of the ophthalmic or central retinal artery may cause a central retinal artery occlusion. Pain, proptosis, chemosis and ophthalmoplegia secondary to orbital involvement are seen.[49,50] Many patients are immunosuppressed or diabetics with ketoacidosis. Therapy consists of correction of the acidosis, débridement of involved orbital and sinus tissues in combination with systemic amphotericin B. The morbidity and mortality of this infection are high.

Nocardia Chorioretinitis

Immunosuppressed patients may develop ocular infections with *Nocardia asteroides,*[51,52] an opportunistic organism that is usually lumped with the fungal infections. Nocardia is not a true fungus but a

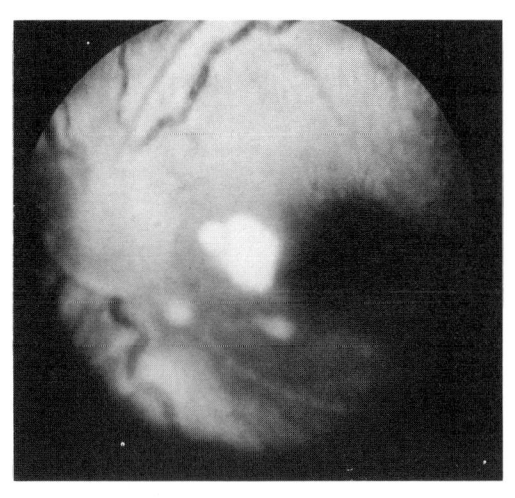

Fig. 17. Candida albicans retinitis. White fluffy preretinal lesions are seen as well as papillitis and retinal venous congestion.

filamentous bacterium. The ocular infection usually begins as a choroidal abscess (*Fig.* 18) with secondary involvement of the overlying retina. It is almost invariably seen in association with systemic involvement (often pulmonary infection or cutaneous abscesses).

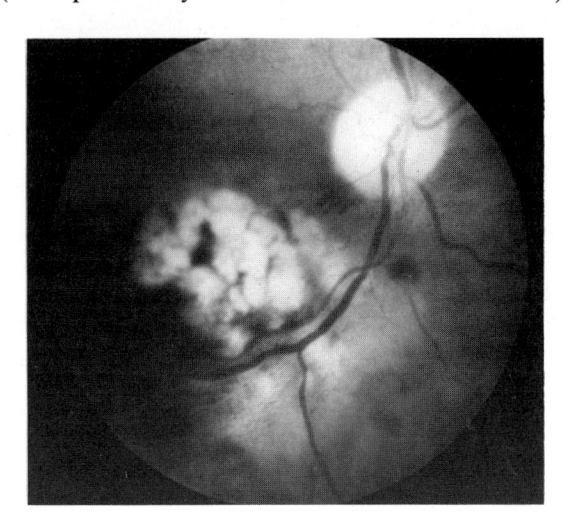

Fig. 18. Nocardia chorioretinitis, right eye. Overlying retinal haemorrhages are seen. (Used with permission of the Ophthalmic Publishing Co.).

Therapy of Nocardia infection includes the use of systemic sulphonamides and other antibiotics. The outcome is usually poor, related to the poor systemic status of the patients and delay in diagnosis. In a few cases, aggressive antibiotic therapy and surgical intervention (vitrectomy) have resulted in resolution of the ocular infection with preservation of vision.

Cryptococcal Chorioretinitis

Cryptococcus is another fungal opportunist that can occasionally cause chorioretinitis.[53,54] Ocular infection is often secondary to central nervous system involvement in immunodebilitated patients. Necrotizing chorioretinitis is seen (*Fig.* 19). The diagnosis is made by the demonstration of the organism in the cerebrospinal fluid, blood or by direct ocular biopsy.

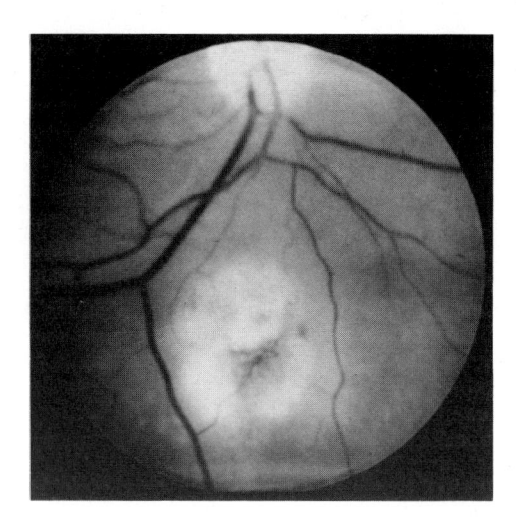

Fig. 19. Cryptococcal chorioretinitis. Choroidal abscess with secondary overlying retinal involvement. (Supplied by Jerry Shields MD.).

Patients with disseminated cryptococcosis in association with chorioretinitis can be treated for presumed cryptococcal retinitis. Therapy consists of systemic administration of amphotericin B, fluorocytosine and occasionally other antifungal drugs.

ACKNOWLEDGEMENT

Fig. 18 was utilized with permission of the Ophthalmic Publishing Co. *Fig.* 19 was kindly supplied by Jerry Shields, M.D.

REFERENCES

1. Schatz H., Maumenee A. E. and Patz A. Geographic helicoid peripapillary choroidopathy. *Trans. Am. Acad. Ophthalmol. Otolaryngol.* 1974; **78**, 747–61.
2. Laatikainen L. and Erkkila H. Serpiginous choroidopathy. *Br. J. Ophthalmol.* 1974; **58**: 777–83.
3. Hamilton A. M. and Bird A. C. Geographic choroidopathy. *Br. J. Ophthalmol.* 1974; **58**, 784–97.
4. Jampol L. M., Orth D., Daily M. J. et al. Subretinal neovascularization with geographic (serpiginous) choroiditis. *Am. J Ophthalmol.* 1979; **88**, 683–9.
5. Ryan S. J. and Maumenee A. E. Birdshot retinochoroidopathy. *Am. J. Ophthalmol.* 1980; **89**, 31–45.
6. Gass J. D. M. Vitiliginous chorioretinitis. *Arch. Ophthalmol.* **99**, 1778–87.
7. Nussenblatt R. B., Mittal K. K., Ryan S. Birdshot retinochoroidopathy associated with HLA-A-29 antigen and immune responsiveness to retinal S antigen. *Am. J. Ophthalmol.* 1982; **94**, 147–58.
8. Fuerst D. J., Tessler H. H., Fishman G. A. et al. Birdshot retinochoroidopathy. *Arch. Ophthalmol.* 1984; **102**, 214–19.
9. Urayama A., Yamada N., Sasaki T. et al. Unilateral acute uveitis with retinal periarteritis and detachment. *Jpn. J. Clin. Ophthalmol.* 1971; **25**, 607–19.
10. Young N. J. A. and Bird A. C. Bilateral acute retinal necrosis. *Br. J. Ophthalmol.* 1978; **62**, 581–90.
11. Fisher J. P., Lewis M. L., Blumenkranz M. et al. The acute retinal necrosis syndrome. Part 1. Clinical manifestations. *Ophthalmology* 1982; **89**, 1309–16.
12. Culbertson W. W., Blumenkranz M. S., Haines H. et al. The acute retinal necrosis syndrome: Part 2. Histopathology and etiology. *Ophthalmology* 1982; **89**, 1317–25.
13. Jampol L. M. Acute retinal necrosis. *Am. J. Ophthalmol.* 1982; **93**, 254–5.
14. Ando F., Kato M., Goto S. et al. Platelet function in bilateral acute retinal necrosis. *Am. J. Ophthalmol.* 1983; **96**, 27–32.
15. Jampol L. M., Sieving P. A., Pugh D. et al. Multiple evanescent white dot syndrome. *Arch. Ophthalmol.* 1984; **102**, 671–4.
16. Colvard D. M., Robertson D. M. and O'Duffy J. D. The ocular manifestations of Behçet's disease. *Arch. Ophthalmol.* 1973; **95**, 1813–17.
17. Winter F. C. and Yukins R. E. The ocular pathology of Behçet's disease. *Am. J. Ophthalmol.* 1966; **62**, 257–62.
18. O'Duffy J. D., Robertson D. M. and Goldstein N. P. Chlorambucil in the treatment of uveitis and meningoencephalitis of Behçet's disease. *Am. J. Med.* 1984; **76**, 75–83.
19. Gass J. D. M. and Braunstein R. A. Further observations concerning the diffuse unilateral subacute neuroretinitis syndrome. *Arch. Ophthalmol.* 1983; **101**, 1689–97.
20. Bos P. J. M. and Deutman A. F. Acute macular neuroretinopathy. *Am. J. Ophthalmol.* 1975; **80**, 573–84.
21. Priluck I. A., Buettner H. and Robertson D. M. Acute macular neuroretinopathy. *Am. J. Ophthalmol.* 1978; **86**, 775–8.
22. Krill A. E. and Deutman A. F. Acute retinal pigment epitheliitis. *Am. J. Ophthalmol.* 1972; **74**, 193–205.
23. Friedman M. W. Bilateral recurrent acute retinal pigment epitheliitis. *Am. J. Ophthalmol.* 1975; **79**, 567–70.
24. Gass J. D. M. Acute posterior multifocal placoid pigment epitheliopathy. *Arch. Opkthalmol.* 1968; **80**, 177–85.
25. Gass J. D. M. Acute posterior multifocal placoid pigment epitheliopathy. A long-term follow-up study. In: Fine S. L. and Owens S. L. (ed.) *Management of Retinal Vascular and Macular Disorders*. Baltimore, Md, Williams and Wilkins, pp. 176–81.
26. Bullock J. D. and Fletcher R. L. Cerebrospinal fluid abnormalities in acute posterior multifocal placoid pigment epitheliopathy. *Am. J. Ophthalmol.* 1977; **84**, 45–9.
27. Deutman A. F. and Lion F. Choriocapillaris non-perfusion in acute multifocal placoid pigment epitheliopathy. *Am. J. Ophthalmol.* 1977; **84**, 652–7.
28. Jampol L. M. and Goldbaum M. H. Peripheral proliferative retinopathies. *Surv. Ophthalmol.* 1980; **25**, 1–14.
29. Spitznas M., Meyer-Schwickerath G. and Stephan B. The clinical picture of Eales' disease. *Albrecht v. Graefes Arch. Klin. Exp. Ophthalmol.* 1975; **194**, 73–85.
30. Elliot A. J. Thirty-year observation of patients with Eales's disease. *Am. J. Ophthalmol.* 1975; **80**, 404–13.
31. Wilkinson C. P. and Welch R. B. Intraocular toxocara. *Am. J. Ophthalmol.* 1971; **71**, 921–30.
32. Santos R., Dalma A., Ortiz E. et al. Management of subretinal and vitreous cysticercosis: Role of photocoagulation and surgery. *Ophthalmology* 1979; **86**, 1501–4.
33. Santos R., Chavarria M. and Aguirre A. E. Failure of medical treatment in two cases of intraocular cysticercosis. *Am. J. Ophthalmol.* 1984; **97**, 249–50.
34. O'Connor G. R. Ocular toxoplasmosis. *Japn. J. Ophthalmol.* 1975; **19**, 1–24.
35. Krill A. E. The retinal disease of rubella. *Arch. Ophthalmol.* 1967; **77**, 445–9.
36. Deutman A. F. and Grizzard W. S. Rubella retinopathy and subretinal neovascularization. *Am. J. Ophthalmol.* 1978; **85**, 82–7.
37. Haltia M., Tarkkanen A., Vaheri A. et al. Measles retinopathy during immunosuppression. *Br. J. Ophthalmol.* 1978; **62**, 356–60.
38. Nelson D. A., Weiner A., Yanoff M. et al. Retinal lesions in subacute sclerosing panencephalitis. *Arch. Ophthalmol.* 1970; **84**, 613–21.
39. Morgan B., Cohen D. N., Rothner A. D. et al. Ocular manifestations of subacute sclerosing panencephlitis. *Am. J. Dis. Childh.* 1976; **130**, 1019–21.
40. Murray H. W., Knox D. L., Green W. R. et al. Cytomegalovirus retinitis in adults, a manifestation of disseminated viral infection. *Am. J. Med.* 1977; **63**, 574–84.

41. Pollard R. B., Egbert P. R., Gallagher J. G. et al. Cytomegalovirus retinitis in immunosuppressed hosts. I. Natural history and effects of treatment with adenine arabinoside. *Ann. Intern. Med.* 1980; **93,** 655–64.
42. Uninsky E., Jampol L. M., Kaufman S. et al. Disseminated herpes simplex infection with retinitis in a renal allograft recipient. *Ophthalmology* 1983; **90,** 175–8.
43. Brown R. M. and Mendis U. Retinal arteritis complicating herpes zoster ophthalmicus. *Br. J. Ophthalmol.* 1973; **57,** 344–6.
44. Folk J. C., Weingeist T. A., Corbett J. et al. Syphilitic neuroretinitis. *Am. J. Ophthalmol.* 1983; **95,** 480–6.
45. Fishman L. S., Griffin J. R., Sapico F. L. et al. Hematogenous candida endophthalmitis – a complication of candidemia. *N. Engl. J. Med.* 1972; **286,** 675–81.
46. Edwards J. E., Foos R. Y., Montgomerie J. Z. et al. Ocular manifestations of candida septicemia: Review of seventy-six cases of hematogenous candida endophthalmitis. *Medicine* 1974; **53:** 47–75.
47. Naidoff M. A. and Green W. R. Endogenous aspergillus endophthalmitis occurring after kidney transplant. *Am. J. Ophthalmol.* 1975; **79,** 502–9.
48. Jampol L. M., Lahav M., Albert D. M. et al. Ocular clinical findings and basement membrane changes in Goodpasture's syndrome. *Am. J. Ophthalmol.* 1975; **79,** 452–63.
49. Bullock J. D., Jampol L. M. and Fezza A. J. Two cases of orbital phycomycosis with recovery. *Am. J. Ophthalmol.* 1974; **78,** 811–15.
50. Schwartz J. N., Donnely E. H. and Klintworth G. K. Ocular and orbital phycomycosis. *Surv. Ophthalmol.* 1977; **22,** 3–28.
51. Jampol L. M., Strauch B. S. and Albert D. M. Intraocular nocardiosis. *Am. J. Ophthalmol.* 1973; **76,** 568–73.
52. Sher N. A., Hill C. W. and Eifrig D. E. Bilateral intraocular *Nocardia asteroides* infection. *Arch. Ophthalmol.* 1977; **95,** 1415–18.
53. Condon P. I., Terry S. I. and Falconer H. Cryptococcal eye disease. *Doc. Ophthalmol.* 1977; **44,** 49–56.
54. Chapman-Smith J. S. Cryptococcal chorioretinitis *Brit. J. Ophthalmol.* 1977; **61,** 411–13.

Retinal Receptor Dystrophies

A. C. Bird

Receptor dystrophies comprise a variety of disparate genetically determined conditions which differ from one another in their mode of inheritance, their pattern of sensory loss and their ophthalmoscopic appearances. Only a small number of distinct disorders have been recognized within the group, and in still fewer is there any clue as to their pathogenesis. Nevertheless, it is possible to subdivide the patients in respect of the various clinical attributes of the disorder. Some patients have symptoms early in disease which imply primary loss of rod function and examination reveals defective vision in the mid-zone of the visual field and morphological changes in the post-equatorial fundus: the diseases in such cases are known collectively as retinitis pigmentosa. By contrast, other conditions which cause loss of visual function related to cones and morphological changes in the central fundus are known as macular degenerations or cone dystrophies.

Such a subdivision is attractive and it is tempting to assume that the pathogeneses of conditions within the retinitis pigmentosa group are related to a disorder of a metabolic function peculiar to rods and conversely that macular dystrophies are due to primary defects of cone metabolism. However, many patients have combined disorders of both rod and cone systems in the early stages of their disease and all retinitis pigmentosa patients have some degree of cone loss, such that the receptor dystrophies comprise a discontinuous spectrum of disorders. It is likely that variation of disease may reflect the effect of different genes but it may be due to observation of the same disorder at different stages of evolution or different phenotypic expression of the same gene. Despite these reservations, receptor dystrophies will be considered in two broad categories – peripheral receptor dystrophies, typified by retinitis pigmentosa, and central dystrophies. Specific attributes of disorders within each group will be sought in order to subdivide the groups and achieve purer samples of disease.

Degeneration of the retina also may occur as part of multi-system disease in a variety of well-described syndromes.

PERIPHERAL RECEPTOR DYSTROPHIES

Retinitis Pigmentosa

Retinitis pigmentosa is a solitary manifestation of several genetically determined disorders characterized by loss of dark adaptation and progressive reduction of peripheral visual fields early in the disease, leading eventually to impairment of central vision. It is likely that each disease entity within this family of disorders has a different fundamental defect.

Inheritance

Retinitis pigmentosa may be inherited as an autosomal dominant, autosomal recessive or X-linked disorder. In the presence of a large pedigree the recognition of X-linked or dominant transmission of the gene is straightforward. As in other disorders, the consanguinity of the parents may indicate autosomal recessive inheritance.

When faced with sporadic cases the problem of identifying the genetic form of the disease is more difficult. The magnitude of the problem is illustrated by one series[1] in which 73.5 per cent of propositi were classified as sporadic. On the basis of the relative frequencies of the different genetic forms of the disease, Roberts[2] considered that such cases are likely to have autosomal recessive disease. However, subsequent experience has questioned the published prevalence[3] and the assumption made by Pearlman and colleagues[1] that all sporadic cases are autosomal recessive may not be justified. The disease may be X-linked if heterozygous females are asymptomatic and affected male relatives are not known to the propositus, or the disease may be autosomal dominant as a result of a new mutation.

Further genetic information may be obtained by examining asymptomatic relatives. In particular, it is useful to examine the mothers of severely affected males because this frequently reveals a mild retinal affection, indicating that she is heterozygous for an X-linked gene.[4]

The severity of the disease may be used as a guide

to the likely inheritance.[3] In general, X-linked and recessive retinitis pigmentosa cause severe disease of early onset, while dominant disease is milder. If these conclusions are correct, severe disease in the female would indicate autosomal recessive inheritance, and mild disease in a male autosomal dominance. Mild disease in a female is compatible with either X-linked or autosomal dominant transmission, whereas severe disease in a male suggests X-linked or autosomal recessive disease. It is unlikely that a severely affected individual will have affected offspring, whereas a mildly affected patient has a risk of producing affected children.

The recorded frequency of the different genetic categories of retinitis pigmentosa varies in different communities. In Finland, Vopio and co-workers[5] have reported that 37 per cent of all cases are inherited in an autosomal recessive fashion, while 19·5 per cent showed autosomal dominance, 4·5 per cent were X-linked and 39 per cent were sporadic. Ammann and colleagues[6] reported that 90 per cent of patients in Switzerland inherited their defect as an autosomal recessive disorder, 9 per cent as autosomal dominant and 1 per cent as an X-linked condition. In a more recent survey in England the calculated prevalence of each genetic type was: autosomal dominant, 26 per cent; autosomal recessive, 51 per cent; and X-linked, 23 per cent.[7]

Ophthalmoscopic Appearances

Typically, the initial ophthalmoscopic changes are seen in the post-equatorial fundus, where depigmentation of the pigment epithelium precedes the migration of pigment-containing cells into the retina. The abnormality becomes more widespread as the disease progresses. In well-established disease the retinal blood vessels are narrow and the optic discs pale, being waxy yellow rather than white (*Fig.* 1). As a rule the disease is remarkably symmetrical.[8]

As yet, studies of the ophthalmoscopic appearance of the diseases have failed to identify individual characteristics that might be used to distinguish one form of retinitis pigmentosa from another. With the possible exception of Leber's amaurosis, ophthalmoscopic differences reflect the extent, duration and severity of the disease rather than distinct types of retinitis pigmentosa. Variation in the amount of pigment has been remarked upon, but it is unlikely that 'retinitis pigmentosa sine pigmento' as first described by Leber[9] is a distinct entity, since patients with visual loss but no pigmentation have been observed to develop pigmented lesions later.[10–12] More recently, it has been shown that patients without migration of pigment-containing cells have a short history of visual loss and have mild disease,[1] and these patients may have early but nevertheless classic retinitis pigmentosa. This conclusion is supported by the histological observation of characteristic pigmentary changes in the outer retina of a patient in whom they had not been detected ophthalmoscopically.[13]

Unilateral retinitis pigmentosa was reported as early as 1865 by Pedralgia[14] and the ophthalmoscopic observations were corroborated by histological examination 25 years later.[15] In 1952, Francois and Verriest[16] reviewed the 56 unilateral cases reported up to that time and concluded that only 10 cases had the typical opthalmoscopic appearance of genetically determined retinitis pigmentosa and were strictly unilateral. Subsequent reports[17,18] have shown that minor changes can be demonstrated in the apparently unaffected fellow eye by sophisticated examination in some cases. Furthermore, Carr and colleagues[17] thought that the lesions in cases described by them and by some previous authors were due to vascular disease and not hereditable. A case report from 1976

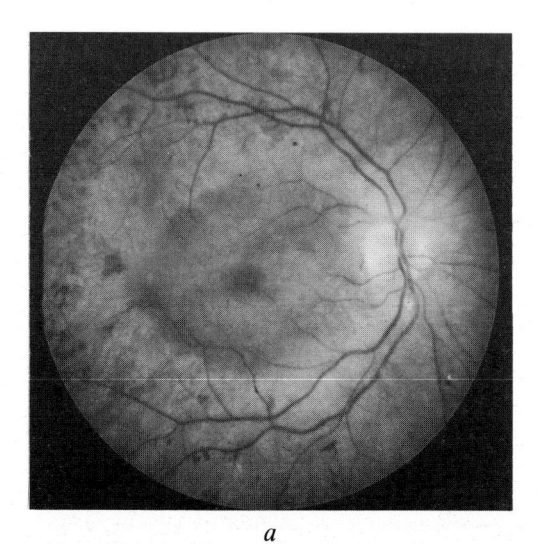

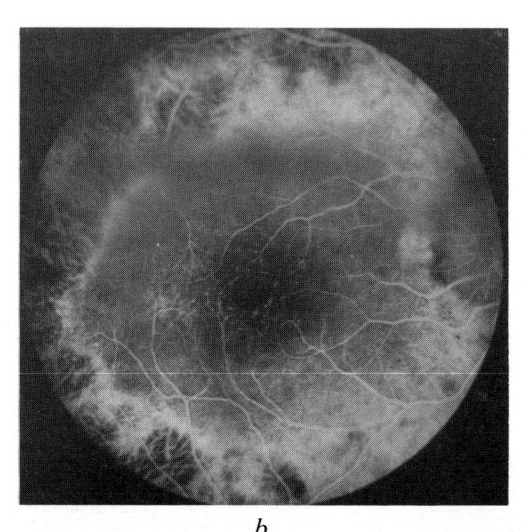

Fig. 1. Fundus photography of a patient with well-established retinitis pigmentosa showing pigment migration, pallor of the optic disc and narrowing of the retinal blood vessels. (*a*). Fluorescein angiography (*b*) confirms the extensive changes in the pigment epithelium and demonstrates dilated retinal capillaries at the macula.

illustrates the difficulty in assessing the significance of such cases. Pearlman and colleagues[19] describe a patient with mild but widespread unilateral outer retinal disease, but present no evidence as to the inheritance of the disease. It should be emphasized that in no case of unilateral retinitis pigmentosa has a family history of eye disease been identified, although, in one patient the parents were consanguineous.[20] Most workers take the view that there is no good evidence that unilateral retinitis pigmentosa represents a distinct hereditable disease.

The disease may involve only one sector of the fundus (*Fig. 2*).[21-22] When this occurs, retinitis pigmentosa usually affects the lower half of the fundus with loss of visual function in the upper field,[23] although rarely the disease affects only the superior,[24] nasal[25] or temporal fundus.[26] In most reported cases with limited sector involvement the inheritance was autosomal dominant and the regional distribution of disease was common to affected members of the family.[22,23,27-29] However, similar cases also appear in families with relatives who have affection of the whole fundus,[30] and some are heterozygous for X-linked retinitis pigmentosa.[4,30] By fluorescein angiography minor changes are often found to be more widespread than might be appreciated by ophthalmoscopy with white light, and the sector of retinitis pigmentosa may be an area of maximum disease rather than of exclusive involvement.[4,30]

By outlining clearly the pigment epithelial changes, fluorescein fundus angiography helps to define the extent of the disease more accurately,[30-32] but rarely reveals outer retinal abnormalities not otherwise apparent by ophthalmoscopy. Fluorescein angiography may also be used to identify the retinal oedema that occurs in some patients (*Fig. 3*).[32-37]

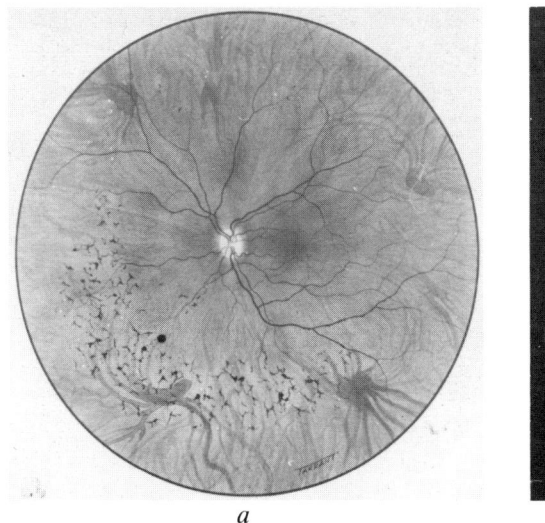

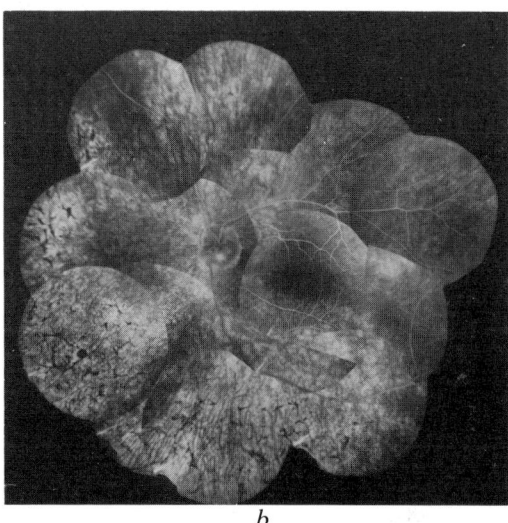

Fig. 2. Fundus painting of an X-linked heterozygote showing apparent sectorial retinitis pigmentosa affecting the inferior and nasal retina (*a*). Fluorescein angiography (*b*) confirms the regional nature of the changes but demonstrates retinal pigment epithelial atrophy in the superior fundus.

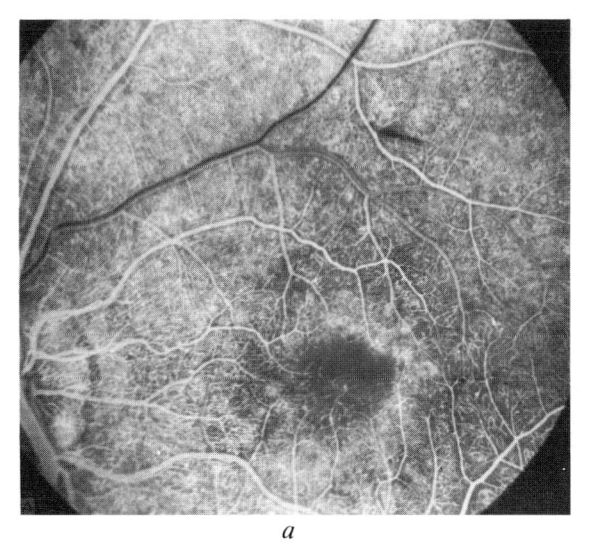

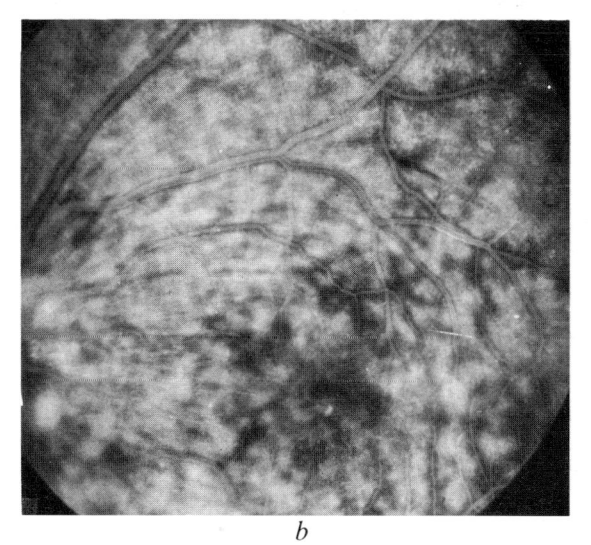

Fig. 3. Fluorescein angiography showing capillary dilatation (*a*) and widespread oedema of the posterior retina (*b*) in a case of retinitis pigmentosa.

Retinal oedema may occur in any of the genetic subdivisions of retinitis pigmentosa. In a small number of patients the vascular changes may be so extreme as to resemble Coats's disease. Oedema, an excess of cells in the vitreous and preretinal fibrosis[38] are probably a secondary response to the primary outer segment degeneration. The pathogenesis of the response is unknown, and no evidence has been found of immunological changes specific to patients developing retinal oedema.[39] Some immunological changes have been documented in retinitis pigmentosa[40] but it is not clear whether or not the abnormalities are purely a secondary response to the disorder and there is no indication to date that they play any part in the pathogenesis of the disease.

A unique fundus appearance was reported by Bietti in three patients who had crystals in the retina and in the peripheral cornea,[51] which has been termed Bietti's crystalline dystrophy. There is progressive atrophy of the retina with prominent atrophy of the pigment epithelium and choroid. As the atrophy supervenes, the intraretinal crystals disappear. The pattern of retinal functional loss is similar to that of retinitis pigmentosa with the initial symptoms usually appearing in the third or fourth decade of life. Patients with a similar fundus appearance but without corneal changes have been described and considered to represent the same disorder.[52-54] No systemic biochemical disorder has been identified and the composition of the crystals is unknown.

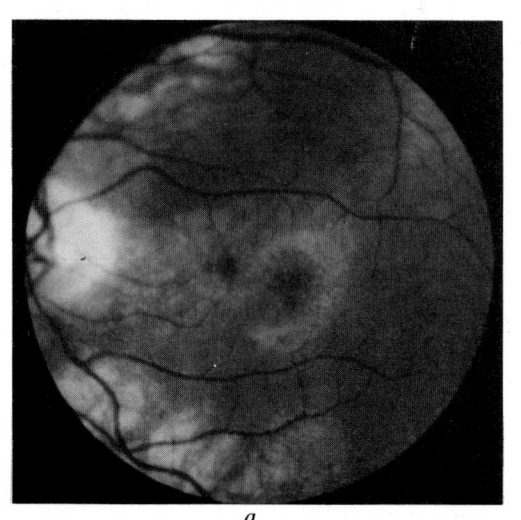

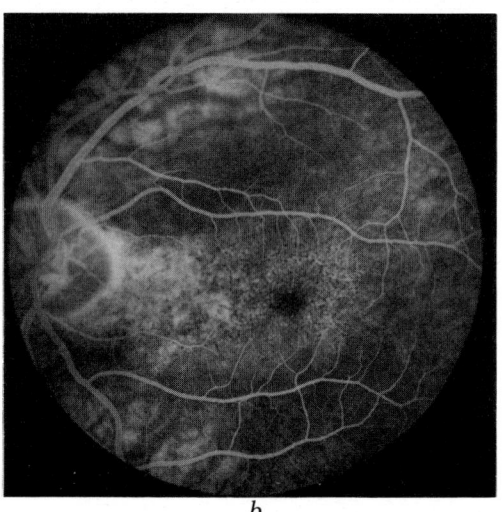

Fig. 4. Punctate reflex in the posterior fundus of an X-linked heterozygote (*a*) and irregularity of the pigment in the pigment epithelium seen on fluorescein angiography (*b*).

White deposits at the level of the pigment epithelium and Bruch's membrane have been identified in many patients with retinitis pigmentosa and the term retinitis punctata albescens has been used to identify this variant of the disease. It is not known whether the deposition indicates a specific pathogenetic mechanism.

As early as 1914, Diem[41] reported abnormal fundus reflexes in females heterozygous for X-linked retinitis pigmentosa, but during the subsequent years similar phenomena were reported in other genetic forms of retinitis pigmentosa and were referred to as 'tapetal reflexes' (*Fig.* 4).[42] An abnormal tapetal reflex has been reported to be the most common expression of the heterozygous state in X-linked disease.[43-49] Ricci and his colleagues found that this reflex could not be seen after exposure of the fundus to light but reappeared after a period of darkness; they called this the 'phenomene de Mizuo inverse'.[47] However, Schappert-Kimmijser[50] could identify this abnormal reflex in females of only one family out of eight and concluded that although this sign is useful when present, its absence does not indicate a normal genotype.

The significance of the ophthalmoscopic variations in terms of the pathogenesis and the recognition of subgroups or variants of retinitis pigmentosa has yet to be evaluated and it is only possible to speculate on the relevance of these variations to the pathogenesis of disease. The presence of disease in the lower half of the fundus in some patients suggests that variation of retinal luminance may play a part in the production of disease. White deposits at the level of the pigment epithelium may be due to a defect in the handling of outer segment debris, which in turn may be due to defective outer segment shedding, phagocytosis or degradation of phagosomes by the pigment epithelial lysosomes. The pathogenesis of the oedema is still not understood.

Certain correlates may be identified between the appearance of the fundus and the temporal characteristics of the disease. A patient with a long history of night blindness but little evidence of progression may have heavy pigmentation of the affected retina. By contrast, rapidly progressive disease of recent onset is associated with a fundus appearance of ill-defined but widespread depigmentation at the level of the retinal pigment epithelium.

Pattern of Visual Loss

The characteristic initial symptom in retinitis pigmentosa is loss of night vision which is followed by an awareness of loss of peripheral visual field. With progression, the visual field will become severely restricted, although visual acuity may be good into very advanced disease. In the late stages of disease patients also have difficulty seeing well in bright light. Visual function may be modified by secondary changes; patients with severe macular oedema may be conscious of loss of visual acuity early in the disease and rarely this is the presenting symptom. Most patients believe that their vision is lost progressively during life but many report step-wise loss of vision. The latter report that vision may remain stable for many months or years with short periods in their life when there is rapid loss of vision. In rare cases vision may remain stable after an initial period of loss in early life.

There is considerable variation in the pattern, rate and severity of disease from one patient to another, although the disease tends to be relatively constant within a single family and to a lesser extent within genetic groups. Whereas males with X-linked disease are severely affected, autosomal dominant disease is relatively mild. Variants of the dominantly inherited diseases may be identified on the basis of sectorial involvement[23] and variable expressivity.[55] The severity of autosomal recessive disease is less constant. Since its original description,[9] Leber's amaurosis has been considered to be a distinct disease. In one study it appeared to be a monofactorial autosomal recessive affection,[56] but in another investigation several forms of the disease seemed to exist, some of which were indistinguishable from autosomal recessive retinitis pigmentosa.[57] These disorders associated with the name of Leber present a unique problem clinically, but for pathogenetic purposes may be considered to represent severe forms of autosomal recessive disease. Some sporadic cases with mild disease are also considered to be included in the autosomal recessive group.

Attempts have already been made to subdivide X-linked retinitis pigmentosa on the basis of differential affection of herterozygotes. In only a few of the early reports was retinal degeneration described in females from families with X-linked disease,[58,59] but profound visual loss in heterozygotes was reported by McKenzie in New Zealand.[60] In 1960 Kobayashi described a family with even more severe involvement of the female members, 5 heterozygous females having retinitis pigmentosa, 11 having some stigmata of the disease and at least 4 being normal.[61] No accurate comparative analysis was made of the severity of the disease between affected men and women, although, he stated that the females were more mildly affected than the males. From this information, it was concluded that there are three separate X-linked conditions: X-linked recessive, X-linked intermediate and X-linked dominant retinitis pigmentosa. However, subsequent experience indicates that there is considerable intrafamilial variability in the severity of the disease in hctcrozygotes and that there is no justification for separating X-linked retinitis pigmentosa into different categories on the basis of the severity of the disease in women.[4]

The initial field defect in retinitis pigmentosa is usually in the mid-zone (*Fig. 5a*), where it corresponds with the ophthalmoscopic changes in the post-equatorial fundus. There is no good explanation for this common distribution of the disease, and although this part of the fundus has a high rod population[62] it is not known to be unique in any other way. Progress to a state with a small residual central field (*Fig. 5b,c*) is assumed to be gradual, but many patients report a stepwise progression of visual loss.

After the discovery that rods subserve night vision,[63–65] it was assumed that these photoreceptors were primarily affected in retinitis pigmentosa. However, visual loss identified under photopic conditions to white light indicates that both rod and cone receptor systems are affected relatively early in the disorder. Several attempts have been made to analyse the quality of the visual loss in order to compare rod and cone function. In the paracentral region, Mandelbaum demonstrated loss of sensitivity of both rods and cones, but the sensitivity interval between the two was reduced.[66] Zeavin and Wald found loss of rod function within 25' of fixation which was complete in some patients, and more peripheral loss of function was detected late in disease.[67] There was also loss of cone function, but it was not clear to them whether the cone loss began at the same time as the rod loss or later. The results of functional studies on foveal cones are at variance. In one investigation the foveal cones remained normal until very late in the disease[68] but this finding is not common to all cases of retinitis pigmentosa.[66,69]

Qualitative visual loss in members of a single family is relatively constant but there is interfamilial variation.[69] In some autosomal dominant pedigrees all members appear to lose rod sensitivity throughout the visual field in the presence of relatively normal cone thresholds, whereas in others there is simultaneous loss of function in both rods and cones in a patchy fashion.[70] Such analyses of retinal function appear to provide further evidence that there are multiple forms of autosomal dominant and recessive retinitis pigmentosa affording a means of subdividing the genetic groups. At least as important is the demonstration that clinical studies can identify the effects of different pathogenetic mechanisms in different forms of RP.

Rhodopsin Metabolism

Our knowledge concerning the nature of the defects within the visual receptors has been greatly enhanced by the study of rhodopsin kinetics by fundus

a

b

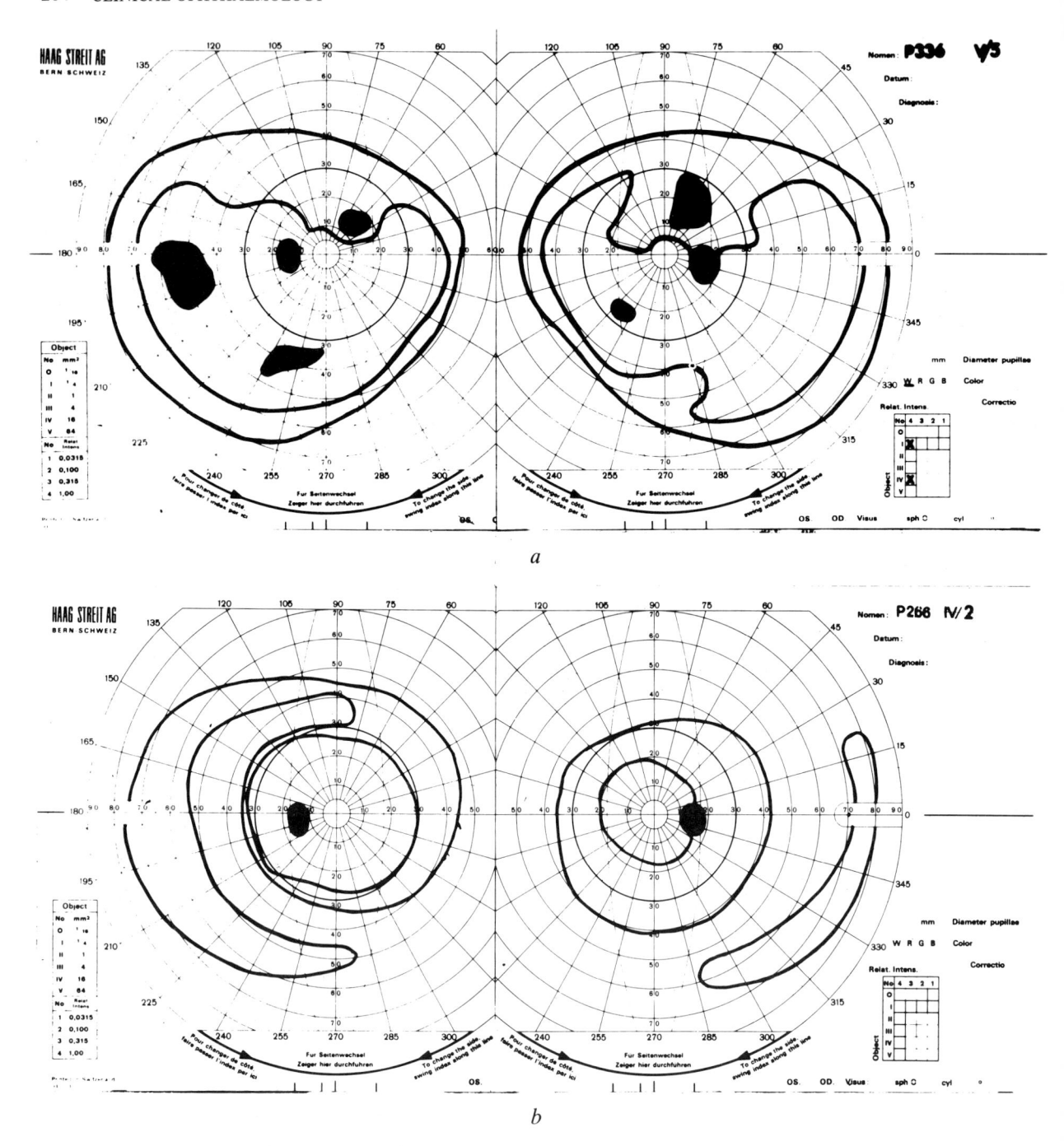

reflectometry and visual thresholds. In one study it was shown that the reduction of light sensitivity in rods can be attributed wholly to a reduced rhodopsin content in the rod outer segment.[71,72] This is in contrast to the relationship of rhodopsin in light adaptation and vitamin A deficiency, which is logarithmic.[72,73] It was with these considerations in mind that Ripps and co-workers postulated that the outer segment membrane function in retinitis pigmentosa is normal and that the reduced quantity of rhodopsin in otherwise normal rods would be best explained by the rhodopsin concentration in the outer segment membranes being normal and the rods having short outer segments. However, the alternative possibility of a reduced population of normal rods does not appear to have been totally excluded. More recently it has been shown that the relationship between rhodopsin concentration in receptors and light sensitivity is linear in some families but in others it is not the case. It has been shown in those with diffuse rod loss and relatively well preserved cone thresholds that loss of rhodopsin does not wholly account for loss of rod function and that some other abnormality of receptor cell function must exist.[74]

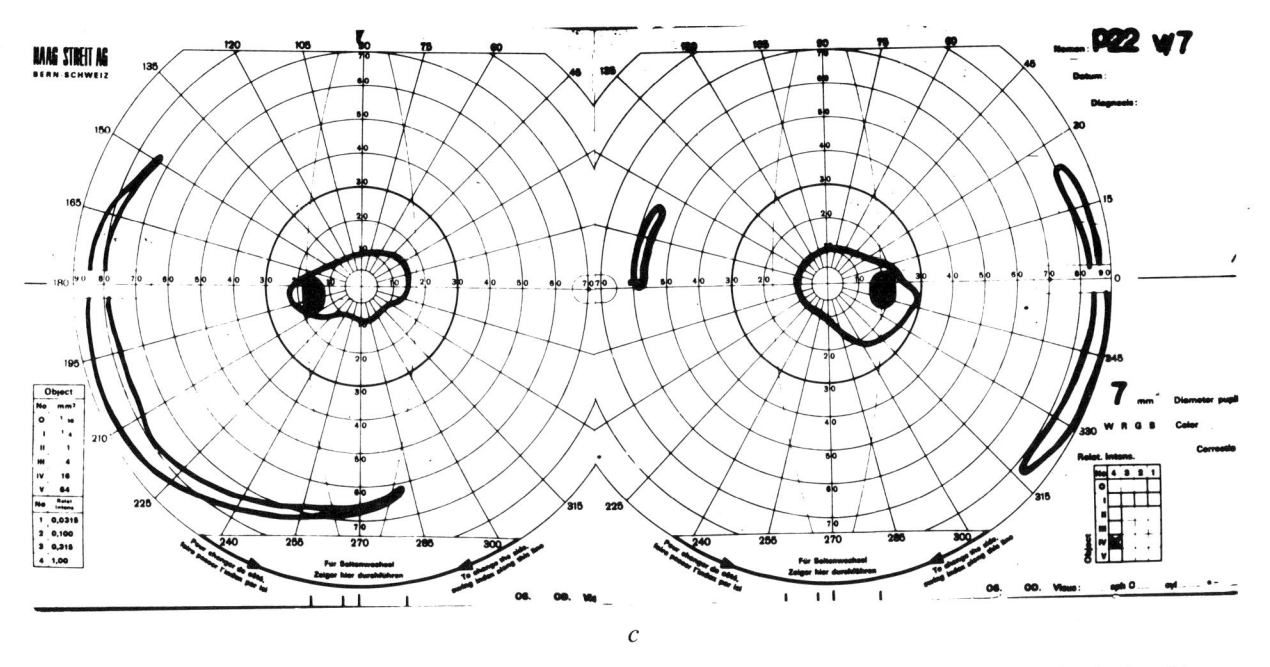

Fig. 5. Visual fields in three different patients with retinitis pigmentosa, illustrating progressive field loss. *a*, Initial defect in the mid-zone in early disease. *b*, Confluent mid-zone loss. *c*, Small central field and peripheral sparing.

Electrophysiology

Soon after the introduction of the electroretinogram (ERG) into clinical practice, its amplitude was found to be reduced in retinitis pigmentosa[75-78] and some patients with relatively good visual function were found to have unrecordable ERGs.[77,79] Riggs believed that receptor cell death alone was insufficient to account for the absence of the ERG and suggested that peripheral receptor degeneration caused short circuiting between the retina and the choroid so that potentials generated in the retina could not be recorded by a distant corneal electrode.[79] He quoted observations by Bush in support of this hypothesis; namely that multiple perforations of the retina caused extinction of the ERG by electrical short circuiting without causing massive retinal destruction.

More recently, however, it has been shown that early in the disease the photopic ERG potential is reduced in the presence of a normal scotopic response[80] and that with better recording systems and averaging techniques, ERG potentials can be recorded in more advanced disease.[81,82] These observations suggest that the reduction of the ERG in retinitis pigmentosa may be due to receptor dysfunction alone.

Using a homogenous light stimulus and an adapting background illumination, qualitative analyses of the ERG in different forms of retinitis pigmentosa have been undertaken. It has been postulated that diminution of the ERG potential in the presence of normal latency implies reduced population of normal receptors, whereas a prolonged implicit time implies widespread receptor dysfunction.[83] The ERG varies in different families with retinitis pigmentosa. For example, in members of a single pedigree with dominantly inherited retinitis pigmentosa, the rod ERG component was reduced in amplitude and in latency while the cone component was normal,[84] whereas in another family with dominantly inherited retinitis pigmentosa with reduced penetrance the cone responses were also abnormal. This finding supports the concept that the difference in penetrance signifies distinct forms of autosomal dominant retinitis pigmentosa and the difference in the influence of the diseases on retinal function implies the presence of distinct pathogenetic mechanisms within this genetic group of retinitis pigmentosa. In X-linked disease both cone and rod responses are delayed and reduced.[85]

The early receptor potential (ERP), which has a short latency period,[86] results from the photochemical reaction induced by light falling on the outer segments[87,88] and depends upon the concentration of visual pigment,[88] the orientation of the outer segments,[89,90] and their morphology. The early receptor potential is reduced early in X-linked disease[88,91] and dominant retinitis pigmentosa[92] and is considered to be caused by a reduction in visual pigment content of the outer segments in the early stages of these conditions.

The light-induced rise in ocular potential as recorded by electro-oculography (EOG) has also been shown to be reduced or abolished early in retinitis pigmentosa when the clinical diagnosis may be in doubt.[93,94] No variation has been recorded between one form of retinitis pigmentosa and another and the changes in the EOG merely reflect the severity of the outer receptor defect.

Histopathology

With few exceptions, all the histopathological reports of the retinal dystrophies are based on inadequately preserved material and describe the most advanced stages of these disorders. These diseases are not life threatening and as visual problems are usually apparent in early adult life the microscopic examination of material 20 years or more after the onset of severe visual handicap or total blindness gives little information about the underlying cause.

The retina has a limited spectrum of responses to injurious agents, and it is not surprising that the histological appearances of advanced cases of retinitis pigmentosa are remarkably similar regardless of the genotype of the disease.[13,14,95–103] Electron microscopical studies have revealed that in advanced autosomal dominant disease[97,104] and possibly in others[100] the only remaining photoreceptor cells in the retina are cones. The surviving cones are located in the posterior pole, are few in number and have an atypical appearance.

Our knowledge of photoreceptor changes associated with the early stages of retinitis pigmentosa are limited to a single specimen, obtained from a 23-year-old male suffering from X-linked disease.[105] This patient had a typical annular zone of pigment distributed in a bone spicule pattern between about 45 and 60' from the fovea. Although all the remaining photoreceptor cells in this patient exhibited abnormalities, there were marked differences between the centre and the periphery. Central foveal cones were reduced in number by about 50 per cent and had shortened and severely distorted outer segments containing vesiculated and disrupted disc membranes similar to the remnants seen in advanced disease. A further similarity was noted in the parafovea, where cones first lost their outer segments and then became progressively more disorganized as the distance from the fovea increased. In the major portion of the zone showing bone spicule formation, only occasional vestiges of cones were noted, these being identified by their swollen tigroid nuclei and in some cases tiny ellipsoids protruding through the outer limiting membrane. On the outermost border of this zone, inner and outer segments of both rods and cones were apparent and these became progressively more organized towards the periphery. Both rods and cones had outer segments at least 25 per cent shorter than those in a comparable location in a normal eye but, whereas the disc membranes of the rods were well ordered and nearly normal in appearance, those of the cones were both disorientated and vesiculated. Thus, the cones in this young patient were similar to those of the very elderly.[106]

Similar photoreceptor changes have been observed in the eyes of an 80-year-old female carrier of X-linked disease. Although all the foveal cones were lost in these eyes, cone nuclei and their fibre components in the layer of Henle could be seen in the macula. A small island of both rods and cones with shortened outer segments was observed in each eye on the nasal side of the disc central to the bone spicule zone. As in the young X-linked specimen reported by Szamier and colleagues,[105] the rods had well-ordered discs in their outer segments, whereas those of the cones were extremely degenerate.

Changes in the pigment epithelium in retinitis pigmentosa may be divided into three main classes, which roughly correspond to the degree of retinal eccentricity.

1. Cells from the central region are typically tall cells with apically displaced nuclei and a cytoplasm crammed with electron-dense inclusions interpreted as lipofuscin[97] or melanolysosomes.[104,105] They contain few melanin granules and occasional phagosomes, the latter having been found only in cells associated with cones possessing vestigal outer segments. Where extensive photoreceptor degeneration has occurred the cells of the pigment epithelium have been identified in various stages of budding or migration from Bruch's membrane.

2. Cells from the central region or bone spicule area may be flattened and devoid of either melanin granules or lipofuscin. These cells may occur in more than one layer and are often found with macrophage-like cells whose processes often penetrate to the mid-layers of Bruch's membrane.

3. In the periphery, in contrast to the centre the pigment epithelial cells contain little lipofuscin but many pigment granules. In some specimens, particularly on the peripheral edge of the bone spicule zone, localized circular regions of epithelial loss with sharply demarcated borders are found, although it is to be noted that similar findings have also been reported in the eyes of the elderly.[107]

One of the most striking features of the retinal dystrophies is the migration of pigment into the retina secondary to photoreceptor degeneration. This is seen as free melanin granules, melanin granules within the cytoplasm of Mueller cells, melanin granules within macrophages and melanin granules within displaced pigment epithelial cells. These cells are most commonly found in large clumps or masses around the retinal vessels and the basement membrane complexes of atrophic vessels, but in some patients they become orientated beneath the inner limiting membrane.[96,103] Fluorescence microscopy gives a strong indication that the pigmented cells responsible for bone spicule formation in the neural retina emanate solely from the peripheral epithelium which is relatively devoid of lipofuscin and is hence non-fluorescent as opposed to the fluorescein lipofuscin-rich epithelium near the fovea.[97] However, electron microscopy reveals that the melanin granules within these cells are predominantly spheroidal and not fusiform like those of normal pigment epithelium.[104]

Degenerative changes in the inner neural retina are highly variable, with retention of relatively unchanged ganglion cell and nerve fibre layers in some eyes long after the eye has become blind, while in others it is frequently impossible to recognize any retinal architecture. In all cases, the retinal vessels show atrophy with loss of endothelium and invasion of basement membrane tubes by both macrophages and glial elements.

With the increasing loss of neurones, secondary changes take place in the retinal glia. In areas of photoreceptor loss, the Mueller fibres increase in size and come to lie in contact with the pigment epithelium. At such regions the complex villi of the Mueller cells interdigitate with those of the apical surface of the epithelial cells, a phenomenon that has been reported in a variety of conditions wherein photoreceptor degeneration has been induced.[108] The outer limiting membrane of the retina is preserved long after photoreceptor cells are lost but becomes less clear in areas where Bruch's membrane is covered by non-pigmented epithelial cells or cells that look like macrophages. There is often a migration of nuclei of Mueller cells into regions between the inner nuclear layer and the pigment epithelium. In some eyes thin pre-retinal membranes thought to be composed of glia have been described forming a single layer of cells with long thin overlapping processes.[104]

Considerable variation has been noted in the condition of the choroid and its vessels, but most studies indicate that any atrophic changes are secondary[95,98,102,109,110] and that the loss of choriocapillaris occurs after the loss of photoreceptor cell.

Hollyfield and colleagues have recently undertaken laboratory functional and histological studies on eyes derived from two members of the same family with autosomal dominant retinitis pigmentosa with advanced visual loss at the time of death.[111] Relatively well-preserved rods were found in certain areas of the retina, which was surprising in view of the poor vision. It was shown that these receptors incorporated proteins and sugars poorly. The demonstration of poor function in the presence of good morphology is reminiscent of dominant disease with diffuse receptor loss in which the rhodopsin content in rods was relatively well preserved, although sophisticated functional studies had not been undertaken during life.

Choroideraemia

Choroideraemia was recorded as a distinct condition by Koenig[112] and the inheritance was recognized as X-linked in 1942.[113,114] Apart from its inheritance, the distinctive feature of this disorder is profound atrophy of the choroid in well-established disease with relative preservation of the inner retina.

The symptoms in affected men are identical to retinitis pigmentosa, with loss of dark adaptation and peripheral fields early which progress to leave a small central field. Visual acuity is maintained at a good level until late in the disorder. The electrophysiological responses are also severely depressed in early disease.

In males the fundus shows redistribution of pigment in the pigment epithelium as early as 2 years of age[115] and by the third decade of life there is confluent atrophy of the pigment epithelium and choriocapillaris in the mid-peripheral fundus. The disease progresses until a small area of choriocapillaris and pigment epithelium survives at the fovea[115] (*Fig. 6a*). Fluorescein angiographic studies demonstrate well the loss of pigment in the pigment epithelium and the associated loss of choriocapillaris (*Fig. 6b*).

Histopathological examination[116,117] confirms the absence of outer retina and inner choroid with relative preservation of the inner retina, although the optic nerve shows signs of atrophy and gliosis.

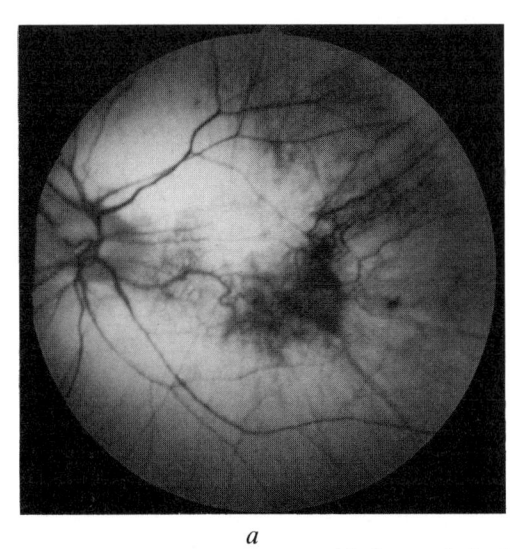

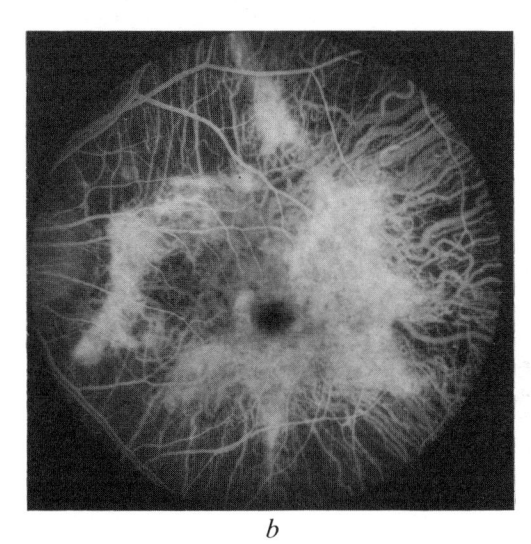

Fig. 6. Confluent atrophy of the pigment epithelium and chorio capillaris with sparing of a small area at the macula in a patient with advanced choroideraemia. Fundus photograph (*a*) and fluorescein angiography (*b*).

The heterozygous females always have abnormal fundi with changes in the pigment epithelium (*Fig. 7*) but functional loss is unusual in the young and mild later in life. Microscopic examination in one case demonstrated abnormalities of the pigment epithelium only.[118]

Choroideraemia is undoubtedly a distinct entity within the group of outer retinal dystrophies, in which the retinal pigment epithelium appears to be primarily affected by the disorder rather than the choroid as the name implies. It is likely that the prominent choroidal atrophy is a secondary response to pigment

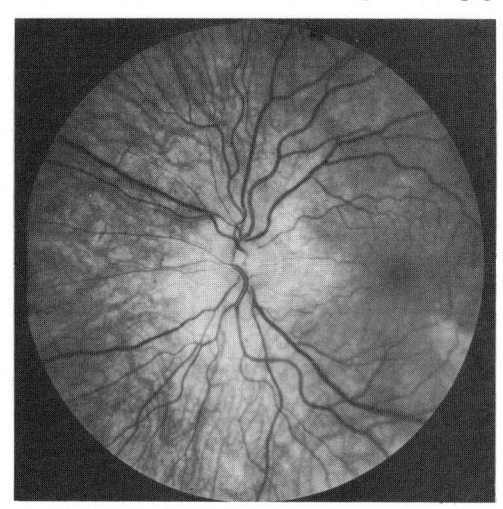

Fig. 7. Fundus photograph of a heterozygote female for choroideraemia showing diffuse changes in the pigment epithelium.

epithelial cell loss. Choroidal atrophy is not unique to choroideraemia, since it has been identified in about half the retinitis pigmentosa eyes subject to histopathological study, but profound atrophy early is unlike retinitis pigmentosa and signifies a pathogenic process different from those in other outer retinal diseases.

RECEPTOR DYSTROPHIES WITH KNOWN METABOLIC DEFECT

In three forms of retinal receptor dystrophy a systemic metabolic defect has been identified and there is reason to believe that, in at least two, treatment has a beneficial effect on the disorder. In a-beta-lipoproteinaemia and in gyrate atrophy of the choroid and retina the diagnosis should be evident because of malabsorption syndrome in the first and characteristic fundus changes in the second. There is little distinctive in the presentation of Refsum's syndrome, which implies that in any patient with possible autosomal recessive disease it is important to exclude the diagnosis by measuring serum phytanic acid.

Refsum's Syndrome

This rare autosomal recessive disorder was first reported in 1945[119] and in 1963 it was identified that affected individuals had elevated levels of serum phytanic acid.[120] This fatty acid is exogenous, being derived from the breakdown of chlorophyll; cultured fibroblasts from skin have defective alpha-hydroxylation of chlorophyll and in heterozygotes the level of activity is about half the normal level although they have no symptoms.[121-3]

Loss of night vision is usually the first symptom occurring before the age of 30 years. The progression and fundus changes are similar to those of retinitis pigmentosa, although loss of central vision and macular changes occur earlier than is usual.

Hypertrophic interstitial peripheral neuropathy is a constant part of the disorder although it is usually not clinically apparent until after the onset of ocular disease. Progressive neurosensory hearing loss, abnormal vestibular responses, anosmia, icthyosis and cardiac conduction defects are commonly found.

Histopathological changes of the eye show accumulation of abnormal material, presumed to be phytanic acid in the pigment epithelium.[124,125]

Treatment consists of reduction of intake of all foods containing chlorophyll, which includes all fat products of herbivores. The principal foods allowed are fish, lean meat, poultry, margarine and grain products.

A-Beta Lipoproteinaemia

This rare autosomal recessive disorder, which was first described in 1950[126] becomes manifest initially with malabsorption syndrome and fat intolerance. It has become clear that the major abnormality is defective fat absorption causing deficiency of vitamins A and E, undetectable beta-lipoproteins[127] and low cholesterol in serum, reduced plasma phospholipids, total lipids, triglycerides and alpha-1-lipoproteins. The intestinal mucosa shows characteristic changes, including packing of the villa with lipid droplets. Some erythrocytes have a curious crenated appearance, termed acanthocytosis.[128]

Fundus abnormalities may become apparent in the first year of life with white dots at the level of the pigment epithelium which is reminiscent of changes seen in dietary vitamin A deficiency. With time the characteristic fundus appearances and histopathological changes of retinitis pigmentosa appear.[129,130]

Progressive neurological disease develops which is usually manifest initially as abnormal gait. Abnormalities include cerebellar ataxia, muscle wasting and sensory loss.

Treatment by restriction of dietary fats and supplementation with large doses of vitamins A and E appears to be effective in preventing the advance of the disease[131,132] and reversal of changes has been reported.[133,134]

Gyrate atrophy

This autosomal recessively inherited disorder was first described in the last century.[135,136] It is typified by well defined and profound atrophy of the outer retina, pigment epithelium and choroid. It has been shown that the disorder is associated with elevated levels of plasma ornithine[137,138] and there is reduced activity of ornithine-d-aminotransferase (OAT) in cultured skin fibroblasts;[139–142] the elevation of serum ornithine levels and deficiency of OAT activity are variable from one patient to another. Abnormally low OAT activity has also been recorded in heterozygotes but they have no clinical manifestations of the disease. Hyperornithinaemia is not always associated with gyrate atrophy and fundus changes typical of gyrate atrophy have been described in patients without hyperornithinaemia;[143] in one case the patient had iminoglycinuria.[144]

The initial symptom is defective dark adaptation, which may be evident as early as 4 years old or may not be noticed until late in the second decade of life. In early disease the pigment epithelium may appear to have irregular pigmentation. Within a short time small patches of well defined atrophy appear which enlarge and coalesce. The changes are seen first in the post-equatorial fundus and progress posteriorly and anteriorly. The macula may have an odd sheen and acuity may be slightly reduced in the young, although profound loss of acuity is unusual before late disease. The optic disc and retinal blood vessels appear normal throughout the course of the disorder. Visual field defects correspond to the visible fundus lesions, being in the mid-zone initially; in the late stages the field is reduced to a small central island. The ERG potentials and light-induced rise in ocular potential are reduced in early disease. Myopia is found in a majority of patients and miosis and cortical lens changes are common. The lens changes appear to be characteristic, occurring along the suture lines posteriorly and are unlike the lens opacities seen in other retinal dystrophies.[145] Short ciliary processes have also been described.

Other systems may be affected, particularly muscles. Type II muscle fibres are affected[146] and this can be recognized clinically as muscle weakness and atrophy but may only become evident on muscle biopsy.[147] The hair may be fine, straight and sparse.[147]

It has been shown in some cases, but not in others, that vitamin B_6 causes OAT activity of cultured skin fibroblasts to increase[140] and serum ornithine in patients to become reduced.[141] It is also the case that the response of fibroblasts gives a good guide of the likely response of the patient.[142] These data demonstrate heterogeneity of the disease. In patients with little or no response to vitamin B_6 the addition of a strict diet in order to reduce arginine intake together with lysine supplementation has been tried with some success,[148–152] although these regimes are hard to sustain. It has yet to be shown that modification of the metabolic state has any influence on the muscle or eye disease.

RETINAL DYSTROPHY AS PART OF MULTISYSTEM DISEASE

Retinal degeneration has been described as a variety of multisystem disorders in many of which the retina is affected as part of a general disease of the central nervous system. In some conditions many abnormalities may be present, although the nature of the association is unknown. With the exception of two, these disorders are rare and are listed at the end of the chapter.

Usher's Syndrome

In this autosomal recessive disorder retinitis pigmentosa is associated with moderate to profound congenital stationary deafness.[153] It accounts for 5–10 per cent of retinitis pigmentosa cases. There may also be vestibular dysfunction which may be manifest by unsteady gait, positional vertigo and mental retardation.[154] The pattern of retinal disease is typical of retinitis pigmentosa although central acuity is usually well preserved into the fifth decade of life unless posterior subcapsular cataract supervenes.[115]

Laurence–Moon–Bardet–Biedl Syndrome

It is not clear how many genetically determined disorders are included within this term. Of the cardinal features – polydactyly, obesity, pigmentary retinopathy, mental retardation and hypogonadism – only the last three were described in the initial report by Laurence and Moon.[156] The syndrome was only fully described by Bardet[157] and Biedl.[158] The expressivity is also variable within a family and from one family to another.[159]

CENTRAL RECEPTOR DYSTROPHIES

A number of genetically determined disorders cause progressive loss of visual functions associated with cones – visual acuity, colour vision and central visual field, and when diffuse, poor vision in bright light. These patients also remark upon difficulty with night vision, but on closer questioning this often relates to a short transient period on first entering a dark environment.

Specific disorders can be identified such as Best's disease, but the remainder comprise a group of entities that cannot be clearly distinguished one from another.

Best's Disease

Clinical Aspects

The typical lesion of Best's disease is a round yellow deposit at the macula (*Fig. 8a*) which may be identified within a short time of birth[160] or which may develop later in a previously normal fundus.[161,162] The abnormal material appears to accumulate at the level of the pigment epithelium. Although flicker fusion studies indicate cone dysfunction much earlier,[163] central cone function remains relatively good in most patients until the second decade of life, at which time there is progressive loss of central vision, associated with disintegration of the central yellow area. The evolution of the lesion during this period is determined by whether or not new blood vessels invade the abnormal deposit from the choroid (*Fig.* 8b). If new vessels invade the lesion, there may be subretinal haemorrhages and fibrosis (disciform response), and the visual outcome is poor.[164] In other patients the yellow material may become partially liquefied, from abnormal handling of receptor outer segment material or, more specifically, cone outer segment material by the cells of the pigment epithelium. Such an accumulation would not necessarily interfere with the metabolic relationship between the pigment epithelium and the outer segment initially and this could account for the relatively good receptor function in the early stages. Krill[118] postulated that the confluent cyst-like nature of the lesion as it disintegrates may be due to lysis of the walls of the retinal pigment epithelial cells. Invasion of the cyst by choroidal vessels is probably a non-specific response common to many macular disorders (*see* pp. 223–37).

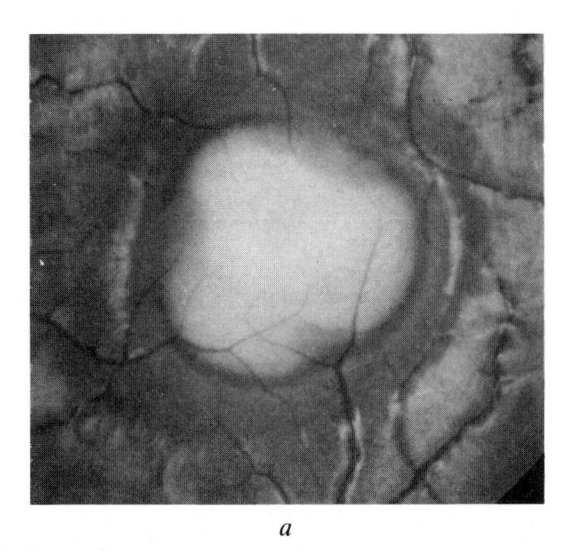

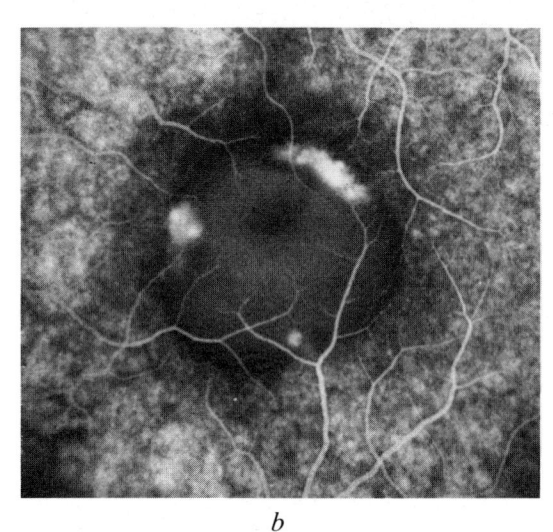

Fig. 8. Best's disease with a well-defined submacular deposit of yellow material (*a*). Fluorescein angiography demonstrates invasion of the material with new vessels (*b*).

forming fluid levels within the subretinal space and eventually the material resorbs, leaving confluent atrophy of the central pigment epithelium and choriocapillaris.

On rare occasions the macular lesion is not seen until later life;[162] the lesion may be extramacular, the disease may be asymmetrical[165] or the fundus may be entirely normal.[118,162] The rise in ocular potential induced by light is always reduced in patients with the abnormal genotype for Best's disease, whatever their clinical status, but ERG potentials are normal.[162,166]

The dominant inheritance of this disorder was first suggested by Best[167] and was substantiated later by further observations on the same family.[168–170]

Pathogenesis

The universal reduction of the light-induced rise in ocular potential even in those patients with normal fundi, indicates a widespread dysfunction of the receptor pigment epithelial complex which has possibly been present from birth. It has been suggested that the abnormal material accumulates within the retinal pigment epithelium[118] and that it may result

Until recently histopathology was confined to eyes from patients with advanced disease.[171,172] Two reports appeared in 1982, one from a 28-year-old[173] and the other from an elderly woman who had very late onset of visual loss.[174] In both studies the retinal pigment epithelium cytoplasm was filled with abnormal material thought to be lipofuscin. In the younger patient macrophages containing the same material were found on either side of the pigment epithelium. In the older patient electron-dense granular material was also found in the receptors and Mueller's cells. These reports appear to support the concept that there is widespread retinal pigment epithelial abnormality.

Butterfly-shaped Dystrophy

In 1970, five members of a family from Holland were described with a unique fundus appearance[175] consisting of patterned hyperpigmentation at the macula. The pigment appeared to be in the pigment epithelium, and fluorescein angiography showed granular hyperpigmentation of the remaining pigment epithelium at the posterior pole (*Fig.* 9). The disorder caused few symptoms since the worst visual acuity was 0·8. The most striking feature was the universal reduction of the light-induced rise in ocular potential to 130 per cent or lower in the presence of good visual function.

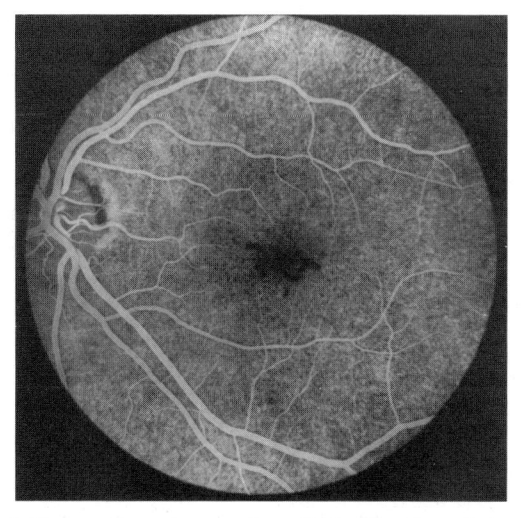

Fig. 9. Fluorescein angiogram of a patient with pattern dystrophy. Fluorescence is blocked by the patterned hyperpigmentation at the macula and the remaining pigment epithelium appears granular.

of the fundus, but no satisfactory categorization of these conditions has yet been devised, and it is likely that each subdivision contains more than one condition. Two broad subdivisions can be identified on the basis of fundus morphology, although the distinction may not be absolute.

Fundus Flavimaculatus

This broad category comprises diseases in which there is deposition of white material at the level of the pigment epithelium; Stargardt's disease[176,177] and fundus flavimaculatus[178,179] have been used to denote these disorders, but there is no evidence that these two terms describe separate conditions. These diseases may be autosomal recessive or autosomal dominant and usually cause rapid loss of central vision during a 6-month period in the first 15 years of life. However, in some cases good visual acuity is maintained until the age of 40 years.

At the time of visual loss confluent atrophy of the outer retina pigment epithelium and choriocapillaris occurs at the fovea, and this area grows slowly during the rest of the patient's life. The white lesions occupy

a   *b*

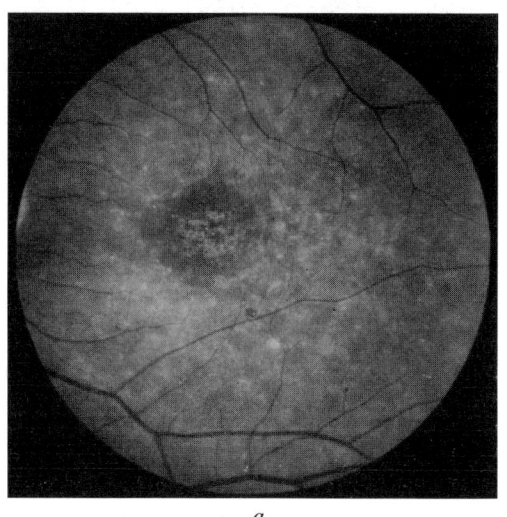

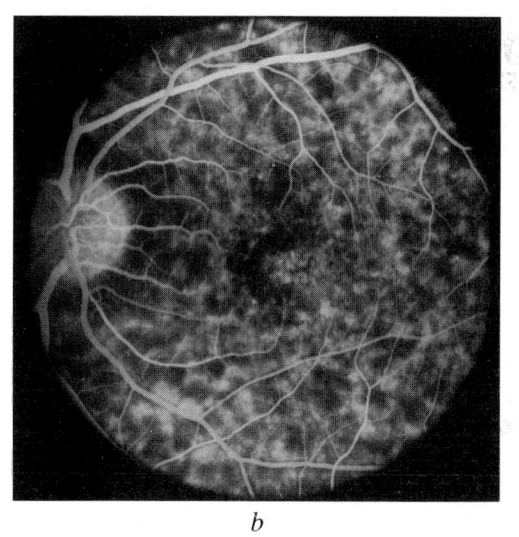

Fig. 10. Atrophic changes at the fovea and scattered white lesions at the level of the pigment epithelium in a patient with fundus flavimaculatus (*a*). Fluorescein angiography shows hyperfluorescence corresponding to the areas of pigment epithelial atrophy and a 'dark choroid' (*b*).

Deutman and colleagues[175] concluded that there was diffuse dysfunction of the retinal pigment epithelium with little associated visual deficit since there was no indication of rod dysfunction as gauged by the electroretinogram and no abnormality of colour vision. In this respect butterfly-shaped dystrophy is similar to Best's disease. The original pedigree is suggestive of an autosomal dominant inheritance, although the disease was identified in only two generations.

The remaining cone dystrophies have been subdivided with respect to inheritance and the appearance

the remaining part of the posterior pole with characteristic sparing of the peripapillary region. These lesions can be identified at the time of the initial visual loss and resolve as additional ones appear elsewhere.[180] At the site of previous white lesions, atrophy of the pigment epithelium occurs. Fluorescein angiography shows multifocal hyperfluorescence, corresponding to the areas of pigment epithelial atrophy.

On fluorescein angiography the choroid appears normal in some patients but it is not seen in others (*Fig.* 10).[181,182] It seems likely that the non-appearance of the choroid signifies an even deposition of abnormal material at the level of the pigment epithelium which absorbs blue–green light. This has been recently confirmed by histopathological studies in which it was demonstrated that the retinal pigment epithelial cells were packed with material thought to be lipofuscin.[183] Previous angiography had shown a dark choroid in this patient. In this regard, it is significant that in one study all patients with dark choroids on angiography had recognizable white deposits in the outer retina.[182] That this may represent a specific attribute of a particular disease process is indicated by the observation that this specific abnormality occurs consistently in affected members of some families with dominant disease[182] but is consistently absent in others.

dystrophy imply that the disorders are clearly separated into two broad groups. Studies of fundus appearances show that in some families the changes are constant, while in others bull's eye dystrophy may be seen in early disease and flavimaculatus lesions seen later.

In none of the conditions within the categories of bull's eye dystrophy or fundus flavimaculatus is the aetiology known, except that it is assumed that there is a metabolic abnormality related in some way to functions specific to cones. The observations of Fish and colleagues[182] suggest a defect in the ability of the retinal pigment epithelium to handle outer-segment material in patients with dark choroids on fluorescein angiography.

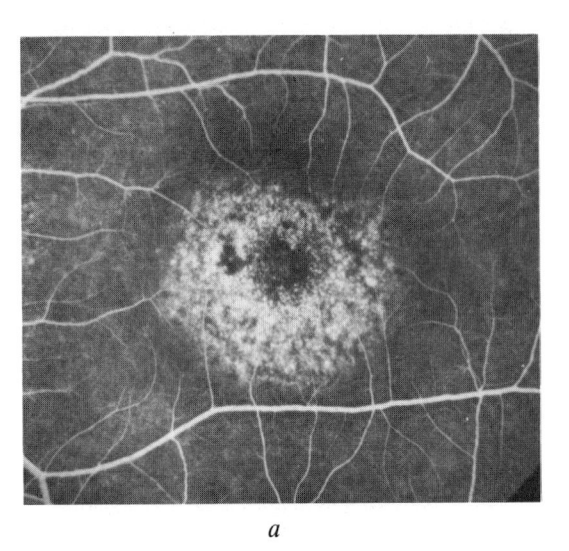

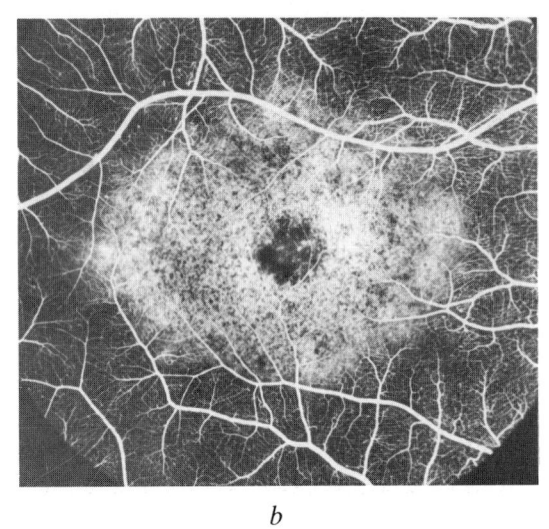

Fig. 11. Fluorescein angiography in Bull's eye dystrophy may show normal choroidal and retinal capillaries (*a*) or retinal capillary dilatation and a 'dark choroid' (*b*).

Bull's Eye Dystrophies

The typical fundus changes consist of one or more concentric rings of pigment epithelial change around the fovea, which gives rise to a characteristic appearance on fluorescein angiography. Visual loss may occur at any time during the second to the fifth decades of life and once started progresses slowly.[184] There may or may not be white deposits at the level of the pigment epithelium. The phenomenon of dark choroid is also seen in some families with bull's eye dystrophy (*Fig.* 11).[182]

The heterogeneity of this group is indicated by its inheritance as an autosomal dominant or autosomal recessive disorder, by the fact that drug-induced phenocopies occur[185,186] and by the presence of peripheral retinal degeneration in some cases. A comparable dystrophy has also been described in hereditary ataxia[187] and fucosidosis.[188]

There is considerable doubt as to whether the fundus changes of fundus flavimaculatus and bull's eye

Central Areolar Dystrophy

Macular dystrophies have been described in which there are features other than simple outer retinal neuroatrophy. The two additional abnormalities that have been described are atrophy of the choroid early in the course of the disease and the disciform response (*see* pp. 223–37). Sorsby and Crick[189] first reported central areolar choroidal sclerosis as an autosomal dominant disorder in which there is bilateral central visual loss during the second decade of life. Electrophysiological responses are usually within normal limits, suggesting that the disorder is localized to the macular region.[190] In established disease there is well-defined atrophy of the retinal pigment epithelium and choroid (*Fig.* 12).

Atrophy of the choriocapillaris or of the whole thickness of the choroid appears to be a common phenomenon at the terminal phase in all outer-retinal dystrophies. It has been described histologically in half the cases of retinitis pigmentosa studied and is a common late feature of most, if not all, central dystrophies, such as Stargardt's disease and bull's eye dystrophy. These observations imply that the choroidal atrophy is a response to absence of the retinal pigment epithelium and retinal receptors. Initially, the choriocapillaris was thought to be primarily affected in central areolar choroidal atrophy[189,191,192] because atrophy of the retinal pigment epithelium and choroid at the macula was apparently the initial or at least the most prominent ophthalmoscopic change when the patient was first seen. However, Ashton[193] demonstrated that the major choroidal blood vessels were normal in a case of central areolar choroidal sclerosis by histopathological examination. It is also evident that Noble[191] could not have been able to comment on the state of the choriocapillaris

according to the three classes of cones: red-sensitive, green-sensitive and blue-sensitive. If colour matching tests demonstrate that one of the three systems is defective but present (trichromats), the terms protanomaly (red), deuteranomaly (green) and tritanomaly (blue) are used and if one is functionally absent (dichromats), the suffix -anopia replaces the suffix -anomaly.

Deuteranomaly, deuteranopia, protanopia and protanomaly are X-linked conditions: deuteranomaly is found in about 5 per cent of the male population of Western Europe and North America and deuteranopia, protanomaly and protanopia each in about 1 per cent.[194] Tritanomaly and tritanopia, which are inherited as an autosomal dominant dis-

a *b*

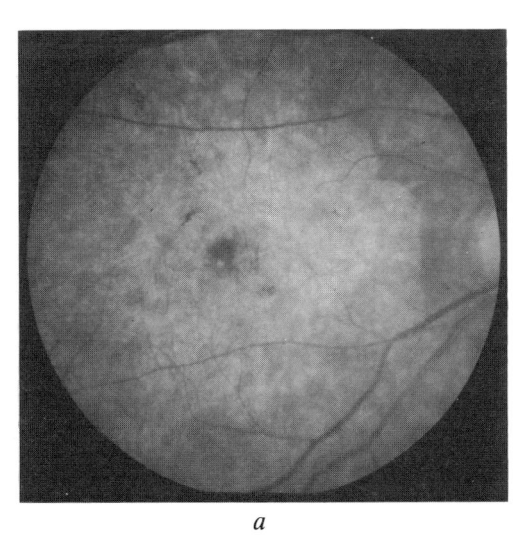

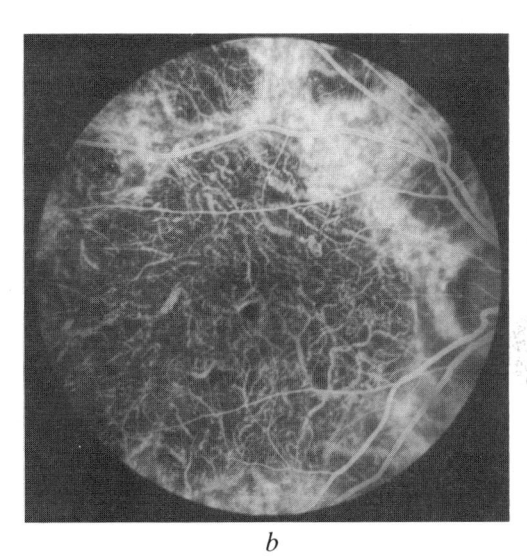

Fig. 12. Fundus photograph (*a*) and fluorescein angiogram (*b*) of a patient with central areolar dystrophy showing well-defined atrophy of the pigment epithelium and choroid.

had the pigment epithelial pigment content been normal. Clearly, there is doubt concerning the primary site of disease in so-called choroidal dystrophies. The two possibilities comprise primary atrophy of the choroid or pigment epithelium, each causing secondary atrophy of the neighbouring tissues.

It is possible that early choriocapillaris closure distinguishes disorders with early pigment epithelial cell death from those in which the disease affects primarily the retinal receptors.

CONGENITAL RECEPTOR DEFECTS

A series of conditions has been recognized in which there is a genetically determined non-progressive visual defect which may be related to either the cone or the rod systems.

Cone Defects

Colour Vision Defects

Defects in colour vision have been classified on the basis of the concept that colour vision is coded

order, are much less common, affecting 0·002–0·007 per cent of the population.[195]

Patients with these abnormalities have normal visual acuities and anomalous trichromats are often unaware of this condition. Apart from the colour defect, the eye is otherwise normal.

It is likely that the defects in anomalous trichromats relate to abnormalities in the visual pigment in the cone system. The finding that more than one photopigment may exist within each class of cones suggests that a defect or absence of one of the pigments within a specific class may account for the colour vision defect.[196–198] In dichromats it is tempting to assume that the relevant cone subsystem is absent and this has been shown in one case of deuteranopia.[199]

Monochromatism

Patients suffering from monochromatism have absent or markedly impaired colour vision. In complete rod monochromatism there is little evidence of cone function, so that visual acuity is poor, the patient has nystagmus and a complaint of poor vision in bright light is usual. The degree of visual disturbance can vary even within the same family, which suggests that there is often more than one functioning receptor system in the retina. The fundi show no gross abnormality, although the foveola may appear abnormal and changes in the central pigment epithelium are sometimes identified.[194] The dark adaptation curve is typically monophasic, fusion frequency is very low and the photopic (cone) ERG is absent but the scotopic (rod) ERG is normal.

Monochromatism may be incomplete, in which case the symptoms are less severe, visual acuity is better and photophobia and nystagmus are absent. In these individuals the dark adaptation curve becomes biphasic, the critical fusion frequency is higher and the photopic ERG is recordable but small.

Two further monochromatic variants have been described. In one there appears to be an intact blue cone system,[200] whereas in the other there is absence of central cones.[118] Complete rod monochromatism is an autosomal recessive condition, but the incomplete disorder is either recessive or X-linked, while blue cone monochromatism is X-linked and central cone achromatopsia autosomal recessive.

Four eyes from individuals with monochromatism have been examined histopathologically.[201-204] These showed a change at the fovea with a reduced number of cones and an abnormality of those that remained.

Rod Defects

Stationary night blindness

The most widely reported form of stationary night blindness is an autosomal dominant disorder.[205] These patients appear to have normal cone function but no detectable rod function. Visual acuity, colour vision and photopic visual fields are normal or are at most mildly abnormal and dark adaptation shows only a cone segment that may be abnormally prolonged;[206] there is no shift from cone to rod characteristics in the dark adaptation curve, and the ERG shows no prolongation of the b-wave implicit time between the photopic and scotopic records. However, fundus reflectometry indicate a normal concentration of bleachable rhodopsin in one case[207] and histological studies have shown no structural abnormalities either in the retina as a whole or in the rods in particular.[208]

The pathogenesis of this form of stationary night blindness is clearly related to a dysfunction within the rod system. The presence of bleachable rhodopsin within the rods suggests an abnormality of rod transduction or bipolar excitation by rods.

Stationary night blindness associated with myopia has been described as an X-linked disorder.[209,210] These patients have similar abnormalities of the rod system to those encountered in the autosomal dominant condition with less than 1 log unit of scotopic function, but in addition there is a greater disturbance of the cones such that the visual acuity is depressed and nystagmus is commonly present. Recently heterozygotes of X-linked disease have been examined and one study has shown that the amplitude of the oscillatory potentials was abnormal.[211] Interaction between receptors also appears to be abnormal in the heterozygotes[212] but reduced rod function has not been found.[213,214]

Three distinct conditions have been described in which the final threshold of dark adaptation is normal but in which the rod phase is abnormally prolonged; the defect in each appears to be static.

Oguchi's Disease

This autosomal recessively inherited disorder with prolonged dark adaptation was first reported in Japan in 1907 by Oguchi[215] and most subsequent reported cases have come from the same country, although some non-Japanese patients have been described.[216,217] In most patients defective night vision is the only complaint, visual acuity being normal. The unique feature of this condition is the abnormal coloration of the light adapted fundus, the outer retina appearing white or cream-coloured (*Plate Xc*). The abnormal colour resolves over a period of 30 min to 8 h in darkness and has been termed the Mizuo–Nakamura phenomenon, after the authors who provided the first description[218,219] (*Plate Xd*). Dark adaptation is characteristically slow and a final rod threshold may be attained only after several hours and even then may be slightly elevated.[220]

Histopathological examination has been undertaken on three eyes. An excess of cones compared with rods together with an abnormal layer of material between the receptors and pigment epithelium was found by Oguchi.[221] Parallel histological studies on the other half of the same eye by another investigator[222] failed to confirm this additional layer. He considered the abundance of round-shaped fuscin granules confined to the apical portion of the pigment cells as the characteristic feature. Histopathological and electron microscopic study of another eye more recently[223] confirmed the existence of an abnormal layer between the outer segments of the photoreceptors and the pigment epithelial cells. However, the constituents were normal components of the retina, consisting of fuscin granules and protrusions of the pigment epithelium with complex interdigitations of the outer segments. There was no abnormal cone distribution. A third histological study[224] is open to question as the patient had reduced vision with retinal pigmentary changes and both parents had retinitis pigmentosa. On electrophysiology, both the a-wave of the ERG and the light rise in the standing potential of the eye were normal, but the scotopic b-wave of the ERG was severely depressed even in the fully dark adapted eye.[225]

The pathogenesis of Oguchi's disease is not understood and although it is tempting to speculate that it is related to a slow regeneration of rhodopsin, this is not substantiated by the single study of rhodopsin kinetics in this disorder, in which rhodopsin regeneration was normal.[225] These observations imply that the primary abnormality is unrelated to light catch and rhodopsin bleaching but is related to other systems of transduction. From the electrophysiology results the region of bipolar cells appears to be the earliest stage in the visual pathway exhibiting signs of defective function. However, the presence of an abnormal layer either on the vitreal side of the pigment epithelial cells or within the apical cytoplasm indicates some abnormality of outer-segment shedding or of the pigment epithelium, whether slow phagocytosis or inadequacy of the lysosomal system.

hyperfluorescence which does not, however, correspond with the punctate white dots.[228]

Although fundus albipunctatus usually involves both eyes, unilateral disease has been reported.[229] Typically, the visual acuity and visual fields are normal, but minor loss of field has been described.[227] In a majority of cases the dark adaptation of both cones and rods is markedly prolonged[17,227,230] and there is delay in the acquisition of scotopic ERG threshold.[227,230,231] Variation from this pattern has been described in which the dark adaptation and ERG are normal[232,233] or dark adaptation shows a cone segment only.[65] It is not clear whether this variation implies various degrees of severity of a single disease or that several disorders have been described which share this fundus abnormality.

Studies of rhodopsin kinetics showed slow rhodop-

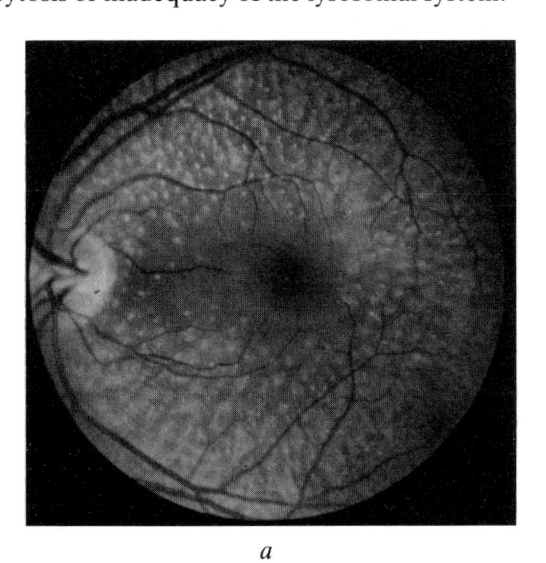

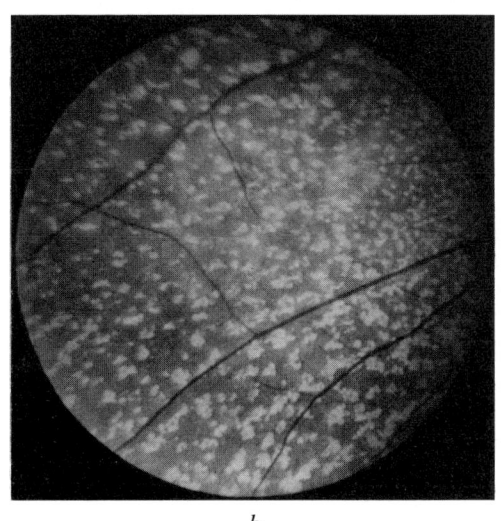

Fig. 13. Widespread distribution of white dots at the level of the pigment epithelium in a patient with fundus albipunctatus.

Fundus Albipunctatus

Fundus albipunctatus is a static autosomal recessive condition in which the only symptoms are related to defective dark adaptation.[226] The condition should not be confused with albipunctate dystrophy (retinitis punctate albescens), which is progressive and which represents a variant of retinitis pigmentosa.

The fundus shows widespread distribution of uniform-sized almost white dots at the level of the pigment epithelium, which are most dense in the post-equatorial fundus; the macula may or may not be involved (*Fig.* 13). Changes in the distribution of the white dots have been described.[227] Diffuse pigmentary changes in the pigment epithelium are unusual. Fluorescein angiography shows punctate

sin regeneration which parallels dark adaptation.[234] This implies that, by contrast with Oguchi's disease, the sensory defect is largely due to abnormal photopigment kinetics in fundus albipunctatus.

Fleck Retina of Kandori

This rare condition, in which there is prolonged dark adaptation giving rise to difficulty with night vision but no other symptoms, has been described only in Japan.[235] Dark adaptation shows a prolonged rod phase reaching normal thresholds within 40 min. The fundus presents large irregular white lesions at the level of the pigment epithelium which are most concentrated in the equatorial region. The photopic ERG is normal and a prolonged interval of dark adaptation is needed to reach scotopic potentials.

REFERENCES

1. Pearlman J. T., Flood T. P. and Seiff J. R. Retinitis pigmentosa without pigment. *Am. J. Ophthalmol.* 1976; **81,** 417–19.
2. Roberts J. A. F. *An Introduction to Medical Genetics.* Oxford, Oxford University Press, 1959, pp. 180–2.

3. Jay B. and Bird A. C. X-linked retinitis pigmentosa. *Trans. Am. Ophthalmol. Otolaryngol.* 1973; **77,** 641–51.
4. Bird A. C. X-linked retinitis pigmentosa. *Br. J. Ophthalmol.* 1975; **59,** 177–99.
5. Voipio H., Gripemburg U., Raittu C. et al. Retinitis pigmentosa: a preliminary report. *Heredita* 1964; **52,** 247.
6. Ammann F., Klein D. and Franceschetti A. Genetic and epidemiological investigations of pigmentary degeneration of the retina and allied disorders in Switzerland. *J. Neurol. Sci.* 1965; **2,** 183–96.
7. Jay M. On the heredity of retinitis pigmentosa. *Br. J. Ophthalmol.* 1982; **7,** 405–16.
8. Biro I. Symmetrical development of pigmentation as a specific feature of the fundus pattern in retinitis pigmentosa. *Am. J. Ophthalmol.* 1963; **55,** 1176–9.
9. Leber T. Uber anomale Formen der retinitis pigmentosa. *Arch. Ophthalmol.* 1871; **17,** 314–41.
10. Nettleship E. On retinitis pigmentosa and allied diseases, III. *R. Lond. Ophthalmol. Hosp. Rep.* 1908; **17,** 333–427.
11. Nettleship E. A note on the progress of some cases of retinitis pigmentosa sine pigmento and of retinitis punctata albescens. *R. Lond. Ophthalmol. Hosp. Rep.* 1914; **19,** 123.
12. Usher C. H. On the inheritance of retinitis pigmentosa with notes of cases. *R. Lond. Ophthalmol. Hosp. Rep.* 1914; **19,** 130–236.
13. Eicholtz W. Histologie der retinopathia pigmentosa cum et sine pigmento. *Klin. Monatsbl. Augenheilkd.* 1974; **164,** 467–75.
14. Pedralgia C. Klinische Berobachtungen. Retinitis pigmentosa. *Klin. Monatsbl. Augenheilkd.* 1865; **3,** 114–17.
15. Deutschmann R. Einseitige typische retinitis pigmentosa mit pathologisch anatomischem Befund. *Beitr. Augenheilkd.* 1891; **1,** 69–80.
16. Francois J. and Verriest G. Retinopathie pigmentaire unilaterale. *Ophthalmologica* 1952; **124,** 65–88.
17. Carr R. E. and Siegel I. M. Unilateral retinitis pigmentosa. *Arch. Ophthalmol.* 1973; **90,** 21–6.
18. Kolb H. and Galloway N. R. Three cases of unilateral pigmentary degeneration. *Br. J. Ophthalmol.* 1964; **48,** 471–9.
19. Pearlman J. T., Saxton J., Hoffman G. et al. Unilateral retinitis pigmentosa sine pigmento. *Br. J. Ophthalmol.* 1976; **60,** 354–60.
20. Cordier J., Reny A. and Seigneur J. P. Rétinite pigmentaire unilatérale. *Bull. Soc. Ophtal. Fr.* 1966; **66,** 224–7.
21. Bietti G. B. Su alcune torme atipiche o rare di degenerazione retinica (degenerazione tappetoretiniche e quadri morbosi similari). *Boll. Oculist.* 1937; **16,** 1159–244.
22. Haase W. and Hellner K. A. Uber familiare bilaterale sektorenformige retinopathia pigmentosa. *Klin. Monatsbl. Augenheilkd.* 1965; **147,** 365–75.
23. Fledelius H. and Simonsen S. E. A family with bilateral symmetrical sectorial pigmentary retinal lesion. *Acta Ophthalmol.* 1970; **48,** 14–22.
24. Ragnetti E. An atypical form of retinitis pigmentosa. *Boll. Ocul.* 1962; **41,** 617–25.
25. Vukovich V. Das ERG bei retinitis pigmentosa (retinopathia pigmentosa) mit bitemporatem Geischstfeldausfall. *Albrecht Von Graefes Arch. Ophthalmol.* 1959; **161,** 27–32.
26. Alezzandrini A. Retinitis pigmentosa in symmetric quadrants. *Am. J. Ophthalmol.* 1965; **60,** 1160.
27. Hommer K. Das ERG bei sektorenformiger retinitis pigmentosa (Retinopathia pigmentosa). *Albrecht Von Graefes Arch. Ophthalmol.* 1959; **161,** 16–26.
28. Kuper J. Familiare sektorenformige retinitis pigmentosa. *Klin. Monatsbl. Augenheilkd.* 1960; **136,** 97–102.
29. Lisch K. Isolierte Entwicklungsstorungen. *Med Wochenschr.* 1960; **14,** 720–25.
30. Krill A. E., Archer D. B. and Martin D. Sector retinitis pigmentosa. *Am. J. Ophthalmol.* 1970; **69,** 977–87.
31. Best M., Galin M. A., Blumental M. et al. Fluorescein angiography during induced ocular hypertension in retinitis pigmentosa. *Am. J. Ophthalmol.* 1971; **71,** 1226–30.
32. Hyvarinen L., Maumenee A. E., Kelly J. et al. Fluorescein angiographic findings in retinitis pigmentosa. *Am. J. Ophthalmol.* 1971; **71,** 17–26.
33. ffytche T. J. Cystoid maculopathy in retinitis pigmentosa. *Trans. Ophthalmol. Soc. UK* 1972: **92,** 265—83.
34. Francois J., De Laey J. J. and Verbraeken H. L'Oedeme cystoid de la macula. *Bull. Soc. Belg. Ophthalmol.* 1971; **161,** 708–21.
35. Metge P., Chovet M., Ebagosti A. et al. Oedeme maculaire cystoide dans las retinopathie pigmentaire. *Bull. Soc. Ophthalmol. Fr.* 1974; **74,** 119–22.
36. Notting J. G. A. and Deutman A. F. Leakage from retinal capillaries in hereditary dystrophies. *Doc. Ophthalmol.* 1976; **7,** 439–45.
37. Spalton D. J., Bird A. C. and Cleary P. E. Retinitis pigmentosa and retinal oedema. *Br. J. Ophthalmol.* 1978; **62,** 174–82.
38. Hansen R. I., Friedman A. H., Garner S. et al. The association of retinitis pigmentosa with preretinal macular gliosis. *Br. J. Ophthalmol.* 1977; **61,** 597–600.
39. Spalton D. J., Rahi A. H. S. and Bird A. C. Immunological studies in retinitis pigmentosa associated with retinal vascular leakage. *Br. J. Ophthalmol.* 1978; **62,** 183–7.
40. Newsome D. and Nussenblatt R. Retinal reactivity in patients with retinitis pigmentosa and Usher's syndrome. *Retina* 1984; **4,** 195–9.
41. Diem M. Retinitis punctata albescens et pigmentosa. *Klin. Monatsbl. Augenheilkd.* 1914; **53,** 371–9.
42. Mann I. *Developmental Abnormalities of the Eye.* Cambridge, Cambridge University Press, 1937, Fig. 105.
43. Falls H. F. and Cotterman C. W. Choroido-retinal degeneration. A sex-linked form in which heterozygous women exhibit a tapetal-like reflex. *Arch. Ophthalmol.* 1948; **40,** 685–703.
44. Francois J. Chorioretinal degeneration of retinitis pigmentosa of intermediate sex-linked heredity. *Doc. Ophthalmol.* 1962; **16,** 111–27.

45. Hussels I. E. Une famille atteinte de retinopathie pigmentaire liee au sexe, de maladie de Parkinson et d'autres troubles neuro-psychiatriques. Thesis No. 3064, Geneva, Medecine de Hygiene, 1967.
46. Krill A. E. X-chromosomal linked diseases affecting the eye: status of the heterozygote female. *Trans. Am. Ophthalmol. Soc.* 1969; **67**, 535–608.
47. Ricci A., Ammann F. and Franceschetti A. Reflet tapetiode reversible (phenomene die Mizuo inverse) chez conductrice de retinopathie pigmentaire recessive liee au sexe. *Bull. Soc. Fr. Ophthalmol.* 1963; **76**, 31–5.
48. Warburg M. and Simonsen S. E. Sex-linked recessive retinitis pigmentosa. *Acta. Ophthalmol. (Kbh.)* 1968; **46**, 494–9.
49. Weiner R. L. and Falls H. F. Intermediate sex-linked retinitis pigmentosa. *Arch. Ophthalmol.* 1955; **53**, 539–53.
50. Schappert-Kimmijser J. Les degenerescences tapetoretiniennes du type X chromosomal aux Pays-Bas. *Bull. Soc. Fr. Ophthalmol.* 1963; **76**, 122–9.
51. Bietti G. Ueber familiares vorkommen von 'retinitis punctata albescens' (verbunden mit 'dystrophia marginalis cristalinea cornea') glitzen des glaskorpers und anderen degenerativen augen veranderung. *Klin. Monatsbl. Augenheilkd.* 1937; **99**, 737–56.
52. Welch R. B. Bietti's tapetoretinal degeneration with marginal corneal dystrophy. Crystalline retinopathy. *Trans. Am. Ophthalmol. Soc.* 1977; **75**, 164–79.
53. Francois J. and de Laey J. J. Bietti's crystalline fundus dystrophy. *Klin. Monatsbl. Augenheilkd.* 1970; **170**, 353–62.
54. Hayasaka S. and Okoyuma S. Crystalline retinopathy. *Retina* 1984; **4**, 177–81.
55. Berson E. L., Gouras P. M., Gunkel R. D. et al. Dominant retinitis pigmentosa with reduced penetrance. *Arch. Ophthalmol.* 1969; **81**, 226–35.
56. Alstrom C. H. and Olson O. Heredo-retinopathia congenitalis monohybrida recessive autosomalis. *Hereditas* 1957; **43**, 1–178.
57. Henkes H. E. and Verduin P. C. Dysgenesis or abiotrophy? A differentiation with the help of the electroretinogram (ERG) and electroculogram (EDG) in Leber's congenital amaurosis. *Ophthalmologica* 1963; **145**, 144–60.
58. Janssen O. Zur Erbbiologie der retinitis pigmentos. Inaugural dissertation, Munster in Westfalen, 1938.
59. McQuarrie M. D. Two pedigrees of hereditary blindness in man. *J. Genet.* 1935; **30**, 147–53.
60. McKenzie D. S. The inheritance of retinitis pigmentosa in one family. *Trans. Ophthalmol. Soc. NZ* 1951; **5**, 79–82.
61. Kobayashi V. A. Genetic study on retinitis pigmentosa. *Japn. J. Ophthalmol.* 1960; **7**, 82–8.
62. Polyak S. L. *The Retina*. Chicago, University of Chicago Press, 1941.
63. Charpentier A. De la vision avec diverses parties de la retine. *Arch. Physiol. Norm. Pathol. 2nd Ser. (Paris)* 1877; **4**, 894–945.
64. Schultze M. Zur Anatomie und physiologie der retina. *Arch. Mikrobiol. Anat.* 1866; **2**, 175–286.
65. Schultze M. Uber Stabchen und Zapfen der retina. *Arch. Mikrobiol. Anat.* 1867; **3**, 215–67.
66. Mandelbaum J. Dark adaptation. Some physiological and clinical considerations. *Arch. Ophthalmol.* 1941; **26**, 203–39.
67. Zeavin B. H. and Wald G. Rod and cone vision in retinitis pigmentosa. *Am. J. Ophthalmol.* 1956; **42**, 253–69.
68. Haig C. and Saltzman S. L. Correlation of visual acuity and absolute luminance threshold in retinitis pigmentosa. *Arch. Ophthalmol.* 1955; **53**, 109–12.
69. Massof R. W. and Finkelstein D. Rod sensitivity relative to cone sensitivity in retinitis pigmentosa. *Invest. Ophthalmol. Vis. Sci.* 1979; **18**, 263–72.
70. Lyness A. L., Ernst W., Quinlan M. P. et al. A clinical, psychophysical and electroretinographic survey of patients with autosomal dominant retinitis pigmentosa. *Br. J. Ophthalmol.* 1985; **69**, 326–9.
71. Highman V. N. and Weale R. A. Rhodopsin density and visual threshold in retinitis pigmentosa. *Am. J. Ophthalmol.* 1973; **75**, 822–32.
72. Ripps H., Brin K. P. and Weale R. A. Rhodopsin and visual threshold in retinitis pigmentosa. *Invest. Ophthalmol.* 1978; **17**, 735–45.
73. Rushton N. A. H. Dark adaptation and the regeneration of rhodopsin. *J. Physiol. (Lond.)* 1961; **156**, 166–78.
74. Kemp C. M., Faulkner D. J. and Jacobson S. G. Rhodopsin levels in autosomal dominant retinitis pigmentosa. *Invest. Ophthal. Vis. Sci. Suppl.* 1984; **25**, 197.
75. Armington J. C. Electrical responses of the light adapted eye. *J. Opt. Soc. Am.* 1953; **43**, 450–6.
76. Bjork A. and Karps G. The electroretinogram in retinitis pigmentosa. *Acta Ophthalmol. (Kbh.)* 1951; **29**, 361–71.
77. Dodt F. and Wadenstein L. The use of flicker electroretinography in the human eye. *Acta Ophthalmol.* 1954; **32**, 165–80.
78. Francois J. L'Electroretinigraphie dans les degenerescences tapeto-retiniennes peripheriques et centrales. *Ann. Ocul.* 1956; **185**, 842–56.
79. Riggs L. A. Electroretinography in cases of night blindness. *Am. J. Ophthalmol.* 1954; **38**, 70–8.
80. Gouras P. and Carr R. E. Primate retinal responses: slow changes during repetitive stimulation with light. *Science* 1964; **145**, 413–14.
81. Armington J. C., Gouras P., Tepas D. I. et al. Detection of the electroretinogram in retinitis pigmentosa. *Exp. Eye Res.* 1961; **1**, 74–80.
82. Henkes H. E., van der Tweel L. and van der Gon J. J. Selective amplication of the electroretinogram. *Ophthalmologica* 1956; **132**, 140–50.
83. Berson E. L., Gouras P. and Hoff M. Temporal aspects of the electroretinogram. *Arch. Ophthalmol.* 1969; **81**, 207–14.
84. Berson E. L., Gouras P. and Gunkel R. D. Progressive cone degeneration dominantly inherited. *Arch. Ophthalmol.* 1968; **80**, 77–83.

85. Berson E. L., Gouras P., Gunkel R. D. et al. Rod and cone responses in sex-linked retinitis pigmentosa. *Arch. Ophthalmol.* 1969; **81,** 215–25.
86. Brown K. T. and Murakami M. A. A new receptor potential of the monkey retina with no detectable latency. *Nature* 1964; **201,** 626–8.
87. Arden G. B. and Ikeda H. Effects of hereditary degeneration of the retina on the early receptor potential and the corneo-fundal potential of the rat eye. *Vis. Res.* 1966; **6,** 121–84.
88. Cone R. A. Early receptor potentials of the vertebrate retina. *Nature* 1964; **204,** 736–9.
89. Brindley G. A. and Gardner-Medwin A. R. The origin of the early receptor potential of the retina. *J. Physiol.* 1966; **182,** 105–91.
90. Cone R. A. and Brown P. K. Dependence of the early receptor potential on the orientation of rhodopsin. *Science* 1967; **156,** 536.
91. Berson E. L. and Goldstein E. B. The early receptor potential in sex-linked retinitis pigmentosa. *Invest. Ophthalmol.* 1970; **9,** 58–63.
92. Berson E. L. and Goldstein E. B. Recovery of the human early receptor potential during dark adaptation in hereditary retinal disease. *Vis. Res.* 1970; **10,** 219–26.
93. Arden G. B. and Barrada A. Analysis of the electro-ocularograms of a series of normal subjects. *Br. J. Ophthalmol.* 1962; **46,** 468–82.
94. Arden G. B. and Kolb H. Electrophysiological investigations in retinal metabolic disease: their range and application. *Exp. Eye Res.* 1964; **3,** 334–47.
95. Cogan D. G. Symposium: primary chorioretinal aberrations with night blindness. Pathology. *Trans. Am. Acad. Ophthalmol. Otolaryngol.* 1950; **54,** 629–61.
96. Gonin J. Examen anatomique d'un oeil atteint de retinite pigmentaire avec scotome zonulaire. *Ann. Ocul.* 1903; **129,** 24–48.
97. Kolb H. and Gouras P. Electron microscopic observations of human retinitis pigmentosa, dominantly inherited. *Invest. Ophthalmol.* 1974; **13,** 489–98.
98. Leber T. Die pigment degeneration der Netzhaut und die mit ihr verwandte Erkankungen. In: Wagenmann A. (ed.) *Graefe–Saemisch Handbuch der gesameten Augenheilkunde,* vol. 5, Leipzig, Wilhelm Engelmann, 1915; p. 1125.
99. Lucas D. R. Retinitis pigmentosa. Pathological findings in two cases. *Br. J. Ophthalmol.* 1956; **40,** 14–23.
100. Mizuno K. and Nashida S. Electron microscopic studies of human retinitis pigmentosa. *Am. J. Ophthalmol.* 1967; **63,** 791–803.
101. Muller H. Anatomische beitrage zur ophthalmologic. *Albrecht Von Graefes Arch. Ophthalmol.* 1858; **4,** 1–54.
102. Verhoeff F. H. Microscopic observations in a case of retinitis pigmentosa. *Arch. Ophthalmol.* 1931; **5,** 392–407.
103. Wolter J. R. Retinitis pigmentosa. *Arch. Ophthalmol.* 1957; **57,** 539–53.
104. Szamier R. B. and Berson E. L. Retinal ultrastructure in advanced retinitis pigmentosa. *Invest. Ophthalmol. Vis. Sci.* 1977; **16,** 947–62.
105. Szamier R. B., Berson E. L., Klein R. et al. Sex-linked retinitis pigmentosa: ultrastructure of photoreceptors and pigment epithelium. *Invest. Ophthalmol. Vis. Sci.* 1979; **18,** 145–60.
106. Marshall J. Ageing changes in human cones. In: Shimizu K. (ed.) *Proceedings of the 23rd International Congress of Ophthalmology,* (Kyoto 1978). Amsterdam, Excerpta Medica, 1979, pp. 375–8.
107. O'Malley P., Allen R. A., Straatsma B. R. et al. Pavingstone degeneration of the retina. *Arch. Ophthalmol.* 1965; **73,** 169–82.
108. Kuwabara T. and Gorn R. A. Retinal damage by visible light: an electron microscopic study. *Arch. Ophthalmol.* 1968; **79,** 69–78.
109. Archer D. B., Krill A. E. and Ernst J. T. Choroidal vascular aspects of degenerations of the retinal pigment epithelium. *Trans. Ophthalmol. Soc. UK* 1972; **92,** 187–207.
110. Carr R. E. Symposium: pigmentary retinopathy. Summing-up. *Trans. Ophthalmol. Soc. UK* 1972; **92,** 289–301.
111. Hollyfield J. G., Frederick J. M., Tabor G. A. et al. Metabolic studies on retinal tissue from a donor with a dominantly inherited chorio-retinal degeneration resembling sectorial retinitis pigmentosa. *Ophthalmology* 1984; **91,** 191–6.
112. Koenig H. Zwei Beobachtungen van mongelhafter Enwichelung der choroidea verbunden mit Hemeralopie. Thesis, Greifswald, Ed. Kunike, 1894.
113. Goedbloed J. Mode of inheritance in choroideraemia. *Ophthalmologica* 1942; **104,** 308–15.
114. Waardenberg P. J. Choroideraemia Erbmerkmal. *Acta Ophthalmol.* (Kbh.) 1942; **20,** 235–74.
115. McCulloch C. and McCulloch R. J. P. A hereditary and clinical study of choroideremia. *Trans. Am. Acad. Ophthalmol. Otolaryngol.* 1948; **52,** 160–90.
116. McCulloch C. Choroideraemia: a clinical and pathological review. *Trans. Am. Ophthalmol. Soc.* 1969; **67,** 142–95.
117. Rafuse E. V. and McCulloch C. Choroideraemia, a pathological report. *Can. J. Ophthalmol.* 1968; **3,** 347–52.
118. Krill A. E. In: Krill A. E. and Archer D. B. (ed.) *Hereditary Retinal and Choroidal Diseases.* New York, Harper & Row, 1977, p. 1036.
119. Refsum S. Heredoataxia hemeralopia polyneuritiformis, a familial syndrome not previously described: preliminary report. *Nord. Med.* 1945; **28,** 2682.
120. Klenk E. and Kahlke W. Uber das Vorkommen der 3,7,11,15-tetramethylhexadecanaure (Phytanaure) in den cholesterinestern und anderen lipoidfraktionen der organe bei einem krankheistfall unbekannter Genese (Verdacht auf heredopatha atactica polyneuritiformis) (Refsum's Syndrome). *Hoppe-Seylers Z. Physiol. Chem.* 1963; **33,** 817.
121. Hutton D. S. and Steinberg D. Localization of the enzymatic defect in phytanic acid storage disease (Refsum's Syndrome). *Neurology* 1973; **23,** 1333.

122. Steinberg D, Herndon J. H., Uhlendorf B. W. et al. Refsum's disease: Nature of the enzyme defect. *Science* 1967; **156,** 1740–2.
123. Herndon J. H., Steinberg D. and Uhlendorf B. W. Refsum's disease: defective oxidation of phytanic acid in tissue cultures derived from homozygotes and heterozygotes. *N. Engl. J. Med.* 1969; **281,** 1034.
124. Toussaint D. and Danis P. An ocular pathological study of Refsum's syndrome. *Am. J. Ophthalmol.* 1971; **72,** 342–7.
125. Levy I. S. Refsum's syndrome. *Trans. Ophthalmol. Soc. UK* 1970; **90,** 181–5.
126. Bassen F. A. and Kornzweig A. L. Malformation of the erythrocytes in a case of atypical retinitis pigmentos. *Blood* 1950; **5,** 318.
127. Salt H. B., Woolff O. H. and Lloyd J. K. On having no beta-lipoprotein: a syndrome comprising a-beta-lipoprotein-aemia, acanthocytosis and steatorrhoea. *Lancet* 1960; **2,** 325.
128. Isselbacher K. J., Scheig R., Plotkin G. B. et al. Congenital beta-lipoprotein deficiency: an hereditary disorder involving a defect in the absorption and transport of lipids. *Medicine* 1964; **43,** 347.
129. Jampel R. S. and Falls H. F. Atypical retinitis pigmentosa, acanthocytosis and degenerative neuromuscular disease. *Arch. Ophthamol.* 1958; **59,** 818–20.
130. Von Sallmann L., Gelderman A. H. and Laster L. Ocular histopathological changes in a case of a-beta-lipoprotein-aemia. *Doc. Ophthalmol.* 1969; **26,** 451.
131. Wolff O. H., Lloyd J. K. and Tonks E. L. A-beta-lipoproteinaemia: with special reference to the visual defect. *Exp. Eye Res.* 1964; **3,** 439.
132. Muller D. P. R., Lloyd J. K. and Bird A. C. Long-term management of a beta-lipoproteinaemia: possible role for vitamin E. *Arch. Dis. Child.* 1977; **52,** 209–14.
133. Gouras P., Carr R. E. and Gunkel R. D. Retinitis pigmentosa in a-beta-lipoproteinaemia: effects of vitamin A. *Invest. Ophthalmol.* 1971; **10,** 784–93.
134. Carr R. E. Vitamin A therapy may reverse degenerative retinal syndrome. *Clin. Trends* 1970; **8,** 8.
135. Cutler C. W. Drei ungewohnliche Falle von retinochoroideal degeneration. *Arch. Augenh.* 1895; **30,** 117–22.
136. Fuchs E. Ueber zweider retinitis pigmentosa verwandte krankheiten (retinitis punctata albescens und atrophia gyrata chorioideal et retinal). *Arch. Augenh.* 1896; **32,** 111.
137. Simell O. and Takki K. Raised plasma ornithine and gyrate atrophy of the choroid and retina. *Lancet* 1973; **i,** 1031–3.
138. Takki K. Gyrate atrophy of the choroid and retina associated with hyperornithinaemia. *Br. J. Ophthalmol.* 1974; **58,** 24–35.
139. Trijbels J. M. F., Sengers R. C. A., Bakkern J. A. J. M. et al. L-ornithine-ketoacid-transaminase deficiency in cultured fibroblasts of a patient with hyperornithinaemia and gyrate atrophy of the choroid and retina. *Clin. Chim. Acta* 1977; **79,** 371–7.
140. Shih V. E., Berson E. L., Mandell R. et al. Ornithine ketoacid-transaminase deficiency in gyrate atrophy of the choroid and retina. *Am. J. Hum. Genet.* 1978; **30,** 174–9.
141. Kaiser-Kupfer M. I., Valle D. and Del Valle L. A. A specific enzyme defect in gyrate atrophy. *Am. J. Ophthalmol.* 1978; **85,** 200–4.
142. Hayasaka S., Saito T., Nakajima Y. et al. Gyrate atrophy with hyperornithinaemia: different types of responsiveness to vitamin B_6. *Br. J. Ophthalmol.* 1981; **65,** 478–83.
143. Jaeger W., Kettler J. V., Lutz P. et al. Differential diagnosis of gyrate atrophy of the choroid and retina: gyrate atrophy with and without hyperornithinaemia. *Metabol. Pediatr. Ophthalmol.* 1979; **3,** 189–91.
144. Hayasaki S., Mizuno K., Yabata K. et al. Atypical gyrate atrophy of the choroid and retina with iminoglycinuria. *Arch. Ophthalmol.* 1982; **100,** 423–5.
145. Kaiser-Kupfer M., Kuwabara T., Uga S. et al. Cataract in gyrate atrophy: clinical and morphological studies. *Invest. Ophthalmol. Vis. Sci.* 1983; **24,** 432–6.
146. Engel W. K., Bishop D. W. and Cunningham G. G. Tubular aggregates in type II muscle fibres: ultrastructure and histochemical correlates. *J. Ultrastructure Res.* 1970; **31,** 507–25.
147. Kaiser-Kupfer M. I., Kuwabara T., Askanas V. et al. Systemic manifestations of gyrate atrophy of the choroid and retina. *Ophthalmology* 1981; **88,** 302–6.
148. Hodes D. T., Mushin A. S., Laurance B. M. et al. Hyperornithinaemia with gyrate atrophy of the choroid and retina in two siblings. *Proc. R. Soc. Med.* 1980; **73,** 588.
149. Kaiser-Kupfer M. I., de Monasterio F., Valle D. et al. Visual results of a long-term trial of a low arginine diet in gyrate atrophy of the choroid and retina. *Ophthalmology* 1981; **88,** 307–10.
150. Berson E. L., Dhih V. E. and Sullivan P. L. Ocular findings in patients with gyrate atrophy on pyridoxine and a low protein, low arginine diet. *Ophthalmology* 1981; **88:** 311–15.
151. Weleber R. G. and Kennaway N. G. Clinical trial of vitamin B_6 for gyrate atrophy of the choroid and retina. *Ophthalmology* 1981; **88,** 316–24.
152. Valle D., Walser M., Brusilow S. et al. Gyrate atrophy of the choroid and retina: biochemical considerations and experience with an arginine restricted diet. *Ophthalmology* 1981; **88,** 325–30.
153. Usher C. H. On the inheritance of retinitis pigmentosa with notes of cases. *R. Lond. Ophthalmol. Hosp. Rep.* 1914; **23,** 130–236.
154. Hallgren B. Retinitis pigmentosa combined with congenital deafness; with vestibulo-cerebelar ataxia and mental abnormality in a proportion of cases: a clinical and genetics-statistical study. *Acta Psychiatr Scand Suppl.* 1959; **138,** 5–101.
155. Fishman G., Vasquez V., Fishman M. et al. Visual loss and foveal lesions in Usher's syndrome. *Br. J. Ophthalmol.* 1979; **63,** 484–8.

156. Laurence J. Z. and Moon R. C. Four cases of retinitis pigmentosa occurring in the same family and accompanied by general imperfections of development. *Ophthalmol. Rev.* 1866; **2**, 32–41.
157. Bardet G. Sur un syndrome d'obesite infantile avec polydactylie et retinite pigmentaire (contributions a l'etude des formes cliniques et l'obesite hypophysaire). Thesis, Paris, 1920.
158. Biedl A. Ein Geschwisterpaar mit adipose-genitale dystrophie. *Med. Klin.* 1922; **18**, 1041.
159. Bell J. The Laurence Moon syndrome. In: *Treasure of Human Inheritance.* London, Cambridge University Press, vol. 15, pt III, 1958.
160. Barkman Y. A clinical study of a central tapeoretinal degeneration. *Acta Ophthalmol.* 1961; **39**, 663–71.
161. Barricks M. E. Vitelliform lesions developing in normal fundi. *Am. Ophthalmol.* 1977; **83**, 324–7.
162. Deutman A. F. *The Hereditary Dystrophies of the Posterior Pole of the Eye.* Assen, Netherlands, Van Gorcum, 1971.
163. Massof R. W., Fleishman J. A., Fine S. L. et al. Flicker fusion thresholds in Best's macular dystrophy. *Arch. Ophthalmol.* 1977; **95**, 991–4.
164. Miller S. A., Bresnik G. H. and Chandra S. R. Choroidal neovascular membrane in Best's vitelliform macular dystrophy. *Am. J. Ophthalmol.* 1976; **82**, 252–5.
165. Maloney W. F., Robertson D. M. and Duboff S. M. Hereditary vitelliform macular degeneration. *Arch. Ophthalmol.* 1977; **95**, 979–83.
166. Deutman A. F. Electro-ocularograph in families with vitelliform dystrophy of the fovea. *Arch. Ophthalmol.* 1969; **81**, 305–16.
167. Best F. Uber eine hereditaire Maculaaffektion: Beitrage zur Vererbungslehre. *Z. Augenheilkd.* 1905; **13**, 199–212.
168. Jung E. E. Uber eine Sippe mit Angeborener macular degeneration. Thesis, Gissen, Seibert, 1936, p. 20.
169. Vossius A. Uber die bestsche familiare macular degeneration. *Albrecht Von Graefes Arch. Ophthalmol.* 1921, **105**, 1050–7.
170. Weisel G. Uber die Bestsche Familiare Maculadegeneration. Thesis, Giessen, 1922.
171. Anderson S. Quoted by A. E. Krill. In: *Hereditary and Choroidal Diseases,* New York, Harper & Row, 1977, p. 697.
172. McFarland C. B. Heredodegeneration of macula lutea; study of clinical and pathological aspects. *Arch. Ophthalmol.* 1955; **53**, 224–8.
173. Weingeist T. A., Kobrin J. L. and Watzke R. C. Histopathology of Best's macular dystrophy. *Arch. Ophthalmol.* 1982; **100**, 1108–14.
174. Frangieh G. T., Green R. and Fine S. L. A histopathological study of Best's macular dystrophy. *Arch. Ophthalmol.* 1982; **100**, 1115–21.
175. Deutman A. F., van Blommestein J. D. A., Henkes H. E. et al. Butterfly shaped pigment dystrophy of the fovea. *Arch. Ophthalmol.* 1970; **83**, 558–69.
176. Stargardt K. Uber familiare, progressive degeneration in der makulagegend des auges. *Albrecht von Graefes. Arch. Ophthalmol.* 1909; **71**, 534–50.
177. Stargardt K. Uber familiare, progressive degeneration in der maculagegend des auges. *Z. Augenheilkd.* 1913; **30**, 95–116.
178. Franceschetti A. Uber tapeto-retinale degeneration in Kindesalter. In: *Entwicklung und Fortschritt in der Augenheilkhunde.* Stuttgart, Enke Verlag, 1963, p. 107.
179. Franceschetti A. and Francois J. Fundus flavimaculatus. *Arch. Ophthalmol. (Paris)* 1965; **25**, 505–30.
180. Hadden O. B. and Gass J. D. M. Fundus flavimaculatus and Stargardt's disease. *Am. J. Ophthalmol.* 1976; **82**, 527–39.
181. Bonin P. Le signe du silence choroidien dans les degenerescences tapeto-retiniennes centrales examinees sous fluoresceine. *Bull. Soc. Ophthalmol. Fr.* 1971; **71**, 348–51.
182. Fish G., Grey R. H. B., Sehmi K. S. et al. The dark choroid in posterior retinal dystrophies. *Br. J. Ophthalmol.* 1981; **65**, 359–63.
183. Eagle R. C., Lucier A. C., Bernardino J. R. et al. Retinal pigment epithelial abnormalities in fundus flavimaculatus; a light and electron microscopic study. *Ophthalmology* 1980; **87**, 1189–200.
184. Grey R. H. B., Blach R. K. and Barnard W. M. Bull's eye maculopathy with early cone degeneration. *Br. J. Ophthalmol.* 1977; **61**, 702–18.
185. Kearns T. P. and Hollenhorst R. W. Chloroquine retinopathy. Evaluation by fluorescein angiography. *Arch. Ophthalmol.* 1966; **76**, 378–84.
186. Krill A. E., Potts A. M. and Johanson C. E. Chloroquine retinopathy. Investigation of discrepancy between dark adaptation and electroretinographic findings in advanced stages. *Am. J. Ophthalmol.* 1971; **71**, 530–43.
187. Bjork A., Lindbalm V. and Wadanstein L. Retinal degeneration in hereditary ataxia. *J. Neurol. Neurosurg. Psychiatry* 1956; **19**, 186–93.
188. Snodgrass N. B. Ocular findings in fucosidosis. *Br. J. Ophthalmol.* 1976; **60**, 508–11.
189. Sorsby A. and Crick R. P. Central areolar choroidal sclerosis. *Br. J. Ophthalmol.* 1953; **37**, 129–39.
190. Carr R. E., Mittl R. N. and Noble K. G. Choroidal abiotrophies. *Trans. Am. Acad. Ophthalmol. Otolaryngol.* 1975; **79**, 796–816.
191. Noble K. G. Central areolar choroidal dystrophy. *Am. J. Ophthalmol.* 1977; **84**, 310–18.
192. Sorsby A. Choroidal angiosclerosis with special reference to its hereditary character. *Br. J. Ophthalmol.* 1939; **23**, 433–44.
193. Ashton N. Central areolar choroidal sclerosis. A histopathological study. *Br. J. Ophthalmol.* 1953; **37**, 140–7.

194. Waardenberg P. J., Franceschetti A. and Klein D. *Genetics and Ophthalmology*, vol. 2, Springfield, Ill., Thomas, 1963, p. 1736.
195. Verriest M. G. Recent progress in the study of acquired deficiencies of colour vision. *Bull. Soc. Ophthalmol. Fr.* 1974; **74**, 595–620.
196. Bowmaker J. K. and Dartnell H. J. A. Visual pigments in rods and cones in human retina. *J. Physiol.* 1980; **298**, 501–11.
197. Bowmaker J. K., Dartnell H. J. A. and Mollon J. D. Microspectrophotometric demonstration of 4 classes of photoreceptors in an Old World primate: *Maccac fasiculus*. *J. Physiol.* 1980; **298**, 131–43.
198. Bowmaker J. K. and Mollon J. D. Primate microspectrophotometry and its implications for colour deficiencies. Proceedings of the 5th Symposium of the International Research Group on Colour Deficiencies. Hilger, Bristol, 1980.
199. Mollon J. D., Bowmaker J. K., Dartnall J. A. et al. In: Verriest G. (ed.) *Microspectrophotometric and Psychophysical Results for the Same Deuteranopic Observer*. The Hague, Junk. 1984, pp. 303–10.
200. Alpern M., Lee G. B. and Spirey B. E. Pi cone monochromatism. *Arch. Ophthalmol.* 1965; **74**, 334–7.
201. Falls H. F., Wolter J. R. and Alpern M. Typical total monochromacy. *Arch. Ophthalmol.* 1965; **74**, 610–16.
202. Glickstein M. and Heath G. G. Receptors in the monochromat eye. *Vis. Res.* 1975; **15**, 633–6.
203. Harrison R., Hoefnagel D. and Hayward J. N. Congenital total colour blindness: A clinicopathological report. *Arch. Ophthalmol.* 1960; **64**, 685–92.
204. Larsen H. Demonstration mikroskopischer Praparate von einem monochromatischen Auge. *Klin. Monatsbl. Augenheilkd.* 1921; **67**, 301–2.
205. Dejean C. and Gassenc R. Note sur la genealogie de la famille Nougaret. Vendemain. *Bull. Soc. Ophthalmol. Fr.* 1949; **1**, 96–9.
206. Krill A. E. and Martin D. Photopic abnormalities in congenital stationary night blindness. *Invest. Ophthalmol.* 1971; **10**, 625–36.
207. Carr R. E., Ripps H., Seigel I. M. et al. Rhodopsin and the electrical activity of the retina in congenital night blindness. *Invest. Ophthalmol.* 1966; **5**, 497–507.
208. Vaghefi H. A., Green R., Kelly J. S. et al. Correlation of clinicopathological findings in a patient: congenital night blindness, branch retinal vein occlusion, cilioretinal artery, drusen of the nerve head and intraretinal pigmented lesion. *Arch. Ophthalmol.* 1978; **96**, 2079–104.
209. Forsius H. and Eriksson A. W. Diferents aspects ophthalmoscopiques de la degenerescence tapetoretinienne chez les habitants d'un archipel. *Ophthalmologica* 1964; **147**, 40–56.
210. Krill A. E. and Martin D. Photopic abnormalities in congenital stationary night blindness. *Invest. Ophthalmol.* 1971; **10**, 625–36.
211. Miyake Y. and Kawase Y. Reduced amplitude of oscillatory potentials in female carriers of X-linked recessive congenital stationary night blindness. *Am. J. Ophthalmol.* 1984; **98**, 208–15.
212. Arden G. Personal communication, 1984.
213. Krill A. E. X-chromosomal-linked diseases affecting the eye. Status of the heterozygote female. *Trans. Am. Ophthalmol. Soc.* 1969; **67**, 535–608.
214. Syversen K. Sex-linked essential nyctalopia in a Norwegian family. *Acta Ophthalmol.* 1974; **145**, 52.
215. Oguchi C. Uber einen Fall von eigenartiger Hemeralopie. *Nippon Gankakai Zasshi* 1907; **11**, 123.
216. Klein B. A. A Case of so-called Ouguchi's disease in the USA. *Am. J. Ophthalmol.* 1939; **22**, 953–5.
217. Winn S., Tasman W., Spaeth G. et al. Ouguchi's disease in Negroes. *Arch. Ophthalmol.* 1969; **81**, 501–7.
218. Mizuo A. On new discovery in dark adaptation in Oguchi's disease. *Acta Soc. Ophthalmol. Japn.* 1913; **17**, 1148.
219. Nakamura B. Uber ein neues phenomen der farberveranderung des menschlichen augenhintergrundes in Ausammenhang mit der fortschreitenden Dunkeladaptation. *Klin. Monatsbl. Augenheilkd.* 1920; **65**, 83–5.
220. Francois J. and Verriest G. La Maladie d'Oguchi. *Bull. Soc. Belg. Ophthalmol.* 1954; **108**, 465–506.
221. Oguchi C. Zur anatomie der sogenannten. Oguchischen Krankheit Albrecht von Graefes. *Arch. Klin. Ophthalmol.* 1925; **115**, 234–45.
222. Yamanaka T. Existiert die Pigmentrerschieburg in Retinalepithel in menschlichen Auge? Der erste Sektionsfall von sogenannter Oguchischer Krankheit. *Klin. Monatsbl. Augenheilkd.* 1924; **73**, 742–52.
223. Kuwabara Y., Ishikara K. and Akiya S. Histologic and electron microscopic studies of the retina in Oguchi's disease. *Acta Soc. Ophthalmol. Japn.* 1963; **67**, 1323–51.
224. Yamanaka M. Histologic study of Oguchi's disease: its relationship to pigmentary degeneration of the retina. *Am. J. Ophthalmol.* 1969; **68**, 19–26.
225. Carr R. E. and Ripps H. Rhodopsin kinetics and rod adaptation in Oguchi's disease. *Invest. Ophthalmol.* 1967; **6**, 426–36.
226. Lauber H. The origin of hyalin formations within the eye. *Ber. Dtsch. Ophthalmol. Ges.* 1924; **44**, 216–20.
227. Marmor M. F. Defining fundus albipunctatus. *Doc. Ophthalmol.* 1977; **13**, 227–34.
228. Gass J. D. M. *Stereoscopic Atlas of Mascular Diseases*. St Louis, Mo, Mosby, 1970, p. 124.
229. Henkes H. E. Unilateral fundus albipunctatus. *Ophthalmologica* 1963; **145**, 470.
230. Krill A. E. and Martin D. Photopic abnormalities in congenital stationary night blindness. *Invest. Ophthalmol.* 1971; **10**, 625–36.
231. Smith B. F., Ripps H. A. and Goodman G. Retinitis punctata albescens. A functional and diagnostic evaluation. *Arch. Ophthalmol.* 1959; **61**, 93–101.
232. Franceschetti A., Dieterle P., Amman P. et al. Une nouvelle forme de fundus albipunctatus cum hemeralopia. *Ophthalmologica* 1963; **145**, 403–10.

233. Francois J., Verriest G. and De Rouck A. Les fonctions visuelles dans les degenerescences tapeto-retiniennes. *Ophthalmologica* 1956; **43** (Suppl. 1), 1.
234. Carr R. E., Ripps H. and Siegel I. M. Visual pigment kinetics and adaptation in fundus albipunctatus. *Doc Ophthalmol. Proc. Ser.* (XI ISCERG Symposium) 1974; **4,** 193–204.
235. Kandori F., Tamai A., Kurimoto S. et al. Fleck retina. *Am. J. Ophthalmol.* 1972; **73,** 673–85.

Macular Disease associated with Elevation of the Retina

Desmond B. Archer

TERMINOLOGY

The macula, in histological terms, represents that part of the retina where the ganglion cell layer is more than one cell thick and includes an area bordered by the superior and inferior temporal vascular arcades, the temporal margin of the optic disc and a point some four to five disc diameters temporal to the optic disc. For clinical purposes the macula is considered a circular area approximately 1·5 mm in diameter the centre of which is located 2 to 2·5 disc diameters (3–4 mm) from the temporal margin of the optic disc. The central part of the macula contained within the retinal avascular zone is referred to clinically as the fovea and corresponds to the histological foveola (330 μm in diameter).

FUNCTIONAL ANATOMY

The macula is the most densely cellular and highly specialized part of the retina and is the site of intense metabolic activity. Retinal photoreceptors are concentrated in the macular area, have a high proportion of cones and are critically aligned and orientated to facilitate optimum absorption of transmitted wavelengths and to provide directional clues about incident light for the purposes of accommodation.

Macular photoreceptors have intricate and highly organized connections with bipolar and horizontal cells, and in the foveal region cones and ganglion cells have a unitary relationship. The retinal neurones are intimately surrounded, supported and insulated by neuroglial fibres and have relatively little extracellular space. The compact retinal neuropile resists extracellular accumulation of fluid, invasion of inflammatory cells and infiltration of vasoproliferative or neoplastic tissue. The internal layers of the macula possess a unique yellow pigment (xanthophyll) which has specific light absorbing properties which may protect the outer macula against noxious wavelengths.

The internal environment of the macula is stabilized by two relatively impermeable layers of cells, i.e. the retinal pigment epithelium (outer blood retinal barrier) and the retinal vascular endothelium (inner blood retinal barrier), which control the movement of fluid, ions and electrolytes from the intravascular compartment into the retinal extracellular space. Strict retinal homeostasis is essential for retinal transparency, receptor photochemistry, neuroconduction and neurotransmitter activity. Fluid and certain ions in the retinal extracellular space can be actively transported to the retinal and choroidal circulations by an anionic pump mechanism located in the retinal vascular endothelium and pigment epithelial cells.

Failure of the blood retinal barriers or their metabolic pumps may result in the accumulation of excessive fluid, protein and metabolic byproducts within the extracellular space of the retina. This accumulation interferes with normal retinal physiology and metabolism and, if persistent, may cause photoreceptor dysfunction and atrophy.

The submacular choroidal vasculature consists largely of a dense network of wide-bore capillaries held in close apposition to the outer retina by virtue of their incorporation into the outer lamellae of Bruch's membrane. The choroidal capillaries are fenestrated, and fluid and some large molecules, e.g. retinol binding protein, can move freely into the extracellular space of the choroid. There is rapid movement and exchange of fluid, protein and metabolic products between the extra- and intravascular compartments of the choroid, and protein tracers, e.g. horseradish peroxidase, are rapidly purged from the choroidal extracellular space after a few minutes of normal perfusion. Water moves from the vitreous body across the retinal parenchyma into the choroid and some fluid passes through the sclera under the driving force of the intraocular pressure (uveo-scleral flow).

PATHOPHYSIOLOGY OF FLUID ACCUMULATION AT THE MACULA

The normal topography of the macula and the critical relationship of its constituent layers are maintained by the inner and outer blood–retinal barriers which preserve normal retinal deturgence and the vertically disposed neuroglial fibres (Mueller) which straddle the entire retina and maintain retinal cohesion. Firm adhesions between the retinal pigment epithelium and Bruch's membrane and the hydrodynamic forces created by the posterior movement of fluid through the retina also oppose forward movement of the retina.

Excessive fluid may accumulate within the macular and submacular tissues from four principal sources:

1. From the choroidal circulation where the extension of fluid into the retina is determined by the integrity of the retinal pigment epithelium.

2. From incompetent retinal capillaries.

3. From abnormal papillary vessels and via defects in optic nerve substance.

4. From the vitreous body through a retinal tear or hole into the subretinal space.

Fluid from these sources tends to accumulate within four main compartments at the macula.

The Choroid

The loosely arranged choroidal lamellae offer little resistance to the accumulation of fluid within their interstices, particularly in the suprachoroidal region. Extravasation of protein-rich fluid from the choroidal circulation may be precipitated by a high vascular hydrostatic pressure, low intraocular pressure, gross impairment of venous return, or where the choroidal vessels have been damaged by inflammation, ischaemia or degenerative processes. Choroidal oedema, folds or 'detachment' may occur without significant structural alteration to the choriocapillaris, Bruch's membrane or outer retina and visual functions are often not seriously or permanently disturbed.

Subretinal Pigment Epithelial Space

The retinal pigment epithelium may become separated from Bruch's membrane by fluid, abnormal cellular deposits, fibrovascular tissue or tumour cells. In most pigment epithelial detachments the basement membrane remains attached to the basal portion of the retinal pigment epithelial cell; however, where the pigment epithelium detaches without its basal lamina it may be more fragile and liable to tear. The separation of retinal pigment epithelial cells from the choriocapillaris places them at a metabolic disadvantage and may impair heat dissipation in this region, compromising the activity of certain heat labile enzymes. Detached retinal pigment epithelial cells may retain barrier functions preventing extension of excessive fluid and protein into the outer retina. Lateral extension of fluid and exudate beneath the retinal pigment epithelium is resisted by reticular fibre connections between the basal lamina and Bruch's membrane, and, as a result, pigment epithelial detachments typically remain discrete, have steep lateral walls and a dome-shaped appearance.

Subretinal Space

The delicate processes of the retinal pigment epithelial cells and the outer segments of the photoreceptors are embedded in a mucopolysaccharide matrix and only loosely adhere to each other by lateral plasma membrane connections. Abnormal fluid and protein entering the retina from the choroidal circulation preferentially collect in this region, detaching the photoreceptor layer from the pigment epithelium and opening the primitive optic vesicle. Fluid may also reach the subretinal space from the optic disc region, e.g. via optic disc pits, from the vitreous via retinal holes and tears and from grossly abnormal or telangiectatic retinal vessels as in Coats's disease, where fluid tracks posteriorly through the retinal neuropile. Resistance to lateral spread of fluid in the subretinal space is low and serous detachments of the retina tend to be low and diffuse with poorly demarcated margins. Bullous retinal detachments also occur and reflect a gross abnormality of the outer blood retinal barrier and choroidal circulation. Movement of fluid (shifting) in the subretinal space can be induced by alterations in head posture, demonstrating that only very tenuous connections exist between the retinal pigment epithelium and receptor layer.

The appearance of a serous detachment of the macula varies according to the quality and quantity of fluid in the subretinal space, and whether blood, fibrovascular tissue or abnormal substances have accumulated in this region. Protein-rich fluid in the subretinal space may impart a turbid or opalescent quality to the detachment.

Separation of the retinal photoreceptor outer segments and processes of the retinal pigment epithelial cells severely compromises retinal photochemistry and metabolism, and if prolonged, leads to dysfunction and atrophy of the outer retina.

If defective blood retinal barriers regain competence or a retinal hole is 'closed', fluid and abnormal metabolic products are rapidly removed from the subretinal space by the active 'pump mechanism' of the retinal pigment epithelium and possibly retinal vascular endothelium. Integrity of the retinal pigment epithelial/receptor axis can be re-established to some degree and limited regeneration of rod and cone outer segments can take place with partial return of visual functions.

Intraretinal Accumulation of Fluid

The compact retinal neuropile offers little facility for fluid accumulation within its layers; however, excess fluid, lipid, plasma-derived protein and cell debris tend to accumulate within the outer plexiform layer, displacing the vertically orientated Mueller cells and retinal neurones. Chronic fluid accumulation at the macula leads to the formation of clear cystoid intraretinal spaces which present a characteristic hyperfluorescent petaloid pattern during the late phases of fluorescein angiography.

Elevation of the macula is usually the result of fluid accumulation in one or more of the above tissue 'spaces'. However, separation of the macula may also follow deposition of abnormal substances within its substance, e.g. lipofuscin, drusen material or the infiltration of the retina by neoplastic, fibrovascular or inflammatory tissue. Traction at the surface of the retina caused by contracting fibrovascular tissue or neuroglial membranes may also cause internal displacement of the macula.

SYMPTOMATOLOGY AND EVALUATION OF VISUAL FUNCTIONS IN CONDITIONS ASSOCIATED WITH MACULAR ELEVATION

The malalignment and disorientation of retinal photoreceptors that follows elevation and separation of macular tissues typically produces metamorphopsia, distortion of vision, micropsia and occasionally monocular diplopia. Blurred vision, alteration in colour discrimination and delayed recovery of visual functions after exposure to a bright light (bleaching) are evidence of impaired metabolism and function at the outer retina. The degree of visual loss varies according to the site, extent and duration of fluid accumulation or severity of associated pathological processes, e.g. macular ischaemia, degeneration or inflammation.

The important tests of visual function are acuity, central visual fields (perimetry or Amsler grid) and pupillary responses. Colour vision tests (Ishihara plates or Farnsworth–Munsell 100-hue test) are often helpful and the photostress test, which measures visual acuity before and after exposure of the macula to a bright light for 10 s, may be useful where subtle fluid accumulation is suspected beneath or within the retina. Special tests of macular function, e.g. contrast sensitivity gratings, pattern reversal visually evoked responses (VER), flicker perimetry and focal electroretinography may be useful in specific instances. Electroretinography, electro-oculography and peripheral visual fields may indicate more widespread retinal pathology as, for example, in vitelliform macular degeneration.

EXAMINATION OF THE MACULA

Ophthalmoscopy and Fundus Biomicroscopy

Elevation of the macular retina can be readily appreciated by direct or indirect ophthalmoscopy (14 dioptre or 20 dioptre lens). The limits of the elevated or detached macula may be evident from abnormal light reflexes occurring at the junction of elevated and non-elevated retina or from discrete alterations in the retinal pigment epithelium at the margin of the lesion. Loss of retinal transparency, alterations in retinal pigment epithelial uniformity, accumulation of abnormal substances or presence of neovascular tissue may give clues as to the site of pathology and sources of macular fluid, blood or retinal deposits.

Fundus biomicroscopy is probably the best method of evaluating macular topography and morphology. A Rhuby lens or Goldmann fundus lens facilitates binocular scrutiny of the macula under high magnification and allows examination of the posterior vitreous for evidence of cellular infiltration, membrane formation and detachment of its posterior face. Detailed examination of the peripheral retina may identify pathological changes, e.g. holes or tears, retinal vascular abnormalities or inflammatory lesions that may have an important bearing on macular oedema.

Fluorescein Angiography

Fluorescein angiography is of primary importance in deciphering the nature and extent of most macular lesions. It allows accurate examination of retinal and choroidal haemodynamics and provides a sensitive measurement of competency of the inner and outer blood–retinal barriers. It is a sensitive marker for intraretinal and subretinal fluid accumulation and on occasions may help trace the pathway of fluid within the retina. Angiography is indispensable for identifying early choroidal neovascularization, tumour circulations and abnormalities of the retinal pigment epithelium.

Vitreous Fluorophotometry

Vitreous fluorophotometry provides a quantitative evaluation of fluorescence in the posterior vitreous cavity and can detect subtle changes in competence of both inner and outer blood–retinal barriers. Vitreous fluorophotometry is not as yet a routine clinical tool but in some cases may be used to supplement information gained from fluorescein angiography.

Ultrasound

Ultrasonography may help identify and elucidate certain lesions causing elevation of the macula, e.g. choroidal oedema, serous detachments, choroidal osteomas and calcium deposits within posterior polar retinoblastomas. Ultrasound is also useful in measuring the progression of macular tumours and differentiating between macular haemorrhages and melanomas. Ultrasonography may also help to exclude retinal detachments, tumours and macular haemorrhages when medical opacities are present, particularly where cataract extraction is being contemplated.

DISEASE PROCESSES CAUSING ELEVATION OF THE MACULA

Macular Diseases Associated with Accumulation of Fluid

Choroidal Vascular Disease (Ischaemia, Stasis, Vasculitis)

Associated with a Systemic Vasculopathy

Systemic vascular disease, such as accelerated hypertension, pre-eclampsia, collagen vascular disease (polyarteritis nodosa) and disseminated intravascular coagulopathy, may cause choroidal arteriolar obstruction or occlusion and impair perfusion of the outer retina. In severe disease the ischaemic outer retina becomes pale and thickened and is often the site of a low serous detachment of the sensory retina (*Fig.* 1).

Fluorescein angiography typically demonstrates lobular filling of the choriocapillaris (a feature of choroidal vascular stasis) and staining of the outer retina at sites of local infarction.

Treatment of the systemic disorder is usually followed by resolution of the serous retinal detachment and improvement in visual functions. Occasionally infarction of the macula may cause severe and permanent loss of central vision.

Local Choroidal Vasculopathy

A group of clinical entities characterized by acute focal lesions of the outer retina show evidence of choroidal vascular stasis and impaired perfusion of the choriocapillaris. Signs of chorioretinal inflammation and serous detachment of the macula may also be present.

ACUTE POSTERIOR MULTIFOCAL PLAQUOID PIGMENT EPITHELIOPATHY

This condition, of unknown aetiology, is described in Chapter 8, p 189. A number of patients with this disorder develop serous detachments of the macula, and fluorescein angiography in the acute phase of the disease process shows abnormal choroidal haemodynamics with impaired perfusion of choriocapillaris units. The disease process may represent a choroidal vasculopathy, occasionally complicating a systemic vasculitis or immune disorder.

SEROUS BULLOUS DETACHMENT OF THE RETINA WITH PIGMENT EPITHELIOPATHY

Patients in this group, usually aged between 20 and 30 years, typically present with acute bilateral loss of vision and multifocal plaquoid grey/white lesions at the level of the retinal pigment epithelium at the posterior pole of the eye (*Fig.* 2a). Serous retinal detachments are also present, but most resolve spontaneously within 1–2 weeks with good recovery of

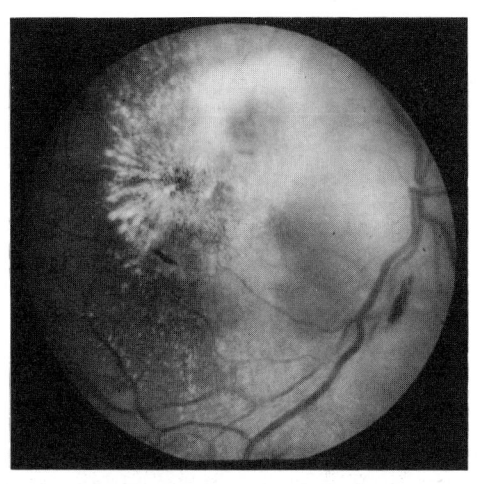

Fig. 1. Right fundus of patient with disseminated intravascular coagulopathy. The optic disc is swollen and fluid accumulates within and beneath the macula.

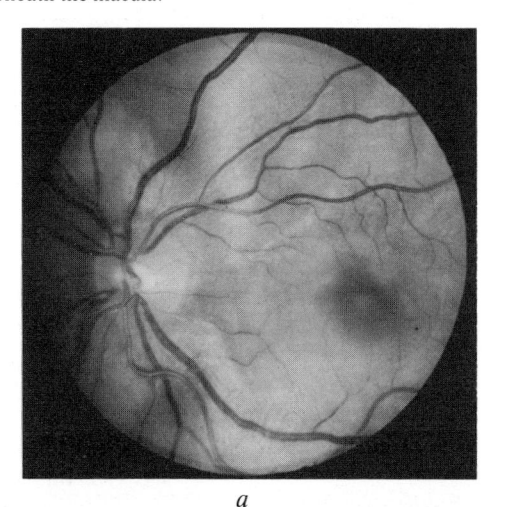

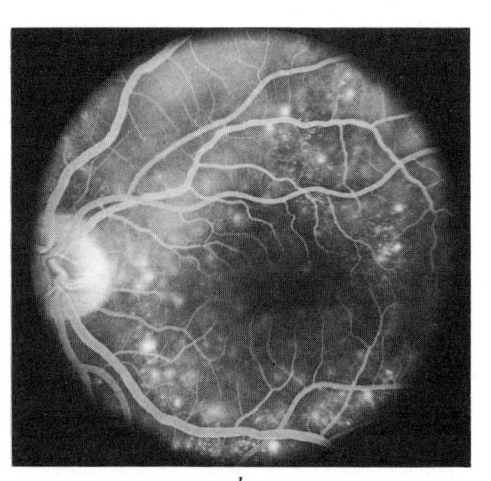

Fig. 2. *a*, Left fundus, 38-year-old female with bullous serous detachments of the retina involving the posterior pole of the eye. Visual acuity 6/36. *b*, Fluorescein angiogram (late venous phase) of fundus shown in (*a*). Multiple punctate hyperfluorescent foci represent sites of retinal pigment epithelial incompetence. Serous retinal detachments are diffusely hyperfluorescent, e.g. superonasal to the macula.

vision. Residual retinal pigment epithelial changes are often indistinguishable from those occurring in the recovery phase of posterior multifocal plaquoid pigment epitheliopathy. Fluorescein angiography may demonstrate choroidal vascular stasis and leakage of dye through focal retinal pigment epithelial defects into the subretinal space (*Fig. 2b*).

These patients differ from those with Harada's disease in that spontaneous reattachment of the retina occurs within 1–2 weeks and none of the systemic abnormalities typical of Harada's disease are present, e.g. tinnitus, alopecia and vitiligo. This condition probably represents a choroidal vasculitis and occupies an intermediate position between acute posterior multifocal plaquoid pigment epitheliopathy and Harada's disease.

HARADA'S DISEASE

Harada's disease, which typically affects young non-Caucasians, causes severe inflammation of the uveal tract, a profound disturbance of the retinal pigment epithelium and widespread accumulation of fluid in the subretinal space (*see* Chapter 1, Biochemistry of the Eye).

Serous detachment of the macula is often persistent, slow to resolve and recurrent; however, resolution may be aided by systemic corticosteroid therapy. Recovery of vision is often incomplete and final visual acuity does not improve beyond 6/60 in a proportion of patients. Fluorescein angiography confirms a widespread disturbance of the retinal pigment epithelium with multiple focal leaking areas through which dye reaches the subretinal space. Abnormal choroidal haemodynamics have been identified in some patients.

CHOROIDAL VENOUS OBSTRUCTION

Experimental obstruction of one or more venae vorticosae systems produces choroidal congestion and occasional haemorrhage in the distribution of the obstructed vein, but marked choroidal effusion or detachment does not commonly occur. Choroidal effusion with or without extension of fluid into the subretinal space, however, has been described in several conditions associated with choroidal venous obstruction, e.g. dural and carotid arteriovenous fistulae, following retinal detachment repair, and in nanophthalmic or normal eyes where an unusually thick sclera or abnormal vortex veins are believed to be the primary cause of the uveal and retinal detachments. Surgical decompression of the venae vorticosae may aid resolution of the uveal and retinal detachments in some patients.

UVEAL EFFUSION SYNDROME

This condition is characterized by the spontaneous development of serous detachments of the ciliary body, choroid and retina. Healthy middle-aged males are predominantly affected and the condition is commonly bilateral. Cilio-choroidal effusions are associated with non-rhegmatogenous bullous detachment of the retina which may occasionally present at the macula. Optic disc swelling, mild anterior uveitis and vitritis, dilated episcleral vessels, small eyes and thickened choroid are associated findings.

Fluorescein angiography confirms choroidal vascular stasis and widespread discrete abnormalities of the retinal pigment epithelium. Spontaneous resolution usually occurs after a protracted course and visual functions are often significantly reduced, i.e. less than 6/12. Sclerectomy with sclerostomy may assist outflow of protein rich exudate through the sclera and assist resolution of the uveal and retinal detachments. The uveal effusion syndrome should be differentiated from other conditions producing bullous rhegmatogenous and non-rhegmatogenous detachment of the retina, e.g. posterior scleritis and infiltration of the choroid by primary or metastatic tumours, e.g. melanomas, or leukaemic or lymphomatous infiltrates.

Choroidal Neovascularization – the Disciform Response

Choroidal neovascularization is the commonest cause of serous macular detachment. It is frequently bilateral and accounts for a high proportion of blind registrations (visual acuity less than 3/60 right and left) in Caucasian communities.

PATHOPHYSIOLOGY

The disciform response is a complication of senile macular degeneration, where new choroidal vessels, and attendant connective tissue, infiltrate Bruch's membrane to gain the subpigment epithelial space. Subsequently the vessels penetrate the retinal pigment epithelium to proliferate and ramify in the subretinal space. Serous exudate, haemorrhage and fibrosis lead to the formation of a circular scar, degeneration of retinal photoreceptors and, in severe disease, atrophy of the nearby retina and choroid (*Fig. 3*). The important constituents of the disciform response are an abnormal Bruch's membrane (microfractures, calcium deposits, collagen degeneration), malfunction and degeneration of the outer retina (pigment epithelial abnormalities, basal laminar deposits, drusen formation) and a reactive choriocapillaris. The precise stimulus for choroidal vasoproliferation is not known; however, displacement of the outer retina from Bruch's membrane (by basal laminar deposits, soft drusen material, serous fluid and blood) and the presence of macrophages and proliferating retinal pigment epithelial cells are probably the important factors. Experimental studies have shown that new vessels extend by proliferation of endothelial cells and pericytes, commonly in association with macrophages and actively proliferating pigment epithelial cells.

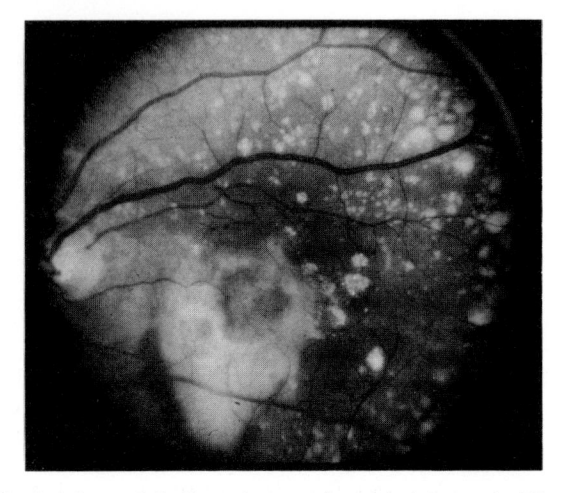

Fig. 3. Advanced disciform degeneration of the left macula. Fibrovascular scar tissue at the macula is associated with inferior subretinal haemorrhage and extensive drusen deposits.

lium, are asymptomatic and clinically occult and are identified only on post-mortem examination. In some patients, e.g. high myopes, disciform lesions may remain discrete, extramacular and produce no serious loss of vision. In most ageing individuals, however, the disease process is progressive, with macular neovascular fronds extending centripetally towards the centre of the fovea.

Fluorescein angiography demonstrates that most choroidal new vessels proliferate vigorously in the subretinal space to form subretinal vascular membranes of widely varying architecture and structure (*Fig.* 4). Occasional anastomoses develop between the new choroidal vessels and the retinal circulation. New choroidal vessels are incompetent and profusely leak fluorescein, protein, lipid and blood into the subretinal space. Occasionally, neovascular membranes atrophy and fibrose but often not before macular functions have been grossly diminished. The

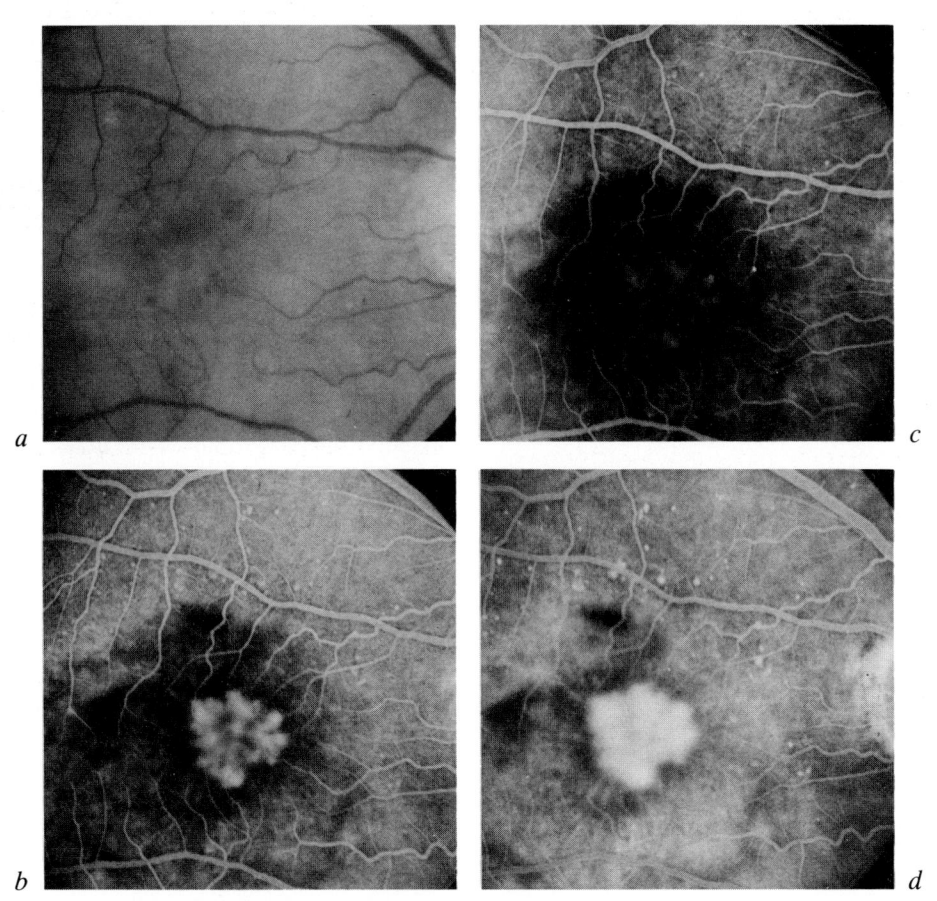

Fig. 4. *a*, Disciform degeneration right macula. Small flecks of subretinal haemorrhage are just visible. *b*, A discrete circular network of new choroidal vessels is outlined during the early phases of angiography. *c*, The new vessels are strikingly incompetent during the late venous phase of angiography. *d*, By the residual phases of angiography dye accumulates in the subretinal space. Widespread retinal pigment epithelial abnormalities are apparent.

NATURAL COURSE

The natural course of choroidal neovascularization is highly variable and often unpredictable. Some new vessels remain beneath the retinal pigment epithe-

fellow eye has a 13 per cent chance per year of developing a similar disciform lesion.

Choroidal neovascularization is a common component of numerous disease processes characterized by abnormalities of Bruch's membrane, the retinal pigment epithelium and outer retina (*Table* I).

Table I. Causes of choroidal neovascularization

Congenital	Rubella retinitis
	Vitelliform degeneration
Traumatic	Choroidal tear
	Photocoagulation
	Retinal detachment surgery
Inflammatory	APMPPE
	Harada's disease
	Toxocara
	Presumed histoplasmosis
	Toxoplasmosis
	Chronic uveitis
Degenerative	Myopia
	Senile macular degeneration – drusen
	Angioid streaks
	Geographic retinal atrophy
	Optic nerve drusen
Neoplastic	Choroidal naevus
	Choroidal melanoma
	Retinal pigment epithelial hamartoma

TREATMENT

To date there are no known pharmacological means of inhibiting or retarding choroidal vasoproliferation, and laser photocoagulation is often impracticable as many neovascular membranes infiltrate beneath the fovea. Laser photocoagulation, however, has been shown to be effective in selected cases of vasoproliferation, and several recent randomly controlled trials have demonstrated that certain neovascular fronds (about 10 per cent of all assessed) can be successfully treated if located 200 μm or more from the centre of the fovea. Argon and krypton laser photocoagulation are both effective, although krypton wavelengths have theoretical advantages when employed near the fovea. The treatment of juxtafoveal lesions may create a positive central scotoma which may be annoying for the patient and additional neovascular membranes may occur at or adjacent to sites of photocoagulation. If the patient has a disciform lesion at one macula he should be instructed to test vision carefully and regularly in the fellow eye using an Amsler chart or fine print and report any alteration in central vision or distortion of acuity to his ophthalmologist.

Impairment of Uveo-Scleral Flow

Posterior uveo-scleral flow can be impeded if there is an acute or chronic reduction in intraocular pressure or if scleral permeability is decreased.

Acute Ocular Hypotony

Acute ocular hypotony occasionally complicates glaucoma procedures or cataract extraction. Fluid commonly accumulates within the interstices of the choroid with a predilection for the suprachoroidal region. Re-establishment of normal intraocular pressure and ocular hydrodynamics results in absorption of fluid without serious consequence to the retina or visual functions. Acute surgical or traumatic decompression of the eye may precipitate severe choroidal haemorrhage, occasionally culminating in an expulsive haemorrhage characterized by acute arterial bleeding into the choroid.

Chronic Ocular Hypotony

Prolonged ocular hypotony is usually the sequela of a severe ocular contusional injury. Diminished uveoscleral flow and the unopposed choroidal intraluminal pressure contribute to the accumulation of fluid

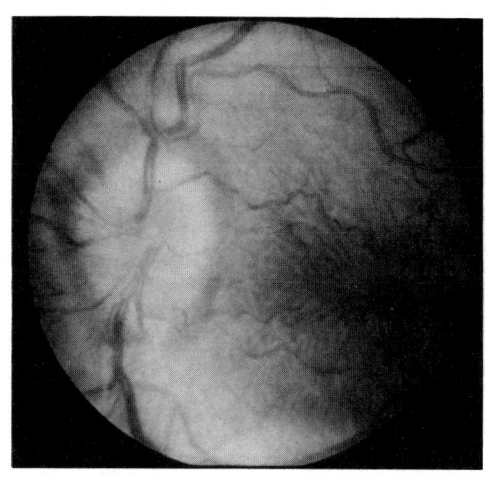

Fig. 5. Left fundus of patient with chronic ocular hypotony following severe contusional eye injury. The optic disc is swollen and numerous macular choroidal folds are present.

and protein within the choroid and development of choroidal folds and oedema (*Fig.* 5). Severe collapse of intraocular pressure may also cause narrowing of the venae vorticosae ampullae and secondary venous obstruction. Visual functions may be preserved for some time as the choriocapillaris/pigment epithelial/receptor axis remains relatively intact. Chronic disc oedema, secondary optic atrophy and retinal pigment epithelial degenerative changes may complicate long standing ocular hypotony and seriously impair visual functions. Re-establishment of intraocular pressure by operative techniques is usually followed by rapid resolution of choroidal oedema and folds and disappearance of optic disc swelling. Residual retinal pigment epithelial defects remain, however, particularly where there have been severe choroidal folds.

Posterior Scleritis

Exudative retinal detachment, macular oedema and optic disc swelling are complications of posterior scleritis. The condition is occasionally bilateral and visual acuity is generally diminished to 6/24 or worse. Yellow/brown subretinal masses may be evident on ophthalmoscopy, associated with severe cellular infiltrate at the posterior vitreous. Systemic corticosteroids may result in prompt relief of pain and resolution of scleritis, although serous detachment of the retina may persist for several months. Visual acuity improves with resolution of macular oedema and detachment.

Fluorescein angiography confirms the presence of disc and macular oedema and may be useful in monitoring the resolution of the disease process.

Lymphocytic infiltration of the choroid with elevation of the overlying retinal pigment epithelium may account for the exudative detachment. Granulomatous infiltration, necrosis and scarring of the sclera may impede uveo-scleral flow and exacerbate the degree of macular detachment. Macular detachment has also been described where the posterior sclera is the site of mucopolysaccharide deposits within its lamellae.

Retinal Pigment Epithelial/Bruch's Membrane/Choroidal Disease

Idiopathic Accumulation of Fluid at the Outer Retina

DETACHMENT OF THE RETINAL PIGMENT EPITHELIUM

Pigment epithelial detachments may be single, multiple, small or large, and preferentially affect the posterior pole of the eye (*Fig. 6a*). It is often difficult to differentiate between small pigment epithelial detachments in the elderly and conglomerates of 'soft' drusen which may harbour neovascular complexes.

If pigment epithelial detachments are small and eccentric to the macula they may be asymptomatic; however, if they are foveal or juxtafoveal the common symptoms are metamorphopsia, micropsia, and a positive scotoma or loss of vision. Acquired hypermetropia with disparity between subjective and objective refraction of the eye may be present. Fundoscopy reveals a slightly depigmented orange-coloured lesion the periphery of which is delineated by a striking light reflex originating from the margins of the elevated retina. The bordering retinal pigment epithelial cells show variations in degree of pigmentation and occasionally impart a yellow/white or orange halo to the detachment. Slit lamp biomicroscopy with a Rhuby lens or Goldmann contact lens confirms a discrete dome-shaped elevation of the retinal pigment epithelium with anterior displacement or bowing of the slit lamp beam. The internal surface of the pigment epithelial dome often displays radiating or stellate lines of pigment which are almost pathognomonic for such a detachment and generally indicate longevity (*Fig. 6*). This pigment probably represents linear accumulations of melanin or lipofuscin granules. If the retinal pigment epithelial detachment is large, wrinkles may occur in the overlying retina.

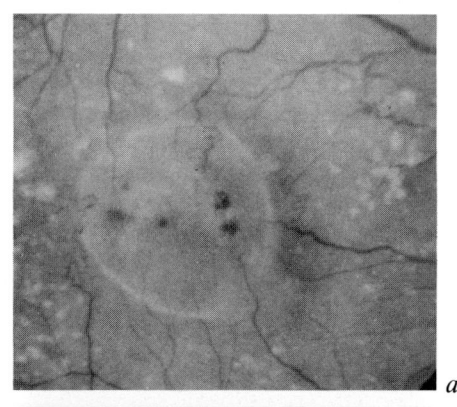

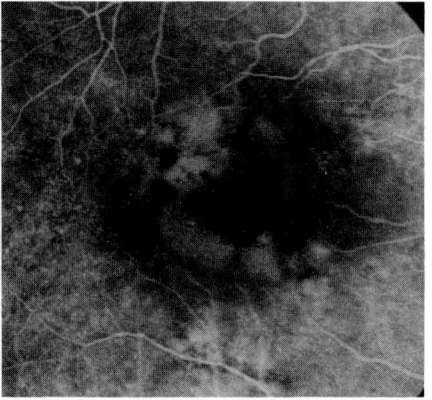

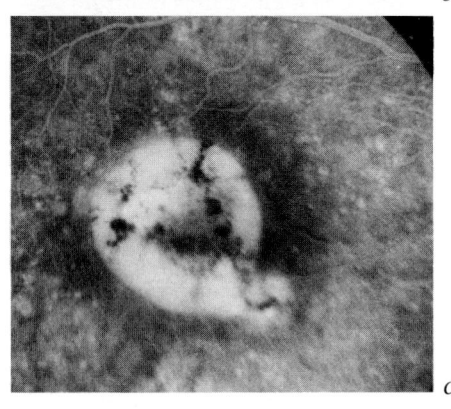

Fig. 6. a, Large pigment epithelial detachment affecting the right macula. The margins are discrete and accumulations of pigment are present over the surface of the detachment. *b*, The pigment epithelial detachment is discretely outlined during the early phases of angiography. Pigment accumulations are observed as hypo- or non-fluorescent regions. *c*, The pigment epithelial detachment is uniformly hyperfluorescent in the residual phases of angiography.

Fluorescein Angiography: Dye from the choroidal circulation outlines precisely the extent of the detachment in the early phases of angiography (*Fig. 6b*). By the later phases of angiography the entire detachment becomes uniformly hyperfluorescent, although variations in intensity may occur due to presence of blood, pigment or retinal deposits which cause focal areas of hypofluorescence (*Fig. 6c*).

Choroidal neovascular complexes beneath the pigment epithelial detachment may fluoresce brightly ('hot spots') and focal areas of expanding hyperfluorescence at the margins of pigment epithelial detachments are highly suggestive of infiltrating neovascular fronds.

In the event of the detached retinal pigment epithelium losing its barrier functions, fluid may accumulate within the subretinal space. If permeability of the retinal pigment epithelium is only slightly affected, fluorescein may not accumulate in sufficient quantity to be detected; however, if diffuse leakage is present, a fluorescent haze or halo may surround the detachment. In the case of a physical defect in the retinal pigment epithelium, fluorescein may rapidly stream through the dehiscence into the subretinal space.

Natural Course: Pigment epithelial detachments in young patients, uncomplicated by retinal degenerative changes or choroidal neovascularization, often resolve spontaneously, although the process may take many months. Some pigment epithelial detachments may develop an overlying sensory retinal detachment and follow a course similar to centroserous retinopathy. Pigment epithelial detachments in the elderly (usually greater than one disc diameter) associated with retinal pigment degenerative changes, e.g. drusen, are commonly complicated by choroidal neovascularization. More than half of such patients develop subpigment epithelial new vessels within 2 years.

Tears may occur in detached retinal pigment epithelium, possibly where it has detached without an intact basement membrane. The retracted pigment epithelium exposes bare sclera and the subsequent hyperfluorescence in this region during angiography may mimic choroidal neovascularization.

Treatment: Pigment epithelial detachments can be flattened by laser or xenon arc photocoagulation, but several studies have shown that pigment epithelial detachments so treated may develop neovascularization or tears of the pigment epithelial layer. At present, in view of the good natural history in young patients and the observation that treatment may cause early visual loss, photocoagulation should be used conservatively and possibly only to destroy new vessels that pose a threat to visual functions and are amenable to laser photocoagulation.

CENTROSEROUS CHORIORETINOPATHY

Centroserous chorioretinopathy is a detachment of the sensory retina of unknown aetiology. It affects males predominantly (80 per cent), is frequently bilateral and commonly occurs in the age range 30–55 years. The condition appears to affect intense, competitive individuals who have occupational stress; however, most patients are in good general health and have no associated extraretinal ocular disease.

Abnormal pigment epithelial changes are commonly present in both the affected and fellow eye (80 per cent). Small extramacular detachments may be asymptomatic and remain undetected; however, most are centrally located and the patient typically complains of distortion of vision (micropsia) and dyschromatopsia and is often aware of a positive scotoma. The presenting acuity is usually between 6/6 and 6/18 and may be improved with a small positive spherical addition. The serous detachment of the retina is usually circular and involves or juxtaposes the fovea (*Fig. 7a*). Less commonly, the detachment may be bullous, measuring several disc diameters in width.

Slit lamp biomicroscopy demonstrates an opalescent area of raised retina with ill-defined edges. Elevation of the retinal veins and anterior bowing of the slip lamp beam are additional clues pointing to separation of the retina. If the condition is long standing, fine, punctate, yellow deposits may be visible on the posterior surface of the detached retina. A range of pigment epithelial abnormalities may also be present, e.g. focal hyper- and hypopigmentation and small detachments of the retinal pigment epithelium.

Fluorescein Angiography: A punctate or discrete hyperfluorescent focus develops during the early phases of angiography at the site of the pigment epithelial abnormality (*Fig. 7b*). During the mid and later phases of angiography the fluorescent area increases in size and intensity as dye accumulates at the outer retina. Dye diffuses into the subretinal space either centrifugally (ink blot pattern) or rises towards the superior limit of the detachment and then expands in a mushroom-like fashion – 'smoke stack' or 'umbrella' type of leak (*Figs. 7c,d*). The sensory detachment of the macula is usually only partially outlined by dye, although its lateral margins may be discernible as a circular hypofluorescent border. Occasionally a small discrete pigment epithelial detachment can be identified beneath the sensory detachment, filling rapidly and uniformly in the early phases of dye transit. The precise factors that determine the movement of fluorescein in the subretinal space are not known, but gravity, convection currents, relative molecular weights of fluorescein and the subretinal proteins may all influence the angiographic pattern. Retinal and choroidal haemodynamics are usually normal.

Natural Course: Most pigment epithelial defects heal spontaneously, although the time taken for functional recovery is highly variable, e.g. 2–3 weeks to longer than 1 year. Most patients (75 per cent) achieve a corrected visual acuity of 6/12 or better, although in many instances the patient is aware of a qualitative difference in vision between the two eyes and occasionally residual distortion. A small proportion of patients have significant and permanent loss of central visual functions, i.e. 5 per cent achieve a visual acuity of less than 6/60. Poor recovery of vision is probably related to the location and duration

Photocoagulation is a relatively innocuous procedure in patients with centroserous retinopathy and complications are few. Subretinal neovascularization, however, may occasionally complicate treatment, especially where leaking sites are parafoveal.

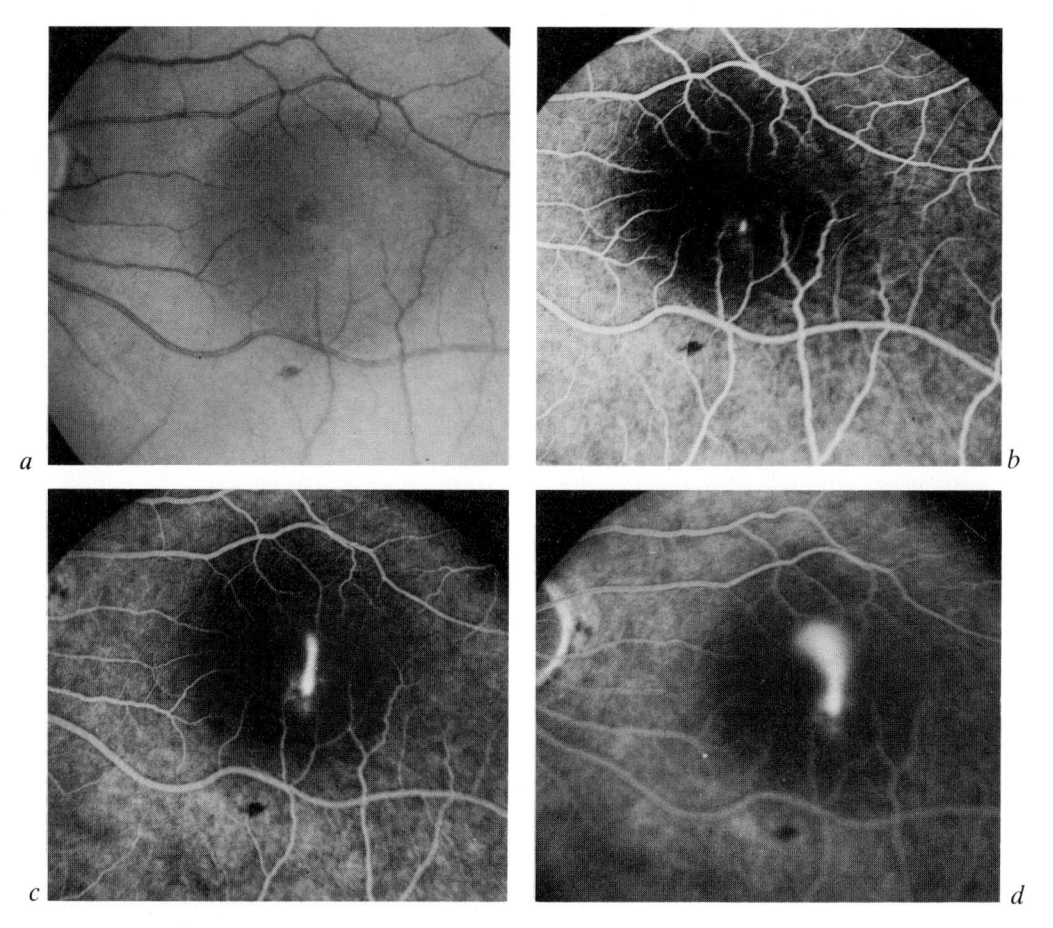

Fig. 7. *a*, Circular serous detachment of the left macula (centroserous chorioretinopathy). *b*, A punctate hyperfluorescent focus develops during early phases of angiography at the inferotemporal margin of the fovea. *c*, During the late venous phase of angiography dye extends superiorly in a typical linear fashion (smoke stack). *d*, Residual angiograms show that dye extends to occupy the superior portion of the serous detachment in a mushroom-like configuration.

of the sensory detachment coupled with atrophic changes in the foveal pigment epithelium. Recurrences are common, usually affecting an independent, although often closely related, area of the macula.

Treatment: Photocoagulation has been shown to shorten the duration of the sensory detachment of the retina, resolution usually occurring within 1–3 weeks of treatment. Whether photocoagulation improves the final visual acuity is not known and at present treatment is usually reserved for punctate leaks that are remote from the fovea, where the detachment persists for longer than 3–4 months and where visual functions show evidence of decline. Should the patient require acute central vision for his work, early photocoagulation may be required.

BULLOUS DETACHMENT OF THE RETINA WITH PIGMENT EPITHELIAL DETACHMENT

Gass in 1973 described an unusual clinical syndrome in healthy young or middle-aged men who presented with rapid loss of vision in one or both eyes. The patients were typically hyperactive and under stress at the time of presentation. Large bullous serous detachments of the retina were present, occasionally extending to the ora serrata. Subretinal shifting of fluid could be demonstrated by changing the position of the patient's head. The retinal detachments were associated with one or more discrete serous detachments of the retinal pigment epithelium which were typically located at the posterior pole of the eye. Fluorescein angiography strikingly outlined the discrete pigment epithelial detachments and often demonstrated focal defects in the retinal pigment epithelial layer through which dye extravasated into the subretinal space.

These patients showed no other evidence of intraocular disease and the serous retinal detachments failed to respond to local or systemic corticosteroid therapy. The natural course was towards spontaneous resolution and improved vision; however, laser or xenon arc photocoagulation was helpful in flattening the pigment epithelial detachment and hastening absorption of fluid.

This condition is probably a variant or exaggerated form of centroserous chorioretinopathy, although it is unusual in the large number and size of pigment epithelial detachments and the extent of serous detachment of the retina. Patients with bullous detachments of the retina require careful fundoscopy and fluorescein angiography, as pigment epithelial detachments may be obscured by cloudy subretinal exudates and the patients may be misdiagnosed as having either a rhegmatogenous detachment with an unidentifiable hole or an exudative detachment due to Harada's disease, leukaemia or collagen vascular disease affecting the choroidal vessels. Retinal detachment surgery may have disastrous results in such patients.

If the solid-appearing retinal pigment epithelial detachments are large and prominent the clinician may suspect a metastatic carcinoma of the choroid, a choroidal haemangioma or melanoma or a focal choroiditis. Fluorescein angiography serves to establish the presence of multiple detachments of the retinal pigment epithelium and indicate a disease process with a relatively good prognosis.

Accumulation of Fluid at the Outer Retina – Inflammatory Conditions

Inflammatory diseases may cause elevation of the retina by creating conditions favourable for the proliferation of new choroidal vessels, by causing decompensation of the outer blood retinal barrier or by impairing choroidal perfusion.

RUBELLA RETINOPATHY

The rubella virus causes a diffuse retinal pigment epitheliopathy which is generally associated with good visual functions and normal or near normal retinal electrophysiological responses. The retinopathy may be complicated by choroidal neovascularization and the development of a dense proliferative macular scar.

PRESUMED HISTOPLASMOSIS CHORIORETINITIS

This condition, commonly found in the mid-west of America, is characterized by inflammatory lesions at the outer retina associated with focal lymphocytic infiltration of the choroid. The clinical picture is one of multifocal chorioretinitis, peripapillary atrophy and a proliferative macular scar. Treatment of macular neovascular membranes by laser photocoagulation is difficult, often unsuccessful and occasionally associated with progression of subretinal vasoproliferation.

SYMPATHETIC OPHTHALMIA

This condition is characterized by a marked thickening of the choroid, a severe papillitis and occasionally serous detachment of the retina. Systemic corticosteroids and immunosuppressive agents have dramatically altered the former unremitting course of the disease process which commonly caused blindness. Intense therapy may lead to resolution of the choroiditis with preservation of near normal visual functions.

TOXOCARA–TOXOPLASMOSIS

Toxoplasmosis retinitis typically results in a dense atrophic chorioretinal scar usually affecting the macular or perimacular area. Occasionally perimacular scars may be associated with choroidal neovascularization and localized detachment of the macula (*Fig. 8*). Toxocara retinitis may provoke a dense proliferative scar and vitreo-retinal traction that may cause severe disorganization and elevation of the retina.

Accumulation of Fluid at the Outer Retina – Degenerative / Traumatic Conditions

A number of non-age-related degenerative conditions may cause elevation of the retina secondary to serous detachment of the retinal pigment epithelium or retina or secondary to proliferative macular scars.

ANGIOID STREAKS

Angioid streaks occur in patients with an abnormality of the elastic component of Bruch's membrane. The patient may have isolated ocular lesions or suffer from pseudoxanthoma elasticum, a systemic condition characterized by generalized abnormalities of elastic tissue principally affecting the media of blood vessels and skin. Patients with angioid streaks develop multiple and often extensive breaks in Bruch's membrane, which predominantly affect the posterior fundi and often involve the maculae (*Fig. 9*). Pigment epithelial and sensory detachments occur in a high proportion of patients and these are commonly complicated by subretinal neovascularization and a disciform scar. Treatment of macular subretinal neovascularization in angioid streaks is usually unrewarding, although occasional good results have been claimed.

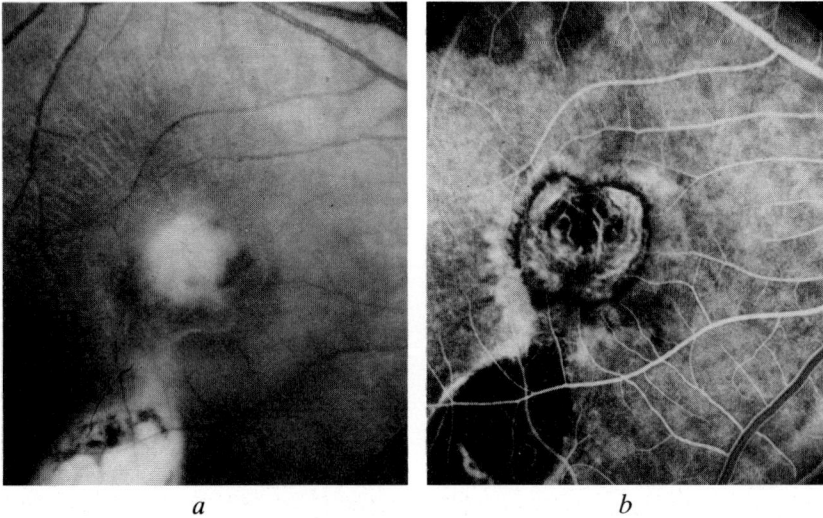

Fig. 8. a, Old toxoplasmosis lesion inferior to the right macula associated with proliferative macular scar. *b*, Early venous phase angiogram demonstrates subretinal neovascular fronds at the macula.

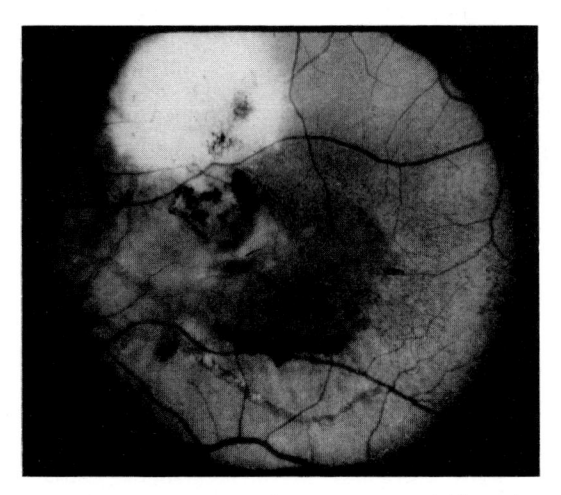

Fig. 9. Left fundus demonstrating numerous angioid streaks and typical pigment epithelial mottling temporal to the macula. A serosanguineous detachment of the macula is present.

MYOPIA

Patients with high degrees of myopia often have breaks in Bruch's membrane (lacquer cracks) and develop pigment epithelial or sensory detachments. These are often complicated by subretinal neovascularization which proceeds to a typical disciform response.

CHOROIDAL TEARS

Choroidal tears may be associated with marked elevation of the macula due to accumulation of blood in the choroid or subpigment epithelial or subretinal spaces. In severe tears blood may dissect through full thickness retina into the vitreous cavity. Most choroidal lacerations heal spontaneously and securely and only about 3–4 per cent of such tears become complicated by progressive subretinal neovascularization or serous detachment. In most instances choroidal neovascularization is short-lived and disciform scars are unusual.

Fluid Extending from the Optic Disc and Papillary Circulation

Congenital Abnormalities of the Optic Disc – Colobomas

Colobomas of the optic disc and nearby retina and choroid may be associated with serous detachment of the macula. Where significant areas of retina are involved in the colobomatous defect, tears and holes can form at the margin of the defect leading to retinal detachment. An unusual type of coloboma, designated 'morning glory syndrome', is associated with retinal vascular abnormalities, glial proliferation and peripapillary degenerative changes. The disc is displaced posteriorly within the depths of a staphlomatous excavation which involves the optic nerve head and peripapillary retina. Serous detachment of the peripapillary retina and macula may occur and extend to involve much of the posterior pole of the eye. Most patients with morning glory syndrome have profound visual loss and other ocular abnormalities, e.g. microphthalmia and anterior chamber cleavage syndrome. Basal encephalocoeles may also be present.

Optic Nerve Pits

Optic nerve pits are congenital defects within the substance of the optic nerve head and may be single, multiple, unilateral or bilateral. The pits may be oval, circular, slit-like or triangular and have steep walls of variable depth. Most occupy the temporal aspect of the optic disc and are grey or blue in colour. Peripapillary pigment epithelial changes are common, particularly when the pit is located temporally (*Fig.*

10a). Most patients with optic nerve pits have visual field defects, e.g. centrocaecal scotomas and enlargement of the blind spot. The commonest complication of optic nerve pits is serous detachment of the macula. Spontaneous resolution may occur; however, if detachment is prolonged, cystoid macular oedema and hole formation may occur.

When subretinal fluid is present fluorescein angiography may demonstrate abnormal papillary vessels at the site of the optic pit which leak dye in the late phases of angiography (*Fig. 10b*). Dye generally does not extend beyond the margin of the optic disc pit or accumulate in the subretinal space in detectable quantities. The source of the fluid is unclear, but it probably arises from the vitreous body. Treatment is often unsatisfactory, although photocoagulation to the rim of the pit may produce a chorioretinal scar and lead to resolution of the serous detachment. The place of photocoagulation in the management of this disease process is as yet unclear.

Optic Disc Degenerative Changes

Drusen of the optic disc and peripapillary chorioretinal degenerative changes may be associated with subretinal neovascularization and occasionally serous or haemorrhagic detachment of the macula with formation of a disciform scar.

Papillary Vascular Anomalies

Diseases affecting the papillary microvasculature, e.g. papilloedema or central retinal vein obstruction, may cause a profuse outpouring of fluid from the papillary vasculature into the retina and, if sufficiently severe, may cause elevation of the retina.

Fluid Originating from the Retinal Circulation

Maculopathies – Macroaneurysm

Advanced diabetic retinopathy, central and branch retinal vein obstruction or parafoveal retinal telangiectasia and macroaneurysms may be associated with fluid, protein and lipid accumulation and haemorrhage within or beneath the macula (*see* pp. 244–7).

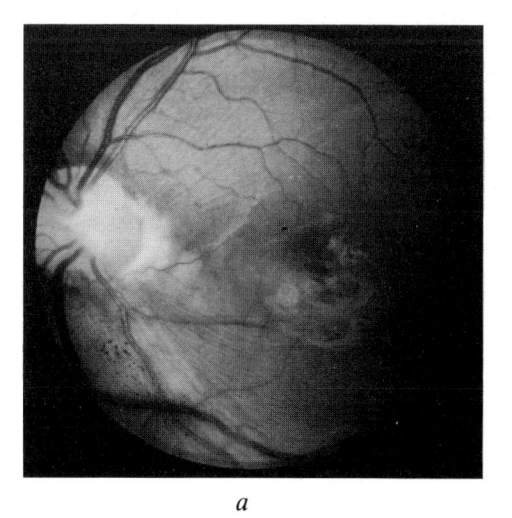

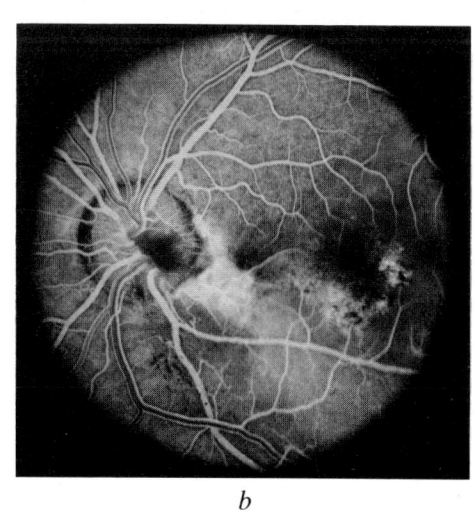

Fig. 10. *a*, Patient with pit at the temporal margin of the left optic disc. A large serous detachment of the macula is present. *b*, Mid-venous phase angiogram of fundus shown in (*a*). Pigment epithelial abnormalities are present temporal to the optic disc and at the macula. The inferior part of the serous retinal detachment is diffusely hyperfluorescent.

Congenital Vascular Abnormalities

Large arteriovenous malformations at the posterior pole of the eye may cause dramatic elevation of the retina. If incompetent, such malformations may cause widespread scarring of the macula with severe loss of vision. Retinal arteriovenous anastomoses may be associated with similar malformations within the brain. Congenital telangiectasia, e.g. Leber's miliary aneurysms or Coats's disease, may result in profuse and widespread extravasation of fluid into the retina, some of which may accumulate within the macular subretinal space. Peripherally located lesions may also cause serous detachment of the macula due to fluid extending posteriorly through extracellular or subretinal spaces (*Fig.* 11). The identification of a serous detachment of the macula or a proliferative macular scar should initiate a careful search of the retinal periphery for such retinal vascular abnormalities. Perimacular or peripheral retinal haemangiomas may also cause detachment of the sensory retina, retinal haemorrhage and proliferative scars. Ablation of small peripheral haemangiomas or telangiectatic lesions may prevent macular oedema. Photocoagulation of macular vascular abnormalities is difficult and often unsatisfactory and may result in extension of a serous detachment with significant loss of vision.

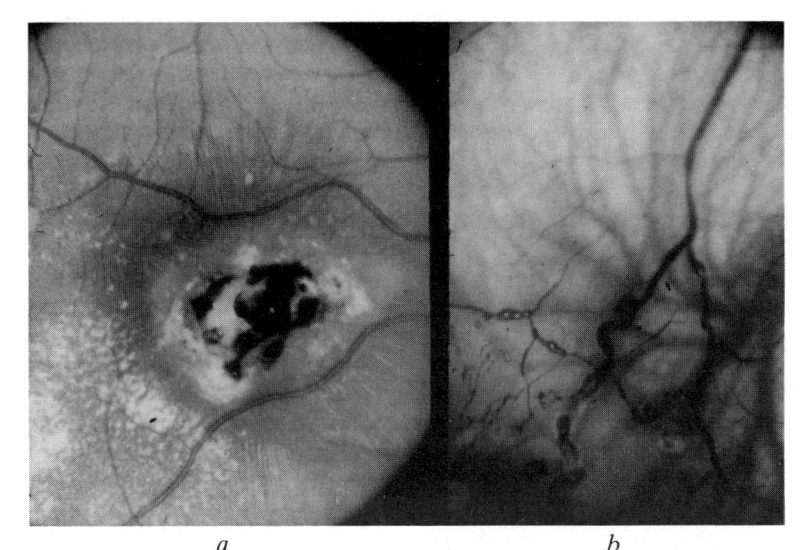

Fig. 11. Proliferative scar and chronic fluid accumulation at the right macula (*a*) of a patient with extensive peripheral retinal telangiectatic vessels (*b*).

Fluid Originating from the Vitreous Body

Detachment of the macula may follow a full thickness macular hole or complicate a peripherally located tear where posterior extension of subretinal fluid has occurred. Rhegmatogenous detachment of the macula typically remains non- or only slightly fluorescent during angiography, as dye only reaches the vitreous and subsequently the subretinal space in low concentration. The management of macular holes with detachments has been facilitated by the introduction of vitreous surgery and techniques of internal retinal tamponade using fluid/gas mixtures or silicone oil.

Macular Separation and Elevation Associated with Abnormal Retinal Deposits

Most degenerative or dystrophic macular deposits occur at the outer retina and are associated with dysfunction of the retinal pigment epithelium, e.g. drusen, fundus flavimaculatus and vitelliform macular dystrophy. Most deposits are small and cause only microscopical displacement of the retina. Vision is impaired where deposits are associated with foveal degeneration or where subretinal neovascularization and serous detachment of the macula occur as secondary phenomena.

Macular Disease Associated with Neoplasia

Primary Tumours

Benign

Choroidal naevi or haemangiomas may cause macular elevation by their physical presence or due to the accumulation of serous fluid beneath or within the retina from incompetent tumour vessels or associated choroidal neovascularization. Hamartomas of the retinal pigment epithelium produce raised proliferative scars with irregular pigmentation (*Fig.* 12) and

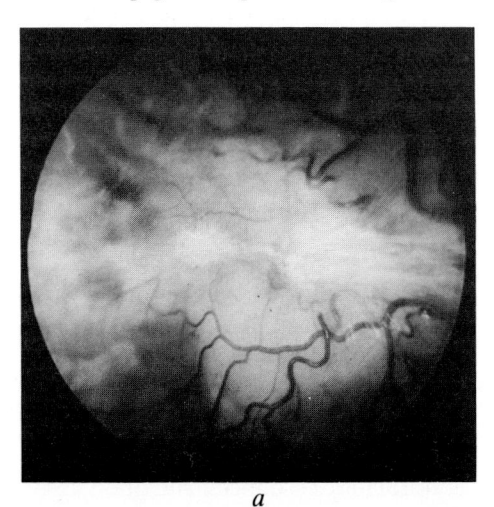

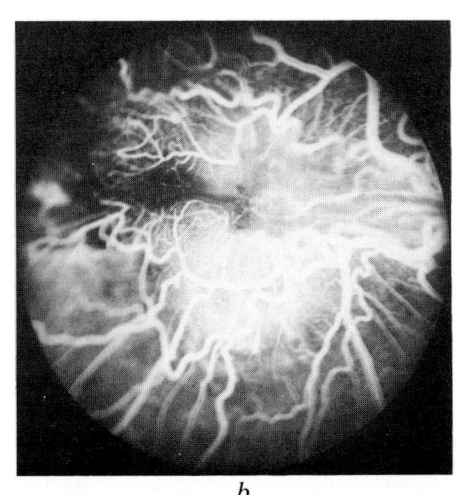

Fig. 12. *a*, Hamartoma of the retinal pigment epithelium, right macula of a one-year-old child. *b*, Fluorescein angiography demonstrates gross irregularity of the macular retinal vasculature and diffuse pigment epithelial abnormalities.

cavernous retinal haemangiomas may be associated with striking intraretinal or preretinal haemorrhage.

Malignant

Choroidal melanomas may directly infiltrate the macula or induce a serous detachment. A tumour detachment of the retinal pigment epithelium may follow infiltration by a reticulum cell sarcoma, which is generally associated with a severe posterior uveitis. Leukaemic infiltrates and retinoblastoma may also cause striking elevation of the retina, and fluorescein angiography and ultrasonography are helpful in determining the size, nature and location of the tumour.

Secondary Tumours

Ocular metastases from distant primary tumours, e.g. breast, stomach, lung and thyroid, may infiltrate the choroid and cause serous detachment of the macula. Fluorescein angiography may be helpful in identifying a tumour circulation and determining the limits of tumour spread. Ultrasonography is useful in demonstrating the nature and physical characteristics of the tumour.

Macular Disease Associated with Traction

Vitreo-retinal Disease

Traction macular detachments may follow extensive vasoproliferation secondary to diabetes, central or branch retinal vein thrombosis or retrolental fibroplasia. Intraretinal or preretinal fibroglial proliferation and retinal elevation may also be the sequel of a toxocaral retinitis. In general, detachment of the macula or impending detachment of the macula is an indication for vitrectomy in diabetes or ischaemic retinal vascular disease, provided that residual visual functions are present or can be realistically retrieved.

Perforating Injuries

Perforating injuries may also occasionally be associated with vitreous bands extending from the site of perforation to the macula and causing dislocation of the macula. Such eyes often respond to excision of the vitreoretinal bands, which allows resolution of the macular detachment.

FURTHER READING

1. Yannuzzi L. W., Gitter K. A. and Schatz H. *The Macula: A Comprehensive Text and Atlas.* Baltimore, Md, Williams and Wilkins, 1978.
2. Gass J. D. M. *Stereoscopic Atlas of Macular Diseases: A Fundoscopic and Angiographic Presentation*, 2nd ed. St Louis, Mo, Mosby, 1977.
3. Fine S. L. and Owens S. L. *Management of Retinal Vascular and Macular Disorders.* Baltimore, Md, Williams and Wilkins, 1983.
4. Macular Photocoagulation Study Group. Argon laser photocoagulation for senile macular degeneration: Results of a randomized clinical trial. *Arch. Ophthalmol.* 1982; **100,** 912–18.
5. Krill A. E. Hereditary retinal and choroidal diseases. In: *Bruch's Membrane Degenerations.* Hagerstown, Md, Harper and Row Medical, 1977.
6. Archer D. B. and Gardiner T. A. Electron microscopic features of experimental choroidal neovascularization. *Am. J. Ophthalmol.* 1981; **91,** 433–57.
7. Wright B. E., Bird A. C. and Hamilton A. M. Placoid pigment epitheliopathy and Harada's disease. *Br. J. Ophthalmol.* 1978; **62,** 609–21.
8. Gass J. D. M. Bullous retinal detachment – An unusual manifestation of idiopathic central serous choroidopathy. *Am. J. Ophthalmol.* 1973; **75,** 810–21.

Vascular Retinopathies
The Management of Diabetic Retinopathy

E. Kohner and A. M. P. Hamilton

INTRODUCTION

Diabetic retinopathy, despite the more frequent use of laser treatment in its management in the United Kingdom, is still the commonest cause of blindness between the ages of 30 and 65. Its frequency is increasing with the greater longevity of diabetic patients. After 10 years of diabetic life, 20 per cent of patients show retinopathy, while after 20 years, this figure increases to some 80 per cent.

Since the introduction of the argon laser by Francis L'Esperance in 1969 considerable progress has been made in the development of techniques that may be used for the treatment of retinopathy. As the basic action of laser therapy is still in doubt, such techniques are empirical and must be established by careful planning and reasonable periods of follow-up.

This section will discuss the methods that have been used in the management of diabetic patients, illustrating the effect of techniques on individual patients at various stages of the development of retinopathy.

A number of different types of laser are available. The argon laser was the first instrument to be used. More recent options comprise the argon laser, with either the blue–green or the green light, and krypton lasers. The YAG laser is also available, with its ability to produce a plasma within any ocular tissue.

This section is almost entirely concerned with the argon green–blue modality, and although the other colours of laser light have a place to play in the management of retinal or macular disease, they have not been established to the same extent in the treatment of diabetic retinopathy. In particular the role of YAG laser in the division of vitreous bands remains to be proved.

The evolution of diabetic retinopathy is extremely varied. In some patients it is slow and progressive, in others rapid. Factors that may have an adverse effect on the progression of retinopathy are poor diabetic control, uraemia, hypertension, oral contraceptives, pregnancy and possibly smoking.

Diabetic retinopathy, a complication of long standing diabetes, may be subdivided into various groups which overlap to a greater or lesser degree. The three main groups are: background retinopathy, maculopathy (pp. 244–7) and proliferative retinopathy.

Diabetic retinopathy is the earliest development of retinopathy, with dilated retinal veins and microaneurysm formation, and the changes are most prominent at the posterior pole. With the passage of time additional lesions may occur and, depending upon the type of change that develops, the pattern of retinopathy alters. It is useful at this stage to enumerate the various lesions that may develop and attribute to them their appropriate importance.

CAPILLARY LESIONS

Microaneurysms

The capillary lesions observed clinically are microaneurysms, which appear as small, round red dots predominantly at the posterior pole inside the temporal vascular arcades. They vary in size from 10 to 25 μm in diameter. They consist of out-pouchings of the walls of the retinal capillaries and therefore may lie at the level of the deep or the superficial capillary plexus. They are seen ophthalmoscopically as round red dots but on fluorescein angiography the dots show a characteristic hyperfluorescence. If the endothelial lining of the microaneurysms is intact there is no leakage of dye, but if the endothelial lining is damaged then there is leakage of fluorescein into the surrounding retina. Many deeper haemorrhages in the retina appear round and the only way to distinguish these from microaneurysms is to carry out fluorescein angiography. The natural history of microaneurysms is variable; some increase in size and develop leakage, while in other areas they may increase in number or spontaneously thrombose and disappear.

Retinal Oedema

At the site of areas of leakage, fluid may accumulate, giving rise to thickening of the retina. In background retinopathy the fluid is confined to the areas of microaneurysms and does not spread into the macular region.

Hard Exudates

At the margin of areas of retinal oedema hard exudates may well precipitate into the outer areas of the retina. They commonly delineate the margin of abnormal capillary permeability and relatively normal capillary bed. These exudates may be small dot-like exudates, many of which are lying within retinal macrophages. As the exudates gradually increase in size they coelesce to form larger plaque-like masses. In background retinopathy these exudates do not encroach on the macula (*Fig.* 1).

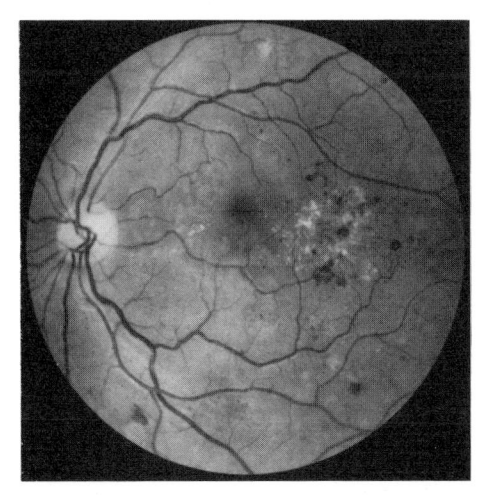

Fig. 1. Microaneurysms and exudates around the macula of the right eye. Some exudates appear as round dots, while others are larger and plaque-like.

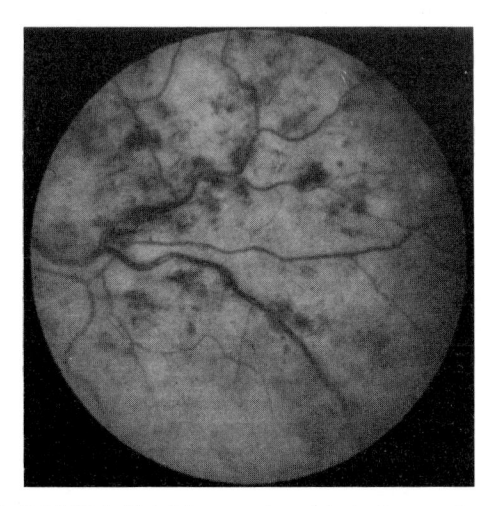

Fig. 2. Multiple blotch haemorrhage (cluster haemorrhages).

Haemorrhage

The common type of haemorrhage that presents in background retinopathy is the round haemorrhage which lies in the reticular layers of the retina and is usually associated with retinal microaneurysms.

Other haemorrhages that may occur are superficial flame-shaped haemorrhages, lying in the nerve fibre layer. Deeper haemorrhages may also occur in the retina, and these have a blotchy appearance similar to ink marks on blotting paper. These deep haemorrhages usually occur in groups or clusters and have been termed cluster haemorrhages (*Fig.* 2). In the areas of these haemorrhages, fluorescein angiography shows variable degrees of capillary closure. The haemorrhages are frequently seen at the margin of large non-perfused areas and indicate the sites of capillary and arteriolar occlusion. Large numbers of such haemorrhages are therefore a very clear indicator of a severe retinopathy.

ARTERIOLAR LESIONS

Cotton-wool Spots

These white fluffy deposits in the superficial retina are often associated with macular insufficiency and represent an accumulation of axoplasmic debris (*Fig.* 3). This intracellular accumulation of material is associated with hypertension and may occur at any stage

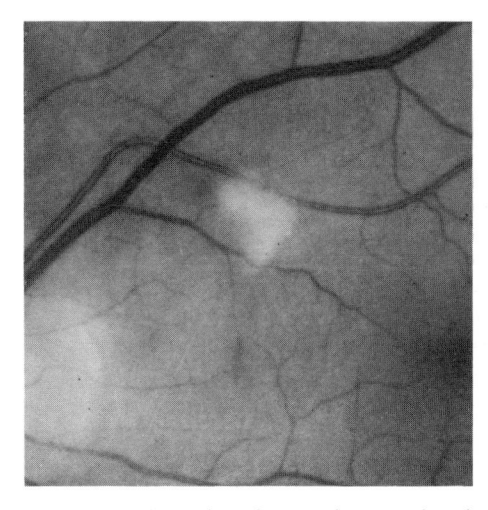

Fig. 3. A cotton-wool spot just above and temporal to the optic disc.

in the development of retinopathy. The presence of cotton-wool spots is of prognostic importance and is an indication of the likely development of sight threatening retinopathy. If there are more than five cotton-wool spots in an eye there is an 80 per cent chance of significant visual loss in 5 years if untreated.

Intraretinal New Vessels

At the site of capillary closure intraretinal new vessels may develop and are visible ophthalmoscopically as hair-pin like protrusions extending from retinal veins or capillaries. These again are an indicator of capillary closure and of severe retinopathy.

White Vessels

Arterioles and venules may become occluded and appear as white streaks within the retina. These white streaks indicate occlusive retinopathy and lie within areas of capillary non-perfusion (*Fig.* 4).

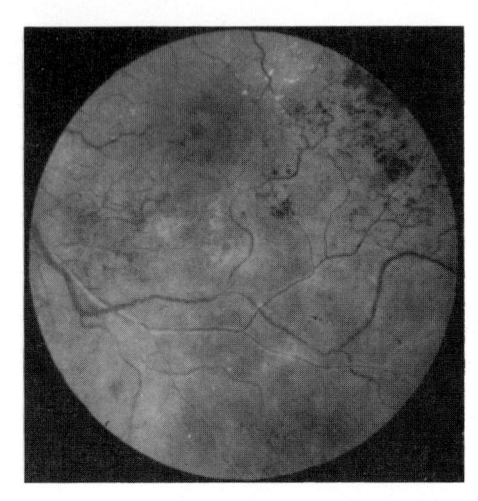

Fig. 4. Inferior temporal region showing white arterioles. In addition there are cluster haemorrhages in the area temporal to the macula.

Venous Changes

Venous abnormalities may be present in background retinopathy. As we have previously mentioned, venous dilatation is one of the earliest signs of retinopathy. With advancement of the retinopathy, venous beading may develop with sausage-like protrusions along dilated retinal veins. In addition, minor venous occlusions may occur which result in the development of collateral channels around the occlusion with the typical diabetic venous loop or reduplication (*Fig.* 5). The venous changes of beading and loop formation only occur in patients with evidence of capillary non-perfusion and are a further indicator of capillary closure within the retina.

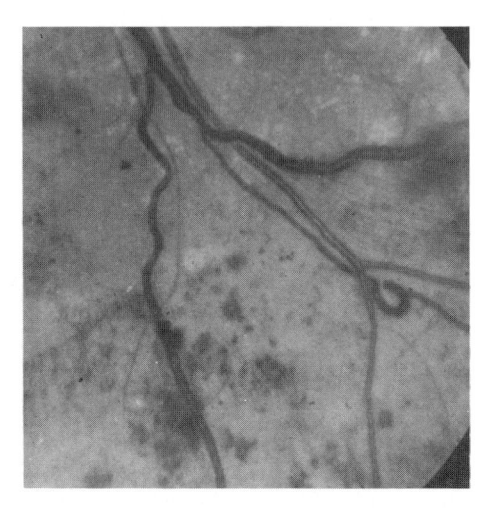

Fig. 5. An area of retina with a venous loop along the vein. The adjacent vein shows some sausage-like dilatation.

Background diabetic retinopathy has some or all of these features, but in background retinopathy none of these features is present directly in the macular area and visual acuity in these patients is normal.

The further these lesions are from the macula, the less the threat to central visual acuity (*Fig.* 6).

The way in which the retinopathy progresses from background retinopathy influences the clinical outcome. If the retinopathy is predominantly confined

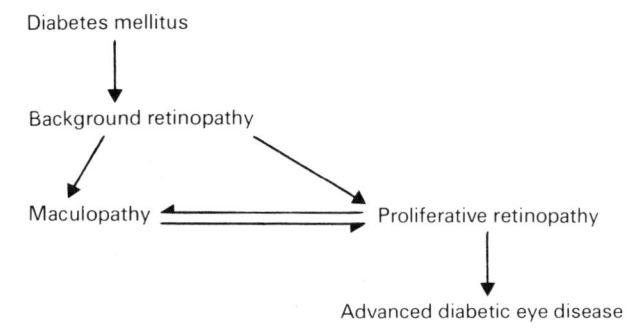

Fig. 6. Classification of diabetic retinopathy.

to the posterior pole with microaneurysms and leakage and exudate formation, then these lesions may spread towards the macular region with oedema and/or exudates damaging macular function and producing slow diminution of central acuity. The patient then passes into the stage of 'maculopathy'. If the changes in the retinopathy are those of progressive capillary non-perfusion, then the patient is likely to develop pre-retinal new vessels and has then moved into the stage of 'proliferative retinopathy'.

In short, maculopathy comprises the features of background retinopathy with oedema or exudates spreading into the macula giving rise to visual loss. Proliferative retinopathy comprises capillary non-perfusion and pre-retinal new vessels. Because of their site these new vessels may give rise to a vitreous haemorrhage and dramatically threaten the patient's visual function. Proliferative retinopathy may pass on to the final stage when the patient is blind as a result of vitreous haemorrhage, retinal detachment or haemorrhagic glaucoma with rubeosis. This stage is known as advanced diabetic eye disease.

PROLIFERATIVE RETINOPATHY

The various stages in the development of proliferative retinopathy are shown in *Table* I.

Table I: Development of proliferative retinopathy

Capillary non perfusion Intraretinal new vessels	Preproliferative
Preretinal new vessels Forward preretinal new vessels Disc new vessels Disc new vessels with retinitis proliferans	Proliferative
Vitreous haemorrhage Retinal traction Macular traction Detachment Rubeosis iridis	Advanced diabetic eye retinal disease

Preproliferative Retinopathy

In this type of eye there are variable amounts of capillary closure and in the long standing cases, intraretinal new vessels. This type of retinopathy may or may not lead to the development of preretinal new vessels. Patients with preproliferative retinopathy have a 50 per cent chance of developing new vessels within a year. Whether laser treatment prevents the development of new vessels or prevents spread of capillary non-perfusion is still in doubt.

As laser treatment is not without risk, no treatment for preproliferative retinopathy is recommended, but the patient must be re-examined at regular intervals to assess the extent of capillary closure and to offer treatment at the first sign of preretinal new vessel formation.

There are two exceptions to this guiding rule. Patients known to be poor compliers either because of their reluctance to attend or because of the distance involved in travelling, should have laser applied to the areas of capillary closure. The second exception applies to patients with a preflorid retinopathy, which occurs in juvenile onset diabetics after 10 years. The course of this disease is best illustrated by the following case history.

Case History

T.W., a 23-year-old butcher, was a diabetic of 10 years' standing. His control was always poor. He had no visual symptoms but his physician found retinopathy on routine examination. When seen, he had preproliferative retinopathy in both eyes, manifested by venous beading and dilatation, intraretinal microvascular abnormalities, cotton-wool spots and cluster haemorrhages (*Fig.* 7). He was advised to improve his diabetic control, which he failed to do. He was then advised to have at least one eye treated by photocoagulation, to which he agreed. *Fig.* 8 shows the untreated eye 4 months after the initial picture was taken. New vessels with fibrous tissue and haemorrhage have developed, causing traction on the internal limiting membrane, which distorts the macula.

Preretinal New Vessels

Once new vessels have formed on the retina there is a threat to the patient's vision due to vitreous haemorrhage and the consequences of associated fibrosis. The new vessels lie on the surface of the retina, having passed through the internal limiting membrane. They are attached with a variable degree of firmness to the posterior vitreous face. In this position they bleed, due to posterior vitreous detachment or as a result of a Valsalva manoeuvre or as a consequence of a hypoglycaemic attack. Once established, new vessels frequently develop adventitial tissue around them which may contract with further bleeding and traction on the retina.

Fig. 9a demonstrates the superior temporal quadrant of the right retina showing extensive new vessels lying in and around the superior temporal vessels.

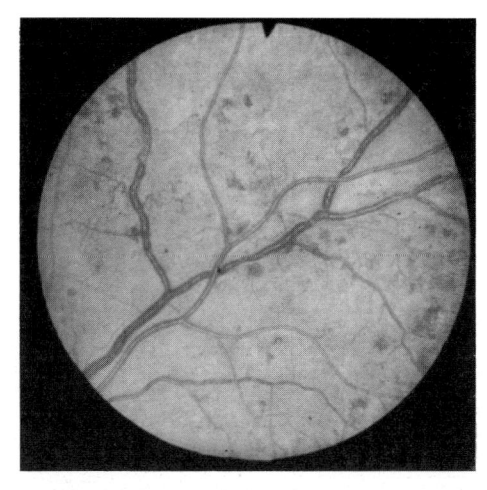

Fig. 7. Superior temporal quadrant with intraretinal new vessels, cotton-wool spots, venous beading and cluster haemorrhages.

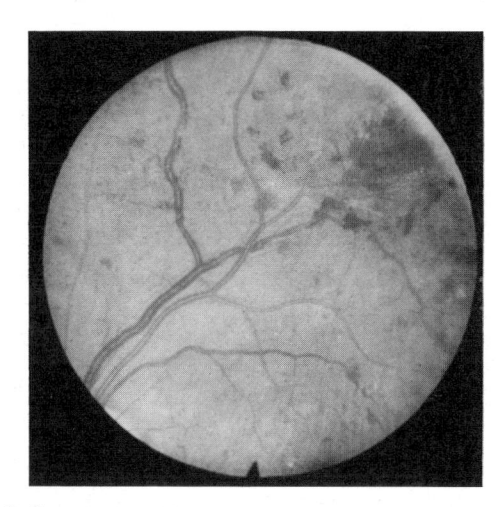

Fig. 8. Same area as *Fig.* 6, with the development of preretinal fibrosis and new vessels.

Fig. 9b demonstrates the effect of laser therapy to the area of new vessels and extensive scatter treatment to the superior temporal quadrant. In patients with extensive new vessels in whom the new vessels are inaccessible by virtue of their closeness to major arcades, treatment should be applied to peripheral areas of non-perfusion. When there are numerous new vessels in all quadrants the patient will receive amounts similar to that of panretinal ablation. Patients with formed new vessels are treated in a similar way. However, if the new vessels persist, it may be necessary to occlude the new vessels directly or occlude the feeding vein.

Disc New Vessels

The presence of disc new vessels indicates a poor visual prognosis if untreated in that 50 per cent of such patients are blind within 5 years. If a quarter of the retina exhibits capillary non-perfusion, development of new vessels on the disc ensues. Initially

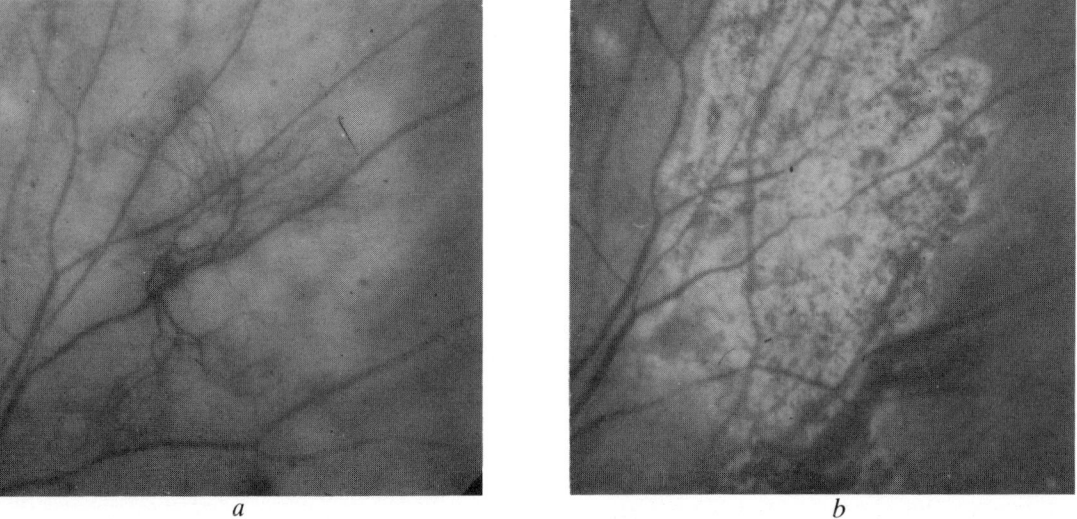

Fig. 9. *a*, The superior temporal quadrant with new vessels around the major vessels. *b*, Following some 450 500 μm burns to the peripheral retina, regression of the new vessels is evident.

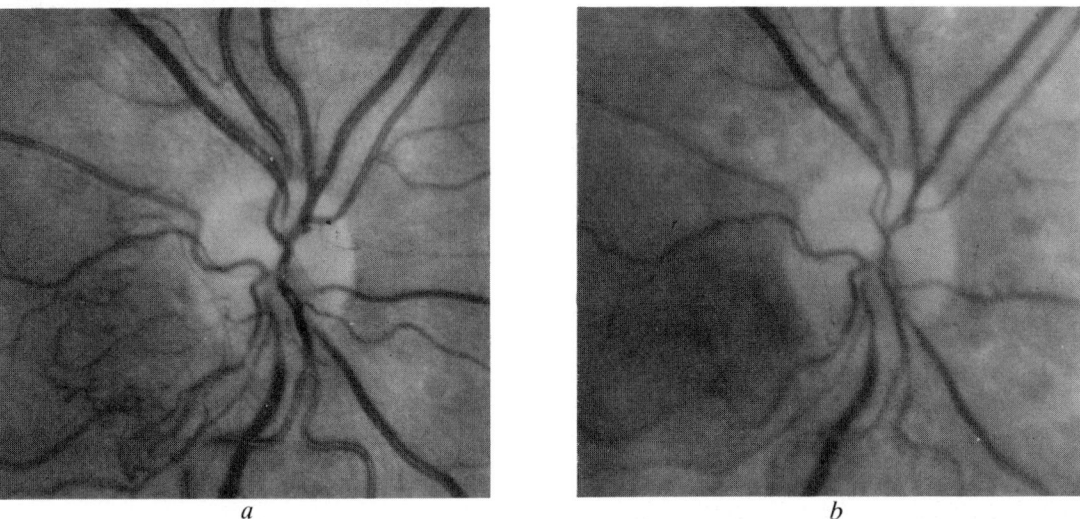

Fig. 10. *a*, New vessels extending from the inferior temporal margin of the optic disc. *b*, The same disc following 2 500 μm burns, showing regression of the new vessels with some resulting pallor of the optic disc.

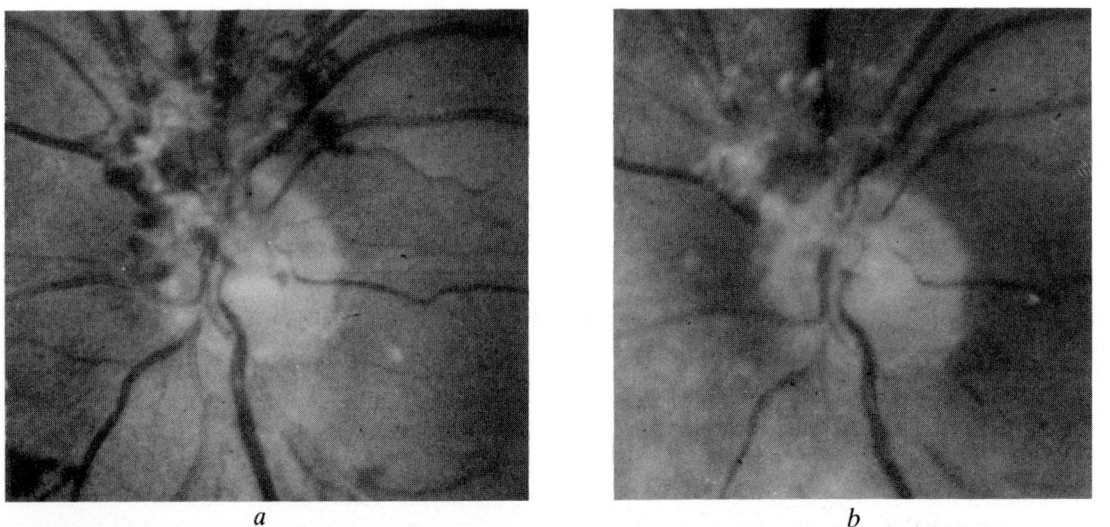

Fig. 11. *a*, New vessels and fibrosis extending from the optic disc of the left eye. *b*, After extensive panretinal photocoagulation, regression of the new vessels can be seen but there is persistence of the fibrosis tissue.

these vessels lie flat on the retina but subsequently may be pulled forwards and attract adventitial fibrous tissue.

Fig. 10*a* shows the right retina of a 39-year-old man with new vessels on the disc. *Fig.* 10*b* demonstrates the same retina following 2500 burns of 500 μm spot size and an exposure time of 0·06 s applied with the argon laser. Burns can be seen adjacent to the disc and superiorly and inferiorly. Burns have also been applied to the area temporal to the macula in the region of capillary non-perfusion. The burns have been placed with a separation of approximately one burn diameter, and have been applied to the peripheral retina as far anterior as the equator. This technique is called panretinal photocoagulation (PRP) or pattern bombing.

Panretinal photocoagulation has altered the prognosis in patients with disc new vessels so that in 80–90 per cent of cases regression is expected. The type of reaction at the time of laser application should be minimal, with just blanching of the pigment epithelium. With this type of burn the side effects are minimal. A small proportion of patients experience a change in refraction associated with shallowing of the anterior chamber and/or macular choroidal detachment. A few patients complain of field changes, mainly constriction of the field, and some develop disturbed colour vision with loss of blue discrimination.

In some eyes new vessels are associated with fibrous tissue. In these cases argon laser is the treatment of choice, but should be used with a gentle burn appropriate to the treatment of the new vessels in the peripheral retina.

Fig. 11*a* demonstrates the retina of a patient of 48 years of age with new vessels peripherally and extensive fibrosis. The peripheral retina showed clinical evidence of capillary non-perfusion. This patient received some 2000, 500 μm burns; a few weeks later there was complete regression of the new vessels with persistence but no increase of fibrosis (*Fig.* 11*b*).

FLORID DIABETIC RETINOPATHY

Florid diabetic retinopathy occurs in diabetics of long years' standing. The diabetes is often unstable and poorly controlled and the patient presents with a lowered visual acuity to the level of 6/24 or 6/18. Fundus examination discloses early new vessels on the disc, marked venous abnormalities, cotton-wool spots, sometimes partial occlusion of a major branch of the central retinal artery, hard exudates and widespread capillary closure. The macular region is usually oedematous with exudates and cluster haemorrhages.

Untreated, nine of ten patients go blind within one year. In the past, the treatment of choice was pituitary ablation. More recently, it has been shown that very extensive photocoagulation with heavy burns throughout the peripheral retina, can arrest progression. The treatment is always urgent and should be done within a week of diagnosis. Because the patients are usually young (often in their 'teens), and somewhat apprehensive, laser treatment may be difficult under local anaesthesia. Xenon arc treatment under general anaesthesia is recommended as a rapid and efficient method of management.

RETINOPATHY IN PREGNANCY

Diabetic retinopathy may be seen for the first time during pregnancy. It frequently deteriorates with the advance of pregnancy and following delivery (or termination of pregnancy) the retinopathy tends to improve. If such a retinopathy is treated adequately by laser therapy subsequent pregnancies rarely cause further problems.

FURTHER READING

Constable I. J. and Lim S. M. *Laser—Its Clinical Uses in Eye Diseases.*
  Edinburgh, Churchill Livingstone, 1981.
Davidson S. I. and Fraunfelder F. T. *Recent Advances in Ophthalmology 7.*
  Edinburgh, Churchill Livingstone, 1985.
Kanski J. J. and Morse P. H. *Ophthalmology 1—Disorders of the Vitreous, Retina and Choroid.*
  Sevenoaks, Butterworths, 1983.
Kohner E. *Diabetic Retinopathy (International Ophthalmology Clinics,* volume 18, no. 4).
  Heidelberg, Winter, 1978.
L'Esperance F. A. and James W. A. *Diabetic Retinopathy—Clinical Evaluation and Management.*
  St Louis, Mosby, 1981.
Morse, P. H. *Practical Management of Diabetic Retinopathy.*
  New York, Appleton-Century-Croft, 1985.
Revue Chibret d'Ophthalmologie. Symposium International sur la Retinopathie Diabetique.
  No. 105, 1985.

The Management of Diabetic Maculopathy

E. Kohner and A. M. P. Hamilton

Diabetic maculopathy is the condition in which visual acuity (VA) is endangered or lost because of 'primary' involvement of the macula, most usually by oedema, but at times by ischaemia or hard plaques of exudate. Macular disease secondary to proliferative retinopathy, e.g. macular traction, is not considered here.

exudates, however, can be reduced by diet or clofibrate. Photocoagulation is the only treatment of proved value in maintaining and occasionally improving vision. It is most effective in the exudative forms of maculopathy but occasionally it is of value in cystoid macular oedema. It prevents development of new vessels in ischaemic maculopathy.

a *b*

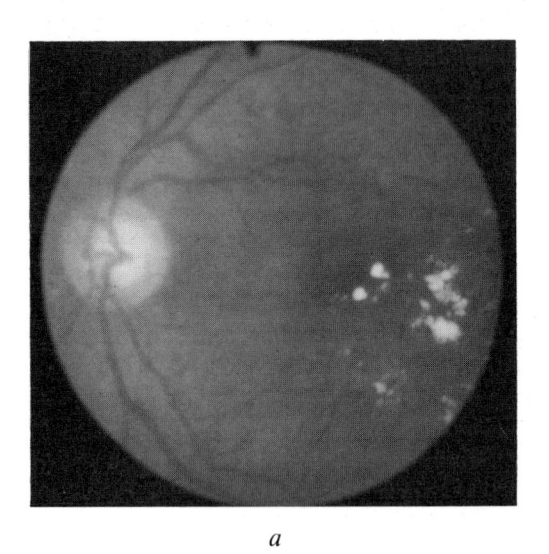

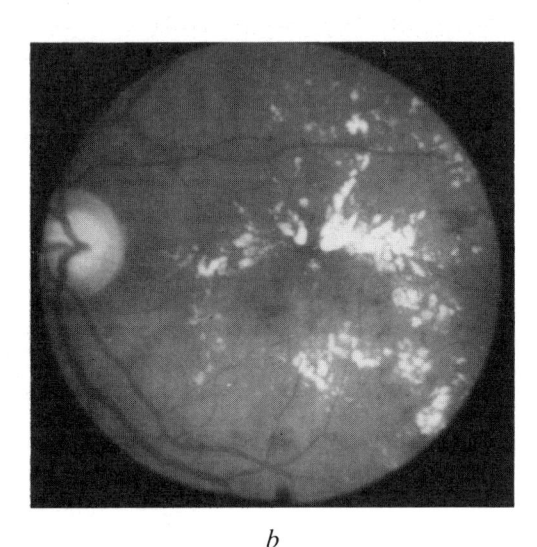

Fig. 1. Example I. Hard exudates left untreated.

Diabetic maculopathy is divided into three major subgroups, which can be further subdivided, according to the type of lesion present.

1. Exudative maculopathy
    (*a*) Hard exudates, small and scattered
    (*b*) Hard exudative rings (circinate maculopathy)
    (*c*) Hard plaques of exudate
2. Oedematous maculopathy
    (*a*) cystoid macular oedema
    (*b*) generalized leakage.
3. Ischaemic maculopathy

None of the maculopathies responds to the medical control of diabetes by improved visual acuity. Hard

EXAMPLE I (*Fig.* 1)

Hard exudates if left untreated tend to increase in number and advance towards the fovea.

Fig. 1*a* shows the left macula of a 54-year-old non-insulin-dependent patient with 4 years' diabetic history. VA = 6/6. There are a few hard exudates, lateral to the macula. The patient was advised to return in 6–12 months for examination, but defaulted and came back 3 years later.

Fig. 1*b* shows the patient at that time. Vision = 6/24. A hard exudative ring has formed involving the macula with microvascular abnormalities within it.

EXAMPLE II (*Fig.* 2)

This example illustrates that hard exudates respond to laser therapy.

Fig. 2*a* shows the left macula of a 58-year-old non-insulin-dependent diabetic patient 5 years after diagnosis of diabetes. VA = 6/12. Hard exudates are scattered and form a ring inferiorly. Many microaneurysms and haemorrhages lie lateral to the macula.

Immediately after treatment with the argon laser (*Fig.* 2*b*), burns of 100 μm size are seen distributed laterally to the macula over microvascular abnormalities. These are light burns aimed at the pigment epithelium.

Fig. 2*c* shows the patient 3 years after laser treatment. VA = 6/6 and only light scars are visible.

In this patient, treatment improved vision, although usually it only preserves what is present.

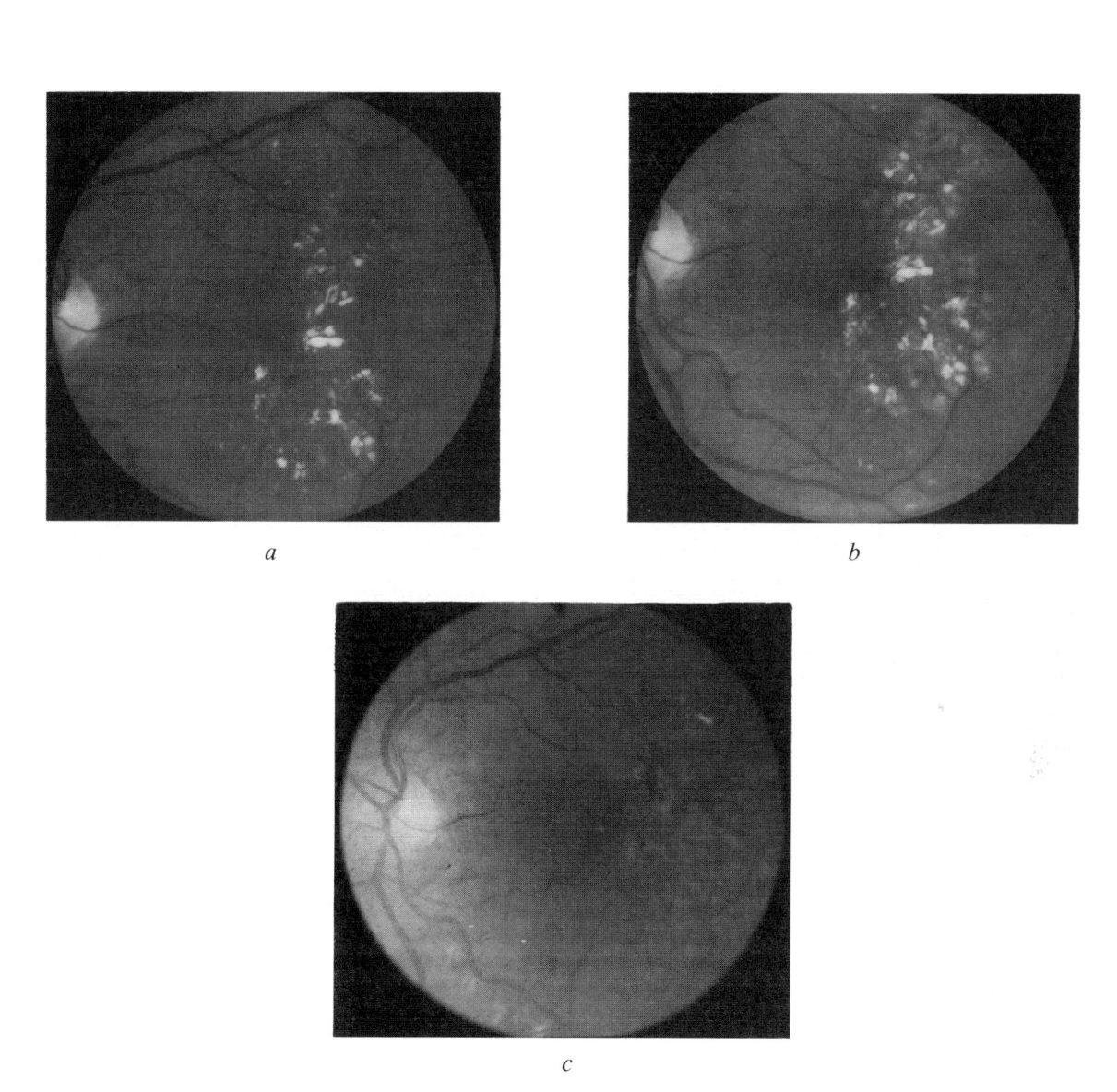

Fig. 2. Example II. Hard exudates respond to laser therapy.

EXAMPLE III (*Fig.* 3)

Treatment of Macular Oedema

This 32-year-old poorly controlled insulin-dependent diabetic patient had an acuity of 6/36. The dark irregular appearance at the macula (*Fig.* 3a) is suggestive of macular oedema. There are some microvascular abnormalities and haemorrhages.

Fluorescein angiogram in the capillary phase (*Fig.* 3b) shows areas of non-perfusion and extensive leakage from all capillaries extending into the foveal area.

Late angiogram confirmed leakage of oedematous maculopathy (*Fig.* 3c).

The macula area was treated, with a grid of 100 μm burns.

Four months later VA = 6/60 and scars of photocoagulation are seen (*Fig.* 3d).

More haemorrhages developed, indicating the development of peripheral ischaemia.

In cases of oedematous maculopathy, a grid over the macula may maintain vision, but it rarely improves it.

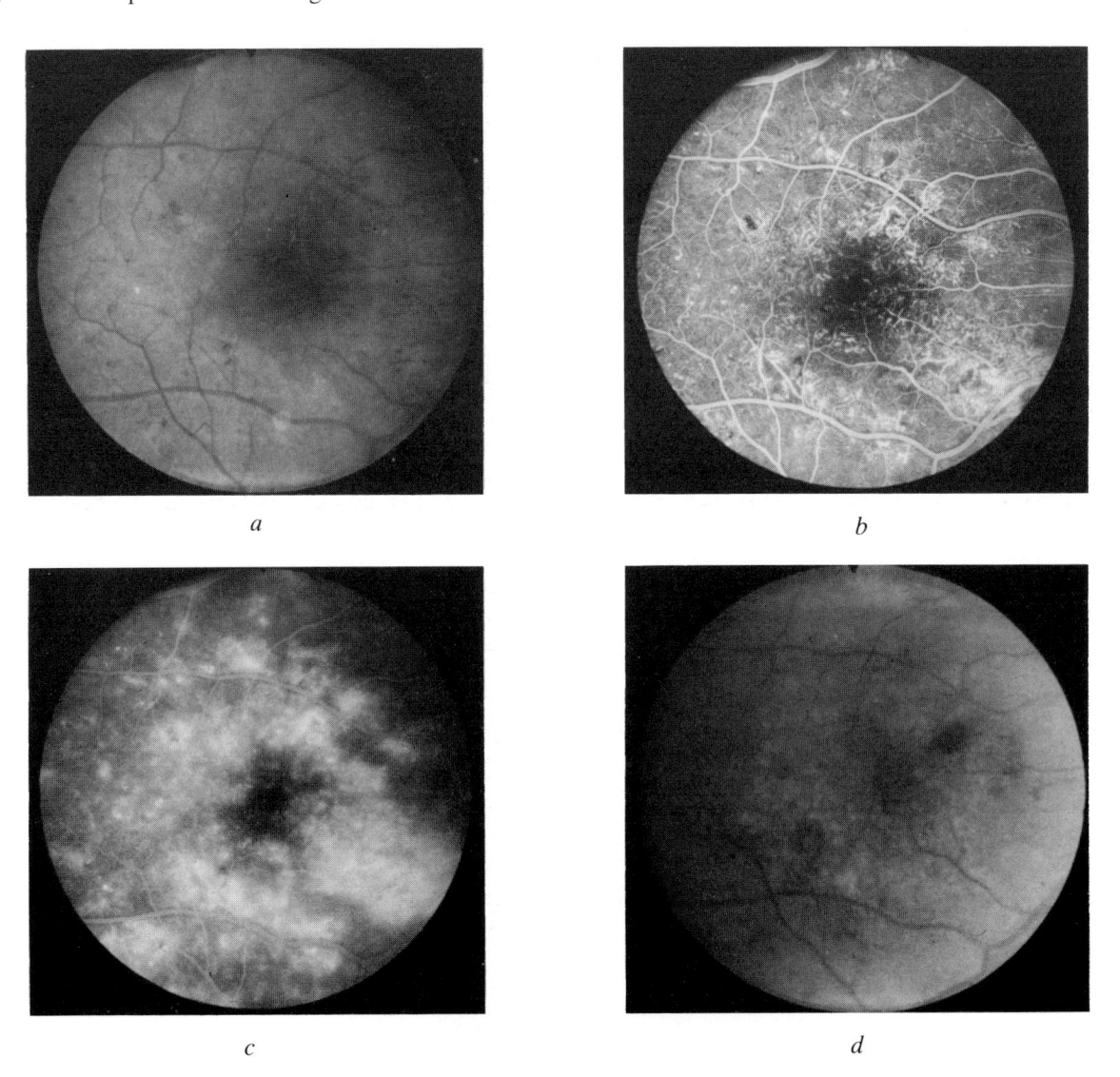

Fig. 3. Example III. Treatment of macular oedema.

EXAMPLE IV (*Fig. 4*)

Treatment of Ischaemic Maculopathy

Fig. 4*a* shows the right eye of a 58-year-old non-insulin-dependent patient with circinate and scattered hard exudates. In addition, there are signs of ischaemia (preproliferative lesions), such as a large venous loop, venous dilatation and a cluster of large blot haemorrhages lateral to the macula.

Initially treatment was applied to the ischaemic area lateral to the macula and to the centre of the hard exudative ring. *Fig.* 4*b* shows light 100 μm burns.

Because of the widespread ischaemia, panretinal photocoagulation (PRP) was also given, to prevent new vessel formation (*Fig.* 4*c*).

The macular area 3 years after completing treatment (*Fig.* 4*d*) reveals only minor residual lesions and photocoagulation scars.

The patient had a mixture of exudative and ischaemic maculopathy. The exudative lesions disappeared and development of proliferative retinopathy was prevented by PRP.

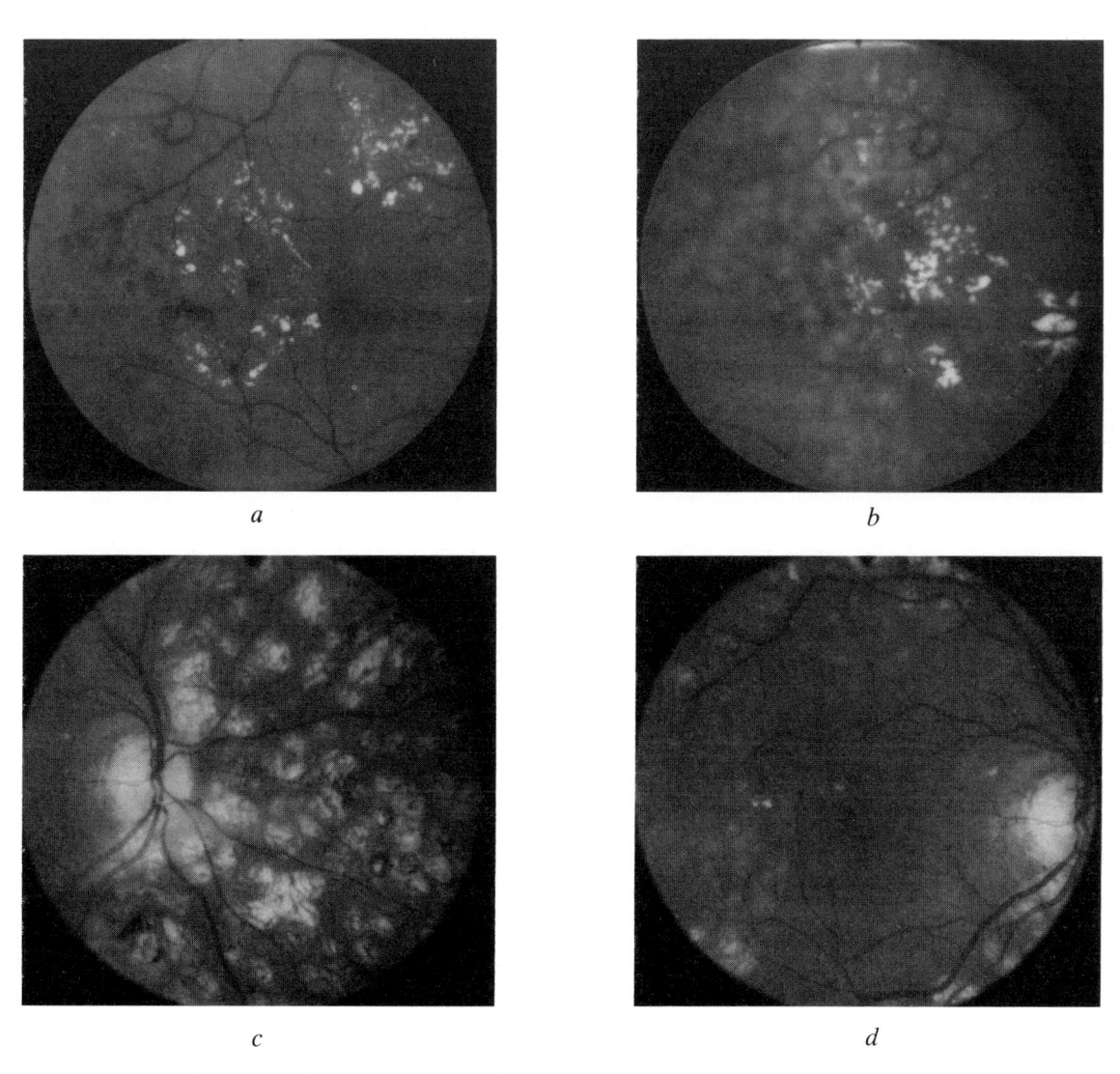

Fig. 4. Example IV. Treatment of ischaemic maculopathy.

Retinal Detachment Surgery

A. H. Chignell

PATHOGENESIS

Retinal detachment is the separation of the photoreceptor and pigment epithelial layers of the retina. In rhegmatogenous retinal detachment the separation has occurred as the result of a retinal hole formation in the photoreceptor layer allowing communication between the vitreal and subretinal spaces. In non-rhegmatogenous retinal detachment there is no such communication.

Retinal Holes

Holes in the retina (which in only some cases lead on to retinal detachment) form in the retina either as a result of intrinsic weakness of the retina itself, or as a result of vitreous pulling on the retina. In many retinal detachment situations encountered, both factors play some part in the production of the retinal hole. Thus vitreous traction resulting, for example, in a horseshoe-shaped tear, may be found in association with underlying retinal degenerative change, e.g. lattice degeneration. Some forms of retinal degeneration leading to weakness in the retina and hole formation (e.g. snail track degeneration) are not associated with vitreous traction.

Vitreous Detachment

Traction on the underlying retina from the vitreous is usually as a consequence of posterior vitreous detachment. If this process is complete, vitreous separates from the posterior retina and from the disc, to which it is usually firmly attached, leaving only its firm attachment at the vitreous base, an area which extends approximately 1 mm on either side of ora serrata. When the detached vitreous is set in motion by the movement of the eye, traction is exerted at the posterior border of the vitreous base, as a result of the whip-like action of the posterior hyaloid. This traction may result in retinal hole formation at the posterior border of the vitreous base (*Fig.* 1) or, on occasions, more posteriorly placed adhesions between vitreous and retina, e.g. along retinal blood vessels. Posterior vitreous detachment may occur as a senile change, as part of the ageing process of the eye, but may occur as a result of more pathological changes occurring in the vitreous body. The most important associated cause is myopia (a situation in which there is also a high incidence of peripheral retinal degenerative change). Thus there is a combination of factors which accounts for the predeliction of myopes to develop retinal detachment.

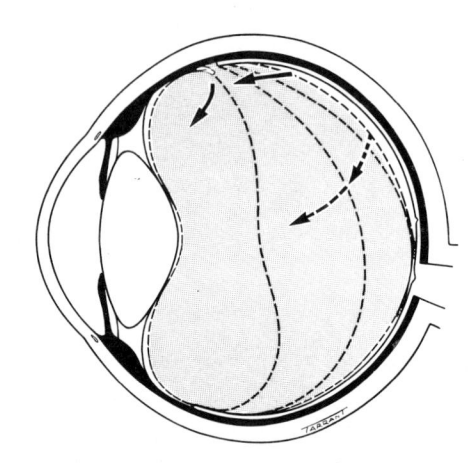

Fig. 1. Progressive posterior vitreous detachment is shown by the dashed arrows. As the posterior vitreous detachment approaches the vitreous base (solid arrows) traction may produce a horseshoe-shaped tear in this area.

Degeneration of the vitreous body may also be induced as a result of its infiltration with white cells (in uveitis) or red cells. Aphakia puts the eye at risk, not only because the intracapsular removal of the crystalline lens almost invariably leads to posterior vitreous detachment, but greater excursion of gel on movement following the intracapsular method accentuates traction on the posterior border of the vitreous base. It has been found that the risk of aphakic detachment is greatly increased if the vitreous has been incarcerated into the cataract section at the time of cataract surgery.[1,2] Use of the extracapsular method of cataract extraction, leaving the posterior segment of the eye intact with less anterior movement of gel, results in a lower incidence of aphakic detachment by altering the pattern of posterior vitreous detachment.[3-5]

Vitreous Traction

Intermittent pulling on the underlying retina as a result of movement of the vitreous gel, i.e. dynamic vitreous traction[6] is the common mechanism by which vitreous traction can result in retinal hole formation. In more complex situations membranes related to the surface of the retina exert a continual tractional force upon it, i.e. static traction. This type of traction may in turn result in secondary retinal hole formation. Static retinal traction may be either mainly vitreo-retinal in its orientation, with contraction of vitreous attachments to the retina, drawing the retina towards the middle of the eye, or the traction may be mainly tangential to the retinal surface and caused by the contraction of membranes on either surface of the detached retina. In many clinical detachment situations a combination of tractional forces is found. In most rhegmatogenous retinal detachments membrane formation succeeds retinal detachment, but sometimes purely tractional retinal detachment situations arise when fibrotic tissue forms in relationship to the retina for other reasons; for example, in proliferative diabetic retinopathy new vessels are converted into a fibrovascular complex, the progressive contraction of which may result first in a traction retinal detachment and later a rhegmatogenous element as retinal holes are produced. Traction retinal detachments may also be produced as a result of contraction of membranes growing in the vitreous cavity as a consequence to penetrating injuries of the posterior segment.

SUBRETINAL FLUID (SRF)

In those cases in which the retinal hole is succeeded by retinal detachment, SRF fluid starts to accumulate between the pigment epithelium and the photoreceptor layers. This fluid itself is derived both from the vitreous cavity and a contribution is probably made from choroidal vessels.[7] In most cases SRF accumulates rapidly (particularly from superior detachments) and the retinal detachment will become total. More rarely, the retinal detachment will become localized and static, but usually this will only happen if the detachment is in the lower half of the retina. If untreated, the eye may become complicated by uveitis, secondary glaucoma and cataract formation and in some cases the eye will become phthisical. On rare occasions spontaneous reattachment of the retina occurs. If retinal detachment has been present for some months, the junction between detached normal retina becomes marked by the presence of a pigmented line (a high-water mark). This line represents activity of the pigment epithelium in response to long term presence of SRF. These pigmented lines take at least 3 months to form and serve as a distinguishing feature between retinal detachment and retinoschisis, as in the latter condition in which the collection of fluid is in the outer plexiform layer of the retina, pigmented lines are never found. With the further passage of time the detached retina itself assumes a thinner and cystic appearance and eventually, after approximately 1 year, secondary intraretinal cysts may form in the outer plexiform layer of the detached retina (*Plate* XI*a*).

MEMBRANES

In response to the presence of a detached retina, cellular membranes derived from both pigment epithelial and retinal glial cells may form on either surface of the retina (proliferative vitreoretinopathy). The preretinal surface is particularly favoured and it is the subsequent contraction of these membranes that causes difficulty in surgical reattachment. Detachments that are particularly likely to be complicated by membrane formation are those that are long standing, aphakic or as a result of giant retinal holes. Surgery which fails to result in reattachment will accelerate the tendency to membrane formation, particularly if the failed surgery has been accompanied by complications of various sorts (e.g. retinal incarceration and choroidal haemorrhage.[8]) The effect of membrane formation on the retina depends on the severity and extent of the membranous process. Early signs of membrane formation are distortion of retinal features, such as blood vessels and retinal holes, and often these preliminary changes are seen before actual whiteness on the surface of the retina is detected. As the membranes become established they become white and readily visible. As contraction of these membranes proceeds the retina becomes folded (often making detection and closure of retinal holes more difficult). The fibrotic process leads to progressive immobilization of normally mobile detached retina. Strong vitreo-retinal adhesions may form and this is particularly seen in the inferior retina at the posterior border of the vitreous base. The progressive contraction of the posterior hyaloid membrane results in high circumferential folds (*Plate* XI*b*). This tends to give the peripheral retina an extremely stretched appearance and the ora serrata may be dragged into view. In some types of periretinal membrane formation distinct morphological patterns (whose behaviour can vary) can be identified. For example, in the retroretinal strands of long standing retinal detachments, there is little tendency for progression. Preretinal membranes, which tend to progress, may be very generalized and widespread, throwing the retina into irregular folds, or may take the form of quite localized epicentres of contracting tissue, producing the clinical appearance of star folding of the underlying detached retina.

Coincidental with periretinal proliferative changes, the vitreous body is also involved. A thin scattering of pigment granules, usually found and associated with retinal detachment, is succeeded by clumps or strands of pigment and the vitreous itself becomes totally collapsed. In the majority of cases remorseless progression of membrane is the rule. The eye progresses to total retinal detachment, which often has a funnel shape configuration with multiple tightly packed adherent retinal folds obscuring the optic disc. When membranes are not well established, successful retinal detachment surgery by closing retinal holes and flattening the retina will halt the fibrotic process. However, when membrane formation is very well established, dense vitreo-retinal and inter-retinal adhesions are present, and conventional surgery will have no chance of reattaching the retina.

PRESENTATION OF RETINAL DETACHMENT

Classic symptoms of retinal detachment include the premonitory symptoms of flashes of light caused by traction on the retina, floating black spots due to vitreous haemorrhage from rupture of a retinal blood vessel at the time that the retinal hole is produced, followed by a field defect resulting from detachment of the retina as it extends posteriorly to the equator. Only about half the patients suffering from retinal detachment will have premonitory symptoms[9] and the symptoms themselves are often variable. For example, vitreous haemorrhage may be absent, may result in a few black spots in the field of vision or may cause substantial reduction of vision due to its severity. As the detachment extends central vision will be lost when the macula has detached. Less commonly, retinal detachment may be discovered when visual acuity is found to be depressed, a depression that is noticed either by the patient or on an ophthalmic examination. Reduced visual acuity may be the method of presentation of retinal detachment in:

1. Children – where the commonest type of retinal hole responsible for retinal detachment is a retinal dialysis. This type of detachment rarely presents with premonitory symptoms.
2. Aphakic retinal detachments – the diagnosis may only be discovered when the patient unexpectedly fails to acquire good visual acuity after cataract surgery.
3. Opacities in the vitreous cavity – these may either be white cells secondary to uveitis or to red cells caused by vitreous haemorrhage and may mask an underlying retinal detachment.

More rarely the patient may be totally asymptomatic with normal visual acuity and a peripheral retinal detachment is detected on an ophthalmic examination.

PREOPERATIVE MANAGEMENT AND ASSESSMENT

Assessment and planning of the operation in the patient with a retinal detachment commences with an initial examination of the anterior segment and anterior third of the vitreous cavity on the slit lamp. An examination of the posterior segment is then performed with indirect ophthalmoscopy with scleral depression, the pupils having been fully dilated with Mydriacyl 1 per cent and Phenylephrine 10 per cent. A retinal chart of the eye that contains the detachment is made by the surgeon who is to perform the operation to familiarize himself fully with the details of the detachment. The examination is completed by three-mirror gonioscopy on a second visit to the slit lamp.

The other eye is similarly examined with the main objective of detecting lesions that may require prophylactic treatment.

The initial slit lamp examination will reveal the presence of any preoperative uveitis or glaucoma which can be brought under control by medical treatment before operation. Bedrest prior to surgery is reserved for those patients presenting with a fresh upper half retinal detachment or those patients in whom there has been vitreous haemorrhage severe enough to obscure details of the fundus. In patients with upper half retinal detachment the use of binocular patching and bedrest placing the retinal hole in the most dependent position (i.e. the patient horizontal) may result in substantial transfer of fluid from subretinal to the retrohyaloid space.[10] The transfer of this fluid may greatly aid the surgeon at the time of the operation, making both the application of cryotherapy and the localization of the scleral buckle easier. This may allow a simple non-drainage operation procedure to be performed. Immobilization of the globe by use of an inferior rectus suture has also been found useful.[11]

There is no advantage in prolonging bedrest for more than 24 hours and it should be avoided in elderly patients with risk of thromboembolic complications. If dense vitreous haemorrhage is present, the patient is immobilized in the sitting position so that the settling of haemorrhage in the inferior vitreous cavity is encouraged and this will allow a view of at least the upper half of the retina to be obtained and provide a good chance of finding the offending retinal hole.[12]

CHOICE OF OPERATION

The purpose of scleral buckling is to relieve vitreo-retinal traction in the immediate vicinity of the retinal holes and, if of sufficient proportions, the buckle will approximate neuro and pigment epithelium. An induced adhesion will then keep the layers in apposition and prevent access of fluid from the vitreous to the subretinal space.

Methods of Adhesion

Cryotherapy has now become the accepted method of achieving adhesion between photoreceptor and pigment epithelial layers of the retina. Indentation with a cryoprobe at the time of surgery can usually approximate the pigment epithelium to the detached retina and freezing of both layers will result in satisfactory intraretinal adhesion. If SRF is too deep to achieve closure at the time of indentation (*Fig.* 2) then cryotherapy should be applied after SRF has been drained and intravitreal injection used to approximate the two layers of the retina. At the time of surgery cryotherapy should only be applied to the immediate vicinity of the retinal hole or to other weak areas of retina. Unnecessarily extensive cryotherapy or refreezing should be avoided as it has been shown that cryotherapy can contribute to the formation of periretinal membranes.[13]

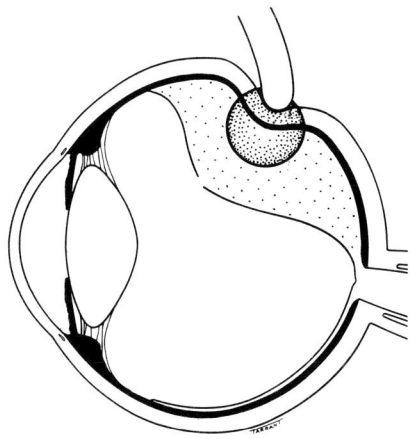

Fig. 2. A bullous detachment in which there is deep subretinal fluid between pigment epithelium and retinal hole. Indentation cannot approximate the layers of the retina.

Type of Buckle

Scleral dissection is now rarely indicated and full thickness scleral buckles are preferred. In encircling procedures these take the form of silicone rubber bands of various widths. For local procedures different sizes of Silastic sponges or solid silicone rubber explants are found to be the most convenient. If it is necessary to increase the height of an encircling element at one point the encircling band may be augmented either by the use of a radially placed silicone Silastic sponge or by an underlying silicone rubber gutter. The latter technique is useful if a long arc of retina needs additional support.

Indications for Local Buckles

Local buckles are suitable for the simple types of retinal detachment while radial implants with little chance of producing postoperative radial fold formation of the retina[14] are particularly favoured. They are used when single holes are present, particularly if these holes are horseshoe-shaped as the hole can be supported in its long axis and traction on the anterior part of the hole relieved. Circumferential buckles are useful when the hole is wide (e.g. in a dialysis) when there are multiple holes close together (*Plate* XIc) or when there is doubt about the presence of a retinal hole, either on the preoperative examination or at the time cryotherapy is applied at surgery.

Indications for Encirclement

Encirclement is preferred in more complicated cases of retinal detachment such as:
1. Multiple retinal holes in separate quadrants (*Plate* XId).
2. When there is uncertainty as to the position of retinal holes if retinal detachment is extensive.
3. If there is widespread static vitreo-retinal traction present.
4. In cases of reoperation where the cause of failure has been impossible to determine.
5. Thin sclera making the placement of local buckling sutures difficult.

In many cases of retinal detachment a combination of situations is present: in aphakia, detection of retinal holes may be difficult due to poor pupillary dilatation and opacities in the media. Thus an encircling procedure will be found necessary in a higher proportion of aphakic than phakic cases.

Complications

The main complication of encircling procedures comes from the raising of high posterior buckles. This is the usual mistake of the occasional retinal surgeon. With the raising of such buckles anterior segment ischaemic syndromes (from vortex vein compression and sometimes interference of anterior or long ciliary artery perfusion) and glaucoma (usually of a closed angle nature due to the production of peripheral choroidal and ciliary body detachment) are the most serious complications seen in the immediate postoperative period. Longer term complications include enophthalmos and severe pain in the eye and periorbital region. Silastic sponge implants may be complicated by infection. These infections may occur any time from weeks to months following surgery and present either as a mucopurulent discharge or as a granuloma protruding from the lips of the conjunctival wound.[15] These infections will only be cured after the sponges have been removed. Such removal will not result in re-detachment of the retina. With passage of time sponges may loosen and become unsightly.

Non-drainage Operations

Non-drainage operations introduced by Custodis[16] and later popularized by Lincoff[17] showed that closure of the retinal hole occurring either at the time the buckle is raised at surgery or sometimes later in the postoperative period will result in absorption of SRF fluid passing towards the sclera from the subretinal space. Thus in many simple cases of retinal detachment in which the holes can be identified and in which the retina has not been immobilized by the presence of periretinal membrane, the non-drainage technique can be safely employed. It offers the outstanding advantage that it converts the retinal detachment operation into an entirely non-invasive extraocular procedure.

If it is not possible to close the retinal hole at the time of surgery when the buckle is raised, the detached neuroepithelium can confidently be expected to sink back against an accurately placed buckle of adequate proportions, if the retina has sufficient mobility to allow such movement. One disadvantage of the non-drainage procedure is that it is often difficult to control the eventual height of the buckle that is to be used. High radial buckles are likely to produce considerable degrees of astigmatism in the postoperative period.[18]

Drainage of Subretinal Fluid

Drainage of SRF involves the least predictable step of the detachment operation.[19]

In the majority of cases it will be possible to decide at the preoperative examination whether drainage of SRF will be necessary. In particular the examination will reveal the degree of mobility of the detached retina that is present and also the relationship between the pigment epithelium and the photoreceptor layers near the retinal hole; thus the deeper the intervening SRF, the more likely is SRF drainage to be necessary.

SRF drainage is indicated:

1. In situations in which it is dangerous to raise the intraocular pressure. These include:
   (*a*) When recent cataract surgery (within 1–2 weeks) or corneal graft (within 1–2 months) may have resulted in an anterior segment wound that is insufficiently strong to withhold the rise of intraocular pressure that occurs during the non-drainage operation.
   (*b*) Poor view of optic disc. If the surgeon is unable to get a good view of the optic disc at the time of surgery, either due to opacities in the media or due to overhanging detached retina itself, then the non-drainage operation cannot be performed as it is essential to observe patency of the retinal arterioles at the optic disc when the pressure rises.
   (*c*) Poor ipsilateral perfusion of the disc (e.g. previous ischaemic optic neuropathy).
2. Difficulty in localization. If there is deep SRF between pigment epithelium and the photoreceptor layer or if the multiplicity of configuration of the retinal holes involved is complicated, then the surgeon has little chance of localizing the holes accurately on the buckle using the non-drainage technique.
3. When vitreous injection is planned the necessary space for the injection has to be made.
4. Retinal immobility. If it is considered that the photoreceptor layer is insufficiently mobile to sink back against the pigment epithelium in the postoperative period, then drainage of SRF is necessary to achieve closure of the hole at the time of surgery. Drainage of fluid may or may not be complemented by intravitreal injection to achieve closure of the hole. In many cases of retinal detachment combined situations may exist, making drainage of SRF necessary (difficulty in localization of the retinal hole combined with a significant degree of periretinal membrane formation rendering the retina partially immobile).

Selection of Site for Drainage

The following points should be borne in mind when selection of site of SRF drainage is made.

1. It is best to drain under a point where SRF is deep. It is wise to check under indirect ophthalmoscopic observation just prior to drainage and to mark on the sclera the exact site that is to be used because during the time the patient is supine on the operating table there may have been a redistribution of fluid, making any preoperative assessment of SRF unreliable.
2. Choroidal vasodilatation is produced by cryotherapy. Areas that have just been treated should be avoided.
3. Drainage should not be performed immediately underneath retinal holes as in the event of vitreous passing through a hole into the drainage site incarceration of the posterior hyaloid may occur. Such incarceration through a retinal hole may make subsequent closure of the hole very difficult.
4. It is better to avoid drainage of SRF under an intended buckle. Tightening of the buckle sutures, which is usually necessary very promptly after drainage of SRF has occurred, makes reopening of the drainage site, if necessary, difficult.

If the above criteria can be satisfied, it is often convenient to drain SRF at the lower border of the lateral rectus. At this site the sclera will be found to be reasonably thin, enabling a satisfactory prolapse of choroid to be achieved, access is easy and transillumination simple.

Technique of Drainage

1. A radial incision is made in the sclera and this incision should be long enough (approximately 3–4 mm) to allow the surgeon good visualization of the choroidal knuckle which is exposed by dissection.
2. When the choroidal knuckle has been exposed a 5·0 Dacron mattress suture is placed across the lips of the incision. This is to enable control of the flow of SRF.
3. Transillumination of the choroidal knuckle is performed by placing a fibreoptic endo-illuminator on the surface of the cornea (*Fig. 3*), thus throwing into relief any substantial choroidal vessel.
4. Actual release of SRF can be achieved in a variety of ways.

One method is to touch gently the protruding lips of choroid with a low heat cautery. This will often produce a flow of SRF as the subretinal space is entered. If cautery does not result in such a flow, however, then the space may be entered by piercing the choroidal knuckle with the tip of a sharp needle.

It is essential for the surgeon to decide prior to drainage of SRF what the drainage is intended to achieve. Thus a correct decision has to be made as to how much SRF needs to be drained (i.e. partial or complete) and whether or not the drainage is going to be supplemented by some form of vitreal injection.

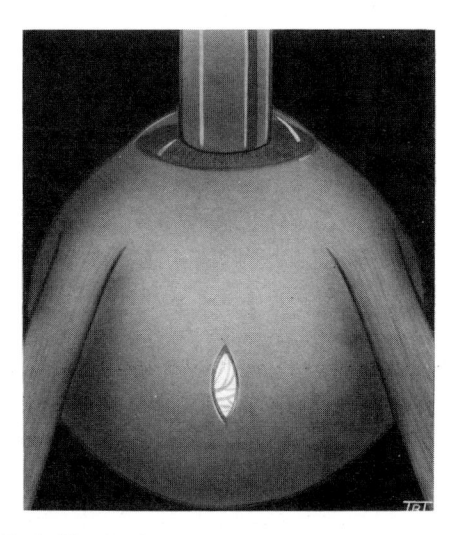

Fig. 3. Endo-illumination on the cornea will allow brilliant transillumination of a choroidal knuckle. Choroidal vessels crossing the sclerotomy site will be thrown into sharp relief.

In cases of mobile retinal detachment it is rarely necessary to drain all SRF from the eye even if a vitreous injection is to be made. In cases of periretinal membrane formation, however, as much SRF will have to be drained from the eye as possible to obtain maximum intraocular injection of gas to encourage prolonged postoperative tamponade of the hole.

COMPLICATIONS OF SRF DRAINAGE

Haemorrhage

Haemorrhage from choroidal vessels is the most serious complication of the drainage procedure, although careful selection of site and good technique makes this occurrence unusual. Bleeding may occur into the suprachoroidal space or there may be subretinal haemorrhage.

The former appears as a black mound beneath the detached retina due to haemorrhagic choroidal detachment. Sometimes a small haemorrhagic detachment will remain localized and will subsequently absorb in the postoperative period. Usually, however, blood will spread from the suprachoroidal into the subretinal space and via the retinal hole into the vitreous cavity. This progressive spread of blood from a choroidal haemorrhage is not immediate at the time of operation and will usually occur during the postoperative few days, resulting in progressive obscuration of the view of the posterior segment.

In subretinal haemorrhage blood introduced into the subretinal space will tend to remain in that compartment and will be deposited at the most posterior aspect of the retinal detachment. If the detachment is total, it will tend to settle in the macular region.

Haemorrhage may also occur from the retinal blood vessels (particularly one crossing a retinal hole), but this is usually slight and occurs either at the time the hole is being localized with an indentor or at the time cryotherapy is applied. Occasionally severe haemorrhage may occur from inadvertent rupture of a retinal vessel at the time of penetration of the eye with a needle during attempted SRF drainage. These haemorrhages are usually severe and are accompanied by the production of an iatrogenic tear in the detached retina.

The surgeon will minimize the risk of choroidal haemorrhage during drainage of SRF if hypotony resulting from drainage of SRF is kept to a minimum. The drainage of fluid should be completed as soon as is reasonably possible and normal intraocular pressure re-established by tightening the buckle sutures and, where necessary, by injection into the vitreous cavity. Undue prolongation of the period of hypotony and excessive manipulation of the globe to squeeze out SRF will increase the risk of haemorrhage. If in the postoperative period the vitreous becomes diffusely infiltrated with haemorrhage, the outcome of the retinal detachment operation will remain in doubt. In these cases regular 'B' scan examinations are made in the postoperative period to establish whether or not the retina is flat. If the retina is detached, pars plana vitrectomy should be performed to achieve reattachment and to frustrate the onset of periretinal membranes.

Vitreous Injections

Injections of fluid or gases into the vitreous cavity may be a useful adjunct to retinal detachment surgery. The indications are:

1. *To achieve Apposition of Retinal Hole and Pigment Epithelium at Surgery*

In cases when depth of SRF between hole and pigment epithelium is deep, simple drainage of SRF will not allow accurate localization and more often will produce only partial settling back, a situation which makes the retina folded. This results in even more difficult localization and also increases the risk of multiple radial retinal folds. In such cases drainage of SRF should be followed by intravitreal injection of air (about 2 ml).[20,21] As SRF is drained from the eye, air is injected via the pars plana and the expanding bubble of gas will gradually push the detached retina back into place against the pigment epithelium. When the holes are opposed or nearly so localization is much easier. Cryotherapy and buckling can then be performed (*Plate* XI*e*). It is not necessary to complete the evacuation of all the SRF during this manoeuvre. Very often posterior fluid will remain and can confidently be expected to reabsorb in the postoperative period after the holes have been sealed.

2. *To achieve Lengthy Tamponade of Retinal Holes*

GASES

When retinal detachment has been complicated by periretinal fibrosis and retinal mobility has been reduced or even lost, it may be judged necessary to close the retinal holes at the time that the retinal detachment operation is performed. If the fibrotic process is in close proximity to the retinal hole, closure of the retinal hole at surgery may not be possible by simple drainage of SRF and the raising of a buckle. It will then be necessary to inject gas into the vitreous cavity to close the hole fully. Progressive traction on the retinal hole in the postoperative period can be resisted by injecting a gas that will have a period of action of at least several days after the operation.

For this purpose a mixture of air and a longer acting gas such as sulphahexafluoride (SF6) can be used. A 3:1 air/SF6 concentration is advised and an injection of approximately 2 ml of such a mixture will usually result in a gas bubble in the vitreous cavity that will tamponade a superior retinal break for at least 4–5 days. In cases of advanced membrane formation it is usually advisable to evacuate all SRF from the eye to allow as large an intravitreal injection as possible and maximize the postoperative effect.

SILICONE OIL

In some situations the use of intraocular gas may be insufficient to cure the retinal detachment, e.g. the treatment of giant retinal tears and advanced periretinal fibrosis. In such cases conventional retinal detachment surgery will fail. The use of very long term agents such as silicone oil will be accompanied by pars plana vitrectomy.[22]

3. *Restoration of Intraocular Pressure*

When a great deal of SRF has been drained from the eye the globe becomes extremely soft. Even after the buckling sutures have been tightened the intraocular pressure may still remain very low. In these situations the intraocular pressure should be restored by intravitreal injection and the temptation to restore intraocular pressure by over-tightening buckling sutures (particularly an encircling element) should be resisted. For restoring intraocular pressure, injection into the vitreous can consist of either a fluid (balanced salt solution) or air. The disadvantage of a fluid is it will tend to pass through the retinal hole into the subretinal space, but is useful in intracapsular aphakia when injection of air into the posterior cavity may result in air bubbles coming forward into the anterior chamber and obscuring the view of the posterior segment.

Technique of Vitreous Injection

Prior to the drainage of SRF, the site for intended vitreous injection is marked in the appropriate position (5 mm from the limbus in front of the insertion of a rectus muscle). When the eye has become softened after drainage of SRF (injection should be commenced before the eye becomes collapsed), a freely running dry glass syringe containing sterile gas on which is mounted a 25 gauge needle is pushed backwards into the centre of the vitreous cavity under indirect ophthalmoscopic observation. Care must be taken to ensure the needle tip is free in the vitreous cavity and not tenting up the non-pigmented part of the pars plana epithelium. Once the needle has gained the vitreous cavity, the globe can be rotated somewhat so that the site of injection is uppermost. The superior position of the needle will result in the bubble of gas remaining close to the tip of the needle. The needle is then withdrawn so that its tip is just visible to the surgeon and injection is begun. By keeping the tip of the needle in the bubble that is forming, a good view of the fundus can be preserved. If the sclerotomy site from which SRF is draining is left open during the vitreous injection, great care must be taken not to overinject as this will result in retinal incarceration.

As the injection proceeds, the retina can be seen to be moving towards the pigment epithelium, and once contact has been achieved the injection should be halted. It is important not to overfill the eye with air or gas, not only to avoid the risk of incarcerating the retina but also to allow enough room for the subsequent buckling procedure.

Complications

1. The tip of the needle may damage either lens or retina.
2. Multiple bubbles may form making view of the posterior segment difficult. As the injection proceeds amalgamation of these bubbles usually occurs and can be encouraged by gentle pressure on the globe.
3. Overinjection may result in incarceration of the retina or closure of the central retinal artery.
4. Contact of gas with the posterior capsular lens (the bubble must be in contact with more than half

the posterior lens capsule) may result in temporary posterior cortical lens opacities. These opacities seen on the first postoperative day are reversed by posturing the patient with head down so that the bubble is not only encouraging tamponade of the hole, but is not in contact with the posterior lens capsule.

Cases not suitable for Conventional Retinal Detachment Surgery and requiring Vitrectomy

Opacities in the Media

These opacities must be dense enough to prevent the surgeon from obtaining a sufficient view of the detached retina to plan a conventional retinal detachment procedure.[23] The decision as to whether or not a conventional detachment procedure can be performed depends upon the severity of the opacities and the capacity of the surgeon to identify the retinal holes clearly.

Difficult Types of Hole

Retinal holes, either because of their size (giant)[24] or position, e.g. holes at the posterior pole of the eye,[24] make conventional buckling techniques difficult or hazardous.

Periretinal Fibrosis

POSITION OF MEMBRANE

If a retinal detachment has been complicated by puckering of the macular region, although conventional retinal detachment surgery may reattach the retina, the subsequent visual result will be poor due to distortion of the macular region. In these cases pars plana vitrectomy and peeling of the preretinal membrane is indicated.

EXTENSIVE MEMBRANES

In cases of periretinal membrane formation where traction on the retina, either tangential or vitreoretinal or both, is very advanced, it may be impossible to reverse the clinical situation by conventional retinal detachment surgery.[24]

OTHER UNUSUAL SITUATIONS

These may include extensive coexisting choroidal detachment.

POSTOPERATIVE MANAGEMENT

Only the operated eye is covered at the time of surgery and the patient is mobilized the day following the operation. The patient is only postured if an intravitreal injection has been used. In these cases the head-down position is used for a few days following surgery.

Failure of Conventional Surgery

The commonest cause of failure in retinal detachment surgery is the inability to close retinal holes.[25] This in turn may be due either to a poor selection of the buckle, which may be inadequate either in width or height, or through failure to detect all the retinal holes. In some cases failure may be due to remorseless progression of preoperative periretinal membrane. This will only happen if the preoperative fibrotic process is severe, as when retinal membranes are less well established reattachment of the retina abolishes the stimulus for the progression of such membranes.

Timing of Reoperation

If inadequately buckled or missed retinal holes can clearly be established as the cause of failure then reoperation should not be delayed, as existing membranes will only become worse or new ones form. Delay in reattaching the macula will worsen the functional result. If, however, the retinal holes appear to have been adequately buckled but there is still residual SRF present, the temptation to reoperate early should be resisted. In some cases absorption of SRF is slow and may take many weeks to occur.

Visual Recovery

All cases of retinal detachment should be operated on as soon as is reasonably possible. It is particularly urgent to reattach the retina in which the macula has not yet become involved, so that central vision will not be affected by the detachment. In cases in which the macula has become detached, reattachment of the retina will result in restoration of at least the peripheral field of vision in the affected eye. Restoration of central vision is less certain and a cautious prognosis should be given. The most important feature in prognosis appears to be the length of time that the macula has been detached prior to operation.[26] Good visual acuity (6/18 or better) can be expected in those patients in whom the macula has only been detached a short time, i.e. a few days. In those in whom the macula has been detached for many weeks or months, the final central vision is much worse. Recovery may take at least 2 years from the time of reattachment.

PROPHYLAXIS

Retinal Holes

In a great majority of cases retinal holes should be treated as it is not possible to anticipate with certainty which holes will proceed to detachment and which will not. Some holes that have almost no risk of leading to detachment need not be treated and these include small round holes in the immediate post-oral region situated in basal gel, and macular holes. Some types of hole have a greater chance of producing retinal detachment than others; thus fresh horseshoe-shaped tears discovered in a patient complaining of flashes and floaters have a much higher chance of causing retinal detachment than a round hole discovered on routine ophthalmoscopic examination in an asymptomatic eye.[27] However, the small risk of complications involved in prophylactic treatment is more than outweighed by the need to make most retinal holes completely safe, making subsequent routine observation of a patient unnecessary.

Retinal Degeneration

Lattice Degeneration (Plate Xe)

Lattice degeneration consists of circumferentially orientated equatorially placed lesions which themselves consist of hyalinized retinal blood vessels, the white appearance of which give the lesions their characteristic appearance.[28] These areas may be quite small or cover up to a quadrant or more in extent, sometimes involving nearly 360° of the retinal circumference. The condition is often bilateral. There are often overlying vitreous abnormalities in association with lattice degeneration, with liquefaction and areas of attachment of the vitreous, particularly to the posterior edges of the affected areas. Lattice degeneration is fairly commonly found and treatment is only indicated in special high risk situations. These are:
  (a) the presence of retinal holes (either round or horseshoe);
  (b) the presence of lattice degeneration in the same or other eye of a patient who has suffered retinal detachment;
  (c) the presence of other high risk factors, e.g. the coincidental presence of lattice degeneration and high myopia in a patient in whom there is a strong family history of detachment.

Sometimes other factors have to be taken into consideration when there is doubt concerning the need for the patient to have prophylactic treatment. For example, there would be a greater tendency to advise prophylaxis in young patients, as there would be in those in whom a posterior vitreous detachment had not yet occurred, as vitreous detachment at a later date will increase the risk of hole formation and detachment.

Snail Track Degeneration (Plate Xf)

This degeneration is similar in distribution to lattice degeneration. It is, however, not found in association with lattice degeneration and overlying vitreous abnormalities are not found, thus horseshoe-shaped tears do not occur. However, the degeneration may be associated with quite large round holes and there is a strong tendency to lead on to retinal detachment.[29]

Prophylaxis of 'Normal Retina'

In patients with giant retinal tears the incidence of involvement of the second eye at some time is known to be high (approximately 50 per cent). In many of the 'second' eyes no clear cut predisposition to detachment in the form of degenerate areas can be seen. In spite of this absence of any abnormality, prophylactic cryotherapy through 360° in the pre-equatorial region is advised. Such treatment appears to reduce the risk of subsequent detachment. It has also been suggested[1] that patients receiving intra-ocular cataract surgery who had previously been myopic, and who had suffered a detachment in their first aphakic eye, should be considered for prophylactic treatment to the second eye as there appears to be a substantial risk to these eyes. It is clear, however, that the use of extracapsular surgical techniques[30,31] in these patients will also result in a greatly reduced risk of detachment.

Methods of Prophylactic Treatment

Cryotherapy

In a great majority of cases when prophylaxis is used it is applied to the 'fellow' eye at the time of retinal detachment surgery. In these cases the patient, who is usually receiving a general anaesthetic, can be treated with transconjunctival cryotherapy. All applications are monitored by indirect ophthalmoscopy. In a great majority of cases the need to perform prophylaxis will have been appreciated preoperatively. Even when such lesions are not detected at the preoperative examination the opportunity should never be lost of examining the other eye at the time of retinal detachment surgery and any necessary treatment carried out. Examination under anaesthesia is particularly valuable in patients in whom the preoperative examination has been unsatisfactory (e.g. nervous or uncooperative patients or children).

Prophylaxis performed on the conscious patient may either be done using transconjunctival cryotherapy or with photocoagulation treatment. In the latter case laser treatment is the method of choice, but it is not suitable for anteriorly placed lesions in which it is difficult to surround the area to be treated with laser burns, or if there are marked opacities in the media as the illumination of indirect ophthalmoscopy is considerably superior to that obtained at the slit lamp. When cryotherapy is to be used topical anaesthesia is all that is necessary (amethocaine drops), but most patients will experience pain if more than a few applications are made.

If a retinal hole is to be treated, the hole must be completely surrounded so that a firm adhesion is obtained. Prophylactic treatment should not be attempted if there is anything more than the slightest amount of SRF around the retinal hole.

REFERENCES

1. Gilbert C. E., Lamb R. J. and Martin B. Aphakic retinal detachment – prophylaxis in the second eye. *Trans. Ophthalmol. Soc. UK* 1983; **103**, 161–4.
2. Le Mesurier R., Booth-Mason S., Vickers S. et al. Aphakic retinal detachment. *Br. J. Ophthalmol.* 1985; **69**, 737–41.
3. Wilkinson C. P., Anderson L. S. and Little J. H. Retinal detachment following phakoemulsification. *Ophthalmology* 1978; **85**, 151–6.
4. Percival S. B., Anand V. and Das S. K. Prevalence of aphakic retinal detachment. *Br. J. Ophthalmol.* 1983; **67**, 43–5.
5. Hurite F. G., Jorr E. M. and Everest W. G. The incidence of retinal detachment following phakoemulsification. *Ophthalmology* 1978; **86**, 2004–6.
6. Scott J. D. Static and dynamic vitreous traction. *Trans. Ophthalmol. Soc. UK* 1971; **91**, 175–88.
7. Chignell A. H., Carruthers M. and Rahi A. H. S. Clinical, biochemical and immunoelectrophoretic study of subretinal fluid. *Br. J. Ophthalmol.* 1971; **55**, 525–32.
8. Chignell A. H., Fison L. G., Davies E. W. G. et al. Failure in retinal detachment surgery. *Br. J. Ophthalmol.* 1973; **57**, 525–30.
9. Morse P. H. and Scheie H. G. Prophylactic cryoretinopathy of retinal breaks. *Arch. Ophthalmol.* 1974; **92**, 297–8.
10. Foulds W. S. Experimental detachment of the retina and its affect on the intraocular fluid dynamics. *Mod. Probl. Ophthalmol.* 1969; **8**, 51–63.
11. Johnston P. B., Maguire C. J. E. and Logan W. L. Management of superior half bullous retinal detachment. *Br. J. Ophthalmol.* 1981; **65**, 618–23.
12. Lincoff H. A. and Kreissig I. The conservative management of vitreous haemorrhage. *Trans. Am. Acad. Ophthalmol. Otolaryngol.* 1975; **79**, 859–64.
13. Laqua H. and Machemer R. Repair and adhesion mechanism of the cryotherapy lesion in experimental retinal detachment. *Am. J. Ophthalmol.* 1976; **81**, 833–46.
14. Lincoff H. A. and Kreissig I. Advantages of radial buckling. *Am. J. Ophthalmol.* 1975; **79**, 955–7.
15. Langston R., Lincoff H. A. and Mclean J. M. Scleral abscess. 2. *Arch. Ophthalmol.* 1965; **74**, 665–8.
16. Custodis E. Bedeutet die plombenanfnahung und die sklera einen fortschritt in der operatiren behaud hung der netzhauta biosurg. *Ber. deutsch. ophth. Gesellsch.* 1953; **58**, 102–5.
17. Lincoff H. A. and Kreissig I. The treatment of retinal detachment without drainage of subretinal fluid. *Trans. Am. Acad. Ophthalmol. Otolaryngol.* 1972; **76**, 1221–33.
18. Goel R., Crewdson J. and Chignell A. H. Astigmatism following retinal detachment surgery. *Br. J. Ophthalmol.* 1983; **67**, 327–9.
19. Cibis P. A. Errors in the management of retinal detachment surgery. *Mod. Probl. Ophthalmol.* 1965; **3**, 284–308.
20. Chawla H. B. and Birchall C. H. Intravitreal air in retinal detachment surgery. *Br. J. Ophthalmol.* 1973; **57**, 60–70.
21. Norton E. W. D. Intraocular gas in the management of selected retinal detachments. *Trans. Am. Acad. Otolaryngol.* 1973; **77**, 85–98.
22. Lean J. S., Leaver P. K., Cooling R. J. et al. Management of complex retinal detachments by vitrectomy and fluid/silicone exchange. *Trans. Ophthalmol. Soc. UK* 1982; **102**, 203–6.
23. Jagger J. D., Cooling R. J., Fison L. G. et al. Management of retinal detachment following congenital cataract surgery. *Trans. Ophthalmol. Soc. UK* 1983; **103**, 103–8.
24. Billington B. M. and Chignell A. H. Treatment of rhegmatogenous retinal detachment uncomplicated by massive periretinal proliferation by pars plana vitrectomy. *Trans. Ophthalmol Soc. UK* 1984; **104**, 120–2.
25. Chignell A. H. *Retinal Detachment Surgery*. Berlin, Springer-Verlag, 1980, p. 159.
26. Kreissig I. Prognosis of return of macular function after retinal reattachment. *Mod. Probl. Ophthalmol.* 1977; **18**, 415–29.
27. Davis M. D. Natural history of retinal breaks without detachment. *Arch. Ophthalmol.* 1974; **92**, 183–94.
28. Straatsma B. R., Peeren P. D., Foos R. Y. et al. Lattice degeneration of the retina. *Am. J. Ophthalmol.* 1974; **77**, 619–49.
29. Aaberg T. J. and Stevens T. R. Snail track degeneration of the retina. *Am. J. Ophthalmol.* 1972; **73**, 370–6.
30. Percival S. P. B., Anand V. and Das S. K. Prevalence of aphakic retinal detachment. *Br. J. Ophthalmol.* 1983; **67**, 43–5.
31. Coonan P., Fung W. E., Webster R. G. et al. Incidence of retinal detachment following extracapsular cataract extraction. *Ophthalmology* 1985; **92**, 1096–101.

Chapter 9

The Vitreous and its Disorders

David McLeod

The vitreous is a vestigial mass of connective tissue with no defined postnatal function. The essential property of the vitreous – transparency – reflects its unique biochemistry (immature collagen fibrils and hyaluronic acid molecules forming an aqueous gel), together with the virtual absence of blood vessels and cells. The structural 'isolation' of the vitreous body is principally maintained by the blood–retinal barrier, although the inner limiting lamina of the retina has a subsidiary protective role. Significant loss of optical clarity (and consequent visual loss) results from cellular and/or molecular invasion of the vitreous secondary to breakdown of these defensive barriers. Disturbances of intrinsic vitreous biochemistry are generally responsible for subtle opacities which only become symptomatic in particular circumstances (e.g. pupillary miosis from brilliant illumination or accommodation and when the opacities are located near the retina). In addition to opacification in the optical axis, other major vitreal causes of visual morbidity include damage to structures with which the vitreous is normally in contact (especially the retina) and displacement of vitreous gel bringing it into contact with the pupil margin or the corneal endothelium.

In the past, the transparency of the vitreous and associated problems of detailed clinical examination resulted in poorly defined concepts of vitreous pathology. However, with improved methods of clinical, ultrasonic and laboratory examination, together with direct clinicopathological correlation at vitrectomy, more specific principles of vitreo-retinal pathophysiology have emerged. It is no longer acceptable, for example, to speak simply of 'traction', 'contraction' or 'organization' of the vitreous: rather it is essential to conform to a standardized nomenclature in respect of both the nature and location of pathological processes. By this means, communication about (and understanding of) vitreous disorders is facilitated and a logical approach adopted to the use of the available repertoire of surgical techniques.

The vitreous gel has a definite internal structure based on its collagen–fibril framework, the physical continuum of which is most evident within its border condensations (the anterior and posterior hyaloid membranes). Thus, normal vitreous cannot be aspirated without danger of damage to the retina with which all gel is eventually connected. The gel structure constitutes a scaffolding or matrix within which cells can proliferate (for example, vascularized epiretinal membranes). Furthermore, the cortical vitreous constitutes a diffusion barrier to large molecules (a 'molecular sieve'), as illustrated in the ischaemic retinopathies where anterior diffusion of vasoproliferative factor (and consequent rubeosis iridis) is facilitated by vitrectomy or intracapsular cataract extraction associated with disruption of the anterior hyaloid face. Changes in the fluid content of the vitreous (normally 99 per cent of the gel) account for most expansions and contractions of vitreous volume, which permit, for example, the growth of intraocular tumours or the expansion of injected insoluble gases. Alternatively, fluid can become redistributed within different compartments either by bulk flow or more gradually, or indeed can transfer out of the vitreous cavity altogether when recruited under the retina.

Surgical access to the contents of the vitreous cavity is usually achieved via more or less watertight incisions in the anterior half of the pars plana. Alternatively, provided the lens is also removed (or in aphakic eyes), a limbal or pars plicata approach can be adopted (e.g. in neonates who have no pars plana, and in retrolental fibroplasia). In contrast to such 'closed' microsurgical techniques, an 'open sky' approach through a large corneal incision or trephination is also possible.

Modern vitrectomy involves the mechanical disruption and subsequent removal of the gel framework using a suction cutter; early in the procedure, the aspirated column of minced gel is viscous and can be observed 'drooling' (as opposed to dripping) into the collection bottle. As tissue is removed, the volume within the scleral envelope (and thus the intraocular pressure) is maintained by simultaneous infusion of a physiological solution under hydrostatic pressure from a supply bottle above the eye, and the aspirated material becomes more fluid. Visualization of surgery requires illumination either remotely (indirect ophthalmoscopy, coaxial or paraxial slit beam), or by reflex-free endo-illumination using fibreoptics. The various devices subserving suction-cutting, infusion and endo-illumination were originally combined in one large instrument (full function probe) but were subsequently separated (e.g. 20 gauge triple-port microsurgery); in future, multiple combined functions through three 19 gauge ports are likely.

Most tissue that can be engaged by suction into the port of a vitreous cutter can be disrupted and aspirated; normal gel is the most difficult to cut and also to visualize (clear gel sometimes requiring fluorescein staining). Engagement problems arise with non-deformable tissues (for example, taut fibrous tissue) or because the tissue to be removed is located upon (and intimately connected with) the retina, thus necessitating peeling, scissors dissection or viscodelamination prior to engagement, cutting and aspiration. The physiological solution replacing the vitreous contents during surgery is itself replaced by aqueous humour postoperatively, the speed of exchange depending upon the integrity of the anterior hyaloid face.

Since an eye tolerates the absence of gel very well, other types of vitreous replacement or substitution are generally unnecessary, though there may be a future role for a stable vitreous substitute which, because of its viscosity and rigidity, mimics normal vitreous and does not pass through retinal breaks. At present, however, most vitreous injections other than infusion fluid are used for 'tamponade' or internal closure of retinal breaks, their surface tension preventing fluid transfer through the retinal break (for example, air, insoluble gases, air–gas mixtures or silicone oil).

The following sections will expand upon these basic concepts of vitreo-retinal pathophysiology and surgery. The underlying processes are common to many different aetiologies and are interrelated, so a mechanistic rather than a primarily aetiological approach will be adopted, together with consideration of surgical implications and principles (but excluding details of surgical techniques).

VITREOUS ADHESIONS

Attachments of the collagenous gel framework to surrounding structures (especially to the retina) are fundamental to most vitreous pathology.

Aetiology

The attachments may form (*a*) as part of normal embryological or postnatal development, or (*b*) they may be acquired.

Vitreolenticular Attachment

The junction of the anterior expanded portion of Cloquet's canal with the anterior hyaloid membrane constitutes a zone of attachment of the vitreous body to the posterior lens capsule (Egger's line or Weiger's ligament) (*Fig.* 1). The strength of vitreolenticular adhesion decreases with age.

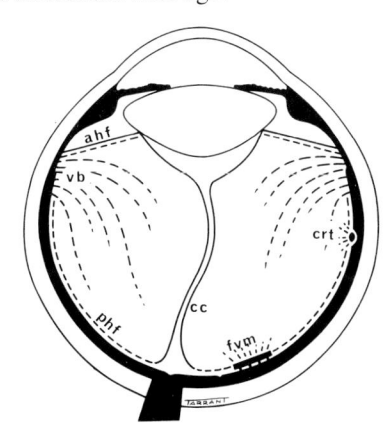

Fig. 1. Vitreous architecture and adhesions. vb, vitreous base; ahf, anterior hyaloid face; phf, posterior hyaloid face; crt, cystic retinal tuft; cc, Cloquet's canal; fvm, fibrovascular membrane.

Sequela

Rupture of the posterior lens capsule may follow blunt trauma, with spillage of lens material into the gel.

Surgical Implications

1. Anterior vitrectomy using strong suction can produce tears of the posterior lens capsule in young eyes.
2. The lens can be peeled from the anterior vitreous face after middle age (intracapsular cataract extraction).

Vitreous Base

This annular zone of vitreous adhesion straddles the ora serrata and divides the border condensation of the gel into two parts – the anterior and posterior hyaloid membranes (*Fig.* 1). The basal vitreous fibrils are indissolubly attached to the multi-layered basement membrane of the non-pigmented epithelium of the posterior pars plana, and are also attached directly to the glial framework of the postoral retina owing to incarceration of gel within 'crypts'. In addition to their perpendicular insertion, the densely packed vitreous fibrils are distributed as annulus in the coronal plane. The anteroposterior dimension of the vitreous base is variable and probably increases with age ('degenerative remodelling').

Sequelae

1. Many vitreous traction systems are founded upon this anterior vitreo-retinal adhesion.
2. Fibroblasts proliferating within the basal gel annulus produce vitreous base traction.
3. Blunt trauma causes vitreous base avulsion ('bucket handle tear').

4. Dialysis and disinsertion of the oral retina result from incarceration of basal gel (e.g. after penetrating trauma).

5. Posterior finger-like protrusions of the vitreous base underlie the production of some flap tears after posterior vitreous detachment.

Surgical Implications

1. The vitreous base area adjacent to pars plana entry sites is especially vulnerable to damage, e.g. from vitreous prolapse and incarceration of gel in instruments during reinsertion, causing retinal breaks.

2. Inefficient suction-cutting (with vitreous 'winding' and traction on the vitreous base) may cause a giant retinal tear during surgery.

Post-basal Vitreo-retinal Juncture

Condensed collagen fibrils constituting the posterior hyaloid membrane are indirectly attached to the retina by a glue-like adhesion to the smooth vitreal surface of the inner limiting lamina of the retina (identified by electron microscopy as the 'superficial electron-dense line'). The strength of the vitreolaminar adhesion decreases with age.

Sequelae

1. Rotational forces (induced by ocular saccades) are transmitted into the vitreous thoughout the area of vitreo-retinal contact.

2. Generalized vitreo-retinal traction is unusual in later life (owing to the tendency to posterior vitreous detachment).

Surgical Implications

1. The cortical gel and posterior hyaloid membrane cannot be stripped readily from the retinal surface during vitrectomy; vitrectomy in the absence of vitreous detachment is therefore termed 'central vitrectomy', and the vitreolaminar adhesion is not disrupted.

2. Excessive traction transmitted to the retina during vitrectomy has been noted to produce photoreceptor damage in experimental animals, and may also cause retinal breaks.

Developmental Post-basal Vitreo-retinal Adhesions

The hemispheric continuum of the vitreo-retinal juncture may be interspersed by exaggerated adhesions between the vitreous and retina, especially in relation to certain focal developmental degenerative lesions (*Fig.* 1). These include ophthalmoscopically identifiable features such as lattice and snail track degeneration, cystic retinal tufts and pigmented patches. In addition to those identified or surmised by simple ophthalmoscopy, other adhesions may be present but are not readily visualized (e.g. equatorial paravascular adhesions and more posterior adhesions, especially in myopia and Stickler's syndrome). There may also be an exaggerated adhesion at the macula.

Sequelae

1. These adhesions (together with posterior extensions of the posterior border of the vitreous base) are important in retinal tear formation and 'retinal erosions' (i.e. partial thickness retinal avulsion), especially after posterior vitreous detachment.

2. Cystoid macular oedema occasionally results from traction on a vitreomacular attachment.

Vitreopapillary Adhesion

The ring of glial tissue overlying the optic disc margin ('epipapillary gliosis') is a primary hyaloid remnant marking the junction of the posterior hyaloid membrane with the posterior expanded portion of Cloquet's canal (*Fig.* 1). The glial tissue is seldom visible except when hyperplastic, as in Bergmeister's papilla.

Sequelae

1. Persistent vitreopapillary adhesion is one basis of incomplete posterior vitreous detachment (funnel-shaped or cone-shaped vitreous detachment).

2. Avulsion of epipapillary gliosis during posterior vitreous detachment produces Weiss' ring.

Acquired Vitreo-retinal Adhesions

Exaggerated adhesion between the vitreous and retina may result from:

1. Trauma (at the site of posterior penetrating injury or the impaction site of an intraocular foreign body).

2. Retinovitreal inflammation (i.e. vitreal extension of focal or multifocal chorioretinitis and retinitis, including the acute retinal necrosis syndrome).

3. Fibrovascular epiretinal membrane proliferation (e.g. in ischaemic retinopathies, *Fig.* 1) and some fibrocellular proliferations.

4. Heavy xenon photocoagulation burns (involving full thickness retina and cortical vitreous).

Sequelae

1. Incomplete posterior vitreous detachment.
2. Retinal tears or traction retinal detachment.

VITREOUS DISPLACEMENT AND INCARCERATION

Aetiology

Displacement of the vitreous from within its natural confines usually follows damage to the corneo-scleral envelope or the lens owing to (*a*) trauma or (*b*) intraocular surgery. In such circumstances, gel is frequently both displaced and incarcerated in the wound (*Fig. 2a*). Vitreous may be displaced without becoming incarcerated, e.g. vitreous protrusion into the anterior chamber around a dislocated lens, and the vitreous volume expansion after intracapsular cataract extraction when the previously concave hyaloid face (patellar fossa) becomes convex behind the iris and in the pupil. If the anterior hyaloid face is broken during or after cataract surgery, formed gel may 'herniate' into the anterior chamber (*Fig. 2b*), prolapse from the eye (vitreous 'loss') and incarcerate in the corneo-scleral section.

8. A route for fibroblastic or fibrovascular ingrowth and invasion is established.

9. Posterior vitreous detachment eventually occurs with exaggerated predisposition to retinal break formation.

Surgical Implications

1. Prophylactic anterior vitrectomy following vitreous prolapse at cataract surgery prevents development of static traction between the section and the vitreous base.

2. Prophylactic cryocoagulation of peripheral retina posterior to pars plana entry sites helps prevent

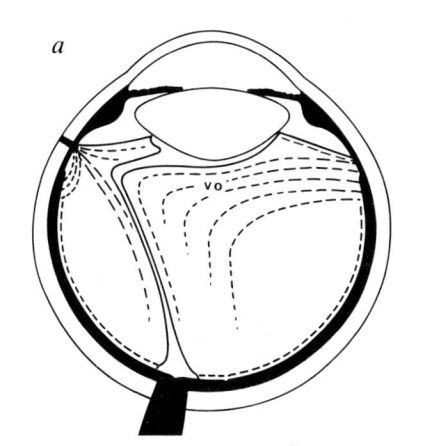

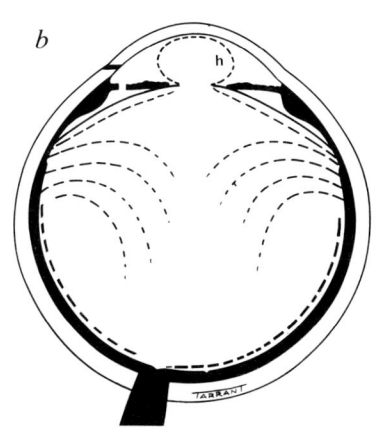

Fig. 2. Vitreous displacement. *a*, After penetrating injury in nasal pars plana: vo, vitreous orientation towards incarceration site *b*, After intracapsular lens extraction through corneoscleral section: h, herniation of anterior gel through hiatus in anterior hyaloid face.

Vitreous displacement and incarceration is manifest on slit lamp examination by the orientation of anterior gel fibrils (tension lines) towards the wound. After acute trauma, these tension lines may not be immediately apparent (owing to hypotony and scleral collapse or choroidal haemorrhage) and are only manifest after restoration of intraocular pressure and/or absorption of suprachoroidal haemorrhage.

Sequelae

1. Contact with (or adhesion to) adjacent structures may cause complications, e.g. pupil block, updrawn pupil and corneal endothelial damage.

2. Anterior transgel traction causes 'purse-string' retinal detachment.

3. Vitreous base traction following basal gel incarceration may lead to disinsertion of the oral retina.

4. Pre-existing tears are distorted by adjacent basal gel incarceration.

5. Endophthalmitis may complicate the vitreous wick syndrome.

6. Associated inflammation causes cystoid macular oedema.

7. Rubeosis iridis in ischaemic retinopathies may result from anterior diffusion of vasoproliferative factor through a broken anterior hyaloid face.

complications of basal gel incarceration; alternatively, prophylactic encirclement is sometimes advocated.

3. Scleral buckling is advisable for most peripheral retinal breaks with unrelieved traction associated with basal gel incarceration.

VITREOUS DEGENERATION

The vitreous gel has a restricted repertoire of pathological change, essentially limited to a breakdown in the physicochemical interrelationship between its constituent macromolecules – hyaluronic acid and collagen. Degenerative destablization of the central gel results in condensation of the collagen fibrils (synersis or vitreous collapse) with increased fluidity and formation of lacunae (with their hyaluronic acid content and collagenous walls). The distribution of such changes is highly variable, but overall a 'compartmentalization' of the gel occurs into 'formed vitreous' and 'fluid vitreous'. The formed vitreous (residual gel) shows an increase in the speed and range of movement following ocular deviations, as seen anteriorly on the slit lamp ('ascension phenomenon'). Ultimately, all vitreous architecture disappears, including the walls of Cloquet's canal. The posterior vitreous cortex may also disappear, especially in front of the macula (*Fig. 3a*); in Stickler's syndrome, several large areas of dehiscence of the posterior hyaloid membrane develop.

Aetiology

1. Normal ageing process.
2. Myopia, where age-related changes in the expanded gel are exaggerated and accelerated.
3. Aphakia, owing to loss of hyaluronic acid through the anterior hyaloid membrane and trabecular meshwork.
4. Following cellular invasion of the vitreous.
5. Following gas injection and temporary vitreous compression peripherally.
6. Yag laser disruption of gel.
7. Retained intraocular foreign bodies ('chemical syneresis').

Sequelae

1. Symptoms of floaters (muscae volitantes) arise from degeneration of posterior gel.
2. Slowly progressive retinal detachment results from passage of fluid vitreous through atrophic holes or traumatic breaks. (Prior to vitreous syneresis, the gel's rigidity and viscosity prevent such subretinal recruitment of fluid.)
3. Retinal tears occasionally complicate the increased vitreous dynamics.
4. Rhegmatogenous posterior vitreous detachment ultimately occurs (*Fig. 3b*).

Surgical Implications

Fluid vitreous may be aspirated.

Asteroid Hyalosis

This is a gel degeneration in which spherules of calcium soaps accumulate within and along the mobile collapsed vitreous fibrils. The spherical bodies are white or yellow by direct illumination, and black by retro-illumination which also highlights their essential relationship to the vitreous fibrils ('string of pearls'). The precise pathophysiology of asteroid hyalosis is unknown; it is slightly more common in diabetes and following congenital cataract surgery, possibly due to exaggerated syneresis in these conditions.

Asteroid hyalosis obscures ophthalmoscopic visualization of the retina, but seldom interferes with vision. Vitrectomy is rarely indicated, except to allow panretinal photocoagulation in proliferative diabetic retinopathy or for identification of retinal breaks causing rhegmatogenous retinal detachment.

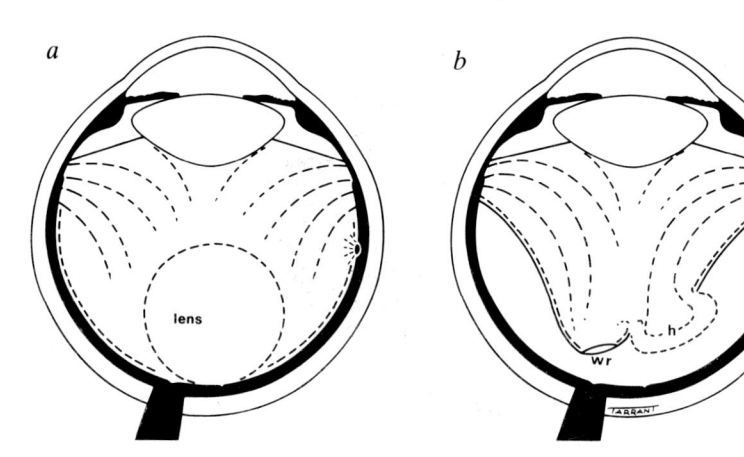

Fig. 3. Vitreous degeneration and detachment. *a*, Formation of lacuna (l) in premacular gel. *b*, Rhegmatogenous complete posterior vitreous detachment: wr, Weiss ring (avulsed epipapillary gliosis); h, herniation of posterior gel through hiatus in posterior hyaloid face; ot, operculated tear from dynamic traction on cystic retinal tuft.

VITREOUS DETACHMENT

The basal gel cannot separate from the posterior pars plana and post-oral retina, but the anterior and posterior hyaloid membranes may detach from surrounding structures. Anterior vitreous detachment is unusual and relatively unimportant; it is seen in Marfan's syndrome, trauma and massive periretinal proliferation. The plane of separation of the posterior hyaloid membrane from the post-basal retina in posterior vitreous detachment is usually situated at the superficial electron-dense line. The posterior hyaloid membrane is thereby separated by fluid vitreous from the smooth vitreal surface of the inner limiting lamina of the retina, and the vitreous cavity is divided into formed gel and fluid (retrohyaloid) compartments.

Aetiology

1. As for vitreous degeneration.
2. Following central vitrectomy.
3. Following vitreous incarceration and/or displacement.
4. Following blunt trauma.

5. Following epiretinal membrane formation with vitreo-membranous incarceration.

There are many variants of posterior vitreous detachment, both in respect of its extent, speed of progression and mechanism, and also in respect of the mobility, structure and integrity of the detached posterior hyaloid membrane. If the gel separates from the entire retina up to the posterior border of the vitreous base, vitreous detachment is said to be 'complete' (*Fig. 3b*). If exaggerated post-basal vitreoretinal adhesions impede this process, but separation occurs except at these sites, vitreous detachment is said to be 'incomplete' and the gel compartment forms a single-point or multi-point 'cone' depending on the number of vitreo-retinal adhesions (*Fig. 4a,b*). The term 'partial' vitreous detachment refers to slowly progressive vitreous detachment, where vitreous separation has yet to be accomplished either up to the posterior border of the vitreous base or up to and around any exaggerated vitreo-retinal adhesions (*Fig. 4c*).

Surgical Implications

1. After complete vitreous detachment, the whole of the gel can be removed except for a frill (or skirt) of basal gel.

2. After incomplete posterior vitreous detachment, posterior adhesions can be readily isolated or 'circumcised' using a suction cutter with relief of anteroposterior and bridging traction.

3. If the vitreous is only partially detached, the residual vitreolaminar attachment may be separated by mechanical peeling or by viscodelamination.

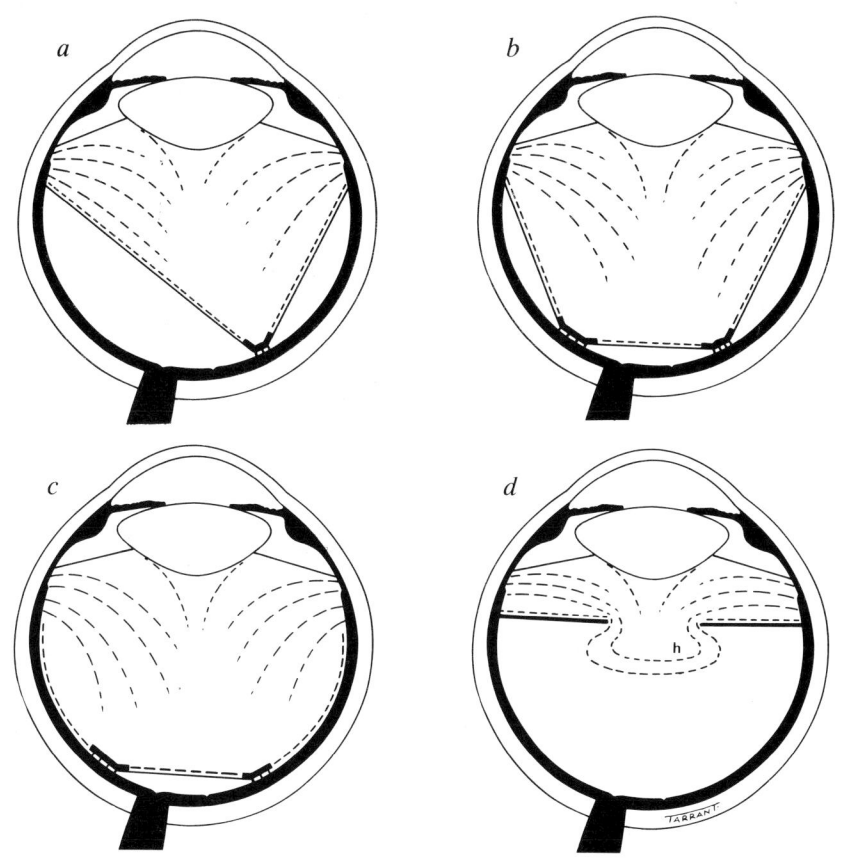

Fig. 4. Posterior vitreous detachment. *a*, Incomplete non-rhegmatogenous posterior vitreous detachment (single-point cone). *b*, Incomplete non-rhegmatogenous posterior vitreous detachment (multiple-point cone). *c*, Partial posterior vitreous detachment. *d*, Complete rhegmatogenous posterior vitreous detachment (vitreous retraction). h, Herniation of gel through posterior hyaloid membrane.

4. Occasionally, vitreous detachment occurs as a dramatic event during the course of a vitrectomy procedure.

Rhegmatogenous Posterior Vitreous Detachment

Following syneresis, fluid vitreous may dissect posteriorly through a dehiscence in the premacular vitreous cortex to strip the posterior hyaloid membrane from the retina ('posterior vitreous detachment with collapse') (*Fig. 3b*). Formed vitreous may also herniate posteriorly into the retrohyaloid space through the hiatus in the detached posterior hyaloid membrane. Progression to complete vitreous separation is usually rapid, and the residual gel and posterior hyaloid membrane become violently mobile with eye movements. The influence of gravity on the relatively dense residual gel may bring the posterior hyaloid membrane very anteriorly within the vitreous cavity during slit lamp biomicroscopy (where the wrinkled posterior hyaloid condensation is visible behind the lens without resort to a fundus contact lens).

Sequelae

1. Symptoms of floaters and photopsiae arise.
2. Dynamic vitreo-retinal traction produces retinal tears, retinal erosions or avulsed retinal vessels (together with haemorrhage and pigment epithelial cell dispersion from Bruch's membrane).
3. Avulsion of epipapillary gliosis produces Weiss' ring and occasionally vitreous haemorrhage; other epiretinal membranes (both fibrocellular and fibrovascular) may also be avulsed from the retinal surface.
4. Epiretinal membrane formation may be induced.
5. Removal of the gel-scaffold prevents new fibrovascular epiretinal proliferations.

Vitreous Retraction

This refers to a complete posterior vitreous detachment with relatively immobile residual gel in an anterior location, the posterior hyaloid interface occupying a coronal pre-equatorial plane (*Fig. 4d*).

Non-Rhegmatogenous Vitreous Detachment

Slowly progressive vitreous detachment may occur with no demonstrable break in the posterior hyaloid interface. There may be no associated syneresis (posterior vitreous detachment without collapse) and the vitreous detachment is usually 'incomplete'; the posterior hyaloid membrane is often rigid owing to vitreous condensation or fibroblastic invasion and synthesis of new collagen. Associated retrohyaloid haemorrhage may be restricted to the fluid vitreous compartment with no penetration into the gel.

Sequelae

1. Static vitreo-retinal traction (anteroposterior and bridging traction) may lead to traction retinal detachment.
2. Haemorrhage arises from avulsion of the edges of fibrovascular epiretinal membranes into which the gel is incarcerated (*Fig. 4a,b*).
3. Retinal breaks may arise adjacent to the vitreo-membranous adhesions with consequent combined traction and rhegmatogenous retinal detachment.

VITREOUS INVASION

The defensive protection provided by the blood–retinal barrier and inner limiting lamina can be breached, and the vitreous thereafter invaded, in a number of circumstances, e.g. by traumatic disruption of the ocular coats, by spontaneous internal disruption of the retina or by outgrowth and proliferation of cells from the retina.

Aetiology

The materials invading the vitreous cavity can be categorized as follows:

1. Foreign or exogenous materials, e.g. IOFB, bacteria and fungi.
2. Large molecules, e.g. amyloid and proteins in inflammatory disorders, retinal vascular diseases and extraretinal neovascularization.
3. Cells, e.g. associated with haemorrhage, inflammation, neoplasia (retinoblastoma and reticulum cell sarcoma) or retinal pigment epithelial cell dispersion via retinal breaks. In addition to diffuse cellular invasion, other cells (particularly of retinal origin) may proliferate on the retinal surface and/or along vitreous scaffolds resulting in vitreous fibrosis (*see below*).

Vitreous Amyloidosis

This is a rare cause of opacification of the vitreous characterized by deposition of amyloid proteins around the collagen framework of the gel. Where there are marked tunica vasculosa lentis remnants in the form of fibrillar attachments to the posterior lens capsule, the deposition produces 'pseudopodia lentis'. Vitreous invasion is associated with the primary or familial (dominantly inherited) form of amyloidosis, and the beta chains probably derive from the retinal circulation. Vitreous opacification is slowly progressive until the time of posterior vitreous detachment, when visual loss can be more precipitate. The 'glass wool' opacities are readily removed (especially after vitreous detachment) by vitrectomy, taking particular care to remove retrolental gel because continuing amyloid deposition can occur in this area with recurrent visual loss. There may be associated chronic open angle glaucoma.

Vitreous Haemorrhage

Vitreous haemorrhage arises from surrounding structures except for bleeding from persistent primary hyaloid vascular remnants (including avulsed epipapillary gliosis). The causes of vitreous haemorrhage are (*a*) traumatic and (*b*) spontaneous.

Spontaneous vitreous haemorrhage may arise: (*a*) by extension from retinal haemorrhage, e.g. submembranous haemorrhage (owing to Terson's syndrome, the Valsalva manoeuvre, venous occlusion etc.) or from macular degeneration ('explosive disciform bleeding' from subretinal neovascularization); or (*b*) as a sequel to posterior vitreous detachment, e.g. during formation of retinal tears or avulsion of fibrovascular epiretinal membranes.

The initial site of haemorrhage depends on the cause. Blood initially clots, but within the next few days undergoes fibrinolysis with dispersion of haemorrhage within the gel or the retrohyaloid space. Thereafter, blood may be absorbed by macrophage activity and passage anteriorly through the anterior hyaloid membrane and the trabecular meshwork. Retained red blood cells undergo a form of haemolysis to produce spheroidal erythroclasts which, unlike erythrocytes, are indigestible by macrophages and non-deformable, thus obstructing the trabecular meshwork. Vitreous containing haemolysing red cells undergoes a number of colour changes (like a bruise); the characteristic colour resulting from bilirubin, biliverdin and other pigmented products is 'ochre'. Clogging of the posterior vitreous cortex by erythroclasts (together with staining by haemoglobin breakdown products) produces an 'ochre membrane'. The cell membranes of erythroclasts may eventually undergo biochemical degradation to cholesterol crystals producing synchysis scintillans (which is a localized form of cholesterolosis bulbi), resulting in dispersion of polychromatic angular crystals throughout the vitreous cavity.

Sequelae

1. Syneresis and posterior vitreous detachment (if not originally causative in haemorrhage formation).
2. Haemosiderosis of the retina and iris.
3. Erythroclastic glaucoma.
4. Complicated cataract.

Surgical Implications

1. Bloodstained vitreous gel is easily disrupted by suction cutters.
2. Unclotted blood in the retrohyaloid space is readily aspirated (vacuum cleaning) following vitrectomy.
3. Residual red cells or erythroclasts in the vitreous frill may leach from the basal gel following vitrectomy to cause temporary recurrent vitreous opacification or post-operative erythroclastic glaucoma.

Vitritis

Vitritis, or invasion of the vitreous by inflammatory cells and proteins, occurs (*a*) in uveitis (e.g. pars planitis, heterochromic cyclitis and sarcoidosis); (*b*) in response to retained reactive foreign bodies (e.g. chalcosis); and (*c*) following bacterial or fungal invasion (endophthalmitis). The white cells may be isolated and dispersed throughout the gel, aggregated in foci ('snow balls') or overwhelmingly concentrated (vitreous abscess).

Sequelae

1. Vitreous syneresis.
2. Posterior vitreous detachment.
3. Vitreous retraction.
4. Vitreous fibrosis (e.g. fibrocellular epiretinal membrane, cyclitic membrane).
5. Extraretinal neovascularization (e.g. disc new vessels or fibrovascular epiretinal membranes following retinal vasculitis, venous occlusion and ischaemia; fibrovascular invasion of retinovitreal abscess in candida endophthalmitis).
6. Fibroglial proliferation in the vitreous base, especially inferiorly ('snow banking') in pars planitis.

Surgical Implications

1. Vitrectomy may be indicated for cytological or bacteriological diagnosis and drainage of a vitreous abscess.
2. Danger of retinal tearing is increased in vitrectomy for endophthalmitis if the vitreous is not detached and the retina is necrotic.

Cellular Proliferation, Contraction and Fibrosis

Vitreous fibrosis is characterized by the production of mature (type I) collagen as distinct from native (type II), fibrils. Although it has been suggested that this 'new' collagen may sometimes be derived from the endogenous vitreous cells (or hyalocytes), its synthesis is generally attributed to fibroblasts or fibroblast-like cells invading from outside the vitreous cavity. Depending on the available routes of invasion, the responsible cells might be (*a*) episcleral fibroblasts, (*b*) choroidal fibroblasts, (*c*) ciliary epithelial cells, (*d*) retinal pigment epithelial cells, (*e*) retinal perivascular fibroblasts, (*f*) retinal glial cells, or (*g*) blood-borne cells, e.g. monocytes.

The collagen-framework of the gel often provides the scaffold or matrix within which invading fibroblasts proliferate; fibrin may provide an alternative scaffolding for proliferation. Proliferation is thought to be stimulated by growth factors and is facilitated by the presence of proteins associated with haemorrhage and inflammation. The glycoprotein fibronectin has an important role in recruiting fibroblasts and in the cohesion of cells to themselves and to scaffolding substrata. Fibroblasts contain contractile proteins (including actin) and are called 'myofibroblasts' when the microfilaments are disposed as 'stress cables' within the cytoplasm (*Fig.* 5). Once the fibroblasts have proliferated and contracted, with consequent tractional effects upon connected structures, the cellular contraction is stabilized or consolidated by the secretion of mature collagen; the collagen itself does not contract. Some of these cohesive contractile systems also have a vascular component.

The causes and consequences of vitreous fibrosis vary according to the site of proliferation and contraction.

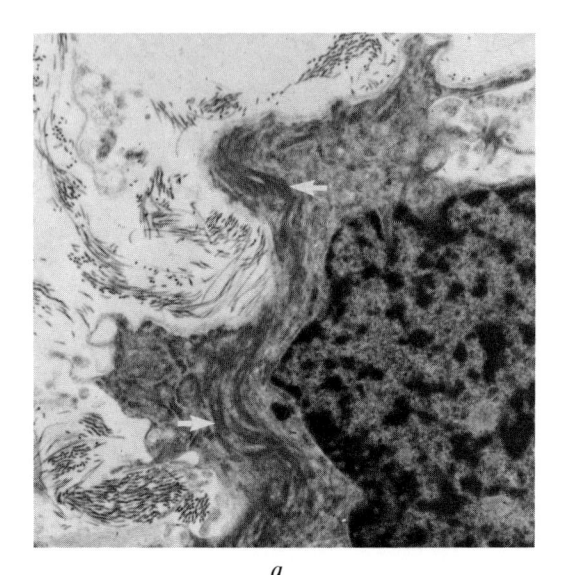

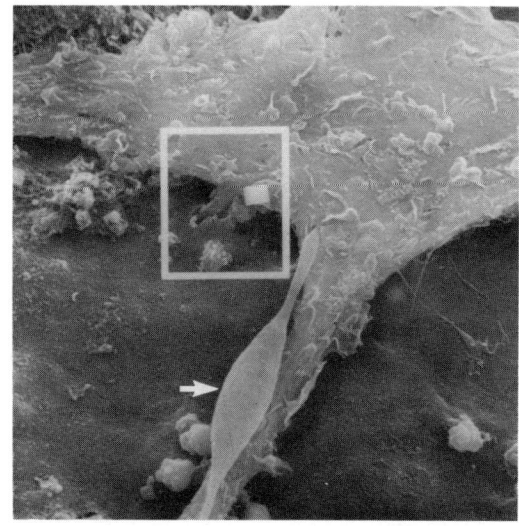

Fig. 5. Epiretinal membrane cells. *a*, Transmission electronmicrograph of myofibroblast and associated collagen fibrils; the cytoplasm shows actin stress cables (arrows). *b*, Scanning electronmicrograph of an epiretinal membrane; outgrowth of glial cell membrane.

Cyclitic Membrane

Fibrocellular or fibrovascular proliferation along the scaffold provided by the anterior vitreous cortex and hyaloid membrane produces a collagenous sheet in a coronal plane at the level of the ciliary body (*Fig. 6a*).

Aetiology

1. Penetrating injury of ciliary body region, especially when accompanied by haemorrhage or inflammation.
2. Severe uveitis.
3. Severe diabetic eye disease, especially after pars plana vitrectomy.

Sequelae

1. Traction upon (and detachment of) the ciliary body with hypotony and phthisis bulbi.
2. Vitreo-retinal traction in the vitreous base area.

Surgical Implications

1. Removal of the membrane in prephthisical stage may prevent phthisis.
2. Fibrinous exudate post-vitrectomy may form a scaffold for reproliferation and recurrence of a cyclitic membrane.

Basal Gel Fibrosis

Fibrous or fibrovascular tissue may proliferate among the densely packed fibrils of the vitreous base region.

Aetiology

1. Gel incarceration and invasion via surgical entry sites or penetrating injuries in the pars plana region (*Fig. 6b*).
2. Severe massive periretinal proliferation.

Sequelae

1. Exaggerated static traction on peripheral retina after basal gel incarceration and purse-string retinal detachment.
2. Anterior vitreous base traction (anterior loop traction) in massive periretinal proliferation.

Surgical Implications

1. Lens removal is necessary for effective vitrectomy in this area.
2. Scleral buckling should be considered for all breaks in this area.

Transgel Fibrosis

The central gel, especially when syneretic, provides a relatively poor scaffolding for cellular proliferation so that central gel fibrosis or 'organization' is rare. Nevertheless, a 'track' of haemorrhage (e.g. along the route of a penetrating foreign body) sometimes encourages proliferation of fibroblasts (with or without blood vessels) across the gel resulting in a transvitreal cord (*Fig. 6c*). However, most central vitreal 'bands' and 'strands' represent condensed gel fibrils with no 'new' collagen content or tractional implications.

Aetiology

1. Double perforating injury.
2. Intraocular foreign body.
3. Intravitreal instrumentation without vitrectomy.

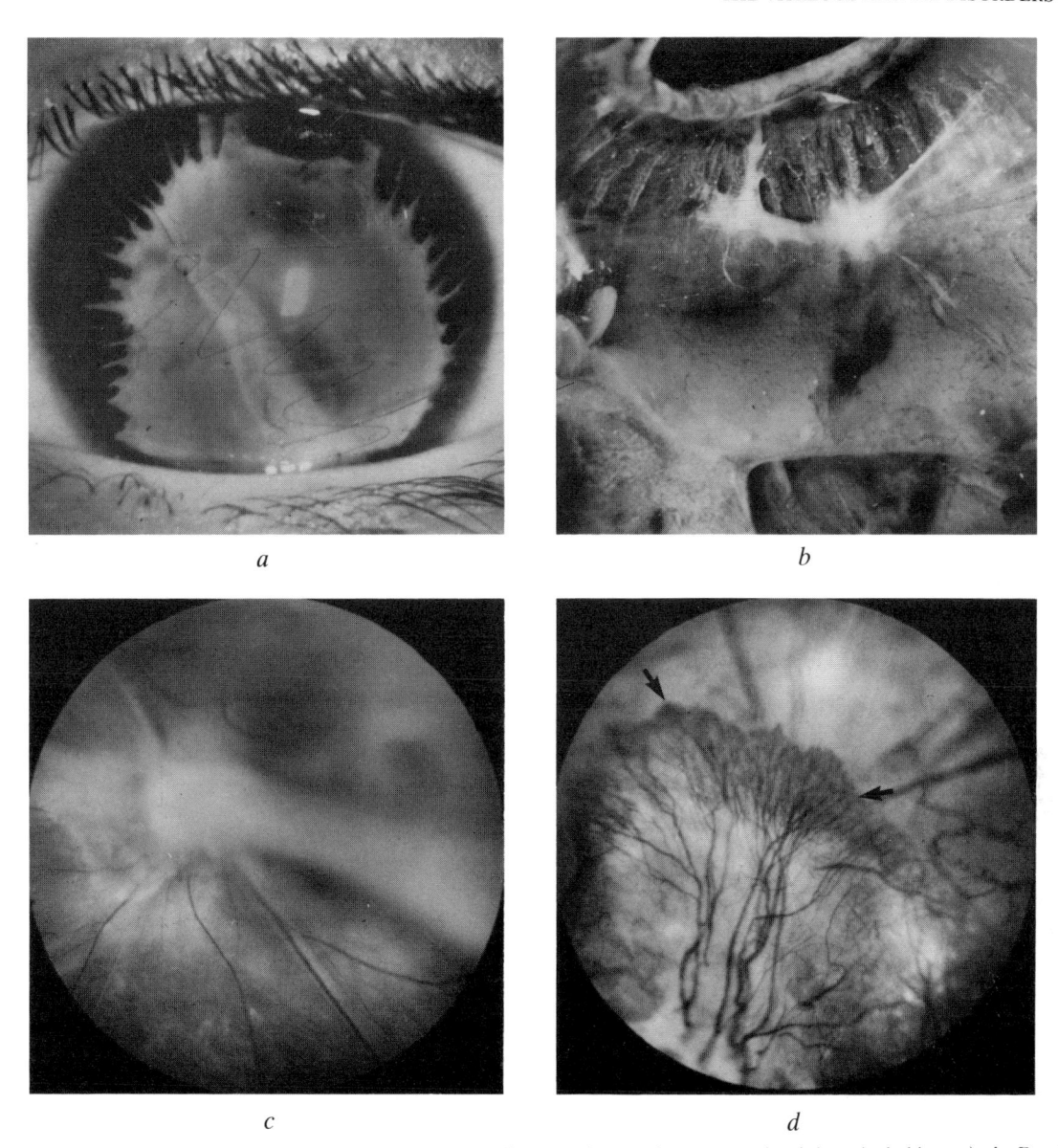

Fig. 6. Proliferations within the vitreous. *a*, Fibrovascular cyclitic membrane after penetrating injury (aphakic eye). *b*, Basal gel fibrosis through pars plana entry sites (post-vitrectomy). *c*, Transgel fibrosis after magnet removal of posteriorly impacted foreign body and clearance of vitreous haemorrhage. *d*, Vascular proliferations (arrows) along detached posterior hyaloid membrane in continuity with fibrovascular epiretinal membrane causing diabetic table-top traction retinal detachment.

Sequela

Transvitreal traction, but retinal detachment is unusual except in association with epiretinal fibrosis, vitreous base fibrosis or retinal breaks.

Surgical Implication

Easy relief of traction by division of cord.

Detached Posterior Hyaloid Membranes

The scaffold provided by the condensed collagenous framework of the detached posterior cortex and posterior hyaloid membrane is frequently the site of fibroblast proliferation and contraction. If the gel is completely detached, the resulting collagenous membrane is located in a coronal plane at the level of the posterior border of the vitreous base ('vitreous retraction'), and traps the retracted gel behind the lens (with or without herniation through a hiatus in the posterior hyaloid membrane) (*Fig.* 4*d*). If the gel is incompletely detached owing to post-basal vitreo-retinal adhesions, the vitreous cavity is compartmentalized by a rigid structure in the form of a single-point cone (e.g. funnel-shaped cone to the disc), or as a more complicated 'multiple-point cone', e.g. to posterior fibrovascular membranes (*see Fig.* 4*b*). If the gel is attached to the margins of an extensive epiretinal membrane, the apex of the cone is said to be 'truncated'. After extraretinal neovascularization and incomplete posterior vitreous detachment, the posterior part of the posterior hyaloid membrane may show fibrovascular proliferation in continuity with the epiretinal membrane (*Fig. 6d*).

Aetiology

1. Proliferative retinopathies.
2. Massive periretinal proliferation.
3. Penetrating trauma.

Sequelae

1. Anteroposterior and bridging elements of traction.
2. Retracted posterior hyaloid membrane immobilizes associated retinal breaks.

Surgical Implications

1. Easy circumcision of posterior vitreo-retinal adhesions by suction cutter.
2. Bipolar diathermy of associated vessels to prevent bleeding.

Fibrocellular Epiretinal Membranes

Non-vascularized membranes grow on the surface of (and in the same plane as) the inner limiting lamina of the retina either (*a*) within the scaffolding of attached vitreous cortex (thus incarcerating vitreous fibrils within their interstices), or (*b*) directly on the retinal surface after posterior vitreous detachment. Such proliferations are especially common in the posterior pole ('epimacular membranes') and may be either (*a*) 'simple' – consisting of a single layer of (glial) cells, or (*b*) 'complex' – forming a multilayered structure often containing several different types of cells including fibroblasts, pigment epithelial cells, glial cells, inflammatory cells and macrophages. The origin of the fibroblasts remains in doubt; they may be transformed hyalocytes, glial cells or pigment epithelial cells, or they may be derived from retinal perivascular fibroblasts. Outgrowth of accessory glia through dehiscences in the inner limiting lamina is a well-established phenomenon, and the resulting glial epiretinal membrane may provide a scaffolding on which other fibroblastic cells proliferate and contract (*see Fig. 5b*).

Aetiology

1. Developmental glial outgrowths through the inner limiting lamina (e.g. over blood vessels).
2. After inflammation via transmigration of white cells through the inner limiting lamina, fibroblast recruitment by macrophage-derived fibronectin or growth factors.
3. After haemorrhage and related to a fibrin-scaffold or associated growth factors.
4. After posterior vitreous detachment and secondary to inner limiting laminar damage after avulsion of simple epiretinal membranes into which the posterior hyaloid membrane was incarcerated.
5. Pigment epithelial dispersion and deposition following retinal break formation.
6. Trauma, e.g. at the impaction site of an intraocular foreign body.
7. Ischaemia, perhaps related to subsurface factors (e.g. cotton-wool spots).
8. Combination of these.
9. Idiopathic.

Sequelae

1. Simple epiretinal membranes are usually asymptomatic and only demonstrable following postmortem retinal autolysis and swelling.
2. Surface wrinkling retinopathy and cellophane maculopathy (inner retinal striation and cystoid retinal oedema).
3. Complex membranes contract to produce full thickness folding of the retina from tangential traction (e.g. macular pucker and 'star-folds' associated with rhegmatogenous retinal detachment).
4. Posterior vitreous detachment is induced (if not originally causative in formation of the epiretinal membrane).
5. Retinal breaks occasionally develop adjacent to contracting fibrocellular membranes.

Surgical Implications

1. Epiretinal membranes must be dissected or peeled from the retina prior to suction cutting and aspiration.
2. Viscodelamination, i.e. separation of extensive membranes from the retina by Healon, methylcellulose or silicone oil injection.

Fibrovascular Epiretinal Membranes

Newly formed blood vessels, arising from retinal veins, penetrate the inner limiting lamina and proliferate on the surface of the retina or optic disc ('extraretinal neovascularization'). The network of blood vessels may be accompanied by fibroblasts, resulting in the same tractional consequences as for fibrocellular epiretinal membranes. Such fibrovascular outgrowths are characteristically associated with inner retinal ischaemia (via production of vasoproliferative factors) though inflammation may also induce neovascularization, especially at the optic disc. Fibrovascular proliferation appears to have a specific dependence on a cortical gel scaffolding; no growth occurs on the retinal surface after posterior vitreous detachment (or proliferation is limited to focal or 'abortive' outgrowths). During proliferation, the gel becomes incarcerated within the interstices of the membrane to produce exaggerated vitreo-retinal adhesions (*see Fig.* 1). The site of neovascularization varies with its aetiology, depending essentially on the location of capillary non-perfusion, i.e. adjacent (usually just posterior) to ischaemic areas or at more distant sites (e.g. the optic disc).

Aetiology

1. Diabetic retinopathy (along the major vascular arcades and at the optic disc).
2. Venous occlusion, especially branch vein occlusion but also central vein occlusion (variable sites including optic disc).
3. Eales's disease or retinal vasculitis (mid-periphery and optic disc).
4. Haemoglobin SC retinopathy (equatorial and optic disc).
5. Uveitis (optic disc).

Sequelae

1. Tangential traction (and traction retinal detachment).
2. Incomplete posterior vitreous detachment and avulsion of edges of vascularized membranes (forward new vessels).
3. Haemorrhage from incomplete or complete avulsion of vascularized epiretinal membranes during vitreous detachment.
4. Retinal tears from avulsion of the edge of an epiretinal membrane during posterior vitreous detachment (and combined traction and rhegmatogenous retinal detachment).

Surgical Implications

1. Scissors dissection (segmentation or delamination technique) to relieve tangential traction.
2. Bipolar diathermy to prevent bleeding.

VITREO-RETINAL TRACTION, RETINAL BREAKS AND RETINAL DETACHMENT

Two broad categories of vitreo-retinal traction are recognized: (*a*) dynamic traction (intermittent traction or 'jactitation'), and (*b*) static traction (sustained or continuous traction).

Dynamic Vitreo-retinal Traction

This is especially associated with rhegmatogenous posterior vitreous detachment with collapse either during the course of vitreous separation or subsequently owing to the relative density (and hence gravitational force) of residual gel or to forces derived from the corporate mobility of the gel induced by eye movements. Whereas the rotational forces generated by saccadic rotations of the globe are normally transmitted into the gel throughout the gel boundary, these transmitted forces are essentially concentrated in the vitreous base and other vitreo-retinal adhesions after posterior vitreous detachment. Dynamic traction is especially liable to cause retinal tearing in relation to focal or irregular vitreo-retinal adhesions (*see Fig.* 3*b*); in the case of giant retinal breaks, however, tearing occurs on a wide front along the apparently smooth posterior border of the vitreous base. Occasionally, breaks arise from dynamic traction independent of posterior vitreous detachment.

Static Vitreo-retinal Traction

This generally results from vitreous fibrosis and/or vitreous prolapse and incarceration (*Fig.* 2*a*). Whereas gel 'contracts' in volume under various laboratory conditions, for example heating, freezing, radiation etc., contraction of the collagen framework of the whole gel is seldom, if ever, the cause of clinically significant static vitreo-retinal traction. Vitreous fibrosis exerts traction either transgel, along the posterior hyaloid interface (anteroposterior and bridging traction), or on the retinal surface (tangential traction). Strictly speaking, not all static traction has a vitreous component, for example, tangential traction from epiretinal membrane contraction subsequent to (and, from the tractional viewpoint, independent of) posterior vitreous detachment.

In certain instances, retinal breaks result from combined static and dynamic traction, e.g. vitreous incarceration complicated by posterior vitreous detachment when dynamic vitreo-retinal traction forces operate on a vitreous base already under the influence of static traction (producing, for example, a giant tear at the posterior border of the vitreous base). Examples include certain aphakic retinal detachments following intracapsular extraction, after penetrating trauma and after central pars plana vitrectomy.

Retinal Breaks

Three broad categories of retinal break are recognized: (*a*) traumatic breaks, (*b*) tractional breaks and (*c*) trophic breaks.

Traumatic Breaks

Traumatic breaks are caused at the moment of (or soon after) blunt trauma to the globe, either at the site of the impaction (e.g. within an area of commotio retinae) or as a result of ocular distortion (e.g. bucket-handle tears, certain giant breaks and certain dialyses and disinsertions at the ora serrata). The terms dialysis and disinsertion tend to be used interchangeably to denote a discontinuity at the ora serrata between the neural retina and the non-pigmented pars plana epithelium (and as such they are not strictly 'retinal breaks'); others reserve the term 'dialysis' for breaks involving more than one oral bay in continuity, while 'disinsertion' denotes multiple breaks within discrete (usually adjacent) oral bays.

Tractional Breaks

These are most frequently a consequence of dynamic vitreo-retinal traction (for example, horseshoe tears, operculated tears, certain giant tears etc.). However, static traction can also result in retinal breaks, e.g. oral dialysis/disinsertion from vitreo-retinal incarceration, and (infrequently) breaks adjacent to contracting epiretinal membranes.

Trophic Breaks

Trophic breaks result from atrophic full thickness retinal disintegration (e.g. round breaks within areas of lattice degeneration). Trophic breaks are generally referred to as 'holes' as distinct from 'tears', which refer to post-oral traumatic or tractional breaks. In lattice degeneration, trophic holes within the lesions and tractional tears around the lesions frequently coexist.

Retinal Detachment

The term 'retinal detachment' is strictly a misnomer in that it refers to separation of the neural retina from the pigment epithelium (rather than separation of the retina and choroid). Such separation implies that the forces and factors maintaining the neural retina in functional apposition to the pigment epithelium (collectively known as the 'pigment epithelial pump') have been overcome. Two broad categories of 'surgical' retinal detachment (i.e. excluding serous and solid detachments) are recognized: (a) traction retinal detachment and (b) rhegmatogenous retinal detachment.

Traction Retinal Detachment

This occurs as a consequence of static vitreo-retinal traction, notably from tangential traction exerted by extensive epiretinal membranes (e.g. macular pucker and diabetic traction detachment). Transgel and anteroposterior traction seldom cause significant retinal detachment in the absence of associated tangential traction or retinal breaks; similarly, most vitreous base traction is associated with oral breaks. Traction detachments are generally slowly progressive, with the greatest retinal elevation at the site of traction and an anterior concavity of the retinal surface resulting from the action of the pigment epithelial pump and the ensuing transretinal pressure gradient. The immobile detachment does not change in configuration with time, rest or position of the patient (*Fig. 7.4a*).

Surgical Implications

1. Vitrectomy is indicated only if the macular retina is distorted or detached with associated visual loss; in extramacular pucker or diabetic extramacular traction detachment, vitrectomy is generally contraindicated.
2. Removal of vitreous and/or epiretinal tractional elements results in retinal reattachment; scleral buckling and internal tamponade are unnecessary.

Rhegmatogenous Retinal Detachment

This category of detachment results from recruitment of fluid vitreous beneath the retina through a retinal break. Frequently, rhegmatogenous detachments result from dynamic vitreo-retinal traction (a) by virtue of tractional retinal breaks and (b) by exerting traction on the adjacent retina (despite relief of traction to some extent by break formation). The factors leading to rhegmatogenous retinal detachment from trophic breaks are not fully understood, though vitreous syneresis is important in allowing subretinal recruitment of fluid vitreous. Rhegmatogenous detachments are typically bullous (i.e. the retina is convex anteriorly since there is no transretinal pressure gradient) and the height and extent of the mobile retinal elevation may vary with time, eye immobilization and posture. The extent of detachment is independent of the size and number of breaks, and the amount of subretinal fluid at any one time represents the result of continuous recruitment of subretinal fluid and absorption through the pigment epithelium (*Fig. 7b*).

Surgical Implications

1. Closure of the retinal break(s) alone is sufficient to allow complete retinal reattachment.
2. With the exception of flapped-over giant retinal breaks, peripheral breaks (oral, pre-equatorial or equatorial) can generally be closed by scleral buckling (with or without subretinal fluid drainage and internal tamponade).
3. Vitrectomy and internal tamponade is generally preferred for posterior breaks (e.g. macular and parapapillary breaks) and flapped-over giant tears.

Combined Rhegmatogenous and Traction Retinal Detachment

Many retinal detachments are associated both with retinal breaks and static vitreo-retinal traction (*Fig. 7c,d*). In some cases, static traction develops subsequent to rhegmatogenous detachment (e.g. massive periretinal proliferation); in others, static traction and break formation are synchronous (e.g. oral dialysis following perforating trauma, vitreous incarceration and basal gel fibrosis); alternatively, a retinal break may occur subsequent to the establishment of static traction (e.g. proliferative diabetic retinopathy and break formation adjacent to fibrovascular epiretinal membranes and secondary to posterior vitreous detachment) (*Fig. 7c*). Apparently rapid progression of traction detachment often reflects merely the development of an open break and conversion of the detachment to a combined traction and rhegmatogenous detachment. The effects of static traction on the retina may be exaggerated by the coexistent rhegmatogenous element such that, after closure of the offending break alone, the retina reattaches and the static traction is hardly discernible.

Massive Periretinal Proliferation (Proliferative Vitreo-retinopathy)

This term is reserved for the progressive immobilization of a (rhegmatogenous) retinal detachment (*Fig. 7b,d*) by proliferation and contraction of fibroblasts (*a*) within the vitreous gel, especially the vitreous

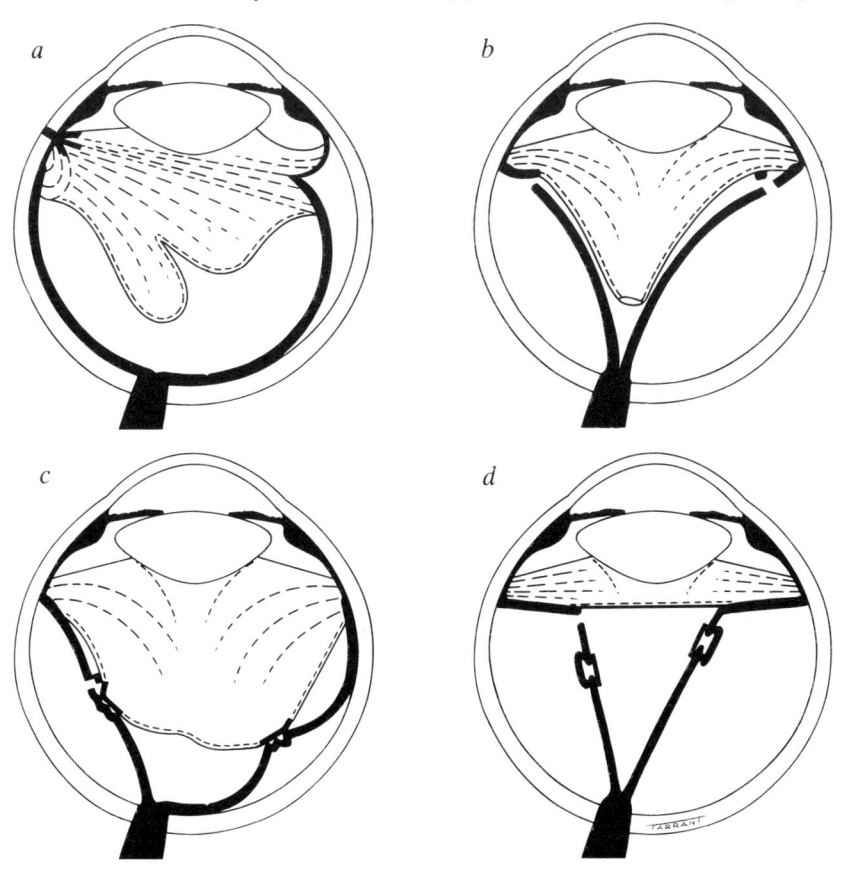

Fig. 7. Retinal detachments. *a*, Purse-string retinal detachment temporally (convex) after nasal pars plana penetrating injury with basal gel incarceration and subsequent basal gel fibrosis and posterior vitreous detachment (cf. *Fig. 2a*). *b*, Rhegmatogenous retinal detachment (concave) after posterior vitreous detachment and formation of two retinal tears (flap tear nasally, operculated tear temporally) (cf. *Fig. 3b*). *c* Combined rhegmatogenous and traction retinal detachment after contraction of two fibrovascular epiretinal membranes, incomplete posterior vitreous detachment and retinal break formation nasally (cf. *Fig. 4b*). *d*, Combined rhegmatogenous and traction retinal detachment with vitreous retraction and post-basal epiretinal membrane contraction (cf. *Figs. 4d* and *7b*).

Occasionally the development of a break apparently has no influence on the configuration of a pre-existing traction detachment (for example, some diabetic detachments).

Surgical Implications

1. Closure of the retinal break(s) alone may be sufficient to allow central retinal reattachment in some cases.
2. Vitrectomy and internal tamponade must be combined with scleral buckling of breaks if all associated traction cannot be eliminated, especially peripherally.

base; (*b*) along the (detached) cortical gel scaffold; (*c*) on the retinal surface (star folds) and/or under the retina (subretinal fibrosis). It occurs as part of the natural history of untreated rhegmatogenous detachments (especially those associated with posterior vitreous detachment and multiple large breaks) and also after failed (or suboptimal) scleral buckling and retinal coagulation. In the early stages, some cases respond to high scleral buckling and internal tamponade. Otherwise, vitrectomy (including epiretinal membrane dissection) and identification and closure of all breaks is indicated. Reproliferation and contraction of fibroblasts frequently causes reopening of retinal breaks and redetachment.

Severe Diabetic Eye Disease

The extent of diabetic neovascularization depends on the degree of inner retinal ischaemia and the timing of posterior vitreous detachment; vitreous separation precludes further vasoproliferation on the underlying retina. Nevertheless, non-vascularized (fibrocellular) epiretinal proliferations may develop both within attached cortical gel and behind detached gel. Posterior vitreous detachment induces bleeding either within the gel or behind the detached gel by complete or incomplete avulsion of fibrovascular membranes. Contraction of fibrovascular epiretinal membranes (with or without anteroposterior and bridging traction along detached cortical vitreous) produces traction retinal detachment (*Fig.* 8) which may involve the macula or may be extramacular, asymptomatic and stable; vitrectomy is not indicated if the macula is not involved. Extramacular traction detachment sometimes progresses rapidly to involve the macula because of retinal break formation (when urgent vitrectomy is indicated). The quintessential strategy of vitrectomy is removal of the whole of the post-basal cortical gel scaffold (plus contained fibrovascular membranes) using a suction cutter, scissors dissection and/or viscodelamination; retinal breaks must be identified, associated traction relieved and the breaks closed by internal tamponade. Panretinal photocoagulation helps to prevent rebleeding and postoperative rubeosis iridis.

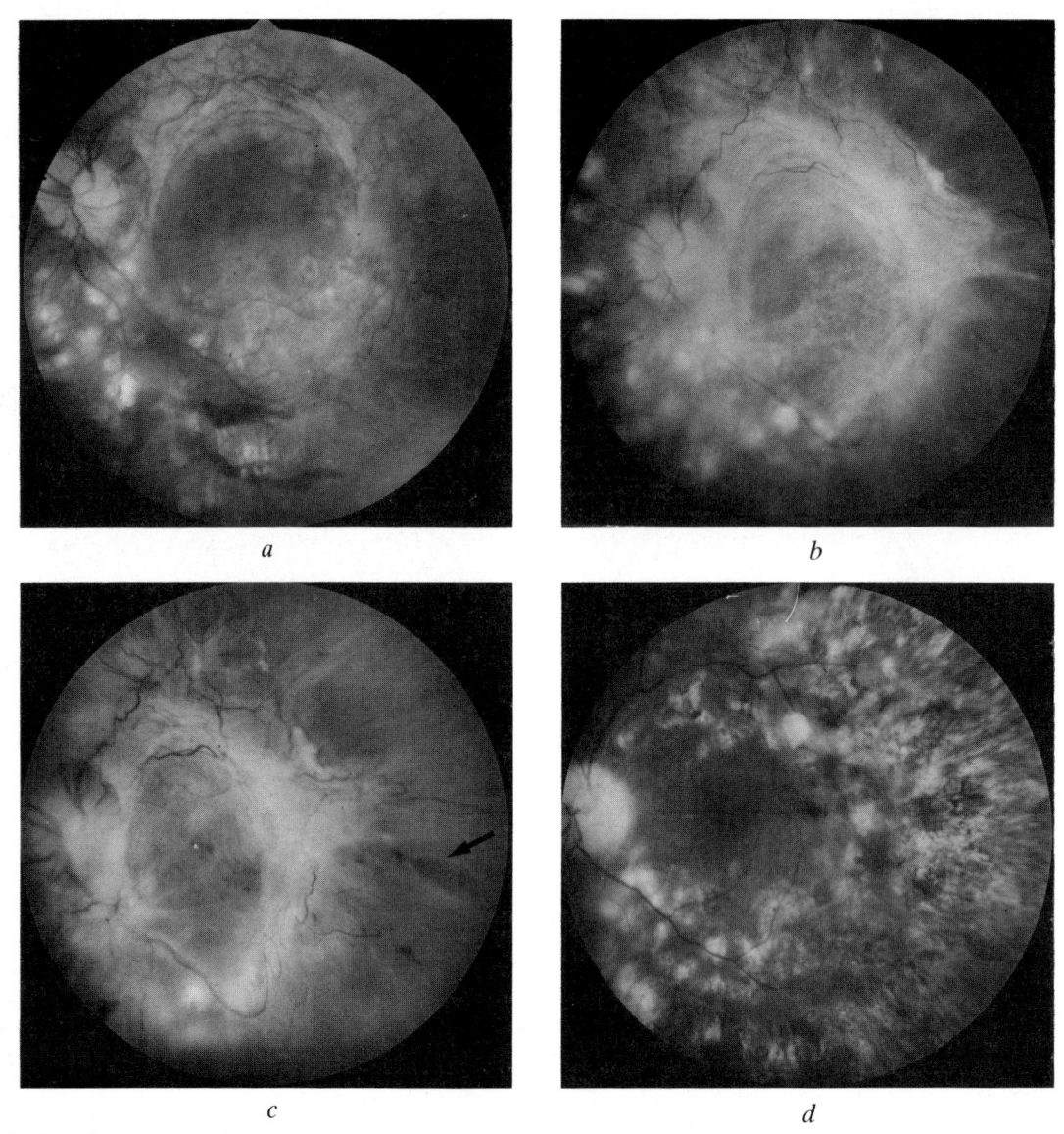

Fig. 8. Pathogenic sequence and treatment of severe diabetic eye disease. *a*, Fibrovascular proliferation along major vascular arcades and mild vitreous haemorrhage (acuity 6/9). *b*, One month later; tangential traction and extramacular traction retinal detachment (acuity 6/9). *c*, Two weeks later; incomplete posterior vitreous detachment owing to retinal break formation (arrow) (acuity 3/60). *d*, One month following vitrectomy, membrane dissection, internal tamponade and cryotherapy to retinal break (acuity 6/12).

VITREOUS SURGERY

Surgical intervention within the vitreous cavity currently ranges in extent and sophistication from 'open-sky' aspiration of fluid vitreous with a wide-bore needle (for vitreous loss at intracapsular cataract extraction), through vitrectomy for opacities within the gel, to highly complex closed microsurgical procedures for complicated retinal detachments. The objectives of such procedures must be carefully defined bearing in mind (a) that every surgical assault on the vitreous potentially endangers surrounding structures (the lens, cornea and especially the retina) both peroperatively and subsequently; (b) that the underlying cause of the vitreo-retinal pathology may obscured. In addition to visual restoration, other manoeuvres are facilitated by removal of opaque gel, for example, endophotocoagulation of ischaemic attached retina, identification of retinal breaks and localization and removal of intraocular foreign bodies. Removal of haemorrhagic or inflammatory debris may also have a beneficial effect in reducing the tendency to fibroblast proliferation and fibrosis. Recurrent opacification occurs transiently after vitrectomy for vitreous haemorrhage (from leeching of erythroclasts from the basal gel frill) or uveitis (owing to fibrinous exudation), but can be serious and persistent in amyloidosis and in the ischaemic retinopathies (owing to rebleeding, e.g. from fibrovascular ingrowth at surgical entry sites).

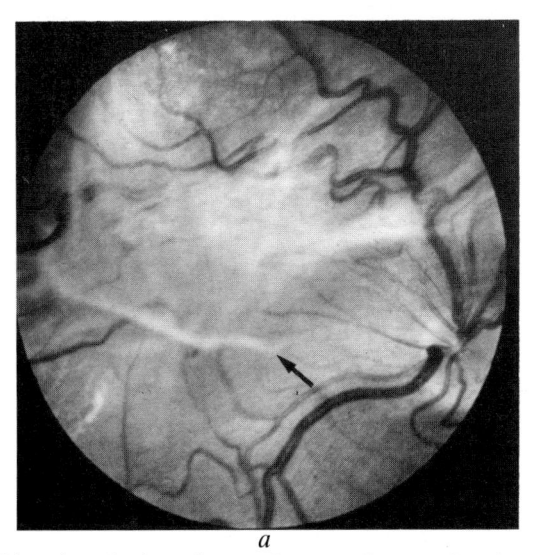

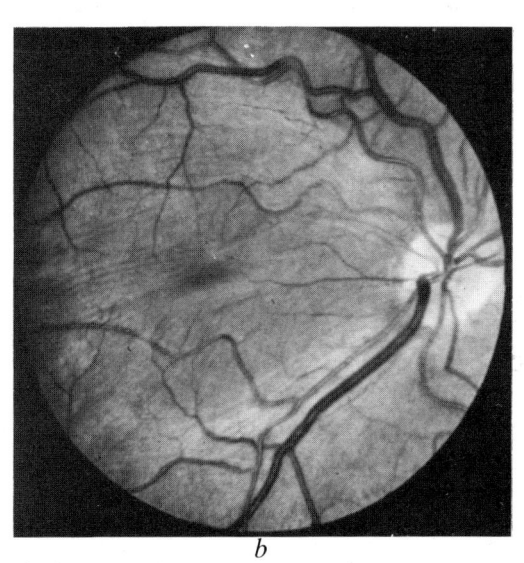

Fig. 9. Dissection of epimacular membrane. *a*, Preoperative photograph of extensive fibrocellular epiretinal membrane; spontaneous avulsion of lower edge of membrane (arrow) and underlying traction retinal detachment (acuity 6/60). *b*, Same eye 2 months after vitrectomy and membrane peeling; residual inner retinal striation (acuity 6/12). (Reproduced with permission from McLeod D., Marshall and Grierson. Epimacular membrane peeling. *Trans. Ophthalmol. Soc. UK* 1981; **101**, 170–80.)

persist (e.g. continuing amyloid deposition, uveitis or the effects of retinal ischaemia); and (c) that the ultimate visual result of surgery often depends on factors other than those directly influenced by the mechanical intraocular manoeuvres (e.g. cystoid macular oedema in uveitis, toxic retinopathy in endophthalmitis, ischaemic maculopathy in diabetes and post-detachment macular atrophy).

The indications for vitreous surgery can be broadly categorized as follows.

Removal of Axial Opacities and Consequent Restoration of a Clear Optical Axis

This is readily achieved by suction cutting of opacified gel, especially if the vitreous is completely detached from the retina or if persistent vitreo-retinal adhesions are both posterior (and therefore readily circumcised) and focal (thus obviating membrane dissection). Residual opacity in the basal gel frill is of little consequence; provided retinal breaks are not

Relief of Vitreo-retinal Traction and Mobilization of Retinal Breaks

This is achieved by removal of incarcerated or fibrotic gel or (most frequently) by dissection of epiretinal membranes (*Fig.* 9). Recurrent (or reparative) epiretinal fibrosis may complicate epiretinal membrane dissection, resulting in post-operative traction retinal detachment or combined traction and rhegmatogenous detachment by formation (or reopening) of retinal breaks. Intensive research is currently in progress to discover pharmacological methods of preventing such recurrent proliferation, adhesion or contraction of cells and subsequent collagen synthesis.

Creation of Space for Intraocular Manipulations or Tamponade

This can be especially valuable in treating complicated retinal detachments, for example, manipulation and repositioning of flapped-over giant retinal breaks and treatment of posterior breaks, e.g. macular holes.

Removal of Gel for Laboratory Diagnosis

This is indicated in bacterial or fungal endophthalmitis (the 'abscess drainage' and precise bacteriological diagnosis facilitating treatment by improving selection and penetration of antibiotics). Cytological examination has proved helpful in the diagnosis of reticulum cell sarcoma.

Prophylactic Vitrectomy

This procedure is frequently advocated in traumatized eyes in order to prevent vitreous fibrosis along gel scaffolds. This objective may be especially difficult to achieve because of the difficulties in completely removing basal gel and attached cortical gel; fibrocellular membranes may also develop on the surface of retina devoid of gel.

CONCLUSION

Vitreo-retinal surgery is applicable to a wide range of intraocular disorders but considerable experience is required in order to identify crucial aspects of pathology and operability, to weigh the risks against the benefits of vitreous surgery, and to detect and successfully manage inadvertent or unexpected complications peroperatively. For these reasons, together with the need for a very wide range of available instrumentation, vitreous surgery (other than for simple objectives) is carried out in regional or supraregional centres. There is no substitute for a planned, protracted surgical apprenticeship for the aspiring vitreo-retinal surgeon.

Chapter 10

The Lens

Pathology of the Crystalline Lens
R. F. Fisher

EMBRYOLOGY AND ANATOMY

The crystalline lens develops from an invagination of the surface ectoderm of the embryo between the time the embryo grows from 4·5 mm to 7·00 mm long. Subsequently the invagination forms a vesicle. The cells of the anterior wall of the vesicle form the lens epithelium, while the cells of the posterior part of the vesicle become elongated, forming the lens fibre system. At the equator of the vesicle the cells retain their germinal activity and continue to contribute lens fibres forwards and backwards in layers to form the adult lens. At an early period the vesicle is surrounded by a capsule which is now known to be formed from the epithelial cells of the vesicle. Because of this the cells which form within the lens capsule are retained throughout life and continually become more compressed as further layers of cells are added. The lens, in consequence, continues to grow. The adult lens fibres form a complex pattern, as shown in *Fig*. 1, and where fibres come in contact with each other a line of demarcation forms, known as a lens suture.

The obvious compression and increased density of the central part or nucleus of the lens was thought to cause a loss of water and a hardening or sclerosis of the lens. However, recently it has been shown that the water content of the normal lens is almost constant throughout life. The adult lens is a transparent, biconvex disc, separating the aqueous and vitreous humours. It is retained in position by a delicate group of radial fibres originating from the ciliary body and inserting into the lens capsule just in front and behind the equator. This ligament is known as the zonule and the separation between the anterior and posterior layers forms a small triangular space known as the canal of Petit. At the time of the onset of presbyopia the lens capsule becomes thickened at the zonular insertion. Before this time the capsule is thickest at the equator of the lens.

The lens fibre forms the essential structural unit of the lens substance. It is hexagonal in cross-section and has recently been shown to be bonded to other fibres by a complex arrangement of ball-and-socket joints which are particularly numerous near the equator of the lens. Recently microfilaments have been demonstrated in the lens fibre but their function is at present uncertain, although they may be related to the elastic properties of the lens substance. The lens capsule plays an important role in acting as an elastic membrane capable of changing the shape of the lens. It also acts as a permeable barrier between the aqueous humour and the lens fibres. In man, if the lens capsule is breached by trauma, the lens rapidly becomes opaque. The function of the lens is to focus the rays of light initially bent on passing through the cornea into the eye and on to the retina to form a perfect image. It thus acts as a fine focusing mechanism, being responsible for about one-third of the focal power of the intact eye. Since the degree of convergence of the rays on the retina varies with the distance of the object from the eye, it is necessary for the lens to alter its refractive power. This is effected mainly by a change in curvature of the anterior surface of the lens and also by a change in the curvature of its nucleus, which has a higher refractive index than the cortex. To enable the lens to

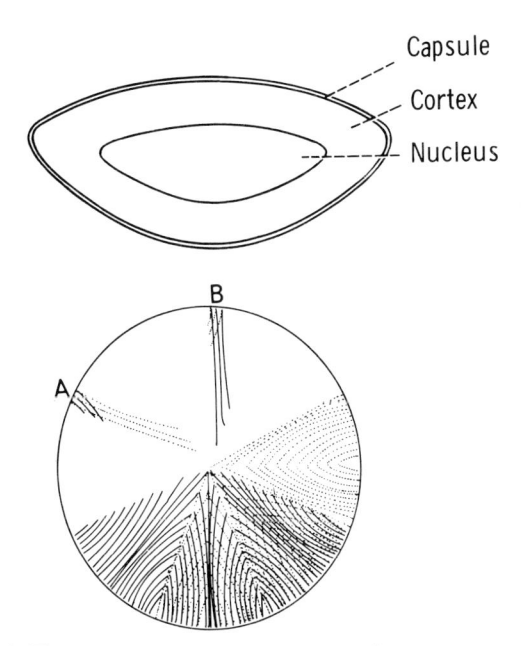

Fig. 1. The arrangement of lens fibres in the human lens. *Above*, the lens in cross-section; *below*, fibres marked A originate near the posterior pole, fibres marked B originate near the anterior pole.

become more spherical in shape and so increase its power, the zonule is relaxed by the contraction of the ciliary muscle.

The lens changes in shape to a marked extent throughout life. In the fetus it is nearly spherical, while in the adult it assumes the form of a biconvex disc. In old age it becomes even flatter and also yellowish in colour. In the ageing lens an accumulation of fine globules between the lens fibres occurs. This process is a precursor of true opacification of the lens, but in its early stages merely shows as a greyish reflection through the pupil of an elderly subject. This may easily be mistaken for cataract.

In association with these changes in light transmission the lens also loses its ability to change shape when the tension in the zonule alters. Recent studies suggest that this loss of accommodation, in the elderly known as presbyopia, is not due to any inability of the ciliary muscle to contract but to a combination of ageing changes in the lens. These changes include weakening of the lens capsule, flattening of the lens and a decrease in the ability of the nuclear fibres to move relative to each other.

DEVELOPMENTAL DEFECTS

Developmental defects of the lens are associated with its anterior and posterior poles and also its equator. A small opacity in the anterior part of the lens is often associated with strands of persistent pupillary membrane. This so-called anterior polar cataract varies in size and often causes little visual disability. Associated with some of the small opacities is the presence of pigment cells which produce small star-shaped areas, and these may be confused with clumps of pigment arising from a previous attack of uveitis. In contrast, a defect of the posterior pole of the lens is usually associated with grave refractive errors. The posterior portion of the lens becomes bowl-shaped and causes myopia and irregular refraction. A defect associated with the equator of the lens is a notch or notches at its border. These are probably produced by a defect of the overlying zonule. Often this condition coexists with a coloboma of choroid or iris and since the suspensory mechanism of the lens is imperfectly developed in one meridian, a high degree of astigmatism results. A more extensive defect of zonular fibres results in the lens becoming markedly displaced, sometimes accompanied by loss of transparency.

Cataract

The word cataract is used to describe the condition of opacification of the crystalline lens of the eye. In the days when various humours were thought to condition the state of health of the body, the white pupil, which is very obvious in advanced cataract, was considered to be due to a humour from the brain falling down behind the pupil.

The term cataract is often used to refer to changes in colour of the lens as well as a decrease in its transparency. Until quite recently this has caused considerable confusion. Because of this much work has been done on the biochemical changes in lenses, some of which might not have seriously interfered with vision. From the clinical point of view, the forward scatter of light from the small portion of the lens adjacent to the posterior pole is all important. Indeed, considerable opacification if confined to the nucleus or anterior cortex, can be surprisingly tolerated with only a small reduction in visual acuity. Slit lamp appearances only show the scatter of the lens at a marked angle to the line of vision. To appreciate the back scatter from the posterior cortex the beam should be so adjusted that a red reflex is produced with the focus of the viewing microscope being at the level of the posterior pole of the lens. Under these circumstances, imperfections of this all-important area are well seen and the reason for reduced vision in an apparently clear lens can be appreciated.

Classification

Ideally cataract should be classified by the aetiological factors which cause the lens to become opaque. Unfortunately, at the present time many of these factors are imperfectly understood and, in consequence, it is necessary to characterize cataract either by its presumed cause or some other factor, such as the appearance of the cataract or the age at which it occurs. For this reason cataract is classified as follows:

Cataract due to Physical Causes

This type of cataract includes traumatic cataract, cataract due to perforating injury or severe contusion of the lens, and irradiation cataract due to exposure of the lens to X-rays, neutrons or gamma rays.

Cataract due to a Biochemical Defect

This type of cataract occurs rarely in infancy due to a defect of galactose metabolism or more commonly in later life in advanced diabetes, where the lens is bathed in an aqueous containing a high concentration of glucose. This group of cataracts also includes those that are caused by cataractogenic agents such as thallium or nitrophenol, which interfere with the metabolism of the lens.

Developmental Cataract

This type of cataract develops at an early stage in the growth of the lens and may be due to a number of factors which are imperfectly understood. These include hereditary, nutritional or inflammatory factors. They produce impaired development of lens fibres, particularly at their ends, and characteristically produce punctate or club-shaped opacities which are seen commonly in coronary cataract. At other times the opacities may be confined principally to the embryonic nucleus of the lens and fibres associated with it, forming the so-called lamellar cataract.

Senile Cataract

This is by far the commonest form of cataract and appears to be an accentuation of some of the normal ageing changes which occur in the lens. It is divided into two main types: a senile opacification of the nucleus of the lens and a senile opacification of the cortex. As might be expected, a large number of senile cataracts possess both nuclear and cortical opacities.

Complicated Cataract

This type of cataract develops initially in the posterior cortex of the lens and is associated with some other disease of the eye such as uveitis, chronic simple glaucoma or retinal detachment.

Cataract associated with Systemic Disease

Often the cataracts in these cases have a strikingly characteristic form. Although an undoubted association with the systemic disease exists, and is presumably a biochemical defect, the causes of these cataracts are at present unknown.

Cataract due to Physical Causes

Traumatic Cataract

Throughout life the complex lens fibre system is subjected to strain during accommodation. On theoretical grounds this has been blamed for the development of senile cataract. More recently, however, it has been shown that the human lens *in vivo*, when subjected to excessive radial strain, shows a pattern of opalescence which is cuneiform in distribution. Moreover, a well-recognized type of cataract is caused either by a perforating wound of the lens capsule or by a contusion of the eyeball without perforation, the latter being known as concussion cataract. A few hours after perforation, the lens becomes cloudy, initially at the seat of the wound, and later throughout the entire lens. The lens substance thereafter begins to be absorbed and in favourable cases, in young persons, this process may continue until there is a clear pupil. More frequently, however, part of the lens remains opaque within the damaged capsule and requires subsequent operation. Occasionally, if the rent in the capsule is small, it may become closed and the opacity of the lens then remains limited. In older persons, when the entire lens matter cannot be rendered soluble by the aqueous, the course is much less favourable. A chronic uveitis results and the swelling of the injured lens may block the filtration angle, or the incompletely absorbed debris of lens fibres may obstruct the trabecular meshwork. In both cases a secondary glaucoma results. Concussion injuries may cause rupture of the capsule with the above results, but more commonly they give rise to circumscribed opacities of two types. The anterior opacity, known as Vossius's ring, is rarely seen. It is ring-shaped, conforming to the pupillary margin, and is due to pigment adhering to the capsule in the area compressed by the pupillary border of the iris after a blow on the cornea. The second type of opacity occurs in the posterior cortex of the lens and produces a rosette or star-shaped opacity. This is probably due to the separation of lens fibres. It may clear considerably in a few weeks or remain permanent, with an ultimate increase of the opacity.

Irradiation Cataract

This type of cataract is caused by exposure of the lens to X-rays, gamma rays or neutrons. It would appear that it is caused by damage to the germinal epithelium of the lens. This is manifested by a latent period and the development of early opacities in the posterior cortex, which slowly extend to the whole lens. The process may take from 4 to 10 years depending upon the degree of exposure. Histologically there is damage to the anterior epithelium of the lens, with the production of subcapsular plaques and the subsequent imperfect development of the lens fibres. These imperfect fibres migrate to the posterior pole, producing feathery and dust-like opacities.

A similar type of cataract may be caused by exposure to infrared rays, which are thought to damage the lens by indirectly heating the heat-absorbent pigment epithelium of the iris. It is seen in glassblowers and those who work for long periods in front of furnaces and ovens. In addition to opacification of the lens, there may be exfoliation of the anterior lens capsule. It has been suggested that exposure to ultraviolet rays may also hasten the development of senile cataract. Recently, it has been shown that the lens protein may be denatured by ultraviolet radiation to form yellow or brown pigment containing substances that may be related to senile cataract formation.

Cataract due to Biochemical Causes

A most significant advance in our understanding of biochemical defects of the lens has been the production of cataract by means of abnormal sugar concentration in the aqueous. In the experimental animals there appears to be an accumulation of polyols within the substance of the lens fibres with a retention of water, separation of the fibres and development of cataract. In the human subject this information has enabled the development of such cataracts to be reversed by giving insulin, in the case of diabetic cataract, or excluding galactose from the diet of an infant, in the case of galactosaemic cataract. Cataract may also occur due to the accumulation of other abnormal substances within the lens, such as homocystine or copper. In the former condition subluxation of the lens also occurs with a subsequent development of cataract, while in the latter (Wilson's disease) a cataract at the posterior pole of the lens with spoke-like opacities develops in a proportion of patients.

Developmental Cataract

Posterior Polar Cataract

This form may result from imperfect regression of the primitive vascular supply of the lens. The remnant of the hyaloid artery may often be seen as a small strand attached to the back of the lens in normal eyes. However, when the remnants of the fibrovascular sheath cause a disturbance of the lens fibres beneath them, a posterior polar opacity results. Since this is near the nodal point of the eye, a considerable disturbance in vision may result. If, after the initial disturbance in early embryonic life, clear fibres are subsequently laid down, a rare and hereditary bilateral discoid opacity between the nucleus and posterior pole may result.

Anterior Polar Cataract

This type of cataract is thought to result from a delayed formation of the anterior chamber and prolonged contact of the lens with the cornea in fetal life. It is usually bilateral. Frequently with this form of cataract small strands of persistent pupillary membrane adhere to the anterior surface of the lens. An acquired form results from perforation of an infantile corneal ulcer. Subsequently, if the anterior chamber is restored, clear lens fibres may be laid down superficial to the original cataractous area.

Lamellar Cataract

This is by far the most frequent variety of cataract in children and almost invariably affects both eyes. The embryonic nucleus of the lens is usually clear and is surrounded by concentric zones of lamellar opacity enveloped by a layer of clear cortex. The anatomical features of the cataract suggest that some hereditary defect or nutritional deficiency occurs during the later development of the lens and causes the subsequent abnormal development of the lens fibres. At the final stage of the disturbance, only individual lens fibres may be affected and this may result in a number of radial striae which run out from the superficial surface of the opacity. Lamellar cataract may remain stationary or the disturbance of the fibres may be so gross that the opacity may continue to increase.

Coronary and Punctate Cataract

These occur due to later and irregular defects of lens fibre growth in childhood or puberty. Since growth is now occurring only in the germinal equatorial portion of the lens epithelium, the defects tend to be confined to the equator of the lens. In the case of coronary cataract a wreath of club-shaped, pear-shaped or oval opacities can be seen in the peripheral cortex and are often obscured by the undilated pupil. Punctate cataract shows a number of small whitish specks again scattered in the anterior cortex, more numerous near the periphery of the lens. They are often semi-transparent and assume a bluish tinge (blue-dot cataract). They rarely interfere with vision and both forms often coexist.

Congenital Complete and Juvenile Complete Cataract

These forms of cataract are infrequent. The lens is uniformly white or bluish-white or it may have a pearly lustre. It is invariably soft and sometimes its contents are fluid and milky. These forms of cataract may occur in eyes that are otherwise healthy or may be complicated cataracts secondary to changes in the retina, choroid and optic nerve. One or both eyes may be affected. The congenital complete cataract is due to a disturbance of development or some intrauterine ocular inflammation. This type of cataract often occurs in cases where maternal rubella has developed during the first three months of pregnancy. In these cases the primary fibres of the lens are affected. They become degenerate and full of swollen droplets and vacuoles. The complete cataract of young people (juvenile) may be hereditary or arise without known cause. In some cases there is a history of convulsions.

Senile Cataract

Senile cataract is the commonest variety of cataract. It is an affection of advanced life, though occasionally it is seen as early as 40 years of age. Sometimes there appears to be a familial tendency to cataract, in which case the condition may occur at an earlier age in succeeding generations; this phenomenon is known as anticipation. As a rule both eyes are involved, but generally one is in advance of the other.

Classification

At present classification of senile cataract is based on morphology, as the relationship between the type of cataract and its cause is obscure. The main types of cataract seen are as follows:

Nuclear Cataract (Fig. 2)

In this type of cataract the nucleus gradually becomes opaque, the cortex being clear. At first it is more refractile and often a degree of myopia of the eye is induced. The cataract appears to involve the nucleus of the lens by forming fine, yellowish, dust-like opacities which are now considered to be aggregations of the crystalline protein of the lens, probably induced by an increased concentration of calcium ions.

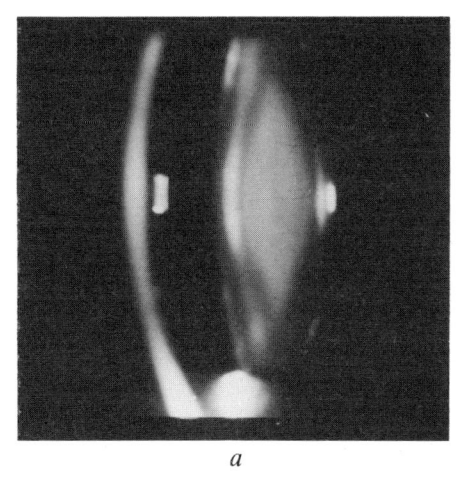

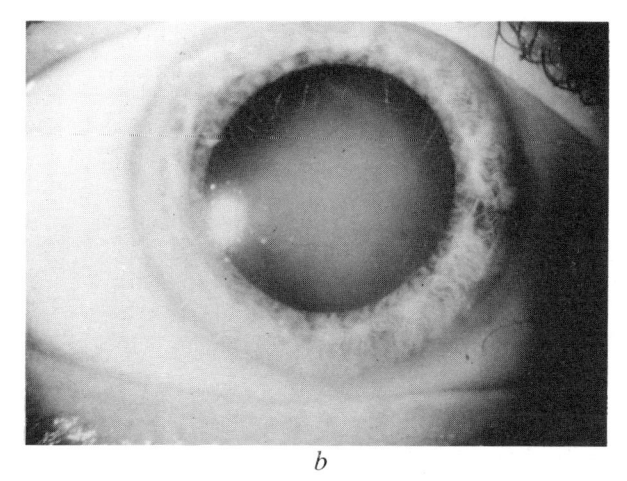

Fig. 2. Slit lamp appearance of early senile nuclear cataract: *a*, oblique illumination; *b*, reflex illumination.

Cortical Cataract (Fig. 3)

In this type of cataract the opacities develop in the cortical fibres and appear to be due to an accumulation of globules and vacuoles between adjacent fibres. The arrangement of these globular areas is characteristically wedge-shaped and since they are initially at the periphery of the lens little disturbance in vision results.

instances the defect in fibre arrangement occurs in the cortex at the posterior pole of the lens. Under these circumstances the effect on vision is severe since the nodal point of the optical system of the eye is situated here and all rays passing to the retina are affected. In these circumstances a good view of the fundus may still be retained while a disproportionate disturbance of vision occurs. At a later stage a much greater disorganization of the lens fibres occurs and the lens becomes totally opaque. From the time when the opacities, whether nuclear or cortical, are first seen to the stage when the cataract becomes totally

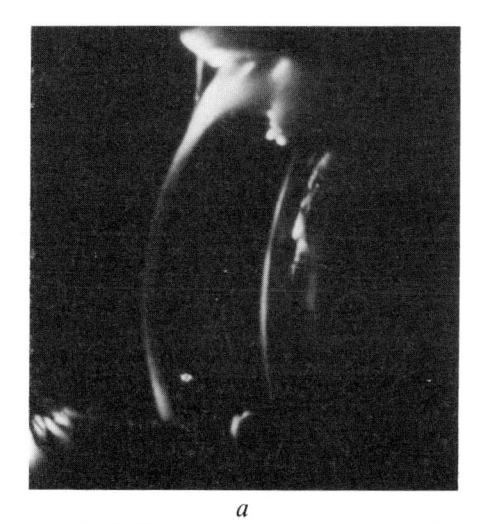

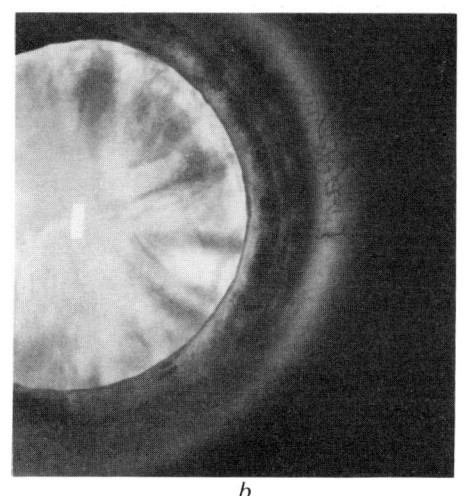

Fig. 3. Slit lamp appearance of early senile cortical cataract: *a*, oblique illumination; *b*, reflex illumination.

This initial defect has recently been shown to be due probably to excessive shear stresses developed between fibres at the onset of presbyopia. At a later stage the damaged lens fibres absorb water and lamellar separation of fibre layers by fluid occurs. This produces a series of water clefts in the lens. It has been shown to be associated with a change in the molecular structure of the lens capsule and this causes an increased permeability of the latter. In some

opaque and hypermature, the cataractous lens is considered to pass through four stages.

INCIPIENT CATARACT

It must be emphasized that, although incipient cataract occurs in two distinct forms, namely nuclear and cortical, over two-thirds of cases show both cortical and nuclear opacities as the cataract develops. Occasionally a frost-like deposit on the anterior lens capsule may occur independently or be associated with cataract. In such cases flakes of similar deposit are also found on the zonular fibres, the iris and the posterior surface of the cornea. It is thought that these deposits represent a degenerative product of the ciliary epithelium. Its recognition is important since it may cause obstruction of the trabecular meshwork and cause a form of glaucoma known as glaucoma capsulare.

of the lens. This occurs normally with ageing, but may be grossly exaggerated so that a dense black cataract may be formed without a gross disturbance in the structure of the lens. These cases present with a dense black pupil. No fundus features can be observed, but fair vision may occasionally be retained. A recent view is that ultraviolet light may degrade the tyrosin-containing proteins of the lens and produce a series of black pigments. A change in the lens apparently associated with infrared radia-

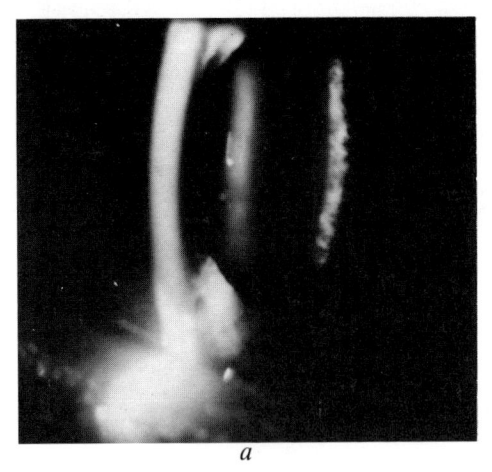

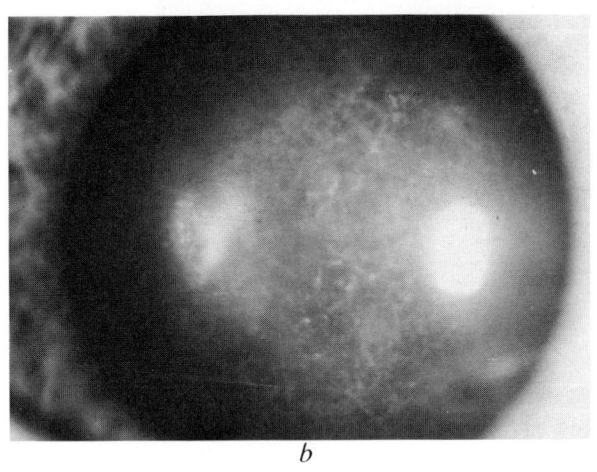

Fig. 4. Slit lamp appearances of posterior cortical cataract: *a*, oblique illumination; *b*, reflex illumination.

THE STAGE OF MATURATION

As the lens fibre system becomes more disorganized, the fibres break up and the lens imbibes increasing amounts of fluid. As a result it swells and the depth of the anterior chamber becomes reduced. The degree of involvement of the cortical fibres can be gauged by the depth of shadow cast by the iris when the eye is illuminated from the side. Occasionally the swelling is so gross that the angle of the anterior chamber becomes obstructed and a secondary glaucoma is induced.

MATURE STAGE

The lens loses some of its fluid, shrinks and becomes a dull grey or amber colour. The original cuneiform clefts may still be recognizable on the surface of this opaque lens.

THE HYPERMATURE STAGE

Further liquefaction of the cortical fibres may occur and with maceration of these fibres a pultaceous fluid is retained within the lens capsule while the more resistant nucleus falls to the bottom of the capsule and can be seen as a dense brown mass (Morgagnian cataract).

Unassociated with these structural changes in the lens fibres there may be an increased pigmentation

tion may likewise occur. Scroll-like exfoliations of the capsular lamellae may be seen, and this is known as true exfoliation of the lens capsule.

Complicated Cataract

Complicated cataract (*Fig.* 4) arises during the course of other eye diseases. The most frequently occurring ocular affections which lead to this type of cataract are uveitis, glaucoma, pigmentary degeneration or total separation of the retina and degenerative myopia. The opacification of the lens usually commences in the fibres adjacent to the capsule in the posterior cortex. A characteristic feature is the presence of polychromatic lustre of the opacity when viewed with the slit lamp. It has been shown recently that this striking display of colours is probably due to interference of light occasioned by the presence of condensed layers of lens fibre membranes in this region of the lens. The greyish, saucer-shaped opacity may remain for a prolonged period of time solely in the posterior region of the lens but ultimately the whole lens becomes opaque. The reason for the predilection of this portion of the lens in this type of cataract is unresolved at the moment, but it is important to establish a diagnosis of complicated cataract when the question of operation arises. The development of such a cataract indicates that there is probably gross disease of the eye usually involving the retina and consequently the improvement of sight by operation may be disappointing. Indeed many cases are unsuitable for operation.

Cataract associated with Systemic Disease

In the case of diabetes and galactosaemia, as mentioned previously, it is well established that the cause of the cataract is a metabolic defect. Cataract also occurs in other endocrine diseases, such as parathyroid dysfunction and thyrotoxicosis. A metabolic defect associated with calcium metabolism is postulated in these cases, but the cause of cataract in other conditions, such as myotonic dystrophy, atopic dermatitis and Down's syndrome, is uncertain. Cataract in diabetics takes two forms. In the young diabetic there may be a sudden development of flocculent, subcapsular deposits which render both lenses rapidly opaque. In early cases a control of the diabetic state may result in a considerable resolution of the cataract. In older patients with glycosuria the characteristic senile cataractous changes appear to occur more frequently and are more rapidly progressive than in non-diabetics.

SYMPTOMS AND SIGNS OF CATARACT

There is a gradual diminution in the acuteness of vision due to the disruption of the regular fibre structure of the lens. In addition, the patient complains of glare due to a progressive increase of light scatter within the lens substance. As the cataractous process may be only apparent in one sector of the lens, a different point of focus may be produced in this sector. As a result, the patient sometimes complains of monocular diplopia or even polyopia.

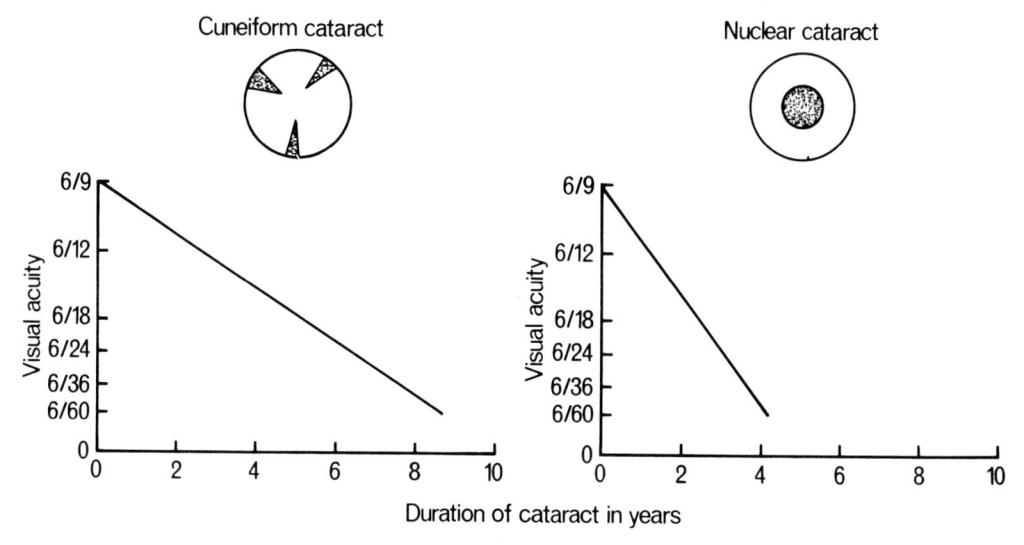

Fig. 5. Time of deterioration of cuneiform and nuclear cataract with an initial visual acuity due to the lens opacities of 6/9.

Examination of the patient by oblique illumination reveals a greyish or whitish opacification in the pupillary area, while with the ophthalmoscope the red fundal reflex outlines the opacities which show up as black areas. If the cataract is mature the pupillary response to light will still remain brisk provided the optic nerve and third nerves are functioning satisfactorily. Visual acuity gradually decreases with the increase of light scattering by the lens. This rate of decrease for nuclear and cortical cataract is shown in *Fig.* 5, the rate of decrease in visual acuity being about twice as great for nuclear as for cortical cataract.

FURTHER READING

1. Bellows J. G. *Cataract and Abnormalities of the Lens.* New York, Grune and Stratton, 1975.
2. Fisher R. F. Presbyopia and the changes with age in the human crystalline lens. *J. Physiol. (Lond.)* 1973; **228**, 765–78.
3. Fisher R. F. and Pettet B. The post-natal growth of the capsule of the human crystalline lens. *J. Anat. (Lond.)* 1972; **112**, 207.
4. Brown N. The change in shape and internal form of the lens of the eye on accommodation. *Exp. Eye Res.* 1973; **15**, 441.
5. Dickson D. H. and Crock G. W. Interlocking patterns on primate lens films. *Invest. Ophthalmol.* 1972; **11**, 809.

Cataract Surgery

Jack J. Kanski

GENERAL PRINCIPLES

Indications for Cataract Extraction

Cataract surgery is performed for one of three reasons.

1. Visual: this is by far the most common indication which varies according to the patient's needs.
2. Medical: occasionally, the presence of cataract is adversely affecting the health of the eye as a whole. This may be due to phacolytic glaucoma, angle closure glaucoma caused by an intumescent lens, or associated posterior segment disease such as diabetic retinopathy or retinal detachment, treatment of which is being hampered by the presence of lens opacities.
3. Cosmetic: very rarely, extraction of a mature cataract is undertaken to obtain a black pupil.

Choice of Technique

Currently the four most common methods of cataract extraction are: intracapsular, extracapsular, phacoemulsification and lensectomy. The choice of technique is governed by the following considerations.

1. The desire to implant a flexible loop posterior chamber lens.
2. Presence of the congenital capsulo-hyaloidal ligament.
3. Hardness of lens nucleus.
4. Fate of the fellow eye, particularly with respect to retinal detachment and aphakic cystoid macular oedema.
5. Associated ocular pathology such as chronic anterior uveitis, persistent hyperplastic primary vitreous and lens displacement.
6. Expense and availability of instrumentation.

Anatomy of the Limbus

The limbus is the transition between the cornea and sclera. It can be divided into an anterior (blue) zone and a posterior (white) zone, each measuring about 1 mm.[1] *Internally* the two zones meet at Schwalbe's line, which is the termination of Descemet's membrane. *Externally* the anterior limit of the limbus is identified as a ridge at which the conjunctiva terminates. The posterior (white) zone overlies the trabeculum and terminates over the scleral spur.[2]

Planning the Incision

Location

The three main locations are posterior limbal, mid-limbal and corneal.[3] The first requires a conjunctival flap, whereas the latter two do not. A corneal incision must be made larger than a posterior limbal incision to provide equivalent working space in the anterior chamber.

Size

An incision longer than necessary is preferable to one too short. For intracapsular extraction the incision should extend for at least five 'clock hours' (i.e. between 150° and 160°), whereas for extracapsular extraction a four clock hour (120°) incision is adequate.

Configuration

This can be either uniplanar or biplanar. Theoretically, the latter improves healing by increasing the surface area of the wound.

Suturing

The purpose of sutures is to keep the incision in apposition while healing is taking place. The sutures may be interrupted or continuous and they may be inserted before or after lens delivery. Continuous sutures may be single 'over-and-over' (i.e. starting at one end of the incision and terminating at the other), or 'shoelace' in which they cross over. Each suture must be placed radially (i.e. from the centre of the cornea) and it must enter and emerge the same distance (about 1 mm) on either side of the incision. When using 10/0 monofilament nylon, the needle should traverse the incision just above Descemet's membrane. In tying the knot, the first portion of the knot utilizes a triple throw, which is then followed by two single throws. The ends of the suture should be cut with a razor knife just on the knot. The knot should be buried within the incision to prevent postoperative irritation.

Superior Rectus (Bridle) Suture

This is necessary for intracapsular cataract extraction in order to keep the globe rotated slightly downwards so that the upper limbus is brought to the most superior position. Closed Lister's forceps are slid gently under the upper eyelid. About 10 mm behind the limbus they are opened and the superior rectus tendon is grasped firmly and transfixed with a black 4/0 silk suture. Spencer–Wells forceps are attached to the cut ends of the suture.

In extracapsular extraction it is also advantageous to have an inferior rectus suture in order to maintain the position of the eye during capsulotomy and aspiration.

INTRACAPSULAR EXTRACTION

Intracapsular extraction is still the most popular method of treating senile cataracts. It involves a large incision and removal of the entire lens with a cryoprobe.

Advantages

1. Since the operation has been performed for many years, the operative and postoperative problems are well known.[4]
2. Postoperative fundus examination is unhampered by an opaque posterior capsule.
3. Instrumentation is relatively inexpensive.

Disadvantages

1. Flexible loop posterior chamber lens implantation is impossible.
2. The operation cannot be performed with safety on patients under the age of 35 years in whom the capsulo-hyaloidal ligament is still intact. If intracapsular extraction is attempted in young individuals, the risk of vitreous loss is unacceptably high. Although the enzyme alpha-chymotrypsin (Zonulysin) dissolves the zonule in a young person, it has no effect on the congenital adhesion between the anterior hyaloid face and the posterior lens capsule.
3. Vitreous related anterior segment complications (e.g. pupil block, vitreous touch syndrome, and vitreous wick syndrome) are more common as compared with extracapsular extraction.[5]
4. The incidence of postoperative cystoid macular oedema and retinal detachment is higher, as compared with extracapsular extraction.

Surgical Technique

Groove (Plate XIIa)

The superior rectus tendon or episcleral tissue is grasped with toothed forceps. A vertical groove is made from 2.30 to 9.30 through two-thirds of corneal thickness.

Completion of Incision (Plate XIIb)

The anterior chamber is entered with a knife at the distal end of the groove and the incision extended for about 5 mm. An adequate opening is essential if inadvertent splitting of the stroma or peeling of Descemet's membrane with the scissors is to be avoided. The inner blade of the scissors is introduced into the anterior chamber. The scissors should be kept as flat as possible (i.e. parallel with the plane of the iris) to ensure correct horizontal bevelling of the second step of the incision. Cutting is commenced without withdrawing the scissors, taking great care not to damage the lens or iris.

Peripheral Iridectomy (Plate XIIc)

This is necessary to prevent postoperative pupil block by vitreous. A traction suture is inserted at 12 o'clock to enable the assistant to retract the cornea. The iris is grasped at 12 o'clock with fine toothed forceps. It is then gently tented upwards and cut cleanly with one cut. The scissors should be held circumferentially with the globe in order to obtain a circular opening in the iris. The patency of the iridectomy is checked with a spatula.

Pre-extraction Suture (Plate XIId)

A continuous 10/0 monofilament nylon suture is run from 2.30 to 12 o'clock. The knot is buried within the incision but the suture is left loose.

Zonulysis (Plate XIIe)

In patients under the age of 60 years, alpha-chymotrypsin is injected through the iridectomy into the posterior chamber.

Lens Delivery (Plate XIIf)

The bridle suture is released and the cryoprobe is tested for normal freezing and thawing. The surface of the lens is dried with a cellulose swab and the iris is retracted with a *dry* swab. The *warm* cryoprobe is gently applied to the superior pre-equatorial region of the lens and freezing is activated by the footswitch. After about 2 s the superior equator is elevated slightly to break the zonule at 12 o'clock and also to ensure that the expanding iceball does not freeze on to the iris. Freezing is continued until an adequate cryoadhesion is formed between the probe and the lens. Lens delivery is performed by a gentle side-to-side sliding motion. Once the iceball is outside the eye, the assistant releases the corneal traction suture. The pupil is constricted by injecting miochol into the anterior chamber. The pre-extraction suture is tightened and the remainder of the incision sutured.

Operative Complications

Freezing of Iris

Freezing of the iris is caused by inadequate retraction (by a wet swab), or undue delay in extracting the lens. If this occurs the surgeon should not panic but merely terminate freezing by releasing the foot-switch. For this reason it is best if freezing is entirely under the surgeon's control and the footswitch is not operated by an assistant or nurse.

Rupture of Capsule

An important sign of imminent capsular rupture is excessive tenting of the capsule. This is due to one of three main causes:

1. Inadequate adhesion between the cryoprobe and the lens due to the fact that extraction is being attempted prematurely.
2. An incision of inadequate size.
3. Strong zonular attachments. If alpha-chymotrypsin has been used then it may be necessary to strip the zonules mechanically with fine forceps.

In the event of capsular rupture, as much of the anterior capsule as possible should be removed with forceps and then the nucleus delivered and soft lens matter cleaned up as in a planned extracapsular extraction (*see below*).

Vitreous Loss

Vitreous loss is undesirable as it is associated with an increased incidence of postoperative complications such as vitreous touch syndrome, vitreous wick syndrome, updrawn pupil, vitreous incarceration in the wound, uveitis, retinal detachment and cystoid macular oedema.

PREVENTION

During surgery vitreous can either be pushed out of the eye by excessive external pressure on the globe or it can be pulled out by the surgeon when attempting to extract a lens with persistent capsulo-hyaloidal attachments. The latter can be prevented by not attempting intracapsular extraction on young patients.

An important clinical sign of impending vitreous loss caused by excessive external pressure is a forward movement of the entire iris–lens diaphragm with prolapse of the iris after the completion of the incision into the anterior chamber. The surgeon should ensure that any undue pressure on the globe by the superior rectus suture or lid speculum is released and that the patient is not performing the Valsalva manoeuvre. If this is ineffective, fluid vitreous should be aspirated through the iridectomy.

If vitreous loss occurred in the fellow eye, measures such as preoperative hyperosmotic agents and ocular massage aimed at reducing vitreous volume should be considered.

MANAGEMENT

The management of established vitreous loss is aimed at clearing the wound and anterior segment of formed vitreous. This can be performed with cellulose sponges and scissors, or a vitreous cutter.

Sponge anterior vitrectomy is easy but tedious and is associated with an increased risk of damage to the corneal endothelium. The apex of a triangular cellulose sponge is applied to the vitreous. The sponge is then gently retracted and the adherent vitreous cut off with scissors. This is repeated until the anterior chamber and incision are free of vitreous and the iris has assumed a concave configuration. Miochol and air are injected into the anterior chamber.

Automated anterior vitrectomy is quicker and safer. It can be performed with a relatively inexpensive vitreous cutter such as the Kaufman vitrector or by one of the more sophisticated and expensive instruments such as the ocutome or SITE. The cutting port is placed in the middle of the pupil, just behind the plane of the iris. A sufficient amount of vitreous is then excised to allow the iris to fall back to its normal position. It is extremely important to ensure that the wound is clear of formed vitreous by checking it with a sponge. Air should be injected into the anterior chamber.

Expulsive Haemorrhage

This extremely rare but very serious complication may occur during the operation or during the immediate postoperative period. It is characterized by spontaneous expulsion of lens followed by vitreous and, in severe cases, also the uvea and retina. Although treatment is unsatisfactory, the surgeon should attempt to drain subchoroidal blood by performing an immediate sclerotomy at the equator.

Postoperative Management

The operated eye should be examined on the first postoperative day and, if all is well, the patient is usually discharged after 3 days. Topical corticosteroids and mydriatics are used until the eye is quiet.

EXTRACAPSULAR EXTRACTION

The renewed interest in extracapsular surgery stems mainly from the increasing popularity of flexible loop posterior chamber intraocular implants. The operation involves excision of a large portion of the anterior capsule followed by expression of the nucleus and cortical clean-up.

Advantages

1. Flexible loop posterior chamber lens implantation is possible.
2. The operation is not influenced by the presence of congenital capsulo-hyaloidal adhesions and is therefore preferred in young adults.

3. Vitreous related complications (e.g. vitreous loss, pupil block, vitreous touch syndrome and vitreous wick syndrome) do not occur *providing the procedure is uneventful.*

4. The incidence of postoperative cystoid macular oedema and retinal detachment is less as compared with intracapsular surgery.

Disadvantages

1. The operation is more difficult to master and is more reliant on instrumentation than intracapsular extraction.

2. Postoperative opacification of the posterior capsule occurs in about 10–50 per cent of eyes after 3–5 years.

3. Extracapsular surgery is contraindicated in eyes with chronic anterior uveitis because the posterior capsule may act as a 'scaffold' along which inflammatory membranes proliferate during the postoperative period. This is undesirable as it not only interferes with vision but contraction of the membrane may detach the ciliary body and be responsible for the development of phthisis bulbi.

Surgical Technique

Groove

A vertical groove is made through two-thirds of the corneal thickness from 2 to 10 o'clock. A small opening is made into the anterior chamber with a Ziegler or Graefe knife.

Anterior Capsulectomy (Plate XIIIa)

This can be performed with an irrigating cystitome or a 22-gauge needle with its tip bent backwards to make a sharp little hook. The infusion is turned on and the cystitome, with its blade turned sideways to avoid catching the wound, is introduced into the anterior chamber.

In using the 'can-opener' technique, multiple small punctures are made in the anterior capsule, just inside the pupillary border, starting at 6 o'clock and extending for 360°.

The cystitome is then used to pull the loose capsule towards the incision, starting at 6 o'clock. The capsule is then pulled through the incision with angled McPherson's forceps and trimmed with scissors. The nucleus is then rocked back and forth with the cystitome in order to dislocate it from within the capsular bag – this manoeuvre is optional.

Completion of Incision

The entry into the anterior chamber is enlarged and the incision completed with scissors. Any large remnants of the anterior capsule are removed with angled McPherson's forceps.

Delivery of Nucleus (Plate XIIIb)

The two steps in delivering the nucleus are tilting and expression. The nucleus is tilted (inferior edge down and superior edge up) by pushing downwards at 6 o'clock just inside the limbus with a lens expressor or lens loop. Expression is performed by retracting the cornea and applying posterior pressure to the sclera at 12 o'clock and at the same time pushing from below. A spatula may be used to 'cartwheel' the nucleus completely from the anterior chamber.

Cortical Clean-up (Plate XIIIc)

Removal of cortical material can be performed with relatively inexpensive aspiration–infusion cannulae (i.e. McIntyre, Simcoe, Gills and Welch), or more sophisticated instruments such as the non-ultrasonic handpiece of the Kelman phacoemulsifier or a vitreous cutter such as the SITE. The procedure involves teasing and stripping cortical lens material from the equatorial regions and the posterior capsule and aspiration into the port. The aspiration port should point upwards or sideways and never posteriorly in order to avoid damage to the posterior capsule. If a vitreous cutter is used residual large fragments of the anterior capsule can be trimmed by activating the cutting mechanism. Cortical clean-up can be performed with an open anterior chamber or after the sutures have been tightened.

Polishing of Posterior Capsule

Small residual areas of cortex adherent to the posterior capsule can be removed by polishing the posterior capsule with a special sandblasted cannula (Kratz scratcher).

Operative Complications

Zonular Rupture during Anterior Capsulotomy

A weak zonule may rupture as the anterior capsule is being pulled by the cystitome. If this is recognized early and vitreous has not presented, the lens can be delivered intracapsularly.

Occasionally, the capsule may tear through the zonule if control over the tearing edge is lost. This may happen without the surgeon's knowledge and vitreous emerges as the nucleus is being expressed. This complication is best managed by excising residual soft lens matter, vitreous and capsule with a vitreous cutter.

Rupture of Posterior Capsule

The posterior capsule may be ruptured during cortical clean-up by aspirating it into the tip of the infusion–aspiration probe, or it may be ruptured during polishing. If vitreous has not herniated through the tear in the posterior capsule and all cortical lens matter has already been removed, then no further action is required. However, if significant amounts of residual cortex remain, the posterior capsule together with residual lens material should be excised with a vitreous cutter. If vitreous has prolapsed through the defect in the posterior capsule, it should be excised together with the posterior capsule and residual cortex.

Postoperative Management

This is similar to intracapsular extraction.

PHACOEMULSIFICATION

The Kelman phacoemulsifier consists of a hollow 1 mm titanium needle which is activated by an ultrasonic mechanism to vibrate at 40 000 times per second in a longitudinal axis.[6] This mechanical vibration transforms the nucleus into an emulsion which can then be aspirated from within the capsular bag and replaced with infusion fluid.

The Shock[7] and Girard[8] units (sometimes referred to as phacofragmentors) are similar apart from the fact that the vibrating needle is only capable of aspiration and a separate incision is required to accommodate an infusion system. The instrumentation is less sophisticated and consequently cheaper than the Kelman unit. It is particularly suitable for removal of opaque lenses in conjunction with pars plana vitrectomy.

Phacoemulsification has most of the advantages and disadvantages of an extracapsular procedure.[9] Additional pros and cons are:

Advantages

The small (3 mm) incision heals rapidly, with few wound-related complications. Refraction is stabilized early following surgery and astigmatism is low.

Disadvantages

1. The technique is relatively difficult to master and is associated with a high incidence of corneal complications, particularly by beginners.[10]
2. Lens material may become mixed with vitreous if the posterior capsule is accidentally damaged. Damage to the iris by the vibrating needle is also fairly common.
3. The procedure is unsuitable for cataracts with grade +3 or more of nuclear sclerosis. Other contraindications are a shallow anterior chamber, cornea guttata and poor pupillary dilatation.
4. The equipment is extremely expensive.

Surgical Technique

Incision

A corneal incision, 3·5 mm in size, is made with a Beaver blade or a diamond knife of suitable size.

Anterior capsulectomy

The technique is the same as in extracapsular extraction.

Emulsification of nucleus

The ultrasonic tip of the Kelman unit is introduced into the anterior chamber. Using between 1 and 2 min of ultrasonic time, the nucleus is emulsified and aspirated. Emulsification can be performed either in the anterior or posterior chamber. Posterior chamber emulsification is associated with an increased risk of damage to the iris and posterior capsule, whereas anterior chamber emulsification is associated with an increased risk of endothelial damage. When performing anterior chamber emulsification, the nucleus is engaged with the cystitome and prolapsed into the anterior chamber with vertical see-saw manoeuvres.

Cortical Clean-up

Residual cortex is removed using the non-ultrasonic handpiece. The pupil is miosed with miochol, a peripheral iridectomy is performed, and the incision sutured. If necessary, a posterior capsulotomy can be performed.

LENSECTOMY

In this procedure the cataract is excised with an automated aspiration-cutting device through a very small incision at the limbus or pars plana.

Advantages

1. The operation is not influenced by the presence of congenital capsulo-hyaloidal adhesions.
2. A combined anterior vitrectomy places the vitreous face posterior to the plane of the pupil. Problems associated with the presence of vitreous in the anterior chamber are therefore eliminated.
3. Excision of the posterior capsule with the cutter is particularly useful in the management of children with cataract in whom postoperative opacification is extremely common and can develop very quickly.[11,12]
4. Lensectomy is the operation of choice for secondary cataracts due to chronic anterior uveitis, especially in children.[13] If necessary the small pupil due to posterior synechiae can be enlarged with the cutter in order to obtain access to the lens. In addition, the total excision of the posterior capsule together with the anterior vitreous eliminates the 'scaffold' along which inflammatory membranes are able to proliferate postoperatively.
5. When performed through the pars plana, lensectomy can be combined with posterior vitrectomy for conditions such as persistent hyperplastic primary vitreous, vitreous haemorrhage and tractional retinal detachment.

6. Lensectomy is the operation of choice in the management of subluxation or dislocation of a soft cataract.

7. The procedure has all the advantages of a small incision closed intraocular microsurgical technique (i.e. control over the level of intraocular pressure during surgery, minimal distortion of the cornea, and virtual absence of surgically induced astigmatism).

Disadvantages

1. The technique is suitable only for soft cataracts in children and young adults. This is because the lens material must be capable of moulding into the small aspiration port prior to excision.

2. Because the procedure is relatively new, long term results and complications, particularly with respect to the incidence of retinal detachment, are lacking. It is possible that the routine violation of the vitreous in infants may result in late complications.

3. The technique is difficult to learn and requires careful case selection.

4. Instrumentation is expensive – the Kaufman vitrector is unsuitable for lensectomy.

Surgical Technique

Incision (Plate XIIId)

An oblique stab incision in clear cornea is made with a Graefe knife. The knife is passed across the anterior chamber and aimed at the centre of the pupil. The anterior capsule is punctured and the knife introduced into the lens nucleus taking care not to damage the posterior capsule. Alternatively, the incision can be made in the pars plicata or pars plana. If the knife does not penetrate the lens nucleus with ease an alternative method of extraction has to be used (i.e. extracapsular or phacofragmentation).

The knife is withdrawn and the soft lens matter is stirrred up with a Ziegler's knife in order to facilitate subsequent removal with the vitreous cutter.

Excision of Lens (Plate XIIIe)

The infusion system is turned on and the tip of the cutter is introduced into the anterior chamber. In eyes with extensive posterior synechiae and small pupils, the pupil can be enlarged with the cutter before proceeding to lens removal.

Soft lens material can be aspirated without activating the cutting mechanism, although harder pieces require both cutting and aspiration. While working within the capsular bag, the nucleus and cortex are removed, great care being taken not to aspirate iris or posterior capsule. When working under the iris the port should be directed sideways and it should never be directed posteriorly until all lens material has been removed. To visualize the tip of the cutter when peripheral lens material is being removed, the intraocular pressure is lowered by turning off the infusion system. The sclera is indented and peripheral lens matter brought into view. At all times the tip of the cutter should be kept well away from the vitreous base in order not to produce a retinal dialysis.

Posterior Capsulectomy and Anterior Vitrectomy

The aspiration port is positioned posteriorly and the posterior capsule together with a variable amount of anterior vitreous excised. In eyes with simple congenital cataracts, the cutter need not pass deeper than the plane of the posterior capsule. However, in eyes with secondary cataracts due to uveitis, a deeper anterior vitrectomy is required.

Anterior Capsulectomy

The anterior capsule is excised taking great care not to damage the iris sphincter. The infusion system is turned off and a small amount of fluid aspirated in order to lower the intraocular pressure prior to removal of the instrument from the eye. This prevents prolapse of intraocular contents through the incision. Air is injected into the anterior chamber and the incision sutured.

Operative Complications

Accidental Iridectomy

Iris can be aspirated and excised if an excessive suction pressure is used while working near the iris.

Posterior Dislocation of Lens Material

The three main causes of posterior dislocation of lens material are: (a) damage to the posterior capsule with the Graefe knife; (b) premature damage to the posterior capsule with the cutter during lens excision; and (c) attempted excision of a hard lens. Small lens fragments may be left alone, but large pieces, especially if composed of hard nucleus, must be removed as they may cause severe inflammation as well as endothelial damage as they usually float into the anterior chamber postoperatively.

Retinal Dialysis

This extremely serious complication is caused by traction on the peripheral retina by aspiration of solid vitreous in the region of the vitreous base.

POSTOPERATIVE COMPLICATIONS

The many complications of cataract extractions may occur during the immediate postoperative period, or days, weeks, or even years later.

Iris Prolapse

This is usually apparent during the immediate postoperative period (most frequently at the first dressing). The pupil is updrawn towards the site of the prolapse. Potential complications of untreated cases include elevation of intraocular pressure, chronic anterior uveitis, epithelial ingrowth, endophthalmitis and, rarely, sympathetic ophthalmitis.

Management

Management is surgical, except when the prolapse is extremely small and covered by conjunctiva. The incision is explored and small prolapses of less than 36 hours' duration may be reposited. If the prolapse is large and long standing it should be abscissed and the wound sutured. Anterior vitrectomy should be performed if vitreous gel is in the wound.

Hyphaema

Most hyphaemas resolve spontaneously and cause no problems. If the hyphaema is large and associated with elevation of intraocular pressure, there is a risk of bloodstaining of the cornea.

Management

The intraocular pressure should be lowered by carbonic anhydrase inhibitors or hyperosmotic agents. If evacuation is deemed necessary, it should be performed through a small limbal paracentesis. The blood can also be removed with an automated infusion–aspiration device.

Striate Keratopathy (Plate XIIIf)

A mild degree of corneal oedema with folds in Descemet's membrane is not infrequently seen during the immediate postoperative period. The most frequent causes are endothelial trauma by instruments, excessive irrigation, swabs, intraocular implants and excessive bending of the cornea.

Management

In most cases the oedema clears spontaneously. In persistent cases with irreversible endothelial damage penetrating keratoplasty may be necessary.

Wound Leak

This is usually evident within the first two postoperative days. The eye is soft and in severe cases the anterior chamber may be shallow or even absent. If the eye remains soft, choroidal detachments invariably develop, frequently accompanied by serous detachment of the ciliary body. The latter causes a reduction in aqueous secretion and exacerbates the ocular hypotony.

Management

The Seidel test should be performed to identify the site of leakage. A drop of fluorescein is instilled into the lower fornix and the patient is asked to blink so that the fluorescein is spread onto the upper part of the cornea. The incision is then examined with a slit lamp using blue light. At the site of leakage the fluorescein will become diluted by aqueous. Initial treatment of mild cases is with a pressure bandage in order to promote spontaneous healing. The pupil should be kept well dilated in order to relieve any associated pupil block. Topical corticosteroids should be used at least four times a day to prevent the formation of peripheral anterior synechiae. If these measures are ineffective after 5 days, the leak should be sutured, choroidal detachments drained, and air injected into the anterior chamber.

Pupil Block

Pupil block is caused by a relative or absolute blockage of the pupil and peripheral iridectomy by formed vitreous. The aqueous entrapped in the posterior chamber leads to iris bombé and shallowing of the anterior chamber. Unless the condition is effectively treated, secondary angle closure glaucoma is the end result. The shallow anterior chamber associated with pupil block usually develops later than that caused by a wound leak. The intraocular pressure is normal or elevated, depending on the severity of blockage.

Management

Management is initially with mydriatics, carbonic anhydrase inhibitors and, in severe cases, hyperosmotic agents. If maximal pupillary dilatation does not break the block, then laser iridotomy or surgical iridectomy should be performed. Very occasionally, anterior vitrectomy is necessary.[14]

Filtering Bleb

This relatively rare complication is due to defective would healing and leakage of aqueous under the conjunctiva.

Management

Surgical intervention is indicated in eyes with chronic irritation, hypotony and in patients wishing to wear a contact lens. Contact lens wear in the presence of a filtering bleb predisposes the eye to intraocular infection. Occasionally the bleb can be treated by cryotherapy. A retinal cryoprobe is used and the bleb is frozen by applying one application for 60 s and then two applications for 30 s. In most cases the only method of treatment is to identify and suture the fistula.

Residual Lens Material

Following inadequate extracapsular cataract extraction or lensectomy, lens material may remain in the eye. In general small pieces can be left as they usually absorb spontaneously. However, large pieces should be extracted as they may cause uveitis and secondary glaucoma. Large pieces of nuclear material may damage the corneal endothelium.

Management

Cortical lens material can be removed with an infusion–aspiration device or a vitreous cutter (not Kaufman vitrector) through a small limbal incision. Large pieces of hard nucleus require an 'open-sky' technique.

Opacification of Posterior Capsule

Following extracapsular extraction the posterior capsule may be opacified due to a residual posterior subcapsular plaque, or opacification may occur sometime following surgery due to proliferation of lens epithelium on to the posterior capsule at the site of apposition of the anterior capsular flap with the posterior capsule.[15]

Management

Management of relatively thin capsules is either by a simple surgical capsulotomy using a Zeigler knife or with the YAG laser. Tough membranes can be excised with a vitreous cutter.

Vitreous Touch Syndrome

This rare complication develops weeks or months following cataract extraction. It is caused by contact of formed vitreous with the corneal endothelium. This interferes with its ability to maintain the cornea in a relatively dehydrated state. Not all eyes with vitreocorneal touch develop corneal oedema. Factors thought to increase the risk of decompensation include the duration and extent of contact as well as the health of the endothelium at the time of contact.

Management

In a substantial number of eyes the corneal oedema may be reversed by anterior vitrectomy.[16] A significant relationship exists between the duration of corneal oedema and the clarity achieved post-operatively.

Vitreous Wick Syndrome

This rare complication is due to prolapse of a small bead of formed vitreous through an oversized suture site or a small wound dehiscence. The eye becomes irritable and a mucus plug is seen within the incision. When the plug is pulled with a cotton bud the pupil will peak.

Management

Management is by anterior vitrectomy, excision of externalized vitreous and closure of the fistula.[17]

Raised Intraocular Pressure

Raised intraocular pressure following cataract extraction may be due to many factors: pupil block, pre-existing primary open angle glaucoma, use of Zonulysin or Healonid, formation of peripheral anterior synechiae due to a flat anterior chamber, hyphaema, steroid induced and epithelial ingrowth.

Epithelial Ingrowth

This very rare but potentially disastrous complication is caused by ingrowth of conjunctival epithelium through a wound defect. The cells invade the anterior chamber and trabeculum, causing intractable glaucoma. Clinical features include persistent uveitis, and the appearance of a scalloped line on the upper corneal endothelium. The pupil is distorted and a fistula can be identified in about 50 per cent of cases.

Management

Management is by identification of the extent of iris involvement by argon laser photocoagulation (iris turns white). The fistula is closed and the involved area of the iris, together with the anterior vitreous, is excised using a vitreous cutter. The anterior chamber is then filled with air and the involved area of the cornea and ciliary body is treated by cryotherapy.[18]

Cystoid Macular Oedema (Irvine–Gass Syndrome)

Although macular oedema is probably the most common 'complication' of cataract extraction, occurring in about 50 per cent of cases, it is usually transient and seldom causes any significant problems.[19] A small minority of patients develop chronic cystoid macular oedema with diminished central vision 1–3 months following cataract extraction. The eye may be otherwise normal or it may show a mild anterior uveitis, vitritis, a ruptured anterior hyaloid and a slight ciliary flush. There is good evidence that this complication is more common following vitreous loss and less common following extracapsular extraction (with an intact capsule) as compared with intracapsular extraction.[20] Fluorescein angiography shows the typical 'flower-petal' pattern due to leakage of dye from the perifoveal capillaries.

Management

Most cases resolve spontaneously within 6 months and require no specific treatment. In those rare cases that do not resolve and cause a significant impairment of central vision, anterior vitrectomy may promote resolution.[21] At present the criteria for vitrectomy are: (*a*) angiographically and clinically significant cystoid macular oedema; (*b*) vitritis associated with adhesion of anteriorly herniated vitreous to the wound with distortion of the pupil; and (*c*) those cases in which the amount of vitreous inflammation and cystoid macular oedema has been lessened by a course of systemic or periocular corticosteroid administration. In these carefully selected cases, anterior vitrectomy has been reported not only to improve visual acuity, but also to decrease the amount of discomfort, which is also frequently seen in these patients.

Retinal Detachment

The incidence of retinal detachment following cataract extraction is about 2 per cent, about half developing within the first year.[22] Risk factors include vitreous loss, high myopia and predisposing vitreoretinal degenerations such as lattice. It appears that an intact posterior capsule protects the aphakic eye from detachment. When compared with phakic retinal detachments, those in aphakic eyes are characterized by the presence of small U-shaped tears just posterior to the vitreous base, early macular involvement, a lower surgical success rate and a greater tendency to bilaterality.

Endophthalmitis

Together with expulsive haemorrhage, endophthalmitis is the most dreaded complication of cataract surgery. It should be suspected in all eyes in which the signs of intraocular inflammation appear to be excessive considering the extent and complications of recent surgery. Severe pain and precipitous decrease in vision are two important symptoms. Most cases become evident within the second postoperative day with chemosis, lid oedema, hazy media and hypopyon.

Management

Successful treatment necessitates identification of the causative organisms, their elimination by the use of broad spectrum antibiotics, and control of host inflammatory response with corticosteroids.

Identification of organisms is done by vitreous aspiration. An aqueous tap is inadequate as it may be negative in the presence of positive vitreous cultures. The aspirate is inoculated on to blood agar, chocolate agar, thioglycolate, and Sabouraud's media, and incubated at 25 °C and 37 °C. Smears are examined by Giemsa and Gram's stain.

Treatment is initially with broad spectrum antibiotics until culture results are available. In order to obtain the highest possible level of antibiotics it is essential to utilize every possible route of administration. It is important to point out that the simultaneous administration of corticosteroids will not interfere with the control of the infection, provided the organisms are sensitive to the antibiotics.

Topical therapy consists of frequent (every 15–30 min) instillation of gentamicin and dexamethasone drops, as well as atropine 1 per cent drops q.i.d.

Subconjunctival therapy consists of gentamicin 40 mg, methicillin 150 mg, cephazolin 125 mg, and dexamethasone 4 mg or betamethasone 4 mg. The injections are given daily for about 5 days according to response.

Systemic therapy is with oral sodium fusidate 500 mg t.i.d. and cephazolin 1 gm q.i.d. In severe cases prednisolone 20 mg t.i.d. should be administered. Treatment should be continued for about 10 days.

VITRECTOMY

The most common causative organism isolated from intraocular contents in eyes with postoperative endophthalmitis is *Staphylococcus epidermidis*. It is an organism of low virulence which can be eliminated successfully by conventional therapy without resorting to intravitreal injections and therapeutic vitrectomy. However, at the initiation of therapy it is frequently impossible to be sure whether the infection is caused by *S. epidermidis* or by more virulent organisms (*S. aureus* and Gram-negative bacteria) which are extremely difficult to eliminate by conventional means alone. For this reason, some authorities advise an aggressive initial approach to all cases of endophthalmitis without waiting 36–48 hours for culture results. A pars plana vitrectomy is performed and antibiotics slowly injected into the vitreous cavity.[23] The recommended doses are gentamicin 100 μg, cephazolin 2·25 mg, each in 0·1 ml volume of saline (not bacteriostatic). Dexamethasone 400 μg can also be used.

Differential diagnosis

Fungal endophthalmitis usually occurs about 8 days after surgery and is characterized by a gradual onset, transient hypopyon and white 'fluff ball' opacities in the anterior vitreous.

Starch endophthalmitis is due to starch or talc particles introduced into the eye from the surgeon's gloves during surgery. It may cause a severe uveitis between the second and eighth days characterized by white focal infiltrates in the anterior vitreous and a diffuse vitreous haze.[24] The response to corticosteroid therapy is good.

REFERENCES

1. Kasner D. Important aspects of surgical anatomy of the limbus. In: Welsh R. C. and Welsh J. (ed.) *New Report on Cataract Surgery*. Miami, Miami Educational Press, 1977, pp. 106–7.
2. Ayoub M. I. and Said A. H. Relationship between limbal incisions and structures of the anterior chamber angle. *Br. J. Ophthalmol.* 1973; **57**, 722–4.
3. Pierce D. The cataract incision. *Trans Ophthalmol. Soc. UK* 1975; **95**, 192–3.
4. Meredith T. A. and Maumenee A. E. A review of 1000 cases of intracapsular extractions. *Ophthalmol. Surg.* 1979; **10**, 32–45.
5. Rich W. Advantages and disadvantages of different methods of senile cataract surgery. *Trans Ophthalmol. Soc. UK* 1982; **102**, 407–9.
6. Kelman C. D. Phacoemulsification and aspiration. *Am. J. Ophthalmol.* 1967; **64**, 23–35.
7. Shock J. P. Phacofragmentation and irrigation of cataracts. *Am. J. Ophthalmol.* 1972; **74**, 187–9.
8. Girard L. J., Nieves R. and Hawkins R. S. Ultrasonic fragmentation and associated surgical procedures. *Trans. Am. Acad. Ophthalmol. Otolaryngol.* 1976; **81**; op 432.
9. Kratz R. P. Phacoemulsification: Difficulties, complications, and management. *Trans. Am. Acad. Ophthalmol. Otolaryngol.* 1974; **78**, op 18.
10. Emery J. M. Phacoemulsification: Personal experience with first 40 cases. In: Emery J. M. and Paton D. (ed.) *Current Concepts in Cataract Surgery*. Selected Proceedings of the Third Biennial Cataract Surgical Congress. St Louis, Mo, Mosby, 1974.
11. Taylor D. S. I. Developments in the treatment of cataract. *Trans. Ophthalmol. Soc. UK* 1982; **102**, 441–53.
12. Taylor D. S. I. Choice of surgical technique in the management of congenital cataract. *Trans. Ophthalmol. Soc. UK* 1981; **101**, 114–17.
13. Kanski J. J. and Crick M. D. P. Lensectomy. *Trans Ophthalmol. Soc. UK* 1977; **97**, 52–7.
14. Kanski J. J. and Ramsay J. H. Vitrectomy techniques in the management of complications of aphakia. *Trans. Ophthalmol. Soc. UK* 1980; **100**, 216–18.
15. McDonnell P. J., Zarbin M. A. and Green W. R. Posterior capsule opacification in pseudophakic eyes. *Ophthalmology* 1983; **90**, 1548–53.
16. Wilkinson C. P. and Rowsey J. J. Closed vitrectomy for the vitreous touch syndrome. *Am. J. Ophthalmol.* 1980; **90**, 304–8.
17. Rice T. A. and Michels R. G. Current surgical management of the vitreous wick syndrome. *Am. J. Ophthalmol.* 1978; **85**, 656–61.
18. Stark W. J., Michels R. G., Maumenee A. E. et al. Surgical management of epithelial ingrowth. *Am. J. Ophthalmol.* 1978; **85**, 772–80.
19. Hitchings R. A., Chisholm I. H. and Bird A. C. Aphakic cystoid macular oedema: incidence and pathogenesis. *Invest. Ophthalmol.* 1975; **14**, 68–72.
20. Jaffe N. S., Clayman H. M. and Jaffe M. S. Cystoid macular oedema after intracapsular and extracapsular extraction with and without intraocular lenses. *Ophthalmology* 1982; **89**, 25–9.
21. Federman J. L., Annesley W. K., Sarin L. K. et al. Vitrectomy and cystoid macular oedema. *Ophthalmology* 1980; **87**, 622–8.
22. Scheie H. G., Morse P. H. and Aminlari A. Incidence of retinal detachment following cataract extraction. *Arch. Ophthalmol.* 1973; **89**, 293–5.
23. Diamond J. G. Intraocular management of endophthalmitis. *Arch. Ophthalmol.* 1981; **99**, 96–9.
24. Aronson S. B. Starch endophthalmitis. *Am. J. Ophthalmol.* 1972; **73**, 570–3.

Intraocular Lens Implantation

Arthur D. McG. Steele and Colin M. Kirkness

The use of intraocular implants has become so much a part of the management of cataract it is now inconceivable that a chapter could be written on the subject of cataract without including discussion of the role of implants for the correction of aphakia. The removal of one of the principal refractive components of the eye has marked optical consequences, in that most eyes are rendered highly hypermetropic. Correction of this hypermetropia to restore a useful level of visual acuity is the seat of difficulty. Three avenues are open: the use of glasses, of contact lenses, or of intraocular implants. The various advantages and disadvantages of these methods of correction are summarized in *Table* I.

Cataract glasses present to the wearer a completely foreign visual environment. High levels of magnification, restriction of field, movement of the field with opposite movements of the head, a large ring scotoma at the periphery of the corrected field and the distortion of images combine together to make this form of correction difficult or impossible to tolerate for many patients. Were this not so, the need for contact lenses and intraocular implants would never have arisen for the majority of patients. Most cataract patients are elderly or at least in late middle age and this is the period of life which renders them less able to cope with the demands of cataract glasses. For those in whom aphakia is uniocular, the wearing of correcting glasses is impossible and such patients must, if they are to retain binocular vision, use a contact lens or be fitted with an intraocular implant.

Most of the optical problems are resolved by contact lens wear. The difficulties here are not optical, despite the remaining theoretical aniseikonia, but are in fact practical problems connected with managing a contact lens: its insertion, its removal and its general care. Once again it is the elderly patient who is least able to cope with these practical difficulties. Younger patients may manage contact lenses sometimes for years but can then develop difficulties with tolerance and often to such a degree that contact lens wear has to be abandoned. Ten years ago, many surgeons

Table I. Advantages and disadvantages of three methods of correction of hypermetropia

Spectacles	*Contact lenses*	*Intraocular lenses*
Advantages		
Surgically safe	Remove most of serious optical disadvantages of spectacles	Effectively and theoretically most natural corrected vision
Simply dispensed	Suitable in unilateral aphakia	Immediate benefit
Alterable	Alterable	
	Relatively easily fitted in healthy eyes	
	Tolerated well by most aphakes	
Disadvantages		
Image magnification	Difficult to manipulate for elderly or infirm or if bilaterally aphakic	Demand higher degrees of surgical exposure
Ring scotoma	Require complicated cleaning routines	Increase rate of complications pre- and postoperatively
Aberration/distortion	Predispose to infection	
Spatial disorientation	Predispose to vascularization of cornea	
Field movement	Soft lens may reduce visual acuity	
Heavy	Late loss of tolerance	
Refraction/haloes/glare	Some patients temperamentally unsuited to contact lens wear	
Inappropriate for unilateral aphakia		
Thick and unsightly		

would have confined their use of intraocular lenses to elderly patients. Since then, however, the designs of implants have been refined and with a return to and refinement of the planned and complete extracapsular extraction techniques, the field of implants in younger patients has expanded.

HISTORY AND DEVELOPMENT

An intraocular implant was first used in the twentieth century by Harold Ridley at St Thomas's Hospital in 1949.[1] The implant was a simple lens with a rimmed edge which was inserted into the posterior chamber after extracapsular removal of the cataract. These lenses were large and heavy (106 mg) and many dislocated into the posterior segment, so that it became necessary to design a different form of lens. A number of patients implanted with Ridley's earlier posterior chamber lenses in the early 1950s, nevertheless, continue to live and see well to the present time.

The next versions of implants were all supported in the anterior chamber. Different lenses were developed by a number of surgeons around the world, including Ridley,[2] Choyce,[3] Sprampelli,[4] Epstein,[5] Barraquer.[6,7] In more recent times, similar lenses have been designed by Kelman and Tenant.[8,9]

Because many early anterior chamber lenses were associated with subsequent corneal decompensation, they failed to find wide favour. Binkhorst, working in Holland, designed a lens that could be supported by the stroma of the iris and this 'Binkhorst clip'[10] gave rise to another generation of implants during the late 1960s and early 1970s. These became very much more popular and the incidence of corneal problems appeared to recede. Lenses supported by the iris stroma, however, tended to be rather more mobile. Again, following Binkhorst's lead, the readoption of extracapsular techniques gave an implant extra stability provided by the retained posterior capsule.[11] The problems of pseudophakodonesis were much lessened. Extracapsular surgery was also associated with a lower incidence of complications in the posterior segment of the eye,[12-15] namely vitreous mobility, retinal detachment and cystoid macular oedema. A major problem, however, with all lenses supported by the iris stroma and using pupillary fixation, was the loss of pupillary mobility. Pupils cannot be widely dilated, either because of synechiae or for fear of giving rise to subluxation of the implant, and this difficulty prohibits adequate inspection of the fundus of the aphakic eye. In those patients who developed retinal detachment with a small fixed pupil and a pseudophakos anterior to the iris, the surgical management became particularly difficult. In addition, in the early days of the return of extracapsular surgery, it was suggested that incomplete removal of the cortex was desirable in order to promote the development of fibrous adhesions between the supporting struts of the implant and the posterior surface of the iris. This retained cortical material increased the likelihood of capsular opacification and made inspection of the peripheral retina even more difficult or impossible.

The next stage was initiated by John Pearce, in England,[16] with his development of a small rigid lens for use entirely within the posterior chamber. These early lenses were secured in the capsular bag below and were sutured to the iris stroma above. Their safe insertion demanded a high degree of surgical skill. The role of the posterior chamber lens was later expanded by Shearing with the development of his style of posterior chamber lens, which has now given rise to a whole new generation of lenses with flexible haptics, all supported by the structures of the posterior chamber behind the iris.[8,17] These lenses can be supported either in the capsular bag or in the ciliary sulcus and leave the pupil free to dilate and constrict with perfect safety. The clean capsule which can be left after a modern microsurgical technique for management of the lens cortex should allow a perfectly clear view of peripheral fundal detail.

Classification of Implants in Current Use

There is now such an enormous variety of implants available that a complete discussion of all is beyond the scope of this text.[8] The authors have selected a few from the wide range and these are classified below into three principal varieties:
1. Anterior chamber lenses.
2. Iris supported lenses.
3. Posterior chamber lenses.

Anterior Chamber Lenses

Such lenses are supported within the eye in the angle of the anterior chamber with the feet of these implants behind the scleral spur. It is claimed that they are the easiest type to insert, following either extracapsular or intracapsular removal of the lens. The ease of insertion of such implants, however, is counterbalanced by a number of disadvantages. First, the anterior chamber is not expandable and the size of the implant needs to be most carefully gauged in order to render it stable.[18] An implant that is too short will be mobile within the anterior chamber and may cause damage to the corneal endothelium. Micromovements of the feet of anterior chamber lenses also promote angle neovascularization and can give rise to a condition similar to the 'UGH' syndrome (see p. 300).

An implant that is too long will stretch the anterior uveal tract, damaging the insertion of the iris and ciliary body, leading to an eye being persistently painful and tender to touch. It may also damage the trabecular meshwork and give rise to secondary glaucoma.[19]

Secondly, the anterior chamber is formed anteriorly by the cornea and any anterior chamber lens is therefore placed extremely close to the precious cells of the endothelium and for many surgeons this degree of proximity continues to be unacceptable. The early anterior chamber lens as developed by Barraquer had flexible supports and many gave rise to late corneal decompensation.[20] More recently, a new group of lenses has been introduced which appears to be very little different from those early lenses and already it would seem that such flexible anterior chamber lenses can still be very hazardous.[21]

Posterior Chamber Lenses

Such lenses can only be used following extracapsular surgery. The advantage of the lens is that it is placed within the eye in the plane from which the original lens has been removed. The lenses are stable and cannot dislocate into the anterior chamber or backwards into the vitreous providing the posterior capsule and supporting zonular ligament remain intact.

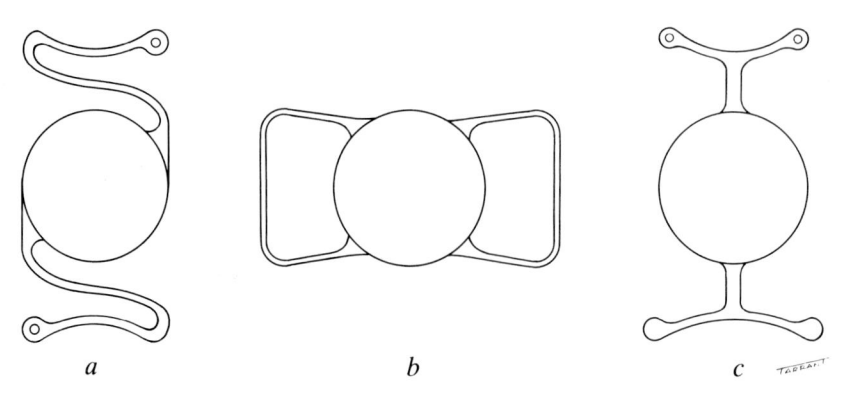

Fig. 1. Examples of anterior chamber lenses. *a*, The Kelman multiflex (P-CQ lathe cut). There is a four point fixation but good vaulting characteristics, semi-flexible. *b*, Rectangular looped Leiske type (available either lathe cut or injection moulded in PMMA / P-CQ). The loops are flexible. Closed loops have inferior vaulting characteristics. *c*, Hessberg lens is similar to the Tennant anchor but with point fixation as opposed to arcuate. (Lathe cut PMMA or P-CQ.) The lens is semiflexible. For the Choyce Mk VIII lens, *see Plate* XIV*a*.

Apart from the ease of insertion, the other great advantage of the anterior chamber lens is that the pupil may be freely dilated behind it and that lenses can be inserted into eyes that have loss of iris substance because the stability of the lens is not dependent on the presence of iris.[22] Conversely there are many recent reports which show that satisfactory anterior chamber lenses are often associated with progressive oval distortion of the pupil.[23] (*Fig.* 1, *Plate* XIV*a*).

Iris Supported Lenses

These have the advantage and initial attraction that they are placed further back in the eye, and in the light of subsequent developments, this would appear to be the only advantage. The principal disadvantage of iris supported lenses is that many of them will not allow the free dilatation of the pupil as they are dependent on sphincter tone or even synechiae for stability.

One variety of iris supported lens which has found greater favour is the small group of lenses (e.g. Severin, Boberg-Ans or Little Arnott[8]) in which the bulk of the lens is placed in the posterior chamber and only some anterior supporting struts remain anterior to the pupil. These lenses have less pseudophakodonesis than other purely iris supported lenses and they have a greater margin for corneal safety (*Fig.* 2, *Plate* XIV*b,c*).

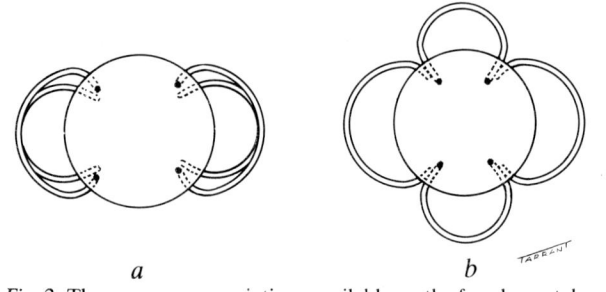

Fig. 2. There are many variations available on the four loop style. The loops are usually polypropylene occasionally nylon with the optic PMMA or P-CQ. Two loops lie anterior to the iris, two posterior. After intracapsular extraction iris fixation suture is mandatory. these implants are now seldom used. *a*, Binkhorst four loop; *b*, Maltese Cross.

The lens placed entirely within the posterior chamber does not depend on the iris sphincter for support and thus the pupil can be widely dilated with impunity to allow a clear view of the peripheral retina.

The principal stated objection to extracapsular surgical treatment, whether using posterior chamber lenses or not, is that a proportion of patients require subsequent treatment for late thickening of the posterior capsule. Figures for the incidence of this complication vary widely and will be discussed in the section on complications.[24]

It is of interest that in 1982 the use of intraocular implants in the United States of America showed that 32 per cent used were purely supported in the anterior chamber and only 2 per cent of those inserted were supported by the pupil and iris stroma alone, the remainder were inserted into the posterior chamber.[25,26] It is the authors' prediction that these proportions will continue to alter in favour of the insertion of posterior chamber lenses with a gradual decline in the popularity of those lenses supported in the anterior chamber. (*Fig. 3, Plate* XIVd).

BIOMETRY

Intraocular implants are manufactured in a wide variety of dioptric power. Clinical guesswork as to the strength of an implant required by an individual patient is now not considered to be good practice and surgery should be preceded by biometry. This includes the measurement of the axial length of the eye from the anterior corneal to the anterior retinal surface together with the measurement of corneal curvature in the vicinity of the visual axis. With these two measurements known, a wide variety of formulae are available to the surgeon for the calculation of the power of the implant required and we quote one as an example, being the most suitable in our practice – the Retzlaff regression formula.[27] These calculations all assume a standard depth of the anterior chamber in the aphakic eye. This assumption, together with the range of human errors in the recording of necessary measurements, can give rise to imperfect final results, but no patient should have a refractive error greater than three dioptres away from the desired level. Most authorities are agreed that aphakic patients are best left very slightly myopic so that they are able to obtain the best use of their acuity at different ranges.

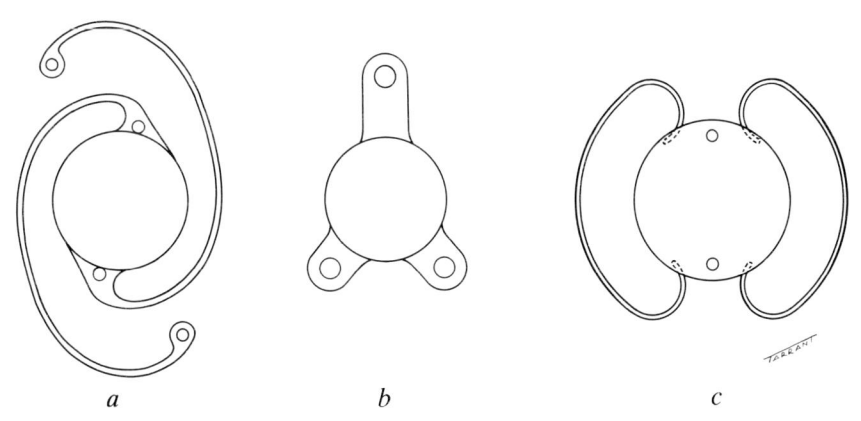

Fig. 3. a, The Arnott type (all P-CQ, lathe cut). Because P-CQ is less flexible the loops need to be longer to allow for compressibility. The lens is uniplanar and ciliary sulcus fixated. All P-CQ has the advantage of lack of biodegradability over polypropylene at the expense of increased fragility. *b,* Pearce tripod. (Solid P-CQ usually.) The smaller inferior feet are capsule fixated, but the upper haptic needs to be iris sutured for stability. *c,* Anis type lens has smaller closed loops (all P-CQ, lathe cut), and is fixated within the capsular bag. Although aesthetically and theoretically appealing, the lens may lack stability owing to difficulty of correctly locating the second loop and ensuring long term placement.

SURGICAL CONSIDERATIONS

Surgical techniques for the management of the cataract are of paramount importance to the role of the implant. Surgeons wishing to use implants are therefore advised to familiarize themselves with the necessary skills for satisfactory cataract management and these have already been dealt with in another part of this book. In this section we will confine discussion to the management of the implant alone.

Anterior Chamber Lens Insertion

These lenses may be inserted into the anterior chamber after either extra- or intracapsular cataract surgery. When using rigid or semi-flexible lenses (e.g. Choyce, Tennant, Kelman), it is necessary to make a careful assessment of the dimensions of the anterior chamber so as to select a lens of the right length. This is customarily defined as 'white to white + 1 mm'. Some authorities believe that this surface measurement is insufficiently accurate and leads to misfits.[18] An alternative, therefore, is to use a measuring dipstick,[28] which can be passed through the surgical wound across the anterior chamber until it comes to rest in the opposite anterior chamber angle. The width of the anterior chamber can therefore be read directly off the dipstick and a lens of suitable length selected accordingly. The proper fitting of the implant is crucial to its success. On introduction, the lens is passed through the wound and across the anterior chamber in the plane of the iris. A common complication at this point is a tendency for the iris on the opposite side of the anterior chamber to become tucked or folded by the leading feet, or edge of the implant. This can be overcome by deepening the anterior chamber prior to the insertion of the implant either by using air or one of the visco-elastic materials available. The use of such techniques has the added advantage of giving extra protection to the posterior corneal surface. When the feet, or the edge of the implant, have engaged the angle of the anterior chamber opposite, the feet at the edge of the wound should still be slightly outside the eye and each foot needs to be carefully placed into the anterior chamber by retracting the posterior edge of the scleral wound. This is the time to check to see whether the implant appears to be correctly sized. Any noticeable degree of implant mobility indicates that the lens is too short and needs to be immediately replaced by a longer lens. Any apparent distortion of the globe by too long an implant should also indicate lens replacement.

Anterior chamber lenses are available which, instead of being rigid or very slightly flexible, are intended to be supported by completely flexible supports. The advantage of such a design is that one does not need a range of implant sizes for every lens power. Such lenses are theoretically attractive, but there is a danger that their flexibility will allow movement both of the lens in the anterior chamber anteroposteriorly and also movement of the flexible feet themselves, giving rise to persistent irritation of the chamber angle. Having said that, however, their mode of insertion is very similar to that described above.

Iris Supported Lenses

One of the major disadvantages of all forms of iris supported lenses is that they are necessarily deeper anteroposteriorly than either anterior or posterior chamber lenses, which are usually uniplanar. The greater thickness of the iris supported lenses is required to allow for both anterior and posterior iris support and the disadvantage is that their insertion means the wound needs to be more widely opened to allow insertion. This in turn is more likely to be associated with damage to the posterior surface of the cornea either by direct touch between the corneal endothelium and the lens surface, or by excessive corneal bending or by stripping of Descemet's membrane at the edge of the wound during the insertion manoeuvre. The use of these lenses therefore requires the greatest surgical care in order to protect the cornea. Here again, insertion is made easier by deepening the anterior chamber either with air alone or with the use of visco-elastic substance such as sodium hyaluronate or methylcellulose. The lens is passed through the wound and is usually grasped by implant forceps either by the lens haptic or by one of the anterior supporting loops. The lens is passed across the anterior chamber until the inferior posterior loop engages the edge of the pupil.

Subsequent manoeuvres necessary to engage the remaining posterior loop will depend upon the degree of mydriasis. If the pupil is still moderately dilated at this stage, it may be possible to displace the lens inferiorly in order to engage the superior posterior loop behind the edge of the iris without releasing the lens. Where a smaller pupil is present, however, it is probably necessary to engage the posterior superior loop by a two-handed technique. The lens is depressed with a spatula held in one hand while the iris is lifted over the edge of the posterior superior loop with the other. These techniques will allow the safe insertion of all varieties of iris supported lenses. It is important to remember that where iris supported lenses are being used following either intracapsular extraction or failed extracapsular extraction such that an intact posterior capsule has not been retained, then these lenses must be sutured to the iris above (and sometimes also below). These iris sutures should be of 10/0 polypropylene as this is the suture material least likely to undergo early biodegradation[29,30] (see Fig. 6). These sutures must not be overtightened to allow the loop of the implant to pass through the suture during dilatation and constriction of the pupil. An overtight suture will give rise to upward displacement of the implant during dilatation of the pupil with increased risk of intermittent corneal touch and inferior loop dislocation. The ends of the suture must be shortened so as to ensure that no touch can occur between the suture and the posterior corneal surface. Failure to suture such lenses can lead to late total posterior dislocation of the implant into the vitreous cavity.

Posterior Chamber Lenses

Like anterior chamber styles these lenses are uniplanar, comprising the optic and usually two supporting flexible loops. Opinions continue to differ as to whether these lenses are best supported in the ciliary sulcus or in the capsular bag itself. Ensuring good capsular bag support is certainly technically more demanding. The advantages and disadvantages of the two modes of support are as yet entirely theoretical. The precise site in the posterior chamber where a supporting loop comes to rest after implant insertion cannot be precisely determined unless the eye is subsequently examined post mortem.[31,32] Early styles of posterior chamber lenses in which the supporting loops were more rigid have been examined post mortem and some were found to have eroded uveal tissue to a varying degree, though none had penetrated major blood vessels. It is improbable that the more flexible loops available on most lens styles now, could significantly erode the ciliary body. Loops for 'in the bag fixation' are, of course, shorter than those used for ciliary sulcus fixation and it is important to ensure that the lens style chosen is appropriate for the particular surgical technique.

The techniques for most styles of posterior lenses are very similar. The principle is to insert the lens in such a way that contact with the posterior surface of the cornea is avoided. The anterior chamber may be maintained either with air, or with one of the viscoelastic materials currently available or using a combination of both whereby a bubble of air is held in place in the anterior chamber by a dam of viscoelastic fluid. The chosen lens, after careful inspection, is grasped with a pair of implant forceps by the lens body and it is then introduced through the wound across the upper part of the anterior chamber until the lower loop is level with the lower margin of the iris. With a slight depressing pressure the lower loop is then passed under the iris and insertion of the lens is continued until the lens occupies the central pupillary area. At this point the lens forceps release the lens and are withdrawn from the anterior chamber. The upper loop may be inserted behind the iris in one of two ways. It is useful to be able to use both, as different eyes lend themselves to different management (*Fig. 4*).

Forceps Placement

The extreme tip of the loop is grasped with the implant forceps and is carried into the anterior chamber and anterior to the optic until the elbow of the loop has passed the pupillary margin. With a slight pronation movement, the elbow of the haptic is then tipped downwards so that it will pass beneath the upper margin of the iris. The tip of the upper loop can then be released and it will spring into the region of the ciliary sulcus. Following this manoeuvre, the lens should then be rotated so that the two posterior loops lie horizontally rather than vertically. This rotation is easily accomplished either by a small hook or by using a bent 27 gauge needle, to engage one of the holes drilled in the lens. A lens placed with its supporting loops aligned horizontally is less likely to become de-centred vertically at a later date.

Dialling

The alternative method for inserting the upper loop after removal of the implant forceps from their hold on the lens is to engage one of the holes in the lens with a small hook or with the tip of a bent needle and then to rotate the lens so as to dial the remaining loop into the posterior chamber. Following the successful dialling procedure, the two posterior loops are then aligned horizontally, as described above.

After any implant insertion technique the cataract wound is closed either with continuous or interrupted sutures taking care to seal the anterior chamber securely without causing suture induced astigmatism.

SECONDARY LENS IMPLANTATION

Any patient who has previously undergone cataract surgery may at some time in the future require the consideration of secondary insertion of an intraocular implant.[33] This may be necessary for a number of reasons, but usually is for spectacle or contact lens intolerance. All secondary implantation techniques carry further surgical risk to the eye. These risks apply both to the anterior segment and to the posterior segment and will be specifically dealt with in the section on complications.

It is important for any surgeon considering the insertion of an implant as a secondary procedure to

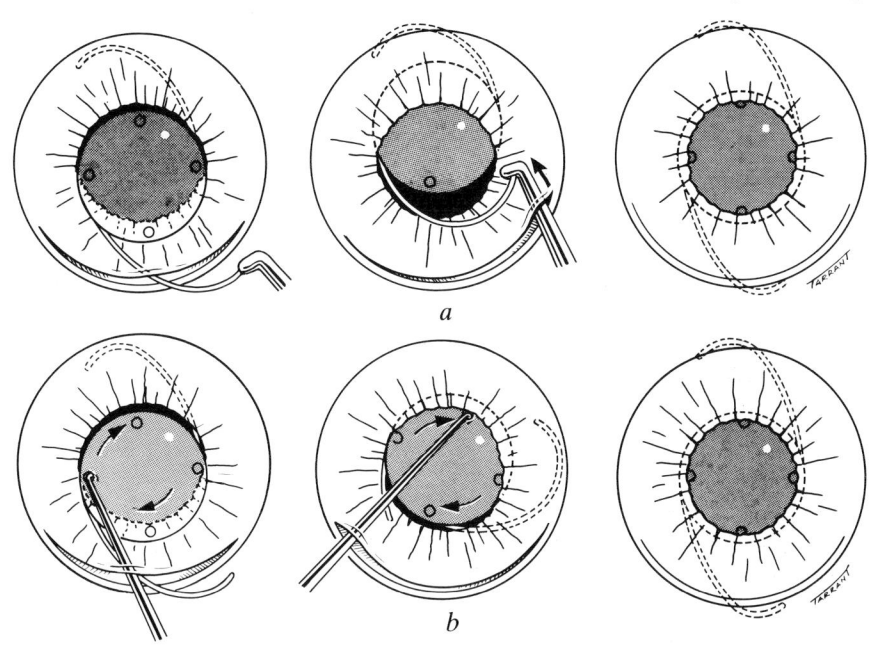

Fig. 4. Techniques for insertion of second loop (Sinskey-type lens): *a*, by direct manipulation with loop forceps; *b*, by dialling. In both cases the lens is subsequently dialled around so that the loops lie horizontally.

satisfy himself that the corneal endothelium has not already suffered severe damage from previous surgical manoeuvres. It will also be apparent that secondary implantation is necessarily safer when the patient has an intact posterior capsule or a capsule which has only a small central capsulotomy through which there is no significant vitreous herniation. Under these circumstances the vitreous can be easily controlled and a posterior chamber lens can be inserted with relative ease. Preliminary separation of any synechiae through a paracentesis may be required. During insertion of the implant lens the anterior chamber can be satisfactorily controlled with air or with visco-elastic fluid.

Where the preceding cataract surgery has involved the removal of the posterior capsule, secondary implantation is necessarily more hazardous, there being considerably greater risk of vitreous loss or disturbance and a higher incidence of cystoid macular oedema. If after consideration of these risks surgery is still indicated, the surgeon must then decide whether he will use an anterior chamber or a pupil supported lens. In both cases, it is advisable to control the vitreous face with air or a visco-elastic fluid during the insertion of the implant. Where there is considerable spillage of vitreous into the anterior chamber the risks of secondary detachment and cystoid macular oedema are significantly greater. Insertion of an implant in these cases is necessarily preceded by an anterior vitrectomy and this should always be performed using one of the vitreous infusion suction cutting instruments and a closed chamber technique.

THE TRIPLE PROCEDURE

The occurrence of cataract is occasionally associated with a considerable degree of corneal opacity. The commonest cause for this combination is Fuch's endothelial dystrophy causing endothelial decompensation associated with cataract. Most corneal surgeons are agreed that the best way of handling this problem is by a combined procedure. After removal of the corneal disc from the recipient, an extracapsular cataract extraction is performed using an open sky technique. Following careful aspiration of all the cortical material, a posterior chamber lens can then be inserted between the intact posterior capsule and the posterior iris surface. The donor corneal button can then be sutured into position, care being taken to keep a layer of visco-elastic fluid between the posterior donor surface and the anterior surface of the posterior chamber implant. After insertion of the implant the pupil can be constricted with acetylcholine and this reduction of the pupil size will further serve to protect the donor button.

INDICATIONS FOR IMPLANT INSERTION

Opinions vary a great deal about this and, therefore, the authors take it upon themselves to state their own views:

1. All patients who have cataract at, or above, the age of 60 years should be considered as candidates for intraocular lens insertion.
2. Younger patients should be considered as candidates for implant insertion if:
   (a) the patient is unwilling to consider the use of a contact lens;
   (b) contact lens intolerance is already established;
   (c) it is the opinion of the surgeon that the patient will never be able to manage a contact lens either by virtue of physical or psychological inaptitude.

It should always be remembered at this stage that the patient, although fit at the time of surgery, may become infirm in the future.

It is the opinion of the authors that, providing these conditions apply, there is no absolute lower age limit for the insertion of an intraocular implant, other than in infancy. (The subject of the implantation of children is a complicated one and is beyond the scope of this text.) It will be seen that the indications for the use of an intraocular implant apply whether the cataract is uniocular or binocular.

Contraindications

1. An implant should never be used in any patient who expresses the slightest reservation about having one.
2. An implant should not be inserted if previous cataract surgery on the other eye has been associated with implant complications, unless the surgeon can completely satisfy himself that the previous complications are of no relevance to the second eye. This would be unusual.
3. An implant should not be inserted into the anterior segment of an eye which is significantly diseased by virtue of:
   (a) previous uveitis;
   (b) uncontrolled glaucoma;
   (c) severe endothelial disease;
   (d) anterior segment neovascularization, and this will include most diabetics who are dependent on insulin for the control of their metabolic state, many of whom will already have significant retinal ischaemia.

It is worth noting that there are no posterior segment ocular contraindications to the use of an intraocular implant.[34] Specifically, when a patient is already known to suffer from macular dystrophy or retinitis pigmentosa, cataract surgery should usually be associated with an intraocular lens so that the patient will obtain maximum benefit from potential acuity and field of vision.

COMPLICATIONS AND THEIR MANAGEMENT

Peroperative Complications

The management of peroperative complications of the cataract technique itself is not included in this section. There are few peroperative complications that can occur during insertion of the implant, but they would include the following.

Difficulty in Maintaining the Anterior Chamber

This is particularly common in the younger patient and in high myopes who have less corneo-scleral rigidity than the usual cataract patient. A collapsing anterior chamber is dangerous when inserting an intraocular implant because of the greatly increased risk of contact between the posterior corneal surface and the structure of the implant. The anterior chamber should be artificially maintained with the use of a visco-elastic fluid. Sodium hyaluronate or 2 per cent methylcellulose have both been found satisfactory by the authors for this purpose.

Anterior Chamber Haemorrhage

This can occur either spontaneously from an iris vessel or more often from an iridectomy. The haemorrhage should be tamponaded by filling the anterior chamber with air. The haemorrhage will then stop within a few moments and the blood clot can then be satisfactorily removed by irrigation and aspiration.

Rupture of the Posterior Capsule

This is a complication that may occur either during the extracapsular technique or even after the insertion of an implant. If the capsular rupture is associated with the displacement of vitreous into the anterior chamber, an anterior vitrectomy will be required and this is usually best managed with a vitreous infusion suction cutting instrument and a closed chamber technique. Repeated corneal bending, which is so damaging to the endothelium, and repeated touching of the iris surface, which is always associated with a severe postoperative uveitis, may thus be avoided. Furthermore, excessive traction on the vitreous and the risk of retinal tears can also be reduced. Whether or not the successful anterior vitrectomy can then be followed by the use of an intraocular implant would depend upon how much the surgeon feels the patient needs the implant. The size and position of the capsular rupture will also influence the decision as to which type of implant to use. Due consideration should also be given to the complications of vitrectomy and the surgeon's subsequent ability to manage them in the presence of a particular intraocular lens. A small capsular tear, which leaves most of the capsule secure can still be used to support a posterior chamber implant. A large capsular rent, however, which may well involve the supporting zonule, is an unreliable support for an intraocular implant in the posterior chamber and the surgeon should then decide whether he is prepared to use a different variety of implant supported either in the anterior chamber or in the pupillary aperture. Such a lens would, of course, be inserted through a bubble of air to ensure total absence of vitreous from the anterior chamber during the insertion manoeuvre.

The Small Pupil

The small pupil may present considerable problems and there are instances where the pupil cannot be adequately dilated preoperatively. The surgeon may then find it necessary to divide the sphincter in order to manage the cataract, either by an intracapsular or an extracapsular technique. When removal of the cataract is to be followed by insertion of either an anterior chamber or a posterior intraocular lens, repair of the sphincter is not mandatory. In cases where division of the sphincter may lead to problems with either cosmesis or photophobia, repair of the sphincter with 10/0 polypropylene sutures can be a kindness, though by no means a medical necessity. Where it is intended by the surgeon to insert a pupil supported lens, repair of the divided sphincter is essential prior to implant insertion.

Postoperative Complications

Corneal Decompensation

This may occur early and may subside spontaneously. This variety of corneal decompensation is often called striate keratopathy, but nevertheless indicates peroperative endothelial trauma. Spontaneous recovery, very much to be hoped for, will always be associated with a significant depletion of the endothelial cell population. Corneal decompensation occurring as a late complication of cataract surgery with or without insertion of an implant will require treatment if the patient suffers persistent corneal discomfort and is unrelieved by the fitting of a soft contact lens, or if the corneal oedema causes such a significant visual impairment that the patient is incapacitated. In either case the treatment is penetrating keratoplasty. Whether this penetrating keratoplasty should be associated with the removal of an intraocular implant will depend entirely on whether the implant can be held responsible for the endothelial destruction.[35] Clearly this would not apply to an eye containing a posterior chamber lens and corneal decompensation is unusual in such eyes anyway. Where corneal decompensation occurs in an eye containing an anterior chamber lens, it would be difficult to support the view that the lens was not directly related to the corneal decompensation. This is true also for most iris supported lenses where the bulk of the implant, and possibly anterior supported loops, are in front of the iris. These lenses often have an unsatisfactory degree of pseudophakodonesis which may permit intermittent endothelial touch.

Anterior Chamber Angle Irritation

This can be caused by anterior chamber supported lenses. The causes are either badly made lens feet with warpage, rough edges or badly polished surfaces. The same anterior chamber irritation can also be seen in eyes in which the anterior chamber lens is too short.[30-38] This gives rise to lens mobility and recurring angle insult. A similar variety of chamber angle irritation has been seen in eyes containing anterior chamber lenses supported by flexible loops. Some of these are not sufficiently firmly fixed and are associated with some mobility, causing chronic irritation of the chamber angle associated with neovascularization, chronic anterior uveitis, glaucoma and spontaneous hyphaema – the so called 'UGH' syndrome. In these cases, where persistent uveitis is associated with the other angle changes, removal of the implant may well be the only satisfactory way of halting the process.

Iris and Pupil Disorder

Anterior chamber lenses may give rise to distortions of the pupil if, during insertion, the feet of the implant cause the anterior stroma of the iris to be tucked into the chamber angle. This complication, though unsightly, does not require surgical intervention. It is also noted that many eyes containing rigid anterior lenses develop a progressive oval distortion of the pupil. This is probably due to sector iris ischaemia and is not associated in most cases with any visible degree of inflammation. Again, this does not require intervention.

Pupil supported implants may produce a variety of iris/pupil complications. Where a pupil supported lens has required long term use of miotics in order to keep the lens stable, synechiae will develop all around the implant struts protruding through the pupil and the pupil will take up a permanently square or hexagonal shape, depending upon how many feet are passing through the pupillary aperture. This is not a serious complication, providing the patient does not develop a retinal detachment. These small fixed pupils give a particularly poor view of the peripheral retina and render essential detachment surgery extremely difficult. It should, however, never be necessary to remove an implant because of this complication.

Chronic Uveitis

Occasionally the insertion of an intraocular implant will be followed by prolonged uveitis which responds unsatisfactorily to steroid therapy and is associated with the development of fibrin around the implant together with keratitic precipitates and similar precipitates on the surface of the implant itself.[39,40] Occasionally, such uveitis can be so severe as to be associated with a hypopyon, multiple synechiae and even the development of pupil block glaucoma. This is particularly important to remember when so many surgeons using posterior chamber lenses after extracapsular extraction see no necessity for the performing of a peripheral iridectomy. If this fails to respond to appropriate topical therapy, it may be necessary to remove the implant as the only way of allowing the inflammation to subside.

Infection

Like any other intraocular operation there is always the risk of postoperative infection and endophthalmitis. This risk is probably increased after cataract extraction when a procedure has included the insertion of an implant. It is not difficult for the surface of an implant to become contaminated if it is not properly handled before insertion into the eye and it is for this reason that we stress the importance of never placing the implant down anywhere in the surgical field. Sterilization techniques used by most manufacturers are now very efficient so that the lenses are only likely to become contaminated after removal from the sterile packet and before their insertion into the eye. The detailed management of postoperative endophthalmitis is beyond the scope of this section, but there may be occasions when the surgeon feels obliged to remove the implant in order to facilitate the control of the endophthalmitis.[41]

Lens Displacement

A mobile intraocular lens of any style is a menace to the eye and is usually a constant source of irritation to the patient. Rigid or semi-rigid anterior chamber lenses, providing they are long enough for the anterior chamber into which they are inserted, seldom become displaced. Occasionally, however, the foot of an implant will produce separation of the ciliary body from the scleral spur and thereby create a cyclodialysis. Such an event may well lead to instability of the implant with consequent damage to the cornea. Very flexible loop anterior chamber implants appear to be capable of considerable movement in almost all directions and this mobility may well pose a serious hazard for the cornea and for the chamber angle structures as previously outlined.

Pupil supported lenses are liable to either anterior or posterior displacement. Anterior displacement, either of an upper or a lower foot, is almost certainly associated with lens–corneal touch and consequent decompensation, albeit only temporarily. The lenses can often be replaced into their proper position by means of dilating the pupil and posturing the patient, followed by miosis. When this manoeuvre fails, it may be necessary to reoperate to manipulate the implant into its proper position. Under these circumstances, the surgeon should give consideration to the need for the insertion of an anchoring suture between the iris stroma and one of the supporting struts of the implant. Such a suture was first described by McCannel[42] as a modification of his technique for the repair of iridodialysis (*see Fig.* 5).

Posterior displacement of an iris supported lens

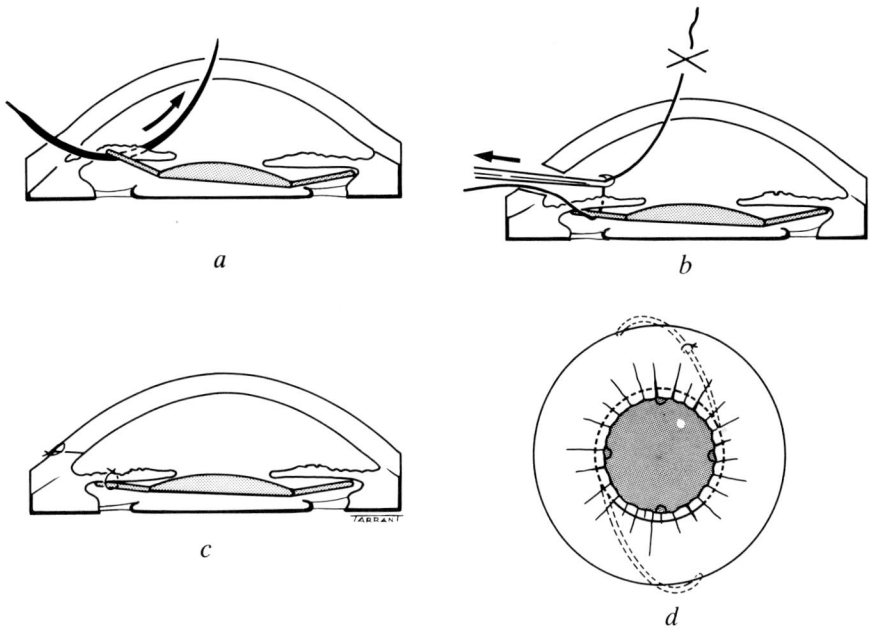

Fig. 5. The McCannel suture. The technique is similar, no matter the type of lens. 10/0 Prolene on 8 mm, 3/8 needle is used. *a*, A needle is passed through the limbal wound engaging iris, loop and iris again and is passed through the cornea. *b*, The needle is cut off. A small hook is passed into the anterior chamber, engaging the suture and pulling it back through the cornea and out through the limbal wound. *c,d*, The suture is tied outside the eye and the ends trimmed short, using intraocular scissors. The limbal wound is then closed.

can only occur following intracapsular extraction. Where the surgeon has sutured one of the haptic loops to the iris stroma, the lens can usually be repositioned by posturing the patient and dilating the pupil as described above. Where the lens has not been previously sutured, an implant is likely to disappear into the posterior segment and it can only be removed or replaced in its proper position by sophisticated vitreous surgical techniques, best performed through the pars plana.[43]

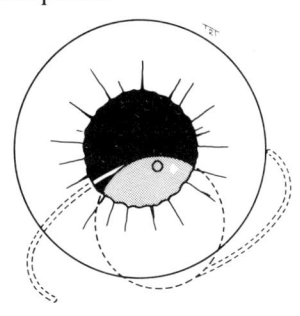

Fig. 6. The setting sun syndrome. The horizontally lying lens is dislocated inferiorly through capsule or zonular rents and only the superior pole of the optic is visible, like the sun setting below the horizon. Ultimately the lens may disappear into the vitreous.

Lenses supported entirely within the posterior chamber may become de-centred. The most commonly described de-centring is where the lens is displaced inferiorly so that part of the pupil can become uncorrected — the so-called 'setting sun' syndrome (*Fig.* 6).

This complication is usually avoided if, after insertion of the implant, the supporting haptics are rotated into the horizontal position. Displacement can be corrected by manipulating the implant and, if necessary, this manipulation can be associated with the insertion of a McCannel suture to stabilize one of the supporting haptics in the desired position.

Another classic complication of this variety is the so-called 'windscreen wiper syndrome' where an implant in the posterior chamber will be mobile and will swing across and out of the pupil depending upon the head posture. Such a mobile lens will need to be fixed with a McCannel suture (*Fig.* 5).

A third variety of displacement of posterior chamber lenses is pupil capture. In this instance the margin of the pupil may contract behind one edge of the implant to produce a cat's eye appearance. This does not usually produce any significant impairment of vision but is unsightly.

Capsular Thickening

Although not technically a complication of implant insertion, fewer capsules would be left in eyes after cataract surgery if intraocular implants were not in use. Some surgeons have reported an incidence of need for a secondary procedure to manage capsular thickening of 50 per cent over a five year period,[28] but individual surgeons report a wide variation of incidence for this complication. Until 1982, it was usually necessary for a patient to be returned to the operating theatre for a surgical capsulotomy performed either through the pars plana or through the limbus. Since the development of the Nd: YAG laser it has become customary for those with such an instrument to divide the thickened capsule by this means. This can occasionally produce pitting of the posterior surface of the intraocular implant but this does not appear to have any significant optical or biological consequences. Nd: YAG laser treatment in the anterior segment of the eye, however, may be complicated by transient glaucoma and varying degrees of endothelial damage.[44]

INTRAOCULAR LENS MATERIAL AND STERILIZATION

When Ridley first decided to insert his first intraocular lens in 1949, he arranged for the lens to be manufactured out of polymethylmethacrylate. He had previously noted this to be a material which appeared to be biologically inert. So far polymethylmethacrylate has proved its worth and has not been bettered. With the need for supporting flexible loops, both open and closed, a variety of other materials was included in implant structure, but over the years some of these have been discarded. Metal loops were found to be very damaging to the sphincter of the pupil and nylon loops were found to be associated with quite obvious biodegradation. At present supporting haptic loops are made either of polymethylmethacrylate or polypropylene. Polypropylene has some tendency to biodegradation, but this would not appear to be clinically significant,[45] at least in the posterior chamber, where it is protected from ultraviolet light.

Lenses are available from manufacturers having been sterilized either by a wet or a dry process. Lenses in dry packets have been sterilized by ethylene oxide and such lenses can be inserted into the eye after removal from the packet and after careful inspection to ensure the absence of any manufacturing defect, without the need for rinsing or soaking. Lenses provided in wet packs, however, have been despatched in a weak solution of sodium hydroxide. These lenses need to be soaked in a provided solution of sodium bicarbonate and for sufficient time to ensure that all traces of the sodium hydroxide have been eliminated. These lenses should then be most carefully washed with normal saline to remove all traces of possible chemical contamination before they are inserted into the eye. Failure to observe these precautions can lead to ferocious postoperative uveitis.

The authors would emphasize the importance of inspecting an implant under the operating microscope after its removal from its sterile container before inserting the implant into the eye. Surface damage or distortion of supporting loops or haptics must be looked for. Failure to recognize these defects, which are by no means uncommon, can lead to long term difficulties for the patient. Most manufacturers will now accept the return of defective lenses and arrange for their replacement without extra cost. As mentioned above, it is important that this inspection be carried out well away from the surface of the eye and great care should be taken by the surgeon that the implant does not become contaminated by touching the surface of the cornea or the eye lashes, lid margins etc. The electrostatic surface properties of polished polymethylmethacrylate are such that they will tend to attract contaminants very easily.[41] No undue time should be lost between removal of the implant from its packet and its subsequent insertion into the patient's eye. These principles apply to all the styles of implant described above, and to the products of any manufacturer.

REFERENCES

1. Ridley H. Intraocular acrylic lenses. *Trans. Ophthalmol. Soc. UK* 1951; **71,** 617–21.
2. Ridley H. Intraocular lenses, ten years development. *Br. J. Ophthalmol.* 1960; **44,** 705–13.
3. Choyce D. P. Correction of uniocular aphakia by means of anterior chamber acrylic implants. *Trans. Ophthalmol. Soc. UK* 1958; **78,** 459–70.
4. Strampelli B. Due anni di esperienza con le lenti camerulari. *Atti Soc. Oftal. Ital.* 1955; **15,** 427–33.
5. Epstein E. Modified Ridley lenses. *Br. J. Ophthalmol.* 1959; **43,** 29–33.
6. Barraquer J. Anterior chamber plastic lenses. Results and complications from 5 years' experience. *Trans. Ophthalmol. Soc. UK* 1959; **79,** 393–424.
7. Barraquer J. The use of plastic lenses in the anterior chamber. Indications – technique – personal results. *Trans. Ophthalmol. Soc. UK* 1956; **76,** 537–52.
8. Colenbrander A., Woods L. and Stamper R. L. Intraocular lens data. *Ophthalmology* (Instrument and Book Supplement) 1983.
9. Tenant J. L. Anterior chamber lenses. In: Rosen E., Haining W. and Arnott E. (ed.) *Intraocular Lens Implantation.* St Louis, Mo, Mosby, 1984, pp. 272–85.
10. Binkhorst C. D. Iris supported artificial pseudophakia. A new development in intraocular artificial lens surgery. *Trans. Ophthalmol. Soc. UK* 1959; **79,** 569–84.
11. Binkhorst C. D., Kats A. and Leonard P. A. M. Extracapsular pseudophakia. Results in 100 two-loop iridocapsular lens implantations. *Am. J. Ophthalmol.* 1972; **73,** 625–36.
12. Wilkinson C. P. A long term study of cystoid macular oedema in aphakic and pseudophakic eyes. *Trans. Am. Ophthalmol. Soc.* 1981; **79,** 810–39.

13. Binkhorst C. D. Five hundred planned extracapsular cataract extractions with iridocapsular and iris clip lens implants in senile cataract. *Ophthalmic Surg.* 1977; **8**, 37–44.
14. Olmos E. and Roy F. H. Results of 1254 intraocular lenses. *J. Ark. Med. Soc.* 1980; **77**, 168–71.
15. Pearce J. L. Modern simple extracapsular surgery. *Trans. Ophthalmol. Soc. UK* 1979; **99**, 176–82.
16. Pearce J. L. A new sutured posterior chamber lens implant. *Trans. Ophthalmol. Soc. UK* 1976; **76**, 6–10.
17. Shearing S. P. A practical posterior chamber lens. *Contact Intra. Lens Med. J.* 1978; **4**, 114–19.
18. Karickhoff J. R. Instruments and techniques for anterior chamber implants. *Arch. Ophthalmol.* 1980; **98**, 1265–7.
19. Clayman H. M., Jaffe N. S. and Galin M. A. *Intraocular Lens Implantation.* St Louis, Mo, Mosby, 1983.
20. Drews R. C. Lens implantation: Lessons learned from the first million. *Trans. Ophthalmol. Soc. UK* 1982; **102**, 505–9.
21. Duffin R. M. and Olson R. J. Vaulting characteristics of flexible loop anterior chamber intraocular lenses. *Arch. Ophthalmol.* 1983; **101**, 1429.
22. Cherry P. M. H. Fixation suture in implantation of flexible anterior chamber intraocular lenses. *Arch. Ophthalmol.* 1983; **101**, 1421–33.
23. Neetens A. and Rubbens M. C. Complications in primary anterior chamber pseudophakic eyes after intracapsular cataract extraction. *Ophthalmologica (Basel)* 1983; **187**, 83–93.
24. Emery J. H. and McIntyre D. J. *Extracapsular Cataract Surgery.* St Louis, Mo, Mosby, 1983.
25. Stark W. J., Worthen D. M., Holladay J. T. et al. The FDA report on intraocular lenses. *Ophthalmology* 1983; **90**, 311–17.
26. Stark W. J., Leske M. C., Worthen D. M. et al. Trends in cataract surgery and intraocular lenses in the United States. *Am. J. Ophthalmol.* 1983; **96**, 304–10.
27. Retzlaff J. Posterior chamber implant power calculation: regression formulas. *Am. Intraoc. Implant Soc. J.* 1980; **6**, 268–70.
28. Leiske L. G. Anterior chamber implants. In: Rosen E., Haining W. and Arnott E. (ed.) *Intraocular Lens Implantation.* St Louis, Mo, Mosby, 1984, pp. 286–305.
29. Drews R. C. Polypropylene in the human eye. *Am. Intraoc. Implant Soc. J.* 1983; **9**, 137–42.
30. Mowbrey S. L., Chang S. H. and Casella J. F. Estimation of useful lifetime of polypropylene fibre in the anterior chamber. *Am. Intraoc. Implant Soc. J.* 1983; **9**, 143–7.
31. Crawford R. C. A histopathologic study of position of Shearing intraocular lens in the posterior chamber. *Am. J. Ophthalmol.* 1981; **81**, 458–61.
32. Hoffer K. J. Pathological examination of a J loop intraocular lens in the ciliary sulcus. *Am. J. Ophthalmol.* 1981; **92**, 268–72.
33. Kraff M. C., Sanders D. R., Lieberman H. D., et al. Secondary intraocular lens implantation. *Ophthalmology* 1983; **90**, 324–6.
34. Stratsma B. R., Petit T. H., Wheeler N. et al. Diabetes mellitus and intraocular implantation. *Ophthalmology* 1983; **90**, 336–43.
35. Taylor D. M., Atlas B. F., Romanchuk K. G. et al. Pseudophakic bullous keratopathy. *Ophthalmology* 1983; **90**, 19–24.
36. Ellingson F. T. The uveitis–glaucoma–hyphema syndrome associated with mark VIII anterior chamber lens implant. *Am. Intraoc. Implant Soc. J.* 1978; **4**, 50–3.
37. Moore C. R. and Steller R. T. Early recognition and proper treatment of the VIP syndrome. *Am. Intraoc. Implant Soc. J.* 1978; **4**, 114–16.
38. McDonnell P. J., Green W. R., Maumanee A. E. et al. Pathology of intraocular lenses in 33 eyes examined post mortem. *Ophthalmology* 1983; **90**, 386–403.
39. Yeo J. H., Jakobiec F. A., Pokovny K. et al. The ultrastructure of an IOL cocoon membrane. *Ophthalmology* 1983; **90**, 410–19.
40. Leonard T. J., Greerson I., Fison P. N. et al. Life on implants. *Trans. Ophthalmol. Soc. UK* 1983; **103**, 164–73.
41. Vafidis G. C., Marsh R. J. and Stacey A. R. Bacterial contamination of intraocular lens surgery. *Br. J. Ophthalmol.* 1984; **68**, 520–3.
42. McCannell M. A. A retrievable suture idea for anterior uveal problems. *Ophthalmic Surg.* 1976; **7**, 98–103.
43. Stark W. J. and Dangel M. Intraocular lens complications. In Steele A.D.McG. and Drews R. C. (eds) *Cataract Surgery*, London, Butterworths, 1984, pp. 309–24.
44. Kerr Muir M. and Sherrard E. S. Damage to the corneal endothelium during Nd:YAG photodisruption. *Br. J. Ophthalmol.* 1985; **69**, 77–85.
45. Apple D. J., Mamalis M., Brady E. S. et al. Biocompatibility of implant materials. A review and scanning electron microscopic study. *Am. Intraoc. Implant Soc. J.* 1984; **10**, 53–64.

Chapter 11

Glaucoma

Roger A. Hitchings

This chapter discusses the primary and secondary glaucomas, emphasizing points in diagnosis and management. Current ideas on pathogenesis are noted, while the reader is referred to the bibliography for reviews providing greater detail and for discussions on controversial aspects.

INTRODUCTION

Glaucoma is the name given to a group of diseases which share three common features: elevated intraocular pressure (IOP); a characteristic enlargement of the optic cup (glaucomatous cupping); and 'nerve fibre bundle' type of visual field loss. Glaucoma may arise directly as a result of a developmental defect or degenerative process occurring within the eye – when it is termed primary – or as a result of other disease processes occurring inside or outside of the eye – when it is termed secondary. The glaucomas are important for three reasons. First, together they form one of the commonest causes of blindness, particularly in the older age groups. Secondly, even in patients not legally blind, they cause considerable visual morbidity; while, thirdly, the cost in human and financial terms of these diseases is considerable.

This chapter will first classify the glaucomas and then for each broad group discuss aetiology, symptoms and signs and management.

Table I. Primary glaucomas

Type	Possible causative factor(s)	Characteristic features
Open angle		
Chronic open angle glaucoma*	Primary trabecular change	Nil
Low tension glaucoma	Primary weakness of optic disc to 'normal' IOP	Dense paracentral field defect. Optic disc haemorrhages
Juvenile glaucoma	Developmental angle anomaly	Onset greater than 3 years
Congenital glaucoma	Developmental angle anomaly	Onset in utero and up to 2 years. Buphthalmos
Pigmentary glaucoma†	Pigment granules blocking trabecular meshwork	Pigment dispersion syndrome
Pseudoexfoliation†	Proteinaceous material blocking trabecular meshwork	Pseudoexfoliative material in the anterior segment
Closed angle		
Acute closed angle	Anatomic predisposition to pupil block; attacks precipitated by stress, drugs, accommodation etc.	Red painful eye with visual loss
Subacute closed angle		Intermittent visual loss
Chronic closed angle	Acute or subacute angle closure with residual PAS. Anatomic predisposition to pupil block	Nil
Combined mechanism		
Mixed glaucoma (Narrow angle glaucoma)	Anatomic predisposition for pupil block. Trabecular damage	PAS in superior angle. IOP higher than extent of PAS would justify

* For the purposes of classification, chronic open angle glaucoma includes patients labelled as having ocular hypertension.
† In some American texts, this glaucoma is classed with the secondary glaucomas. However, as the disease process is limited to causing glaucoma, the older classification as a primary glaucoma is maintained.

PLATE I

Chapter 1

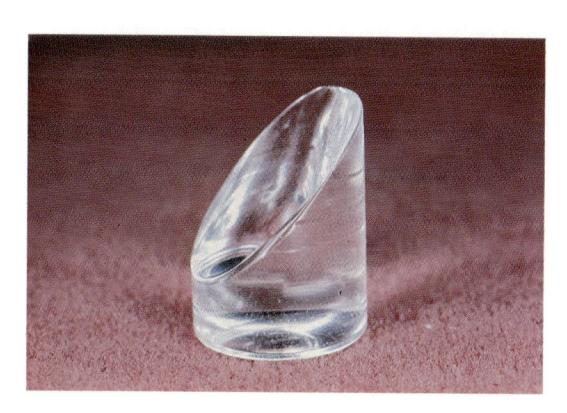

a, A simple direct gonioscope made for the author by the contact lens department at Moorfields Hospital. This prism is similar to Lister's goniolens.

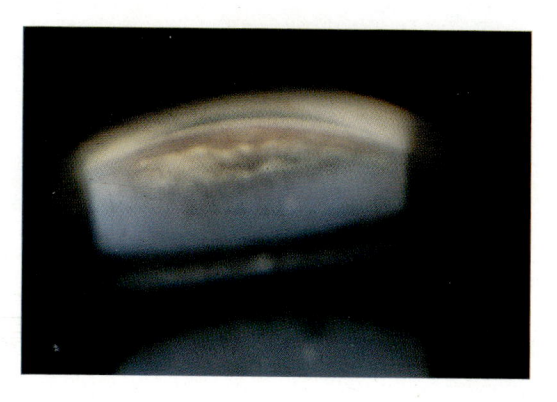

b, Early rubeosis. Note the blood vessels crossing the trabecular band.

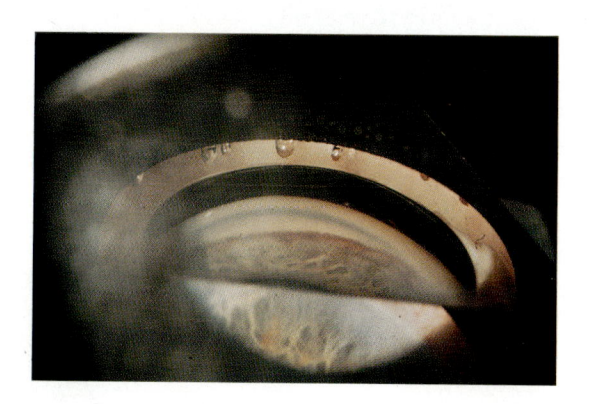

c, Neovascular glaucoma. A densely vascularized angle with free blood inferiorly.

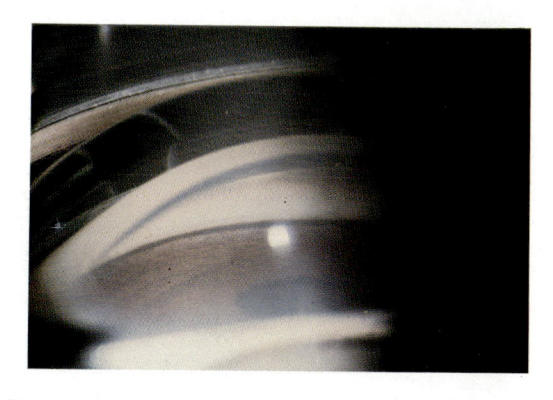

d, Pigmentary glaucoma. Note the heavily pigmented trabecular zone.

PLATE II
Chapter 4

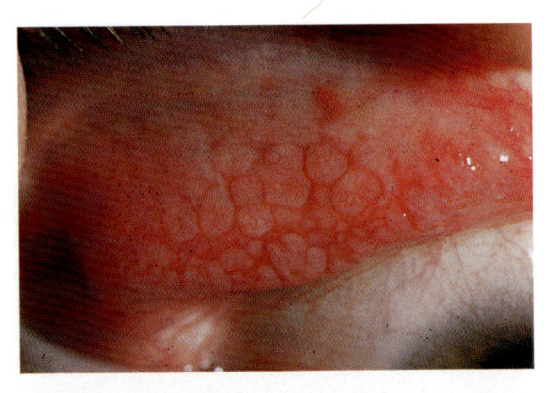

a, Compound hypertrophic papillae in vernal conjunctivitis.

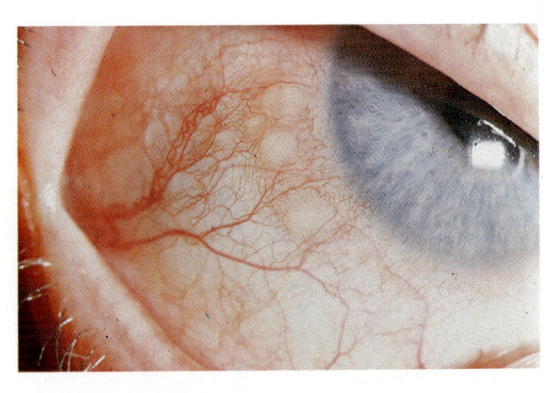

b, Bulbar follicles in response to drops of acetyl cysteine.

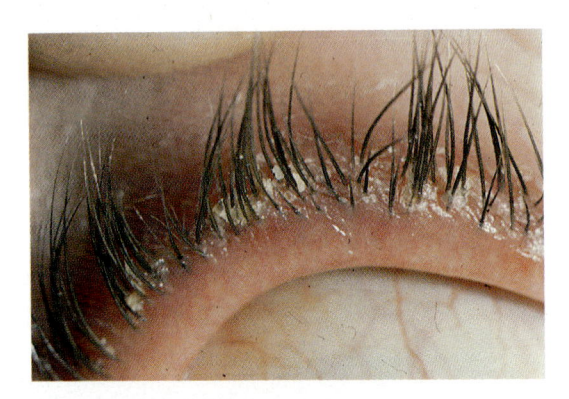

c, Seborrhoeic blepharitis.

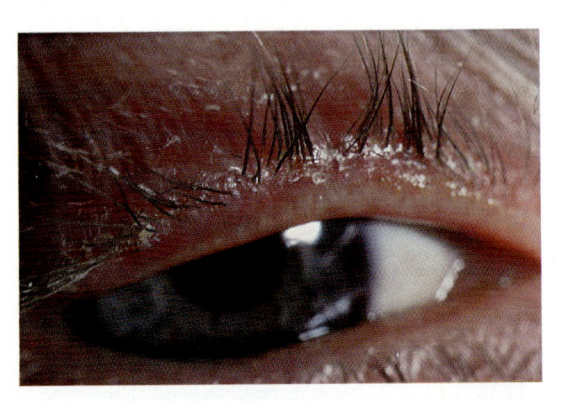

d, Staphylococcal folliculitis with damage to follicles and loss of lashes.

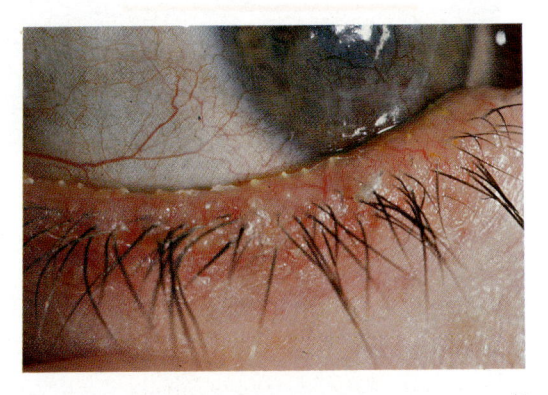

e, Staphylococcal meibomitis with obstructed meibomian orifices, hyperaemia and metaplasia of the lid margin.

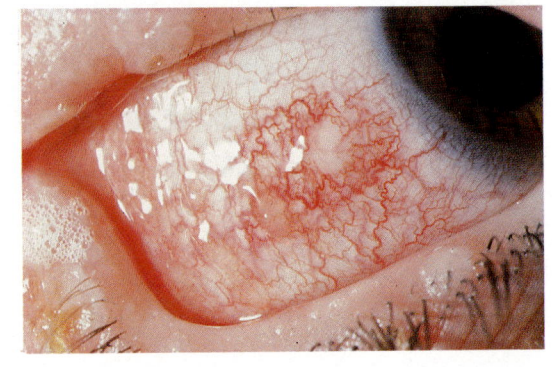

f, Phlycten and bulbar follicles associated with staphylococcal folliculitis.

PLATE III
Chapter 4

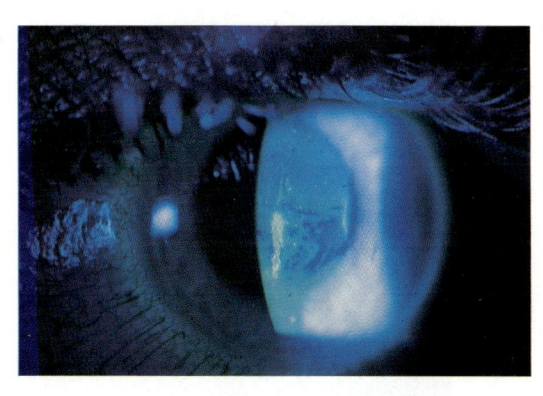

a, Break up of the precorneal tear film.

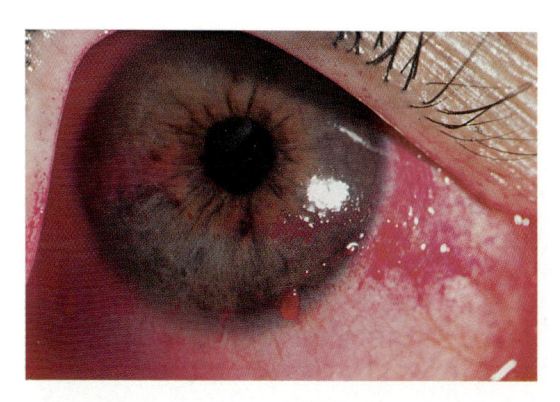

b, Mucus deposition and filament in a dry eye.

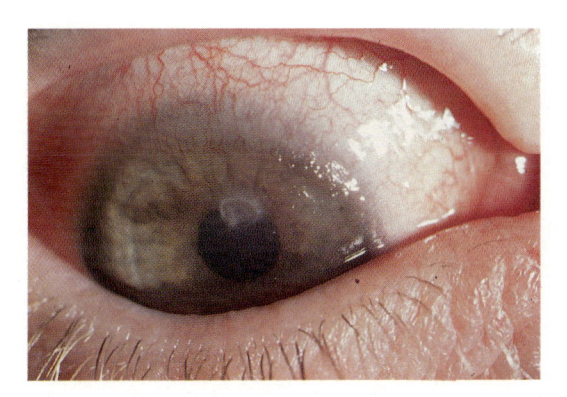

c, Active vernal keratitis with vernal plaque.

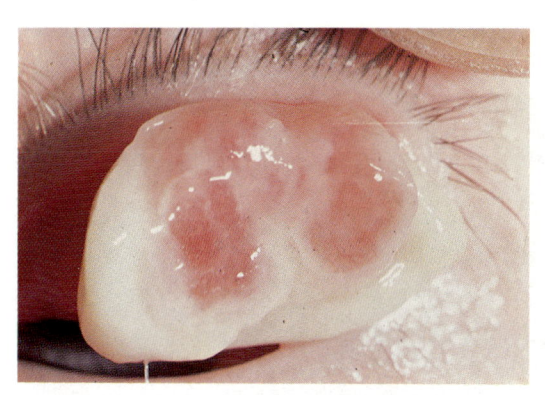

d, Ligneous conjunctivitis affecting upper tarsal conjunctiva in an 8-month-old baby following chlamydial ophthalmia neonatorum.

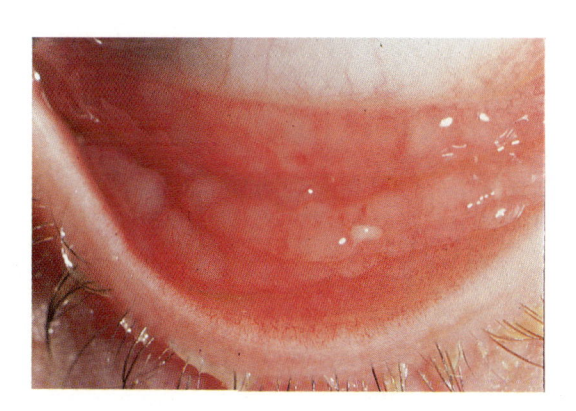

e, Acute follicular conjunctivitis.

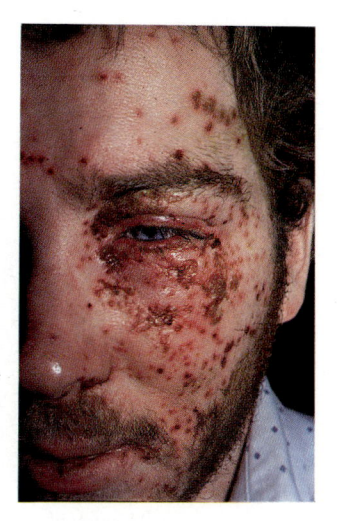

f, Primary herpes simplex.

PLATE IV

Chapter 4

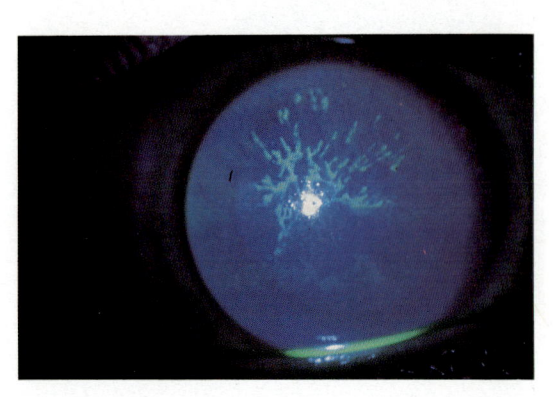

a, Multiple dendritic figures in primary ocular herpes simplex.

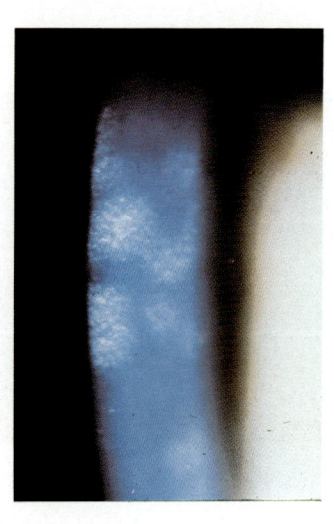

b, Epithelial and subepithelial keratitis in adenovirus 19 infection.

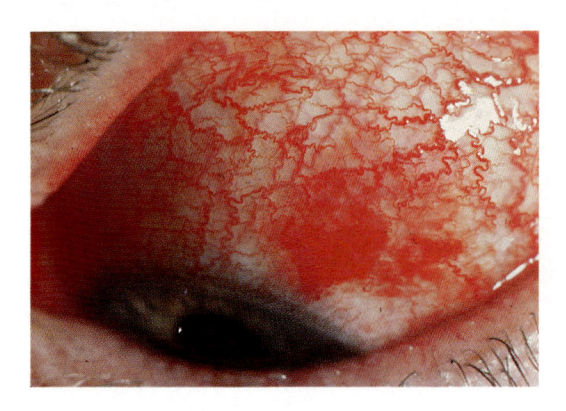

c, Epidemic haemorrhagic conjunctivitis (picorna virus).

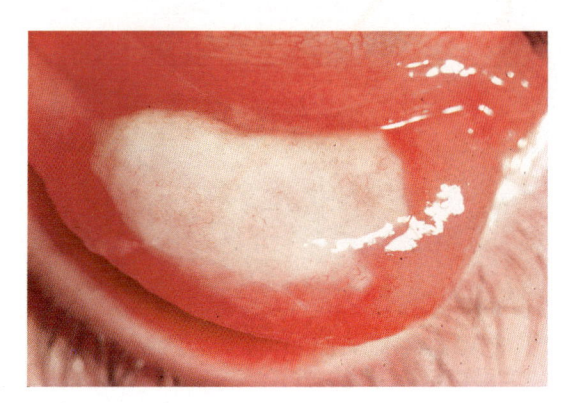

d, Parinaud's syndrome due to Epstein–Barr virus.

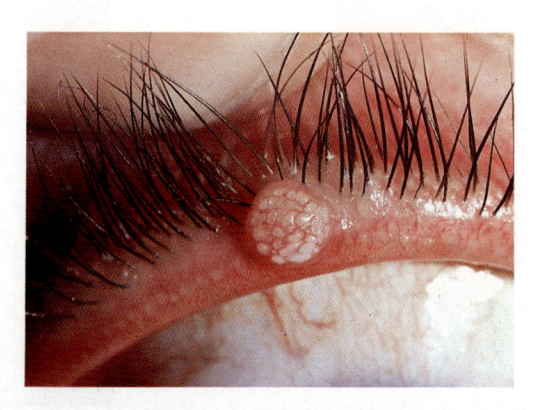

e, Molluscum contagiosum of the lid margin causing chronic follicular conjunctivitis.

PLATE V
Chapter 4

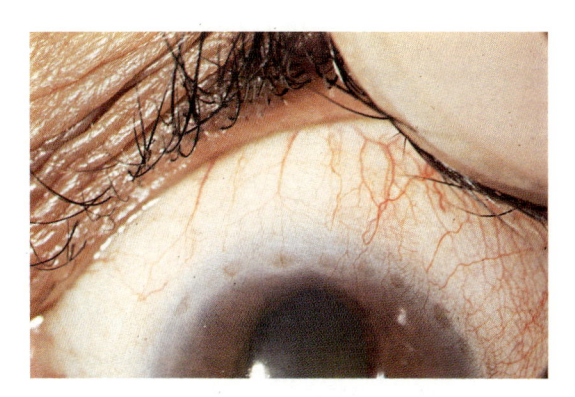

a, Herbert's pits.

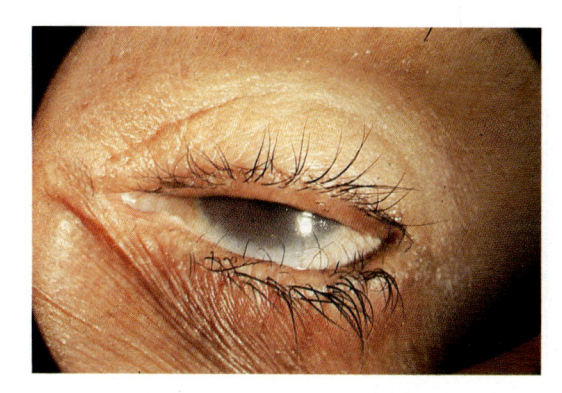

b, Trachomatous cicatricial entropion.

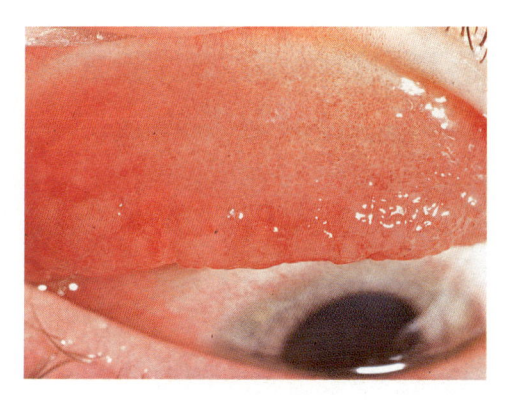

c, Follicles in upper fornix (TRIC).

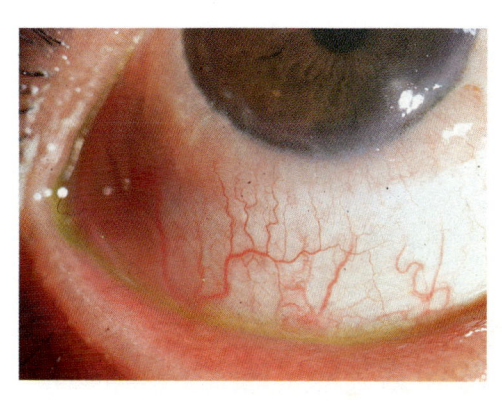

d, Limbitis and bulbar follicles after pilocarpine drops.

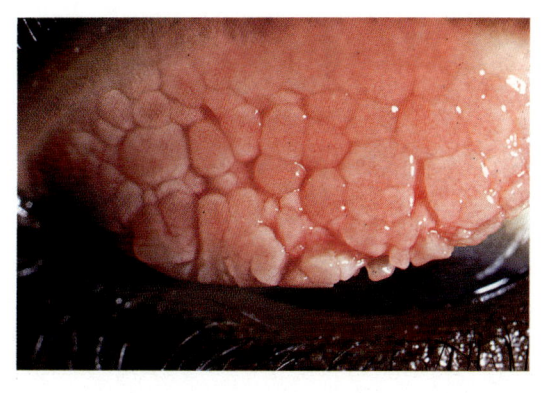

e, Palpebral vernal conjunctivitis, inactive.

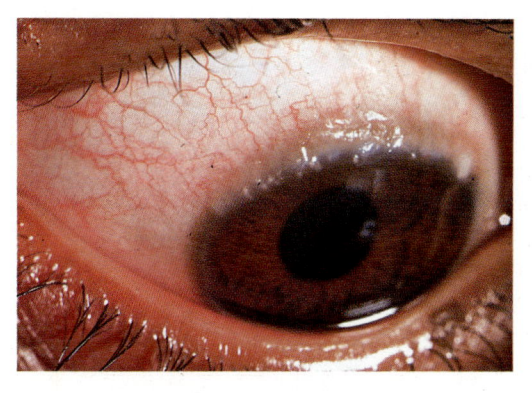

f, Limbal vernal with Trantas' dots.

PLATE VI
Chapter 4

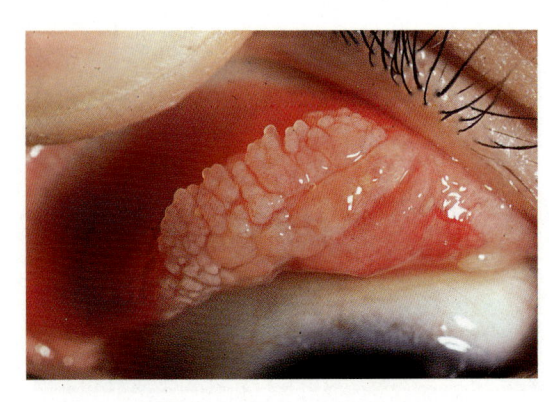

a, Inactive hyalinized papillae in vernal.

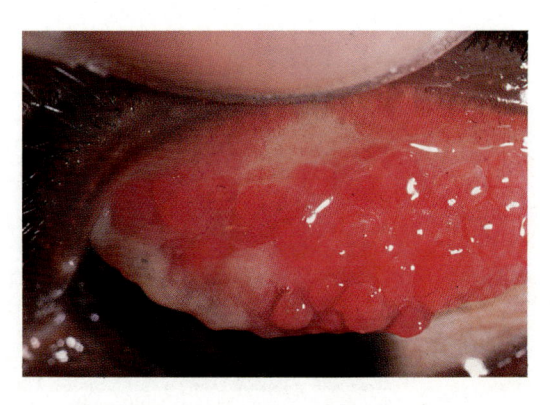

b, Active palpebral vernal conjunctivitis (same patient as *Plate* V*e*).

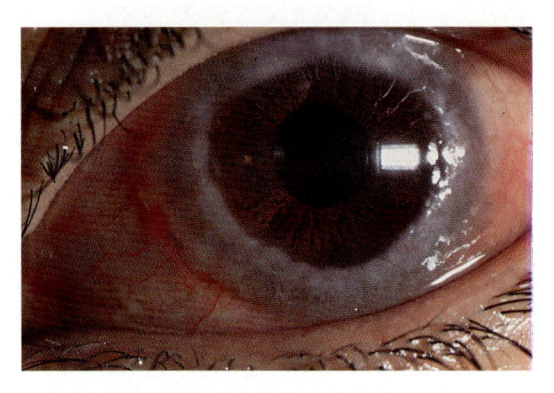

c, Confluent limbal form of bulbar vernal.

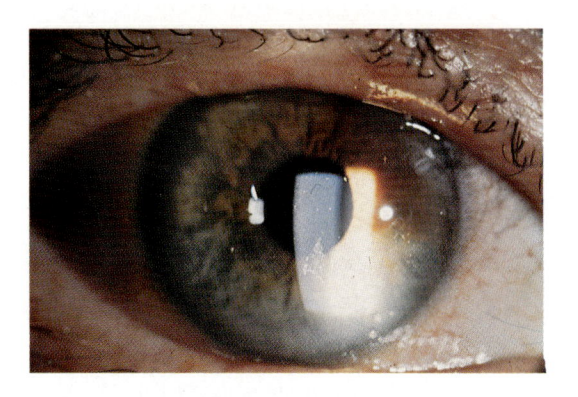

d, Mucus and debris in precorneal film of patient with dry eye.

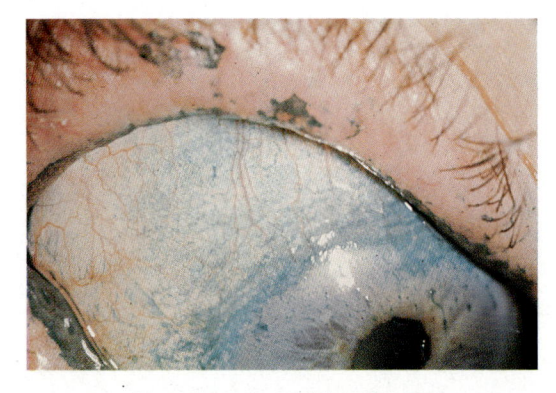

e, Lissamine green staining of dry eye.

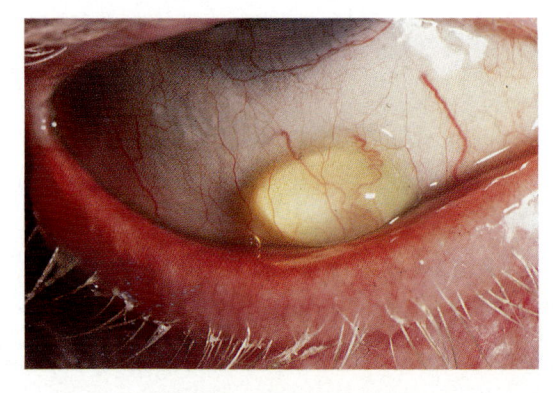

f, 'Lacrisert' in lower fornix.

PLATE VII
Chapter 4

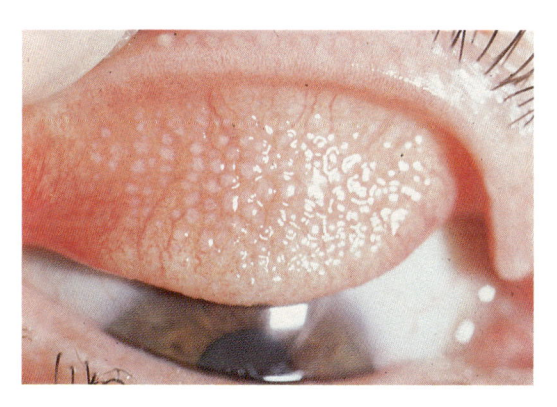

a, Giant papillary conjunctivitis associated with the use of CAB contact lenses.

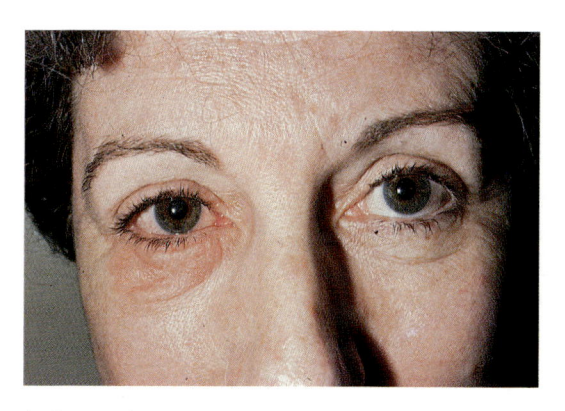

b, Contact dermatitis of the right lids caused by neomycin.

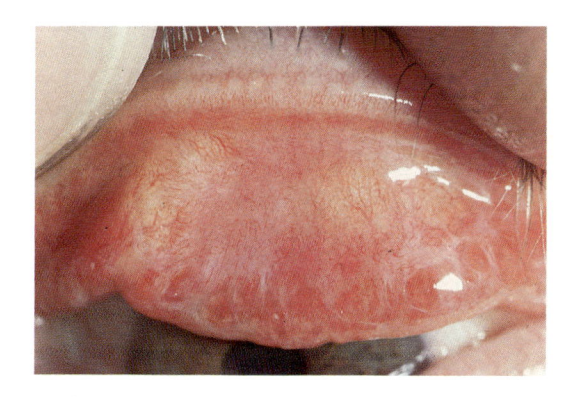

c, Conjunctival scarring following severe adenovirus conjunctivitis.

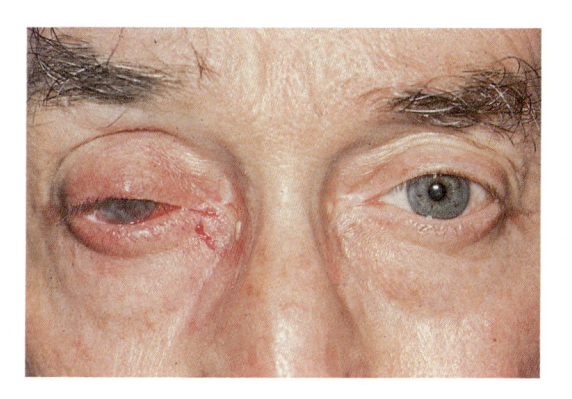

d, Unilateral chronic conjunctivitis with scarring and dryness subsequently shown to be due to mucous membrane pemphigoid.

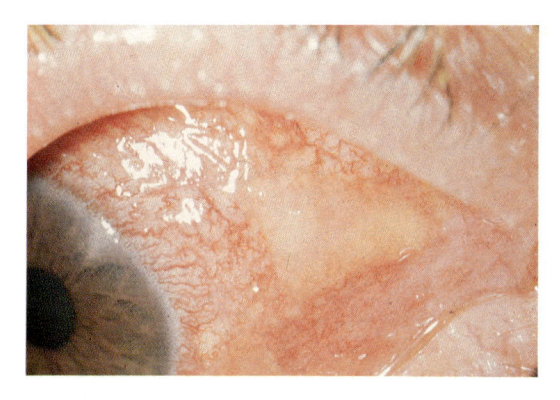

e, Loss of inner canthal architecture and conjunctival ulceration in mucous membrane pemphigoid.

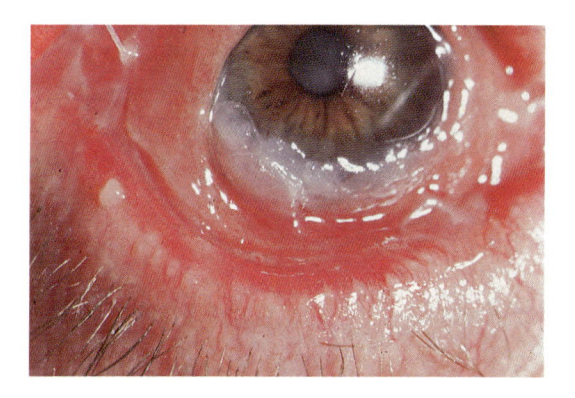

f, Loss of lower fornix and advancing fleshy pannus in mucous membrane pemphigoid.

PLATE VIII

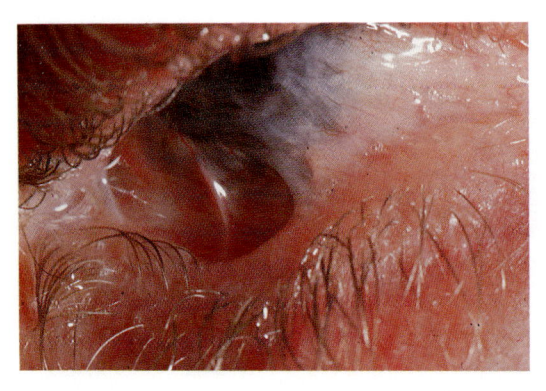

Chapter 4

a, Conjunctival involvement in linear IgA disease.

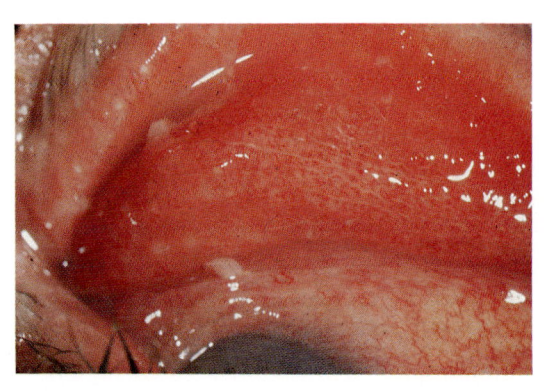

b, Conjunctival reaction in early stage of Stevens–Johnson syndrome.

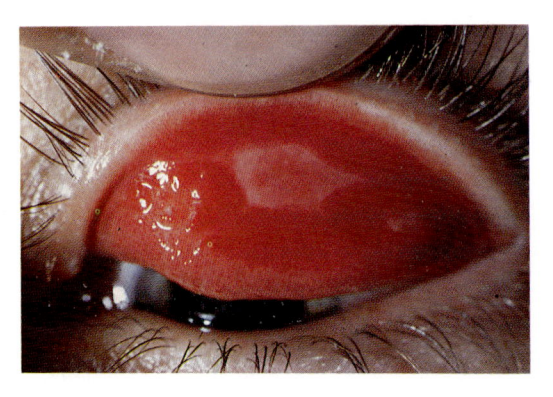

c, Conjunctival reaction in Stevens–Johnson syndrome has progressed to infarction.

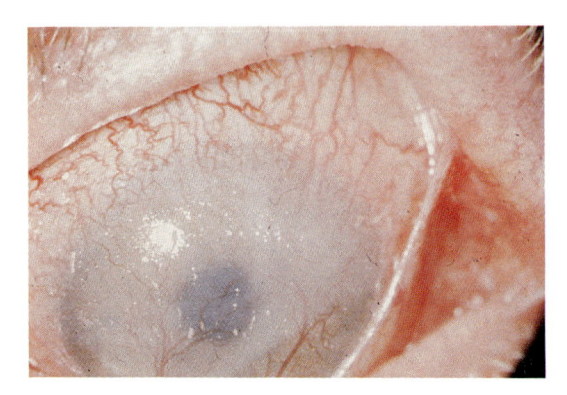

d, Soft conjunctival adhesions, corneal vascularization and dry eye as late complications in Stevens–Johnson syndrome.

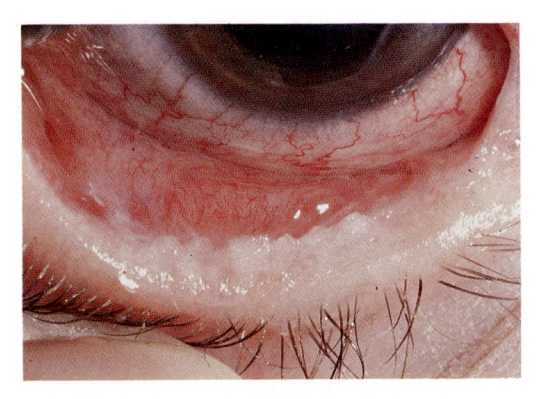

e, Keratinization of conjunctiva adjacent to lid margin in Stevens–Johnson syndrome.

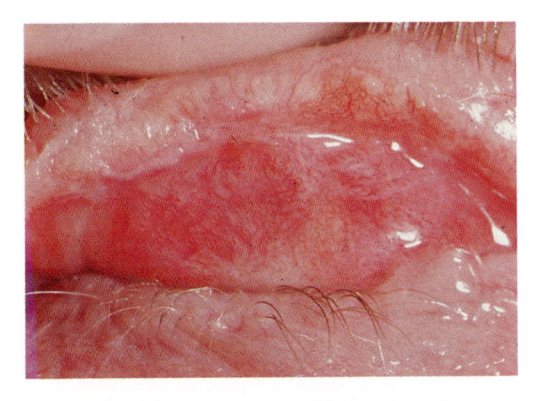

f, Pseudopemphigoid – scarring and inflammation of upper tarsal conjunctiva following prolonged use of miotics.

PLATE IX
Chapter 6

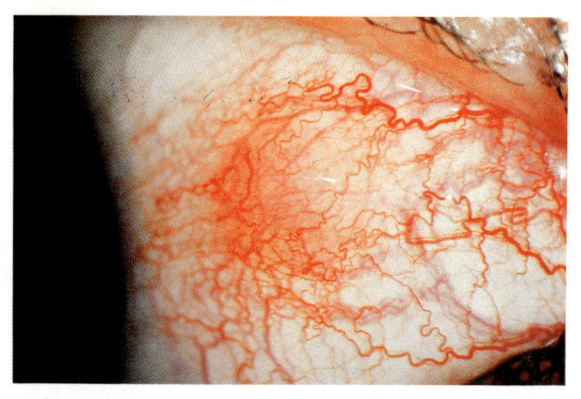

a, Nodular episcleritis. The episclera is oedematous, congested and infiltrated 2 mm from the limbus. Although there is dilatation of all the capillary bed at the site of inflammation the vessels retain their normal architecture and the underlying sclera is not swollen.

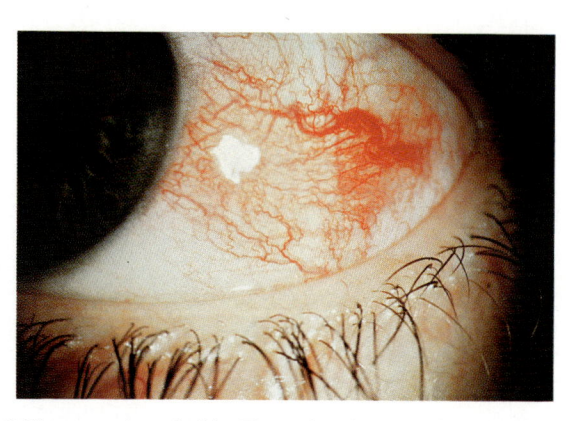

b, Diffuse anterior scleritis. The patient had complained of intermittent redness of the eye associated with severe ocular and periocular pain which spreads to the temple over a period of 4 months. The sclera is swollen, the episcleral vessels are congested and there is a prominent vessel at the site of inflammation. The vascular configuration is normal. (See Fig. 4.)

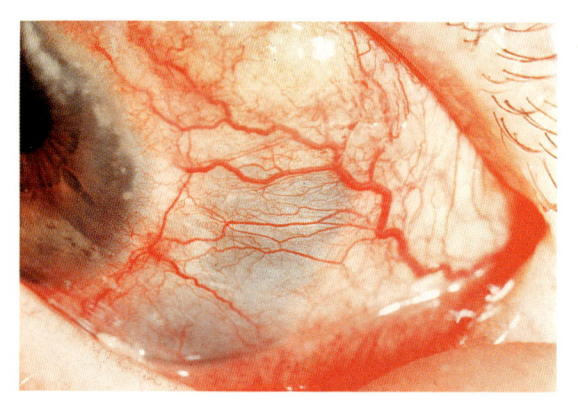

c, Necrotizing scleritis. This patient had had a severe scleritis which had been inadequately treated for 9 months. The sclera has become translucent between 6 and 3 o'clock but there is no loss of tissue. There is an avascular area at 2 o'clock with early necrotic changes. The vascular pattern has become grossly distorted and the upper part of the cornea infiltrated and vascularized.

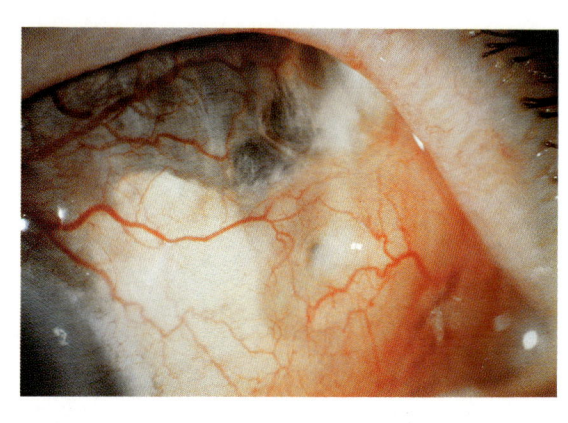

d, Necrotizing scleritis with scleral lysis and early sequestrum formation. Severe necrotizing scleritis which followed trabeculectomy in a patient with periarteritis nodosa. The sclera at 12 o'clock has been completely removed. An area above the horizontal vessel is pale yellow and avascular and about to be removed. There is an area at 2 o'clock from which the conjunctiva is absent. The sclera around this is swollen and inflamed. The vascular pattern is irregular and distorted.

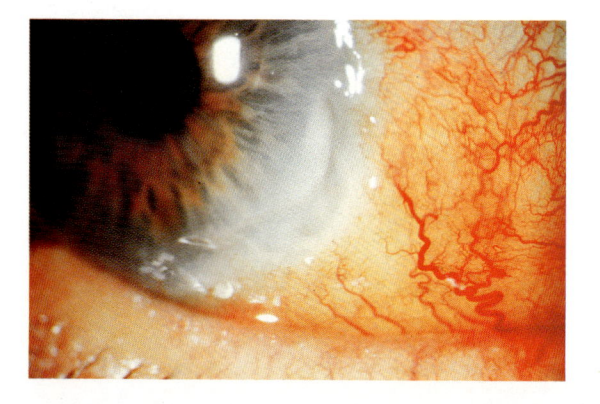

e, Acute necrotizing sclerokeratitis. A deep peripheral corneal gutter in a patient who later proved to have Wegener's granulomatosis. The eye is congested and the gutter transgresses the limbus. The cornea centrally is infiltrated.

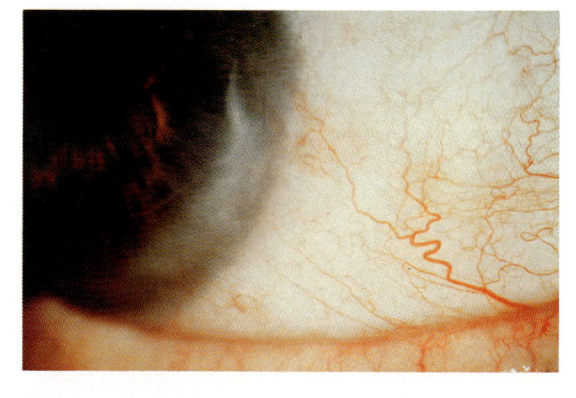

f, Acute necrotizing sclerokeratitis. Healing of the ulcer after treatment with cyclophosphamide.

PLATE X

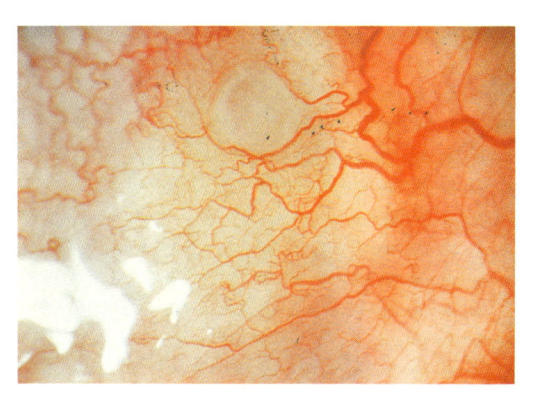

Chapter 6

a, Necrotizing scleritis. An area of early scleral necrosis in which the conjunctiva has become involved and ulcerated. However, closer inspection shows much of the surrounding area to be affected with a yellow discoloration showing through the overlying inflamed episcleral tissue.

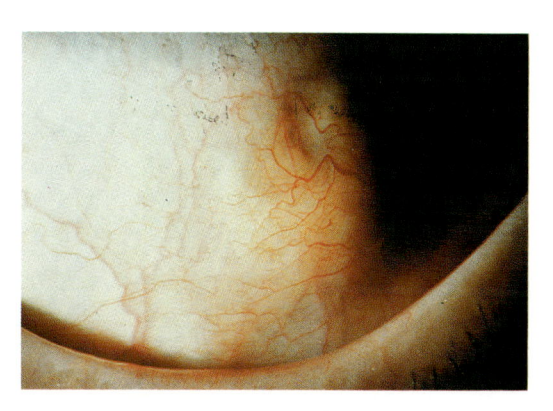

b, Necrotizing scleritis. The same area after treatment with pulsed steroid and cyclophosphamide therapy. The ulcer is completely healed, its base being transgressed by new vessels. The surrounding area is still discoloured but beginning to whiten.

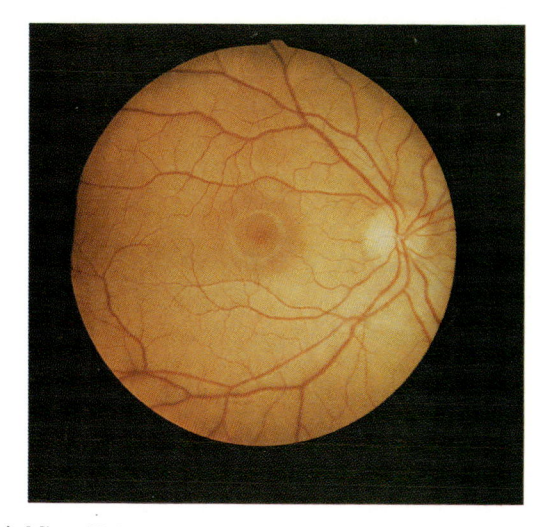

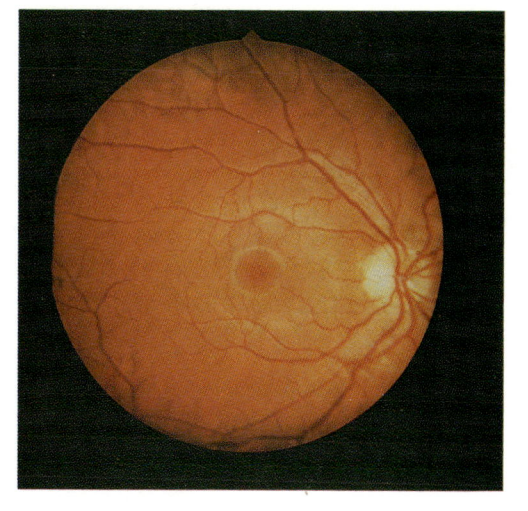

c, d, Mizuo-Nakamura phenomenon in a patient with Oguchi's disease. Golden-cream coloration of the light-adapted fundus (*c*) resolves to normal fundus colour (*d*) after 4 hours' dark adaptation.

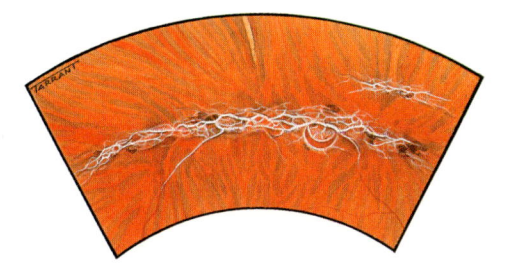

e, Lattice degeneration with retinal pigmentation and an associated horseshoe-shaped tear rising from the posterior edge of the lattice is seen. Round holes are also present.

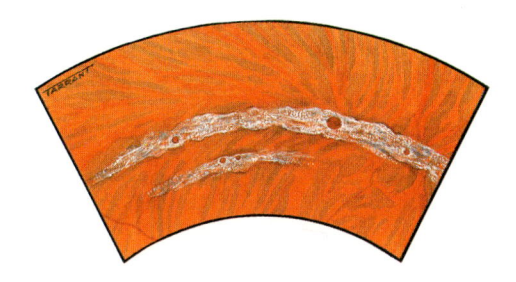

f, Snail track degeneration associated with round holes.

PLATE XI
Chapter 8

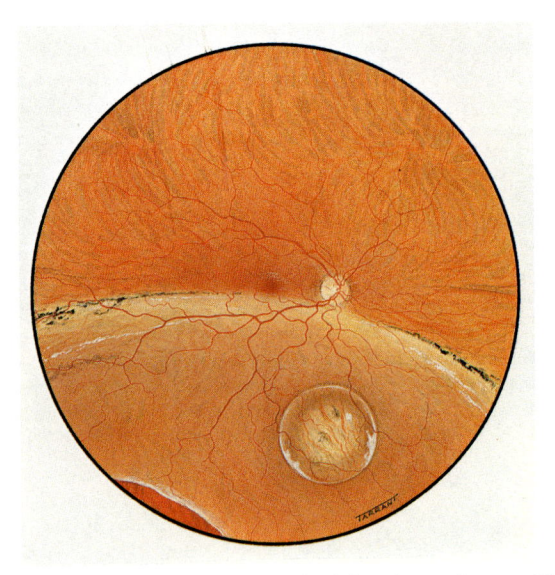

a, A long standing inferior half retinal detachment is seen. Pigmented water marks limit the upper edge of the detachment and a secondary intraretinal cyst is present. Retinal dialysis is present in the inferior temporal quadrant of the retina.

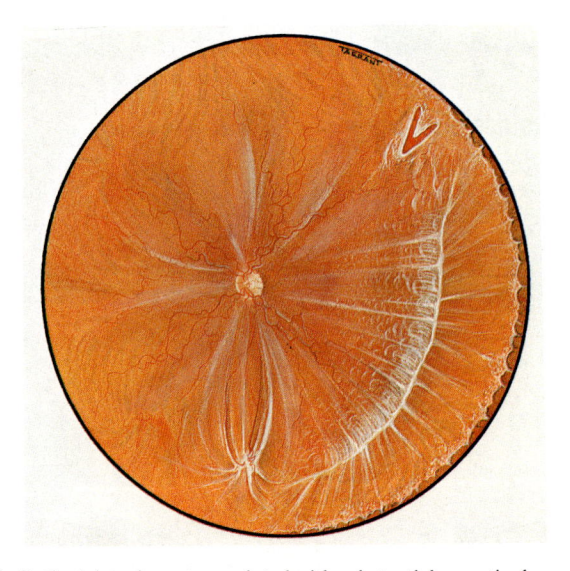

b, Retinal detachment associated with substantial preretinal membrane formation is present. A star-shaped fold is seen at 6 o'clock which has caused distortion of neighbouring blood vessels. Preretinal membrane formation in the vicinity of the horseshoe-shaped tear has resulted in excessive elongation of the tear. In the temporal quadrant of the retina, traction of the posterior hyaloid face has resulted in the raising of a high circumferential retinal fold: this has caused stretching of peripheral retina and has dragged the ora serrata into view.

PLATE XI

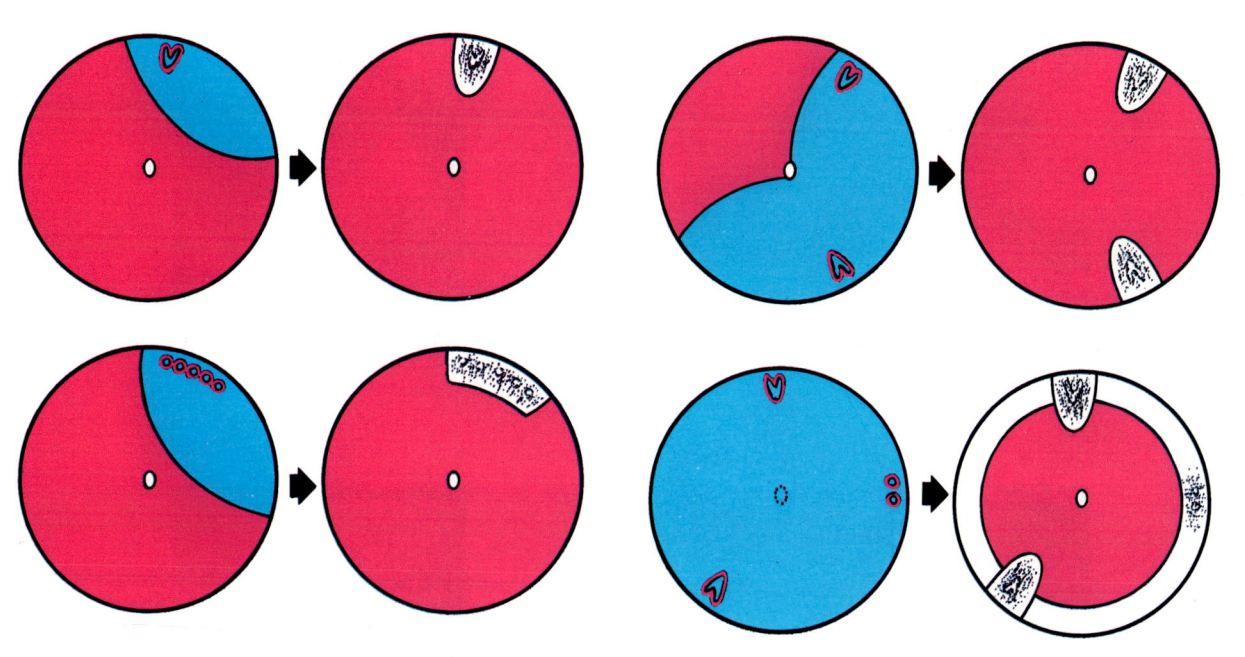

Chapter 8

c, The use of a radial buckle to close a horseshoe-shaped tear, and the use of a circumferential buckle to seal a row of small round holes.

d, Two radial sponges may be used to seal horseshoe-shaped tears in separate quadrants. Multiple holes in separate quadrants are treated with an encircling procedure augmenting the encirclement with a local buckle.

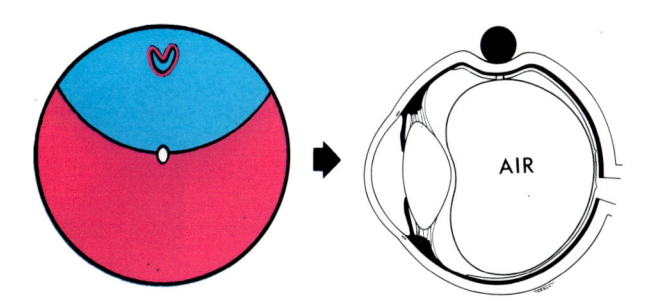

e, Bullous retinal detachment is present with a large horseshoe-shaped tear. Drainage of subretinal fluid followed by intravitreal injection of air, cryotherapy and buckling is the treatment of choice.

PLATE XII

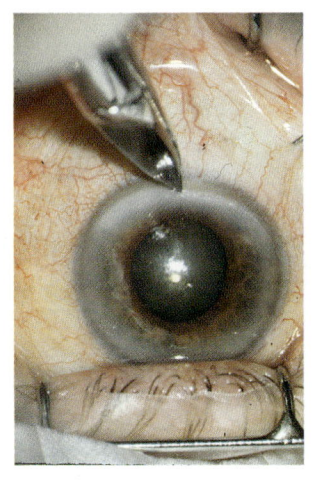

Chapter 10

a, Groove in clear cornea.

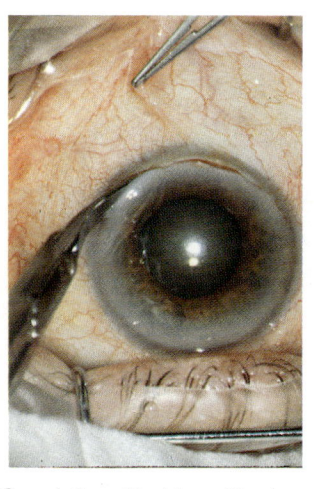

b, Completion of incision with scissors.

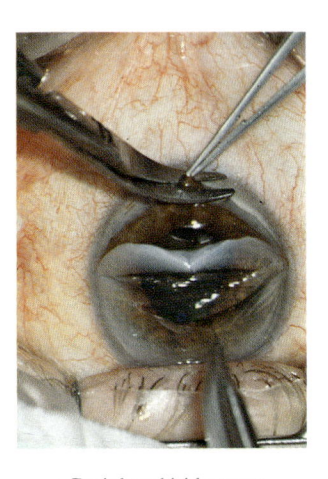

c, Peripheral iridectomy.

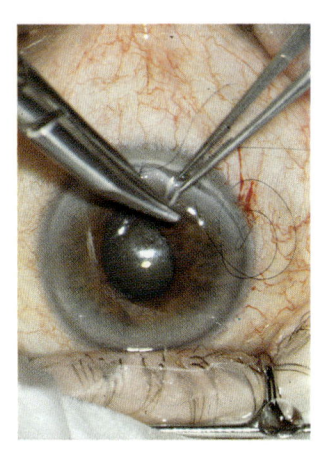

d, Insertion of pre-extraction continuous suture.

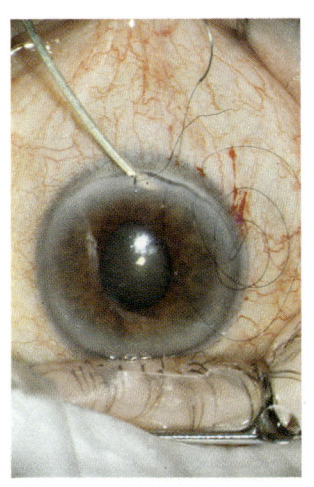

e, Injection of alpha-chymotrypsin into posterior chamber.

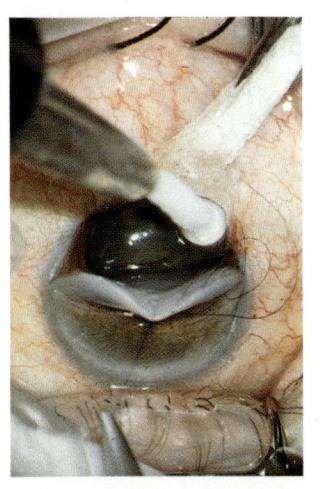

f, Extraction of lens with cryoprobe.

PLATE XIII
Chapter 10

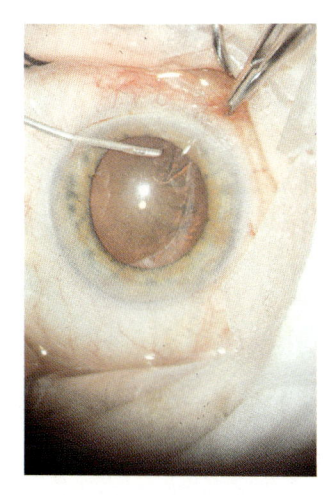

a, Anterior capsulotomy.

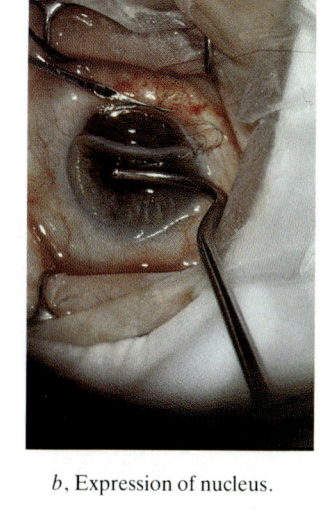

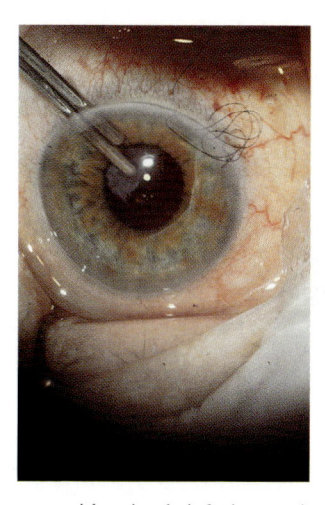

b, Expression of nucleus.

c, Cortical clean-up with a simple infusion–aspiration cannula.

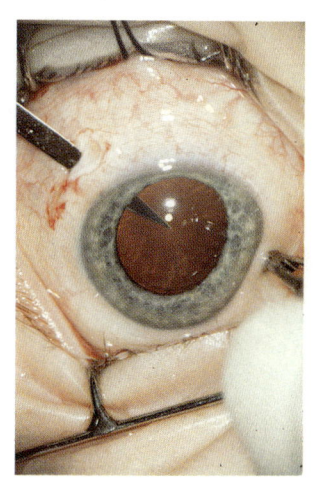

d, Insertion of knife into lens through pars plana.

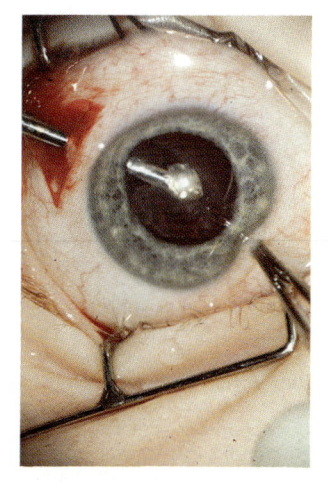

e, Excision of lens with vitreous cutter (lensectomy).

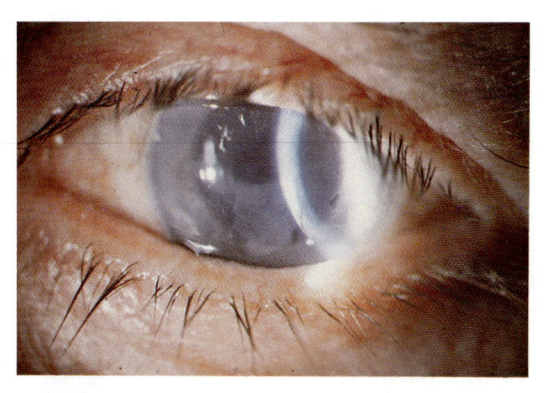

f, Aphakic bullous keratopathy.

PLATE XIV

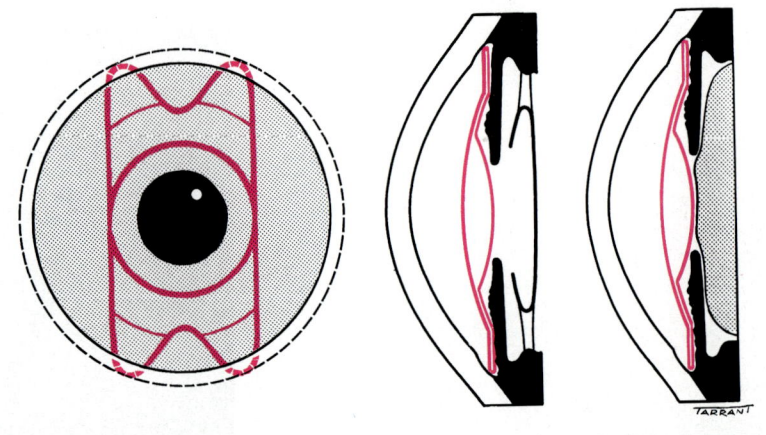

Chapter 10

a, The Choyce Mk. VIII. For many years this lens was the mainstay of anterior chamber intraocular lenses. The correctly sized lens is resting on the scleral spur without distorting the eye. The pupil is freely mobile behind it and there is no iris tuck. An intracapsular extraction may be performed. NB: No iridectomy is shown. (All PMMA or P-CQ, either lathe cut or injection moulded.)

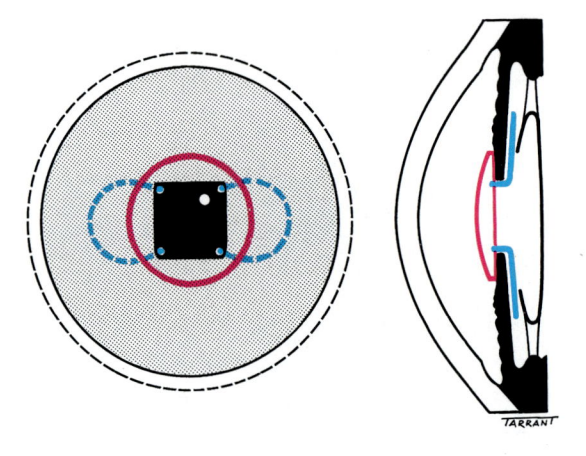

b, The Binkhorst two loop (polypropylene/nylon P-CQ/PMMA) lens is intended for extracapsular extraction and irido-capsular fixation. This type of implant is also losing favour, although it outlasted the four loop variety.

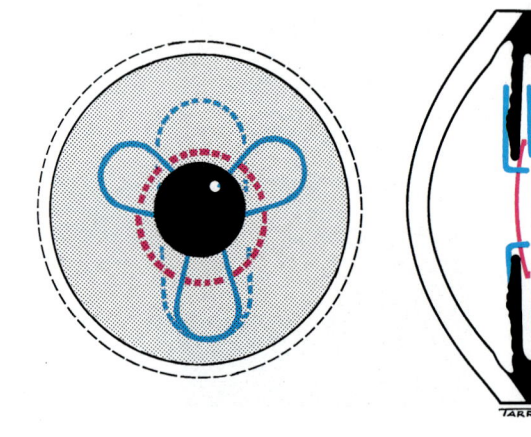

c, The Severin style lens. (PMMA injection moulded optic, Prolene haptic.) This style has the advantage that the optic is placed in the posterior chamber and only the Prolene loops lie anterior to the iris plane. An iris suture is mandatory if the lens is inserted following intracapsular extraction.

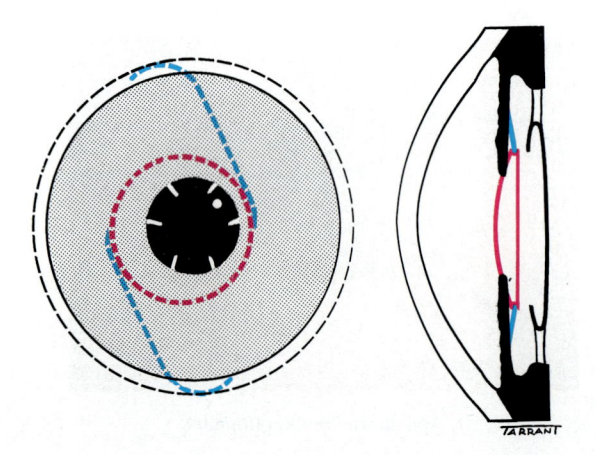

d, The posterior chamber intraocular lens for ciliary sulcus fixation. There are a multitude of variations, either uniplanar or with loops angled at 10° to hold the optic back from the iris. The usual design is convex-plano but biconvex and plano-convex are also made. The Kratz J-loop is shown here, but *see* Fig. 4 (p. 00) for what is probably the most popular – the Sinskey lens. Other refinements include a haptic rim for extracapsular optic clearance, UV filters and oval optics. An extracapsular extraction leaving an intact zonule is essential. (PMMA / P-CQ optic, polypropylene loops.)

PLATE XV

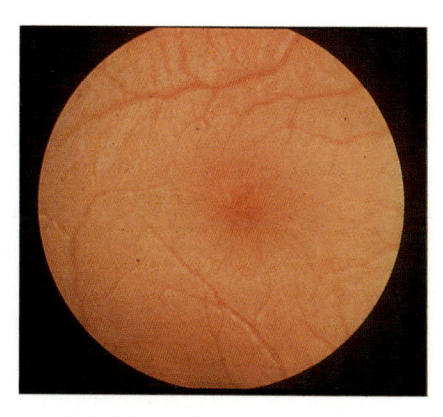

Chapter 19

a, The macula in X-linked retinoschisis, showing the characteristic radial folds.

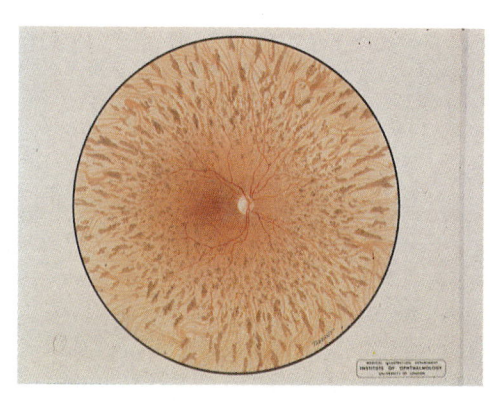

b, c, Fundus of a heterozygote for X-linked ocular albinism. *b*, Fundus painting showing small areas of hypopigmentation and hyperpigmentation, particularly in the retinal periphery.

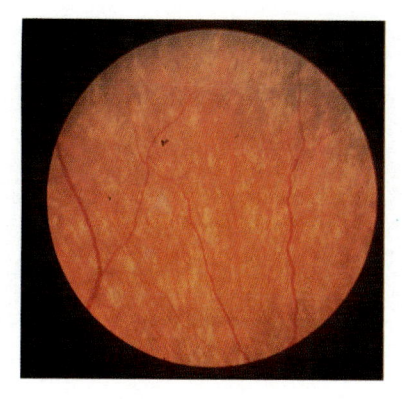

c, Periphery of fundus showing the small areas of hypopigmentation characteristic of this heterozygous state.

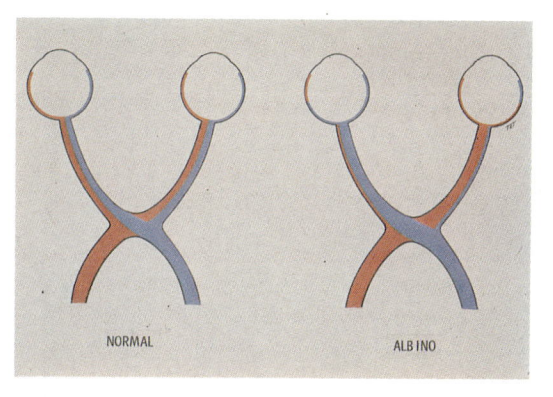

d, Abnormality of visual pathways in albinism. In the human albino about 90 per cent of the fibres cross the optic chiasm. Only those derived from the temporal periphery of the retina remain uncrossed.

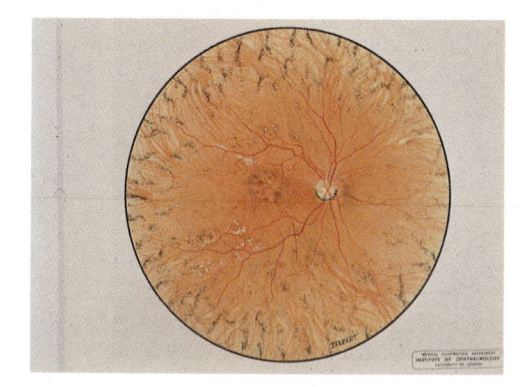

e, f, Fundus of a heterozygote for choroideremia. *e*, Fundus painting showing disturbance of the retinal pigment epithelium, particularly in the periphery of the fundus, with fine pigmentation and some white spots within the retina.

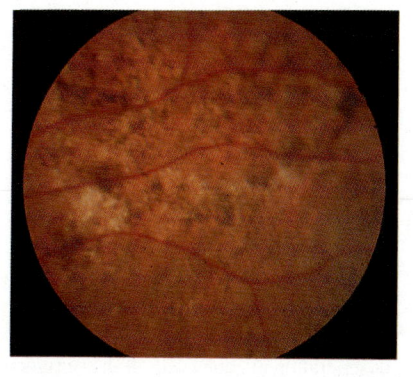

f, Periphery of the fundus, showing the abnormality of the retinal pigment epithelium, and the pigment migration typical of this heterozygous state.

PLATE XVI

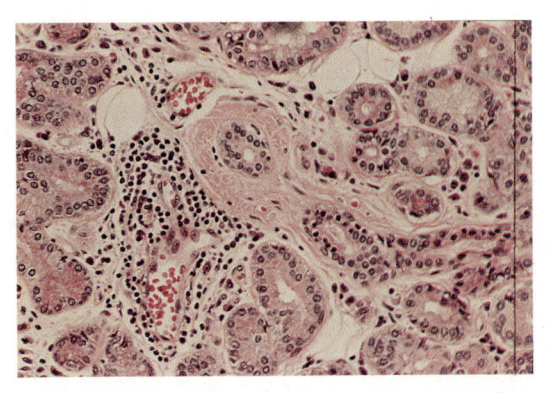

Chapter 21

a, Periductal inflammation in an 'ageing' normal lacrimal gland.

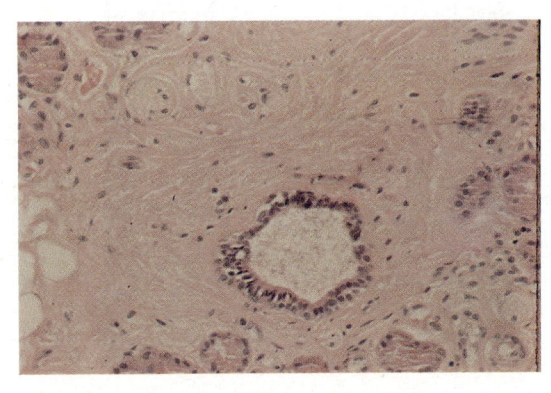

b, Obliteration of nutrient blood vessels and replacement fibrous tissue in the lacrimal gland.

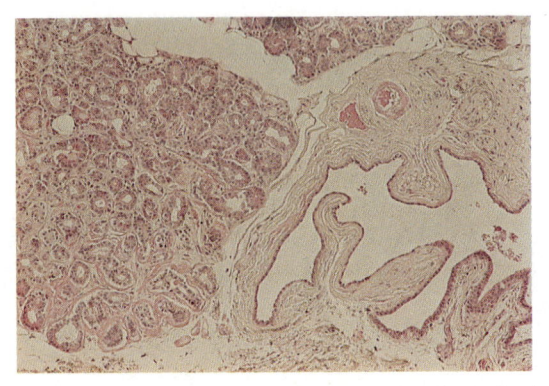

c, Acinae of duct atrophy with cystic dilatation in the lacrimal gland.

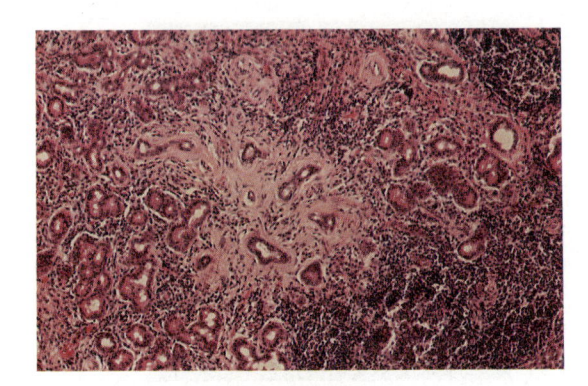

d, Massive lymphoid infiltration in lacrimal gland in secondary Sjögren's syndrome.

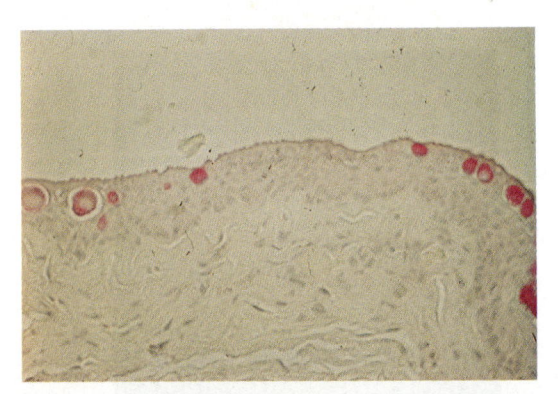

e, Hyaline degeneration in goblet cells of the conjunctiva.

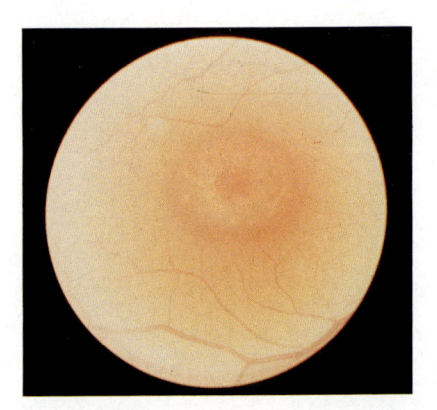

f, Chloroquine maculopathy.

PLATE XVII

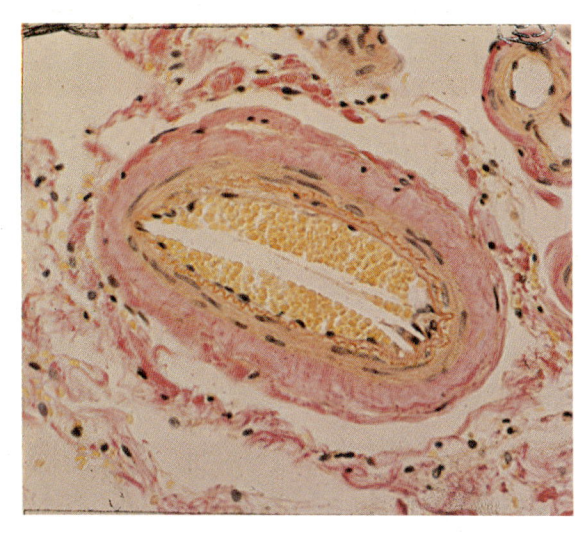

Chapter 21

a, Cross-section of a leptomeningeal artery containing a cholesterol crystal from a patient with ulcerating atheroma in the internal carotid artery.

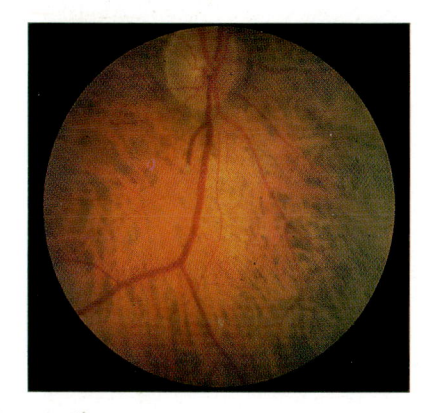

b, Calcific embolism impacted permanently in the retina from a patient with chronic rheumatic heart disease (mitral stenosis).

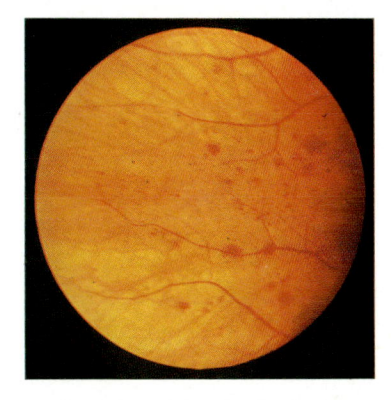

c, Small haemorrhages in peripheral retina in a patient with carotid artery occlusion.

CLASSIFICATION

Primary glaucomas are classified in *Table* I and secondary glaucomas in *Table* II. It should be noted that ocular hypertension (*see below*) has been included as a primary glaucoma. It should also be noted that to diagnose a secondary glaucoma, it is only necessary to identify an elevated IOP secondary to other disease – cupping and field loss need not coexist. However, with continued elevation of IOP, all secondary glaucomas will develop these additional signs.

EPIDEMIOLOGY

Total population surveys of selected areas in the United Kingdom provide information as to the prevalence of glaucoma in this country. From these surveys, it has been found that chronic glaucoma affects approximately 0·8 per cent and ocular hypertension approximately 9 per cent of the over 45s. The prevalence of these two conditions increases with each successive decade. The proportion of the different types of glaucomas seen in the general population has been set out in *Fig.* 1. It is considered that in the United Kingdom, there are 125 000 cases of glaucoma, of which one-third are diagnosed. Fourteen per cent of blind registrations (13 000 people) have glaucoma (although other disease may have contributed, e.g. cataract and macular degeneration) while a similar number have serious visual loss, although not legally

Table II. Secondary glaucomas

Site of block	Mechanism		Example
Open angle			
Pre-trabecular	Membrane overgrowth	'New' blood vessels	– thrombotic glaucoma
		Fibrous tissue	– post uveitis
		Epithelial cells	– epithelial downgrowth
		Endothelial cells	– ICE syndrome
Trabecular	Degeneration	Trauma	– angle recession
		Iron	– haemosiderosis
		Peptides etc.	– topical steroids
	Clogging	Pigment } Protein }	– laser iridotomy, uveitis
		RBCs	– hyphema
		Macrophages	– lens induced glaucoma
		Tumour	– melanoma
Post-trabecular	Raised episcleral venous pressure		Sturge–Weber syndrome Extradural A/V shunt

Closed angle with pupil block			
Precipitating factor	*Cause of angle closure**		*Example*
Forward movement subluxed or dislocated lens	Shallow AC with pupil block		Spontaneous, e.g. Marfan's syndrome. Post-traumatic, e.g. concussion injury
			Degenerative, e.g. old uveitis and secondary cataract
Occlusio pupillae	Marked iris bombé with iris/lens adhesions		Post uveitis

Closed angle without pupil block			
Forward movement lens/iris diaphragm	Angle crowding	Loss of AC	– fistulizing surgery
			– penetrating injury
		Posterior segment disease	
			– encircling buckle
			– pan-retinal laser, tumours
			– choroidal effusion
			– posterior scleritis etc.
		Retrolenticular aqueous	– 'malignant' glaucoma
Intumescent lens	Angle crowding		
Cellular overgrowth of angle	Iris root/trabecular† adhesions	Inflammatory cell	– uveitis sarcoid
		Endothelial cell	– ICE syndrome
		Epithelial cell	– downgrowth
		Neovascularization	– thrombotic glaucoma

* See Fig. 5.
† It should be noted that cellular overgrowth may cause raised IOP with an open angle or the membrane may contract producing angle closure.

blind. Chronic simple glaucoma occurs frequently in some families, making screening of close relatives useful.

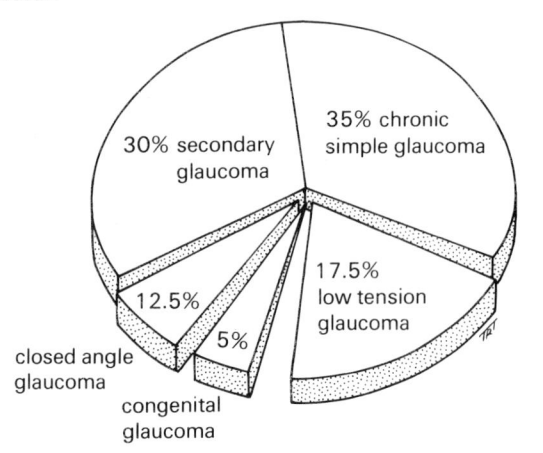

Fig. 1. Pie chart illustrating the relative occurrence of the different types of glaucoma.

PRIMARY GLAUCOMAS

Open Angle

Chronic open angle glaucoma will be described in detail. Variations of primary open angle glaucomas will then be described emphasizing points of special distinction.

Pathogenesis

Current ideas on the pathogenesis of this disease suggest that a progressive degenerative change takes place in the outflow pathways. In man, approximately 75 per cent of aqueous leaves the eye through the trabecular meshwork to Schlemm's canal, the so-called 'conventional' outflow pathway, while the remaining 25 per cent leaves by passing through iris root, ciliary body and sclera – the so-called 'non-conventional' pathway. Under normal conditions, two-thirds of the outflow resistance in the conventional route is found in the outer one-third of the trabecular meshwork and the remainder in the endothelial lining of Schlemm's canal.

It is suggested that in primary open angle glaucoma increased outflow resistance occurs both from loss of trabeculocytes lining the trabecular meshwork struts and from deposition of extracellular material in the intertrabecular spaces which together form channels leading to Schlemm's canal. The former allows hydration of the struts reducing the diameter of these spaces while the latter occludes some or all of these channels. Fluid passes from the trabecular meshwork into Schlemm's canal in giant vacuoles within the endothelial cells. This passive process is dependent upon the amount of aqueous reaching the endothelium and is reduced in chronic glaucoma (*Fig.* 2).

The importance of the non-conventional or uveo-scleral outflow in health and in glaucoma is uncertain. A progressive increase in outflow resistance results in an intermittent and, eventually, a persistent elevation of IOP. It is this change in intraocular pressure which causes glaucomatous cupping and visual field loss.

The optic disc is a three-dimensional structure, so enlargement of the cup may be caused by an increase in the dimensions of the orifice of the cup (C/D ratio), an increase in the depth of the cup and, possibly, alterations in the inclination of its walls. Such an enlargement could result initially from compression of component parts, but is eventually caused by tissue loss. Thus glial cells, neurones and blood vessels all disappear. Neuronal loss will be associated with a nerve fibre bundle type of visual field defect and ophthalmoscopically visible defects (grooves) in

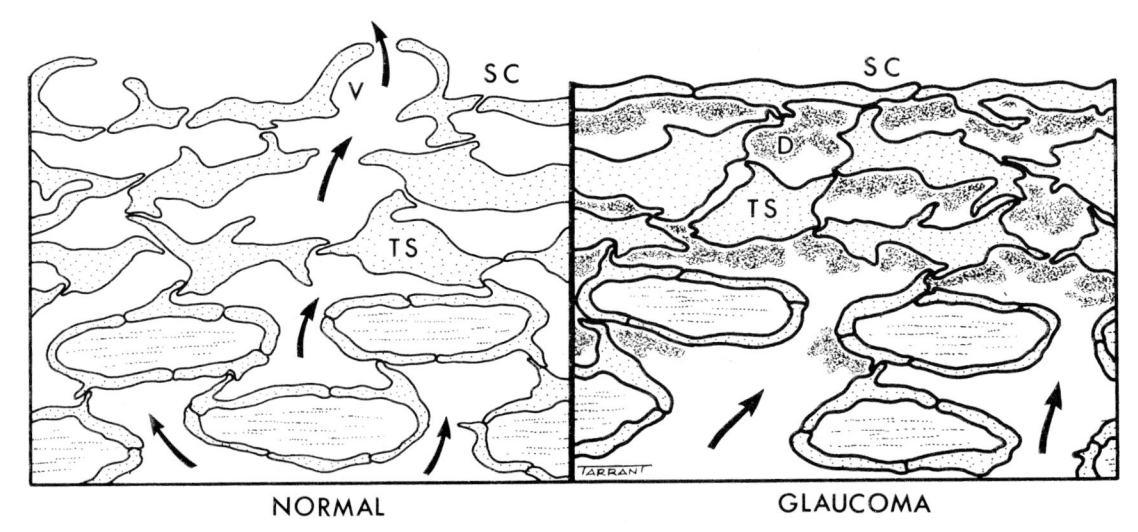

Fig. 2. 'Normal' and 'glaucomatous' trabecular meshwork. Notice that the glaucomatous meshwork shows a reduction in the size of the intertrabecular spaces and deposition of extra cellular material. SC, Canal of Schlem; TS, intertrabecular space; D, intertrabecular deposit; V, giant vacuole.

the retinal nerve fibre layer. These changes in the optic disc may be a direct mechanical effect of elevated intraocular pressure producing distortion of the lamina cribrosa and compressing neurones at the optic disc, a pressure-related reduction in the blood flow to the optic disc, or a combination of both. The reader is referred to the bibliography for recent reviews that discuss factors important in the development of glaucomatous cupping.

Symptoms and Signs

Symptoms are typically few and late. Ocular discomfort is frequent in people who know they have glaucoma but rarely reflects an increase in intraocular pressure. However, rapid increases of IOP in the young may be associated with a non-specific ocular discomfort and may arise from stretching of the deep sensory plexus in the cornea.

Visual disability may involve difficulty with focusing (which by tradition is ascribed to reduced effectiveness of the ciliary muscle in eyes with elevated IOP), although presbyopia is a common symptom of this age group.

Self-awareness of a visual defect occurs late in the disease. The speed of recognition depends on the extent of self-awareness in the patient, the closeness of the defect to fixation, the density of the defect and the rapidity of onset. Total loss of vision in one eye may remain unnoticed in some patients – who only present with visual loss in the second eye. It is the slow development of a defect many degrees from fixation which is difficult to detect; in contrast, the sudden development of a dense paracentral defect is usually noted.

It should be remembered that glaucoma patients have many visual symptoms arising secondary to their treatment or other ocular disease. Pilocarpine causes visual 'constriction', 'darkening' of vision and myopia. Sympathomimetics and occasionally timolol cause blurring of vision. Coincidental cataract or macular degeneration will cause visual disturbance too.

Signs diagnostic for chronic open angle glaucoma are singularly lacking, there are no specific diagnostic signs. The signs seen in chronic open angle glaucoma are shared with chronic glaucoma from any cause. These are set out in *Table* III.

Glaucomatous cupping must be distinguished from other conditions associated with a large optic cup (*Table* IV) (*Figs.* 3–11). This may be congenital or be found in myopia and optic disc colobomata. It may be acquired as a result of an ischaemic optic neuropathy, optic nerve poisons – e.g. methyl alcohol – and in chiasmal tumours. In most instances, glaucoma can be correctly diagnosed if the enlarged optic cup coexists with preservation of a neuroretinal rim which is pink, at least in part. However, advanced

Table III. Signs of chronic simple glaucoma

Sign	Normal	Chronic glaucoma
IOP	8–21 mmHg range	>21 mmHg some or all of the time Up to 50+ mmHg
	Diurnal variation 0–5 mmHg	0–20 mmHg
	Postural change 0–4 mmHg	0–15 mmHg
Optic disc		
Cup	Central or upper temporal	Initial concentric enlargement *Fig.* 12
	Circular	Vertical extension of cup orifice with field defect
		Posterior bowing of laminar cribosa
	Vertical C/D ≤0.3	C/D = 0.9+ in late stages
	Symmetrical cups	Asymmetrical cups
Rim	Pink	Pale and atrophic in late stages
	Thickest at upper and lower poles	Diffuse thinning
		Notching of rim at upper and lower poles of disc
Blood vessels	Smooth and undulating course over disc	Angulated or kinked
		Flame-shaped haemorrhages
Nerve fibre layer	Intact or invisible	Grooves or defects precede visual loss
Anterior chamber angle	Varying amounts of pigmentation at trabecular meshwork and Schwalbe's line	360° mid-trabecular band with pigment dispersion syndrome
Visual field		'Nerve fibre bundle' defects
		Nasal step only outside central 15°, in 10% of patients
		(Defects respect horizontal meridian, See Chapter 3)
Anterior chamber	Unless pseudoexfoliation or pigment dispersion is present, there is no difference from age-related normal eyes	

glaucoma with considerable atrophy of the neuro-retinal rim may be extremely difficult to differentiate from ischaemic optic neuropathy or chronic chiasmal compression. For these cases, a careful neurological examination and CAT scan are helpful. Points of differentiation between glaucomatous cupping and other conditions of the optic nerve are set out in Table IV.

Any disease of the optic nerve may give rise to a similar type of 'glaucomatous' visual field defect. Points of differentiation between the visual field defects seen in glaucoma and other eye conditions are set out in Table V.

Table IV. Differential diagnosis of glaucomatous cupping

Condition	Points of differentiation
Congenital:—	
Coloboma	Irregular cup orifice, cup depth
	Abnormal course disc blood vessels
	Optic disc asymmetry
	Associated neurological conditions
Pit	Temporal with serous retinal detachment
	Polar differentiation may be impossible as similar appearance in glaucoma
Megalopapilla	Large optic disc
Acquired:—	
Ischaemic optic neuropathy	Diffuse pallor of rim
	Cup shallow often without being vertically oval
	Large optic cup with atrophy – similar appearance to advanced glaucoma
Chiasmal compression	Visual field defect may coexist with normal looking disc
	Diffuse atrophy of neuroretinal rim

Table V. Differential diagnosis of glaucomatous field defects

Condition	Features
Congenital	
Myopia	Refractive scotoma, 'irregular' defects which go with myopic condition
Coloboma	Irregular defect
Acquired	
Retinal	Associated retinopathy
Optic nerve	Nerve fibre bundle loss as for glaucoma
Chiasmal and retrochiasmal	Haemianopic defects

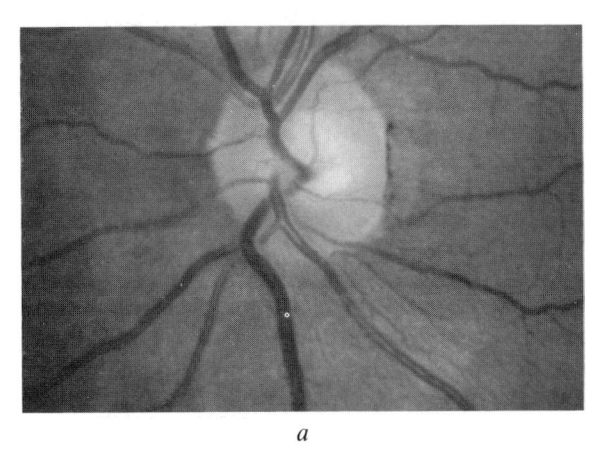

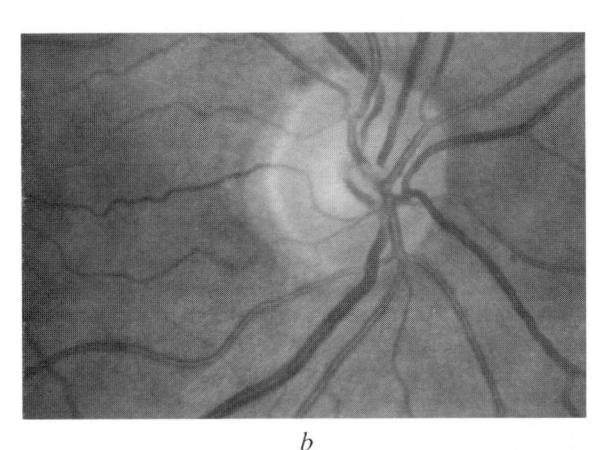

Fig. 3. Photographs of two optic discs of one patient. *a*, Left eye; *b*, right eye. Notice that the central cups are of equal size. A normal circumlinear vessel is visible in the right eye together with a normal appearance to the retinal nerve fibre layer.

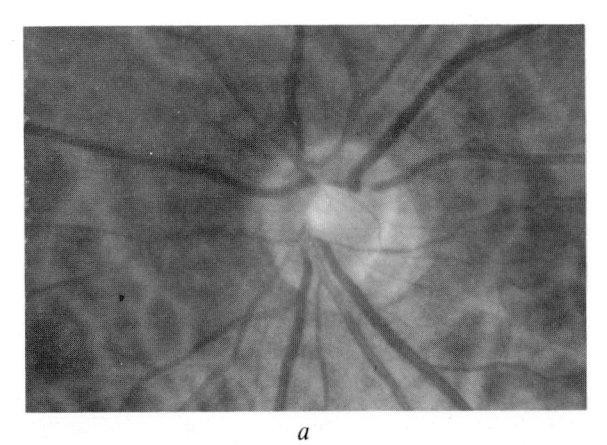

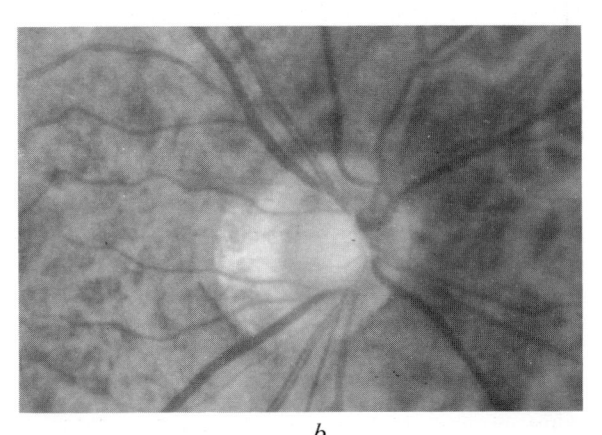

Fig. 4. Normal optic discs. *a*, Left eye; *b*, right eye. In this case note the small infero-temporal crescent and the unequal size of the scleral canals. The optic cup appears larger in the right eye and this eye also has the larger optic disc.

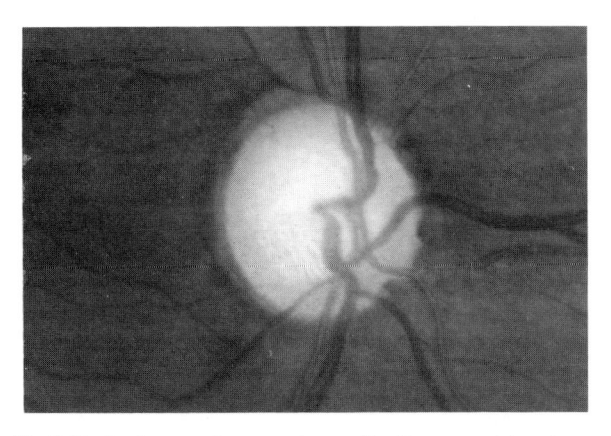

Fig. 5. Early glaucomatous cupping, notice the concentric enlargement to the optic cup, baring of the circumlinear vessel superiorly together with preservation of a pink neuroretinal rim.

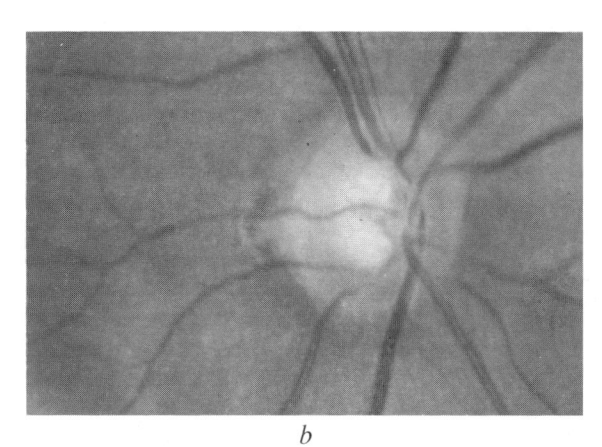

Fig. 6. Focal notching of the neuroretinal rim. A left (*a*) and right (*b*) eye of the same patient are shown; the right eye is normal. The left eye shows focal notching of the neuroretinal rim at 6 o'clock.

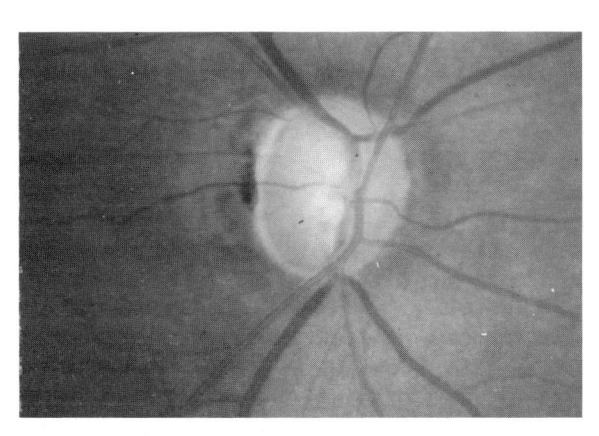

Fig. 7. Advanced glaucomatous cupping. In this instance notice deviation of the retinal vessels at the upper and lower pole as they pass over the edges of the enlarged optic cup.

Treatment

The aim of treatment is to lower IOP to a level where (further) visual loss does not occur. Frequently, the success of treatment is only recognized retrospectively. Increasing sophistication in visual field analysis allows earlier recognition of progressive visual damage. The management plan depends on whether or not visual loss exists at the outset of treatment. Two groups of patients may be identified: those with and those without detectable visual field loss. The latter group have ocular hypertension.

Ocular hypertension was the term given to patients without recognizable visual field loss having chronic elevation of IOP. This term has been criticized because it suggested a more benign condition than chronic glaucoma. Since its introduction, ophthalmologists have a better understanding of what constitutes glaucomatous cupping and visual field loss. Many of the patients originally diagnosed as having ocular hypertension would, if they presented now, be considered to have chronic glaucoma.

The prevalence of ocular hypertension is approximately ten times that of chronic open angle glaucoma and, although it is one of several risk factors in the development of this disease, a high proportion of ocular hypertensives will not progress to develop chronic open angle glaucoma. Recognition of this fact allows retention of the term. Treatment will be discussed separately for ocular hypertension and elevated IOP with visual field loss.

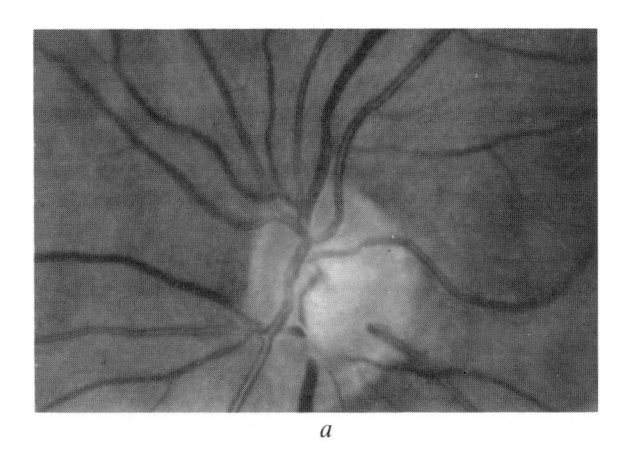

Ocular Hypertension

The risk of visual field loss occurring in the untreated patient is approximately 10 per cent in 10 years. The risk increases with the height of the intraocular pressure and with the presence of other risk factors. These risk factors have been set out in *Table* VI.

The aim of treatment in this group is to lower intraocular pressure from a level where it is considered likely that visual damage will occur, in time, to a level where it is considered unlikely. It will be seen from *Table* VI that the 'starting' IOP may vary considerably. These patients are being treated prophylactically so that they should *not* be rendered symptomatic as a result of treatment. Although it is often sufficient to lower IOP to the low 20s, in some instances it is considered advisable to reduce

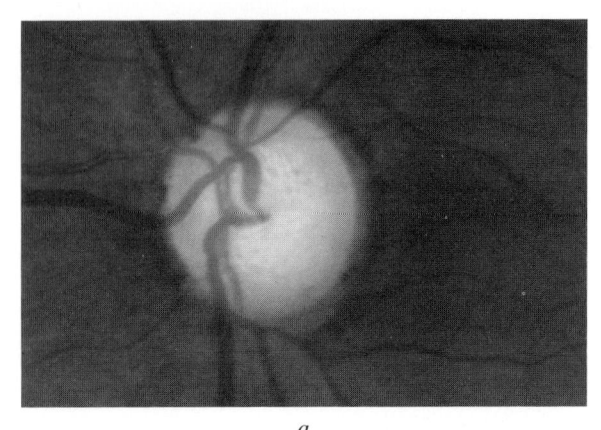

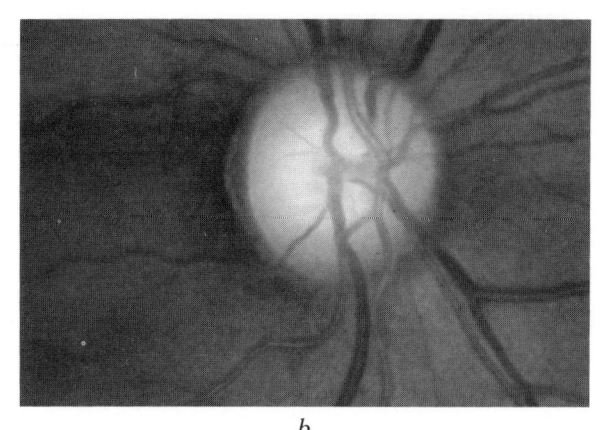

Fig. 8. Ischaemic optic neuropathy. The right eye (*b*) is normal but the left eye (*a*) has suffered an ischaemic optic neuropathy. Note that in the left eye there is diffuse pallor of the neuroretinal rim together with concentric enlargement of the optic cup.

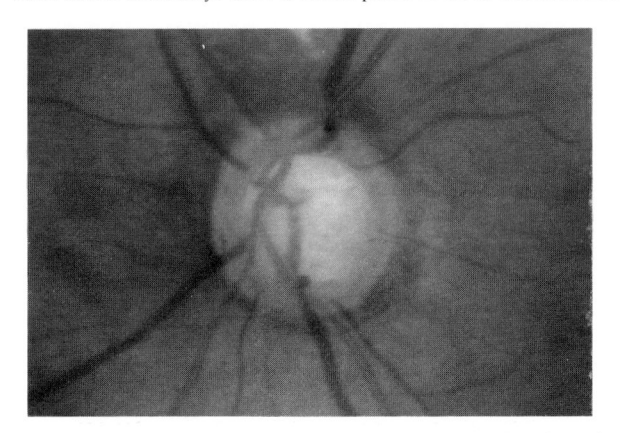

Fig. 9. Optic disc pit. In this instance the optic cup is enlarged as evidenced by baring of the circumlinear vessel superiorly. Note the small blue–grey coloured oval pit in the optic cup at the 5 o'clock position of the optic disc.

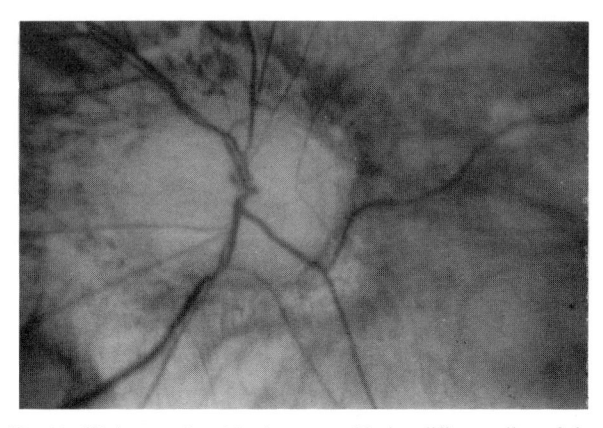

Fig. 11. High myopia with glaucoma. Notice diffuse pallor of the optic discs together with peri-papillary atrophy. The outline of the optic cup is indistinct but angulation of the infero-temporal retinal vein is present as it crosses the cup orifice at the 7 o'clock position.

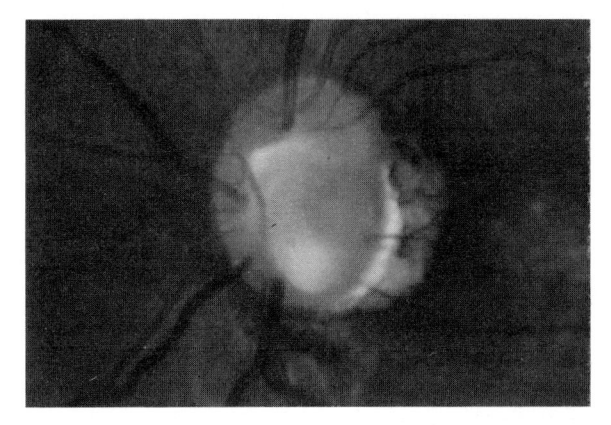

Fig. 10. Coloboma of the optic disc. In this case notice the irregular orifice of the optic cup together with colour variation indicating an irregular base to the cup. In addition, the retinal vessels take an anomolous course as they cross the surface of both the optic disc and cup.

IOP to below 21 mmHg. The treatment methods are outlined below, in the section on chronic open angle glaucoma.

The long term progress of these patients is monitored by sequential photographs of the optic disc and visual field tests. Tests of contrast sensitivity, colour vision and visual evoked potential may play a role in detecting very early defects in visual function. They have not been universally adopted at this time.

Elevated IOP with Visual Field Loss

The aim of treatment is to reduce IOP to below 21 mmHg all the time. In patients with advanced glaucoma, it is advisable to reduce the pressure to 18 mmHg or below and, in patients in low tension glaucoma, *for whom treatment is considered necessary*, the pressure may need to be reduced to less than 15 mmHg. It should be remembered that diurnal variation in IOP occurs; 70 per cent of patients have their peak pressures between the hours of 10 and 2 o'clock and this is the optimum time to check IOPs in long term management. It should also be remembered that the intraocular pressure may rise considerably when the patient lies down. This postural hypertension may be the cause of progressive visual field loss in apparent low tension glaucoma or in patients who are considered well controlled on treatment.

Table VI. Risk factors in patients with ocular hypertension

Type	Risk factors	Management plan
Moderate risk	Disease in contralateral eye Glaucoma Ischaemic optic neuropathy Central retinal vein occlusion 'High' steroid responder ($<pHpH$)	Reduce IOP <21 mmHg
High risk	IOP >28 mmHg Elderly patient C/D >0·6 Positive family history of glaucoma Pigment dispersion Pseudoexfoliation	Reduce IOP at least to low 20s
Low risk	Diabetes Myopia	

Table VII. Topical and systemically applied anti-glaucoma medications

Type	Strength	Duration of action	Mechanisms of action	Side effects
Parasympathomimetics				
Pilocarpine drops	$\frac{1}{2}$–10%	2–8 h	Ciliary muscle contraction rotates scleral spur and opens trabecular meshwork	Bow ache Myopia Miosis
Ocuserts	P20 = Pilo $\frac{1}{2}$, 1% P40 = Pilo 2%	7 days	Outflow resistance reduced	Dark vision Anecdotal association with retinal detachment
Gel	(Piloplex)*	12 h		
Sympathomimetics				
Adrenaline	$\frac{1}{2}$–1%	12 h	Alpha conventional outflow ↑	Mydriasis, blurring
Alpha beta agonists			Beta 1, beta 2 non-conventional outflow ↑ Beta aqueous production ↑	Cystoid macular oedema in aphakia Hyperaemia Brow ache
(Prodrug: Dipivalyl adrenaline)*		12 h		Lower incidence of side effects affecting external eye
Guanethidine and adrenaline (Ganda)	1 and 0·2% to 5 and 1%	12 h	Guanethidine potentiates alpha effect of adrenaline	The same as, but more pronounced than adrenaline
Salbutamol* 2% beta agonist	2%	12 h	Aqueous production ↑ Non-conventional outflow ↓	?
Sympatholytics				
B-blocker Timolol	0.25–0.5%	12 h+	Aqueous production ↓ Non-conventional outflow ↑	Blurred vision keratitis Asthma, bradycardia Hypotension
Betaxolol*	0·5%	12 h	Selective B_1-blocker May be of use in patients with reversible airways disease	
Carbonic anhydrase inhibitors				
Diamox	250 mg tabs 500 mg tabs	6 hourly 12 hourly	Aqueous production ↓	GI upsets Anorexia
Daranide (Oratrol)	50 mg	12 h		Depression Renal stones Parasthesiae

* This preparation is not currently available in the United Kingdom.
↑, raised; ↓, lowered.

The treatment of chronic open angle glaucoma may be subdivided into stages. The first line treatment is medical. This should be restricted to a regime which is both tolerable and practical for the individual patient. The working adult frequently fails to instil medicines during the day while the arthritic, elderly patient may be incapable of instilling drops at all. Many patients find it impossible to instil more than two different types of medicines on a regular and long term basis. Non-compliance or poor control of intraocular pressure merits laser trabeculoplasty or surgery. A list of the commonly used topical medicines is set out in *Table* VII. The noted side effects are a frequent cause of intermittent non-compliance.

The first choice medicine for the working adult is a drop that need only be instilled twice a day, while miotics that need to be instilled four times a day are best for the retired patient. Axial lens opacities preclude the use of pilocarpine in many patients; here a sympathomimetic, causing slight mydriasis, is often beneficial. An increase in the hypotensive effects of pilocarpine occurs when increasing the strength from 0·50 to 2 per cent (or 4 per cent in eyes with heavily pigmented irides). A similar increase in the hypotensive effect occurs when changing from adrenaline to the higher strengths of Ganda (guanethidine). Timolol 0·25 per cent and 0·50 per cent have a similar hypotensive effect. An additive effect is seen between the different classes of medicines outlined in *Table* VII, with the exception of adding adrenaline to timolol. A history of reversible airways disease (bronchitis or asthma) would usually preclude the use of timolol, although a selective β-blocker would appear not to cause this effect.

The second line of treatment is surgical, to which – recently – laser trabeculoplasty has been added.

Laser trabeculoplasty should be considered if the measures outlined above are insufficient. Laser trabeculoplasty has an additive effect to the drugs noted above. Its hypotensive effect is caused by increasing outflow facility, possibly by producing collagen shrinkage on the inner aspect of the trabecular meshwork and opening the intertrabecular spaces. It has been shown to lower intraocular pressure by a mean of 8–10 mmHg in patients on medical treatment and by a mean of 14 mmHg in patients who are not receiving medical treatment. Laser treatment should be reserved for patients who are not controlled on maximally tolerated medical treatment and who would otherwise be considered for glaucoma surgery. The treatment regime (*Fig.* 12) usually employed consists of placing 50 spots on the anterior half of the trabecular meshwork over 180°.

The spot size should cover the anterior half of the trabecular meshwork. This may be recorded as a spot 50–150 μmin size. The burns should last for 0·1 s and be of sufficient intensity to cause transient blanching. A power of approximately 0·75 watts usually suffices to do this. Should large gas bubble formation or permanent blanching be produced, then the energy level is too high and the hypotensive effect less certain. Complications include short lived ocular hypertension, which can be prevented by pre-treatment with pilocarpine and/or Diamox, and inflammation, which can be lessened by giving topical steroids for 3–4 days afterwards. Less commonly, haemorrhage, uveitis, PAS formation and reduced accommodation occur.

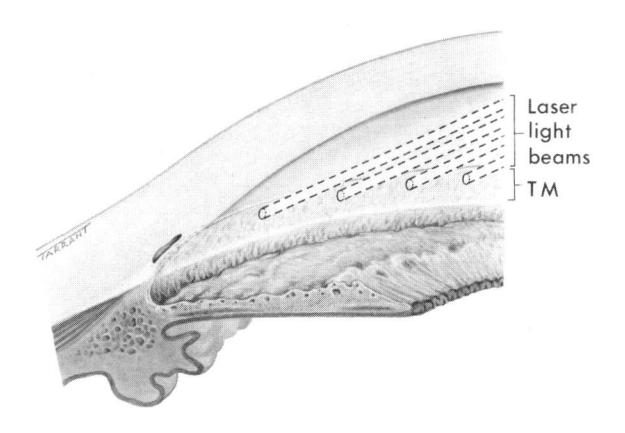

Fig. 12. Schematic three-dimensional view of inclination and placement of laser beams during argon laser trabeculoplasty.

Surgical treatment is, in most instances, fistulizing surgery. The guarded sclerostomy (trabeculectomy) operation under a fornix or limbal based flap is safe, 85 per cent successful in lowering intraocular pressure to below 21 mmHg and has little long term effect on vision. It should be considered if medical treatment and laser trabeculoplasty have failed to control intraocular pressure. As with any intraocular operation, complications include infection, haemorrhage and cataract formation. There are specific complications that follow filtration surgery. These have been set out in *Table* VIII.

Malignant glaucoma is the term given to a form of secondary glaucoma with a shallow or absent chamber that occurs in phakic eyes in the early postoperative period. The name was given because the glaucoma did not respond to pilocarpine. Typically it follows the trephine or unguarded sclerostomy (Scheie) operation. In these eyes bulk outflow of aqueous is high in the immediate postoperative period. The adoption of the guarded sclerostomy (trabeculectomy) has reduced the frequency of this complication. The mechanism is considered to be an initial shallowing of the anterior chamber followed by retrolenticular pooling of aqueous. Occlusion of the sclerostomy is followed by marked elevation of intraocular pressure (*Fig.* 13). The condition seems more likely to occur in eyes with a shallow anterior chamber preoperatively, together with an increase in lens mobility. A patient who suffers from malignant glaucoma in one eye runs an appreciable risk of developing it in the second eye.

Continued obstruction to the forward movement of aqueous may come from close apposition of the

Table VIII. Postoperative complications of trabeculectomy

Symptoms and signs	Probable cause	Treatment
Early		
Blurring of vision	Refractive change with forward movement of the lens	Spontaneous resolution
Shallow anterior chamber c̄ hypotony		
Large pale bleb	Excess outflow through sclerostomy	Spontaneous resolution after 4–5 days
Small inflamed bleb some pain and congestion, choroidal effusion	Excess outflow through uveo-scleral pathway	Topical steroids and spontaneous resolution 1–4 weeks *but* reform AC if lens–cornea contact.
c̄ hypertension (malignant glaucoma)	Ciliolenticular or lens sclerostomy block	Cycloplegics, Chandler's operation or cataract extraction
Raised IOP	Inflammation around sclerostomy	Topical steroids – massage
Late		
Raised IOP	Keloid scar in bleb wall	Incise
Cystic bleb		
Infection	Opportunistic bacteria	Antibiotics/steroids
		Reform bleb
Leak	Progressive atrophy bleb wall	Leave unless AC shallow
Cataract	Coincidence or complication	Cataract extraction through a transcorneal incision
		Bleb may need revision too

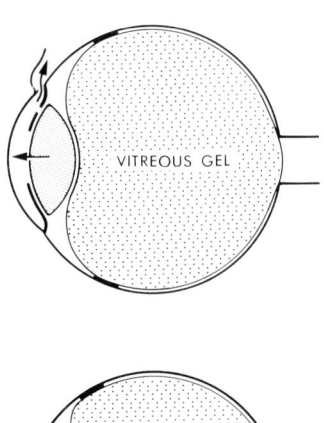

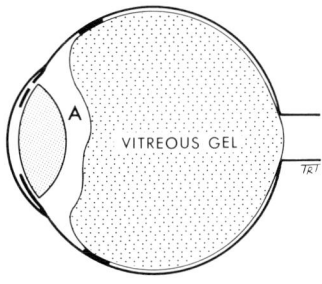

Fig. 13. Accumulation of aqueous in the retrolenticular space in malignant glaucoma. A, Retrolenticular aqueous.

ciliary processes to the lens equator, giving rise to the alternative name of cilio-lenticular block (and, indeed, treatment by shrinking the ciliary processes with a laser has been tried). An alternative explanation for the development of the glaucoma is closure of the sclerostomy internally by the lens and externally by fibrous tissue proliferation (*Fig.* 4).

The treatment of malignant glaucoma consists initially of both cycloplegic and hypotensive agents. Should the anterior chamber fail to reform and the pressure not fall, then surgery is necessary. Surgical treatment may be Chandler's operation – reformation of the anterior chamber combined with aspiration of fluid vitreous (and again it used to be considered that aqueous accumulated within or behind the vitreous although in the intact vitreous gel there is no reason for this bulk flow of aqueous to occur; aqueous may well remain in the retrolenticular space in these eyes). An alternative approach is to reform the anterior chamber and release retrolenticular aqueous through a pars plana incision or, should that prove impossible, a pars plana vitrectomy. Finally, should all these fail, then intracapsular cataract extraction associated with an anterior vitrectomy should be carried out.

Fistulizing surgery may fail early (within the first 1–2 months) or late. The former is seen with failure to establish fistulizing bleb in the immediate postoperative period. Histological examination of such eyes shows a marked inflammatory reaction around the fistula. At the present time recognition of marked inflammation clinically merits treatment with intensive steroids. Late failure is seen months or years after an apparently successful fistulizing operation. A gradual rise in IOP occurs. This is associated with thickening of the walls of the bleb. If required, the bleb in these eyes can be revised by incising the thickened wall.

Should the trabeculectomy operation fail to control the intraocular pressure, then alternative approaches include reoperation, cyclodialysis or implantation of a silicone tube. The reader is referred to the bibliography for techniques and results.

The long term management of chronic glaucoma consists not only of monitoring intraocular pressure but also checking the appearance of the optic disc and visual field. The optic disc should be photographed at the onset of treatment for use in subsequent comparative observations. Sequential photographs are rarely justified for perimetry is a more sensitive indicator of change. Sequential perimetry should be undertaken, at least 6-monthly, using the most sophisticated technique that the facilities, time and the patient's concentration permit. Progressive field loss merits a search for non-glaucomatous causes (cataract, CRVO, etc.) before concluding that the intraocular pressure is 'too high for the eye' and should be further lowered.

Low Tension Glaucoma

This diagnosis is considered when glaucomatous cupping and field loss coexist with an intraocular pressure less than 21 mmHg. The diagnosis is confirmed when the IOP remains less than 21 mmHg not only throughout the 24 hour period and when the patient lies flat, but also when no other cause for the visual loss can be found. The disease is usually bilateral, occurs in middle age and affects women more frequently than men. Progression of the disease is seen with recurring optic disc haemorrhages which are followed by further visual loss. The pattern of visual field loss is 'stop-go', the occurrence of dense paracentral defects interspersed with periods of many years of non-progression. Treatment, if justified at all (because of the difficulty in assessing progression), is to lower IOP to less than 15 mmHg. This usually requires fistulizing surgery.

Juvenile Glaucoma

Typically, this condition is often undiagnosed, from failure to consider glaucoma in children without buphthalmos. Not infrequently, an apparent angle anomaly is visible. Treatment is as for the adult disease except that trabeculotomy could be considered safer than trabeculectomy.

Congenital Glaucoma

Primary buphthalmos may be sub-divided into trabeculodysgenesis, where a visible angle anomaly or tissue remnants (the so called 'morning mist') are visible. Examples of this are seen in Axenfeld's anomaly. Secondly, it may be called 'irido-trabeculodysgenesis' where both iris and trabecular anomalies may be seen (e.g. Rieger's anomaly, and, thirdly, corneo-irido-trabeculodysgenesis such as Peters' anomaly. Goniotomy carries a good prognosis only for the first of these 3 sub-divisions.

Secondary buphthalmos may be diagnosed where other extra-ocular development anomalies co-exist (*Table* IX).

Fifty per cent are present at birth, 70 per cent are diagnosed in the first 6 months of life and 80 per cent by 1 year. Buphthalmos needs to be differentiated from other causes of large corneae, cloudy corneae and patients with photophobia and lacrimation (*Table* X). It may be seen in a number of systemic conditions (*Table* XI). Management consists, first, of examination under anaesthetic (EUA) and measurement of IOP under anaesthesia without muscle relaxants, e.g. (ketamine), together with gonioscopy and fundoscopy. Goniotomy is the treatment of choice, failing this trabeculectomy or trabeculotomy.

Table IX. Classification of buphthalmos

Primary	No other associated ocular abnormality
Secondary	Cleavage syndromes – Axenfeldt's, Rieger's or Peter's anomaly
	Aniridia
	Sturge–Weber, von Recklinghausen's disease
	Infection – Rubella (+cataract)
	Metabolic – Lowe's syndrome (+cataract)

Table X. Differential diagnosis of buphthalmos

Large corneae	Megalocorneae, high myopia
Cloudy corneae	Hereditary corneal dystrophy, idiopathic corneal oedema, cystinurea, mucopolysaccharridoses
Photophobia and lacrimation	Interstitial keratitis, blepharitis, conjunctivitis and kertatitis
	Corneal ulceration
Tears in Descemet's membrane	Birth injury, keratoconus
Secondary glaucoma in neonates	Inflammation, trauma, tumours and others

Table XI. Associated systemic conditions in buphthalmos

Mesodermal	Marfan's, Marchesani's syndrome
Metabolic	Lowe's syndrome, homocystinurea, sulphite oxidase deficiency.
Hamartoses	von Recklinghausen's disease, von Hippel–Lindau's disease, naevus of ota, Sturge–Weber syndrome
Others	Down's syndrome, Hallerman–Strieff syndrome, Werner's syndrome, Conradi's syndrome, Pierre-Robin syndrome

Follow-up examinations require repeated EUAs until the child is able to be applanated with topical anaesthesia. Careful watch needs to be kept for an increase in the C/D ratio as evidence of disease progression and the development of amblyopia.

Closed Angle Glaucoma

The angle of the anterior chamber is formed by the meeting of an imaginary radial line passing along the peripheral iris with a similar line passing through the peripheral cornea. This circular zone lies 1–2 mm behind the limbus. The trabecular meshwork lies at the apex of the angle. Under normal conditions, this angle has a width of approximately 40°. The angle may be more acute in eyes having a shallower axial anterior chamber depth and/or a greater anterior convexity to the peripheral iris than normal. Angle closure is present if part or all of the iris root lies in contact with the trabecular meshwork. This closure may be iris trabecular apposition or adhesion; only the former is reversible.

The width of the anterior chamber angle may be graded. Numerous quantitative schemes exist. Observer error and inter-observer variation reduce their validity. A simple clinical scheme is outlined below:

Grade 1: Open angle, unlikely to close under any condition.
Grade 2: Narrow angle, angle closure could occur.
Grade 3: Angle possibly closed.
Grade 4: Angle closure present, at least in part of the angle.

Examination of the anterior chamber angle by indirect gonioscopy should be performed with both a Goldmann lens and a Zeiss four-mirror lens. The former, when placed on the eye and held with the eye in the primary position, allows an appreciation of angle width and permits the grading scheme outlined above. With the eye rotated in the direction of the gonioscopy lens, it is frequently possible to see into the depths of the anterior chamber angle. However, even with this manoeuvre, anterior iris convexity may not allow visualization of the whole of the trabecular meshwork. To do this, indentation gonioscopy is required (See Chapter 3, p.67).

Indentation gonioscopy is carried out with the Zeiss four-mirror gonioscopy lens. The glass surface that comes into contact with the cornea has a greater radius of curvature than the cornea. This means that the apex of the cornea comes into contact with the contact lens first, removing the need for gonioscopy fluid. This is in contrast to the Goldmann lens, which has a smaller radius of curvature and requires a fluid interface to prevent air bubble formation. The Zeiss lens may indent axial cornea, displacing aqueous towards the periphery of the chamber, and artificially separate iris from the cornea, thus widening the angle. This manoeuvre distinguishes between angle closure from iris trabecular apposition and iris trabecular adhesion, for, in the latter condition, the *false* angle is widened but angle closure persists. Careful gonioscopy allows identification of the junction between angle closure and the open angle by this manoeuvre. Recognition of peripheral anterior synechiae allows the correct diagnosis to be made as well as suggesting the possible prognosis.

Pathogenesis

The factors that could produce angle closure are summarized in *Table* XII and *Fig.* 14. The dimensions of the anterior chamber appear the same in the fellow eye of patients suffering an acute attack of angle closure glaucoma as in eyes with sub-acute and chronic angle closure glaucoma. Characteristically, all these eyes have an axial anterior chamber depth of <2·5 mm (usually <2·1 mm) and a slit-like angle appearance on gonioscopy. For the angle to remain

Table XII. Mechanisms producing angle closure

Increase in iris bombé	Increase in pupil block (Reduction in iris tone) (Increase in aqueous production)
Shallowing of the anterior chamber	Increase in lens size with age Forward movement of lens Miotics Accommodation
Crowding of the angle	Mydriasis (even in presence of iridectomy)

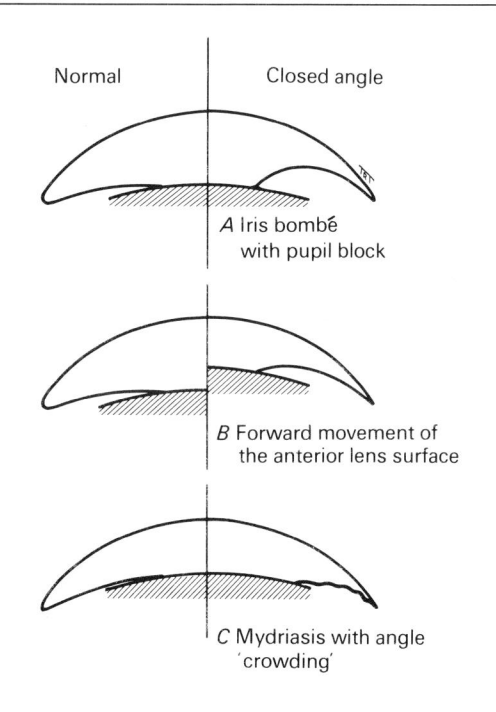

Fig. 14. Mechanisms of angle closure.

slit-like in eyes with an anterior chamber depth varying between 1·5 and 2·5 mm, there has to be a varying degree of anterior iris convexity (iris bombé). The deeper the anterior chamber before iridectomy, the wider the angle afterwards, suggesting that a greater than average degree of iris bombé existed beforehand. The effects of an iridectomy on a group of fellow eyes and a comparison of iris profile in eyes with similar anterior chamber depth is shown in *Fig.* 15.

Physiological pupil block is considered to be present in all eyes. It exists with a pressure differential of 1–2 mmHg between the posterior and anterior chambers. Iris 'tone' may vary so that the same pressure difference may cause a greater degree of iris bombé in eyes with less iris tone.

With advancing age (and also with accommodation) the anterior lens surface moves forwards, thus shallowing the anterior chamber. This occurs with age from progressive growth of the lens and with accommodation by relaxation of the zonular fibres. Shallowing of the anterior chamber is associated with shallowing of the angle – either by pushing the peripheral iris forward, towards the cornea and/or by an increase in pupil block. The difference between these two is seen in eyes having a shallow anterior chamber (<1·8 mm axially) who may or may not develop significant widening of the angle after an iridectomy.

The conditions under which maximum mydriasis occurs are: dim illumination and/or maximum physiological stress.

Acute Closed Angle Glaucoma

Closure of most or all of the anterior chamber angle produces a rapid rise in intraocular pressure. In acute closed angle glaucoma, this rapid increase is sufficient to infarct one or more of the radial iris vessels, resulting in a breakdown of the blood–aqueous barrier, prostaglandin release and the development of the signs of inflammation. Most of the symptoms and

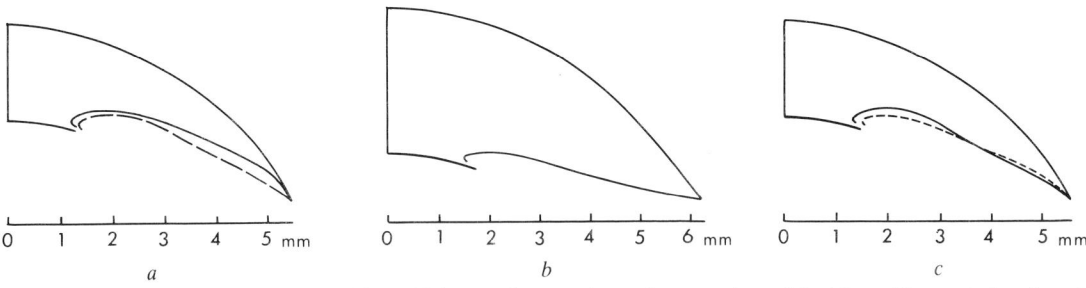

Fig. 15. Anterior chamber profiles constructed from slit image photographs. *a*, A comparison of the iris profile seen before (continuous line) and after iridectomy (dotted line). Showing that the only dimension of the anterior chamber to change is the iris periphery. *b*, Anterior chamber profile in age-matched normals. *c*, Anterior chamber profile after iridectomy (dotted line) and anterior chamber depth matched normals (continuous line). (After Coakes R., Lloyd-Jones D. and Hitchings R. A. *Trans. Ophthalmol. Soc. UK* 1979; **99**, 78–81.)

Eyes having a shallow anterior chamber are also at risk following mydriasis, even after an iridectomy, for dilator muscle contraction may 'thicken' the iris sufficiently to close the angle (crowding of the angle).

The radius of corneal curvature is steepest superiorly and here the angle is narrowest. Eyes with raised intraocular pressure and narrow angles frequently develop peripheral anterior synechiae superiorly, suggesting that chronic contact between the iris and trabecular meshwork may produce adhesions. Iridectomy in these eyes widens the angle (by removing pupil block) and prevents further closure. As a peripheral iridectomy frequently lowers intraocular pressure as well, it suggests that the raised IOP was due to appositional angle closure.

Acute and subacute angle closure are characterized by a very high intraocular pressure. The very high pressure follows closure of most or all of the angle. This degree of closure will be produced by a sudden change in the dimensions of the anterior chamber, either forward movement of the anterior lens surface or an increase in the degree of pupil block (and iris bombé).

To date (with the rare exception of reading-induced angle closure in young adults), there is no evidence that transient shallowing of the anterior chamber occurs in these eyes. It seems more likely that an increase in pupil block occurs. Theoretically pupil block is greatest in the mid-dilated position of the iris. The semi-dilated pupil is characteristically found in an attack of acute closed angle glaucoma.

signs of acute closed angle glaucoma are caused by this combination of raised intraocular pressure and anterior segment inflammation.

Symptoms

A history of haloes or intermittent blurring may be elicited, occurring before the acute attack. Ocular inflammation causes pain, redness and endothelial decompensation, the latter producing the symptoms of blurred vision.

Signs

1. Raised intraocular pressure: This may be as high as 70 mmHg.
2. Ocular inflammation: Circumcorneal congestion, also anterior chamber inflammation, rarely hypopyon or hyphema. Endothelial decompensation occurring as a result of inflammation and raised IOP will result in corneal oedema. The epithelial oedema of the cornea causes diffraction of light and is responsible for the perception of haloes. As a general rule the more severe the inflammation the worse the prognosis.
3. Semi-dilated oval pupil: Iris ischaemia causes paralysis of part of the sphincter pupillae muscle: unequal contraction of the remaining muscle causes the pupil to assume an oval shape. Characteristically, sphincter paralysis occurs in the 3 and/or 9 o'clock position of the pupil thus producing a vertically oval and partially dilated pupil.

4. Glaukumfleken: These subcapsular lamellar cortical lens opacities are caused by foci of cortical fibre necrosis. They are associated with high IOP and anterior chamber inflammation.

5. Disc swelling: In predisposed individuals, a rapid increase in the intraocular pressure will infarct part or all of the optic disc. This causes disc swelling and haemorrhages, the appearance of which, in time, will resolve into a flat white disc indistinguishable from that seen in ischaemic optic neuropathy.

6. Fellow eye: Characteristically, the anterior chamber of the contralateral eye is shallow, a useful differentiating point between primary and secondary acute closed angle glaucoma for, in the latter condition, transient shallowing of the anterior chamber has occurred from some other cause. The main problems in differential diagnosis lie in those hypertensive eyes who have a shallow anterior chamber. Points of differentiation are set out in *Table* XIII.

Treatment

PROPHYLAXIS

It is accepted that a prophylactic iridectomy to the uninvolved eye should be carried out, for 60 per cent of individuals will develop an acute attack in the fellow eye in 5 years, the majority of these within 6 months after the first attack.

THE INVOLVED EYE

The majority respond to intravenous Diamox and one drop of 4 per cent pilocarpine instilled at the time of initial examination and every 3–4 h afterwards. There is little indication for intensive pilocarpine and no indication for eserine. The pupil will *not* respond to pilocarpine until the intraocular pressure has been lowered. Pilocarpine enters the eye easily through the oedematous cornea. Intensive pilocarpine and eserine may give rise to symptoms of parasympathetic overactivity such as nausea and vomiting. Should the eye not respond to intravenous Diamox and pilocarpine, then oral hypoglycaemic agents (glycerol 1·5–3 ml of a 50 per cent solution per kilogramme, or 1–1·5 g/kg) or intravenous agents (mannitol 20 per cent solution, urea 30 per cent solution 1–2 g/kg) should be given. Topical steroids, e.g. guttae predsol 0·5 per cent four times a day, probably help in most cases, although eyes with severe inflammation should be given a proportionate increase in topical steroids.

A small proportion of eyes will, at the time of initial presentation, still have a pupil that responds to light. As these eyes have considerably less inflammation in the anterior chamber, the prognosis is correspondingly better. These eyes often respond to topical pilocarpine alone.

Subsequent management of the acutely inflamed eye depends upon the response to initial treatment. As soon as the cornea has cleared sufficiently, indentation gonioscopy should be carried out to see how much of the angle has been permanently closed by peripheral anterior synechiae. At the same time, optic disc analysis should be carried out.

The further management as well as the prognosis depends on the findings on examination after the cornea has cleared. There are three main possibilities. First, the angle may be openable throughout its extent and the optic disc appear normal. For these eyes, the prognosis is excellent and peripheral iridectomy or laser iridotomy is usually curative. Secondly, there may be a variable extent of peripheral anterior synechiae located in the upper half of the trabecular meshwork, and frank glaucomatous cupping is present. These changes have not been caused by the acute attack but have been caused by chronic angle closure, upon which an acute attack has been superimposed.

Even though the eye may not show much evidence of inflammation, the response to simple peripheral iridectomy is questionable. However, the eye may remain normotensive on medical treatment, so that following resolution of the acute attack an iridectomy should be carried out. The patient should then be followed as a case of mixed glaucoma, or narrow angle glaucoma (*see below*) and given medical treatment as required.

Thirdly, considerable anterior segment inflammation may be present. In these eyes, patchy or confluent peripheral anterior synechiae are found throughout the extent of the trabecular meshwork and the optic disc may show signs of infarction. The visual outcome depends first, and in the short term, on the extent of optic disc damage suffered both at the time and after the acute attack. As it is considered

Table XIII. Differential diagnosis of the red painful eye with visual loss, raised intraocular pressure and a shallow anterior chamber

	Contralateral AC depth	Iris	AC inflammation	Posterior segment
Primary angle closure glaucoma	Same depth	Spiralling with oval pupil	Often	May have disc changes
Secondary angle closure glaucoma	Normal depth	Round pupil	Minimal	Causative lesion
Hypertensive uveitis	Same depth	Reactive or fixed with iris bombé	Definite	May have inflammation

that such damaged optic discs are more susceptible to persistent ocular hypertension than the normal disc, every effort should be made to maintain normal ocular tension after the acute attack. Secondly, and in the long term, the prognosis depends upon the extent of peripheral anterior synechiae. Although it is difficult to predict in these eyes how successful medical control will be, the acutely inflamed eye is not a good candidate for primary filtration surgery; therefore, a peripheral iridectomy should be carried out followed by medical treatment. Should medical treatment prove insufficient to control IOP, then filtration surgery will need to be performed. In these eyes, filtration surgery should be deferred if at all possible for a period of at least 1 month after the eye has become free from inflammation. In rare instances failure to control IOP at acute presentation will necessitate primary filtration surgery.

All patients who have suffered from acute closed angle glaucoma should be followed indefinitely. The trauma sustained by the trabecular meshwork at the time of the acute attack may cause chronic elevation of intraocular pressure at any time in the future.

The Place of Laser Iridotomy in the Management of Closed Angle Glaucoma

Continuous wave (argon) or pulsed (Nd:YAG or DYE) laser iridotomy has supplanted surgical iridectomy in some clinics. There can be no doubt that this approach is preferred by most patients. Because of this preference, a number of points should be considered. First, continuous wave laser iridotomy can be an extremely time-consuming approach and is not always effective. Also, there is a theoretical risk from heat generation causing damage to the adjacent lens capsule. Laser iridotomy is of little use when the cornea is oedematous, for diffraction dissipates the beam.

The recent introduction of Nd:YAG and DYE laser iridotomy has allowed a full thickness iridotomy to be made in most eyes with one to two burns. A number of eyes undergoing pulsed laser iridotomy suffer appreciable endothelial cell loss from iris particles hitting the cornea. Although this is not usually of clinical significance, it could be in eyes that have suffered an attack of acute angle closure, for these eyes suffer significant loss of endothelial cells during the acute attack.

Pulsed laser iridotomy may cause a considerable rise in intraocular pressure. This is especially likely in eyes with coincidental damage of the remaining open angle. It should, therefore, be used with caution in patients with optic disc infarction or glaucomatous cupping, for these eyes have already suffered significant loss of endothelial cells.

Despite the preceding cautionary remarks, pulsed laser iridotomy has been a real advance in the treatment of closed angle glaucoma. It would appear to be an approach preferable to continuous wave laser. It can be used with apparent safety to create a prophylactic peripheral iridectomy and, perhaps, in selected cases of acute primary closed angle glaucoma.

Subacute Closed Angle Glaucoma

Subacute closed angle glaucoma should be suspected in any patient with a shallow anterior chamber who gives a history of intermittent blurring of vision with or without haloes. A lycopodium disc should be used to demonstrate haloes to the patient. To differentiate between haloes produced by corneal epithelial oedema and lens opacities, the patient should be asked to look at an ophthalmoscope light at a time when the IOP is known to be normal. Provocative tests (prone provocative test, prone dark room test, mydriatic test), have such a high false-positive and false-negative rate that they cannot be relied upon in uncertain cases. Occasionally, there is a role for a provocative test in an asymptomatic individual with a shallow anterior chamber, who has been found to have considerably raised intraocular pressure. Such asymptomatic attacks of angle closure should be suspected in eyes with heavily pigmented irides, for these seem less likely to develop iris infarction. Young adults with shallow anterior chambers may have subacute attacks precipitated by reading – as accommodation causes forward movement of the anterior lens surface.

Identification of subacute angle closure attacks means a recommendation for prophylactic peripheral iridectomy to both eyes. Pilocarpine can only be used as a temporizing measure. When it is used, pilocarpine should be given as pilocarpine 1 per cent twice a day, for stronger strengths given more frequently may cause sufficient shallowing of the anterior chamber to make the patient run the risk of developing angle closure.

Chronic Closed Angle Glaucoma

Chronic closed angle glaucoma may develop as a sequel to an acute angle closure attack. It is also found in patients with shallow anterior chambers who have no symptoms nor signs suggestive of an acute or subacute attack. Such individuals present with the same lack of symptoms as individuals with chronic open angle glaucoma. An element of angle closure should be suspected in any individual who is considered to have 'chronic simple glaucoma' but who has a shallow anterior chamber.

In addition, a small number of such patients have a plateau iris. This term is given to the cross-sectional appearance of the iris profile where, despite an axial anterior chamber depth of near normal and a lack of iris bombé, the angle is slit-like or closed. This condition is considered to develop without iris bombé and is not helped by a peripheral iridectomy. (In some American texts the term is restricted to the cross-sectional appearance of the angle after peripheral iridectomy when the angle remains narrow.) Identation gonioscopy is essential for the identification of peripheral anterior synechiae; these, when present, will be found where the angle is narrowest – superiorly. It should be noted that the absolute depth of the anterior chamber is no guide as to the presence or absence of peripheral anterior synechiae, all glaucoma patients with an anterior chamber depth of less than 2·5 mm axially should undergo indentation gonioscopy to rule out the presence of PAS.

The management of chronic closed angle glaucoma has the same aims as for chronic open angle glaucoma, where intraocular pressure is concerned. The intraocular pressure should be reduced to a level at which it is considered that further loss of visual field will not occur. In eyes with a very shallow anterior chamber, sympathomimetic induced mydriasis may precipitate an acute angle closure attack. Pilocarpine should be used with caution for it can produce considerable shallowing of the axial anterior chamber depth. Laser iridotomy or peripheral iridectomy should be used as a preliminary treatment in these patients for, by deepening the periphery of the anterior chamber, it will render mydriasis, sympathomimetics and miotics safer to use. All patients with chronic angle closure glaucoma who have not had an acute attack should be warned of this possibility and, if possible, shown the appearance of haloes with a lycopodium disc.

Mixed Glaucoma

Patients with shallow anterior chambers and peripheral anterior synechiae may have coincidental angle damage. This may be due to coincidental open angle glaucoma or occur secondary to an attack of acute angle closure glaucoma. Mixed glaucoma is the term given to the former group. The diagnosis is suspected when the intraocular pressure is higher than one would expect from the extent of the peripheral anterior synechiae. As it can be difficult to differentiate between these two types of glaucoma, there is a case to be made for calling both groups narrow angle glaucoma (NAG). The principles in management are the same as for chronic closed angle glaucoma. Should troublesome ocular hypertension persist after laser iridotomy, there is a definite place for laser trabeculoplasty to the remaining open angle.

SECONDARY GLAUCOMAS

The secondary glaucomas were classified in *Table* II (*see* p. 305). From this classification, it will be seen that glaucoma may arise secondary to many other ocular diseases. As noted above, to make this diagnosis it is not necessary for glaucomatous cupping or visual field loss to be present.

The symptoms and signs will depend on the aetiology of the secondary glaucoma. Acute secondary closed angle glaucoma shares many of the symptoms and signs of 1° acute angle closure glaucoma. It will, in addition, provide evidence for the precipitating cause. Chronic secondary open angle glaucoma will have symptoms and signs as for chronic open angle glaucoma, and, again it will have evidence for the precipitating cause.

The management of a case of secondary glaucoma aims to treat both the precipitating cause and the raised intraocular pressure. The principles of the antiglaucoma treatment are based on a number of premises; first, the optic disc may be assumed to be healthy at the outset of the disease and as such can withstand a higher intraocular pressure than the glaucomatous optic disc. If, therefore, the secondary glaucoma is likely to be short-lived (weeks or months), it is not necessary to lower intraocular pressure to the same levels as in chronic open angle glaucoma.

Secondly, in many of the chronic secondary open angle glaucomas, pilocarpine is ineffective. In these instances, drugs that lower aqueous production are essential.

Thirdly, topical steroid treatment is required in many instances. Topical steroid treatment is beneficial in treating the primary inflammatory condition as the risk of inducing steroid glaucoma is slight.

Fourthly, fistulizing surgery in those secondary glaucomas with coincidental inflammation is much less successful than in primary open angle glaucoma. Similiarly, laser trabeculoplasty, too, is ineffective. Many of the chronic secondary glaucomas for whom fistulizing surgery has been found to be ineffective require insertion of a silicone tube.

There is one variety of secondary glaucoma which merits individual description here: acute aphakic pupil block. Acute aphakic pupil block occurs usually days after an intracapsular cataract extraction with or without insertion of an intraocular lens. In this condition vitreous gel has blocked the pupillary aperture while the iridectomy is occluded also. Aqueous accumulates in the retro-iridic region and the anterior chamber shallows. Intraocular pressure rises precipitiously following closure of the anterior chamber angle (*Fig.* 16). Treatment of this condition, in the first instance, is intensive mydriasis to try to break the pupillovitreous adhesions and produce deepening

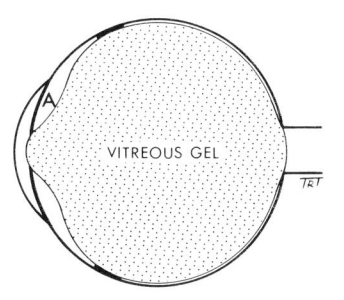

Fig. 16. Aphakic pupil block. Retro-iridic aqueous (A) accumulates when vitreous gel plugs the pupil at a time when there is no functioning iridectomy.

of the periphery of the anterior chamber. Usually, however, by the time the diagnosis has been made, this is insufficient. Should initial mydriasis fail to cause spontaneous deepening of the anterior chamber, then an iridotomy is required. Laser iridotomy is the treatment of choice. This creates a new channel between the anterior and posterior chambers and is followed by immediate, spontaneous, deepening of the anterior chamber. Unless the condition is broken days after the onset of the attack, irreversible peripheral anterior synechiae may give rise to chronic closed angle glaucoma in aphakia.

CONCLUSION

It will be seen from the foregoing discussion that the glaucomas are a group of widely differing diseases. The acute glaucomas may be approached as for any short-lived disease and treatment be arranged accordingly. Management of the chronic glaucomas, particularly in the elderly patient with severe and increasing visual restriction, may be extremely trying for both the patient and the physician. For the greatest degree of success, it is essential that the patient understand, as far as is possible, the nature of the disease and the reasons for the treatment he has been given. It is essential to discuss all possible side effects as they occur so that patients will not be put off by the medicines they are asked to use. By encouraging the patient to live with this long term disease, he can be supported and come to terms with it. Such individuals are in the best possible position to comply with treatment and to make the regular follow-up attendances that are so necessary in preventing further visual loss.

ACKNOWLEDGEMENTS

I would like to thank Mrs Kay Mills for her patience in typing the manuscript and Terry Tarrant for the illustrations. *Figs.* 3–11 are reprinted by permission of G. L. Spaeth, MD.

FURTHER READING

Grierson I., Wang Q., McMenamm P. G. et al. The effect of age and antiglaucoma drugs on the meshwork cell population. *Res. Clin. Forums* 1982; **4,** 69–92.
Hayreh S. S. Pathogenesis of optic nerve damage and visual field defects. In: Heilman K. and Richardson K. T. (ed.) *Glaucoma: Conceptions of a Disease:* Part 3. Philadelphia, Saunders, 1978, pp. 104–37.
Maumanèe A. E. Causes of optic nerve damage in glaucoma. *Ophthalmology* 1983; **90,** 741–57.
Rich R. and Sheilds M. B. (ed.) *The Secondary Glaucomas.* St Louis, Mo, Mosby, 1982.
Spaeth G. L. (ed.) *Ophthalmic Surgery: Principles and Practice.* Philadelphia, Saunders, 1982.

Chapter 12

The Visual Pathways

Diseases of the Optic Nerve

Joel S. Glaser

The optic nerve—that relatively simple hyalinated fibre tract of the central nervous system—is the site of an extraordinary range of disease states. These disorders may be listed as in *Table* I.

Table I. Optic nerve disorders

Developmental dysplasias
Hereditary atrophies/abiotrophies
Nutritional and toxic neuropathies
Neuritides
    demyelinative
    post-viral infections
    contiguous inflammations
Vascular disorders
    ischaemic optic neuropathy
    giant cell arteritis
    acute blood loss
Intrinsic tumours
Extrinsic tumours and vascular compressive lesions
Papilloedema and disc swelling

SYMPTOMS AND SIGNS

Acquired optic nerve disease is usually heralded by acute or subacute progressive dimming of central vision. In cases of nutritional amblyopia, heredo-familial optic atrophies or toxic optic neuropathies, visual loss is always bilateral though not necessarily symmetrical. On the other hand, as a rule, optic neuritis or ischaemic optic neuropathy provides a more apoplectic pattern of dysfunction, most commonly in one eye. Pain is not generally a symptom of optic nerve disease, with the important exception of the orbital and brow ache that commonly accompanies inflammations of the optic nerve, as in idiopathic or demyelinative optic neuritis. This discomfort may be exacerbated by eye movement or by percussion of the globe itself.

In many ways the optic nerve may be functionally considered as a structure principally carrying information from the cone cells of the retina. As such, defects in colour sensation are regularly encountered. In the evaluation of patients with diminished visual function certain relatively simple basic principles may be applied. Colour vision testing may be confined to gross comparison between the two eyes, and the use of colour vision plates.

As a rule, subtle lesions of the fundus that reduce visual acuity do not grossly interfere with colour perception, although sophisticated testing will show mild defects. In fact, relatively large chorioretinal scars or serous separations with vision reduced to the 6/60 level will not interfere with gross recognition of colours, although scotomatous areas for certain colours may be demonstrated. Conduction defects of the optic nerve (e.g. optic neuritis), however, reduce colour perception; this colour reduction may precede, or be disproportionately greater than, the reduction in visual acuity. This phenomenon may be attributed to a generalized elevation of threshold due to diminished conduction, affecting primarily the small calibre myelinated nerve fibres subserving the cone system. This defect may be conceived as a 'high frequency filter' that acts as a barrier to conduction in the optic nerve and to which the nerve fibres associated with cone (colour) function are preferentially sensitive. On the other hand, a focal fundus lesion will correspond only to an isolated hole in the colour-sensitive screen of the retina.

A rapid comparison for brightness value of a coloured object may be performed quite simply. A red disc or any other suitable brightly coloured test object may be used. The eyes are alternately covered, and the patient is asked whether the object is 'just as red' with one eye as with the other, or 'just as bright'. Although the image may be blurred when viewed by an eye with, for example, a small serous separation at the fovea, the intensity of the colour will compare favourably with the intensity perceived by the intact eye. Recall that we are discussing cases in which the appearance of the fundus is equivocal; obviously, with an extensive macular lesion this test is superfluous.

In response to the colour-intensity test, the patient with reduced central acuity due to an optic nerve lesion will usually report that the coloured object is dimmer when compared with that seen by the normal eye. In other words, the colour is desaturated or washed-out and appears yellow, white, or grey. In the absence of pathological change in the fundus, a positive response to this alternate eye colour comparison test is evidence of an optic nerve lesion. Of course, the individual subjective response must be evaluated; but in a reasonably intelligent patient even a subtle difference may be significant.

For alternate eye colour comparison (and light brightness comparison) it is important that the two retinae be in a similar state of light adaptation. Therefore, comparison testing should not be done immediately after photostress or ophthalmoscopy. A minute's interval in a well-lit room is sufficient to light adapt both eyes.

It is of value in some patients to do a more formal examination of colour vision, in which case a series of pseudoisochromatic plates (AOHRR, Ishihara) is helpful. Optic nerve lesions classically produce red–green defects of variable intensity. In addition, the colour plates may be used individually for alternate eye comparison to elicit subtle defects even if the coloured figures have been successfully identified.

The subjective impression of the quantity of light perceived during alternate-eye stimulation is a helpful method of differentiating optic nerve disease from fundus disease when ophthalmoscopy is inconclusive. Optic nerve lesions tend to cause a generalized depression of light sensitivity, so that 'things look dimmer' or 'it is as if someone turned the lights down'. On the other hand, a subtle macular defect or even a large circumscribed lesion will not give the general impression of 'less light getting into the eye' when the fundus is diffusely illuminated.

This test may be performed by directing a bright light alternately into the pupils and asking the patient whether the light is just as bright in each eye. If a difference is reported, the response can be semi-quantitated by repeating the alternate stimulation while asking, 'If the light is worth "so much" in this eye [the intact eye], what is it worth in this eye [the abnormal eye]?'

Obviously the light brightness comparison test is a subjective parallel to the alternate pupil response to light, the so-called 'swinging flashlight' test, popularly misnamed the Marcus Gunn test.

Special attention is called to a simple macular photostress test[1] using a hand light. The test is conducted as follows:

1. Best corrected visual acuity is recorded for each eye.
2. The normal eye is subjected to photostress by having the patient fix with one eye a penlight held 3–5 cm from the cornea, for a period of 10 s.
3. Recovery time is recorded from the time the light is removed until the patient can again begin to read optotypes on the line just greater than the initial acuity.
4. The second eye is subjected to the same procedure.

Macular lesions (e.g. central serous choroidopathy, disciform degeneration etc.) usually show prolonged photostress, while optic nerve lesions do not. This phenomenon may be attributed merely to a delay in regeneration of visual pigments after light bleaching of the fovea. With optic nerve disease the defect is one of conduction, which is not affected by bleaching and regeneration of visual pigments. This same photostress may be employed to elicit or reinforce a central scotoma while visual fields are recorded or the Amsler grid is used.

A practical technique for determining whether reduced acuity is due to a long standing functional amblyopia or to an organic lesion (of the macula or the optic nerve) is the use of a neutral density filter. If a two-log unit filter (Kodak no. 96, ND 2·00) is placed before a normal eye, vision will be reduced by approximately two lines (e.g. from 6/6 to 6/12). With an optic nerve conduction defect such as retrobulbar neuritis, vision will usually be drastically reduced when a neutral density filter is used (from 6/18 to 6/60 or less). The effect of such reduced contrast testing on functional amblyopia is of great interest, for vision in such eyes will decrease only minimally or not at all. Thus, the use of neutral density filters can distinguish between a functional amblyopia and an acquired retrobulbar lesion. If amblyopia is severe, this test is difficult to interpret.

Another subjective but useful test is the Amsler grid. Professor Mark Amsler of Zürich designed a series of line and patterned grids for testing the central 20° of field at reading distance (14 in, 0·33 m). Although designed for analysis of maculopathies, this technique is especially helpful in elucidating all central and paracentral scotomas. The manner in which the patterns are altered (curvilinear metamorphopsia in serous retinal separations, scotoma in optic nerve disease) may provide further diagnostic clues.

Pulfrich described the following stereo-illusion: when a subject binocularly views an object swinging in a frontal plane, and one eye is covered with a lens that reduces light intensity (e.g. neutral density filter), the target appears to oscillate in an elliptical orbit. This situation is mimicked by the patient with a unilateral neural conduction defect, who has an acquired 'filter' that reduces light intensity (or delays transmission of visual signals). This phenomenon may be used as a simple test to detect residual conduction defects; it also explains the paradoxical complaints of patients with 'fully recovered' optic neuritis who are plagued by abnormal depth perception of moving objects (tennis balls, underground station platforms).

Ophthalmoscopically, optic disc pallor or swelling are compelling signs of nerve disease. Neither finding may be particularly striking and often no specific aetiological cause is suggested by fundus findings alone. These subjects will be considered in greater detail under subsequent specific discussions.

The characteristic deficits of visual function with optic nerve disease may be summarized as follows:

1. Monocular deficits are the rule unless both optic nerves are involved. Hereditary atrophies and toxic nutritional neuropathies are bilateral.
2. Defects in central field function include

diminished acuity, colour perception, light sensation, pupillary light reaction.
3. Field defects include central depression and nerve fibre bundle defects. The altitudinal defect is usually vascular in origin.
4. Optic atrophy depends on the nature of the lesion and the distance from the optic disc.

Acute onset of visual dysfunction, with a normal appearing optic disc, is highly suggestive of retrobulbar neuritis, especially if accompanied by dull orbital pain or discomfort of the globe itself. Slowly progressive monocular visual loss typifies chronic compression of the optic nerve in its prechiasmal portion. Insidious bilateral central or caecocentral scotomas are hallmarks of intrinsic optic nerve disease, either of a heredofamilial nature or due to nutritional or toxic states. In cases where a central field defect is found in one eye, careful search of the temporal field of the contralateral eye is mandatory to rule out the possibility of junctional (nerve and chiasm) compression.

DEVELOPMENTAL DYSPLASIAS

The congenital variations and anomalies may produce mild to severe defects in visual acuities and visual fields. In some instances, disc hypoplasia (*Fig. 1*) may go undiagnosed and, therefore, masquerade as an acquired cause of visual loss. Variable degrees of nystagmus may accompany hypoplasia, and also hidden forebrain anomalies should be sought. The de Morsier syndrome[2] septo-optic dysplasia is more than just a fundus curiosity since endocrine disturbances of diabetes insipidus and growth retardation are reversible. Likewise, dysplastic colobomas of the optic nerve heads may indicate the presence of congenital herniations of brain substance, such as transsphenoidal encephalocoele.[3] Inferior disc crescents (*Fig. 2*), with and without significant nasal fundus ectasia, may show relative superior temporal field depressions, superficially simulating chiasmal disease.[4]

The most important congenital disc abnormality is pseudopapilloedema. Anomalous elevation of the optic nerve head, with or without ophthalmoscopically detectable drusen (*Fig. 3*) is a major cause of unnecessary alarm and misdirected diagnostic procedures. Because the funduscopic appearance resembles papilloedema, patients have been subjected to cerebral arteriography, pneumoencephalography, and even craniotomy for innocent headaches, vertigo or more trivial symptoms. Nowhere in neuro-ophthalmology is funduscopic differentiation more critical, because, once a pronouncement of 'papilloedema' has been made, a course of invasive neurodiagnostic procedures becomes inevitable.

Congenitally elevated discs have been called pseudopapilloedema or pseudoneuritis. It is very likely that the majority of cases of anomalous elevation are associated with nerve head drusen. These intrapapillary refractile bodies are unrelated to choroidal drusen. Not uncommonly, drusen progressively become visible as they enlarge towards the disc surface margins. Children with anomalously elevated discs do not commonly have detectable buried drusen, but emergence of drusen is frequent by the early 'teens.

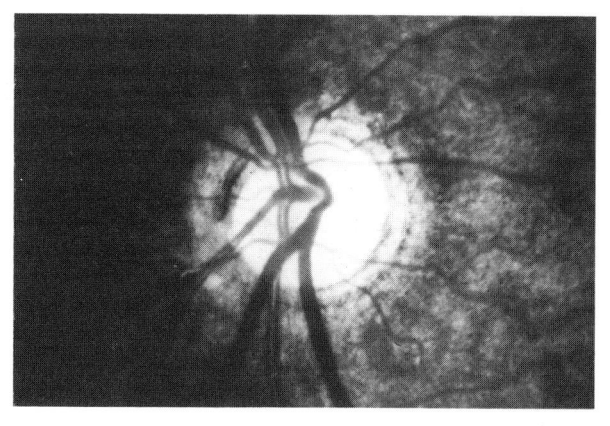

Fig. 1. Disc hypoplasia. Note small diameter of nerve head relative to vessel size. Also double pigment ring is typical, as well as mild pallor. Vision 6/36 with nystagmus.

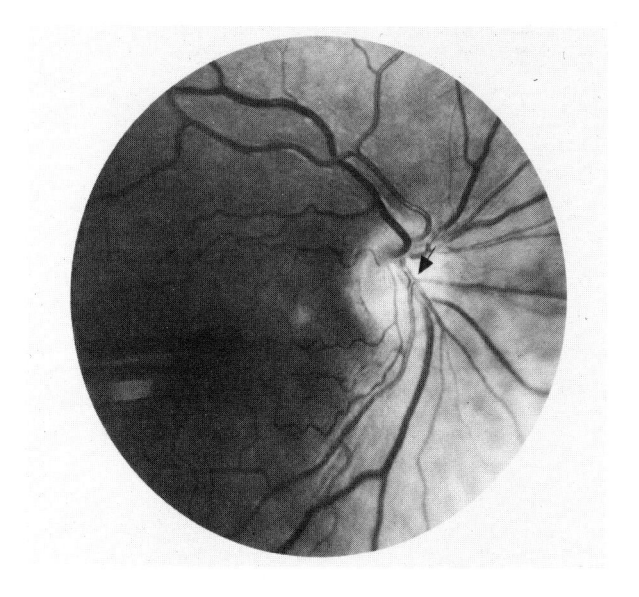

Fig. 2. Inferior scleral crescent. Lower border of hypoplastic right disc indicated by arrow. Note hypopigmented inferonasal segment of retina. Vision 6/9.

The occurrence of overt disc drusen in the parents of children with anomalously elevated discs, but without apparent drusen, attests to both the progressive and the heredofamilial nature of disc drusen. Some family members may be observed to have visible drusen, while others have only elevated discs without ophthalmoscopically distinct drusen. The fact that these conditions are frequently familial makes examination of family members mandatory when the distinction between true and pseudo-papilloedema is in doubt. Disc drusen are inherited as an irregular

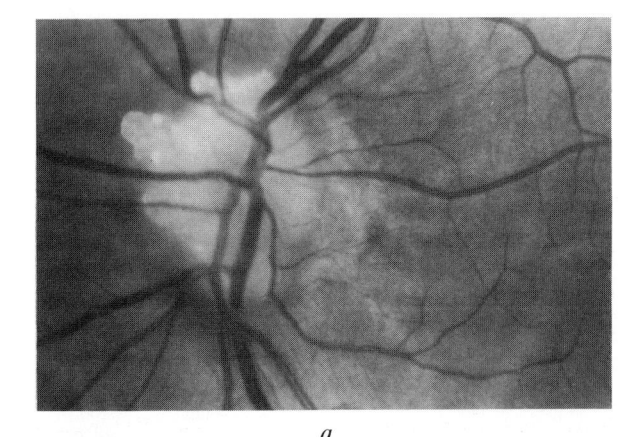

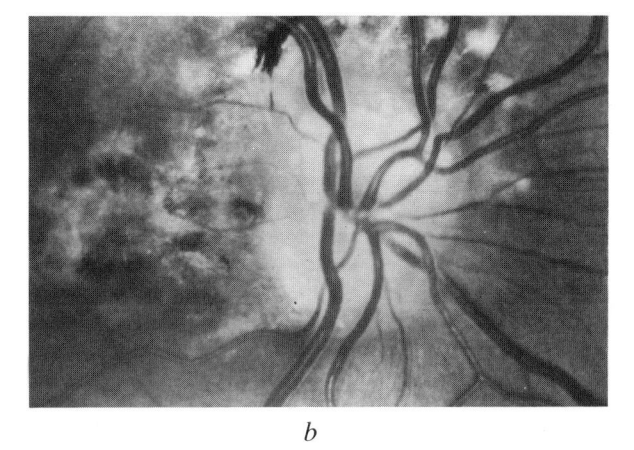

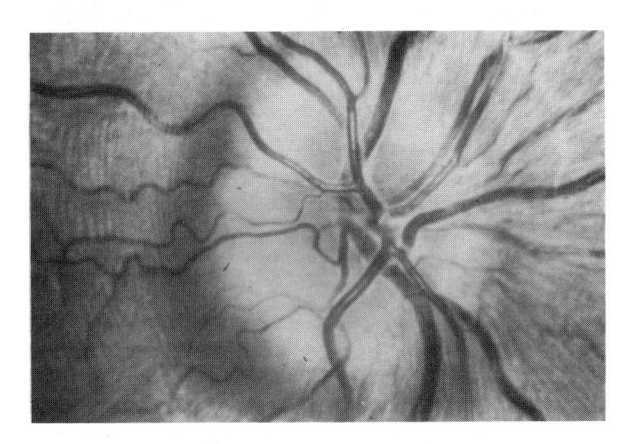

Fig. 3. Pseudopapilloedema. *a*, Hyaline bodies of disc. Note absence of cup, small disc diameter. *b*, Vascular anomalies, hyaline bodies, peripapillary pigment epithelial derangement. *c*, Anomalous disc elevation without visible hyaline bodies. Note absence of cup, hypervascularity and temporal circumferential retinal folds.

autosomal dominant trait; however, in addition, there would appear to be a distinct tendency for occurrence of drusen in fair Caucasians.

Although one disc may be more elevated than the other, with or without apparent drusen, there is a tendency towards some degree of bilaterality. In some 15 per cent of cases, ophthalmoscopically visible drusen are present unilaterally.[5] Also, there is no significant relationship between disc drusen and refractive error. With the possible exception of the tapetoretinal degenerations, there would appear to be no statistically significant association of disc drusen with the numerous and diverse ocular and neurological disorders (including tuberous sclerosis) with which drusen have been described.

Drusen may become symptomatic either by virtue of field loss or spontaneous haemorrhage. Field defects usually take the form of arcuate or other nerve fibre bundle patterns, or irregular peripheral contractions. These deficits typically progress very slowly. Enlarged blind spots may be found in both pseudopapilloedema and true papilloedema.[6] Loss of central field, i.e. diminished acuity, should not be attributed to disc drusen unless it is due to haemorrhagic complications or associated with profound loss of peripheral field as well.

It is not uncommon to elicit a history of transient obscurations of vision in patients with disc drusen. These episodes may last seconds to hours, and vision may be profoundly affected during the episode. This symptom, although infrequent, may serve to confuse the clinical differentiation from true papilloedema.

Ophthalmoscopic criteria of pseudopapilloedema are as follows:

1. Central cup absent but spontaneous venous pulse present.
2. Vessels arise from the central apex of the disc.
3. Anomalous branching of vessels; increased number of major disc vessels.
4. Disc may be transilluminated, with glow of drusen when present.
5. Disc margins irregular with derangement of peripapillary retinal pigment epithelium.
6. Absence of superficial capillary telangiectasia.
7. No haemorrhages (rare exceptions).
8. No exudates or cotton-wool spots.

If difficulty in fundus diagnosis persists, the following rules may prove valuable: (*a*) a spontaneous venous pulsation militates strongly against papilloedema; (*b*) serial observations, looking for changes, are more valuable than hasty pronouncements; (*c*) if the patient is otherwise thriving, the disc condition is probably not papilloedema; and (*d*) if, in the last analysis, a conclusion cannot be reached, the course of action should be based on other symptoms and signs.

HEREDITARY ATROPHIES AND ABIOTROPHIES

Among the causes of insidious, bilateral and symmetrical loss of central vision, the heredodegenerative optic atrophies must be considered. While seemingly a simple task to uncover familial incidence, in many cases such patterns cannot be established.

quently discovered before the patient is 3–4 years of age. Severe visual impairment is the rule, but nystagmus is variable. The optic disc is quite pale, and attenuation of arteries may suggest a tapetoretinal degeneration. However, electroretinography will distinguish between the two conditions, being normal in optic atrophy. Consanguineous parentage is uncovered in more than half of the patients.

Table II. Heredofamilial optic atrophies

	Dominant	*Recessive*			*Indeterminate*
	Juvenile (infantile)	*Early infantile (congenital); simple*	*Behr's type; complicated*	*With diabetes mellitus ± deafness*	*Leber's disease*
Age at onset	Childhood (4–8 years)	Early childhood† (3–4 years)	Childhood (1–9 years)	Childhood (6–14 years)	Early adulthood (18–30 years, up to sixth decade)
Visual impairment	Mild/moderate (20/40–20/200)	Severe (20/200–HM)	Moderate (20/200)	Severe (20/400–FC)	Moderate/severe (20/200—FC)
Nystagmus	Rare‡	Usual	In 50%	Absent	Absent
Optic disc	Mild temporal pallor ± temporal excavation	Marked diffuse pallor (± arteriolar attenuation)§	Mild temporal pallor	Marked diffuse pallor	Moderate diffuse pallor, disc swelling in acute phase
Colour vision	Blue–yellow dyschromatopsia	Severe dyschromatopsia/achromatopsia	Moderate to severe dyschromatopsia	Severe dyschromatopsia	Dense central scotoma for colours
Course	Variable, slight progression	Stable	Stable	Progressive	Acute visual loss, then usually stable, may improve/worsen

HM, Hand motions; FC, Finger counting.
† Difficult to access in infancy, but visual impairment usually manifests by the age of 4 years.
‡ Presence of nystagmus with poor vision and earlier onset suggests separate congenital or infantile form.
§ Distinguished from tapetoretinal degenerations by normal electroretinogram (ERG).
From: Glaser J. S. Heredofamilial disorders of the optic nerve. In: *Goldberg's Genetic and Metabolic Eye Disease*, Renie W. (ed.), 2nd ed. Boston, Mass., Little Brown, 1986.

Optic abiotrophies may occur as monosymptomatic isolated events or accompanying other nervous system lesions. Optic atrophy may also occur secondarily in heritable neurolipid storage disorders, in which accumulation of abnormal material in retinal ganglion cells results in consecutive atrophy (e.g. Tay–Sachs disease). Retinal dystrophies, including Leber's congenital amaurosis, and tapetoretinal abiotrophies, show variable degrees of optic atrophy, but the primary disorder is retinal.

Simple or complicated optic atrophy occurs with various patterns of transmission and graded symptomatology, such that a vast and heterogeneous literature has accrued. *Table* II is an attempt at pragmatic classification but should not be considered complete.

Recessive

Simple

Optic atrophy of recessive inheritance represents a relatively rare entity, noted occasionally in the neonate and, therefore, termed congenital. It is fre-

Complicated

Complicated optic atrophy is also called infantile recessive atrophy or Behr's syndrome. In 1909, Behr described six boys in whom optic atrophy was associated with mild mental deficiency, spasticity, hypertonia and ataxia. Subsequent studies have indicated no sex predilection. The disorder has its onset in childhood (1–9 years) and stabilizes after a variable period of progression. Pallor of the disc tends to be temporal; nystagmus is present in half of the patients and strabismus in two-thirds. It is generally thought that Behr's infantile complicated optic atrophy may represent a transitional form between simple hereditary optic atrophy and the hereditary cerebellar ataxias of the Marie type.

Recessive Optic Atrophy and Juvenile Diabetes

Rose et al.[7] reviewed the association of optic atrophy and juvenile diabetes, and Rorsman and Söderström,[8] added a family of four involved siblings. The latter authors discuss the frequency of bilateral nerve deafness and the lesser occurrence of Friedreich's ataxia. Lessell and Rosman[9] have reviewed the literature on this form of genetically determined optic atrophy, and reported nine additional cases. A variety of associated manifestations were recorded, including: sensorineural hearing loss, ptosis, ataxia, nystagmus, seizures, mental retardation, abnormal ERG, elevated CSF protein and cells, and small stature.

In essence, autosomal recessive optic atrophy is quite rare, and, in fact, several authors have pointed out that patients previously categorized as having autosomal recessive congenital or infantile optic atrophy may indeed have retinal dysplasia.

to 6/60); temporal pallor of optic discs; centrocaecal enlargement of the blind spot; full peripheral fields to white targets; inverted peripheral fields to colour; and acquired blue–yellow dyschromatopsia.

Kjer noted that many of his patients were ignorant of the familial nature of their disease and that many had noticed no symptoms. These phenomena attest to the insidious onset in childhood, mildly progressive course and usual mild degree of visual dysfunction. There is some evidence for progression, since patients less than 15 years old did not show vision below 6/60, while 10 per cent of patients 15–44 years old and 25 per cent of patients 45 years old or more had visual function below 6/60. No patient had vision

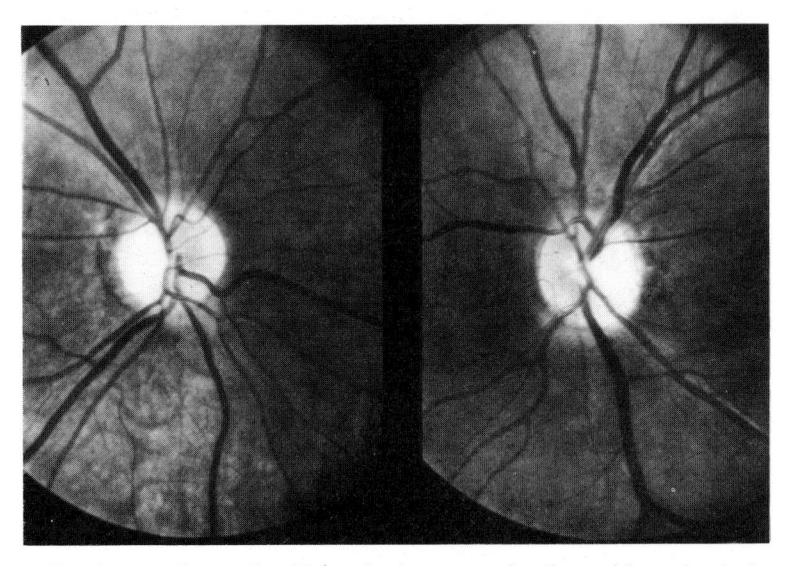

Fig. 4. Dominant optic atrophy. Note selective temporal pallor and loss of retinal nerve fibre layer in papillomacular bundle.

Dominant

Kjer's study[10] defined the clinical parameters of dominant optic atrophy and provided further evidence for distinction from Leber's disease, with which it had previously been confused. Kjer distinguished two dominant forms, separated primarily by the presence of nystagmus, but Waardenburg takes exception, commenting that 'nystagmus is too unspecific a symptom to be used as a reliable criterion for differential diagnosis'. Waardenburg mentions the possibility of separate genotypes for a form of dominant infantile optic atrophy with severe visual loss versus the more benign form with moderate visual dysfunction. However, since there is considerable interfamilial and intrafamilial variability as regards vision, this point remains unsettled.

Damien Smith[11] provided an admirable review of dominant optic atrophy and defined diagnostic criteria and clinical variants. Smith's analysis revealed eight major clinical manifestations: dominant autosomal inheritance; insidious onset between the ages of 4 and 8 years; moderately reduced visual acuity (6/20

reduced to hand motion or light perception levels. Kline and Glaser[12] noted that acuity could be strikingly asymmetrical in any individual case, e.g. 6/9 in one eye and 6/60 in the other, and that pattern reversal visual evoked responses were characterized by diminished amplitudes and prolonged latencies.

Optic disc changes may take the form of temporal pallor or may show a peculiar pie-shaped excavation of the temporal sector (*Fig.* 4). Still other discs demonstrate diffuse pallor with sharp margins.

Regarding visual fields, Kjer states that the characteristic defect is a centrocaecal scotoma, which may be quite minimal. Subtle scotomas can enlarge the blind spot vertically and superficially resemble depression of the temporal field. Especially with coloured targets, a pseudo-hemianopic temporal defect may be simulated. The field for blue may fall within that for red – a phenomenon called 'inverted' colour fields by both Kjer and Damien Smith – simply reflecting preferential diminution of blue perception. The peculiar acquired tritan dyschromotopsia of this disorder has been adequately documented and, although at times subtle, should be considered a characteristic and relatively constant finding. Eventually, achromatopsia may ensue.

Regarding nystagmus, interestingly, none of Kjer's patient's was unequivocally demonstrated to have the combination of optic atrophy and nystagmus. Hoyt[13] reported pendular nystagmus in 4 of 31 patients, and all of these also had neural hearing loss. Therefore, the presence of nystagmus with early severe visual loss may constitute either a separate nosological entity of congenital dominant optic atrophy or may represent the extreme degree of a single genetic disorder with great symptomatic variability.

Sufficient case material has accrued to indicate that dominant (juvenile onset) optic atrophy is the most

dition, the existence of families with apparent Leber's disease complicated by neurological complications suggests the possibility of a slow virus mechanism (as in the kindred encephalitis reported by Wallace[15]), in which the expression of the disorder may be dependent on genetically determined resistance.

The hereditary pattern of Leber's disease may be summarized as follows:
1. Males are predominantly affected (males and females are equally affected in Japan).
2. There is no transmission in the male line, i.e. an affected male does not transmit to his issue, unlike transmission in x-linked disorders, in

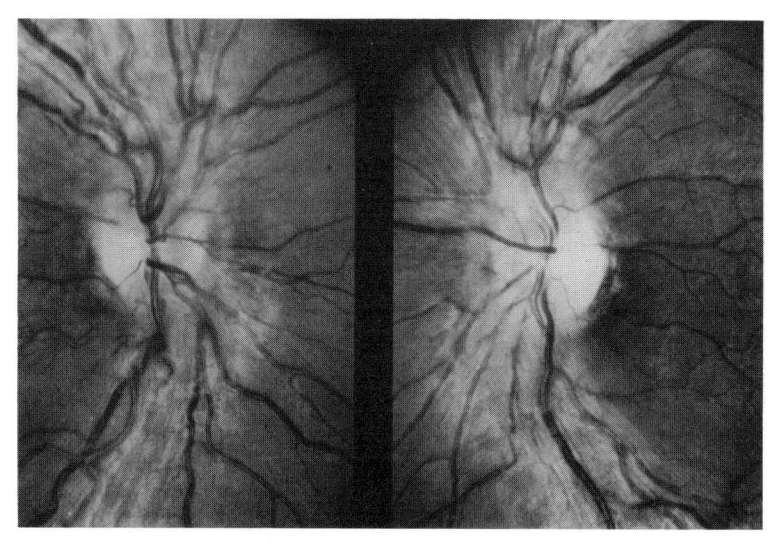

Fig. 5. Leber's optic neuropathy. Acute 'neuritic' phase shows pseudoedema of arcuate nerve fibre bundles and tortuous vessels. Absence of cup is typical. Vision 6/60 OU.

common heredofamilial monosymptomatic optic atrophy. Visual dysfunction in this disorder is considerably more mild than in either Leber's optic neuropathy or recessive optic atrophy. As a rule, progression is minimal and prognosis good.

Leber's Disease

In 1871, Leber described a nosologically distinct hereditary form of optic neuropathy that now bears his name. This entity is characterized by sudden loss of central vision occurring in the second and third decades of life and non-direct transmission with male preponderance.

Although the disorder has been classically considered x-linked recessive, pedigrees of indisputable Leber's disease do not conform to rigid Mendelian rules. For example, there is absence of transmission through males, and passage occurs from the female to most of her offspring. According to Nikoskelainen,[14] the pattern of strict maternal inheritance argues strongly in favour of vertical transmission of cytoplasmic (mitochondrial) DNA. Mitochondrial DNA is derived exclusively from the mother. In ad-

which an affected male transmits through his daughters.
3. The heterozygous female can transmit the trait to sons and the carrier state to daughters.
4. There is no genotypic difference between a female carrier and a manifestly affected woman.
5. According to Lundsgaard,[16] 50 per cent of sons and approximately 10 per cent (expected, 50 per cent) of daughters are manifestly affected.
6. According to Seedorff,[17] all women born in pedigrees with only females affected are carriers, i.e. the 'carrier rate' is 100 per cent.

Combined data indicate the age at onset to be usually in the second or third decade, typically in the late 'teens to middle 20s, ranging from 5 to 65 years of age. Lundsgaard[16] feels that there are insufficient data to support a different age-onset incidence in females, but she points out the remarkably constant age at onset for members of the same sibship. Asymmetry of onset is difficult to assess because of patient subjectivity, but some interval of days to weeks would appear to be the rule. Entirely unilateral cases are distinctly rare and, at the time of Lundsgaard's review, only found in females.

Loss of central visual function progresses rapidly to levels of 6/60 or finger-counting, although more benign and more severe loss is not infrequent. During the acute neuritic phase, elevation of the optic disc and swelling of nerve fibre bundles may be observed (*Fig.* 5). Of great interest is the observation that asymptomatic family members in the female line have pre-morbid peripapillary telangiectatic microangiopathy, very much resembling the fundus findings during visual loss of the acute 'neuritic' phase.[18] Typical thickening of the arcuate nerve fibre layer, however, was absent. Three asymptomatic boys with angiopathy subsequently developed classic symptomatic Leber's disease. Headaches may accompany the onset of visual loss and are construed as meningeal signs by advocates of an arachnoidal aetiology. Progressive atrophy ensues, leaving a flat pale disc. The visual fields show large dense central scotomas at the fixational area.

Although relative stability of visual function following initial loss is anticipated, gradual decline or sudden improvement after years of stationary vision has been reported. Such spontaneous variation after stationary intervals makes objective studies of treatment difficult, and ultimate visual outcome cannot be forecast with certainty. The family reported by Brunette and Bernier[19] is of great interest, with spontaneous recovery to normal vision in 6 of 51 affected members. Four other members recovered vision of 6/15 in at least one eye. Certainly, this high recovery rate must be kept in mind in evaluating suggested forms of therapy, including neurosurgical intervention, which will be discussed below.

Although the hereditary nature and aetiology of Leber's disease remain obscure, therapeutic measures have been suggested. Wilson and colleagues feel that failure to detoxify cyanide may be the basic heritable defect in Leber's disease and suggest the therapeutic use of hydroxocobalamin.[20] This theory of cyanide toxicity in Leber's disease, as well as in tobacco and nutritional amblyopias, is very much undecided, despite enthusiastic advocates.

NUTRITIONAL AND TOXIC OPTIC NEUROPATHIES

Insidious and slowly progressive bilateral loss of function in the central fields, with resultant diminished acuity and central scotomas, should alert the physician to the possibility of intrinsic optic nerve disease related to dietary deficiencies, exposure to toxins, or adverse reaction to pharmaceuticals. Atypical centrocaecal field loss with glaucoma, macular cone dystrophy and primary hereditary optic atrophy must also be considered. A differential diagnosis is outlined in *Table* III. No distinction is made between central and caecocentral defects.

Vitamin Deficiencies and Tobacco Alcohol Amblyopia

Regarding the aetiology of nutritional neuropathies,

Table III. Causes of bilateral central scotomas

1. Deficiency states
   Thiamine ('tobacco–alcohol amblyopia'); B_{12} (pernicious anaemia; ? 'tobacco amblyopia')
2. Drugs/toxins
   Ethambutol; chloromycetin; streptomycin; isoniazid (INH); chlorpropamide; digitalis; chloroquine; Placidyl (Serenesil – ethchlorvynol); antabuse; heavy metals
3. Hereditary optic atrophies
   Dominant (juvenile); Leber's; associated with heredodegenerative neurological syndromes; recessive, associated with juvenile diabetes.
4. Demyelinative syndromes
5. Graves's orbitopathy
6. Atypical glaucoma
7. Macular dystrophies

the great weight of clinical evidence overwhelmingly favours a dietary deficiency of B-complex vitamins (predominantly thiamine) rather than the direct toxic effects of tobacco or chronic alcoholism. In the United Kingdom, where 'tobacco amblyopia' is claimed to be the common variety of abuse optic neuropathy, multiple factors seem to converge:[21] the patients are often elderly and have diets poor in protein and B vitamins; many patients have pernicious anaemia with defective B_{12} absorption; alcoholic consumption is minimal; all patients smoke pipe tobacco.

Of greater practical importance, there are no clinical differences between 'tobacco amblyopia', 'tobacco–alcohol amblyopia', optic neuropathy in chronic alcoholism, or malnutrition optic neuropathy. It would appear that dietary deficiency is the common denominator, and thiamine improves the condition in spite of continuing abuse of alcohol or tobacco.

It goes without saying that alcoholics tend not to disclose accurate daily consumption figures, and history-taking from relatives and friends may be more reliable, including details of diet. Normal body weight, much less obesity, is uncommon in this group.

Bilateral, relatively symmetrical centrocaecal scotoma, with preservation of the peripheral field, is the characteristic field defect encountered in nutritional toxic neuropathy. Although minor variations in the scotomas have been said to distinguish between 'alcohol' and 'tobacco' amblyopia, Carroll[22] believes that no such difference exists. The defects are characterized by 'soft' margins that are difficult to define for white stimuli but are larger and easier to plot for coloured targets, especially red. A dense 'nucleus' may at times be found between the blind spot and the fixational area, but nerve fibre bundle defects do not occur. Visual acuity is usually reduced to 6/60 levels but may be surprisingly good despite a symptomatic central defect, in which case the scotoma may be demonstrable with red targets only.

On occasion, bilateral caecocentral scotomas may mimic the bitemporal depression of chiasmal interference. The following features should distinguish the field of nutritional neuropathies from that of chiasmal interference: visual acuity is diminished; the defects extend across the vertical meridian, especially demonstrable with red targets; there is no peripheral hemianopic depression; and as the defects progress, they appear more caecocentral and less hemianopic.

As a rule, the fundus appears perfectly normal, but a small percentage of patients may show splinter retinal haemorrhages on or off the disc or very minimal disc oedema.

Prognosis for recovery is excellent for all but the most chronic cases. Treatment consists of a well-balanced diet and B-complex vitamin supplement. Among the least expensive preparations is yeast, either in powder form (Fleischmann's Dried Yeast) or tablets (500 mg, 20 tablets per day, Squibb). Intramuscular thiamine may also be used.

In elderly patients especially, the possibility of B_{12} or folate deficiency should not be overlooked. Central scotoma disease may precede the classic neurological syndrome of subacute dysfunction of the dorsal and lateral spinal columns, and, in fact, optic nerve and neurological deficits may be well established before macrocytic anaemia is present. Haematologic consultation, including elucidation of B_{12} absorption, is warranted in the investigation of cases of bilateral progressive central scotoma, especially in the presence of normal haematocrit. The field defects of pernicious or prepernicious anaemia are identical to those of the other toxic nutritional optic neuropathies.

Toxic Optic Neuropathies

Insidiously progressive central field defects may occur as complications of medical therapy or exposure to specific toxins. The catalogue of neurotoxic substances of ophthalmic significance compiled by Grant in his *Toxicology of the Eye*[23] should be consulted for more complete indices. Leibold[24] has provided a well-referenced monograph entitled *Drugs Having a Toxic Effect on the Optic Nerve*, and has included pertinent discussions of agents currently in use, including: chloramphenicol, ethambutol (Myambutol), isoniazid, streptomycin, sulphonamides, digitalis, chlorpropamide (Diabinese) and ergot.

Previously undocumented is the association of a commonly used non-barbiturate hypnotic, ethchlorvynol (Placidyl, Serenesil), with progressive central scotoma. Haining and Beveridge[25] reported a patient who used 1000 mg nightly for many months, developed central visual loss and recovered rapidly when the ethchlorvynol was discontinued. The authors pointed out the value of colour vision testing in such cases. Ethchlorvynol has also been incriminated as a cause of chiasmal-type field defects.[26]

Extensive clinical and epidemiological evidence, primarily from Japan, has linked a neurological syndrome which includes optic atrophy (subacute myelo-optic neuropathy, SMON) with the halogenated hydroxyquinolines.[27] These preparations include Entero-vioform (clioquinol), Diodoquin (di-iodo-hydroxyquinoline) and clioquinol, the utilization of which should probably be reserved for acrodermatitis enteropathica or asymptomatic amoebiosis. Certainly, the use of these agents is to be deprecated in inflammatory bowel disease or non-specific diarrhoea, especially in children.

With regard to ethambutol, there is some evidence that the optic chiasm is the site of involvement.[24,28] Field defects may take the form of true bitemporal hemianopias that resolve on discontinuance of the drug.

A most peculiar, relatively rapid, bilateral optic atrophy termed 'Jamaican optic neuropathy' afflicts young West Indian blacks. This paradoxical disorder defies characterization in terms of an infectious, hereditary, toxic or nutritional aetiology. Vision is reduced to 6/60 levels and dense central scotomas are demonstrable. Carroll has pointed out an occasional association with nerve deafness, ataxia or spasticity.[29] A similar syndrome exists in young Bahamians, Cubans, Puerto Ricans and Jamaicans who have lived in the United States for several years preceding loss of sight. They are well-nourished, non-intoxicated and non-reactive (FTA-ABS test), with inconsequential family histories. No form of therapy affords relief.

The greatest care and attention must be exercised to probe for factors possibly related to the onset of central scotomata. As well as drug and family history, the patient should be carefully questioned regarding exposure to toxins (heavy metals, fumes, solvents). In the absence of any identifiable specific aetiology, the investigation of bilateral central scotomas, excluding maculopathies, should include the following: family history; medical history; drug history; diet history; work history; serum B_{12}, folate; serum lead; haemogram, including mean corpuscular volume; haematology consult; B_{12} absorption tests; skull X-ray and computerized tomography when indicated.

All previous medications should be discontinued; the patient should be placed on a high protein diet with supplementary B-complex vitamins. If pernicious anaemia is suspected, the aid of a competent haematologist should be sought before any parenteral medications are administered.

Finally, while radiological studies are not anticipated to be of help (where the history-taking and evaluation of visual function are properly performed), plain skull series with visualization of the sinuses and sella turcica are advisable. Progressive visual loss, as determined by sequential perimetry, should be investigated appropriately, based on the emerging pattern of field loss (e.g. bitemporal progression indicates chiasmal interference).

OPTIC NEURITIDES

The term 'optic neuritis' is best reserved for primary inflammation of the nerve, including that accompanying demyelinative disease or contiguous spread of inflammation from meninges, orbital tissues, or paranasal sinuses. Where the optic nerve is damaged by vascular, compressive, or unknown mechanisms, the more general term 'optic neuropathy' is preferable. 'Papillitis' (*Fig.* 6) refers to the intraocular form of optic neuritis in which disc swelling in variable degrees is observed. The clinical distinction between 'papilloedema', i.e. passive disc swelling associated with increased intracranial pressure, and papillitis is discussed subsequently. As previously noted, papillitis is the typical form of optic neuritis in childhood, while unilateral retrobulbar neuritis is the common form in adults.

The clinical characteristics of optic neuritis may be summarized as follows:

1. There is relatively acute impairment of vision, progressing rapidly for hours or days; visual function usually reaches its lowest level by one week after onset, but may actually be improving by that time.

2. The typical episode involves one eye only, although in children, especially, it is not unusual for bilateral neuritis (with disc swelling) to be associated with viral illnesses, including measles, mumps and chicken pox.

3. Tenderness of the globe and deep orbital or brow pain, especially with eye movements, may precede or coincide with visual impairment.

4. Visual field defects usually involve the central field with diminution of acuity, but the fixational area may be spared such that normal or near-normal acuity is found in 20–25 per cent of neuritic cases.[30]

5. In the majority of cases, visual function begins to improve in the second or third week, and many patients enjoy normal or near-normal vision by the fourth to fifth week; in others, following a fairly rapid improvement to modest levels of acuity, vision slowly but steadily improves over several months.

6. In a small percentage of cases, vision does not improve to functional levels and, even more rarely, vision does not improve at all after the initial precipitous loss.

7. Some patients experience light flashes (photopsias) during acute and chronic phases.

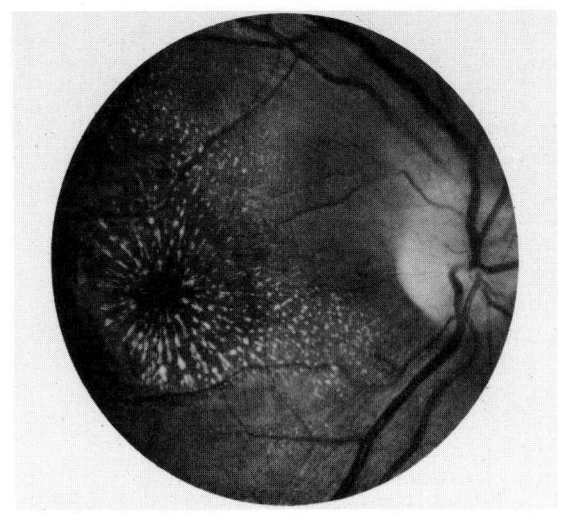

Fig. 6. Papillitis (neuroretinitis) with extensive deposition of exudates in outer retinal layers, forming 'star' figure around fovea. Vision 6/18.

Table IV. Clinical characteristics of optic neuritis, papilloedema and ischaemic optic neuropathy

	Optic neuritis	*Papilloedema*	*Ischaemic neuropathy*
Symptoms			
Visual	Rapidly progressive loss of central vision; acuity rarely spared	No visual loss; ± transient obscurations	Acute field defect, commonly altitudinal; acuity variable
Other	Tender globe, pain on motion; orbit or brow ache	Headache, nausea, vomiting; other focal neurological signs	Usually none; cranial arteritis to be ruled out
Bilateral	Rarely in adults; may alternate in MS; frequent in children, especially papillitis	Always bilateral, with extremely rare exceptions; may be asymmetrical	Typically unilateral in acute stage; second eye involved subsequently with picture of Foster Kennedy syndrome
Signs			
Pupil	No anisocoria; diminished light reaction on side of neuritis	No anisocoria; normal reactions	No anisocoria; diminished light reaction on side of disc infarct
Acuity	Usually diminished	Normal acuity	Acuity variable; severe loss (inc. NLP) common in arteritis
Fundus	Retrobulbar: normal; papillitis: variable degree of disc swelling, with few flame haemorrhages; cells in vitreous variable	Variable degrees of disc swelling, haemorrhages, cytoid infarcts	Usually pallid segmental disc oedema with few flame haemorrhages
Visual prognosis	Vision usually returns to normal or functional levels	Good, with relief of cause of increased intracranial pressure	Poor prognosis for return; second eye ultimately involved in one-third of idiopathic cases

Ophthalmological findings are summarized in *Table* IV.

Optic neuritis is a syndrome and not a primary disorder. Associated aetiologies are diverse and numerous, but the largest proportion of cases of optic neuritis present as a monosymptomatic event without identifiable underlying cause. Such cases may follow a non-specific upper respiratory infection and, therefore, a viraemia or immunopathy may be implicated. Only on rare occasions is a specific aetiology detected (*Table* V).

Table V. Causes of optic neuritis

Unknown aetiology
Multiple sclerosis
Viral infections of childhood (measles, mumps, chicken pox) with or without encephalitis
Viral encephalitis
Postviral, paraviral infections
Infectious mononucleosis
Herpes zoster
Contiguous inflammation of meninges, orbit, sinuses
Granulomatous inflammations (syphilis, tuberculosis, cryptococcosis, sarcoidosis)
Intraocular inflammations

In the patient with optic neuritis, the history should include questions regarding the following points: symptoms of a preceding viral illness (e.g. upper respiratory or gastrointestinal infection, febrile illness); previous or co-existing neurological signs and symptoms (e.g. paraesthesiae, clumsiness of limbs, ataxia, diplopia); sinus symptoms; concurrent viral illness in family (especially children) or other close contacts.

Visual symptomatology in optic neuritis is related to the nature of conduction defects. In addition to diminished central acuity and field loss, the following symptoms may be reported: drabness (desaturation) of coloured objects; apparent reduction of light intensities (e.g. room lighting appears dim when viewed with affected eye); impairment of depth perception, especially with moving objects; increase in visual deficit with exercise or other elevations of body temperature (Uhthoff's symptom). All these visual symptoms may persist after return of acuity to normal levels and, thus, patients continue to be visually symptomatic in spite of good acuity and field.

The extent of investigation to which the patient with monosymptomatic optic neuritis should be submitted is controversial. If skull X-rays are obtained, it is probably more profitable to determine the status of paransal sinuses (especially ethmoid and sphenoid) than the optic canals. In an otherwise asymptomatic patient, neuroradiological procedures and lumbar puncture are so infrequently productive as to be considered unnecessary. Therapeutic considerations will be discussed subsequently (p. 333).

It must be noted that optic neuritis, usually with some degree of disc swelling, may accompany inflammation of the uvea or retina. The ocular signs and symptoms, including cellular debris in the vitreous, are sufficient to establish a local, if non-specific, cause of the neuritis. In such cases, cystoid macular oedema may be the cause of reduced central vision rather than the papillitis, or both processes may be contributory.

Primary Demyelinative Disease

The association of optic neuritis, usually of the retrobulbar type, with demyelinative disease is well recognized. In fact, optic neuritis and internuclear ophthalmoplegia are the two most common ocular complications of multiple sclerosis (MS). In the individual patient with a first episode of monosymptomatic optic neuritis, it is not possible to predict the future development of demyelinative disease. According to Bradley and Whitty,[31] approximately 20 per cent of patients with first episode optic neuritis will develop one or more neurological symptoms of relapsing or remitting character, together with two or more signs of multiple lesions of the nervous system ('definite multiple sclerosis'); in addition, another 30 per cent will develop a sign indicating a separate neurological lesion without a history of relapsing symptoms ('probable multiple sclerosis'). In that series, recurrent episodes did not predict a statistically significantly higher incidence of subsequent disseminated disease. Those authors also noted that, of the patients with 'definite multiple sclerosis', the disease almost always declared itself by 4 years.

In a prospective study[32] of 60 patients with complicated optic neuritis followed for at least 5 years (mean 7·1 years), 17 patients (28 per cent) developed definite MS and four (7 per cent) developed probable MS; 6 of the 17 patients who developed definite MS did so within the first year. Nineteen of 42 women (45 per cent) but only 2 of 18 men (11 per cent) developed MS. There was an overall increased risk of MS between the ages of 21 and 40, and with recurrent optic neuritis. The course of MS appeared relatively benign during the period of observation. Also, from the Moorfields Clinic in London it was calculated that some 60 per cent of patients with optic neuritis developed multiple sclerosis after 8 years.[33]

Neuromyelitis optica (Devic's disease) is most likely an acute variant of MS with a propensity for occurrence in children and young adults. This syndrome is characterized by rapid, severe bilateral visual loss accompanied by paraplegia. Unlike typical MS, full recovery of vision is less predictable.

Attempts have been made to identify specific immunological profiles in patients with MS utilizing histocompatibility antigens (e.g. human lymphocyte antigens HLA-3 and HLA-7). It has been suggested that spinal fluid protein electrophoresis, along with histocompatibility titres, genetic determinant LD-7a typing and circulating B-lymphocyte levels, may prove helpful in predicting the risk of MS in patients presenting with isolated optic neuritis. Of further interest is the infrequent association of MS with uveitis or retinal vein sheathing. Atypical immune responses or latent viral infections have been suggested as aetiological possibilities in both MS and uveitis, but conclusions to date are speculative.

It is an error to consider a monosymptomatic episode of optic neuritis as a harbinger of multiple sclerosis, and a grave injustice to the patient to make pronouncements in this regard. It is poor judgement to raise the spectre of demyelinative disease for the following reasons: very few patients are sufficiently well informed of the mild non-disabling form of MS; it is currently not possible to predict the subsequent development of MS in the individual patient; no therapeutic or preventive modalities are available.

Contiguous Inflammations

As opposed to intrinsic demyelinative reaction, the optic nerve may be secondarily involved by various inflammatory lesions of adjacent tissue including the orbit, paranasal sinuses and meninges.

With orbital cellulitis or non-specific inflammatory orbital pseudotumour it is not clear whether a true optic neuritis is present or visual deficits are caused by pressure effect. In orbital pseudotumour, visual loss is frequently accompanied by variable degrees of disc swelling, which suggests an actual neuritis; rarely is visual impairment an initial symptom, and other clinical signs usually have evolved before vision is disturbed. Systemic steroids are frequently beneficial.

Decades ago, many cases of optic neuritis were attributed to acute or chronic sinusitis. This popular concept was not far-fetched, especially when the close anatomic relationship of the optic nerve to the ethmoid and sphenoid sinuses is considered. The pendulum has now swung far in the other direction and, indeed, rarely can the paranasal sinuses be directly incriminated in cases of optic neuritis. In a survey of 104 consecutive patients with optic neuritis, purulent maxillary sinusitis was observed in 3 patients, thickened membranes of the maxillary sinus in 3, maxillary sinus cyst in 3 and large ethmoidal air cells in 3.[34] Six of these 12 patients experienced otolaryngological signs at the time of the appearance of the optic neuritis. In only 1 patient who had acute left maxillary sinusitis at the time of the left optic neuritis was the infection thought to be directly related; in 6 patients MS was the suggested aetiology.

Mucocoeles of the sphenoid sinus may be associated with chronic progressive visual loss and ocular motor nerve palsies. However, on rare occasions a clinical picture consistent with optic neuritis may be encountered.

Optic neuritis may accompany acute meningitis in children or adults. Purulent leptomeningitis spreads to involve the optic nerve sheaths, primarily in the optic canal, or the substance of the nerve itself. Disc swelling may be present. Optic atrophy can follow severe neuritis but, as a rule, vision returns to functional levels, even after several months. In cases complicated by hydrocephalus or opticochiasmatic arachnoiditis, field loss may be progressive.

The optic nerves may also be involved in granulomatous and fungal meningitis, including syphilis, tuberculosis and cryptococcosis. The therapy is that of the primary infectious process, but ultimate visual outcome is guarded.

Optic neuritis is not rare in the viral disorders of childhood. As a rule, disc swelling is seen and the condition is bilateral. Both viral and bacterial meningitis may be complicated by transient cortical blindness. Therefore, visual loss in meningitis may fall into three groups: (*a*) papillitis – retrobulbar interstitial or perineuritis (leptomeningitis); (*b*) cortical blindness (?cortical venous thromboses); and (*c*) progressive optic atrophy as a result of optico-chiasmatic arachnoiditis or hydrocephalus.

On rare occasions, herpes zoster ophthalmicus may be associated with optic neuritis, either in the retrobulbar form or with severe ischaemic papillitis. Poor visual outcome is the rule. Optic neuritis may accompany or precede the polyradiculopathy syndrome of Guillain-Barré and is an infrequent ocular complication of infectious mononucleosis. Although more closely akin to an ischaemic optic neuropathy, visual loss due to 'optic neuritis' is a rare occurrence in systemic lupus erythematosus.

Papillitis is disc swelling caused by a local inflammatory process of the nerve head; it is usually acute and almost always associated with moderate to severe loss of vision. Papillitis may be thought of as an intraocular form of optic neuritis, although aetiological considerations are not parallel. It is difficult to establish the percentage of acute optic neuritides that present with disc swelling versus a normal fundus appearance. According to Bradley and Whitty,[35] of 78 eyes with 'acute optic neuritis', 17 per cent showed 'papilloedema or blurred discs with haemorrhage' and 24 per cent had 'blurred discs only'; the age spectrum was the same in those patients with 'papilloedema' as in those with normal discs. This study included patients through the seventh decade, and it is possible that ischaemic optic neuropathy falsely elevated the incidence of papilloedema in the adult group of patients. Disc oedema is relatively uncommon in adults with inflammatory or demyelinative optic neuritis.

In children, papillitis is the common form of neuritis. Also, simultaneous bilateral neuritis is much more common in children than adults. This latter point may be attributed to two factors: children with unilateral visual loss are less likely to be symptomatic than those with bilateral visual loss; and the incidence of viral diseases (mumps, chicken pox, non-specific fevers and upper respiratory infections) is high in childhood, and these systemic disorders may be more prone to produce symmetrical optic neuritis than other demyelinative or inflammatory aetiologies. It is likely that some degree of encephalomyelitis exists in such patients, as evidenced by the frequency of headache, nausea and vomiting, and spinal fluid lymphocytosis.

Papillitis is distinguished from papilloedema by the following criteria:
1. Rapid loss of vision (on occasion good acuity may be retained).
2. Ocular or orbital pain.
3. Afferent pupil defect.
4. Cells in the vitreous, especially just anterior to the disc.
5. Obliteration of the central cup.
6. Deep retinal exudates or macular star figure (see Fig. 6).

This last-named characteristic of some cases of papillitis is best termed neuroretinitis. Although neuroretinitis is a non-specific entity usually encountered in young patients, this fundus appearance is not likely to be associated with subsequent disseminated sclerosis. In certain patients, especially following febrile illnesses, a viral agent may be suspected.

Visual prognosis with papillitis or uncomplicated neuroretinitis is surprisingly good, even in the presence of massive disc oedema and haemorrhages, or with initial severe loss of visual function. However, progressive atrophy may ensue regardless of therapeutic intervention and good visual outcome should not be guaranteed. In the hope of favourably influencing visual results, corticosteroids are sometimes used, either orally or by sub-bulbar depot. As with retrobulbar neuritis, there is no substantive evidence that eventual visual function is affected by steroid therapy. However, in patients with neuroretinal oedema or cellular debris in the vitreous, the use of steroids seems reasonable.

An inflammatory condition somewhat related to papillitis has been termed papillary retinal vasculitis. The following features are characteristic:
1. Usually involvement of one eye only.
2. Occurrence in otherwise healthy young adults.
3. Vague visual symptoms with generally good vision (except where the macula was directly involved by haemorrhage or oedema).
4. Enlarged blindspot.
5. Marked disc oedema with dilated and tortuous veins and papillary–peripapillary haemorrhages.
   Although the course may be protracted (up to 18 months), the outcome is benign and apparently unaltered by corticosteroid therapy.[36]

Therapeutic Considerations

The need for treatment of primary optic neuritis is a controversial subject. The natural course of acute idiopathic neuritis or even recurrent neuritis associated with demyelinative disease tends to be rather benign with good prognosis for return of vision to normal or near-normal levels. Therefore, the alleged efficacy of any therapeutic agent must be compared against the spontaneous return of vision afforded by observation without intervention.

Bird et al.,[37] using single-blind control techniques, have investigated the efficacy of retrobulbar injections of corticosteroids for optic neuritis. Functional parameters included corrected acuity, Friedmann field-analyser score and Farnsworth–Munsell colour vision test. It was concluded that retrobulbar instillation of corticosteroids did not improve the natural course of neuritis. Bowden et al.[38] reported the outcome of a double-blind study in which 27 patients with acute unilateral optic neuritis were treated with daily subcutaneous injections of corticotropin for 30 days; a similar number of patients were given an inert control. Utilizing parameters such as visual acuity, Friedmann field-analyser score, macular light threshold and colour vision, no significant differences were found between the treated and control groups at any time within a 2-year follow-up. In fact, if patients seen within 14 days of onset of visual deterioration are considered, there were still no significant differences.

Therefore, to date, there are no controlled studies which convincingly demonstrate that any form of therapy significantly alters the course of optic neuritis. At best, ocular and orbital pain may be diminished. While clinical trials do indicate a modest trend towards more rapid recovery with treatment, this indication should be considered marginal. In patients with simultaneous bilateral neuritis, or when one eye has previously defective vision, corticosteroids may be justified. Taking the adverse effects of systemic corticosteroids into account or the potential for perforation of the globe during sub-bulbar or retrobulbar injection, there seems little to defend the treatment of monocular neuritis on a routine basis. Moreover, there is certainly no evidence that withholding therapy adversely alters the ultimate visual outcome.

Chronic Optic Neuritis

While it is true that certain inflammatory conditions such as syphilis, tuberculosis or sarcoidosis may be responsible for a chronic and progressive loss of vision, the diagnosis of 'chronic optic neuritis' is clinically rarely applicable. It is exceptional for demyelinative optic neuritis to run a relentless course; the majority of patients harbour a compressive lesion such as a meningioma (intracanalicular or tuberculum sellae), pituitary tumour, or paraclinoid aneurysm. Incipient optic nerve compression with progressive monocular signs and symptoms may be characterized by progressive dimming of vision, minimally decreased visual acuity, afferent pupillary light defect (the Marcus Gunn pupil), striking dyschromatopsia and a normal-appearing optic disc. However, the major clue to accurate diagnosis is documented progression (visual acuity and field). The value of modern computerized tomography of the optic canals and chiasmatic cisterns cannot be over-emphasized.

On occasion, a salutary visual response to systemic corticosteroids may be interpreted as positive evidence of inflammatory optic neuritis where a mass lesion actually exists. It is worthwhile to restate that a favourable and prolonged response to corticosteroids does not confirm a diagnosis of optic neuritis, and such patients should be followed with serial field examinations where any doubt exists.

The cautionary comment of Cogan bears repetition: 'Probably no branch of neuro-ophthalmology has to its discredit the abundance of erroneous diagnoses as has optic neuritis'.[39]

VASCULAR DISORDERS

A variety of vascular diseases affect the anterior portion of the optic nerve. The vascular components of glaucoma, radiation effect, retinal vasculitis, trauma or infections will not be discussed here.

Infarction of the anterior portion of the optic nerve, unrelated to inflammation, demyelinization, or compression by mass lesion, is a poorly understood, but well-recognized and unfortunately common cause of sudden loss of vision in the presenescent and elderly population. In contrast to inflammatory or demyelinative optic neuritis, ischaemic optic neuropathy characteristically involves the intraocular (prelaminar) portion of the optic nerve and has a rather constant ophthalmoscopic appearance of disc swelling (*Fig.* 7); there is little or no tendency to recovery of vision. In fact, absence of optic disc swelling in the situation of acute monocular loss of vision makes untenable the diagnosis of primary ischaemic infarction. The rare exception to this rule is retrobulbar ischaemic neuropathy associated with cranial arteritis. Otherwise, abrupt visual loss in the elderly patient

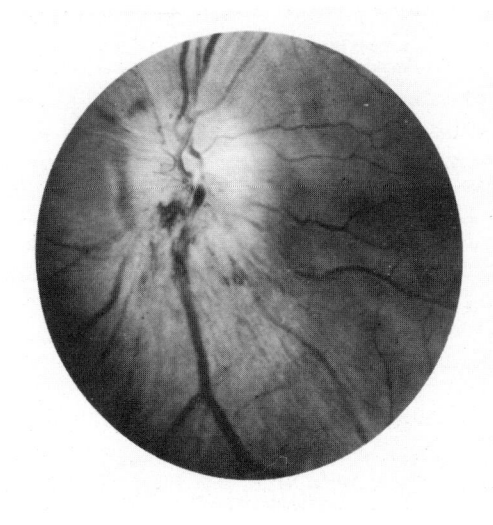

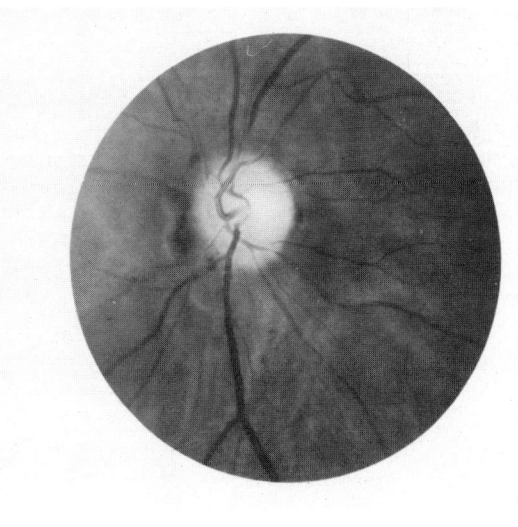

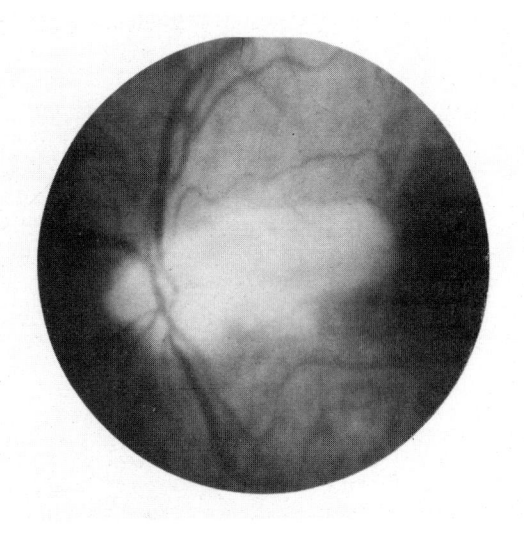

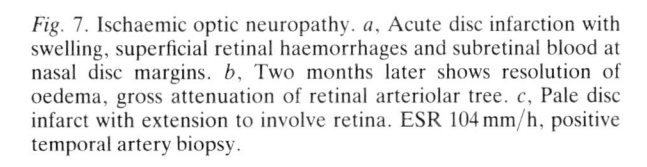

Fig. 7. Ischaemic optic neuropathy. *a*, Acute disc infarction with swelling, superficial retinal haemorrhages and subretinal blood at nasal disc margins. *b*, Two months later shows resolution of oedema, gross attenuation of retinal arteriolar tree. *c*, Pale disc infarct with extension to involve retina. ESR 104 mm/h, positive temporal artery biopsy.

with a normal optic disc should bring to mind the possibility of a rapidly expanding basal tumour (e.g. pituitary adenoma) or carcinomatous infiltration of the optic nerve sheaths.

Ischaemic optic neuropathy (ischaemic 'papillopathy') assumes an infrequent arteritic form or an all-too-common idiopathic ('arteriosclerotic') form (*Table* VI). Idiopathic ischaemic optic neuropathy (ION) may be characterized as follows:

1. Peak incidence at age 60–70 years, but on rare occasions ION occurs even in the late forties.
2. Onset of altitudinal or other field defects is sudden and usually, but not invariably, involves the central fixational area with reduction of visual acuity.
3. The deficit is usually maximal at onset, but visual deterioration may progress for several days.
4. Unlike infarction with cranial arteritis, transient premonitory visual obscurations do not occur.
5. Subsequent improvement in visual function is distinctly rare, regardless of therapy.

Table VI. Ischaemic optic neuropathy

	Idiopathic (arteriosclerotic)	*Cranial arteritis*
Age peak	60–65	70–75
Visual dysfunction	Minimal–severe	Usually severe
Second eye*	Approximately 40%	Approximately 75%
Fundus, acute	Swollen disc, often segmental	Swollen disc, normal disc, or central artery occlusion
Systemic	Hypertension approximately 50%	Malaise, weight loss, fever, polymyalgia, head pain
ESR (mm/h)	Up to 40	Usually high (50–120)
Response to steroids	None	Systemic symptoms +; return of vision ±

* Simultaneous bilateral visual loss is highly suggestive of arteritis and practically excludes idiopathic type. Acute massive blood loss with hypotension may produce bilateral nerve infarction.

The optic papilla is swollen to some degree (usually in a sector) and shows small flame haemorrhages. The swelling usually extends only a short distance beyond the border of the disc. Pain or other nonvisual symptoms are atypical. Optic atrophy ensues as disc oedema resolves. More than one episode per eye is extremely rare, and one-half to one-third of patients will experience a similar occurrence in the remaining eye at intervals of months to many years. When the second eye is involved, a 'pseudo-Foster Kennedy syndrome' is observed (i.e., optic atrophy in one eye with disc swelling in the other), which is easily distinguished from true papilloedema (with increased intracranial pressure) by clinical setting of acute visual deficit. There is no evidence that any form of therapy (corticosteroids, anticoagulants, vasodilators) in any way alters the course of the disorder.

It is worth reiterating that ischaemic optic neuropathy, because it occurs first in one eye and then the other, produces a 'pseudo-Foster Kennedy syndrome'. It is vital that these patients are not subjected to invasive neurodiagnostic procedures. In fact, plain skull films or optic canal views make little sense if the clinician is attuned to this clinical situation.

An arteritic form of ischaemic optic neuropathy occurs with onset in a slightly older age group (70–80 years); this form usually produces devastating visual loss. As pointed out by Wagener and Hollenhorst,[40] arteritis may result in a retrobulbar form of nerve infarction or may produce a picture similar to central retinal artery occlusion. These authors also noted an appreciable incidence of fleeting premonitory visual symptoms similar to amaurosis fugax of carotid embolic episodes.

It is critical to discover, when possible, those instances of ischaemic optic neuropathy due to cranial (temporal) arteritis because prompt steroid therapy may prove efficacious in restoring some degree of vision, averting visual deficit in the other eye, and improving long-term systemic morbidity and mortality. Patients with cranial arteritis may complain of weakness, weight loss and fever. Myalgia of the large muscle masses of the shoulders, neck, thighs and buttocks is common. These symptoms constitute polymyalgia rheumatica, which really cannot be clinically or histologically distinguished from cranial arteritis.[41] Other common complaints include pain in the jaw muscles precipitated by eating or talking (masseter claudication), chronic suboccipital headache, and pain or tenderness of the scalp of the forehead or temples. A palpable but often non-pulsatile temporal artery should be sought as a likely biopsy site.

The erythrocyte sedimentation rate (ESR) is the most consistently helpful laboratory test to confirm the diagnosis of arteritis. Cullen,[42] in comparing arteritic versus 'arteriosclerotic' (idiopathic) ischaemic optic neuropathy, found only 3 of 19 patients in the latter group with an ESR greater than 30 mm/h (mean 26 mm), while only 3 of 25 patients with biopsy-positive arteritis had ESRs of 50 mm and below (mean 84 mm; 70 mm or above in 80 per cent). Cullen has also pointed out the rare occurrence of arteritis with a normal ESR.

It is clear from the papers of Boyd and Hoffbrand[43] and Milne and Williamson[44] that ESR increases with age and is 'elevated' (greater than 20 mm/h) in apparently healthy elderly subjects. It was demonstrated that in at least 50 per cent of persons with an ESR greater than 50 mm, no obvious reason was found.[44] Furthermore, taking 20 mm as the upper limit of normal, bacteriuria, ischaemic heart disease and chronic respiratory symptoms show no association with a raised ESR. In the elderly 35–40 mm/h (Westergren) should be regarded as the upper limit of normal.

The affirmation provided by a positive artery biopsy is helpful when instituting long term corticosteroid therapy in an elderly patient, but a negative biopsy in no way militates against diagnosis of arteritis. The concept that a negative temporal biopsy in effect makes a diagnosis of arteritis is untenable, or that steroid therapy should be based on repeated biopsies. Klein et al.[45] have seemingly established the presence of 'skip lesions' in temporal artery biopsies from patients with unequivocal cranial arteritis. They have also pointed out that a temporal artery that is normal to palpation may show histological signs of inflammation and that patients with 'skip lesions' do not have a more benign form of the disease. Therefore, it may be argued that arterial biopsy is superfluous since diagnosis or treatment is not altered by the results. Furthermore, biopsy of a branch of the superficial temporal artery complex may destroy a major source of cranial arterial anastomoses.

In the appropriately aged patient with systemic or cerebral signs or symptoms and an elevated sedimentation rate, systemic steroid therapy should be instituted immediately (e.g. prednisone, 80–100 mg daily). In addition, retrobulbar depot steroid on the side of the acutely involved eye is a reasonable procedure. In the patient with suspected arteritis, therapy should not be delayed for results of ESR or biopsy. Symptomatic response to steroids, excluding vision, may be dramatic within 24 hours with relief of headache and malaise. Prolonged therapy should be dictated by symptomatic response to steroid and depression of the sedimentation rate. It is suggested that a high dosage be maintained for approximately 4 weeks and then tapered, so long as the patient remains symptom free and the ESR is below 40 mm/h (an arbitrary but practical figure). Complications of prolonged steroid usage are well known and include gastric ulcers, osteoporosis and recrudescence of tuberculosis.

Carroll[46] has called attention to a form of ischaemic optic papillopathy that occurs after uncomplicated cataract extraction; this form involves sudden visual loss from 4 weeks to 15 months postoperatively. He cautions that 50 per cent of patients with involvement of the first eye may anticipate visual loss following operation on the second eye. Two additional points regarding pathophysiology are worth noting: first, three patients were in their fifties, and secondly, the syndrome occurs with both retrobulbar and general anaesthesia. In Carroll's series, no patient experienced a loss of vision in the second eye unless it was subjected to cataract extraction. Carroll also concluded that neither corticosteroids nor anticoagulants provide effective therapy.

It would seem that optic neuropathy following cataract extraction represents a distinct variant of the ischaemic optic neuropathy syndrome, characterized by a circumscribed time course and high incidence of bilaterality when the second eye is operated on (even in the sixth decade) to the point of predictability.

Pathological material is strikingly deficient in the idiopathic form of ischaemic neuropathy. The relationship to carotid occlusive disease is tenuous, at best, but approximately half of these patients do have some degree of hypertension. On the other hand, cranial arteritis has been extensively studied, including the eye and orbit, and the pattern of involvement of extradural portions of the cranial vessels.[47]

Salient features of idiopathic ischaemic optic neuropathy may be summarized as follows:

1. The syndrome occurs primarily in patients aged 55–70 who, for the most part, are otherwise well.
2. Mild hypertension is present in about half of the patients, but does not determine a separate variant of the disorder.
3. There is no significant direct association with extracranial carotid occlusive disease.
4. Over long follow-up periods, there does not appear to be an increased incidence of stroke.
5. The syndrome should be easily recognized on the basis of clinical findings, including sudden or rapidly progressive monocular visual deficit associated with optic disc swelling, with stable visual defects of variable degree.
6. After an interval of months to many years, the second eye becomes involved in about 40 per cent of patients (old optic atrophy coupled with contralateral fresh disc infarction may be confused with the Foster Kennedy syndrome).
7. No form of therapy has proved efficacious.
8. Pathophysiological mechanisms remain speculative.

It is the responsibility of the physician to distinguish the patient with occult arteritis (by history, physical examination, sedimentation rate, arterial biopsy) and institute immediate high-dosage corticosteroid therapy. It is also incumbent on the clinician to refrain from unnecessary and unrewarding diagnostic procedures, particularly cerebral angiography, when confronted with a case of non-arteritic ischaemic optic neuropathy.

While diabetes mellitus represents an increased-risk factor in non-arteritic, adult ischaemic optic neuropathy, there is a rarer form of what must be a vascular-dependent disc swelling in juvenile diabetics.[48] As a rule, such patients are in the second or third decade of life, with a 10–15 year average duration of diabetes. Acuity may be minimally lowered and, indeed, disc swelling may be asymptomatic, even when bilateral. There does not appear to be a positive correlation with degree of diabetic retinopathy, and recovery generally occurs spontaneously. Visual fields may show retained arcuate nerve fibre bundle defects. Florid disc swelling is found and, occasionally, cystoid macular oedema.

Graves's disease may also be associated with an optic neuropathy that shows variable degrees of disc swelling, although 'ischaemia' as such is probably not the principle pathological mechanism. Typical congestive signs always precede visual loss, which is usually gradual in onset and bilateral.[49] Systemic corticosteroids, radiation therapy and, if necessary, orbital decompression provide therapeutic modalities. The possibility of spontaneous improvement of visual deficits is problematic. Apparently such a course is not unique, but very few physicians (or their patients) are likely to elect a passive course of observation only, especially if vision is greatly diminished. The physician should be careful not to attribute a disproportionate visual loss to minor corneal complications and ignore the presence of an optic neuropathy. The functional tests for clinical diagnosis of optic nerve defects once again apply.

Otherwise, especially in younger patients, rare forms of ischaemic optic neuropathy may accompany lupus erythematosus or other collagenoses, migraine, syphilis, or massive blood loss.

TUMOURS

Intrinsic Tumours

A wide variety of tumourous lesions may involve the optic nerves along their course to the base of the brain. These include neoplasms of the nerve itself (gliomas) or its sheaths (meningiomas) or tumours arising in adjacent tissues of the orbit, paranasal sinuses, pituitary gland and parasellar structures, and at the base of the middle cranial fossa. In addition, distant malignancies may metastasize to the nerve and its coverings. Saccular and fusiform aneurysms of the internal carotid artery also simulate neoplastic masses, as do basal infiltrative and inflammatory lesions.

Primary astrocytic tumours of the anterior visual pathways assume two major clinical forms: the relatively benign gliomas of childhood and the rare malignant glioblastoma of adulthood. With the exception of visual loss and anatomical location, these two groups have little in common, and the assumption that the progressive malignant form stems from the static childhood form is untenable. The major clinical characteristics of these tumours are contrasted in Table VII.

With regard to the benign glioma of childhood, clinical presentation depends on location and extent of the tumour. Strictly, intraorbital gliomas present as insidious proptosis of variable degree, and, although vision is usually diminished, remarkably good visual function is not uncommon. Strabismus, disc pallor or disc swelling may be observed. Progressive proptosis, even if abrupt, or increased visual deficit does not imply aggressive activity of the tumour, haemorrhage or necrosis.[50]

Table VII. Primary gliomas of nerve and chiasm

	Childhood	Adulthood
Age at onset of symptoms	4–8 years	Middle age
Presentation	Visual defects, proptosis	Rapid, severe unilateral visual loss (mimics neuritis)
Course	Relatively stable, non-progressive	Rapid bilateral visual deterioration; other intracranial signs
Prognosis	Compatible with long life	Death within months to 2 years
Neurofibromatosis	Related in large percentage of cases	No relationship
Histology	Non-invasive, pilocytic astrocytoma	Invasive, malignant astrocytoma (glioblastoma); may metastasise

Approximately 70 per cent of orbital gliomas involve the anterior aspect of the optic canal, which is seen on X-ray as a uniform round enlargement without erosion of the bony margins. Involvement of the intracanalicular nerve without evidence of enlarged canal is a distinct rarity. Paradoxically, an enlarged canal does not categorically imply gliomatous change of the intracanalicular nerve but may represent arachnoidal proliferation, which Taveras terms 'a bulky nerve'.

Regarding the concept of 'extension' of orbital gliomas to involve the intracranial visual pathway, or aggressive orbital and transcranial surgery to prevent such 'extension', the following points must be made:

1. Incomplete resection of gliomas leads to no recurrence (although rarely arachnoidal hyperplasia may mimic regrowth of tumour), and such patients do spectacularly well over long periods of observation.

2. Incomplete excision is not accompanied by malignant transformation, and it must be considered extremely rare that childhood gliomas ever undergo malignant degeneration.

3. There is only a single published documented case wherein a previously normal optic canal subsequently enlarged[51] (large canals probably represent congenital bony changes in concord with congenital large optic nerves).

4. Subsequent visual symptoms in the opposite eye, or of a chiasmal nature, do not imply 'extension' since many gliomas initially reside in one nerve plus chiasm, or chiasm plus both intracranial nerves.

Chiasmal gliomas are more common than the isolated orbital type. These tumours present to the ophthalmologist as unilateral or bilateral visual loss, strabismus, 'amblyopia', optic atrophy or nystagmus. The nystagmus may mimic spasmus nutans complete with head nodding, or may show a gross bilateral mixed horizontal rotary pattern, especially when vision is severely defective.

Children with extensive basal tumours also show hydrocephalus and signs and symptoms of increased intracranial pressure. Hypothalamic signs include precocious puberty, obesity, dwarfism, hypersomnolence and diabetes insipidus. As a rule, the non-visual complications of extensive gliomas occur in infancy or early childhood, and onset of obstructive signs or hypothalamic involvement much beyond the age of 5 is uncommon.

Visual fields with chiasmatic gliomas[52] show no consistent relationship between the pattern of field defects and the location, size, or extent of tumour; in 12 of 20 patients the putative bitemporal pattern of chiasmal involvement was absent. Central scotoma or measurable depression of the central field occurred in 70 per cent of the eyes; therefore, absence of bitemporal hemianopia or one of its variants cannot be interpreted as a sign that the glioma does not involve the chiasm.

The radiological investigation of potential gliomas is now refined to the extent that 'neuroradiological biopsy' may obviate tissue diagnosis. For some clinicians, the demonstration of typical dysplastic changes of the sella turcica and canals, coupled with computerized tomographic evidence of intrinsic chiasmal mass, suggests so strongly the diagnosis of glioma that histopathological affirmation is superfluous and hazardous. There is no authoritative consensus in this regard, and many clinicians would insist on craniotomy for direct observation of the tumour, if not biopsy. Biopsy, however, may produce further field loss.

Radiological investigation of visual loss in infancy and childhood includes evaluation of the optic canals, the bony structures of the sella turcica and clinoids, and position of the intracranial optic nerves, chiasm and anteroinferior floor of the third ventricle. Changes typical of optic glioma include large optic canals, so-called J-shaped or gourd sella, and suprasellar mass with elevation and flattening of the anterior aspect of the third ventricle. On rare occasions the optic canal may be widened by processes other than by glioma; but other destructive changes of the parasellar structures are usually evident as, for example, with craniopharyngioma.

Gliomas of the optic nerves and chiasm are distinctly associated with neurofibromatosis; the patients have either other characteristic stigmas or affected relatives. The frequency of this association cannot be established with accuracy and it is far more common than generally recognized. The review by Hoyt and Baghdassarian[53] includes 36 cases of patients with anterior visual pathway gliomas, of which 21 were associated with neurofibromatosis; in one family, two siblings had optic gliomas, and in a second family, a mother and child had gliomas. In the child with proptosis or diminished vision, the clinician should search for any of the stigmas of neurofibromatosis, in family members as well. These signs include café au lait spots, axillary freckling, iris fibromas and peripheral nerve tumours.

Considerable controversy exists regarding the natural course, growth potential and efficacy of therapy in optic gliomas. In 1922, Verhoeff remarked that, since the great majority of optic gliomas become manifest in early childhood, it is highly suggestive that these tumours 'are really congenital in origin and due to some more or less localized abnormality in the embryonic development of the neuroglia of the nerve'. Furthermore, Verhoeff felt that a glioma 'does not increase in size by invading or destroying ... but by causing pre-existing neuroglia in the vicinity of the growth to proliferate'. Taking into account their occurrence in infancy and early childhood, their natural course, growth characteristics, histopathological picture and association with neurofibromatosis, it is not unreasonable to consider gliomas of the anterior visual pathways as hereditary congenital hamartomas.[54]

Primary malignant gliomas (glioblastoma) of the anterior visual pathways are rare tumours of adulthood, not to be confused with the relatively frequent indolent optic gliomas of childhood (*see Table* VII). Hoyt et al.[55] have reviewed the subject and recorded 5 new cases. They synthesize a syndrome of malignant optic glioma of adulthood comprised of the following:

(*a*) usually involves middle-aged (majority in 40s and 50s, range 22–59 years) males (10 of 15 cases);

(*b*) begins with signs and symptoms mimicking optic neuritis (rapid monocular loss of vision, retro-orbital pain, disc oedema, transient improvement with steroid therapy);

(*c*) progresses within 5–6 weeks to total blindness (may pass through chiasmal syndrome with contralateral temporal hemianopia, then bilateral blindness);

(*d*) terminates fatally within several months (3 months to 2 years).

Pathologically, this syndrome represents the occurrence of a common brain tumour (gliobastoma) in an uncommon location. No known therapy has any effect, with spread of tumour to hypothalamus and midbrain.

The optic nerves may be involved by diffuse infiltrative lesions of diverse aetiology, including sarcoidosis, the lymphoma-reticuloendothelioses, the histiocytoses, plasmacytomas and others.

Infiltrative disorders more or less share a common clinical profile of subacute or rapid visual loss in one or both eyes. Disc swelling is seen on occasion indicating infiltration of the nerve head itself. Two cases of patients with visible optic disc involvement with sarcoid, without visual deficits, have been recorded. In the first instance, small whitish lesions evolved on the surface of one disc; the second case demonstrated bilateral disc swelling similar to chronic papilloedema, which resolved dramatically during steroid administration.[56]

Leukaemia may produce disc swelling via several mechanisms. These include meningeal infiltrate or intracranial haemorrhagic diatheses resulting in obstruction of cerebrospinal fluid and increased intracranial pressure, pseudotumour cerebri syndrome associated with prolonged corticosteroid therapy, disc oedema associated with severe anaemic retinopathy, and actual leukaemia infiltration of the disc tissue. As a rule, vision is reduced only in the latter situation. Ellis and Little[57] have defined the pathology of pallid disc oedema due to massive neoplastic infiltrates in the nerve heads of a child with acute leukaemia. An earlier review[58] indicates that such disc swelling tends to occur only in the acute forms of leukaemia, and that, in general, the distal portion of the optic nerve is chiefly involved in such disorders. Reticulum cell sarcoma has been reported to involve the intracranial optic nerve.[59] The syndrome of posterior uveitis associated with reticulum cell sarcoma (microgliomatosis) of the brain has become well established.

Infiltration of the optic nerves occurs infrequently in multiple myelomatosis[60] and with solitary plasmacytoma.[61] Leptomeningeal infiltration by metastatic systemic cancer is an infrequent cause of acute or subacute visual loss. This disorder presents as 'retrobulbar neuritis' with a normal fundus appearance, but usually the second eye is rapidly and relentlessly involved. Where the systemic illness is previously diagnosed, abrupt visual loss not attributable to fundus lesions is *prima facie* evidence of meningeal carcinomatosis. In two reviews of carcinomatosis,[62,63] the incidence of ocular symptoms is striking; either as the presenting complaint or as a subsequent development, visual loss or double vision comprised the largest group of symptomatic cranial nerve deficits. Adenocarcinoma of the breast and lung are the most frequent tumours to metastasize diffusely to the leptomeninges and subarachnoid space. Lymphoma, including reticulum cell sarcoma, and melanoma are also relatively common sources of meningeal seedings.

Altrocchi et al.[64] have reviewed the pathophysiological concepts of visual loss with meningeal carcinomatosis; these include 'tumour-cuffing' in the perioptic meninges accompanied by localized demyelination, direct tumour infiltration into the substance of the nerve, or demyelination out of proportion to sparse tumour cell infiltrate. This latter mechanism is of interest with regard to the concept of optic myelopathy as a remote complication of distant malignancy. In such situations it is problematic whether miniscule seeding has escaped detection. The outcome of carcinomatosis of the meninges is uniformly grim, with death ensuing within months. However, a substantiated diagnosis precludes unnecessary and uncomfortable neurodiagnostic studies, such as arteriography and contrast cisternography.

Extrinsic Tumours

A wide spectrum of masses may potentially compress the optic nerve in its orbital, intracanalicular and basocranial course. These lesions include: orbital tumours or inflammations; nerve sheath, canalicular or sphenoidal meningiomas; pituitary adenomas; sphenoidal mucocoeles; aneurysm of the supraclinoid portion of the internal carotid artery; metastases and lymphoma-related infiltrations. Of these external compressive masses, only meningiomas bear discussion here.

Meningiomas arise from meningothelial cells of the arachnoid, at multiple intracranial sites, in the optic canals and from the intradural tissue that invests the optic nerves in the orbit. There is a distinct female predilection for meningiomas, and the intracranial variety occurs predominantly in adults. However, orbital perioptic meningiomas tend to occur at an earlier age. Karp et al.[65] noted that 10 of 25 primary intraorbital meningiomas occurred in patients under 20 years of age, and 6 patients were in the first decade. Meningiomas presenting in youth may be associated with neurofibromatosis.

Meningiomas of the anterior and middle cranial fossae, along with those arising in the orbit and optic canal, are of major neuro-ophthalmological interest because of the signs and symptoms with which these lesions consistently present. The optic nerves may be involved via several mechanisms, as follows.

Intraorbital meningiomas arising from the nerve sheath produce very slowly progressive axial proptosis and/or loss of vision. The retrobulbar mass may be further manifest by increasing hyperopia and the appearance on ophthalmoscopy of retinochoroidal striae. At first, the disc may appear normal, but optic atrophy or chronic disc swelling ensues (*Fig.* 8).

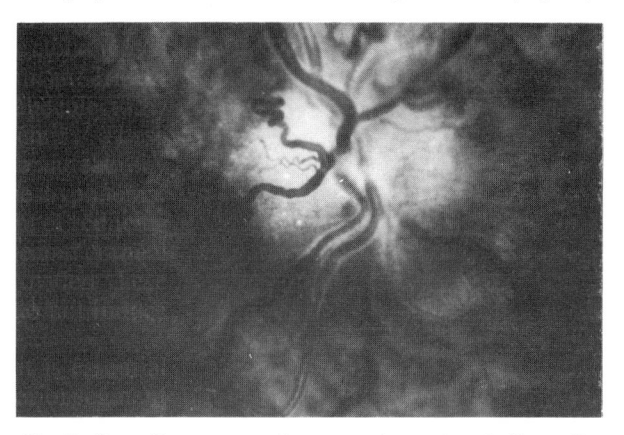

Fig. 8. Optociliary venous shunt vessels on chronically swollen disc due to perioptic nerve sheath meningioma. Vision 6/24, gross field constriction.

Frisen et al.[66] have suggested that the presence of optociliary venous shunts on the disc, when accompanied by disc pallor and visual loss, is highly suggestive of indolent nerve sheath meningiomas, even in those cases without proptosis when the posterior aspect of the optic canal is principally involved. Defective ocular motility usually indicates extension of tumour to the orbital apex or dural penetration with invasion of orbital tissues. Radiologically, unless the posterior aspect of the tumour involves the orbital apex or optic canal, no bony abnormalities are seen on plain X-ray views. In adults, delay in diagnosis is the rule, and any surgical procedure is ineffective with regard to preservation of vision. With indolent tumours there may be no advantage to any form of surgical intervention, either by an orbital approach or by transfrontal craniotomy. Alper[67] has analysed 55 cases of 'primary' optic nerve sheath meningiomas. He concludes that only those tumours occurring under the age of 20 behave 'aggressively'.

Intracanalicular meningiomas usually represent extensions either of posterior orbital tumours, or invasion into the canal by periforaminal meningiomas arising in the area of the anterior clinoids or tuberculum sellae. Strictly mid-canalicular meningiomas are extremely rare.

Posterior periforaminal and tuberculum sella meningiomas comprise the majority of meningiomas producing prechiasmal (optic nerve) visual deficits. The monotonous presentation is a complaint of slowly progressive monocular loss of vision, with all the signs and symptoms of an optic nerve conduction defect. With suprasellar extension these tumours produce chiasmal interference, with variations on a bitemporal theme. Pallor of the disc is usually less than that anticipated in view of the visual deficit. With relatively early diagnosis, surgical intervention offers arrest of visual loss, if not reversal, and prevention of involvement of the chiasm or contralateral nerve. Suprasellar meningiomas usually present as slowly progressive, asymmetric visual loss in the form of the chiasmal syndrome.

Meningiomas of the sphenoidal wing present as proptosis and reactive hyperostosis evident even on plain skull films. These slow-growing tumours may involve the optic nerve early in their course, if medially located, and as a relatively late complication if the mass predominantly involves the lateral aspect of the sphenoid ridge and middle cranial fossa (pterional meningioma). Along with computerized tomography, arteriography is helpful in determining the size of tumour and involvement of major cranial arteries. Bony hyperostosis alone may be misleading. Decompression of the posterior orbit or optic canal is a hazardous neurosurgical undertaking that is a temporizing measure at best and may actually serve to increase morbidity by providing the tumour access into additional tissue spaces.

Stern has analysed meningiomas of the cranio-orbital junction and suggests that these lesions represent an anatomical continuum rather than specific syndromes.[68] The surgical management is outlined, but the author rightly points out that unless radical operative procedures are curative, they cannot be justified on the basis of short-term evaluation, since many of these tumours grow very slowly. Despite enthusiastic advocates, radiation therapy is as yet an unproved therapeutic modality and there is little evidence that it should be considered as a primary attack on meningiomas anywhere along the length of the optic nerves.

PAPILLOEDEMA AND THE 'SWOLLEN OPTIC DISC'

While admittedly an arbitrary decision, in this discussion the word papilloedema will be reserved for the following situation: passive disc swelling associated with increased intracranial pressure, almost always bilateral, and without visual deficit (at least in those stages of development that precede atrophy). For the ophthalmologist, the finding of papilloedema constitutes an emergency, and computerized tomography is mandatory within the shortest possible interval.

The pathogenesis of papilloedema is a confused and controversial issue. Elevation of intracranial pressure in acute and chronic experiments has provided variable results and conclusions. It is very likely that intracranial pressure elevation is transmitted in the vaginal sheaths of the optic nerves with resultant (or attendant?) stagnation of the venous return from the retina and nerve head. That nerve sheath pressure is critical has been demonstrated by Hayreh,[69] who showed that disc swelling is reversed by opening of the nerve sheath. By nerve sheath ligation, Rios-Montenegro et al.[70] demonstrated that pressure in the central retinal vein within the nerve and eye becomes elevated when pressure rises in the subarachnoid space of the nerve sheath itself and not in the intracranial space.

No simple mechanistic explanation serves to include other circumstances in which papilloedema develops. Patients with cyanotic congenital heart disease may show papilloedema with markedly tortuous retinal vessels, in the absence of elevated cerebrospinal fluid pressure. Decreased arterial oxygen saturation and/or polycythaemia are felt to be aetiological factors. Albeit rare, spinal cord tumours may also produce papilloedema, as may inflammatory polyneuritis.

The clinical picture of chronic unilateral disc swelling most commonly results from obstruction of the subarachnoid space of the ipsilateral nerve by an intraorbital process such as sheath meningioma (with no visual loss in early stage and normal CSF pressure). However, on rare occasions true unilateral papilloedema does evolve from increased CSF pressure. In such instances the side of the papilloedema has no consistent lateralizing value with respect to mass lesions. Previous optic atrophy may prevent disc swelling of one side, with papilloedema developing on the other (the so-called Foster Kennedy syndrome, attributed to subfrontal masses). It has also been speculated that a congenital nerve sheath anomaly may obstruct transmission of pressure such that the disc remains flat despite elevated intracranial pressure.

Although usually associated with slow growing or subacute mass lesions, papilloedema may develop within hours from subarachnoid or intracerebral haemorrhage. Once the intracranial space is decompressed, venous congestion of the disc will diminish rapidly, but disc swelling, haemorrhages and exudates will resolve more slowly. Well-developed papilloedema will take from 6 to 10 weeks to regress following lowering of intracranial pressure.

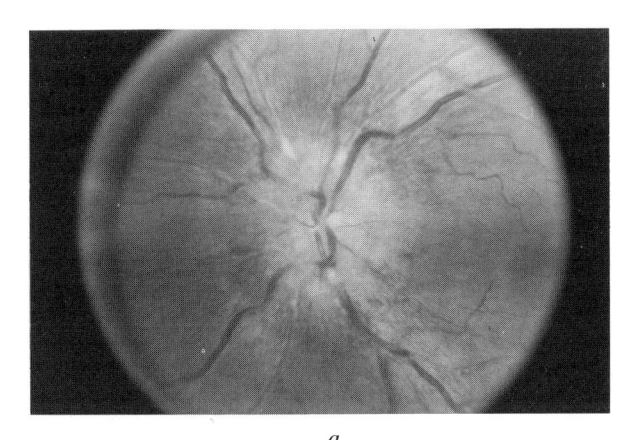

changes in posture may precipitate such obscurations or they may occur spontaneously. The cause of these visual disturbances is unknown but is probably related to transient fluctuations in nerve head perfusion as determined by the influence of increased intracranial pressure on cerebral blood flow mechanisms. It has been suggested that mild pressure on the globe may reproduce these obscurations. Obscurations are unrelated to the location or nature of space-occupying lesions and occur with regularity in the pseudotumour cerebri syndrome. The frequency of obscurations appears to be most closely correlated with high intracranial pressure (at least at the moment of the obscuration) and advanced degree of disc swelling. Prognosis of ultimate visual function is not related to the frequency or intensity of these

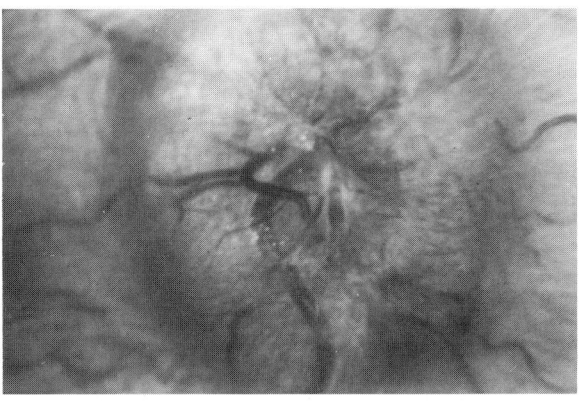

Fig. 9. Papilloedema. *a*, Relatively early phase. Note nerve fibre layer oedema involves principally disc margins, sparing cup area; venous engorgement minimal. *b*, Chronic papilloedema (enlarged). Note relative preservation of disc centre; major vessels are buried in nerve fibre layer; glittering inspissated exudates superficially simulate hyaline bodies.

Early and even well-developed papilloedema may not be symptomatic. Neither visual field nor acuity are affected unless retinal haemorrhage or oedema involves the macular area. Enlargement of the blind spot is of no help in early diagnosis since ophthalmoscopically overt disc swelling precedes this field change. The major clinical concept that separates papilloedema of intracranial origin from other forms of acquired disc swelling is that visual acuity, field and pupillary reactions are typically normal, whereas visual function (acuity, field, pupillary reaction) is almost always defective with papillitis (neuritis) or ischaemic optic neuropathy. When papilloedema has existed for many weeks or months, nerve fibre attrition results in progressive field loss in the form of irregular peripheral contraction and nerve fibre bundle defects. This is the atrophic stage of chronic papilloedema, which can ultimately lead to severe visual loss and even blindness.

Patients with well-developed papilloedema may note very brief transient obscurations of vision. 'Grey-outs', 'black-outs', or other momentary dimming of vision usually involve one eye at a time, last for a few seconds and clear completely. Sudden

episodes. The clinical aspects of such paroxysmal phenomena with brain tumours have been elaborated by Ethelberg and Jensen,[71] but their conclusions regarding transient interference with circulation through the posterior cerebral arteries are somewhat speculative.

Other signs and symptoms with papilloedema are related to the basic underlying pathological process that has caused the increased intracranial pressure. Headache, nausea and vomiting, and lateral recti weakness, are typical but non-specific symptomatology associated with raised CSF pressure, while hemiparesis, hemianopias or other field defects, seizures or specific ocular motility disturbances all have localizing value.

It is often helpful to 'stage' papilloedema ophthalmoscopically, which on occasion has considerable clinical value. As suggested by Jackson in 1871, papilloedema may be classified into four temporal types: early, fully developed, chronic, and atrophic (*Fig.* 9).

The early phase of papilloedema refers to the incipient disc changes that occur before the development of obvious disc swelling. Blurring of the nerve fibre layer with obscuration of the superior and inferior disc margins are early changes which may actually precede venous engorgement. A spontaneous venous pulsation is anticipated in approximately 80 per cent of eyes, and its presence strongly militates against a diagnosis of papilloedema. According to Walsh, spontaneous venous pulsation ceases when intracranial pressure exceeds 200 ± 25 mm H_2O.[72] The veins of the retina ultimately become engorged and dusky, but this sign does not constitute a major sign of papilloedema, unless accompanied by other features or seen to change progressively on serial observations. In fact, multiple careful observations are the keystone to diagnosis of papilloedema in its incipient form.

The occurrence of splinter haemorrhages in the nerve fibre layer at, or just off, the disc margin is a major sign, especially in the course of repeated observations. However, as noted previously, haemorrhages may on rare occasions occur with intrapapillary drusen or for no apparent reason in older individuals.

In early papilloedema, as well as in the more fully developed stage, the optic cup is retained. Therefore, absence of the central cup is much more likely to be seen in pseudopapilloedema than in incipient disc swelling. In the more chronic stage of papilloedema the central cup is very likely to be obliterated.

As oedema progresses, the surface of the disc becomes elevated above the plane of the retina. Disc margins are obscured and vessels are buried as they pass off the disc. At this stage, i.e. fully developed papilloedema, disc elevation is consistently accompanied by multiple flame haemorrhages, nerve-fibre layer infarcts ('cotton-wool' spots), serpentine tortuosity of veins and marked disc hyperaemia and hypervascularity attributable to dilatation of the superficial capillary bed of the disc surface.

Swelling in the nerve fibre layer extends laterally into the retina, so that the area of the nerve head appears enlarged. Circumferential retinal folds (Paton's lines) may be seen around the swollen disc, and these may extend to the macula. Rarely, retinal exudates may radiate from the fovea in the form of a star (or half-star between the disc and fovea).

If intracranial pressure remains elevated, the acute haemorrhagic and exudative components resolve, and the disc progressively takes on the appearance of the dome of a champagne cork. The central cup remains obliterated, but peripapillary retinal oedema resorbs. Small, round glistening 'hard exudates' in the disc substance may simulate buried hyaline bodies. This stage of chronic papilloedema indicates that disc swelling has been present for months. Nerve fibre attrition is predictable, leading to progressive field loss. As the disc detumesces, pallor slowly emerges, with apparent 'sheathing' of vessels but no real loss of disc substance. Although the disc usually has a milky grey appearance due to reactive gliosis ('secondary optic atrophy'), at times it may be remarkably crisp and white. Even with fairly rapid detumescence of preatrophic papilloedema, changes in the pigment epithelium at the fovea may produce mild but permanent reduction in central acuity.

Bird and Sanders[73] have described choroidal folds in association with papilloedema and have suggested that these striae are likely related to distension of the most distal portion of the optic nerve sheath (recently confirmed by ultrasonography).

The appearance of the disc, sequence of changes and ultimate visual outcome is dependent on variations of intracranial pathology, surgical interventions and obscure haemodynamic events involving both the disc and visual pathways. At times, decompression of chronic papilloedema is followed by visual loss which may be abrupt or progressive. These tragic events are neither understood nor predictable. Keane has reported blindness following ventriculography in the situation of high-grade papilloedema.[74] This event may be related to hypotension caused by intracranial decompression or even an increase in CSF pressure precipitated by anaesthesia.

Much has been written regarding the use of fluorescein angiography in the diagnosis of papilloedema, but basically the 'well-tempered' ophthalmoscope is still the primary diagnostic tool. In instances of ophthalmoscopically definable papilloedema, fluorescein angiography is superfluous. In eyes where disc changes are truly debatable, fluorescein angiography is usually inconclusive. Under no circumstances should the interpretation of the fluorescein angiogram be considered the single indication for invasive diagnostic studies.

A condition of benign intracranial hypertension (pseudotumour cerebri) is a diagnosis of exclusion, although in obese females it may be an anticipated cause of well-developed, often florid, papilloedema and headaches. Other neurological deficits, with the exception of non-specific signs of increased intracranial pressure (including unilateral or bilateral sixth nerve palsies), are inconsistent with a diagnosis of pseudotumour cerebri. Although a variety of factors may play a role in the production of this syndrome, most cases reveal no clearly identifiable underlying cause. In the large idiopathic group there is a distinct female preponderance and age distribution from the 'teens through the fifth decade. A series of papers in the journal *Brain* provides a detailed discussion of the pseudotumour cerebri syndrome.[75-77]

As a rule, the treatment of papilloedema is related to relief of the underlying process by which intracranial pressure is elevated. Therefore, therapy is usually in the hands of the neurologist or neurosurgeon. However, in instances when irresectable tumours or unrelenting pseudotumour cerebri sustain papilloedema with progressive visual loss, the ophthalmic surgeon may play a vital role. Although described more than 100 years ago by de Wecker and documented experimentally by Hayreh,[69] relief of papilloedema by incision of the orbital optic nerve sheath has only recently been revitalized by Davidson,[78] and Galbraith.[79] In appropriate patients, the medial orbital approach as detailed by Galbraith is a relatively simple route to the retrobulbar space where nerve sheath incision may produce dramatic relief of papilloedema. Progressive visual loss may be averted and improvement of visual function can ensue.

Differential Diagnosis of the 'Swollen Disc'

The causes of disc 'swelling' are legion, as outlined in *Table* VIII. It is imperative to separate papilloedema, i.e. disc swelling due to increased intracranial pressure as defined in the preceding section, from all other causes of acquired disc oedema. Disc swelling is usually interpreted as such a compelling sign of intracranial mass lesion that diagnostic studies often take an inappropriate course.

The distinction of congenitally elevated discs from papilloedema has already been elaborated. It should be recalled that true papilloedema, even in the fully developed form, does not reduce acuity or present with field defects other than enlarged blindspots. Therefore, confusion should not arise in distinguishing papilloedema from papillitis or ischaemic optic neuropathy, two common causes of disc oedema which regularly are associated with acute loss of acuity and/or field, and diminished direct light reaction of the ipsilateral pupil.

Local ocular disease, including uveitis, vein occlusion, and postoperative hypotony should represent no diagnostic problem. Primary nerve head tumours (melanocytoma, glioma, astrocytic hamartoma, haemangioma) are rare and usually definable by ophthalmoscopy. Metastatic disc tumours, other than those arising in the adjacent choroid and retina, are extremely infrequent and are characterized by massive haemorrhagic elevation of the disc and peripapillary retina, and drastic reduction of vision. Occasionally the optic nerve head may be infiltrated by a leukaemic or similar haematological process, usually with rapidly progressive visual loss.

Orbital mass lesions usually produce proptosis but may present as very chronic disc swelling due to a perioptic mass lesion in the orbit (e.g. nerve sheath meningioma). On extremely rare occasions papilloedema from increased intracranial pressure, including pseudotumour cerebri,[80,81] may be strictly unilateral. In this dilemma computerized tomography may prove valuable, after thorough history-taking and examination.

Table VIII. Aetiology of the 'swollen' disc

Congenital
  Anomalous elevation
  Hyaline bodies (drusen)
  Gliotic dysplasia
Ocular disease
  Uveitis
  Hypotony
  Vein occlusion
Metabolic
  Dysthyroidism
  Juvenile diabetes
  Proliferative retinopathies
Inflammatory
  Papillitis
  Neuroretinitis
  ? Papillophlebitis
Infiltrative
  Lymphoma
  Reticuloendothelial
Systemic disease
  Anaemia
  Hypoxaemia
  Hypertension
Disc tumours
  Haemangioma
  Glioma
  Metastatic
Vascular
  Ischaemic neuropathy
  Arteritis, cranial
  Arteritis, collagen
Orbital tumours
  Perioptic meningioma
  Glioma
  Sheath 'cysts'
  Retrobulbar mass
Elevated intracranial pressure
  Mass lesion
  Pseudotumour cerebri
  Hypertension

REFERENCES

1. Glaser J. S., Savino P. J., Sumers K. D. et al. The photostress recovery test in the clinical assessment of visual function. *Am. J. Ophthalmol.* 1977; **83**, 255.
2. Brook C. G. D., Sanders M. D. and Hoare R. D. Septo-optic dysplasia. *Br. Med. J.* 1972; **30**, 811.
3. Pollock J. A., Newton T. H. and Hoyt W. F. Transsphenoidal and transethmoidal encephaloceles: A review of clinical and roentgen features of 8 cases. *Radiology* 1968; **90**, 442.
4. Riise D. The nasal fundus ectasia. *Acta Ophthalmologica* 1975; Suppl. 126.
5. Rosenberg M. A., Savino P. J. and Glaser J. S. A clinical analysis of pseudopapilloedema. Part I. Population, laterality, acuity, refractive error, ophthalmoscopic characteristics, and coincident disease. *Arch. Ophthalmol.* 1979; **97**, 65.
6. Savino P. J., Glaser J. S. and Rosenberg M. A. A clinical analysis of pseudopapilloedema. Part II. Visual field defects. *Arch. Ophthalmol.* 1979; **97**, 71.

7. Rose F. C., Fraser G. R., Friedman A. I. et al. The association of juvenile diabetes mellitus and optic atrophy: Clinical and genetic aspects. *Q. J. Med.* 1966; **35**, 385.
8. Rorsman G. and Söderström N. Optic atrophy and juvenile diabetes mellitus with familial occurrence. *Acta Med. Scand.* 1967; **182**, 419.
9. Lessell S. and Rosman N. P. Juvenile diabetes mellitus and optic atrophy. *Arch. Neurol.* 1977; **34**, 759.
10. Kjer P. Infantile optic atrophy with dominant mode of inheritance: A clinical and genetic study of 19 Danish families. *Acta Ophthalmol. (Kbh.)* 1959; Suppl. 54.
11. Smith D. P. Diagnostic criteria in dominantly inherited juvenile optic atrophy: A report of 3 new families. *Am. J. Optom. Physiol. Opt.* 1972; **49**, 183.
12. Kline L. B. and Glaser J. S. Dominant optic atrophy. The clinical profile. *Arch. Ophthalmol.* 1979; **97**, 1680.
13. Hoyt C. S. Autosomal dominant optic atrophy. A spectrum of disability. *Ophthalmology* 1980; **87**, 245.
14. Nikoskelainen E. The clinical findings in Leber's hereditary optic neuropathy. *Trans. Ophthalmol. Soc. UK* 1985; **104**, 458.
15. Wallace D. C. A new manifestation of Leber's disease and a new explanation for the agency responsible for its unusual pattern of inheritance. *Brain* 1970; **93**, 121.
16. Lundsgaard R. Leber's disease: A genealogic, genetic and clinical study of 101 cases of retrobulbar optic neuritis in 20 Danish families. *Acta Ophthalmol. (Kbh.)* 1944; Suppl. 21.
17. Seedorff T. Leber's disease: V. *Acta Ophthalmol. (Kbh.)* 1970; **48**, 186.
18. Nikoskelainen E., Hoyt W. F. and Nummelin K. Ophthalmoscopic findings in Leber's hereditary optic neuropathy. I. Fundus findings in asymptomatic family members. *Arch. Ophthalmol.* 1982; **100**, 1597.
19. Brunette J. and Bernier R. G. Study of a family of Leber's optic atrophy with recuperation. In: Brunette J. and Barbeau A. (ed.) *Progress in Neuro-Ophthalmology*. Amsterdam, Excerpta Medica, 1969, pp. 91–8.
20. Wilson J., Linell J. C. and Matthews D. M. Plasmacobalamins in neuro-ophthalmological diseases. *Lancet* 1971; **1**, 259.
21. Potts A. M. Tobacco amblyopia. *Survey Ophthalmol.* 1973; **17**, 313.
22. Carroll F. D. Nutritional amblyopia. *Arch. Ophthalmol.* 1966; **76**, 406.
23. Grant W. M. *Toxicology of the Eye*, 2nd ed. Springfield, Ill., Thomas, 1974, pp. 49–54.
24. Leibold J. E. Drugs having a toxic effect on the optic nerve. *Int. Ophthalmol. Clin.* 1971; **11**, 137.
25. Haining W. M. and Beveridge G. W. Toxic amblyopia in a patient receiving ethchlorvynol as a hypnotic. *Br. J. Ophthalmol.* 1964; **48**, 598.
26. Reynolds W. D., Smith J. L. and McCrary J. A. Chiasmal optic neuritis. *J. Clin. Neuro-Ophthalmol.* 1982; **2**, 93.
27. Oakley G. P. The neurotoxicity of the halogenated hydroxyquinolines. *JAMA* 1973; **225**, 395.
28. Lessell S. Toxic and deficiency optic neuropathies. In: Smith J. L. and Glaser J. S. (ed.) *Neuro-Ophthalmology*. St Louis, Mo, Mosby, 1973, vol. 7, pp. 21–37.
29. Carroll F. D. Jamaican optic neuropathy in immigrants to the United States. *Am. J. Ophthalmol.* 1971; **71**, 261.
30. Trobe J. D. and Glaser J. S. Quantitative perimetry in compressive optic neuropathy and optic neuritis. *Arch. Ophthalmol.* 1978; **96**, 1210.
31. Bradley W. G. and Whitty W. M. Acute optic neuritis: Prognosis for development of multiple sclerosis. *J. Neurol. Neurosurg. Psychiat.* 1968; **31**, 10.
32. Cohen M. M., Lessell S. and Wolf P. A. A prospective study of the risk of developing multiple sclerosis in uncomplicated optic neuritis. *Neurology* 1979; **29**, 208.
33. Compston D. A. S., Batchelor J. R., Earl C. J. et al. Factors influencing the risk of multiple sclerosis developing in patients with optic neuritis. *Brain* 1978; **101**, 495.
34. Tarkkanen J. and Tarkkanen A. Otorhinolaryngological pathology in patients with optic neuritis. *Acta Ophthalmol.* 1971; **49**, 649.
35. Bradley W. G. and Whitty W. M. Acute optic neuritis: Its clinical features and their relation to prognosis for recovery of vision. *J. Neurol. Neurosurg. Psychiat.* 1967; **30**, 531.
36. Miller N. R. The big blind spot syndrome. Unilateral disc oedema without visual loss or increased intracranial pressure. In: Smith J. L. (ed.) *Neuro-Ophthalmology Update*, New York, Masson, 1977, pp. 163–9.
37. Bird A. C., Leaver P. K., Gould E. et al. Assessment of intraconal steroids in the treatment of retrobulbar neuritis. In: Glaser J. S. (ed.) *Neuro-Ophthalmology. Symposium of the University of Miami.* St Louis, Mo, Mosby, 1977, vol. 9, pp. 154–9.
38. Bowden A. N., Bowden P. M. A. and Friedman A. I. A trial of corticotropin gelatin injection in acute optic neuritis. *J. Neurol. Neurosurg. Psychiat.* 1974; **37**, 869.
39. Cogan D. G. *Neurology of the Visual System*. Springfield Ill., Thomas, 1966, p. 157.
40. Wagener H. P. and Hollenhorst R. W. The ocular lesions of temporal arteritis. *Am. J. Ophthalmol.* 1958; **45**, 617.
41. Hamilton C. R., Shelley W. M. and Tumulty P. A. Giant cell arteritis: Including temporal arteritis and polymyalgia rheumatica. *Medicine* 1971; **50**, 1.
42. Cullen J. F. Ischaemic optic neuropathy. *Trans. Ophthalmol. Soc. UK* 1967; **87**, 759.
43. Boyd R. V. and Hoffbrand B. I. Erythrocyte sedimentation rate in elderly hospital in-patients. *Br. Med. J.* 1966; **1**, 901.
44. Milne J. S. and Williamson J. The ESR in older people. *Gerontol. Clin.* 1972; **14**, 36.
45. Klein R. G., Campbell R. J., Hunder G. G. et al. Skip lesions in temporal arteritis. *Mayo Clin. Proc.* 1978; **51**, 504.

46. Carroll F. D. Optic nerve complications of cataract extraction. *Trans. Am. Acad. Ophthalmol. Otolaryngol.* 1973; **77**, 623.
47. Wilkinson J. M. S. and Russell R. W. R. Arteries of the head and neck in giant cell arteritis. *Arch. neurol.* 1972; **27**, 378.
48. Barr C. C., Glaser J. S. and Blankenship G. Acute disc swelling in juvenile diabetes. Clinical profile and natural history of 12 cases. *Arch. Ophthalmol.* 1980; **98**, 2185.
49. Trobe J. D., Glaser J. S. and Laflamme P. Dysthyroid optic neuropathy. Clinical profile and rationale for management. *Arch. Ophthalmol.* 1978; **96**, 1199.
50. Anderson D. R. and Spencer W. H. Ultrastructural and histochemical observations of optic nerve gliomas. *Arch. Ophthalmol.* 1970; **83**, 324.
51. Spencer W. H. Primary neoplasms of the optic nerve and its sheaths: clinical features and current concepts of pathogenetic mechanisms. *Trans. Am. Ophthalmol. Soc.* 1972; **70**, 490.
52. Glaser J. S., Hoyt W. F. and Corbett J. Visual morbidity with chiasmal glioma: Long-term studies of visual fields in untreated and irradiated cases. *Arch. Ophthalmol.* 1971; **85**, 3.
53. Hoyt W. F. and Baghdassarian S. A. Optic glioma of childhood: Natural history and rationale for conservative management. *Br. J. Ophthalmol.* 1969; **53**, 793.
54. Borit A. and Richardson E. P. The biological and clinical behavior of pilocytic astrocytomas of the optic pathways. *Brain* 1982; **105**, 161.
55. Hoyt W. F., Meshel L. G. Lessell S. et al. Malignant optic glioma of adulthood. *Brain* 1973; **96**, 121.
56. Laties A. M. and Scheie H. G. Evolution of multiple small tumours in sarcoid granuloma of the optic disc. *Am. J. Ophthalmol.* 1972; **74**, 60.
57. Ellis W. and Little H. L. Leukemic infiltration of the optic nerve head. *Am. J. Ophthalmol.* 1973; **75**, 867.
58. Allen R. A. and Straatsma B. R. Ocular involvement in leukemia and allied disorders. *Arch. Ophthalmol.* 1961; **66**, 490.
59. Walsh F. B. and Shewmake B. J. An unusual case of reticulum cell sarcoma. *Am. J. Ophthalmol.* 1972; **74**, 741.
60. Gudas P. P. Optic nerve myeloma. *Am. J. Ophthalmol.* 1971; **71**, 1085.
61. Kamin D. F., Hepler R. S. Solitary intracranial plasmacytoma mistaken for retrobulbar neuritis. *Am. J. Ophthalmol.* 1972; **73**, 584.
62. Olson M. E., Chernik N. L. and Posner J. B. Infiltration of leptomeninges by systemic cancer: A clinical and pathologic study. *Arch. Neurol.* 1974; **30**, 122.
63. Little J. R., Dale A. J. D. and Okazaki H. Meningeal carcinomatosis: Clinical manifestations. *Arch. Neurol.* 1974; **30**, 138.
64. Altrocchi P. A., Reinhardt P. M. and Eckman P. B. Blindness and meningeal carcinomatosis. *Arch. Ophthalmol.* 1972; **88**, 508.
65. Karp L. A., Zimmerman L. E., Borit A. et al. Primary intraorbital meningiomas. *Arch. Ophthalmol.* 1974; **91**, 24.
66. Frisen L., Hoyt W. F. and Tengroth B. M. Optociliary veins, disc pallor and visual loss: A triad of signs indicating spheno-orbital meningioma. *Acta Ophthalmol.* 1973; **51**, 241.
67. Alper M. G. Management of primary optic nerve meningiomas: current status-therapy in controversy. *J. Clin. Neuro-Ophthalmol.* 1981; **1**, 101.
68. Stern W. E. Meningiomas in the cranio-orbital junction. *J. Neurosurg.* 1973; **38**, 428.
69. Hayreh S. S. Pathogenesis of oedema of the optic disc (papilloedema): A preliminary report. *Br. J. Ophthalmol.* 1964; **48**, 522.
70. Rios-Montenegro E. N., Anderson D. R. and David N. J. Intracranial pressure and ocular haemodynamics. *Arch. Ophthalmol.* 1973; **89**, 52.
71. Ethelberg S. and Jensen V. A. Obscurations and further time-related paroxysmal disorders in intracranial tumors; Syndrome of initial herniation of parts of brain through tentorial incisure. *AMA Arch. Neurol. Psychiat.* 1952; **68**, 130.
72. Walsh T. J., Garden J., Gallagher B. et al. Obliteration of retinal venous pulsations. *Am. J. Ophthalmol.* 1969; **67**, 954.
73. Bird A. C. and Sanders M. D. Choroidal folds in association with papilloedema. *Br. J. Ophthalmol.* 1973; **57**, 89.
74. Keane J. R. Sudden blindness after ventriculography. *Am. J. Ophthalmol.* 1974; **78**, 275.
75. Johnston I. and Paterson A. Benign intracranial hypertension: I. Diagnosis and prognosis. *Brain* 1974; **97**, 289.
76. Johnston I. and Paterson A. Benign intracranial hypertension: II. CSF pressure and circulation. *Brain* 1974; **97**, 301.
77. Boddie H. G., Banna M. and Bradley W. F. 'Benign' intracranial hypertension: A survey of the clinical and radiologic features, and long-term prognosis. *Brain* 1974; **97**, 313.
78. Davidson S. I. A surgical approach to plerocephalic disc oedema. *Trans. Ophthalmol. Soc. UK* 1969; **89**, 669.
79. Galbraith J. E. K. and Sullivan J. H. Decompression of the perioptic meninges for relief of papilloedema. *Am. J. Ophthalmol.* 1973; **76**, 687.
80. Kirkham T. H., Sanders M. D. and Sapp G. A. Unilateral papilloedema in benign intracranial hypertension. *Can. J. Ophthalmol.* 1973; **8**, 533.
81. Sher N. A., Wirtschafter J., Shapiro S. K. et al. Unilateral papilloedema in 'benign intracranial hypertension' (pseudotumour cerebri). *JAMA* 1983; **250**, 2346.

Diseases of the Chiasm and Posterior Visual Pathways

C. J. Earl

ANATOMICAL FEATURES

Fibres of the optic nerves become reorganized in the optic chiasm, fibres from the nasal retina crossing to join fibres from the temporal retina on the opposite side. Fibres from the macula are similarly 'split'. As a result of this a lesion of the centre of the chiasm involves the central field first and may then be more difficult to detect unless it is suspected and the central fields examined carefully with this in mind. Such bitemporal central defects will often produce more prominent complaints of visual disturbance than loss of the periphery, which is often discovered accidentally. Fibres from the macular region lie in the posterior part of the chiasma and are affected by compressive lesions, e.g. pituitary adenomas, when the chiasm is 'pre-fixed' (i.e. the optic nerves are relatively short) or when the mass lies posteriorly. the posterior part of the chiasma and are affected by compressive lesions, e.g. pituitary adenomas, when the chiasm is 'pre-fixed' (i.e. the optic nerves are relatively short) or when the mass lies posteriorly. Patients with peripheral bitemporal defects may be remarkably unaware of them until they encroach on the central field but some complain of loss of lateral vision or realize that it is lost as a result of accidents, for example when driving. As the condition progresses central vision is involved and acuity impaired, usually one eye being affected before the other. In the end, if the cause is untreated, total blindness may follow. The optic discs may become pale, but this is often a late sign.

Some patients complain of diplopia without ocular palsy, most often observed during reading. This is due to failure of binocular fusion on account of the field defect. Some with complete bitemporal hemianopia become aware of an area of blindness beyond the point of fixation, when they are looking at objects close to the eyes. This is due to an 'overlap' of the blind temporal field of each eye in these circumstances.

PITUITARY ADENOMA

Compressive lesions are by far the most common cause of disturbance of chiasmal function and of these pituitary adenomas with suprasellar extension form a high proportion. Most are not 'endocrinologically active' and the endocrine abnormalities if present are those of hypopituitarism. Of those which are 'active', the most common are those producing growth hormone or prolactin. ACTH-producing tumours are less common and when they occur are usually confined to the sella. Treatment is usually surgical and in recent years more and more tumours are being removed by the trans-sphenoidal route rather than by craniotomy. Partial or full recovery of field is the rule except in late cases and the recovery may occur very rapidly (*Fig.* 1). In many instances a course of postoperative radiotherapy is given.

Pituitary Apoplexy

Occasionally pituitary tumours become haemorrhagic and their size increases rapidly with a rapid onset of visual failure. Although there is more severe loss in the temporal fields the nasal fields are often affected. These haemorrhagic tumours often extend laterally into the cavernous sinus as well as upwards towards the chiasm and involve the IIIrd, IVth and VIth cranial nerves to produce a picture of loss of vision and extra-ocular muscle paralysis. The onset is usually with acute severe headache, sometimes mimicking that of subarachnoid haemorrhage, and there may be leakage of blood into the subarachnoid space. The syndrome is associated with acute severe pituitary failure which needs urgent treatment with hydrocortisone.

Occasionally pituitary tumours may extend laterally into the cavernous sinus even when they are not haemorrhagic and they may then cause ocular palsies. They may also spread more widely in the skull, particularly in the middle fossa or over the back of the sella down into the posterior fossa. Such adenomas have been described as 'invasive'.

CRANIOPHARYNGIOMA

These tumours arise from cellular remnants of Rathke's pouch. They may be solid, but often contain cysts which may be large. The tumours occur in childhood and in adult life. In childhood they tend to

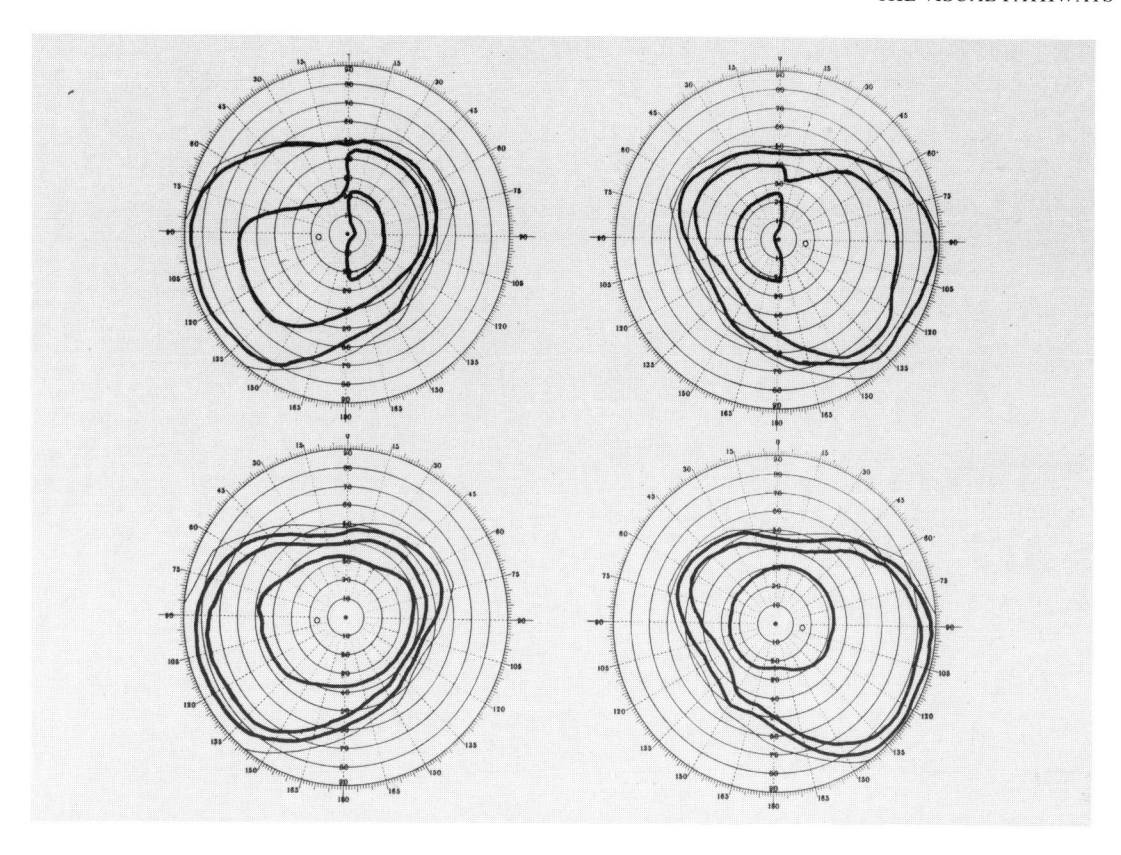

Fig. 1. Pituitary adenoma. Partial bitemporal field defect (3, 10W and 10R / 330); before operation and 4 days after operation.

extend upwards into the hypothalmus and third ventricle, causing hypothalmic functional disorders, obstruction of the third ventricle and hydrocephalus. In adult life their symptomatology tends to be visual, with associated hypopituitarism. The visual field defects are bitemporal and are often asymmetrical. Some cases show remarkable spontaneous variations in vision, presumably due to fluctuations in the size of the cystic elements. This variation may give rise to difficulties in diagnosis. Complete surgical excision is rarely possible without causing serious postoperative neurological deficits and is often limited to decompression of the chiasm by aspiration of cysts. Hydrocephalus, if present, may be treated by shunting and radiotherapy may be given postoperatively. However, these tumours have a very long natural history and patients may survive many years with minimal symptoms following palliative treatment and treatment of endocrine deficiencies if necessary.

MENINGIOMAS

Meningiomas which compress the chiasm produce very insidious loss of vision. Although meningiomas arising from the tuberculum sellae may produce symmetrical chiasmal defects, more often they produce a picture of combined chiasmal and optic nerve involvement and the field defects produced may be very variable. One well known pattern of loss is related to compression of one optic nerve adjacent to the chiasm and the field loss is characteristic with monocular failure of vision and optic atrophy in the eye on the side of the tumour. Another is depressed visual acuity and central field loss, combined with a loss of the temporal field in the opposite eye, usually beginning in the upper quadrant. This early involvement of the upper quadrant is due to the fact that fibres from the lower nasal retina of the opposite eye loop for a short distance into the proximal portion of the optic nerve of the other side before turning back into the optic tract, and may therefore be involved in a compressive lesion at the posterior end of the nerve. Meningiomas can frequently be completely removed surgically but the success of operation is largely dependent on early diagnosis. Recovery of vision may be less satisfactory than that following removal of a pituitary adenoma.

INTRACRANIAL ANEURYSMS

Intracranial aneurysms may also compress the chiasm.

OPTIC NERVE GLIOMAS

Gliomas may arise in the optic nerves and spread to the chiasm or may arise in the chiasm itself. They may invade the hypothalmus and in some cases hypothalamic gliomas may spread to involve the chiasm. It is sometimes difficult to tell in which situation the tumour has originated. These tumours produce less symmetrical field defects than external compressive lesions. They frequently arise in association with neurofibromatosis. Their natural history is very variable. Some may be present for many years with little or no increase in symptoms or signs.

CHIASMATIC ARACHNOIDITIS

This condition may have been diagnosed too frequently in the past. When it occurs it produces visual failure with field loss suggestive of chiasmal involvement. It certainly may occur in sarcoidosis involving the central nervous system and as a complication of treated tuberculous meningitis, and more rarely as the result of other forms of mengingitis. Arachnoiditis may be associated with the formation of arachnoid cysts in the region of the chiasm which may cause chiasmal syndromes and which can be relieved by decompression. Sometimes surgical division of the compressive adhesions can also be successful even when there is no cyst present. Diagnosis may be very difficult except where there is evidence elsewhere of underlying disease, and it may be made only at operation.

EMPTY SELLA SYNDROME

This may follow treatment for pituitary tumour but sometimes arises for no apparent reason. In some cases it is a sequel to benign intracranial hypertension and it is interesting that even among those patients who have no past history of this condition there is a high proportion of obese females. There is a similar high proportion of obese females among those suffering from benign intracranial hypertension. Occasionally bitemporal field defects occur, the exact mechanism of which is uncertain but it has been thought that the cause may be downward displacement of the optic chiasm into the sella.

HEAD INJURY

The chiasm may also be damaged in closed head injury. This may be due to physical disruption of the crossing fibres but in some cases it is thought to be due to ischaemia of the central part of the chiasm as a result of movement of intracranial structures at the moment of impact with damage to nutrient vessels. A complete bitemporal hemianopia may result, which does not recover.

OPTIC TRACT AND GENICULATE BODY

Proved lesions of the optic tract or geniculate body are rare, although the tract may be involved in lesions described above which more commonly affect the central part of the chiasm, and there may then be involvement of the chiasma and optic nerves as well, with a correspondingly complex pattern of field loss. Where the tract alone is affected a homonymous hemianopia results which, if partial, may show marked incongruity. Theoretically the presence of Wernicke's hemianopic pupillary reaction should give a clue to the presence of a tract lesion causing a hemianopia but it is difficult to elicit reliably by ordinary methods of clinical examination.

Although rare, intrinsic demyelinating lesions do occur in multiple sclerosis, but unless there is other evidence of the disease, the diagnosis cannot be established. Large aneurysms of the internal carotid lying on the lateral side of the chiasm may compress the optic tract and malignant tumours of the third ventricle may extend laterally to involve it. Medial extension of similar tumours in the temporal lobe may have a similar effect.

The lateral geniculate body may be involved in intracerebral gliomas but involvement will be difficult to confirm. It may also be involved in vascular lesions, but again only rarely will proof be possible.

OPTIC RADIATION

Lesions of the optic radiation are frequent causes of visual disturbance. The fibres in the lower part of the radiation loop forward from the geniculate body into the temporal lobe before turning back to the occipital lobe, passing deeply in the parietal lobe to join the fibres of the upper part of the radiation. As a result, lesions of the temporal lobe may produce an upper quadrantic homonymous field defect on the opposite side. In the non-dominant temporal lobe this may be the only physical sign of a lesion in the temporal lobe. On the dominant side it will usually be associated with some degree of speech disturbance. The visual field defect may be congruent or show some degree of incongruity, the inequality being shown by more extensive involvement of the field of the eye on the side of the lesion. Lesions in the parietal lobe may cause a lower homonymous field defect from involvement of the upper part of the radiation but more often affect both upper and lower fields.

Parietal lesions may be associated with other evidence of contralateral sensory disturbance, disturbances of speech (when the dominant hemisphere is involved) and other disturbances of higher cerebral function such as topographical disorientation and apraxia. There may also be a disturbance of ocular motor function with abnormalities of fixation (spasticity of gaze). Even where such abnormalities of ocular motor function are not present, optokinetic nystagmus may be asymmetrical with loss or impairment of the normal response when the drum is rotated towards the abnormal hemisphere. This is often a valuable localizing sign, and is not found where the hemianopia is due to a lesion of the optic tract or occipital cortex.

The optic radiations are frequently involved in ischaemic lesions, being supplied for the most part by one of the deep penetrating branches of the middle cerebral artery. The resultant hemianopias are usually complete and are associated with hemiplegia and hemi-anaesthesia from simultaneous involvement of the internal capsule. The chances of recovery of the hemianopia are poor. Temporal lobe infarction or haemorrhage may produce a superior quadrantic homonymous defect and involvement of the inferior part of the parietal lobe may produce quadrantanopia involving the lower half of the field of vision. Tumours of the parietal lobe will also produce homonymous field defects. Gliomas or metastatic tumours are the commonest types encountered. Extracerebral compressive lesions may also affect the optic radiation. Meningiomas in the parietal region or the occipital region may therefore produce homonymous hemianopic disturbance of vision, as may subdural haematomas. In such cases visual disturbances are almost always associated with other contralateral signs of disease in the cerebral hemisphere. The hemianopia in cases of this sort may usually be distinguished from hemianopia of vascular origin by the suddenness of the onset of symptoms in the latter, although occasionally symptoms from a tumour may develop suddenly. Intracerebral angiomas may also involve the optic radiation and produce clinical signs as a result of haemorrhage or infarction.

OCCIPITAL LOBE, VISUAL CORTEX

Lesions of the occipital lobe may involve the terminal portion of the optic radiation or the occipital cortex itself. The visual cortex lies on the medial side of the occipital lobe and much of it is buried in the calcarine fissure. The cortex above the fissure is concerned with vision in lower fields and the cortex below with the upper fields. The posterior cortex receives fibres concerned with central vision, the more anterior is related to vision in the peripheral parts of the field. The cortex on the superficial surface (unburied) is related to vision closer to the vertical meridian, while the cortex deep in the fissure is concerned with vision close to the horizontal meridian. These relationships were described accurately by Holmes more than 60 years ago and have been confirmed since then.

Occipital lesions are frequently vascular and the hemianopia is often an isolated finding without other neurological signs. In particular optokinetic nystagmus is normal in contrast to the findings in hemianopia related to a lesion of the optic radiation in the parietal lobe (q.v.). In vascular lesions there may also be true 'macular sparing'. This is due to the pattern of blood supply to the occipital cortex. The medial surface of the cortex is supplied by the terminal branch of the posterior cerebral artery, while the cortex at the very tip of the occipital lobe (concerned with central vision) may be supplied by a long posterior branch of the middle cerebral, so that the occipital pole may remain intact when the posterior cerebral artery is occluded. True macular sparing of this sort may be easily confused on casual examination with apparent macular sparing related to shift of fixation. True macular sparing can be demonstrated only by using more than one target object simultaneously in testing fields on the Bjerrum screen. One object is brought along the horizontal meridian into the central field and the other at about 10° above or below. If there is true macular sparing the object on the horizontal meridian will be seen before the object 10° above or below. With apparent macular sparing due to shift of fixation, both objects will be seen simultaneously.

The posterior cerebral arteries arise as terminal branches of the basilar artery, and blood flow in both posterior cerebral arteries may be interrupted simultaneously as a result of occlusion of the basilar artery. Where the basilar artery is stenosed or where there is failure of flow in the vertebral artery, flow in the posterior cerebral artery may be intermittently reduced. Patients may then experience episodes of brief loss or other disturbance of vision together with other appropriate symptoms of brain stem ischaemia such as vertigo, impairment of balance, slurred speech and sensory disturbance in the hands or limbs. Such episodes may occur frequently over weeks or months and may then clear spontaneously or they may be followed by a persistent loss of vision, either complete or hemianopic, with patchy and particularly central sparing.

Sometimes as a result of vascular disease, or more rarely as a result of a penetrating injury or other lesion, the visual cortex may be affected on both sides and the picture of complete cortical blindness may result. The pupils react normally to light. Where the lesion is ischaemic and there is a sparing of the central fields a small area of useful vision remains and acuity is preserved, but there is a serious visual disability which is often poorly understood by the patient. Occasionally patients appear quite unaware of the visual defect and may confabulate in great detail about what they can see. Most ischaemic lesions of the visual cortex are due to occlusion of terminal branches of both posterior cerebral arteries, but may occur as a result of cerebral anoxia.

DISORDERS OF HIGHER VISUAL FUNCTION

Alexia without Agraphia

This syndrome of acquired word blindness occurs as the result of a lesion in the dominant parieto-occipital region associated with interruption of fibres in the posterior part of the corpus callosum. There is loss of ability to read in spite of preservation of other speech functions, including writing. The syndrome appears to be due to a disconnection of the surviving (non-dominant) visual cortex from the 'speech centres' in the dominant hemisphere so that visual information, while correctly interpreted in other ways, cannot be interpreted as speech. The responsible lesion is usually ischaemic.

Visual Agnosia

This has been defined as an inability to identify objects by sight alone when vision is apparently normal otherwise and where the object may be identified through some other sensory channel. The problem is a complex one and the pathology uncertain, but in most cases the syndrome is associated with right hemianopia.

to destruction of the anterior wall of the sella and a lower part of the anterior clinoid process. Meningiomas may cause hyperostosis of the tuberculum sellae or the sphenoid wing.

CT scanning has assumed a very important and safe role in the diagnosis of tumours in the region of the chiasm. Suprasellar extensions of pituitary adenomas may be readily seen, particularly when images in the sagittal plane can be produced (*Fig.* 2). Suprasellar meningiomas can be similarly demonstrated unless they are very small. Craniopharyngiomas may be identifiable by the presence of calcification in a suprasellar mass on CT scanning even when this is not present on plain radiographs, and areas of low

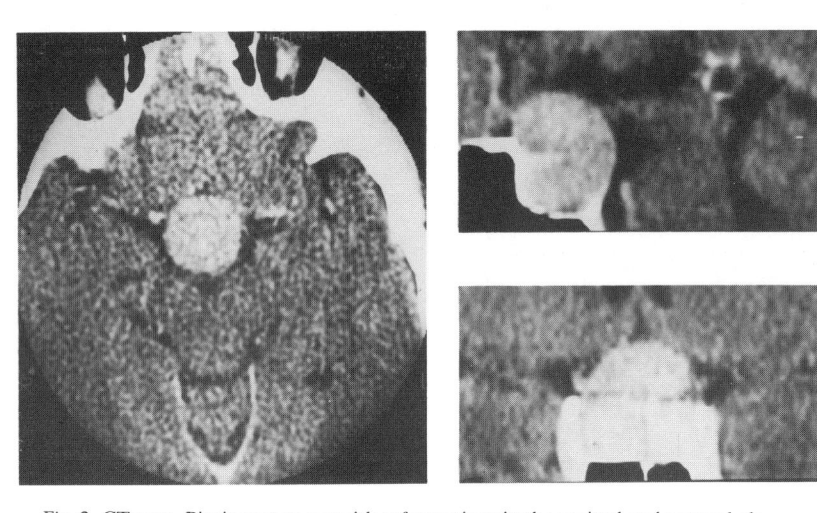

Fig. 2. CT scan. Pituitary tumour with reformations in the sagittal and coronal planes.

Visual Hallucinations

Visual hallucinations are most commonly 'toxic' or metabolic in origin but occasionally may occur in cerebral lesions and arise in the blind half field in hemianopia. They may also occur in patients with cortical blindness. Transient visual hallucinations are common in epilepsy arising in temporal or occipital lobes and in classic migraine, but they have also been described as rare manifestations of lesions of the anterior visual pathways.

INVESTIGATION OF THE OPTIC CHIASMA

Plain radiographs with special views of the sella turcica and the optic nerve canals will often give a strong clue as to the nature of a chiasmal lesion. Pituitary adenomas usually cause enlargement of the sella, which is often asymmetrical, and the floor may be eroded. Craniopharyngiomas may show speckled calcification in the suprasellar region (particularly in children) and large aneurysms may show a ring of calcification in the wall. Chiasmal gliomas that have extended into the optic nerve will cause enlargement of the optic nerve canals, best seen on tomography. The sella may have the characteristic J-shape due

density may suggest the presence of cysts. Optic nerve gliomas may reveal themselves with enlargement of the chiasm and optic nerves and hypothalamic tumours invading the chiasm will be readily visible. Chiasmatic arachnoiditis may be suspected as a result of failure to demonstrate the chiasmatic cisterns clearly, particularly where there is an associated local enhancement of the meninges with contrast. Large aneurysms will be readily identified. Pneumo-encephalography, previously a most useful investigation, is now hardly ever necessary although occasionally encephalography with a positive contrast medium, such as Metrizamide, may give useful information. Angiography remains essential in some cases and certainly as a preliminary to surgery it is often necessary to demonstrate the situation of major vessels in relation to the tumour. Endocrine studies will be helpful diagnostically in some cases and are certainly necessary before embarking on surgical treatment, in establishing whether or not there is endocrine activity in the tumour, or whether there is evidence of hypopituitarism.

Vascular lesions in the cerebral hemisphere may be associated with heart disease or narrowing of the carotid or vertebral arteries, of which there may be evidence on clinical examination and which may be confirmed by echocardiography and angiography. Hypertension may give rise to haemorrhage deep in the cerebral hemisphere which is likely to affect the optic radiation. Arteriovenous malformations may be associated with bruits heard over the carotid artery, the skull or the eyeball and occasionally malformations in the occipital region may be fed by a prominent occipital artery.

The presence of a cerebral infarct or a cerebral haemorrhage may be readily demonstrated on CT scanning, and the diagnosis of an intracranial tumour affecting the visual pathways behind the chiasm can almost always be established by appropriate CT scans (*Fig.* 3), although where surgery is to be undertaken cerebral angiography may be necessary in addition.

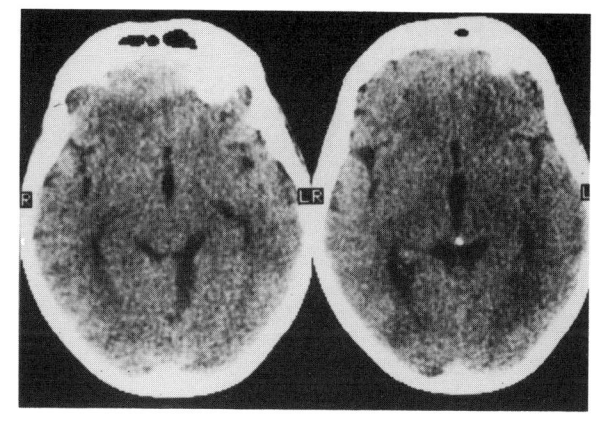

Fig. 3. CT scan. Posterior cerebral territory infarction with involvement of visual cortex.

FURTHER READING

Cogan D. W. *Neurology of the Visual System.* Springfield, Ill., Thomas, 1966, Ch. 11–15.
Glaser J. S. *Neuro-ophthalmology.* Hagerstown Md, Harper and Row, 1978, Ch. 6, 7.
Huber A. (trans. Blodi F.) *Eye Symptoms in Brain Tumours.* Ch. 3, 'Local symptoms in brain tumours'. St Louis, Mo, Mosby, 1977.
Walsh F. B. and Hoyt W. F. *Clinical Neuro-ophthalmology.* Baltimore, Md, Williams and Wilkins, 1969.

Chapter 13

The Management of Ocular Tumours

M. A. Bedford

During the past 20 years there has been a complete change in the management of ocular tumours, from the almost automatic enucleation of an eye containing such a neoplasm to a more cautious approach with consideration of conservative therapy or planned procrastination. Such changes have been engendered by earlier precise diagnosis and the use of sophisticated therapeutic techniques when necessary.

Ocular tumours may be subdivided into epibulbar and bulbar tumours.

EPIBULBAR TUMOURS

Benign

The most common benign lesion arising from the conjunctiva is a small pigmented area usually adjacent to the limbus or on the caruncle. These lesions may vary from a fraction of a millimeter to several millimeters across; the limbal lesions in particular show adjacent cystic changes in the conjunctiva. They may be removed for cosmetic reasons or may be observed, as they occasionally may enlarge at an alarming rate, having changed their nature (*see below*).

Malignant Tumours

These are rare and may classically be divided into non-pigmented and pigmented.

Non-pigmented Malignant Tumours

LOCAL

Classically they are squamous cell carcinomas presenting as a single vascular nodule varying from a few millimeters to many millimeters in diameter. Less commonly basal cell carcinomas are seen. Treatment is an excision biopsy.

DIFFUSE

Bowen's disease presents as confluent gelatinous areas with many fine branching blood vessels (*Fig.* 1). The diagnosis is established by a biopsy and wherever possible the lesion is best simply excised. If this is impossible, however, it may be necessary to treat it by radiation or even exenteration. A diffuse

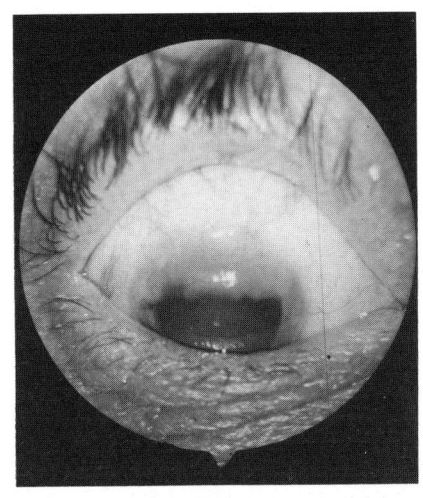

Fig. 1. Bowen's disease. Showing the typical gelatinous area with many fine branching blood vessels. Treatment is preceded by a biopsy to establish the diagnosis, and wherever possible, the lesion is simply excised.

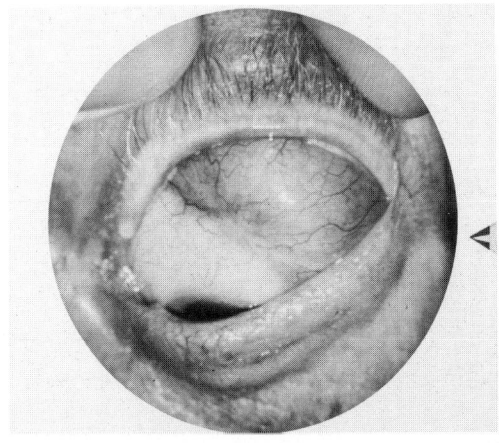

Fig. 2. The characteristic salmon pink swelling of a lymphoma. These usually melt away with radiation but can be associated with systemic manifestations.

subconjunctival 'salmon pink' swelling is characteristic of a lymphoma (*Fig.* 2). It may be associated with dissemination and lymphosarcomatous changes, when chemotherapy is necessary. If confined locally, radiation produces a dramatic cure. Occasionally a diffuse malignant melanoma of the conjunctiva may be non-pigmented (*see below*).

Pigmented Malignant Tumours

LOCAL

These may arise from pre-existing naevi (*Fig.* 3), therefore such benign lesions are best observed until they develop signs of thickness, large feeder vessels or inflammatory signs, such changes indicating a malignant alteration in character (*Fig.* 4). The lesion is best removed by local excision (*Fig.* 5).

DIFFUSE

These lesions pose very difficult therapeutic problems. Pigmented patches which are flat and light brown may be observed over a period of many years – 'precancerous melanosis' (*Fig.* 6). A biopsy need

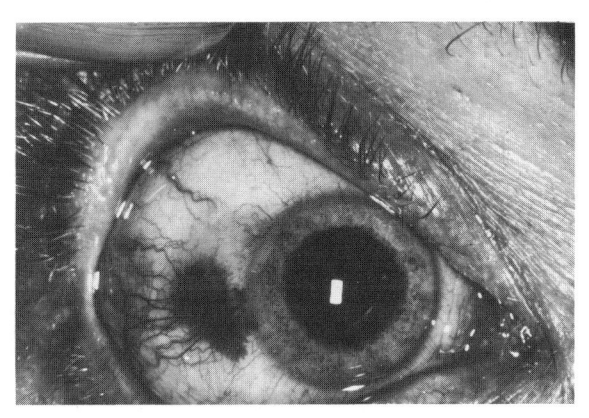

Fig. 3. A naevus. A brown patch which has been present for many years and has shown signs of slight enlargement.
(From M. A. Bedford, 'A Colour Atlas of Ocular Tumours' London, Wolfe Medical, 1979.)

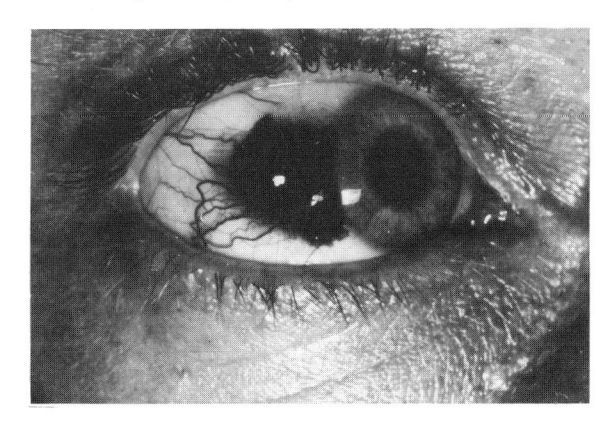

Fig. 4. A malignant melanoma arising from a pre-existing naevus. The same case as *Fig.* 3.
(From M. A. Bedford, 'A Colour Atlas of Ocular Tumours' London, Wolfe Medical, 1979.)

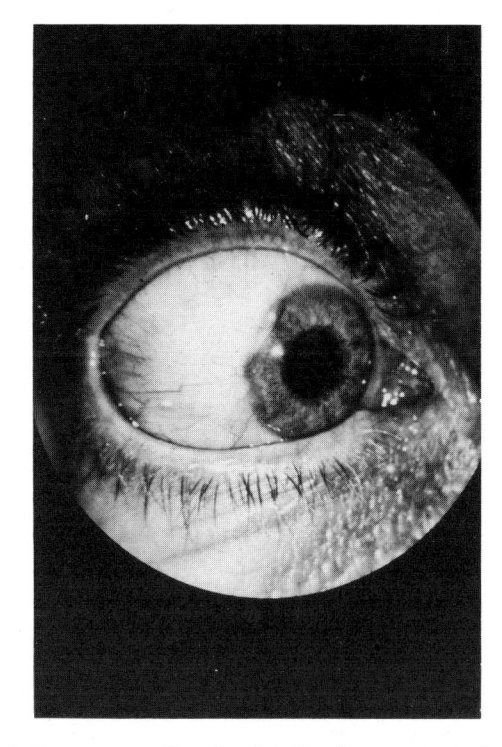

Fig. 5. Same case as *Figs.* 3 and 4. Excellent result obtained by local removal of a localized malignant melanoma.
(From M. A. Bedford, 'A Colour Atlas of Ocular Tumours' London, Wolfe Medical, 1979.)

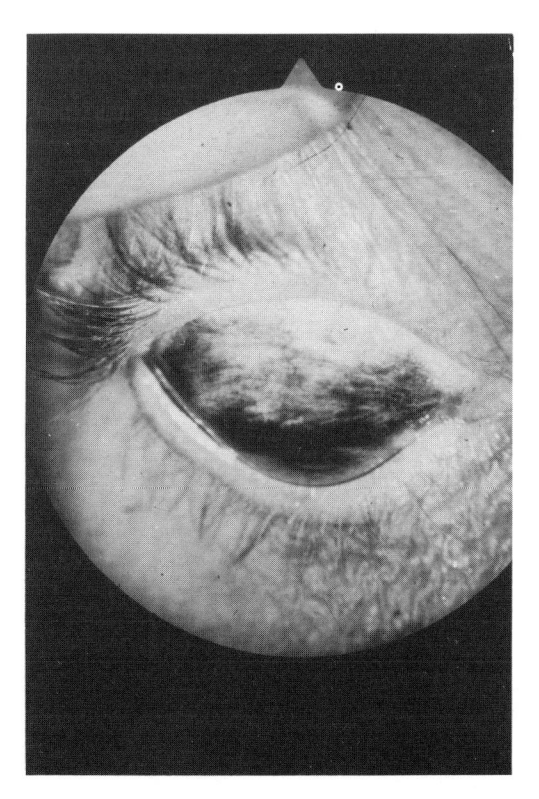

Fig. 6. 'Precancerous' melanosis showing the fine brownish scattered and flat pigmentation typical of this condition.
(From M. A. Bedford, 'A Colour Atlas of Ocular Tumours' London, Wolfe Medical, 1979.)

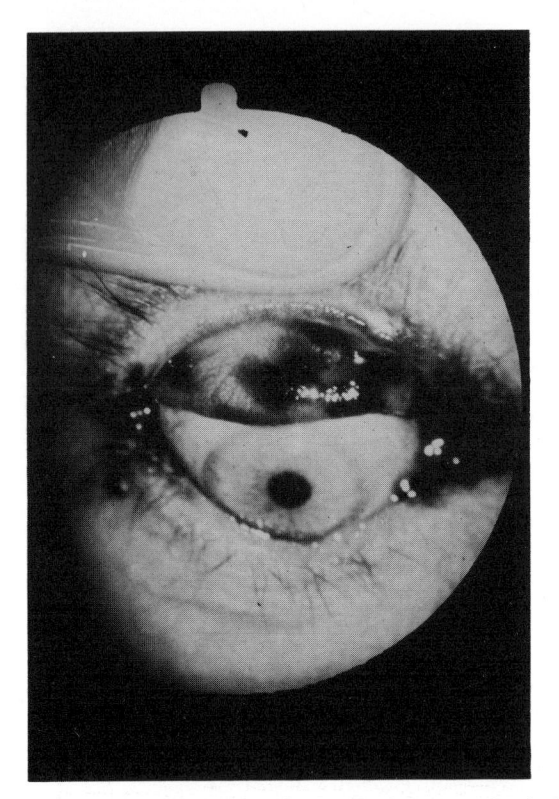

Fig. 7. Heavier pigmentation with much congestion associated with a diffuse malignant melanoma. The diagnosis is proved by biopsy and, in a case like this, the treatment is exenteration.
(From M. A. Bedford, 'A Colour Atlas of Ocular Tumours' London, Wolfe Medical, 1979.)

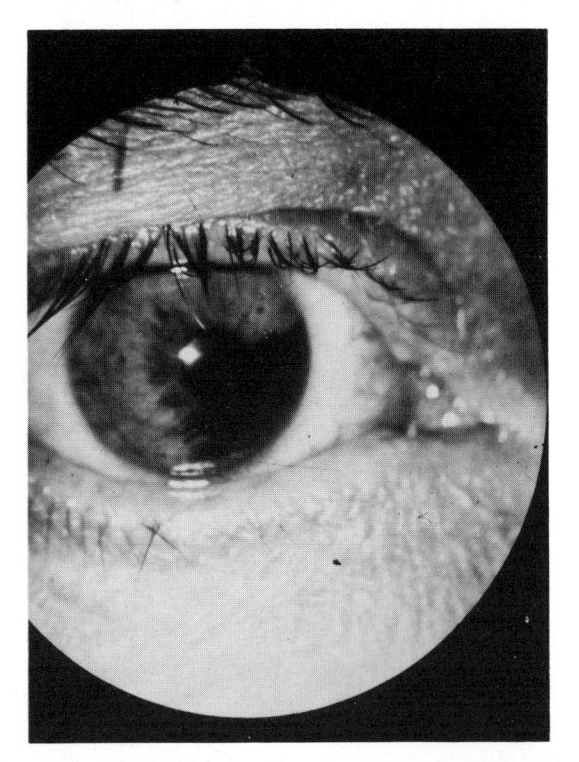

Fig. 8. A typical iris malignant melanoma producing distortion of the pupil.
(From M. A. Bedford, 'A Colour Atlas of Ocular Tumours' London, Wolfe Medical, 1979.)

not be done as the histology can be difficult to interpret and may be unnecessarily worrying. If the lesion becomes raised, develops large feeder vessels or shows inflammatory signs, then a biopsy should be carried out (*Fig.* 7). If the presence of an outright malignant melanoma is noted histologically, the treatment will depend on the site of the lesion. If it is on the globe, beta irradiation may be applied, but if bulky and down in the fornix or involving the back of the lids, then exenteration will be necessary (perhaps with conservation of the skin of the lids). Cryosurgery can sometimes be very helpful in selected cases or recurrences.

BULBAR TUMOURS

The most common tumours seen at Moorfields Hospital, London, are uveal tumours, usually in adults, of a primary or secondary variety, and retinal tumours seen in children. Uveal tumours may be classified on an anatomical basis – iris, ciliary body, choroid.

Uveal Tumours

Iris

Benign

The most common lesion of the iris seen is a naevus. These are of variable size and may be surprisingly large. They are usually pigmented, flat and circumscribed, showing no nutrient vessels or capillary dilatation. Observation is all that is required as they may occasionally undergo malignant change. In babies a fleshy vascular tumour, naevoxanthoendothelioma, may cause recurrent hyphaemas, which necessitate urgent treatment with a small dose of X-rays and/or steroids. The eye lesion may be associated with cutaneous manifestations of the xanthomas.

Malignant

These are the least common of the uveal malignant melanomas but are usually diagnosed much earlier, as they tend to be noted because of their superficial position. They present as a single or multiple, spreading, bulky vascularized lesion of the iris producing pupillary distortion (*Fig.* 8). They spread around the angle, producing secondary glaucoma and may rarely extend outside the globe with a subsequent worsening of prognosis. The treatment is iridectomy or iridocyclectomy if the ciliary body is involved secondarily, while the presence of secondary glaucoma necessitates enucleation. Their prognosis in terms of life is excellent. Secondary tumours may be seen, usually from breast or bronchus, and these may be single or multiple, perhaps associated with secondary glaucoma.

Ciliary Body

Benign

Benign cysts and hyperplasia of the ciliary body are thought to be common pathologically but are rarely a clinical worry.

Malignant

Unfortunately most malignant melanomas of the ciliary body do not present until they are too large for convenient removal by iridocyclectomy. The expanding lesion tends to spread forwards, backwards, inwards or outwards before it presents (*Fig.* 9). If,

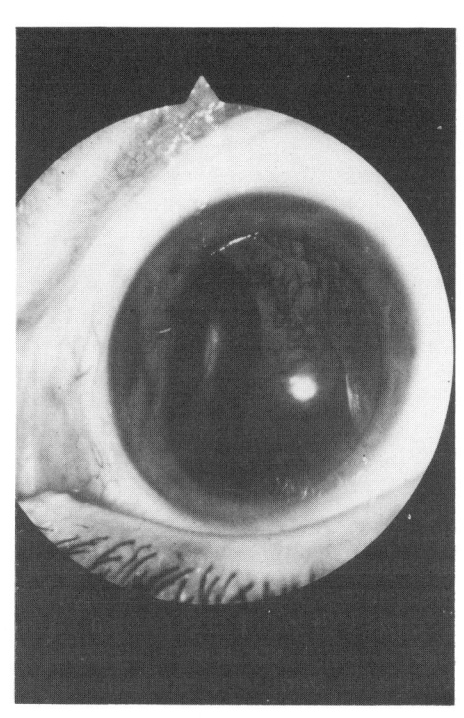

Fig. 9. A large ciliary body malignant melanoma extending into the angle, distorting and displacing the lens and producing a cataract.
(From M. A. Bedford, 'A Colour Atlas of Ocular Tumours' London, Wolfe Medical, 1979.)

however, a small tumour is noted before any extension occurs, then local removal is indicated either by an iridocyclectomy or cyclectomy. The earliest signs of a ciliary body tumour are slight hypotony, an unaccountable loss of visual acuity with dilated episcleral veins in the quandrant containing the tumour.

Choroid

Benign

NAEVI

Naevi are commonly seen in the choroid, often noted accidentally. They are classically flat with feathered edges, a dark grey colour, and perhaps with overlying colloid bodies. They should be noted and observed, as there is no doubt that they can undergo malignant change.

HAEMANGIOMA

Haemangiomas present as a raised, salmon pink swelling at the posterior pole of the eye. A serous detachment may be present as the fluid escapes from the deeper large vascular spaces, the overlying retina having a crinkled cystoid appearance (*Fig.* 10). At their first appearance they can be easily missed unless the fundus is examined by the indirect ophthalmoscope. Fluorescein angiography may be characteristic.

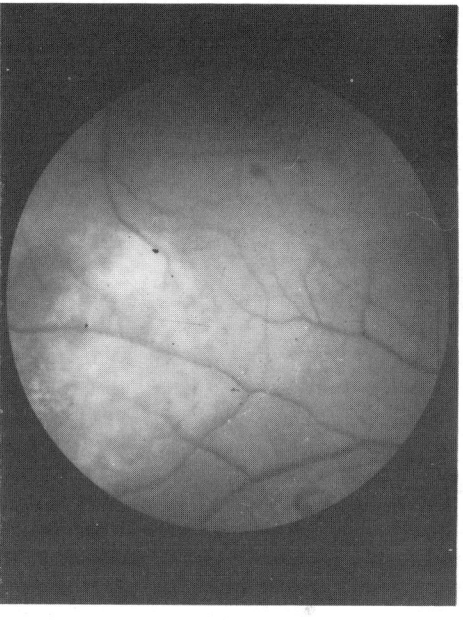

Fig. 10. A haemangioma of the choroid showing the ill-defined pinkish swelling with large vascular spaces. The overlying retina is crinkled and cystic.
(From M. A. Bedford, 'A Colour Atlas of Ocular Tumours' London, Wolfe Medical, 1979.)

MELANOCYTOMA

These lesions are only locally invasive but never metastatic. They present as a jet black tumour around the optic disc, typically in non-Caucasians (*Fig.* 11). No treatment is indicated except observation. It is worth remembering they can occur elsewhere in the eye.

Malignant

Malignant melanoma is the most common primary malignant tumour occurring in the eye in adults. It may be seen in all races but rarely occurs in Negroes. Historically the characteristic stages are quiescent, glaucomatous, extraocular extension and metastatic, but these are of little use nowadays as the diagnosis is made much earlier than hitherto and the prognosis is therefore correspondingly better.

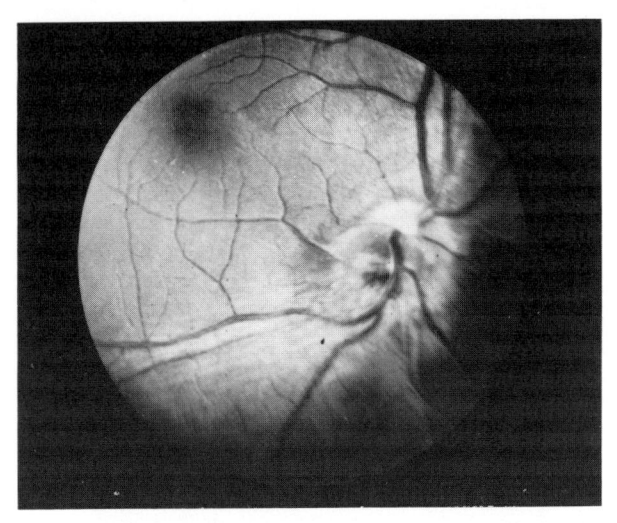

Fig. 11. A heavily pigmented lesion adjacent and overlapping the optic disc. This is typical of a melanocytoma.
(From M. A. Bedford, 'A Colour Atlas of Ocular Tumours' London, Wolfe Medical, 1979.)

The lesion may start as a flat, slate-grey area indistinguishable from a naevus. The earliest pathognomonic sign at this stage is the appearance of 'orange patches' in the pigment epithelium. The lesion becomes thicker and penetrates Bruch's membrane, producing a serous retinal detachment. This extension of the tumour grows inwards, producing the upper portion of the typical 'collar-stud'. The inner portion of the tumour is usually non-pigmented, the outer portion keeping the grey colour. The non-pigmented inner portion has ribbon-like wide vessels coursing over its surface (*Fig. 12*). The detachment deepens as the growth enlarges and the eye gradually fills with tumour, producing a blind eye with secondary glaucoma. The final stage of proptosis due to extraocular extension is very rarely seen nowadays. The differential diagnosis is important as at one time the error in diagnosis of an enucleated eye with a presumed melanoma was 20 per cent. The single most important step is the examination by indirect ophthalmoscopy.

Differential diagnosis may be considered: (*a*) in a lesion without an overlying serous retinal detachment; (*b*) in a lesion with an overlying serous retinal detachment.

In lesions without an overlying serous retinal detachment, the diagnosis is between naevus (*see above*), melanocytoma (*see above*) and hyperplasia

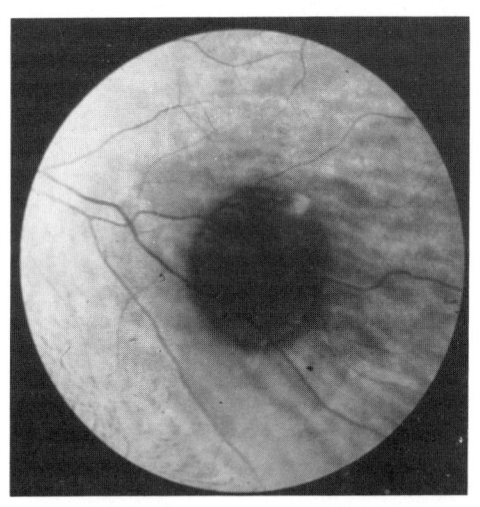

Fig. 13. Hyperplasia of the pigment epithelium showing a characteristic dark area with a surrounding halo.
(From M. A. Bedford, 'A Colour Atlas of Ocular Tumours' London, Wolfe Medical, 1979.)

of the pigment epithelium – presenting characteristically as dark splodges of black pigment with a characteristic surrounding halo (*Fig. 13*).

In lesions with an overlying serous retinal detachment there are three possibilities to consider. The first is haemangioma (*see above*). Secondly, simple retinal detachment. Classically a simple retinal detachment is caused by a retinal hole or holes and a good working rule says that if there is a hole present then there is no tumour. However, there are known exceptions to this rule. An examination with the indirect ophthalmoscope will always show a tumour below the detachment. Thirdly, secondary deposits should be considered. These are more common than supposed and are characteristically fluffy, pale, multiple and perhaps bilateral. The lesions usually occur in someone with known metastatic disease, typically from breast or bronchus (*Fig. 14*). Fluorescein angiography may be useful but there is a considerable overlap in the photographic appearances of these tumours, haemangiomas and malignant melanomas.

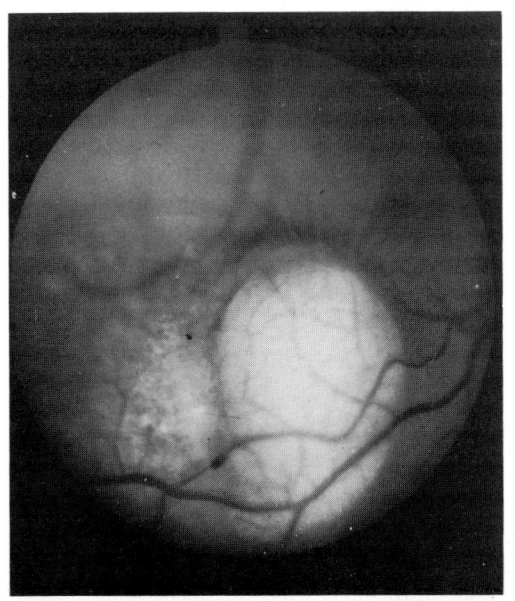

Fig. 12. The typical pale extension of malignant melanoma through Bruch's membrane with its ribbon-like vessels on the surface. The base of the tumour below the retina is below and to the left.

The routine use of fluorescein angiography, ultrasonography, P_{32} test etc. is of limited use diagnostically but may be of more use to judge the progress of a lesion over a period of months, perhaps after the use of some form of therapy (*see below*). Most cases are easily diagnosed by a clinician well versed in the use of the indirect ophthalmoscope.

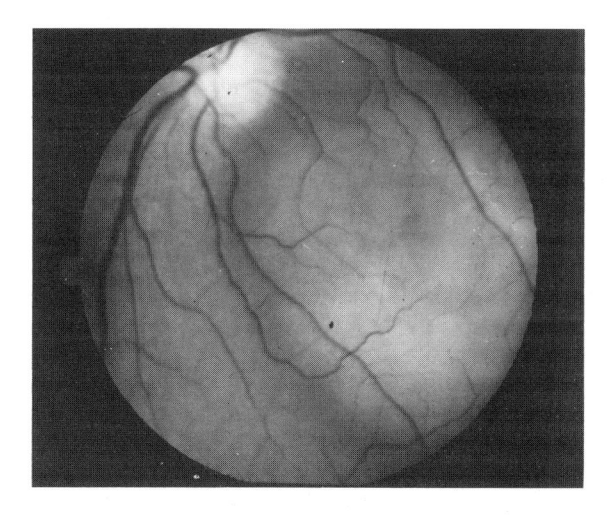

Fig. 14. A pale fluffy area adjacent to the optic disc involving the macula caused by a metastasis from a carcinoma of the breast. (From M. A. Bedford, 'A Colour Atlas of Ocular Tumours' London, Wolfe Medical, 1979.)

Treatment of Malignant Melanoma

The classic treatment of an eye harbouring a malignant melanoma was an urgent enucleation. However, over the last few decades workers throughout the world have shown varying degress of success with several types of therapy aimed at conserving the eye with useful vision. Cobalt plaques emitting gamma radiation have been advocated, beta radiation has been tried, external radiation with a proton beam or helium ion irradiation, light-coagulation, cryosurgery and even local removal have been advocated in certain cases. Doubts have even been cast over the efficacy of enucleation. Most clinicians in this field, however, seem to adopt an attitude of conservation tempered with the use of some or all other forms of therapy; including enucleation. Thus, if a lesion is found to be a 'malignant melanoma' with all current diagnostic techniques and the lesion is small, say under 7 mm in diameter, and posteriorly situated and shows no evidence of change over a period of months, then there would appear to be little use in proceeding to urgent enucleation. If the advent of a serous detachment threatened vision, however, then conservative therapy, as listed above, might be indicated, ideally in a unit used to the application of such therapies.

Should the neoplasm grow rapidly or be anteriorly situated, most clinicians would probably agree that a simple enucleation (done carefully with a minimum amount of pressure transmitted to the globe) is probably necessary. In view of the rapidly changing views on therapy it is difficult to prognosticate in a given case but it would certainly appear that the smaller, slower growing neoplasms have an excellent prognosis so that no therapy is needed. The difficulties arise in a given case when it is decided that some form of therapy is needed, i.e. to enucleate or not and if not, what form of conservative therapy is to be adopted. It must be borne in mind that these guidelines are of necessity very vague as at present they are under review by many authorities throughout the world.

Retinal Tumours

Retinoblastoma

Incidence

Moderately large series have been reported from many parts of the world, giving an incidence of approximately 1 in 20 000 live births. One excellent summary has shown that the incidence is becoming more common because of increasing therapeutic success, and also the spontaneous rate is increasing. Since the early 1960s interest has been directed towards the chromosomes of patients with retinoblastoma, and in 1966 the association was noted with retinoblastoma patients suffering from multiple congenital abnormalities with partial deletion of the X-group of chromosomes. Work has continued over the years in this area of increasing complexity and it is now known that it may also be associated with other systemic changes. The fact that a maternal defect was present in one case may herald an exciting entry into the discovery of children at risk. Similarly, the linkage of the gene with human esterase *D* in children at risk is an exciting prospect. At present, though, there is no certain way of predicting the potential development of the disease in all children at risk.

From a clinical point of view the following practical points may be of help.

1. The hereditary type of the disease: autosomal dominant with a variable penetrance. Typically occurs at an early age, usually involving both eyes, but not necessarily simultaneously. A gonadial mutation can produce a similar clinical picture but with no family history.

2. The spontaneous type: i.e. no previous family history, a somatic mutation. Cases occur later, usually between the age of 3 and 5, with only one eye being involved. Unfortunately, 20 per cent of these are incompletely expressed gonadial mutations and therefore the disease can be passed on.

3. The type associated with multiple congenital abnormalities and chromosomal abnormalities. In this type one or both eyes may be affected.

The following guidelines may be cited:
1. Healthy parents with one affected child have a low risk of producing more affected children (6 per cent).
2. Patients with unilateral retinoblastoma should remain under medical control, since the tumour can always become bilateral.
3. Brothers and sisters of a person with retinoblastoma should undergo regular ophthalmoscopic examination.
4. Affected offspring of retinoblastoma survivors run a high risk of developing the tumour bilaterally, even when a parent was affected unilaterally.
5. When there are already two affected children in a sibship further brothers and sisters run a high risk of being affected because one of the parents must be a carrier, and 50 per cent of the children are likely to be affected at least genetically (although only 40 per cent may show the disease clinically).
6. A retinoblastoma survivor who himself has proved hereditary retinoblastoma has a 50 per cent chance that some of his children will be affected (though only 40 per cent will be affected clinically).
7. The children of a sporadically affected person have a 25 per cent chance of being affected.
8. Apparently healthy persons who come from retinoblastoma stock may carry the gene and pass the disease on to their offspring.

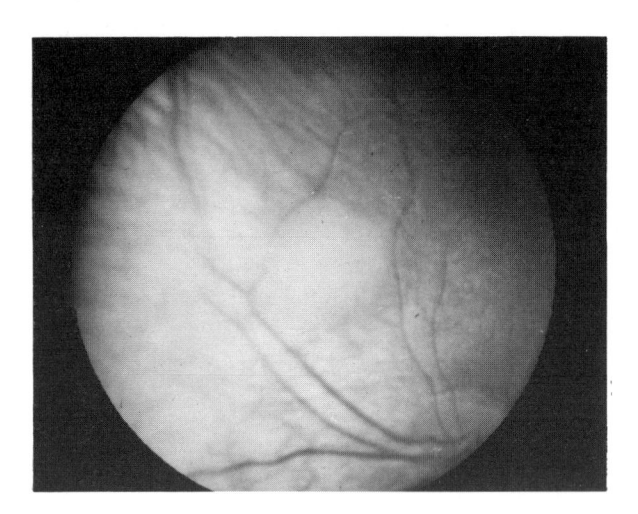

Fig. 15. An early retinoblastoma showing as a minute gelatinous nodule obscuring the pattern of the choroid beneath it.
(From M. A. Bedford, 'A Colour Atlas of Ocular Tumours' London, Wolfe Medical, 1979.)

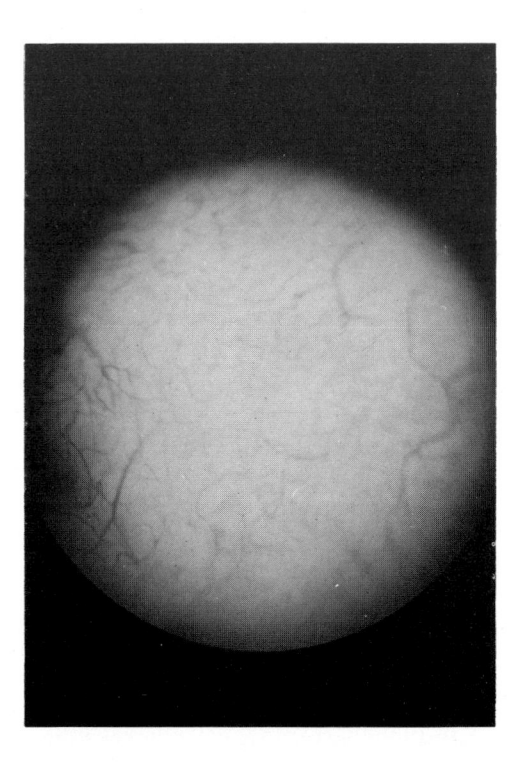

Fig. 16. The surface of a large retinoblastoma with fine blood vessels on its surface.
(From M. A. Bedford, 'A Colour Atlas of Ocular Tumours' London, Wolfe Medical, 1979.)

Signs and Symptoms

The tumour is composed of rosettes or clusters of small, densely packed, round cells with a tendency to necrosis. The smallest tumours appear clinically as a minute gelatinous nodule (*Fig.* 15) which gradually grows larger, showing fine blood vessels on its surface (*Fig.* 16). Over a period of months it may produce a total retinal detachment or else break into the vitreous as a series of round seedlings which may produce satellite growths (*Fig.* 17). Alternatively, it may break into the vitreous as a confluent white mass with ill-defined margins showing as a dense white pupil. The neoplasm then tracks up the optic nerve and seeds in the subarachnoid space. Small tumours at the macula present as a squint early in life before proceeding to these signs. Other presenting signs are those of an endophthalmitis, glaucoma, hyphaema or pseudohypopyon. Long standing cases present with unilateral or bilateral extraocular extension showing clinically as a lesser or greater degree of proptosis. Occasionally some children present with bilateral ocular disease and signs of a mid-brain expanding lesion (trilateral retinoblastoma).

Differential Diagnosis

Provided the child is subjected to examination with the indirect ophthalmoscope, under full general anaesthesia, with scleral indentation, the diagnosis is self evident in the majority of cases. However, a uniocular congenital cataract, persistent primary hyperplastic vitreous, Coats's disease or a toxocara infestation are the commonest errors in diagnosis. Other diagnostic methods are of restricted use, e.g.

ultrasonogram, fluorescein angiogram, VMA excretion, lactic acid dehydrogenase estimation and CT scan are rarely indicated. Vitreous aspiration or outright ocular biopsy are of course contraindicated because of the lethal potentialities.

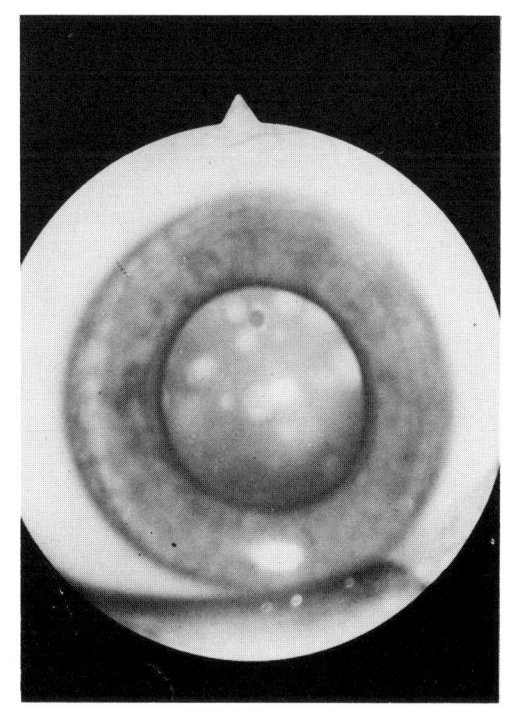

Fig. 17. Multiple growths of retinoblastoma floating free in the vitreous.
(From M. A. Bedford, 'A Colour Atlas of Ocular Tumours' London, Wolfe Medical, 1979.)

Treatment

Nowadays there are many forms of treatment which may be used in the large centres specializing in combating this disease. The modality used is that which will produce the least side effects while at the same time dealing effectively with the tumour. Thus, the whole eye may be irradiated for a large tumour, either anteriorly with a cobalt beam unit, with the consequent development of a radiation cataract, or transversely with the linear accelerator to spare the lens (and perhaps the danger of missing anteriorly floating malignant cells). Medium-sized tumours may be eradicated with radioactive discs, while light coagulation may be used for the posterior small tumours and cryosurgery for small peripheral ones. The only real indication for enucleation nowadays is involvement of the optic nerve. The fact that intensive radiation therapy to the eye and orbit in the treatment of this emotive disease may give radiation-induced sarcomas locally is well known. However, there is an increased incidence of other primary malignant tumours occurring in these unfortunate children. The most common is an osteogenic sarcoma of one of the long bones, appearing later in life.

PRECISE INDICATIONS FOR SPECIFIC FORMS OF THERAPY

All Tumours up to 3 mm: A single small tumour could be treated by any of the forms of therapy listed above, but the type of therapy is not so much dictated by size as by its situation. It would appear unnecessary deliberately to irradiate the whole eye either with the betatron or the cobalt beam unit, as these forms of therapy ideally are only given once, as repeated doses will give an increased chance of a radiation-induced sarcoma. A small single tumour can be treated focally and if during the initial examination it can easily be seen on the dimple produced by the scleral depressor, then cryosurgery would be indicated as it is quick and effective. If the tumour is further back, light coagulation would be indicated. However, if the lesion is adjacent to the optic disc or macula, then the field defects induced would prohibit this form of therapy. This situation would appear to be the ideal indication for the betatron used temporally to spare the lens.

Tumours from 3 mm to 10 mm: These would appear to be too large for certain cure with light and 'cryo' so focal radiation techniques appear to be indicated, either by cobalt plaque, giving γ-radiation, or a ruthenium plaque emitting β-radiation. Should the tumour be adjacent to the optic disc or macula, however, then again there would appear to be an excellent case for betatron therapy from the side, as this would prevent the late vascular complications inherent with the use of high doses of radiation given by focal means. It must be remembered that all forms of focal technique emit radiation laterally and posteriorly as well as anteriorly to the lesion. The complications that can develop must be borne in mind.

Tumours Larger than 10 mm: These would appear to be best treated by whole-eye irradiation by either the betatron or cobalt beam unit. The presence of vitreous seedlings, however, would seem to indicate anterior cobalt beam therapy (with the subsequent development of a radiation cataract).

Multiple Tumours: Two tumours in one eye can be treated by the focal methods listed above provided that the largest tumour is not greater than 10 mm. If it is, then the whole eye must be irradiated. Below this size two tumours can be treated by a combination of focal irradiation to one and light or 'cryo' to the other, or light to one and 'cyro' to the other. It is probably unwise to put two focal radiation plaques on one eye at one time because of the ensuing vascular complications and long term risks of a radiation-induced sarcoma. All other types of multiple tumour are best treated by whole-eye irradiation bearing in mind the criteria listed above.

Indications for Enucleation: There would appear to be a move away from the opinion that the excision of the worst-affected eye is necessary (or one eye in a unilateral case). In view of the success of the techniques described above, it is probably worth while treating all cases, provided that the optic nerve can be seen to be free of the tumour. Thus, involvement of the optic nerve would appear to be the only indication for enucleation, and this can be seen by direct examination, or it has to be assumed because of the presence of opaque media.

Recurrent Orbital Disease: Some success had been claimed with the administration of intra-arterial triethylene melanine (TEM) in these cases, perhaps combined with exenteration.

Metastatic Disease: At present it would seem that the administration of a combination of vincristine and cyclophosphamide offers some hope.

Secondary Tumours: These tumours are secondary to systemic changes classically seen with the phacomatosis, e.g. von Hippel–Lindau disease, Sturge–Weber syndrome, neurofibromatosis and Bourneville's disease. Now they are usually easily differentiated because of their other systemic manifestations.

In broad terms it would seem that there is now a move towards a more conservative approach, to the rapid referral of patients to large centres which are equipped with many, if not all, of the therapeutic approaches listed above.

FURTHER READING

Conjunctiva

Fraunfelder T. T., Farris M. E. Jun. and Wallace T. R. Cryosurgery for ocular and periocular lesions. *J. Dermatol. Surg. Oncol.* 1977; **3,** 422.
Jakobiec F. A., Braunstein S., Albert W. et al. The place of cryotherapy in the management of conjunctival melanoma. *Ophthalmology* 1982; **89,** 502.

Malignant Melanoma

Boniuk M. A crisis in the management of patients with choroidal melanoma. *Am. J. Ophthalmol.* 1979; **87,** 840.
Casebow M. B. The calculation and measurement of exposure distribution from ^{60}Co ophthalmic applicators. *Br. J. Radiol.* 1971; **44,** 618.
Chang M., Zimmerman L. E. and McLean I. The persisting pseudomelanoma problem. *Arch. Ophthalmol.* 1984; **102,** 726.
Foulds W. S. Experience of local excision of uveal melanomata. *Trans. Ophthalmol. Soc. UK* 1977; **97,** 412.
Fraunfelder F. T., Boozman F. W., Wilson R. S. et al. No-touch technique for intra-ocular malignant melanomas. *Arch. Ophthalmol.* 1977; **95,** 1616.
Gragoudas E. S., Goitein M., Koehler A. et al. Proton irradiation of choroidal melanomata. Preliminary results. *Arch. Ophthalmol.* 1978; **96,** 1583.
Gragoudas E. S., Goitein M., Verhey L. et al. Proton beam irradiation. An alternative to enucleation for intraocular melanomas. *Ophthalmology* 1980; **87,** 571.
Lommatzsch P. K. B-irradiation of choroidal melanomas with ^{106}Ru/^{106}Rh applicators. *Arch. Ophthalmol.* 1984; **101,** 713.
Macfaul P. A. Local radiotherapy in the treatment of malignant melanoma of the choroid. *Trans. Ophthalmol. Soc. UK* 1977; **97,** 421.
Meecham W. J., Char D. H., Chen G. T. Y. et al. Correlation of visual field, treatment fields and dose in helium ion irradiation of melanoma. *Am. J. Ophthalmol.* 1975; **100,** 658–65.
Packer S., Torman M., Fairchild R. G. et al. Irradiation of choroidal melanoma with iodine 125 ophthalmic plaques. *Arch. Ophthalmol.* 1980; **98,** 1453.
Shields J. A., Augsburger J. J., Brady L. W. et al. Cobalt plaque therapy of posterior uveal melanomas. *Ophthalmology* 1982; **89,** 1201.
Zimmerman L. E. The changing concepts concerning the management of ocular tumours. *Arch. Ophthalmol.* 1967; **78,** 166.
Zimmerman L. E. Clinical pathology of iris tumours. *Am. J. Ophthalmol.* 1963; **56,** 183.

Retinoblastoma

Abramson D. H. Retinoma, retinocytoma and the retinoblastoma gene. *Arch. Ophthalmol.* 1983; **101,** 1517.
Abramson D. H., Ellsworth R. M. and Zimmerman L. E. Non-ocular cancer in retinoblastoma survivors. *Trans. Am. Acad. Ophthalmol. Otolaryngol.* 1976; **81,** 454.
Bedford M. A. Treatment of retinoblastoma. *Adv. Ophthalmol.* 1975; **31,** 2.
Brownstein S. et al. Trilateral retinoblastoma. *Arch. Ophthalmol.* 1984; **102,** 257.
Burke R. M. Esterase D and hereditary retinoblastoma. *Am. J. Ophthalmol.* 1984; **97,** 779.
Ellsworth R. M. The management of retinoblastoma. *Jap. J. Ophthalmol.* 1978; **22,** 389.

François J., De Bie S. and Matton van Leuven M. T. Genesis and genetics of retinoblastoma. *Jap. J. Ophthalmol.* 1978; **22,** 301.

Howard G. M. and Ellsworth R. M. Differential diagnosis of retinoblastoma. *Am. J. Ophthalmol.* 1965; **60,** 610.

Sang D. N. et al. Retinoblastoma: Clinical observations and histopathological studies. *Int. Ophthalmol. Clin.* 1982; **22,** 72.

Shields J. A. and Augsburger J. J. Current approaches to the diagnosis and management of retinoblastoma. *Surv. Ophthalmol.* 1981; **25,** 347.

Williams I. G. 'Let there be Light'. The treatment of advanced retinoblastoma by external radiation. *Proc. R. Soc. Med.* 1967; **60,** 189.

Chapter 14

Ocular Injuries

Robert J. Cooling

INTRODUCTION

In recent times, ocular trauma in its many guises has been the subject of considerable basic research effort and clinical development. Fundamental changes in clinical management have taken place with the emergence of more rational and comprehensive treatment regimes, displacing many traditional and often empirical approaches. New methods of diagnostic evaluation of the injured eye and the exploitation of innovative surgical techniques have improved the prospects for visual recovery and the prevention of visual loss in many categories of injury.

Rather than attempt to provide a comprehensive account dealing with all types of ocular injury, this chapter considers some of the more recent and major advances in the field of ocular trauma and the important principles underlying modern management.

CONTUSION INJURIES

Blunt ocular injuries characteristically result in a spectrum of damage involving multiple intraocular structures, often in continuity. The extent of damage can often be predicted from the nature of the injury and the site of impact.[1] The effects of mechanical distortion or displacement upon the vulnerable intraocular tissues may include tearing, separation, or even frank necrosis in addition to microvascular damage and the disruption of ocular barriers. Shear forces may also be created between anatomically related tissues with differing elasticities. Damage may be localized to the point of impact or develop at distant sites in response to deformation of the globe. Remote effects may also result from the transmission of energy across the globe to inflict damage at various tissue interfaces – the contre-coup theory.[2]

Anterior Segment Sequelae

In the majority of contusional injuries, damage is likely to be inflicted upon anterior segment structures with involvement of the iris, drainage angle, lens and supporting zonule. Fortunately, the majority of eyes are likely to recover good central vision unless accompanied by overt posterior segment damage. None the less, psychophysical testing, including contrast sensitivity studies, often reveals evidence of subclinical retinal damage.

Cornea

Deformation of the cornea may cause focal or generalized oedema from endothelial decompensation. Depletion of the endothelial cell population, identified by specular microscopic studies,[3] can be correlated with the severity of injury. Associated ocular hypertension or uveitis may lead to further endothelial cell loss whereas the mere presence of hyphaema appears to have little effect, as shown by serial specular microscopy in patients with subtotal hyphaema (unpublished observations). Despite significant endothelial damage, corneal oedema is usually reversible. The occurrence of single or multiple ruptures of Descemet's membrane is generally confined to the neonatal cornea from maladjusted forceps, causing compression of the globe during delivery. Although the oedema is self-limited, possible sequelae include high astigmatism, axial myopia and amblyopia.[4]

Characteristic annular opacities of the corneal endothelium may result from the impact of multiple small epithelial foreign bodies following blast injuries.[5] These transient appearances are due to endothelial cell swelling with adherence of fibrin and leukocytes and result from axial displacement of the corneal stroma with radial distension of the endothelium.[6]

Hyphaema

The presence of macroscopic hyphaema is almost invariably associated with anterior segment structural damage. Although variable in amount, most hyphaemas occupy less than half the anterior chamber volume. Haemorrhage is usually derived from tributaries of the greater arterial circle disrupted by a tear of the anterior face of the ciliary body or iris root. In general, clearance through the trabecular meshwork occurs over a period of 7 days.

The reported incidence of secondary haemorrhage occurring between the second and sixth day following injury ranges from 9 per cent to 38 per cent.[7] To some extent, the risks of secondary bleeding are related to the initial size of the hyphaema and the severity of associated structural damage. The pathogenesis is thought to be related to fibrinolysis and clot retraction involving the original disrupted vessel. Secondary haemorrhage is often greater in extent than the original bleed, with increased risks of secondary glaucoma and a consequent worsening of the visual prognosis. Total hyphaema may lead to stagnation of the aqueous circulation with raised intraocular pressure and deoxygenation of the clotted hyphaema as indicated by a change of colour to brown or black (eight-ball or black-ball hyphaema). Uncontrolled rise of intraocular pressure carries significant risks of ischaemic optic neuropathy or corneal blood staining from stromal impregnation of haemoglobin products. Often rapid in onset, blood staining usually develops in the presence of a healthy corneal endothelium and clearance from the periphery may take years to complete.

Management

The aims of immediate management are to promote clearance of blood from the anterior chamber, to prevent secondary haemorrhage and associated complications and to identify coexisting structural damage.

Controlled studies have shown that time-honoured measures including bedrest, patching and sedation do not influence the incidence of secondary haemorrhage. Furthermore, the necessity for routine hospital admission is open to question. Although no definite policy has emerged, admission of high risk groups including young children, large hyphaemas (in excess of half the anterior chamber volume) and the presence of an unstable intraocular pressure should be considered.

Various topical and systemic agents, including miotics, mydriatics and corticosteroids, recommended for the treatment of hyphaema have not been shown to reduce the incidence of secondary haemorrhage. There is, however, evidence from a number of studies[8-10] that the use of antifibrinolytic agents may substantially reduce the incidence of re-bleeding. Aminocaproic acid, a potent antifibrinolytic agent, competitively inhibits the conversion of plasminogen to plasmin (fibrinolysin) preventing or retarding clot dissolution. Oral administration is necessary in a recommended dosage of 100 mg/kg every 4 hours for a 5-day period to a maximum daily dose of 30 g. Prominent adverse reactions include nausea and vomiting and the drug must be used with caution in patients with renal, cardiac or hepatic disease. In a randomized, double-blind, controlled trial of aminocaproic acid in a series of 49 eyes, the incidence of re-bleeding in the treated group was 4 per cent as compared with 33 per cent in placebo-treated eyes. Similar experiences have been reported in European studies with the use of the antifibrinolytic agent tranexamic acid.[11,12] Interestingly, a topical preparation of tranexamic acid is available and is currently under investigation. Antifibrinolysis may, however, delay the absorption of hyphaema with the accumulation of ghost cells and obstruction of the trabecular meshwork. Delayed absorption may also increase the risks of complications in patients with sickle haemoglobinopathies prone to develop glaucoma from an increased percentage of sickled erythrocytes in the anterior chamber compared with peripheral blood.[13]

Elevated intraocular pressure may accompany large initial hyphaemas but is most likely to develop following secondary haemorrhage or total hyphaema. Normal intraocular pressure or hypotony in the presence of total hyphaema should suggest the possibility of occult scleral rupture. Raised intraocular pressure in the presence of subtotal hyphaema may respond to medical treatment including acetazolamide, oral glycerol or intravenous mannitol supplemented by topical beta-blocking agents. In the presence of an eight-ball hyphaema, however, medical treatment often fails to restore aqueous circulation, leading to a dramatic and sustained pressure rise.

Many surgical techniques have been advocated for the treatment of secondary glaucoma accompanying total hyphaema. These have included paracentesis, enzymatic clot dissolution and aspiration, clot expression through a large incision and, most recently, the use of vitrectomy instrumentation in a closed chamber technique. To a varying degree, these methods pose risks of damage to the corneal endothelium, iris or lens and may provoke further intraocular haemorrhage. As the simplest procedure, limbal paracentesis may release sufficient lysed blood to reinstate aqueous flow. The effect is often temporary but the procedure can be repeated. Methods of clot dissolution and aspiration, including intracameral injection of fibrinolysin or urokinase, have been widely used in the past but have now been largely abandoned. The use of small-gauge suction-cutters offers a more controlled method of clot evacuation and favourable results have been described in several reports.[14,15] However, in many cases it would appear that pupil block is an important if not the principal mechanism of secondary glaucoma and that extensive clot removal is unnecessary to eliminate this mechanism. Iridectomy alone or in combination with trabeculectomy offers a more rational surgical approach.[16,17] These methods may restore aqueous circulation and thereby promote spontaneous absorption of the hyphaema. Earlier surgical intervention with the aim of reducing the high incidence of optic nerve damage and corneal blood staining may be preferable, provided these potentially less hazardous procedures do not induce further haemorrhage.

Following resolution of hyphaema, it is essential to document associated anterior or posterior segment damage and in particular to exclude changes affecting the peripheral retina.

Early gonioscopy may identify haemorrhages or

full-thickness tears of the trabecular meshwork in addition to clefting of the ciliary body.[18] Trabecular damage, often difficult to identify with early remodelling, may account for transient glaucoma during the first few months of injury, which may prove resistant to medical treatment. Reduction of intraocular pressure may follow recanalization of the damaged meshwork improving outflow facility. The rare occurrence of delayed open angle glaucoma many years following injury can be correlated with the extent of angle recession and appears confined to those cases showing involvement of three quadrants or greater.[19] In many patients, the discovery of mild ocular hypertension in the fellow eye and the response to steroid provocation suggests genetic predisposition to glaucoma is a necessary co-factor.

The development of chronic ocular hypotony with visual loss from optic disc and macular oedema may be caused by traumatic cyclodialysis or aqueous hyposecretion accompanied by ciliochoroidal effusion.[20] Restoration of normal intraocular pressure and visual improvement has been reported following surgical reattachment of the ciliary body in these cases.[21]

Lens Opacity and Displacement

Concussional damage to the lens or its supporting zonule is a common sequel invariably accompanied by damage to other intraocular tissues. Although many different forms of lens opacity have been described, including glaucomflecken and zonular or localized cortical cataract, rosette-shaped opacity restricted to the anterior or posterior subcapsular region is most commonly encountered. Opacification probably reflects diffuse concussional damage to the lens epithelium with impaired cation transport and hydration of the subcapsular cortex.[22] The evolution of lens opacity is extremely variable, including the possibility of complete regression, but often becomes localized and non-progressive. The likelihood of progression is in part age-related and pre-existing cataract is likely to be accentuated.

Concussional damage may also result in dehiscence of the lens capsule with immediate hydration and swelling of adjacent lens fibres. Proliferation of the lens epithelium and subsequent fibrous metaplasia may seal small capsular defects, resulting in a localized subcapsular cataract. Extensive dehiscence causes rapid and diffuse opacification and the possible release of hydrated cortical fibres into the anterior chamber. This may undergo uncomplicated absorption but in older patients phacoallergic uveitis or secondary glaucoma (phacolytic) commonly supervenes. Disruption of the anterior or equatorial capsule is readily visible, whereas a defect of the posterior capsule may be obscured by diffuse opacity. Extensive tears may develop at the attachment of Weiger's ligament with liberation of lens material into the anterior vitreous cavity. Such an event, suggested by the presence of a flattened contour to the anterior lens capsule (*Fig.* 1), carries important implications in terms of the surgical approach.

In those eyes showing progressive cataract, lens extraction is generally required within a period of 18 months.[23] The choice of surgical technique and the methods of optical correction are determined by the extent of associated damage, especially the integrity of the posterior capsule and supporting zonule and other factors, including the age and occupation of the individual.

Extracapsular extraction or pars plana lensectomy may be indicated with provision of contact lens correction or, in suitable cases, the insertion of an anterior or posterior chamber lens implant. Recovery of binocular vision following contact lens correction of unilateral traumatic aphakia is often disappointing with problems of aniseikonia, many patients ultimately discontinuing lens wear. In selective cases, insertion of improved designs of intraocular lens currently available can provide excellent functional results and possible reduction of the high incidence of stimulus deprivation amblyopia accompanying traumatic aphakia in childhood.

Minor displacement of the lens from localized disruption of the zonule is not uncommon and is frequently associated with lens opacity, tearing of the iris root (iridodialysis) and changes within the borders of the contiguous vitreous base. Irido- and phacodonesis with irregular deepening of the anterior chamber may be accompanied by forwards displacement of vitreous gel through the area of zonular dehiscence with the possibility of intermittent pupil block (*Fig.* 2). Pars plicata vitreous surgery offers a controlled approach for the removal of subluxated lenses with minimal nuclear sclerosis causing visual distortion and instability or multiple imagery.[24]

It is rare for the lens to dislocate into the anterior chamber but this may occur in response to minor injury with inherent abnormalities of the zonule or microspherophakia. Although developmentally abnormal lenses may be repositioned without recourse to surgery, lens extraction in conjunction with anterior vitrectomy is otherwise required with the inevitable development of pupil block glaucoma and endothelial damage.

Posterior lens dislocation gives rise to few immediate complications. Removal using bimanual vitrectomy techniques may be required in the event of lens-induced uveitis or phacolytic glaucoma. The development of open angle glaucoma is, however, more commonly attributable to contusion angle deformity requiring treatment on its own merits.[25]

Posterior Segment Manifestations

Contusional damage to posterior segment structures often carries an unfavourable visual prognosis and in the majority of instances co-existing anterior segment damage, however subtle, can be identified. The

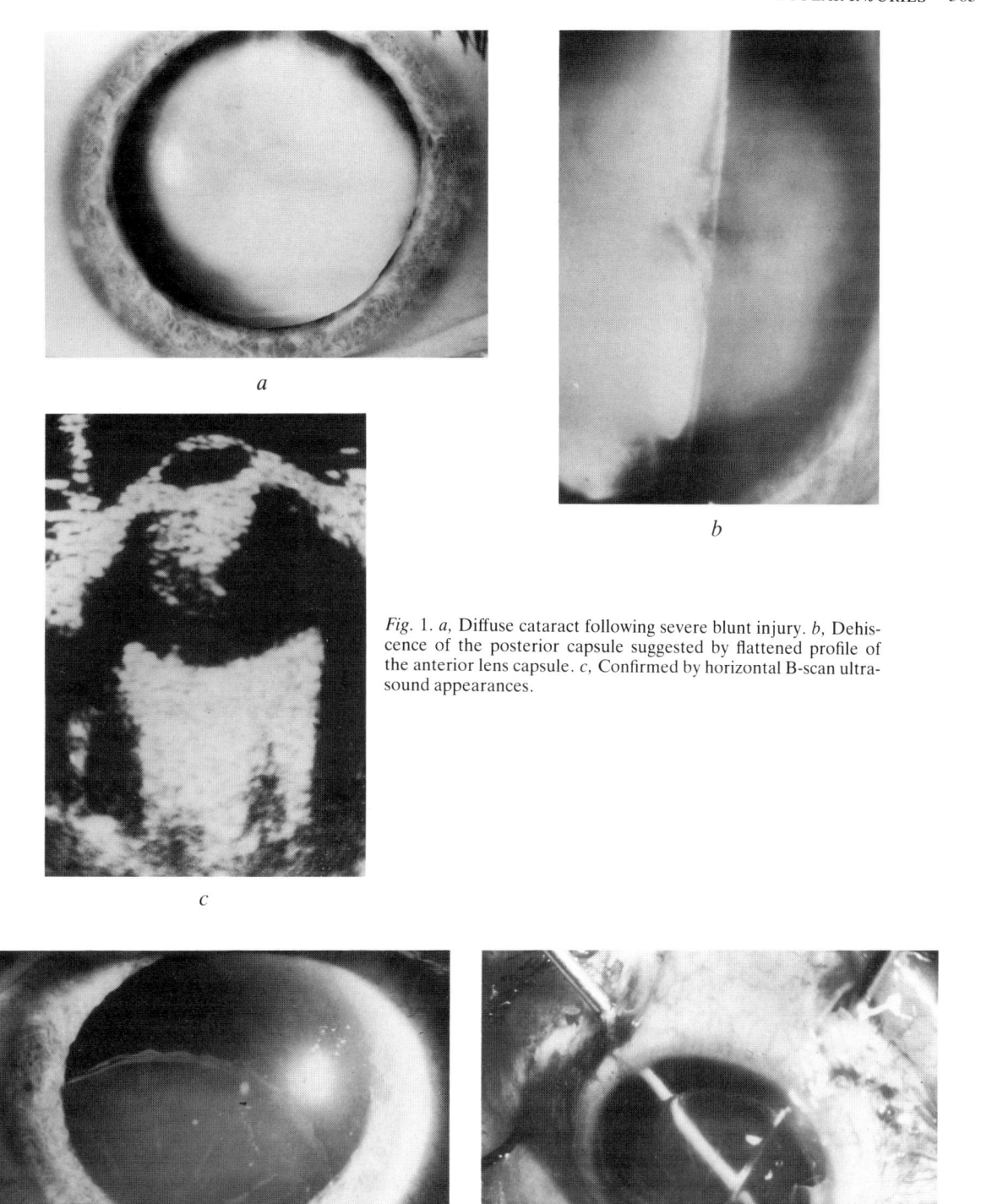

Fig. 1. *a*, Diffuse cataract following severe blunt injury. *b*, Dehiscence of the posterior capsule suggested by flattened profile of the anterior lens capsule. *c*, Confirmed by horizontal B-scan ultrasound appearances.

Fig. 2. *a*, Multiple sphincter ruptures, lens subluxation, glaucomflecken and anterior gel prolapse; associated pupil block glaucoma. *b*, Managed by pars plicata lensectomy and vitrectomy.

ultimate extent of visual loss is impossible to predict on the basis of the initial findings but visual recovery may continue over a prolonged period following injury.

Commotio Retinae

Transient retinal opacification or commotio retinae is a common response to compression or distortion of the globe. Immediate and profound depression of central vision is followed by complete recovery. The opacity appears to be located at the level of the outer sensory retina or retinal pigment epithelium with preferential involvement of the macula following diffuse impact.

The pathophysiological basis of acute traumatic retinal opacity is uncertain. Fluorescein angiography shows an intact blood-retinal barrier at the level of the retinal capillaries.[26] Incompetence of the retinal pigment epithelial barrier may be identified and suggests irreversible tissue damage with implications for visual recovery. From experimental studies[27,28] the most prominent histopathological feature is the disruption of photoreceptor outer segments in the absence of extracellular oedema. Intracellular glial oedema and axonal swelling have also been described and may cause a transient conduction block accounting for reduced vision. Functional changes in the underlying pigment epithelium and the accumulation of extracellular oedema have been described in an unconfirmed report using horseradish peroxidase tracer techniques.[29] The ultimate visual recovery may therefore depend upon the extent of photoreceptor outer segment damage and the potential for recovery of the retinal pigment epithelial barrier.

Following resolution of macular commotio, there may be permanent structural damage affecting the inner or outer retina with incomplete visual recovery. This may be manifested by protracted intraretinal oedema with lamellar hole or cyst formation and focal or diffuse rarefaction of the underlying pigment epithelium with clumping and migration of pigment into the outer retina. Similar pigmentary changes may also affect the fundus periphery and on occasions are sufficiently extensive to resemble sector retinitis pigmentosa closely.[30,31]

Retinal Breaks and Detachment

The overwhelming majority of retinal breaks caused by blunt injury develop at the moment of impact. Characteristically, breaks are located at sites of maximal scleral displacement in the region of the vitreous base or at the site of scleral impact. There are likely to be other manifestations of significant contusion injury affecting the peripheral or posterior fundus or anterior segment structures. Identification of the retinal break is often delayed by intraocular opacity. The latent interval between injury and the development of retinal detachment is unpredictable but in the majority the detachment is delayed in onset and slowly progressive. This may be explained by the absence of posterior vitreous detachment with limited recruitment of subretinal fluid and the absence of persistent vitreo-retinal traction.

The following types of retinal break may be encountered:

1. Retinal breaks are most commonly located at or within the borders of the vitreous base in the form of oral disinsertion or dialysis of variable circumferential extent. Multiple breaks may be identified in one or more quadrants and most reported series show predilection for the superonasal quadrant. Giant retinal breaks located at the posterior border of the vitreous base may also occur.

Avulsion of the vitreous base, pathognomic of contusion injury, occurs in approximately 25 per cent of all cases of contusion detachment. This lesion is readily identified by the presence of a garland of pigmented or non-pigmented ciliary epithelium suspended in the vitreous cavity integrally attached to the vitreous base (*Fig.* 3).

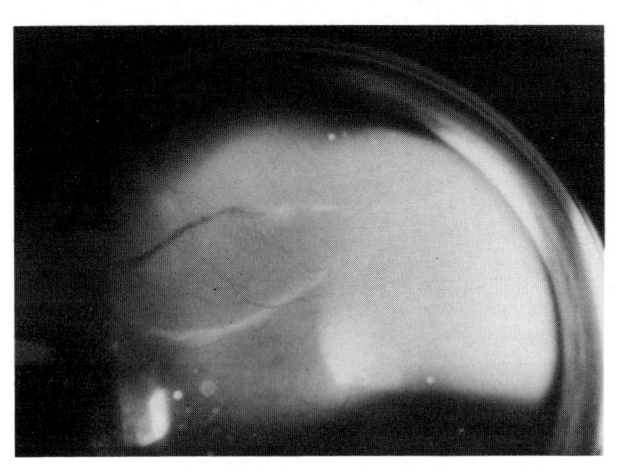

Fig. 3. Contusion retinal detachment and vitreous base avulsion: panfundoscope photograph of avulsed pigmented ciliary epithelium and superior retinal detachment.

2. Atrophic breaks occurring at the point of anterior scleral impact range from single or multiple small round holes to large irregular areas of retinal dissolution which may occupy an entire quadrant.[32,33] Retinal fragmentation is usually immediate but it is possible that breaks may develop as a delayed consequence in areas of severely contused retina. Intraretinal, choroidal and vitreous haemorrhage are common associated findings. Retinal detachment may be immediate or delayed in onset and in some instances extensive disruption of the choroid and pigment epithelium results in spontaneous retinal reattachment.

3. Equatorial traction tears at the site of anomalous vitreo-retinal adhesions are uncommon and develop at the time of delayed posterior vitreous detachment. The latter may result from the direct effects of contusion injury upon the gel framework or from blood-induced syneresis.

4. Posterior retinal breaks appear to develop from the effects of rapid deformation of the posterior pole. Full thickness macular breaks are most commonly encountered but rarely lead to progressive retinal detachment (*Fig.* 4). Extensive slit tears, often paravascular in distribution, may also develop following severe global compression and incomplete posterior vitreous separation.

The majority of retinal detachments caused by contusion injury are managed by standard repair techniques using cryotherapy and segmental explants to support the anterior retina. Vitrectomy techniques with gas tamponade may be indicated for the removal of associated lens or vitreous opacity or to control large or posterior retinal breaks.

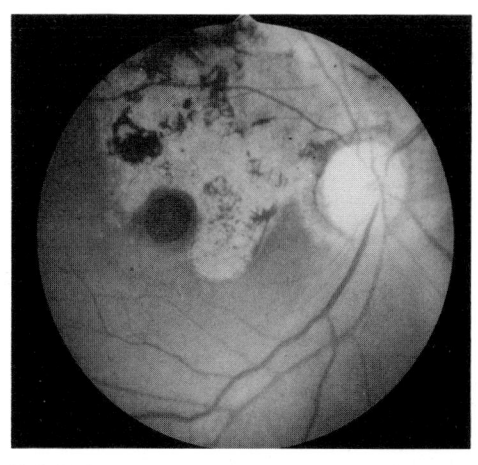

Fig. 4. Full thickness macular break, extensive RPE atrophy and optic atrophy following blunt injury.

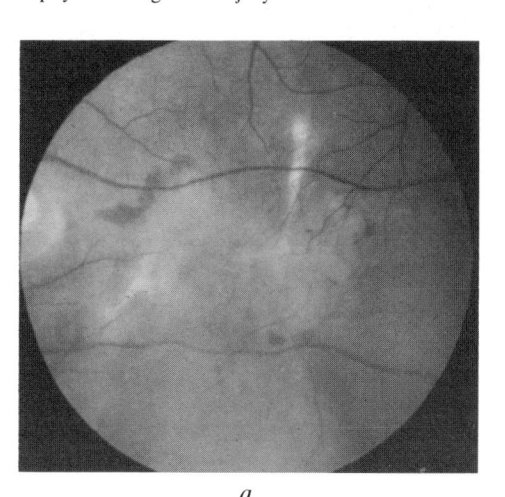

Incomplete recovery of acuity or residual field defects result from associated retinal contusion damage.[34] Delayed subretinal neovascularization at the site of previous choroidal rupture is an uncommon development and if paramacular in location and progressive requires laser photocoagulation[35] (*see Fig.* 5).

Peripheral chorioretinal rupture (retinitis sclopetaria) in the absence of scleral rupture most commonly results from the impact of high velocity missiles. Gross tissue disruption results in an exuberant connective tissue response fusing choroid and retina and preventing the development of retinal detachment. Extensive areas of retinal capillary nonperfusion affecting the surrounding retina have also been documented.[36] Following resolution of associated vitreous haemorrhage, associated oral breaks should be carefully excluded.

Optic Nerve

Contusional injuries of the optic nerve caused by blunt trauma to the globe or closed head injury typically result in severe and irreversible visual loss. Considerable mechanical forces are often involved with associated fractures of the facial skeleton or base of

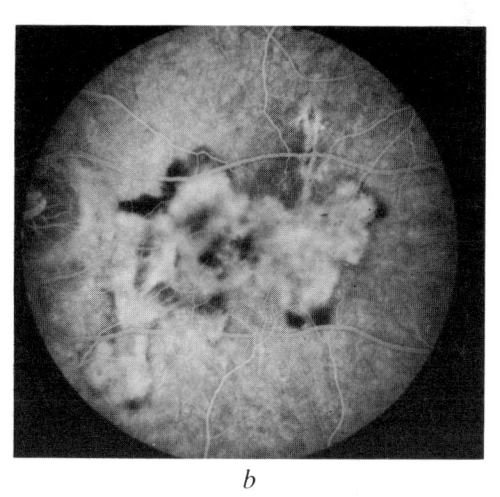

Fig. 5. a, Indirect choroidal tears complicated by delayed subretinal neovascularization. *b,* Fluorescein angiographic appearances (mid-venous phase).

Choroidal Tears

Peripheral or posterior choroidal tears develop in response to severe concussional forces. The tear is usually limited to the choriocapillaris and Bruch's membrane but may involve all layers of the choroid, the overlying pigment epithelium and rarely the neuroretina. Associated subpigment epithelial or subretinal haemorrhage may initially obscure all or part of the rupture. Indirect tears at the posterior pole may be single or multiple appearing as curvilinear defects often disposed concentrically about the optic disc. With the exception of submacular choroidal tears, improvement of central vision is to be expected.

skull in a high proportion of cases. For anatomical reasons, damage to the anterior optic nerve is most likely to occur at the optic foramen or lamina cribrosa but the precise location of damage is often difficult to determine and the pathological mechanisms open to speculation. Immediate evaluation is often precluded by intraocular haemorrhage and the opportunities for clinicopathological correlation are limited.

Damage to the intrascleral optic nerve may cause swelling of the optic disc and haemorrhage which may be accompanied by juxtapapillary choroidoretinal damage. These appearances may reflect damage to the superficial nerve fibres, obstructed axoplasmic transport or most likely damage to the intrinsic microvasculature. The development of segmental or diffuse optic disc swelling has been ascribed to posterior ciliary artery ischaemia following ocular contusion – traumatic anterior ischaemic optic neuropathy.[37,38]

Damage to the lamina cribrosa results in disorganization and variable displacement of the optic nerve head. This may result from the extension of peripapillary choroidoretinal and scleral tears following severe displacement of the globe.[39] Partial or complete avulsion of the optic nerve, a rare event, causes complete disconnection of optic nerve fibres and is usually accompanied by dense intraocular haemorrhage with vitreous incarceration into the optic disc cavity. These features may be readily identified by B-scan ultrasound. Avulsion may result from forcible dislocation of the globe with retropulsion of the nerve, extreme torsional forces or gross intraocular pressure rise causing explusion of the nerve. In the absence of intraocular haemorrhage, early fluorescein angiography reveals normal filling of the choroidal circulation, indicating preservation of the posterior ciliary vessels. Surprisingly, perfusion of the retinal vessels is maintained but with evidence of venous stasis and the formation of collaterals with the peripapillary choroidal vessels.[40]

Indirect damage to the intracanalicular optic nerve following blunt forehead trauma is a well-recognized pattern of injury. Various mechanisms have been proposed, including primary neural ischaemia and optic nerve infarction or ischaemia secondary to compression within the confines of the optic canal. The reported incidence of associated optic canal fracture varies widely, although even with modern radiographic techniques, including tomography, identification of the fracture may prove impossible.[41] Recent studies using holographic techniques suggest that sufficient forces may be generated to produce skeletal distortion in the region of the optic nerve causing optic nerve damage in the absence of fracture.[42] Complete visual loss immediately following injury indicates irreversible optic nerve damage but delayed or progressive loss of vision due to secondary ischaemia may respond to high doses of systemic steroids. There is no convincing evidence that delayed visual loss may be reversed by immediate surgical decompression of the optic nerve, including a transantral–ethmoidal approach.[43]

PENETRATING OCULAR TRAUMA

Penetrating ocular injuries cause an infinite spectrum of damage with variable effects upon vision and the life of the individual. The extent of the initial structural damage is of paramount importance and is largely determined by the nature and severity of the injury. However, there appear to be many different factors that may influence the prospects for visual recovery or survival of the globe in any individual injury. A number of surveys have been undertaken to determine the final visual outcome of different types of injury[44–47] from which the following prognostic factors can be abstracted (*Fig. 6*).

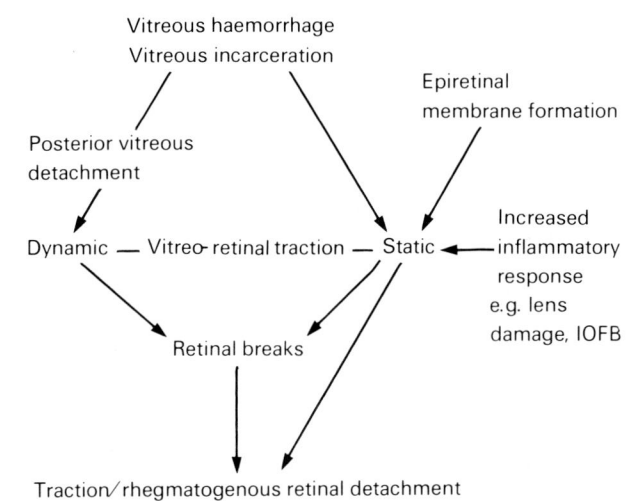

Fig. 6. Vitreo-retinal sequelae of posterior penetrating trauma.

Characteristics of the Penetrating Wound

The size and location of the penetrating wound is not unexpectedly a principal determinant of the visual outcome. Extensive gaping wounds are likely to be accompanied by major intraocular damage or loss of contents. Scleral wounds extending posterior to the rectus muscle insertions are particularly unfavourable, with the risk of expulsive choroidal haemorrhage or major retinal prolapse. By contrast, corneal lacerations in the absence of lens damage carry a favourable outlook, in which significant astigmatism is confined to lacerations exceeding one-third of the corneal diameter.

Contusional Component

Penetrating injuries with a major contusional component carry a significantly worse visual prognosis related to extensive choroidal damage and expulsion of intraocular contents. Most penetrating injuries include some degree of contusion damage occurring in its purest form in cases of global rupture resulting from indirect scleral tears from severe blunt injury. Large foreign bodies or high velocity missiles often resulting in double penetration of the globe also inflict major contusion damage with a poor visual outcome.

Initial Visual Acuity

Although dependent upon many interrelated factors, the initial visual acuity is considered to be one of the important factors in the prediction of ultimate vision irrespective of the type of injury and the extent of intraocular damage.

Afferent Pupil Defect

The presence of a marked afferent pupil defect immediately following injury is generally indicative of major posterior segment damage with a poor visual prognosis (*Fig. 7*).

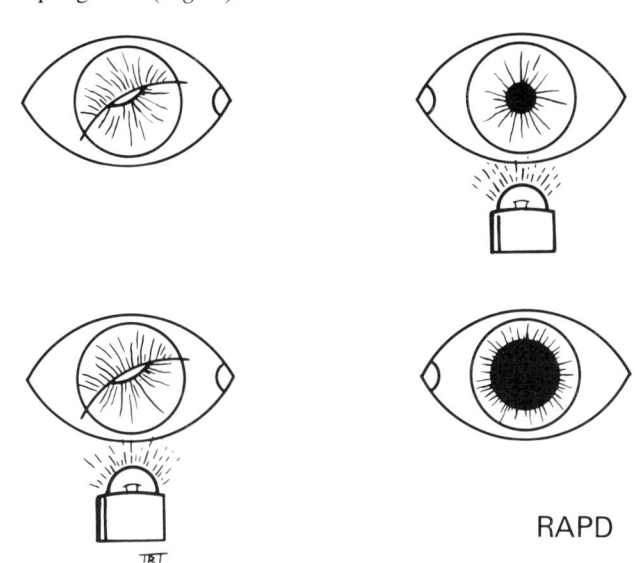

Fig. 7. Diagrams to show right afferent pupil defect (RAPD) as indicated by left pupillary escape.

Intraocular Damage

In eyes with visual potential following injury, the extent of the initial mechanical damage to intraocular tissues determines the likelihood of complications leading to ultimate visual loss.

Injuries resulting in expulsion of the lens carry significant risks of major collapse of the posterior segment and primary retinal displacement.

Dense vitreous haemorrhage obscuring all fundus details implies a guarded prognosis and in conjunction with major vitreous incarceration within the wound poses significant risks of secondary retinal detachment (*Fig. 8*). Primary displacement or major incarceration of the retina are common findings in those eyes requiring enucleation.

Immediate Surgical Repair

Without doubt, the ultimate visual outcome is often directly related to the quality of primary surgical repair. In particular, failure to achieve the principal objectives of initial repair may jeopardize or delay the opportunities for early secondary intraocular reconstruction.

Primary Surgical Repair

Although most penetrating ocular injuries require prompt surgical repair, experience has shown that it is often preferable to defer surgery for a limited period until conditions favour comprehensive and expert reconstruction. At the earliest opportunity, the nature and extent of intraocular damage should be determined to decide the objectives and sequence of repair. Planning of the surgical repair requires thorough preoperative evaluation, including detailed biomicroscopic examination following dilatation of

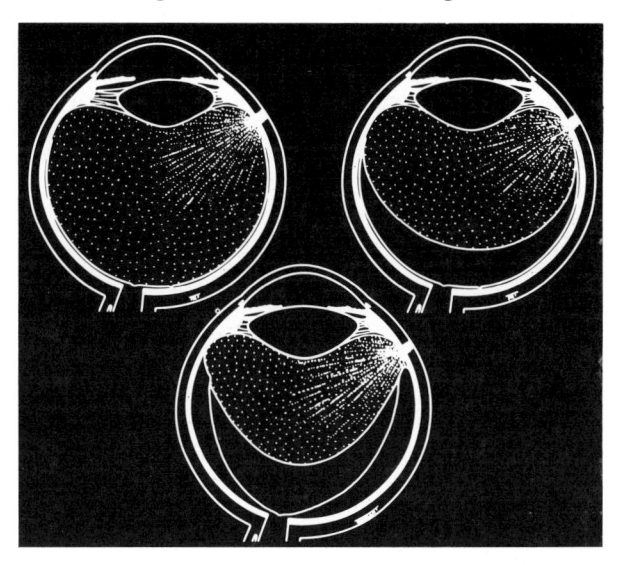

Fig. 8. Diagrams illustrating possible vitreo-retinal sequelae of anterior scleral penetration. *Top left*, anterior scleral wound and vitreous haemorrhage; note lens shift towards incarceration site. *Top right*, delayed posterior vitreous detachment. *Bottom middle*, traction / rhegmatogenous retinal detachment due to oral break.

the pupil, indirect ophthalmoscopy and testing of the pupillary responses.

The important principles governing the repair of penetrating injuries are as follows.

Microsurgical Wound Repair

Accurate alignment and closure of the wound with avoidance of distortion and tissue incarceration are essential to promote orderly wound healing and to facilitate any subsequent intraocular reconstruction. Adequate exposure of scleral wounds to determine the posterior extent requires reflection of the conjunctiva and possible detachment of extraocular muscles. Continuous or interrupted monofilament nylon sutures $(8/0-10/0)$ are used to appose corneal and scleral wounds placed sufficiently deep to avoid internal gaping. Extensive corneo-scleral lacerations with a collapsed globe require the preliminary insertion of a limbal suture to orientate the wound. Irregular or stellate wounds with severely oedematous or macerated edges may prove difficult to appose. Often a single purse-string suture will suffice but alternatively cyanoacrylate tissue adhesive or, rarely, donor tissue replacement is required. Posterior exit wounds of double penetrating injuries are in general self-sealing and attempted repair is likely to induce further choroidal bleeding and tissue extrusion. All devitalized tissues and foreign material are meticulously removed from the wound prior to closure. Prolapsed vitreous gel is carefully excised with avoidance of undue traction, bearing in mind gel incarceration within scleral wounds cannot be completely eliminated.

Repositioning of Prolapsed Intraocular Tissues

Wherever possible, prolapsed uveal tissue is replaced depending upon tissue viability and the time elapsed since injury. Preservation of an intact iris diaphragm and functioning pupil improves the ultimate functional and cosmetic results and may prevent adhesion of the iris to the wound and obliteration of the chamber angle. Where abscission is required, the iris diaphragm may be reconstituted by the insertion of a polypropylene or nylon suture as part of the primary procedure. Preliminary paracentesis of a spontaneously reformed anterior chamber facilitates disengagement of the iris from the wound using a cyclodialysis spatula. Replacement of prolapsed ciliary body may require gentle bipolar cautery to produce tissue shrinkage. Haemorrhage from damaged uveal tissue is often difficult to control and, although hypotensive anaesthesia may be helpful, haemostasis relies upon wound closure and restoration of intraocular pressure. In the absence of major intraocular haemorrhage, limited retinal prolapse may be freed from the wound and replaced during closure of the scleral wound.

Reformation of Compartments to Restore Normal Ocular Contours

Reformation of all compartments of the globe is essential to restore normal anatomical relationships. Early reformation of the anterior chamber using inert visco-elastic materials, in particular sodium hyaluronate, confers a number of advantages throughout the repair.[48] Chamber depth is maintained despite wound manipulation in contrast to air or fluid replacement. Reopening of the anterior chamber angle is achieved at an early stage and capillary bleeding into the anterior chamber is prevented or confined. Visualization of internal structures is improved and any subsequent intracameral manipulation facilitated.

Posterior wounds with loss of vitreous gel may require careful injection of physiological fluid or air via the pars plana avoiding the area of scleral wounds.

Reconstruction of Intraocular Damage

Aspiration of a disrupted lens with release of flocculent material into the anterior chamber is an important objective of the initial repair to reduce the subsequent inflammatory response and to prevent adhesion of the lens to the wound.[49] In the absence of major posterior segment damage, lensectomy can be undertaken via the pars plana or alternatively through the limbus with avoidance of the penetrating wound. Similarly, attempts should be made to clear incarcerated gel from the inner aspect of corneal wounds using a suction-cutter with linear suction control. These techniques present considerable hazards in the presence of major intraocular haemorrhage with difficulties of identification of damaged tissues, the possibility of elevated retina and risks of renewed haemorrhage. Although there may be indications for immediate posterior segment intraocular microsurgery, e.g. infectious endophthalmitis, toxic intraocular foreign body, in the majority of cases definitive repair of vitreo-retinal damage is undertaken as a secondary procedure for reasons outlined below.

Prophylactic Cryotherapy and Scleral Explants

These measures are of limited application in the initial repair of posterior penetrating injuries. There is no place for unmonitored application of cryotherapy or radial buckling of scleral wounds. Cryotherapy in the vicinity of the wound may precipitate or increase choroidal haemorrhage and may also enhance surface retinal proliferation.[50] In the presence of clear media or minimal opacity, the use of a wide circumferential explant to indent the ora serrata on either side of the wound can be considered in conjunction with cryotherapy to the post-oral retina to prevent subsequent retinal detachment. These prophylactic measures may be considered at a later stage either alone or in conjunction with vitrectomy.

Prevention of Infection and Immediate Management of Suspected Endophthalmitis

Prevention of infectious endophthalmitis relies upon topical and subconjunctival broad spectrum antibiotics rather than routine systemic antibiotic cover. Suspicion of early endophthalmitis is raised by disproportionate intraocular inflammation and requires immediate aqueous and vitreous samples for Gram-staining and culture. The response to treatment depends upon the virulence of the pathogen and the duration of infection. Encouraging results have been reported with intraocular antibiotic injection and in selected cases, core vitrectomy.[51]

With few exceptions, reconstruction of a severely injured eye should be undertaken in preference to primary enucleation. At the time of presentation, it is impossible to determine the existence of overwhelming posterior segment damage and it is not unknown for eyes that were initially deemed unsalvageable to recover useful levels of vision.

Secondary Reconstruction

As previously indicated, many eyes sustaining major intraocular damage following penetration require some form of secondary procedure to restore useful vision or to prevent or control secondary complications. This may reflect the extent of structural damage precluding definitive reconstruction at the time of primary repair or as a consequence of the inflammatory response and reparative processes possibly enhanced by inadequate initial repair.

Revision of anterior segment damage may include penetrating keratoplasty for severe axial corneal scarring, repair of an iris sector coloboma resulting from abscission by closed chamber techniques (McCannel suture), lens extraction and possibly secondary intraocular acrylic lens insertion (*Fig.* 9) or dense pupillary and cyclitic membranes requiring surgical branes or dense vitreous haemorrhage is essential to restore form vision and to allow identification of retinal damage.

Prevention or Relief of Vitreo-Retinal Traction: Complete rather than central (core) vitrectomy is required to eliminate trans-gel traction and indirectly to limit surface proliferation within the vitreous base (in conjunction with anterior encircling explants). Surface traction involving the posterior retina may also be relieved by dissection of epimacular membranes.

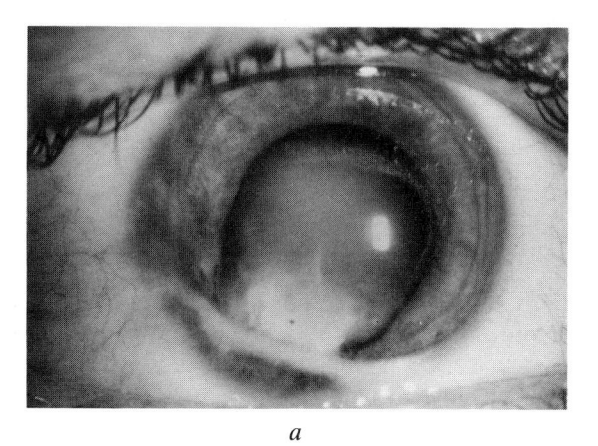

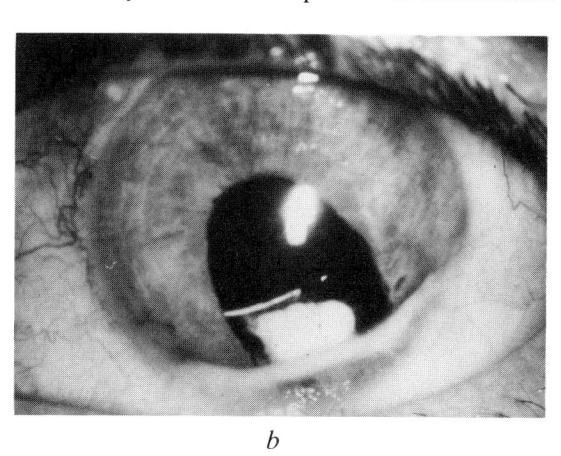

Fig. 9. a, Healed transverse corneal laceration and associated cataract. *b,* Appearances following extracapsular extraction and posterior chamber intraocular lens; visual acuity 6/9 unaided.

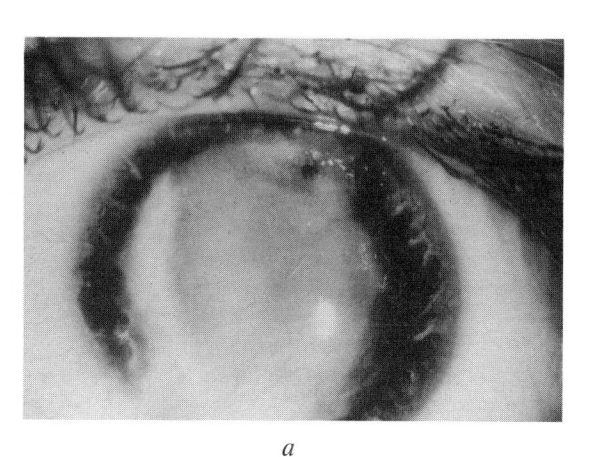

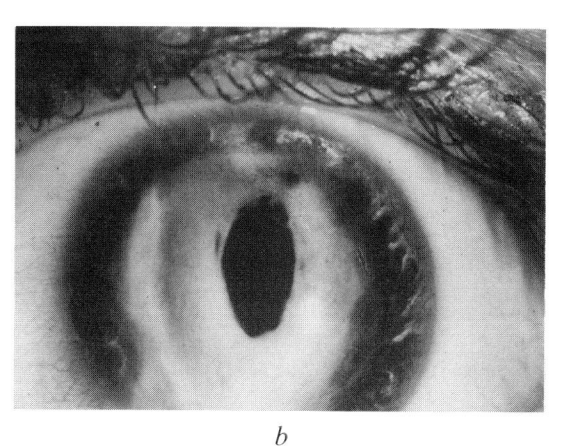

Fig. 10. a, Vascularized cyclitic membrane following combined anterior and posterior penetrating injury. *b,* Appearances following Nd: YAG laser membranotomy.

excision or short-pulsed laser photodisruption (*Fig.* 10).

In view of the important sequelae of posterior segment damage and the implications for visual recovery or survival of the globe, posterior segment intraocular microsurgical techniques have been at the forefront of interest over recent years. These techniques, often complex in nature, may be indicated in order to achieve the following broad objectives.

Clearance of Intraocular Opacities: The removal of a disrupted or displaced lens, fibrotic pupillary mem-

Control of the Inflammatory Response and Reduction of Intraocular Cellular Proliferation: Reduction of fibrocellular proliferation is achieved by the removal of intraocular haemorrhage, lens–vitreous admixture and elimination of anterior segment or post-basal gel incarceration within the wound.

Identification of Retinal Damage: Primary retinal damage or the effects of subsequent vitreo-retinal traction must be identified and treated appropriately to prevent retinal detachment. The ora must be visualized to exclude retinal breaks or predisposing changes and to allow monitoring of cryotherapy and accurate placement of scleral explants.

Repair of Retinal Detachment: This may include mobilization of the retina by relief of vitreo-retinal traction and in most cases of progressive or total detachment, identification and control of the responsible retinal break. Closure of retinal breaks often requires a combination of external and internal tamponade.

Control of Secondary Glaucoma: Normal aqueous dynamics may be restored by the removal of accumulated ghost cells within the vitreous gel, an intumescent lens or flocculent lens material, possibly in combination with trabeculectomy. Similar considerations apply in cases of lens-induced glaucoma.

Removal of Retained Intraocular Foreign Bodies

Exploration of the Posterior Segment: Exploratory vitrectomy should be undertaken to confirm overwhelming structural damage to vital posterior segment tissues as a prelude to enucleation for the prevention of sympathetic ophthalmitis.

In the view of most authorities, these important objectives are more readily achieved with reduced risks of operative complications by secondary intervention within a period of 1–3 weeks following injury. Although in any individual case many different factors enter into the decision, the major considerations governing the timing of vitrectomy include:
1. The unpredictable risks accompanying early secondary intervention of major operative choroidal or ciliary body haemorrhage from extensive scleral wounds or posterior foreign body exit sites.
2. Accompanying anterior segment wounds or residual hyphaema in the presence of a clear lens may seriously compromise visualization and control of intraocular manoeuvres.
3. The development of spontaneous or intraoperative posterior vitreous detachment confers important technical advantages and facilitates complete vitrectomy.
4. Spontaneous fibrinolysis of choroidal haematoma is necessary before drainage of the suprachoroidal compartment can be accomplished and so allow controlled surgical access to the vitreous cavity.
5. The likelihood of occult retinal damage and the risks of retinal break formation or progressive detachment in the presence of opaque media.

Increasing surgical experience and the reported results of vitreous surgery in posterior segment trauma appear to support the concept of early secondary intraocular reconstruction,[52-54] and that surgery undertaken prior to the development of retinal detachment substantially improves the prognosis for ultimate visual recovery.

INTRAOCULAR FOREIGN BODIES

Intraocular foreign body injuries vary widely in their effect depending upon the dimensions, composition and ultimate location of the foreign body, the mechanical damage to intraocular tissues during penetration and the compounding effects of surgical removal of the foreign body. Despite successful removal of the foreign body, the long term results of traditional management often prove disappointing,[55] even for small magnetic foreign bodies with an initially favourable prognosis.

It is well recognized that the majority of reactive intraocular foreign bodies are small metallic fragments predominantly composed of ferrous materials endowed with sufficient momentum to reach the posterior segment. Damage occurs at the site of entry, along the trajectory of the foreign body and at sites of retinal impaction or ricochet. Traversal of the lens causes localized peripheral cataract or diffuse opacity of rapid onset. Retinal impaction of the foreign body may cause localized damage to the retina and adjacent tissues of mechanical or possibly thermal origin. Retinal vascular damage may occur either in the form of arteriolar or venous occlusion or, more commonly, haemorrhage extending into the vitreous often disposed along the foreign body tract. In addition, impaction results in the incarceration of vitreous gel and the development of an exaggerated posterior vitreo-retinal adhesion. Similar changes may occur at ricochet sites which may be single or multiple, the foreign body being deflected ultimately to lie within the inferior vitreous cavity. Ricochet damage may also give rise to full thickness retinal tears which may subsequently give rise to retinal detachment. Larger metallic fragments or high velocity missiles are more likely to undergo double penetration, inflicting severe contusion damage to the posterior choroid and retina. The existence of vitreous haemorrhage generally implies the presence of primary retinal damage. These factors are of crucial importance in the development and disposition of subsequent vitreo-retinal traction leading to retinal detachment.

In addition to the mechanical effects of injury, there may be risks of specific chemotoxic damage depending upon the precise composition and location of the foreign body. In view of their prevalence, iron and steel fragments or copper-containing foreign bodies are of particular importance. Distinctive clinical appearances result from the rapid oxidation and the diffusion of ions throughout the globe.[56]

Generalized siderosis resulting from the dissemination and intracellular accumulation of ferrous ions causes insidious damage, particularly affecting those tissues with limited ability to detoxify iron. The earliest clinical manifestations result from the deposition of iron in the lens epithelium to cause siderotic cataract and in the iris with the development of heterochromia and a fixed dilated pupil (which may be reversible). Retinal degeneration is the most serious consequence resulting in progressive visual field constriction, dyschromatopsia (particularly blue–yellow), reduced acuity and early extinction of the electroretinogram. Although functional loss was originally ascribed to retinal vascular damage, experimental studies suggest direct cytotoxic damage to the photoreceptors (*Fig.* 11).[57]

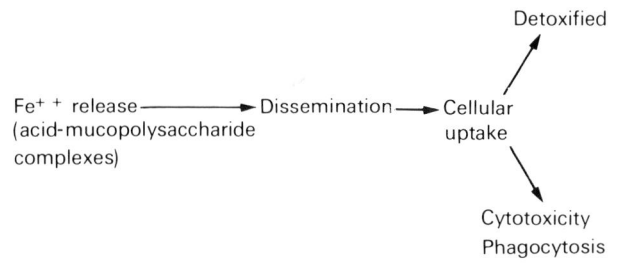

```
                                           Detoxified
                                              ↗
Fe⁺⁺ release ─────────→ Dissemination ──→ Cellular
(acid-mucopolysaccharide                   uptake
complexes)                                    ↘
                                           Cytotoxicity
                                           Phagocytosis
```

Fig. 11. Siderosis bulbi.

Copper-containing foreign bodies may provoke an acute suppurative inflammatory response depending upon their location and exact composition. Pure copper foreign bodies sequestered in the mid-vitreous fail to initiate a chemotactic response but this may develop following migration towards the surface of the retina.[58] Alternatively, slow release of copper ions with preferential involvement of basement membranes results in the development of a sunflower cataract, Kayser–Fleischer ring and potentially reversible maculopathy.

Organic materials often induce an intense granulomatous response and may also introduce fungal or bacterial pathogens. This is in contrast to metallic foreign bodies in which the incidence of microbial endophthalmitis is approximately 5–10 per cent.

Certain other materials, including silicates, precious metals and polymerized plastics, appear remarkably inert and may be retained indefinitely without adverse effects provided they remain immobile or become encapsulated.

Evaluation

At an early stage, clinical examination will often reveal the characteristics of the foreign body including its precise location and the extent of associated intraocular damage. In the presence of opaque media, indirect methods of foreign body localization are required, although the need for accurate preoperative localization has to some extent been reduced with the advent of vitrectomy techniques. Innumerable methods of radiographic localization have been described, many of which are now of historical interest only. Sutured limbal rings and contact lenses incorporating radio-opaque markers are more reliable but have largely been superseded by tomography (*Fig.* 12). Computerized tomographic scans with axial and coronal projections offer considerable accuracy and are of particular value in distinguishing intramural foreign bodies from those located immediately outside the globe.[59] Bone-free plain films using a dental cassette at the inner canthus may aid the identification of selected anterior segment foreign bodies. Even though non-biological materials give rise to the highest echo amplitudes, diagnostic ultrasound is of limited value in terms of localization and is principally used to identify the extent of intraocular damage.

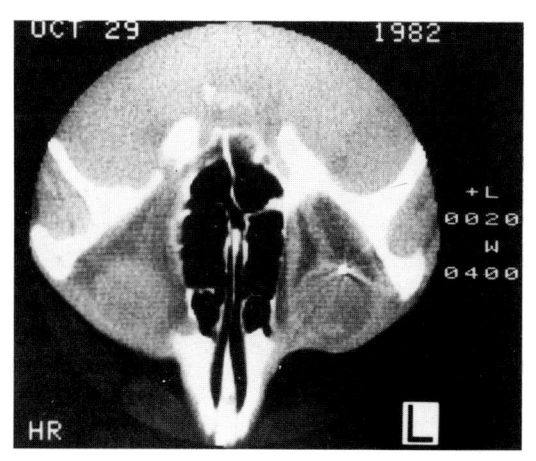

Fig. 12. Axial computerized tomographic scan showing foreign body impacted within the posterior coats of the globe.

Again, in the context of modern surgical management, the use of electro-acoustic localization is of limited application but may be helpful in the discrimination of magnetic from non-magnetic materials.

Management

Foreign bodies retained within the anterior chamber or impacted in the iris, which are often of smaller dimensions, are approached through a clear corneal incision of sufficient size to allow direct visualization during removal. Maintenance of the anterior chamber with visco-elastic materials is often helpful. Removal may be accomplished using a hand-held electromagnet or suitable microforceps.

Intralenticular foreign bodies can remain in situ with no risk of generalized metallosis provided the lens capsule is intact. Associated cataract is treated on its own merits and the foreign body removed at the time of elective extracapsular extraction.

Pars plana electromagnet extraction remains the treatment of choice for small, visible, magnetic foreign bodies located within the vitreous gel in the absence of major retinal damage. A direct approach through a scleral trap-door incision is used for intra-retinal foreign bodies located in the region of the equator or peripheral retina. To minimize gel prolapse and subsequent incarceration, the foreign body is extracted through the intact uvea. Failure of the foreign body to exit from the wound generally requires enlargement of the sclerotomy with incision of the uvea. Pre-placed monofilament sutures are tied and monitored cryotherapy applied to the post-oral retina in relation to the sclerotomy.

Closed vitrectomy techniques may be indicated to facilitate the removal of retained material or for the surgical repair of intraocular damage at varying intervals following penetration.[60] These techniques are used to extract large magnetic foreign bodies in the presence of a clear lens and those impacted or encapsulated within the posterior retina in which a direct trans-scleral approach presents difficulties of access. The foreign body is mobilized from the retinal surface following incision of the overlying capsule and retrieved with appropriate microforceps through an enlarged pars plana sclerotomy. Various designs of intraocular microforceps are available to accommodate foreign bodies of differing dimensions and materials and to reduce the risks of displacement during delivery.[61] Large foreign bodies, for example glass fragments, are preferably removed through a clear corneal incision following lensectomy. These techniques are of obvious application in the management of non-magnetic materials, although these continue to represent less than 10 per cent of all retained intraocular foreign bodies.

Perhaps the most important concept in the modern management of intraocular foreign bodies is the ability to undertake removal under direct visualization following clearance of associated lens opacity or vitreous haemorrhage. Early application of these methods may prevent the development of vitreoretinal sequelae with reduced risks of early or delayed retinal detachment. It is important to appreciate that these injuries present many of the surgical problems common to any posterior penetrating injury and in which removal of the foreign body may be of subsidiary importance in the overall surgical management.

SYMPATHETIC OPHTHALMITIS

Sympathetic ophthalmitis, a rare and unpredictable chronic inflammatory disorder possibly unique to the human eye, develops exclusively following accidental or surgical penetration of the globe. The clinical course of the condition and the response to treatment are extremely variable. The rarity of the disorder and the lack of an experimental model have hampered understanding of the pathogenesis and the possibility of definitive treatment or prevention.

Although a decline in the incidence is generally stated, no reliable figures to support this view are available since the disorder was recognized as a pathological entity. Indeed, there is continuing concern that more radical surgical treatment of injured eyes may lead to an increased incidence and that the risks are cumulative. A number of surveys report an approximate incidence of 0·2 per cent following accidental penetration.[62,63] Approximately one-third of all cases of sympathetic ophthalmitis are attributable to previous surgery with an incidence of 1 in 10 000 intraocular procedures. There is a bimodal age distribution but no particular age group is more susceptible to the disorder. It is rarely encountered in certain ethnic groups and the geographical variations in the reported incidence may reflect differing genetic susceptibility.

The usual onset of the disorder (as determined by inflammation in the contralateral eye) is between 1 and 3 months following injury. In cases reported to have developed many years following the initial injury, the possibility of mild intercurrent inflammatory episodes cannot be excluded. The injured or exciting eye is likely to show indolent, low-grade inflammation, often dating from the time of injury, the significance of which may be difficult to determine in the context of a severely injured eye. A limited response to anti-inflammatory treatment or the appearance of features suggestive of a granulomatous uveitis including mutton-fat keratic precipitates may be early diagnostic pointers. Prodromal symptoms in the sympathizing eye, including photophobia and transient visual disturbance, give way to symmetrical intraocular inflammation of variable degree. Although often generalized, inflammatory changes may preferentially affect the anterior or posterior segment. In a significant number of cases, diffuse choroidal thickening with optic disc and macular oedema are prominent features often accompanied by small, discrete subretinal lesions located in the midperiphery of the fundus corresponding to Dalen–Fuchs nodules. There may be associated serous retinal elevation which can progress to total detachment. Systemic manifestations including cutaneous pigmentary disturbances, auditory defects and meningeal inflammation are rarely encountered.

The clinical features reflect diffuse and often massive lymphocytic infiltration of the uveal tract with foci of epithelioid cells containing giant cells. The choroidal infiltrate is predominantly composed of T lymphocytes with a minor contribution of immunoglobin-producing B-lymphocytes as shown by recent immunopathological studies.[64] Dalen–Fuchs nodules, located beneath the retinal pigment epithelium, appear to be composed of histiocytes and transformed retinal pigment epithelial cells. Contrary to previous reports, associated retinal inflammation with perivasculitis, optic neuritis and obliteration of the choriocapillaries are not uncommon findings and may be correlated with the severity of choroidal inflammation.[65]

Immunopathogenesis

There is now considerable evidence to show that cell mediated immune mechanisms are of fundamental importance in the pathogenesis of sympathetic ophthalmitis.[66] Originally, uveal pigment was believed to be the responsible antigen but in its pure state melanin appears immunologically inert. Of the various intraocular antigens, interest has largely centred upon those of retinal origin and, in particular, retinal soluble antigen (S antigen). Experimental immunization with photoreceptor membrane antigen produces a dose-dependent inflammatory response which may resemble sympathetic ophthalmitis. Localization of the inflammatory response to extra-retinal tissues from the activation of cytotoxic-suppressor T lymphocytes does not therefore preclude a retinal origin for the antigenic determinant. It is possible that shared cell surface antigens may play an adjuvant role and this may explain the significance of associated phacoallergic uveitis in reported cases.[67] *In vitro* studies of circulating antibodies reveal inconsistent results whereas lymphocyte transformation in the presence of uveo-retinal antigens in most but not all cases of sympathetic ophthalmitis underscores the importance of cell mediated hypersensitivity. The significance of a penetrating wound may relate to the exposure of uveo-retinal antigens to conjunctival and regional lymphatics or contaminating adjuvant factors triggering an immunopathological response. The degree of inflammation and the possibility of contralateral involvement may depend upon the antigenic load or the level of responsiveness of the immune surveillance system.[68]

At the present time, immunological investigations are of no value in the prediction or definitive diagnosis of sympathetic ophthalmitis.[69] The burden of proof rests with histopathological examination of the excised eye or possibly choroidal biopsy.

Treatment

The principal aim of treatment is the suppression of intraocular inflammation as early as possible in the course of the disease. High initial levels of systemic steroids are required commencing with 100 mg Prednisolone daily or greater in adults for a period of several days with subsequent titration of the dose according to the level of inflammation. In this respect, posterior segment manifestations, including optic disc and macular oedema or serous retinal detachment, are useful parameters. Once the threshold level of systemic steroids is achieved, treatment should be continued for a period of 6 months to prevent recurrence of inflammation. Alternate day regimes of systemic steroids are unlikely to achieve adequate suppression. Anterior segment inflammation requires appropriate levels of topical steroids. Systemic steroids in combination with immunosuppressive agents, including cyclophosphamide and azathioprine, can be considered in cases of intractable inflammation or in patients with significant adverse effects of steroid therapy. The place of agents known selectively to inhibit T-cell function, such as cyclosporin A either alone or in combination with oral steroids, has yet to be evaluated.

Data from retrospective studies suggest that enucleation of a blind exciting eye within a short period of onset of the disorder reduces inflammation and improves the visual outcome in the sympathizing eye.[65,70]

Enucleation of an eye damaged beyond repair within 2 weeks of penetrating injury offers the only known prevention of sympathetic ophthalmitis. There is no evidence that immunosuppression using currently available agents can prevent the onset of the disorder but topical application of T-cell inhibitors, possibly in combination with steroids, holds some promise.

CHEMICAL OCULAR BURNS

Chemical burns of the eye range in their effects from self-limited surface defects to widespread cellular destruction throughout the anterior segment. Severe chemical burns pose a stern therapeutic challenge in which a protracted clinical course often culminates in blindness. However, considerable laboratory research has identified some of the biochemical events underlying tissue damage with the advent of new pharmacological approaches which may hopefully influence the dismal natural history of these injuries.

The major factors determining the extent and severity of chemical injury are the duration of contact and, by implication, the efficiency of immediate dilution, the concentration of the chemical and the inherent toxicity, including pH and the nature of the cation.

Weak acid radicals precipitate surface protein upon contact with limited tissue penetration. By contrast, alkalis react with lipid cellular constituents to form soluble compounds resulting in rapid penetration and access to intraocular structures. Cell lysis is accompanied by denaturation of structural and enzymatic proteins and vascular obliteration. Rapid and persistent elevation of aqueous pH causes disruption of ocular barriers and damage to the outflow pathway, iris, lens and ciliary body. Dramatic pressure rise caused by collagen shrinkage may be compounded by prostaglandin release.[71] Anterior choroidal and retinal damage resulting from direct scleral penetration of alkali has also been described.[72]

Various classifications have been devised based upon evaluation of the extent of damage and the prognostic implications of certain clinical features identifiable during the early phase. The circumferential extent of limbal damage and in particular ischaemia of the deep vascular plexus (*Fig.* 13) is of considerable importance, with the likelihood of delayed resurfacing and vascularization of the cornea and risks of tissue melting.

Management

While immediate irrigation and removal of particulate chemical reduces the extent of damage, it is doubtful whether prolonged irrigation over many hours confers additional benefits. Paracentesis and intracameral phosphate buffer irrigation, recommended for severe burns with persistent rise of

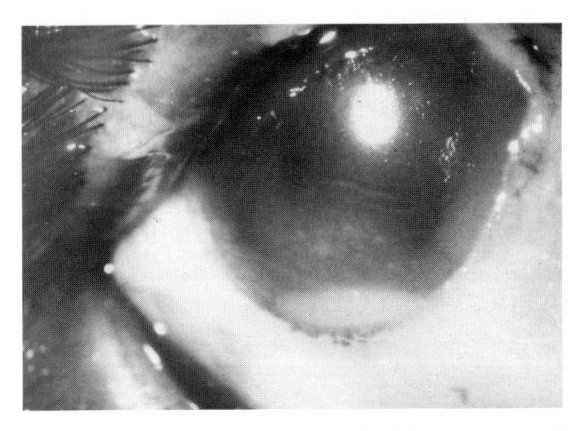

Fig. 13. Severe alkali burn 1 week following injury; note extensive ischaemia, mild corneal haze and hypopyon.

aqueous pH, has not been shown to improve the ultimate outcome.[73]

Universal indicator paper may be helpful in the identification of the chemical and as a guide to the effectiveness of irrigation. Important early measures include the relief of pain, reduction of elevated intraocular pressure and the prevention of secondary infection by topical antibiotics. In the presence of extensive conjunctival damage, mechanical lysis of fibrinous adhesions and the insertion of methacrylate conformers have been widely used but do not appear to reduce the risks of symblepharon formation and conjunctival shrinkage. Corneal exposure from damage to the lids requires energetic treatment with the possibility of early lid reconstruction to achieve adequate cover.

Suppression of the inflammatory response and other measures to limit the recruitment of polymorphs in damaged tissues have assumed increasing importance. On the basis of recent studies, polymorphs appear to play a central role in tissue degradation and collagenolysis. During the first week of treatment, intensive topical steroids are used to reduce inflammatory cell infiltration and combat the effects of intraocular inflammation. At a later stage, steroids may augment collagenolysis and retard collagen synthesis and it is usual to limit steroid therapy and introduce topical enzyme inhibitors. Other mediators of inflammation, including prostaglandins, may play an important subsidiary role but the value of prostaglandin synthetase inhibition is presently unknown. The efficacy of other steroid preparations, including medroxyprogesterone and anabolic agents in the prevention of corneal ulceration, is unclear.

The possible value of supplementary ascorbate in the prevention of corneal breakdown was raised some years ago following observations in a rabbit model of alkali burns.[74] Levels of aqueous ascorbate, normally concentrated by active transport mechanisms, were found to be reduced and reversal of this deficiency by immediate systemic or topical ascorbate lowered the incidence of corneal ulceration and subsequent perforation. The effect was initially ascribed to the correction of a scorbutic state and the promotion of collagen synthesis during repair. Further experimental studies have suggested that ascorbate may prevent tissue damage caused by free superoxide radicals derived from damaged epithelium or the degranulation of polymorphs.[75] Oral ascorbic acid 1000 mg daily is given in combination with hourly 10 per cent topical sodium ascorbate until re-epithelization is complete and maintained at a reduced level for several weeks. Recent studies have also indicated that citric acid may have similar effects by chelation of calcium ions and cellular inhibition of polymorphs.[76] Controlled clinical studies to determine the possible benefits of ascorbate and citrate therapy are currently in progress.

Various compounds have been used to inhibit proteolytic enzymes responsible for corneal ulceration.[77] Many of these agents have been shown clinically to confer little advantage but there is some evidence in favour of L-cysteine.[78]

Re-establishment of the corneal epithelium and the prevention of recurrent breakdown pose major problems reflecting underlying stromal damage or abnormalities of the basement membrane. Resurfacing may be promoted by improvement of the tear film, the avoidance of preservatives and the possible use of extended-wear contact lenses. New avenues of approach include transplantation of autologous conjunctiva from the fellow eye in conjunction with superficial keratectomy.[79]

Despite reports of improved long term results of penetrating keratoplasty, a high incidence of complications is to be expected including recurrent epithelial breakdown and stromal lysis, vascularization and allograft reaction. Preliminary correction of associated lid and conjunctival abnormalities and improvement of the tear film are essential in addition to complete regression of inflammatory changes.

REFERENCES

1. Eagling E. M. Ocular damage after blunt trauma to the eye. *Br. J. Ophthalmol.* 1974; **58,** 126–40.
2. Wolter J. R. Coup-contrecoup mechanism of ocular injuries. *Am. J. Ophthalmol.* 1963; **56,** 785–96.
3. Slingsby J. G. and Forstot S. L. Effect of blunt trauma on the corneal endothelium. *Arch. Ophthalmol.* 1981; **99,** 1041–3.
4. Angell L. K., Robb R. M. and Berson F. G. Visual prognosis in patients with ruptures in Descemet's membrane due to forceps injuries. *Arch. Ophthalmol.* 1981; **99,** 2137–9.
5. Cibis G. W., Weingeist T. A. and Krachmer J. H. Traumatic corneal endothelial rings. *Arch. Ophthalmol.* 1978; **96,** 485–8.

6. Maloney W. F., Colvard D. M., Bourne W. M. et al. Specular microscopy of traumatic posterior annular keratopathy. *Arch. Ophthalmol.* 1979; **97**, 1647–50.
7. Wilson F. M. Traumatic hyphaema. *Ophthalmology* 1980; **87**, 910–19.
8. Crouch E. R. and Frenkel M. Aminocaproic acid in the treatment of traumatic hyphaema. *Am. J. Ophthalmol.* 1976; **81**, 355–59.
9. McGetrick J. J., Jampol L. M., Goldberg M. F. et al. Aminocaproic acid decreases secondary haemorrhage after traumatic hyphaema. *Arch. Ophthalmol.* 1983; **101**, 1031–13.
10. Bramsen T. Traumatic hyphaema treated with the antifibrinolytic drug tranexamic acid. *Acta Ophthalmol.* 1977; **55**, 616–20.
11. Missotten L., de Clippelier L., van Tornout I. et al. The value of tranexamic acid (Cyclokapron) in the prevention of secondary bleeding: a complication of traumatic hyphaema. *Bull. Soc. Belge Ophtalmol.* 1977; **179**, 47–52.
12. Bramsen T. Fibrinolysis and traumatic hyphaema. *Acta Ophthalmol.* 1979; **57**, 447–54.
13. Goldberg M. F. The diagnosis and treatment of secondary glaucoma after hyphaema in sickle cell patients. *Am. J. Ophthalmol.* 1979; **87**, 43–9.
14. McCuen B. W. and Fung W. E. The role of vitrectomy instrumentation in the treatment of severe traumatic hyphaema. *Am. J. Ophthalmol.* 1979; **88**, 930–4.
15. Diddie K. R., Dinsmore S. and Murphree A. L. Total hyphaema evacuation by vitrectomy instrumentation. *Ophthalmology* 1981; **88**, 917–21.
16. Parrish R. and Bernardino V. Iridectomy in the surgical management of eight-ball hyphaema. *Arch. Ophthalmol.* 1982; **100**, 435–7.
17. Weiss J. S., Parrish R. K. and Anderson D. R. Surgical therapy of traumatic hyphaema. *Ophth. Surg.* 1983; **14**, 343–5.
18. Herschler J. Trabecular damage due to blunt anterior segment injury and its relationship to traumatic glaucoma. *Trans. Am. Acad. Ophthalmol.* 1977; **83**, 239–48.
19. Kaufman J. H. and Tolpin D. W. Glaucoma after traumatic angle recession: a ten year prospective study. *Am. J. Ophthalmol.* 1974; **78**, 648–54.
20. Dotan S. and Oliver M. Shallow anterior chamber and uveal effusion after nonperforating trauma to the eye. *Am. J. Ophthalmol.* 1982; **94**, 782–4.
21. Shea M. and Mednick E. B. Ciliary body reattachment in ocular hypotony. *Arch. Ophthalmol.* 1981; **99**, 278–81.
22. Fagerholm P. P. and Philipson B. T. Experimental traumatic cataract 1. a quantitative microradiographic study. *Invest. Ophthalmol.* 1979; **18**, 1151–9.
23. Canavan Y. M. and Archer D. B. Anterior segment consequences of blunt ocular injury. *Br. J. Ophthalmol.* 1982; **66**, 549–55.
24. Peyman G. A., Raichand M., Goldberg M. F. et al. Management of subluxated and dislocated lenses with the vitrophage. *Br. J. Ophthalmol.* 1979; **63**, 771–8.
25. Rodman H. I. Chronic open-angle glaucoma associated with traumatic dislocation of the lens. *Arch. Ophthalmol.* 1963; **69**, 445–54.
26. Hart J. C. D. and Frank H. J. Retinal opacification after blunt nonperforating concussional injuries to the globe. *Trans. Ophthalmol. Soc. UK* 1975; **95**, 94–100.
27. Blight R. and Hart J. C. D. Structural changes in the outer retinal layers following blunt mechanical non-perforating trauma to the globe: an experimental study. *Br. J. Ophthalmol.* 1977; **61**, 573–87.
28. Sipperley J. O., Quigley H. A. and Gass J. D. M. Traumatic retinopathy in primates. *Arch. Ophthalmol.* 1978; **96**, 2267–73.
29. Gregor Z. and Ryan S. J. Blood–retinal barrier after blunt trauma to the eye. *Albrecht von Graefe's Arch. Klin. Exp. Ophthalmol.* 1982; **219**, 205–8.
30. Cogan D. G. Pseudoretinitis pigmentosa. *Arch. Ophthalmol.* 1969; **81**, 45–53.
31. Bastek J. V., Foos R. Y. and Heckenlively J. Traumatic pigmentary retinopathy. *Am. J. Ophthalmol.* 1981; **92**, 621–4.
32. Bloome M. A., Ruiz R. S., Russo C. E. et al. Acute retinal necrosis. *Ann. Ophthalmol.* 1979; **11**, 723–8.
33. Cox M. S. Retinal breaks caused by nonperforating trauma at the point of impact. *Trans. Am. Ophthalmol. Soc.* 1980; **78**, 414–66.
34. Hart J. C. D., Natsikos V. E. Raistrick E. R. et al. Indirect choroidal tears at the posterior pole: a fluorescein angiographic and perimetric study. *Br. J. Ophthalmol.* 1980; **64**, 59–67.
35. Smith R. E., Kelley J. S. and Harbin T. S. Late macular complications of choroidal ruptures. *Am. J. Ophthalmol.* 1974; **77**, 650–8.
36. Hart J. C. D., Natsikos V. E., Raistrick E. R. et al. Chorioretinitis sclopetaria. *Trans. Ophthalmol. Soc. UK* 1980; **100**, 276–81.
37. Wyllie A. M., McLeod D. L. and Cullen J. F. Traumatic ischaemic optic neuropathy. *Br. J. Ophthalmol.* 1972; **56**, 851–3.
38. Hedges T. R. and Gragoudas E. S. Traumatic anterior ischaemic optic neuropathy. *Ann. Ophthalmol.* 1981; **13**, 625–8.
39. Archer D. B. and Canavan Y. M. Contusional injuries of the distal optic nerve. *Trans. Ophthalmol. Soc. NZ* 1983; **35**, 14–23.
40. Hillman J. S., Myska V. and Nissim S. Complete avulsion of the optic nerve. *Br. J. Ophthalmol.* 1975; **59**, 503–9.
41. Ramsay J. H. Optic nerve injury in fracture of the canal. *Br. J. Ophthalmol.* 1979; **63**, 607–10.
42. Anderson R. L., Panje W. R. and Gross C. E. Optic nerve blindness following blunt forehead trauma. *Ophthalmology* 1982; **89**, 445–55.

43. Kennerdell J. S., Amsbaugh G. A. and Myers E. N. Transantral-ethmoidal decompression of optic canal fracture. *Arch. Ophthalmol.* 1976; **94**, 1040–3.
44. Johnston S. Perforating eye injuries: a five year survey. *Trans. Ophthalmol. Soc. UK* 1971; **91**, 895–921.
45. Barr C. C. Prognostic factors in corneo-scleral lacerations. *Arch. Ophthalmol.* 1983; **101**, 919–26.
46. Hutton W. L. and Fuller D. G. Factors influencing final visual results in severely injured eyes. *Am. J. Ophthalmol.* 1984; **97**, 715–22.
47. Sternberg P., De Juan E., Michels R. G. et al. Multivariate analysis of prognostic factors in penetrating ocular injuries. *Am. J. Ophthalmol.* 1984; **98**, 467–72.
48. Roper-Hall M. J. Visco-elastic materials in the surgery of ocular trauma. *Trans. Ophthalmol. Soc. UK* 1983; **103**, 274–6.
49. Roper-Hall M. J. Immediate management of iris and lens in perforations of the eye. *Trans. Ophthalmol. Soc. UK* 1982; **102**, 221–2.
50. Cooling R. J. Immediate management of posterior perforating trauma. *Trans. Ophthalmol. Soc. UK* 1982; **102**, 223–4.
51. Peyman G. A., Carroll C. P. and Raichand M. Prevention and management of traumatic endopthalmitis. *Ophthalmology* 1980; **87**, 320–4.
52. Ryan S. J. and Allen A. W. Pars plana vitrectomy in ocular trauma. *Am. J. Ophthalmol.* 1979; **88**, 483–91.
53. Brinton G. S., Aaberg T. M., Reeser F. H. et al. Surgical results in ocular trauma involving the posterior segment. *Am. J. Ophthalmol.* 1982; **93**, 271–8.
54. Miyake Y. and Ando F. Surgical results of vitrectomy in ocular trauma. *Retina* 1983; **3**, 265–8.
55. Percival S. P. B. Late complications from posterior segment intraocular foreign bodies. *Br. J. Ophthalmol.* 1972; **56**, 462–8.
56. Neubauer H. Ocular metallosis. *Trans. Ophthalmol. Soc. UK* 1979; **99**, 502–10.
57. Burger P. C. and Klintworth G. K. Experimental retinal degeneration in the rabbit produced by intraocular iron. *Lab. Invest.* 1974; **30**, 9–19.
58. Rosenthal A. R., Appleton B. and Hopkins J. L. Intraocular copper foreign bodies. *Am. J. Ophthalmol.* 1974; **78**, 671–8.
59. Lobes L. A., Grand M. G., Reece J. et al. Computerizied axial tomography in the detection of intraocular foreign bodies. *Ophthalmology* 1981; **88**, 26–9.
60. Cooling R. J., McLeod D., Blach R. K. et al. Closed microsurgery in the management of intraocular foreign bodies. *Trans. Ophthalmol. Soc. UK* 1981; **101**, 181–3.
61. Hickingbotham D., Parel J. M. and Machemer R. Diamond-coated all-purpose foreign-body forceps. *Am. J. Ophthalmol.* 1981; **91**, 267–8.
62. Liddy N. and Stuart J. Sympathetic ophthalmia in Canada. *Can. J. Ophthalmol.* 1972; **7**, 157–9.
63. Gass J. D. M. Sympathetic ophthalmia following vitrectomy. *Am. J. Ophthalmol.* 1982; **93**, 552–8.
64. Jakobiec F. A., Marboe C. C., Knowles D. M. et al. Human sympathetic ophthalmia. *Ophthalmology* 1983; **90**, 76–95.
65. Lubin J. R., Albert D. M. and Weinstein M. Sixty-five years of sympathetic ophthalmia. *Ophthalmology* 1980; **87**, 109–19.
66. Rao N. A. and Wong V. G. Aetiology of sympathetic ophthalmitis. *Trans. Ophthalmol. Soc. UK* 1981; **101**, 357–60.
67. Marak G. E. Recent advances in sympathetic ophthalmia. *Surv. Ophthalmol.* 1979; **24**, 141–56.
68. Rao N. A., Robin J., Hartmann D. et al. The role of the penetrating wound in the development of sympathetic ophthalmia. *Arch. Ophthalmol.* 1983; **101**, 102–4.
69. Rahi A., Morgan G., Levy I. et al. Immunological investigations in post-traumatic granulomatous and non-granulomatous uveitis. *Br. J. Ophthalmol.* 1978; **62**, 722–31.
70. Reynard M., Riffenburgh R. S. and Maes E. F. Effect of corticosteroid treatment and enucleation on the visual prognosis of sympathetic ophthalmia. *Am. J. Ophthalmol.* 1983; **96**, 290–4.
71. Paterson C. A. and Pfister R. R. Intraocular pressure changes after alkali burns. *Arch. Ophthalmol.* 1974: **91**, 211–18.
72. Smith R. E. and Conway B. Alkali retinopathy. *Arch. Ophthalmol.* 1976; **94**, 81–4.
73. Burns R. P. and Hikes C. E. Irrigation of the anterior chamber for the treatment of alkali burns. *Am. J. Ophthalmol.* 1979; **88**, 119–20.
74. Levinson R. A., Paterson C. A. and Pfister R. R. Ascorbic acid prevents corneal ulceration and perforation following experimental alkali burns. *Invest. Ophthalmol.* 1976; **15**, 986–93.
75. Nirankari V. S., Varma S. D., Lakhanpal V. et al. Superoxide radical scavenging agents in the treatment of alkali burns. *Arch. Ophthalmol.* 1981; **99**, 886–7.
76. Pfister R. R. The effects of chemical injury on the ocular surface. *Ophthalmology* 1983; **90**, 601–9.
77. Brown S. and Hook C. W. Treatment of corneal destruction with collagenase inhibitors. *Trans. Am. Acad. Ophthalmol.* 1971; **75**, 1199–1207.
78. Wright P. The chemically injured eye. *Trans. Ophthalmol. Soc. UK* 1982; **102**, 185–7.
79. Thoft R. A. Conjunctival transplantation as an alternative to keratoplasty. *Ophthalmology* 1979; **86**, 1084–92.

Chapter 15

The Lids: Diseases and Treatment

J. R. O. Collin

FUNCTIONAL ANATOMY

The eyelids are composed of two layers, an anterior lamella of skin and orbicularis muscle and a posterior lamella of tarsus and conjunctiva (*Fig.* 1). The skin is thin, mobile and free of fat. The usual skin structures are present but at the lid margin the hair follicles are specialized to form cilia with their associated oily glands (the glands of Zeis). The orbicularis muscle,

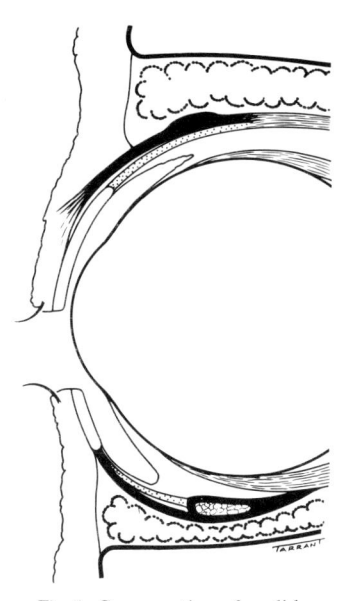

Fig. 1. Cross-section of eyelids.

innervated by the VIIth nerve, is responsible for eyelid closure. It is composed of 'twitch' muscle fibres responsible for blinking and found mainly in the palpebral part of the muscle, and other fibres capable of prolonged contraction, responsible for forced eyelid closure and found mainly in the orbital part of the muscle. The tarsus gives stability to the lid, especially to the lid margin, and contains the meibomian glands. These produce an oily secretion which reduces the evaporation of the tear film. Mucus, which helps to spread the tear film, is produced by goblet cells in the conjunctiva. Tear fluid is produced by the accessory lacrimal glands in the conjunctiva as well as the main lacrimal gland.

The eyelids are opened by their retractors which are similar in the two lids and consist of a main retractor muscle with its associated aponeurosis and smooth muscle. In the upper lid the levator palpebrae superioris muscle extends forward from the apex of the orbit and divides into two layers, the aponeurosis and the superior tarsal or Mueller's muscle which inserts into the upper border of the tarsal plate. The aponeurosis becomes continuous with the fibrous tissue on the posterior surface of the orbicularis muscle, the post-orbicular fascia. This insertion is responsible for the skin crease and for elevating the anterior lamella of the eyelid. The posterior lamella of the eyelid is elevated mainly by the superior tarsal (Mueller's) muscle. The frontalis muscle acts as an accessory upper lid retractor through its insertion into the eyebrow and skin. The main lower lid retractor is the inferior rectus muscle. A sheet of fibrous tissue extends forwards from the sheath of the inferior rectus muscle, splits to enclose the inferior oblique muscle, and extends forwards to the lower border of the inferior tarsal plate with fibrous attachments to the post-orbicular fascia. There are smooth muscle fibres associated with this inferior aponeurosis, the inferior tarsal muscle, which is analogous to the superior tarsal (Mueller's) muscle in the upper lid. Both these muscles are innervated by the sympathetic nervous system via the perivascular plexi. Denervation, as in Horner's syndrome, results in about 2 mm of upper lid ptosis and 1 mm of lower lid elevation. The orbital septum extends as a firm sheet of fibrous tissue from the orbital margin and blends with the superior and inferior aponeurosis. The pre-aponeurotic fat pad in both the upper and lower eyelids lies behind the orbital septum and anterior to the aponeurosis, providing a distinctive anatomical landmark of great help in identifying these structures during eyelid surgery.

EYELID MALPOSITION

Entropion

An entropion is defined as a condition in which the eyelid margin turns inwards against the globe. It can be either congenital or acquired, and the acquired forms are involutional or cicatricial.

Congenital Entropion

The congenital form is said to be due to a hypertrophy of the subcutaneous tissues and orbicularis muscle. Mild degrees of this are very common in young babies and usually resolve with age. Rarely the child gets symptoms of photophobia and irritation with conjunctival injection, superficial punctate erosions on the cornea and recurrent attacks of conjunctivitis. In these rare circumstances operative correction of the entropion is justifiable. An ellipse of skin, subcutaneous tissue and orbicularis muscle is excised from the medial part of the lower eyelid and the skin edges are sutured to the inferior border of the tarsal plate with fine absorbable sutures such as 6/0 collagen. This operation is best done bilaterally in the interests of a symmetrical scar.

An epicanthic fold or epiblepharon is a fold of tissue not associated with inversion of the lid margin but which, like a congenital entropion, usually resolves with time. It may give rise to the false appearance of a convergent squint.

Involutional Entropion

Involutional entropion of the lower eyelid is caused by ageing changes which affect all the lid tissues simultaneously, although various factors can be identified separately. The palpebral part of the orbicularis muscle in front of the orbital septum (the preseptal muscle) overrides the lower border of the tarsus. The lower lid retractors become lax. The tarsus atrophies and buckles on itself. The lid does not fit tightly against the globe due to laxity of the orbicularis muscle and its medial and lateral canthal tendons, and in addition there is some enophthalmos of the globe induced by atrophy of the orbital fat. These factors all contribute to inversion of the lid margin. Various operations have been described to correct an involutional entropion. The simplest of these is to pass double-armed sutures through the lid from the conjunctival surface just below the lower border of the tarsus and to tie them on the skin of the eyelid. These sutures create a barrier to the upward movement of the preseptal muscle. A more permanent cure can be obtained by cutting through the lid horizontally just below the tarsus and passing double-armed everting sutures from the conjunctival surface below the lid transection which pick up the lower lid retractors, pass behind the orbicularis muscle and in front of the tarsus above the lid transection, and emerge through the skin just below the lash line (*Fig.* 2). When these sutures are tied they tighten the lower lid retractors and transfer their pull to evert the eyelid margin. The lid transection heals and creates a fibrous tissue barrier which prevents the upward movement of the preseptal muscle. If there is marked lid laxity, this procedure can be combined with a horizontal lid shortening procedure.

If the entropion recurs the probable cause is that the lower lid retractors have not been shortened adequately. They can be approached directly via an incision through the skin and orbicularis muscle at the lower border of the tarsus. The orbital septum is incised and the pre-aponeurotic fat pad reflected to

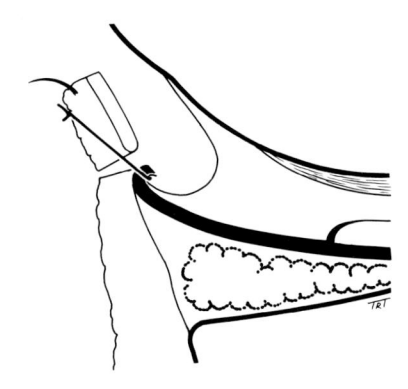

Fig. 2. Horizontal lid transection and everting sutures.

expose the lower lid retractors. These can be shortened as required with a suture which passes from the inferior skin edge, through the lower lid retractors, through the lower border of the tarsus and out through the upper skin edge (*Fig.* 3). The point at which the lower lid retractors are picked up governs the amount of the retractor shortening and the extent of the eversion of the lid margin achieved.

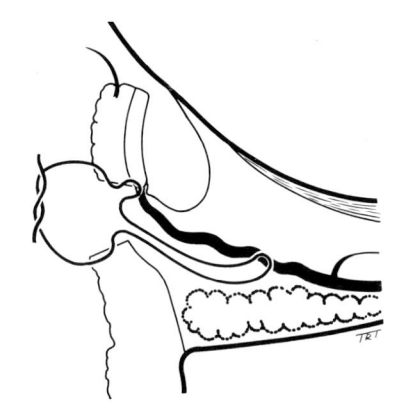

Fig. 3. Lower lid retractor plication.

Cicatricial Entropion

Cicatricial entropion can affect either upper or lower lids and is caused by anything that leads to scarring and contraction of the posterior lamella of the lid, such as trachoma, chronic conjunctivitis, chemical injuries and pemphigoid. The contraction pulls the lid margin posteriorly against the globe causing first an entropion and then lid retraction. In the lower lid, if the lid retraction is mild, the entropion can be corrected with a tarsal 'hinge' procedure. The tarsus is split horizontally leaving the skin and orbicularis muscle intact. Everting sutures are then passed through the lid to hinge the lid margin into eversion

(*Fig. 4a*). If the lid retraction is more severe the same incision is made but a graft is sutured between the cut edges of the tarsal plate in order to lengthen the posterior lamella. The graft can be of mucous membrane, sclera, cartilage, or nasal septal cartilage with its mucoperichondrium, and everting sutures are required to evert the lid margin (*Fig. 4b*).

line to a depth of about 2 mm. If the eversion is still not adequate because the tarsus is thickened, scarred, and buckled, a wedge can be cut out of the anterior surface of the tarsus. When this is closed the tarsus will be straightened and the effect of the grey line split and anterior lamella repositioning will be enhanced (*Fig. 5b*). Mild degrees of upper lid retrac-

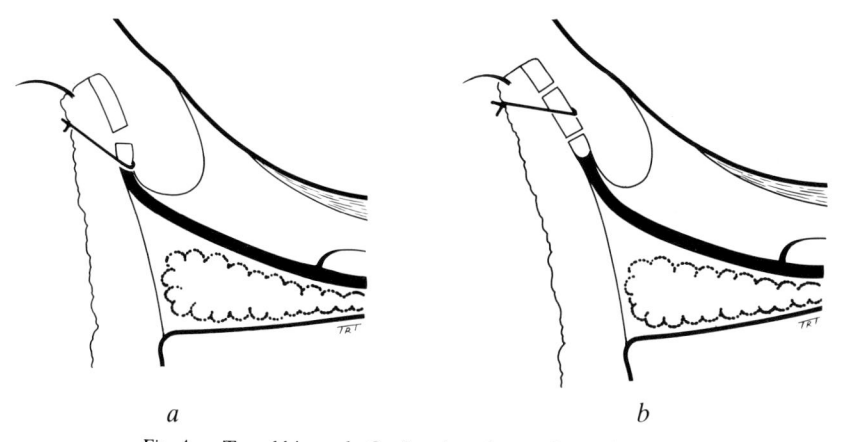

Fig. 4. a, Tarsal hinge. *b*, Graft to lengthen and evert lower tarsus.

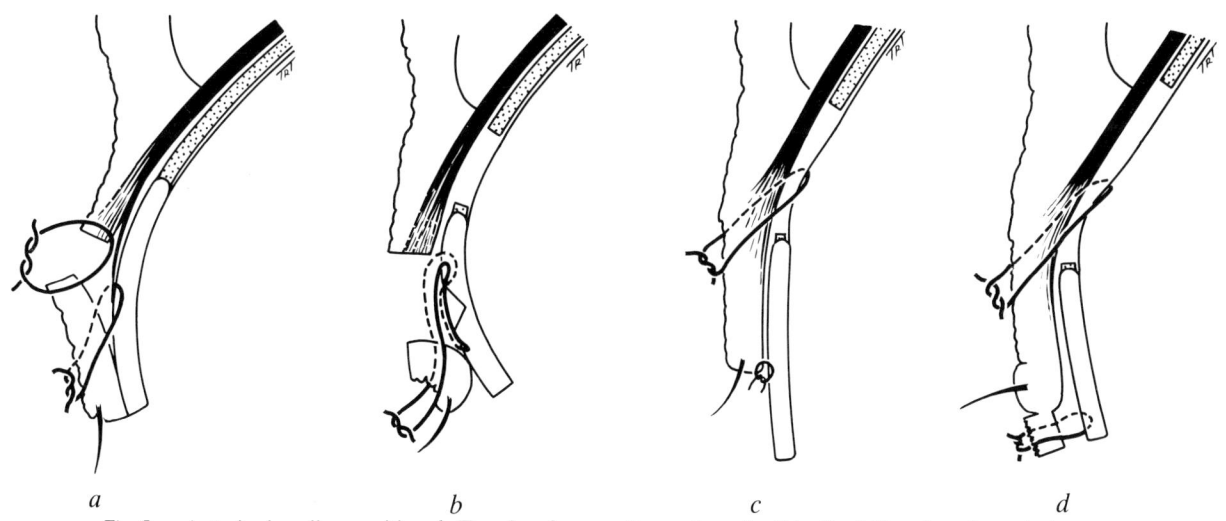

Fig. 5. a, Anterior lamella reposition. *b*, Tarsal wedge resection. *c*, Lamellar lid split. *d*, Rotation of terminal tarsus.

Upper Lid Entropion

This is always cicatricial. As with a cicatricial lower lid entropion the degree of lid retraction is important but in addition surgical correction is influenced by the severity of the entropion, the thickness of the tarsal plate and the state of the tarsoconjunctiva lining the lid margin. If the entropion is mild, a skin crease incision is made and the tarsal plate exposed. The anterior lamella of skin and orbicularis is then pulled upwards to evert the lashes and repositioned, i.e. fixed to the tarsus at a higher level with long acting absorbable sutures tied on the skin (*Fig. 5a*). If this simple repositioning procedure does not produce sufficient eversion of the lid margin and lashes, the eversion can be increased by splitting the grey-

tion can be corrected by dissecting Mueller's muscle from the conjunctiva and recessing it. The skin is closed with interrupted sutures which pick up the underlying aponeurosis. This ensures that the anterior lamella and eyelashes are maximally everted on upgaze.

If the tarsus is very thin, as in some patients with Steven's–Johnson syndrome, there is no point in attempting to cut a wedge out of the tarsus. In these patients the lid can be split at the grey line into its anterior and posterior lamellae. The posterior lamella is advanced and Mueller's muscle recessed. The anterior lamella is then sutured to the posterior lamella leaving the anterior surface of the tarsal plate bare to granulate or it can be covered with a mucous membrane graft if preferred (*Fig. 5c*). If the tarsoconjunctival surface of the lid margin in contact with the globe is keratinized or has metaplastic hairs, this terminal fragment of the tarsus must be rotated away from the globe and the remaining posterior lamella advanced with a full recession of Mueller's muscle. The two lid lamellae are then sutured together and the cut surface of the tarsus forms the new lid margin (*Fig. 5d*). If the degree of lid retraction is greater than can be corrected by a simple recession of Mueller's muscle, the posterior lamella of the lid must be lengthened with a graft of mucous membrane, sclera, cartilage, or nasal septal cartilage with its mucoperichondrium as described for the lower lid.

cryotherapy to the posterior lamella. The anterior lamella with the normal lashes is then sutured to the posterior lamella leaving 2–3 mm of bare tarsus exposed to prevent the subsequent development of an entropion. This type of surgery is more effective in the upper than the lower lid and it may be better to treat the whole of the lower lid with cryotherapy and destroy all the lashes.

Ectropion

Ectropion is a condition in which the eyelid margin is everted away from the globe. It can be congenital

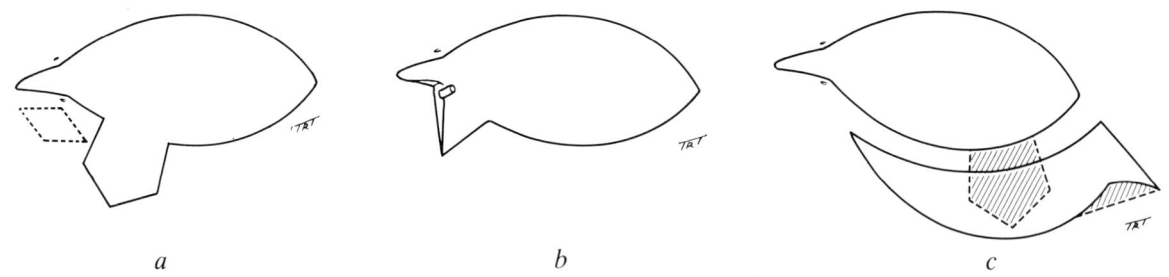

Fig. 6. a, 'Lazy-T', horizontal lid shortening plus punctal inversion. *b*, Horizontal lid shortening at medial canthus. *c*, Khunt–Zymanowski, horizontal lid shortening and blepharoplasty.

It is essential to ensure that the lids close completely on any patient undergoing entropion surgery on whom it is proposed to carry out a corneal graft.

Trichiasis

Abnormal lashes may be associated with any chronic lid margin or conjunctival inflammation, or may occur idiopathically. If there is an entropion this should be managed as discussed previously and if there is a localized lid margin abnormality, e.g. a notch after trauma, this may be excised. Single lashes may be treated with electrolysis but there is a high recurrence rate and it may cause scarring of the lid substance affecting other lashes if it is used repeatedly. Cryotherapy is effective for treating larger areas of trichiasis since lash follicles are more susceptible to cold than other lid tissues with the exception of melanocytes. Ideally the lash roots should be exposed to a temperature of approximately −20 °C with a double freeze–thaw cycle. This can be achieved using specially designed nitrous oxide probes or using liquid nitrogen. The ordinary retinal cryoprobe using carbon dioxide has an unacceptably high failure rate since it does not reach a low enough temperature. Oedema, which may persist for several days, and depigmentation, which may never recover, are likely to follow cryotherapy. Its use in pigmented patients is therefore limited and surgery may have to be attempted instead.

Distichiasis is a congenital condition in which a second row of lashes emerges from the meibomian gland orifices. It is possible to destroy these lashes by splitting the lid into two lamellae and applying

or acquired and the acquired causes are involutional, mechanical, cicatricial and paralytic.

Congenital Ectropion

This is relatively rare except in young babies in whom it may be induced by spasms of crying. If it requires surgical correction it is due to a shortage of skin which may occur in association with such conditions as Down's syndrome and the blepharophimosis syndrome. The treatment is to insert skin as a graft or preferably as a flap.

Involutional Ectropion

This is caused by laxity of all the lid tissues. If the lid starts to evert, the tarsoconjunctiva becomes thickened and mechanical and gravitational factors aggravate the ectropion. The prime treatment is to shorten the lid and tighten it in the area of maximum lid laxity. If this occurs centrally a central full-thickness horizontal lid shortening is sufficient. If the lid laxity involves the lateral canthal area, the lid shortening can be carried out laterally with re-attachment of the cut tarsus to the periosteum of the orbital wall. If the ectropion is primarily medial a horizontal lid shortening can be carried out just lateral to the lacrimal punctum and the punctum inverted by excising a diamond of tarsus and conjunctiva from below the punctum (*Fig. 6a*). Laxity of the medial canthal tendon can be treated by plicating the medial canthal tendon, but in extreme cases such as may occur with advanced paralytic ectropion, a horizontal lid shortening can be performed to include the lacrimal punctum and part of the canaliculus (*Fig. 6b*). The lid is then reconstituted by suturing it to the posterior limb of the medial canthal tendon with marsupialization of the inferior canalicular stump. If the involutional ectropion is associated with excess skin, the horizontal lid shortening is carried out under a blepharoplasty flap and the excess skin excised laterally, as in the modified Kuhnt–Zymanowski procedure (*Fig. 6c*).

Mechanical Ectropion

Mechanical ectropion can be caused by any lump on an eyelid, such as a meibomian cyst or tumour. The treatment is to excise the lump.

Cicatricial Ectropion

This is caused by any condition that leads to a shortage of the anterior lamella of the lid, such as trauma, burns, surgical excision, scleroderma, and other skin conditions. If the shortage of skin is localized, as with some post-traumatic scars, the ectropion can be corrected with a Z-plasty to the skin coupled with a full-thickness lid resection if necessary. If the skin shortage is generalized, the skin must be replaced with a skin flap or graft, again coupled with a horizontal lid shortening if necessary.

Paralytic Ectropion

Paralytic ectropion is caused by a VIIth nerve palsy. The cause should be established and no repair of the ectropion carried out if there is a reasonable chance of recovery. If the ectropion is mild and surgery is required, the lid can be tightened with a lateral canthal sling. In this procedure the lower limb of the lateral canthal tendon is divided, the amount of horizontal lid shortening is assessed, but instead of excising this part of the lid the tarsal stump is cleaned, passed through a button hole in the intact upper limb of the lateral canthal tendon and sutured to the periosteum of the lateral orbital wall (*Fig.* 7). In this way the lateral canthal angle is reformed, there is no horizontal shortening of the palpebral aperture, the lower lid is held posteriorly against the globe by its passage through the upper limb of the lateral canthal tendon, and the raised position on the lateral orbital rim to which the tarsal remnant is sutured gives gravity a chance of aiding tear drainage.

A small degree of medial ectropion can be improved with a medial canthoplasty or tarsorrhaphy. Probes are passed into the upper and lower canaliculus. The lid is split into two lamellae anterior to the probes. The posterior lamellae are sutured together with long acting absorbable sutures, taking care to avoid the canaliculi, and the skin is closed anterior to this with the excision of any excess skin (*Fig.* 8). If the paralytic ectropion is of long standing and there is excessive medial canthal tendon laxity, a horizontal lid shortening is carried out to include the inferior lacrimal punctum and part of the canaliculus, as previously described for extreme involutional medial ectropion (*see Fig. 6b*).

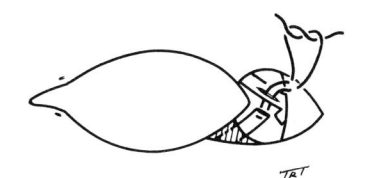

Fig. 7. Lateral canthal sling.

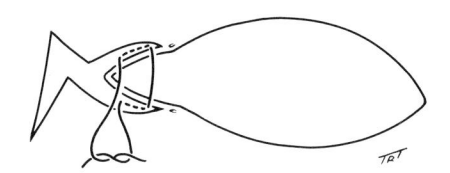

Fig. 8. Medial tarsorrhaphy.

Ptosis

Causes

Blepharoptosis is a condition in which the eyelid level is lower than normal, i.e. lower than 1–2 mm below the upper limbus. It must be differentiated from contralateral lid retraction. Ptosis may be either congenital or acquired. The usual cause of congenital ptosis is an isolated dystrophy of the levator muscle but it may also occur with a congenital IIIrd nerve palsy, or aponeurotic weakness. These other causes are usually considered with the acquired group, which include aponeurotic, neurogenic, myogenic, myasthenic and mechanical defects. Aponeurotic defects may be congenital but are more often acquired, either as a result of trauma or of ageing changes (involutional senile ptosis). Neurogenic ptosis is caused by any condition affecting the IIIrd nerve, its brain stem connection, such as with a Marcus Gunn jaw-winking ptosis, or the sympathetic system. Involvement of the sympathetic system, as in Horner's syndrome, results in about 2 mm of ptosis due to denervation of Mueller's muscle. Myogenic ptosis is caused by any myopathy which affects the levator muscle itself, such as chronic external ophthalmoplegia. Myasthenic ptosis is due to an abnormality at the neuromusclar junction. Mechanical ptosis can be caused by an eyelid tumour, a laceration, injury or scarring, affecting the lid retractors or severe cicatrizing conditions such as pemphigoid. Trauma may cause a ptosis by directly injuring the upper lid retractors, damaging the nerve supply, or weakening the aponeurosis through oedema. It is therefore included as a cause of mechanical, neurogenic and aponeurotic defects, and is not considered separately. A pseudoptosis is any condition which creates a false impression of a ptosis, such as may be associated with enophthalmic conditions, e.g.

microphthalmos and anophthalmos, or with excess lid skin, or with a hypotropia in the primary position of gaze.

Assessment

The assessment of a patient with ptosis must establish the diagnosis, cause and possibilities of treatment. The presence of ptosis is confirmed and the degree measured by noting the extent to which the lid covers the limbus and comparing the distance between the lid margin and the fixation corneal light reflex on the two sides. The levator function is a measurement of the maximum excursion of the eyelid between full up-gaze and full down-gaze with the frontalis muscle prevented from acting by pressure over the brow. The lid position on down-gaze is important, since if there is relative lid lag on down-gaze this suggests that the levator muscle is dystrophic and cannot either contract or relax properly as in most cases of congenital ptosis, provided there is not some other cause of mechanical restriction. The depth of the skin crease gives some idea of the extent of the levator function and is especially useful in very young children who present with a ptosis. The position of the skin crease depends on the aponeurosis and is raised with a 'disinsertion'. Bell's phenomenon gives an assessment of the ability of the eye to protect itself if the eyelid is raised. Other features which may be relevant to the cause of the ptosis include jaw-winking, the miosed pupil of Horner's syndrome and the pigmentary retinopathy associated with some ocular myopathies.

Management

The management of ptosis depends on its cause and the assessment. Surgical correction in a child is usually best performed at about the age of 4 years when an accurate assessment is possible and before the child goes to school. If the lid level is interfering with the pupillary axis and preventing the development of normal vision, the eyelid needs to be lifted as an emergency with a brow suspension procedure to prevent amblyopia. The levator function is the prime factor in the assessment, and governs the choice of ptosis operation, but the procedure will be modified depending on the cause and other factors in the assessment primarily affecting corneal protection, e.g. Bell's phenomenon, IIIrd nerve palsy, dry eyes, VIIth nerve palsy, myasthenia and ocular myopathies. The main types of ptosis operation are a Fasanella Servat procedure, aponeurosis surgery, a levator muscle resection and a brow suspension procedure.

The Fasanella Servat Operation

The procedure involves the excision of the upper border of the tarsal plate and the lower border of conjunctiva with its attached Mueller's muscle (*Fig.* 9). It is an effective procedure for correcting a mild degree of ptosis (1–2·5 mm) provided there is good levator function (10 mm or more). A stab incision is made in the skin crease laterally, extending through skin and orbicularis muscle. The eyelid is then everted and two small curved artery forceps applied to the upper border of the tarsal plate. One needle of a double-armed 6/0 absorbable suture is passed through the eyelid below the clamps starting at its medial extremity and finishing laterally. Both ends of this suture are then held and the clamps removed.

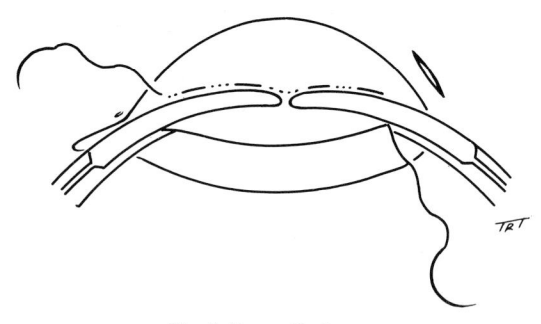

Fig. 9. Fasanella Servat.

The superior border of the tarsal plate with its attached conjunctiva and Mueller's muscle is then excised by cutting along the clamp marks. The second needle of the double-armed 6/0 suture is then used to close the lips of the wound. Both needles are then passed through the lid and made to emerge from the lateral stab wound. A knot is tied and buried under the skin.

Aponeurosis Surgery

Such a procedure can be carried out via an anterior or posterior approach. It is indicated in conditions in which there is a suspected aponeurotic weakness. Such an aponeurotic weakness can occur anywhere in the aponeurosis. The usual cause is ageing changes (involutional senile ptosis) which leads to a generalized weakness of the aponeurosis. The insertion of the aponeurosis into the post-orbicular fascia governs the skin crease. If the aponeurosis becomes thinned and 'disinserts' but the levator muscle is working normally, the remnant of the aponeurosis and the orbital septum are pulled back into the orbit by the levator muscle and the skin crease rises. Eventually the patient is left with a ptosis, a raised skin crease and a deep upper lid sulcus, but still has good levator function (*Fig.* 10). In some extreme cases the lid may be so thin that the colour of the cornea can be seen through the lid substance above the tarsal plate.

If the aponeurotic defect does not involve the lower portion of the aponeurosis responsible for the skin crease, the patient will have a normal skin crease associated with a ptosis and good levator function. Aponeurosis surgery via the anterior approach involves an incision through the skin in the position of the desired skin crease. The orbicularis muscle is opened and the aponeurosis inspected. If necessary, the orbital septum is opened and the pre-aponeurotic fat pad retracted to aid in its identification. Healthy looking aponeurotic tissue is then advanced and sutured to the anterior surface of the tarsus. The skin edges are closed with sutures that pick up the underlying aponeurosis to reform the skin crease. The operation can be performed equally well via the posterior approach. An incision is made through the tarsal plate at the height of the desired

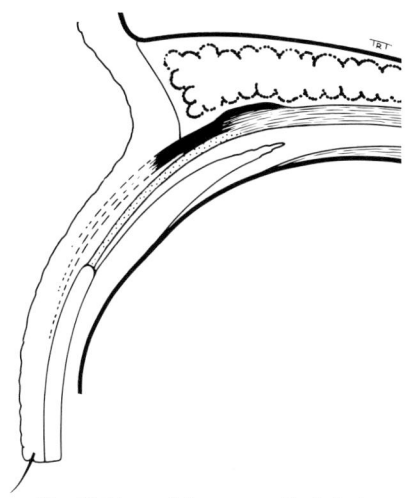

Fig. 10. Upper lid aponeurotic defect.

skin crease above the lid margin. The fragment of tarsus with its attached Mueller's muscle and conjunctiva is reflected until healthy looking aponeurotic tissue is identified. The tarsal fragment and lower border of Mueller's muscle is then excised and double-armed sutures passed from the conjunctiva through the cut edge of Mueller's muscle and through the healthy looking aponeurotic tissue. The sutures then pass through the tarsal plate about 1–2 mm below its cut edge and emerge through the skin in the position of the skin crease where they are tied (*Fig.* 11). All aponeurosis surgery is preferentially performed under local anaesthesia so that the eyelid level can be more easily assessed and adjusted at operation. The benefit of the anterior approach is that any excess skin can be excised, the aponeurosis can be examined directly, and the surgery does not interfere with the posterior lamella of the eyelid. The advantage of the posterior approach is that pull-out sutures are used and the timing of their removal gives better postoperative control of lid height and contour.

Levator Muscle Resection

This procedure is indicated if the levator function is between 4 and 10 mm. A graded resection is performed depending on the preoperative levator function and the lid level achieved at operation. If the levator function is 7 mm preoperatively, the lid may be expected to stay approximately where it is positioned at operation. If the levator function is better than this the lid will rise postoperatively and if it is worse, the lid will fall postoperatively.

Either an anterior or a posterior approach may be used, with the same relative merits for each approach, as described for aponeurosis surgery. The exposure via an anterior approach is easier for a major levator resection but a posterior approach would be preferred in conditions in which problems of corneal exposure might be anticipated. The surgical approaches are similar to those described for apo-

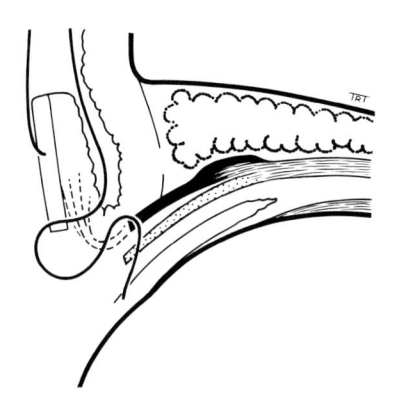

Fig. 11. Posterior approach repair of aponeurotic defect.

neurosis surgery but the dissection is carried more extensively into the orbit as required. This may involve cutting the medial and lateral horns of the levator muscle and advancing it. It is preferable to maintain Whitnall's ligament (the so-called superior suspensory ligament of the globe) as this will give some superior and anterior support to the advanced and resected levator muscle.

Brow Suspension Procedure

This is indicated if there is less than 4 mm of levator function preoperatively. Under these circumstances there is no point in attempting to resect the levator muscle since it will be so atrophic that even if the lid level were initially raised the ptosis would recur with subsequent stretching of the atrophic muscle remnants. The frontalis muscle is an accessory eyelid elevator and this action can be enhanced by attaching the eyelid to the eyebrow with strips of tissue. Various autogenous and non-autogenous substances have been used such as nylon and Supramid sutures, silicone rods, stored ox and human fascia, but the best results are obtained with autogenous fascia lata. This can be taken from the lateral aspect of the leg via a small incision just above the knee. Various techniques of insertion have been described, e.g. double triangles (*Fig.* 12), rhomboids and pentagons, but whatever substance is used must pass deep to the orbicularis muscle and superficial to the tarsal plate and be tied in and/or above the brow such that the lid elevating function of the frontalis muscle is enhanced.

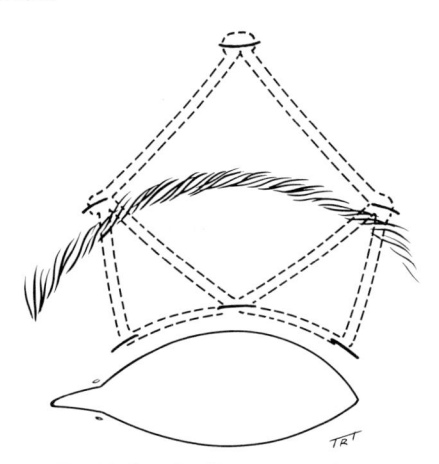

Fig. 12. Crawford brow suspension.

Complications

The complications of ptosis surgery can be considered under the headings of corneal protection, poor lid level, poor technique and routine risk of lid surgery. If the eyelid has been raised certain routine measures will be required until the cornea has 'acclimatized' to the new lid level. These include the use of a lower lid traction suture at the time of operation, which can be pulled up and taped to the brow to protect the cornea. When this is removed the patient will require lubricant drops and ointment for a variable period until the cornea has 'acclimatized'. If the lid level is too high and/or the cornea cannot tolerate the degree of exposure, the eyelid must be lowered. If pull-out sutures have been used, as with a posterior approach procedure, these can be removed and the eyelid lowered as required by gentle traction on the eyelashes, by eversion over a Desmarre's retractor, or by spreading open the posterior wound. After an anterior or posterior approach procedure massage may be helpful but if these simple remedies are not effective the eyelid must be lowered with one of the lid lowering procedures described in the treatment of lid retraction. If the eyelid is too low postoperatively reoperation is required, which should be delayed while there is a chance of a late rise in lid level, which may occur several weeks or even months after surgery.

Complications due to poor technique include an asymmetrical skin crease due to an inadequate assessment preoperatively and inadequate surgery, ectropion due to the levator muscle complex being inserted too low on to the anterior tarsus, entropion, usually due to the excision of too much tarsal plate or loss of cilia due to dissecting too far down the anterior surface of the tarsal plate. Complications that are inherent in any eyelid procedure include haemorrhage, infection and even blindness, thought to be due to interference with the pial vascular supply to the optic nerve as a result of traction on the fat pads and fibrovascular septa in the orbit.

Lid Retraction

A disturbance of the lid retractors themselves occurs most commonly with thyroid eye disease and may be due to either primary sympathetic stimulation, or secondary to inferior rectus tethering, or infiltration and fibrosis of the orbital structures. There are other conditions which affect the lid retractors such as tumour infiltration, scarring from trauma, including ptosis surgery, and anything which stimulates the IIIrd nerve nucleus. If there is a VIIth nerve palsy the eyelids will be retracted since the normal lid closing action of the orbicularis muscle is defective. If the globe is proptosed the lids will be relatively retracted. It is obviously necessary to establish the cause of any lid retraction and treat this where possible. The cornea can be protected with lubricant drops and ointment and the palpebral aperture reduced vertically, by lowering the upper lid or raising the lower lid, and horizontally, with medial or lateral tarsorrhaphies. A medial tarsorrhaphy has been described under paralytic ectropion (*see Fig.* 8).

Upper Lid Lowering Procedures

Posterior Approach

TENOTOMY OR TARSOTOMY

The upper lid retractors can be lengthened simply by everting the lid over a Desmarre's retractor and

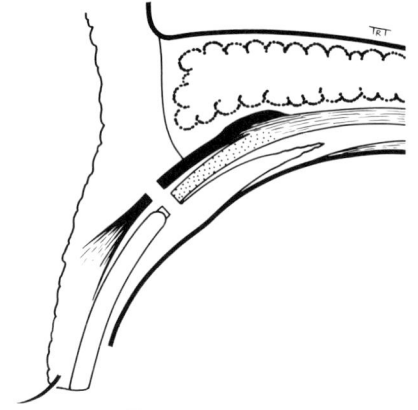

Fig. 13. Tenotomy.

making a horizontal incision through, or just above, the tarsus (*Fig.* 13). The incision is deepened until the lid is lowered by twice as much as it was previously retracted, i.e. if there was 2 mm of lid retraction the lid should be lowered by about 4 mm. The eyelid is then pulled down with a traction suture which is taped to the cheek and the eye is kept padded for 48 h. The suture is then removed and when the lid regains a symmetrical level it can be maintained at this height with massage. This may be required throughout the time there is active wound healing, i.e. for up to 6 months. Such a procedure will usually correct approximately 2 mm of lid retraction.

RETRACTOR RECESSION

If there is more than 2 mm of retraction the lid lowering will be enhanced if the retractors are held recessed with a continuous absorbable or pull-out nylon suture. Essentially the same procedure is used as for a tenotomy, but the conjunctiva and lid retractors are sutured to the preseptal orbicularis to maintain a larger raw area in the posterior lamella, delay healing and thereby increase the effect of the recession.

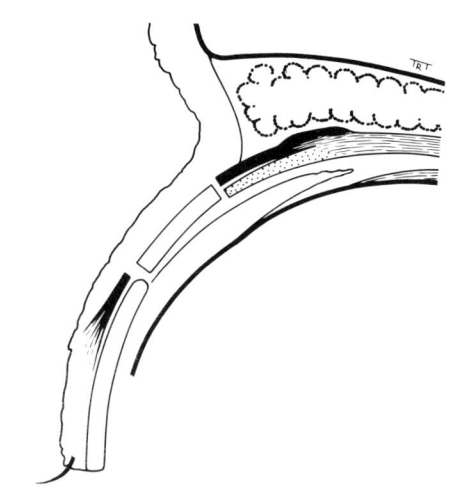

Fig. 14. Scleral graft to lengthen upper lid retractors.

SCLERAL GRAFT

The lid can be even more effectively lowered if a scleral graft is inserted between the retractors and the tarsus (*Fig. 14*). This can be inserted with a similar posterior approach procedure and the sclera left bare to fill the raw area in the posterior lamella or it can be covered with conjunctiva if this is fully mobilized.

Anterior Approach

All the previously discussed posterior approach procedures lower the lid effectively but by disinserting the upper lid retractors the skin crease rises, which is not always desirable. If the lid retractors are approached via an incision in the skin, they can be lengthened, either with a simple recession, or a Z-myotomy, or a scleral graft can be inserted between the retractors and the tarsus. The Z-myotomy involves a horizontal cut through each side of the retractors at different levels (*Fig. 15*). In all cases the skin crease is reformed by suturing the skin edge to the underlying retractors but it will end up high unless the original skin incision has been made deliberately low to compensate for this.

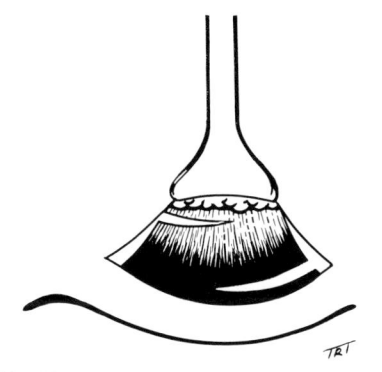

Fig. 15. Z-myotomy to upper lid retractors.

Lower Lid Raising Procedures

The lower lid retractors can be lengthened in a similar way to the upper lid retractors but the effect is less marked since the result is limited by the height of the medial and lateral canthus and the lid must be raised against gravity. A scleral graft is generally required between the lower lid retractors and the tarsus and it is more comfortable for the patient if the conjunctiva is mobilized to cover this graft (*Fig. 16*). Traction for 48 h is necessary.

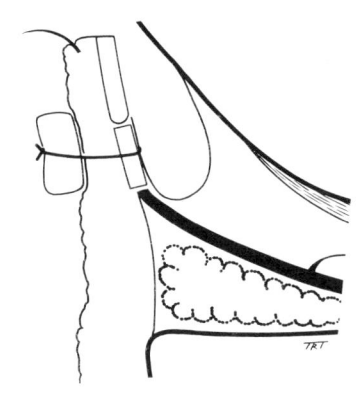

Fig. 16. Scleral graft to lengthen lower lid retractors.

Lateral Tarsorrhaphy

Suturing the lids together will primarily reduce the horizontal palpebral aperture but will also limit the vertical distance between the upper and lower lids. A tarsorrhaphy is either permanent or temporary, in which case it is theoretically possible to undo it and reconstitute a reasonably normal lid margin. This is useful in conditions where corneal protection is required but which might improve spontaneously, e.g. a Bell's palsy.

Temporary Tarsorrhaphy

A useful technique involves removing the lid margin epithelium from the posterior lamella of both upper and lower lids and suturing the raw areas together

(*Fig.* 17). Mattress sutures tied over bolsters hold the lids in good apposition and should be left for at least 2 weeks to allow the raw areas to adhere. The lash margin of both upper and lower lids should be left undisturbed so that if the adhesion is subsequently divided the lid margins will be as normal as possible and trichiasis avoided.

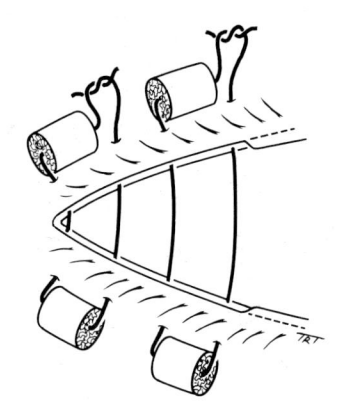

Fig. 17. Temporary lateral tarsorrhaphy.

Permanent Tarsorrhaphy

If there is no possibility of opening the tarsorrhaphy, a better adhesion between the two lids can be obtained by excising skin and orbicularis with the lash margin from the lower lid and partial thickness tarsal plate from the upper lid. The lids are then overlapped and sutured together. If this 'permanent' tarsorrhaphy is opened, the lid margin will always be irregular and there will be no lower lid lashes, but the cosmesis and effectivity of the tarsorrhaphy is considerably better than with a temporary tarsorrhaphy. A small permanent tarsorrhaphy is often beneficial in dysthyroid eye disease and proptosis. It can be combined with lid retractor surgery for a better cosmetic and functional result. If there is difficulty in obtaining a proper adhesion between the lids, the lid retractors should be freed first with a cut above the tarsus as described for a tenotomy (*see Fig.* 13).

Central Tarsorrhaphy

A central or para-central tarsorrhaphy is sometimes required for corneal protection. If there is any chance of undoing it in the future it is essential that as little permanent damage as possible is done to the lid margin. A useful technique is to make a small split in the grey line of the upper and lower lids in the area of the proposed tarsorrhaphy and to increase the eversion of the split with two small relieving cuts at either end of the incisions making a letter H (*Fig.* 18). The posterior lamellae are then sutured together with a long acting absorbable suture. The raw areas are brought into closer contact with a mattress suture tied over a bolster on the skin and the cut edges of the anterior lamellae are also sutured together. The tarsorrhaphy can either be left permanently or undone, in theory without complications, since no actual tissue has been removed from the lid margins.

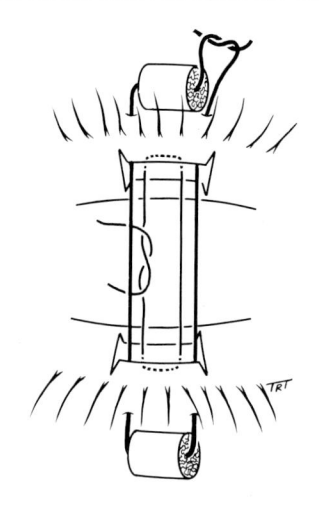

Fig. 18. Central tarsorrhaphy.

VIIth Nerve Palsy

A facial palsy may present with corneal exposure, a paralytic ectropion or the cosmetic defect of lid retraction and ectropion. If the palsy is acute and the cornea cannot be adequately protected with simple lubricants or taping the lids if necessary, a temporary lateral tarsorrhaphy may be indicated (*see Fig.* 17). Chronic corneal exposure, lid retraction and the cosmetic defect are best managed with a combination of upper and lower lid retractor lengthening (*Figs.* 13–16) supplemented with a lateral (*Fig.* 17) and/or medial tarsorrhaphy (*Fig.* 8) as required. Lid closure can be improved with various more ambitious static mechanical techniques such as burying a weight or wire spring in the upper lid and by encircling the lids with a band of silicone (file d'Arion) under sufficient tension to allow lid closure unless the upper lid retractors are voluntarily activated. There is, however, a risk of extrusion of foreign materials implanted in the lids and these techniques are seldom required. Dynamic methods of improving lid closure involve a cross-face nerve anastomosis, in which a donor nerve graft (e.g. sural nerve) is used to connect branches of the VIIth nerve from the normal side of the face to the facial nerve on the paralysed side. In another technique muscle grafts, such as the extensor digitorum brevis muscle from the foot, can be laid on the normal orbicularis muscle and the tendons passed through a hole in the nose to encircle the paralysed eyelids. A cross-face nerve anastomosis is effective following an acute section of the facial nerve, e.g. after the removal of an acoustic neuroma, but is less effective in chronic cases where muscle atrophy has occurred. Most cases of VIIth nerve palsy do not require these more extensive mechanical and dynamic techniques. Management of paralytic ectropion has already been described.

EYELID LESIONS

Eyelid Infections and Inflammations

Blepharitis and inflammation of the lid margin is common and usually associated with chronic staphylococcal infection of the lash roots. Management involves regular mechanical cleaning of the lid margin and lash roots using a lotion such as sodium bicarbonate if desired followed by the application of a local antibiotic ointment. A steroid may be incorporated in this antibiotic ointment since there is often an allergic element to the inflammation. The lid margin inflammation is rarely severe enough to warrant systemic antibiotics unless there is an associated chronic meibomianitis in which case a long term low dose tetracycline may be helpful. Primary infections of the lid skin do occur, e.g. after trauma, primary herpes simplex, or the small whitish umbilicated lesions of molluscum contagiosum. Usually infection is secondary to some other cause, e.g. dacryocystitis, dacryoadenitis or an infected meibomian cyst, and will be enhanced by any reduced resistance of the patient, e.g. leukaemia, cytotoxic therapy etc.

Meibomian Cyst

A meibomian cyst starts in the tarsal plate with an obstruction to drainage of a meibomian gland. In the acute phase it may become painful, red, swollen and infected. It may discharge spontaneously and the resolution can usually be hastened with applications of local heat and antibiotics. In a proportion of cases a chronic granulomatous reaction persists and the patient develops a small, firm, rounded tumour in the tarsus. The standard treatment is incision and curettage but good results have been reported with intralesional injections of steroid.

Eyelid Tumours

Eyelid tumours can arise from any of the structures in the eyelid. Common benign epithelial lesions include a squamous papilloma, which may develop a cutaneous horn, a basal cell papilloma or seborrhoeic keratosis, which is usually raised, fissured, sometimes cheesy and usually pigmented, as opposed to a senile keratosis which is usually a flatter dry scaly lesion which may occasionally undergo malignant change into a squamous cell carcinoma. These lesions can be simply excised but senile keratoses usually respond very well to cryotherapy. A cyst of Moll is a benign, clear, fluid-filled cyst in a sweat gland near the lid margin, and a cyst of Zeis is a yellowish white cyst due to obstruction in a sebaceous gland associated with a lash follicle. Both can be excised and/or marsupialized. A xanthelasma is a cholesterol plaque developing in the skin. It can occur in hypercholesterolaemic states, which should be excluded. Diet may reduce the size of the lesion but eradication usually involves surgery or applications of trichloroacetic acid etc. Naevi are usually benign but any rapid growth or the development of satellite lesions suggest the possibility of malignant change, when an excisional biopsy is indicated. Keratoacanthomas are rapidly growing umbilicated lesions with a central crater, which is usually filled with a keratin plug. They normally involute spontaneously after about 3 months but a small proportion develop into a squamous cell carcinoma and continue to grow, in which case they should be excised.

The most common malignant lesions of the eyelid skin are basal cell and squamous cell carcinomas but malignant melanomas do occur. Of all malignant eyelid lesions, 95 per cent are basal cell carcinomas, which occur most commonly on the lower eyelid and in the medial canthal region and present in many forms. The basic clinical distinction is between a relatively benign, localized, usually nodular lesion, often with a pearly margin laced with blood vessels, and the much more diffuse infiltrating more malignant variety which spreads under the epithelium and whose margin is difficult to define. Treatment involves surgery, radiotherapy or cryotherapy. Histological confirmation of surgical clearance can be obtained before repair with rapid standard histology or frozen sections. Frozen section control can be used at the time of surgery, or routine paraffin sections can be cut postoperatively. If the margins are clear, the 5-year cure rate with surgery approaches 100 per cent, but even if the margins are not clear, only about 50 per cent recur. Radiotherapy has almost as good cure rates as surgery but is contraindicated for lesions on the upper eyelid, where it might induce keratinization of the tarsal conjunctiva overlying the cornea. It is not always easy to define the extent of lesions involving the medial canthus and fornices, and radiotherapy is relatively contraindicated in these sites. Cryotherapy is especially good for small lesions around the canaliculi since the lacrimal drainage apparatus is relatively resistant to freezing and can be damaged with surgery or radiotherapy. Squamous cell carcinomas occur most commonly on the upper lid in the older age group. They may present as a discoloured patch on the skin, carcinoma in situ, as malignant change in a senile keratosis or keratoacanthoma, or as a raised skin ulcer sometimes with everted edges. Management is similar to that of a basal cell carcinoma. A malignant melanoma of the eyelid skin is rare, but mainly occurs either as a flat superficial spreading lesion or as a nodule. Pigmentation is variable. Lesions at the lid margin have a worse prognosis than those on the eyelid skin itself. Wide surgical excision is the treatment of choice.

Tumours involving the deeper structures of the eyelid are, with the exception of meibomian cysts, much less common than skin tumours. They include benign tumours of blood vessels – haemangiomas – which are important as they may induce occlusion amblyopia if they occur on the upper lid in young children and are large enough. They may also lead to astigmatism. Various methods of treatment have been tried, including surgery, radiotherapy, freezing, photocoagulation and injections with sclerosing agents. Promising results have been reported with injections of intralesional steroid and with laser and photocoagulation. Benign tumours of nerves, neurofibromas, often occur in association with von Recklinghausen's neurofibromatosis and can lead to an enormous enlargement and deformity of the lid. This may be improved by surgical debulking but the results depend on the extent of the condition. Adenocarcinomas of the lid usually start in a meibomian gland and can present in many different ways. The commonest presentation is either an enlarging mass in the tarsus, which may be confused with a recurrent meibomian cyst, or as a blepharoconjunctivitis, which is resistant to treatment. If it is suspected, a deep or full thickness biopsy of the eyelid should be performed and part of the tissue submitted for frozen section as it may be difficult to diagnose the carcinoma on routine histology if the sebaceous material has been removed by the fixative. The lesion should be treated with a wide surgical excision and possibly radiotherapy but despite aggressive treatment the 5-year survival rate is poor and in some series is below 60 per cent. Lymphomatous infiltration of the eyelid is not uncommon and responds to radiotherapy with a good prognosis if the lesion is localized. Primary conjunctival tumours are not included in this chapter.

Principles of Lid Repair

Surgical repair of eyelid defects is only urgent if the cornea is prejudiced. Congenital upper lid colobomas should only be repaired in the first 3 months of life if there are signs of progressive corneal damage despite lubricants. Burns involving the eyelid may lead to skin contracture, lagophthalmos and rapid corneal deterioration unless the skin is replaced urgently. This usually requires split skin, since a lot of skin is required, the graft bed and 'take' are prejudiced by the burn and the usual full thickness skin donor sites, e.g. post-auricular, may have been involved and not be readily available. Provided the cornea can be preserved, the repair of lid lacerations and defects, whether traumatic or surgical, can safely be delayed for up to 48 h if this will improve the facilities available. Following trauma it is important to preserve all possible tissue as the excellent blood supply to the lids ensures a remarkable degree of tissue survival. All dirt and foreign bodies should be removed to prevent tatooing and the anatomy should be reconstructed as accurately as possible.

Post-enucleation Lid Problems

When an eye is enucleated for whatever cause there is a loss of orbital contents. This may be partially replaced with a buried orbital implant and the remaining volume deficit is made up with the artificial eye. This eye is partly supported by the lower lid, which tends to sag under its weight. As the artificial eye drops it does not support the upper lid as effectively. The upper lid therefore becomes ptotic and develops a hollow and sunken appearance which increases the more the lower lid sags. These factors of a lax lower lid, ptosis, deep upper lid sulcus and enophthalmos constitute the features of the post-enucleation socket syndrome. Although the ptosis, deep upper lid sulcus and enophthalmos can be improved with a larger artificial eye, this improvement is temporary since the increased weight further depresses the lower eyelid. The volume of the orbital contents needs to be increased as much as possible with either a larger orbital implant and/or an orbital floor implant. The artificial eye should be as thin and light as possible. The lower lid can then be tightened if necessary and finally the ptosis corrected if required. Correction of the presenting eyelid defect without a systematic approach to the syndrome is unlikely to be satisfactory.

Entropion and lid retraction associated with an anophthalmic or post-enucleation socket is likely to be caused by a deficiency or contraction of the conjunctiva or socket lining. This may require correction with mucous membrane or other grafts. Expansion of a contracted socket with conformers is only likely to be helpful immediately after an injury or enucleation or with an anophthalmic socket which presents early in life.

FURTHER READING

Beard C. *Ptosis*. St Louis, Mo, Mosby, 1981.
Callahan M. A. and Callahan A. *Ophthalmic Plastic and Orbital Surgery*. Birmingham, Ala., Aesculapius, 1979.
Collin J. R. O. *A Manual of Systematic Eyelid Surgery*. Edinburgh, Churchill Livingstone, 1983.
Reeh M. J., Beyer C. K. and Shannon G. M. *Practical Ophthalmic Plastic and Reconstructive Surgery*. Philadelphia, Lea and Febiger, 1976.
Soll D. B. *Management of Complications in Ophthalmic Plastic Surgery*. Birmingham, Ala., Aesculapius, 1976.

Chapter 16

The Lacrimal Drainage Apparatus

Richard A. N. Welham

INTRODUCTION

Epiphora

Among patients attending eye clinics in the United Kingdom, some 3–4 per cent complain of a surfeit of tears.[1] These moist-eyed patients usually have epiphora; that is, tears flowing onto their cheeks. This annoying symptom occurs either when the volume of tears produced exceeds the normal drainage capacity of the excretory passages (lacrimation) or more commonly, when there is an obstruction in the tear drainage apparatus (obstructive epiphora). The vast majority of patients with obstructive epiphora have an anatomical obstruction in the membranous tear drainage passages, but occasionally, a functional defect is responsible.

Not only is the presence of a watery eye a cause of annoyance and embarrassment to the afflicted patient, the overful tear film may impair vision and the persistent watering cause excoriation of the skin of the cheek. The invasion of the obstructed tear passages by pathogenic organisms causes either acute or chronic dacryocystitis and a reservoir of such contaminated tears represents a hazard to the patient's vision, should any form of intraocular surgery be contemplated.

Most patients with obstructive epiphora can be completely and permanently relieved of their symptoms by the construction of a mucosa-lined passageway to the nose. In that small number of patients in whom there is extensive damage to the canaliculi or in whom the lacrimal pump is defective, recourse may have to be made to the insertion of an artificial tear drainage system which, although effective in controlling watering, suffers the disadvantage of requiring indefinite maintenance.

The Secretory Apparatus

Tears have a complex composition and variations in the quality of the constituents may produce abnormalities that are dealt with elsewhere in this book.

In a normal person, some 5–10 µl is present in the precorneal tear film and conjunctival sac. Most of this volume (some 95 per cent) is secreted by the main lacrimal gland and about 50 small accessory glands of Krause and Wolfring. These are sometimes referred to as 'primary glands', to distinguish them from the secondary mucin-producing goblet cells of the conjunctiva and oil-producing glands of Meibomius and Zeis, which are the principal constituents of the other two layers in the three-layered film.

The main lacrimal gland is divided into an orbital and palpebral lobe by the aponeurosis of the levater palpebrae superioris. The secretions of the orbital lobe have to traverse the palpebral lobe to reach the upper conjunctival fornix where both lobes emit their secretions via some 14 or so ductules.

The volume of tears produced by the lacrimal gland is controlled by the autonomic nervous system. Although innervated by both sympathetic and parasympathetic fibres, for all practical purposes, the volume of tears being produced is controlled by the parasympathetic lacrimal nucleus.

This group of general visceral efferent cells lies close to the caudal end of the facial nucleus in the brain stem in the floor of the IVth ventricle. It is an intimate relation of the superior salivary nucleus.

These parasympathetic preganglionic connector neurones run a complicated course, first in the intermediate nerve (of Wrisburg) to the geniculate ganglion and then, passing via the greater superficial petrosal nerve, join the nerve of the pterygoid canal (Vidian nerve) and synapse in the sphenopalatine ganglion, which is situated in the pterygoid palatine fossa. The post-ganglionic fibres are conveyed in the maxillary and zygomatic nerves, passing by its anastomotic branch to join the lacrimal branch of the ophthalmic nerve from whence they are distributed to the lacrimal gland.

It is generally supposed that a basic secretion of tears comes from the accessory lacrimal glands. This volume is small and amounts to about 1 µl/min.[2] Most of this is lost by evaporation so that in the resting state it is doubtful whether any tears drain via the lacrimal passages. How the secretion of the accessory lacrimal glands is controlled is not clear.

The main gland produces lacrimal fluid in response to activity in the lacrimal nucleus. This autonomic nucleus is under the influence of higher neurological centres located principally in the frontal cortex and anterior part of the limbic lobe. Tear production in response to such stimulation is referred to as 'psychic weeping'.

Reflex stimulation of the lacrimal nucleus is largely mediated by the trigeminal nerve, particularly through its terminals in the cornea and conjunctiva, but may be produced by stimulation of the retina by light. Adverse environmental factors such as a smoky atmosphere or cold wind are accompanied by an increase in tear production and this may be more spectacular in the presence of a corneal ulcer or foreign body. Although these reflex causes of lacrimation are usually self-evident, more subtle causes of trigeminal irritation should always be sought.

These operations are, however, unpredictable in their results and may occasionally produce the potentially dangerous complication of a dry eye. Such operations are best avoided, but may occasionally be indicated in the treatment of crocodile tears or watering in the presence of anophthalmos. They do not give as effective results as surgery to the drainage apparatus in obstructive epiphora.

Crocodile Tears

This interesting example of aberrant reinervation, described by Antonelli in 1902,[9] may occur in lesions

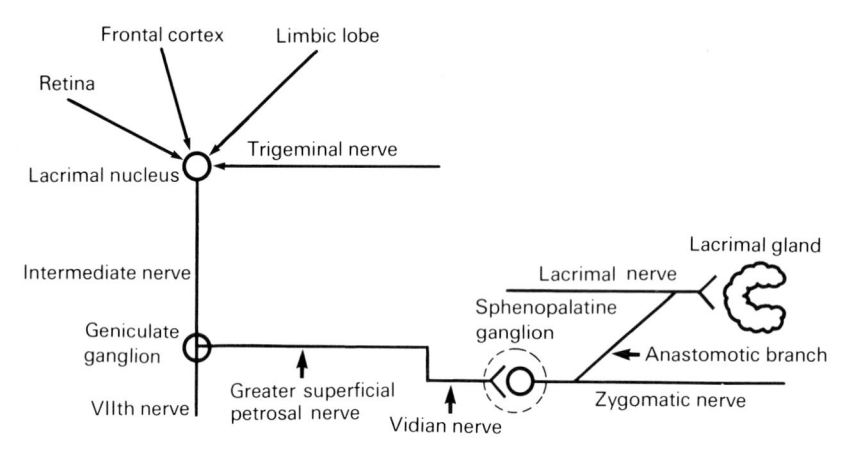

Fig. 1. Innervation of the lacrimal gland.

Chronic inflammatory disease of the lids (blepharitis) is frequently overlooked. This, and other less obvious sources of trigeminal stimulation by diseases of the teeth or paranasal sinuses, should always be considered in a watering-eyed patient as control of the source of irritation may produce a dramatic improvement in a patient's symptoms even in the presence of obstructed drainage passages (*Fig.* 1).

Rarely irritative lesions of the brain stem directly involve the nucleus, as occurs in the tabetic crisis of Pel.[3]

That the reflex component of lacrimal secretions decreases with age, having reached a maximum in young adulthood, was shown by de Roetth.[4] This fact should always be borne in mind when surgery is contemplated in older patients who, with advancing years, are not only likely to spend more time in a protected environment, but are less capable of producing tears in response to provocation by it.

Operations to Limit Tear Secretion

A variety of operations has been described with the objective of controlling epiphora by interfering with the secretory mechanism. Thus, dacryoadenectomy, either total or partial,[5] division of the lacrimal ductules,[6] division of the lacrimal branch of the zygomatic nerve[7] and Vidian neurectomy[8] have all been recommended.

of the facial nerve proximal to the geniculate ganglion. Secretomotor fibres destined for the salivary glands regenerate into the greater superficial petrosal nerve and excitation of these gustatory fibres produces paradoxical weeping.

The Excretory Mechanism

The lacrimal drainage passages consist of the canaliculi, tear sac and the nasolacrimal duct (*Fig.* 2).

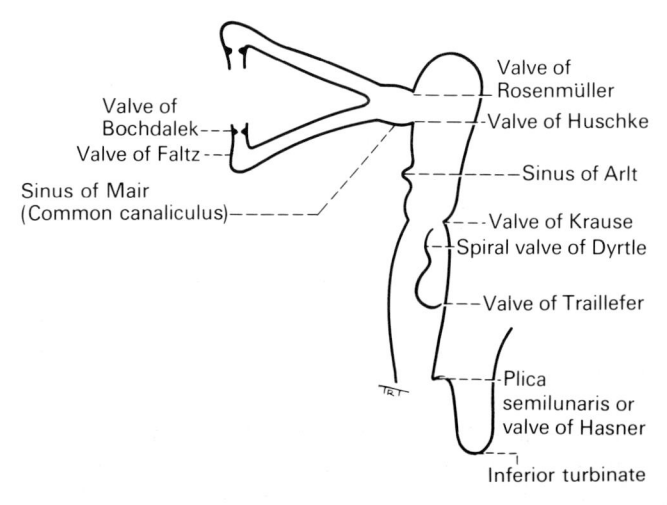

Fig. 2. The membranous tear drainage passages.

Various valves have been described in the membranous passages, the function of which is presumably to prevent reflux of tears. Competence of these valves is, however, not essential as in otherwise normal patients air can occasionally be demonstrated to escape from the puncta on nose blowing.

Each canaliculus has a vertical part consisting of punctum and ampulla and a horizontal part. The punctum is found on the summit of the lacrimal papilla, a tiny prominence situated on the posterior margin of each lid between its ciliary and lacrimal parts. Their orifices are directed slightly inwards towards the eye, the lower one being some 0·5 mm lateral to the upper.

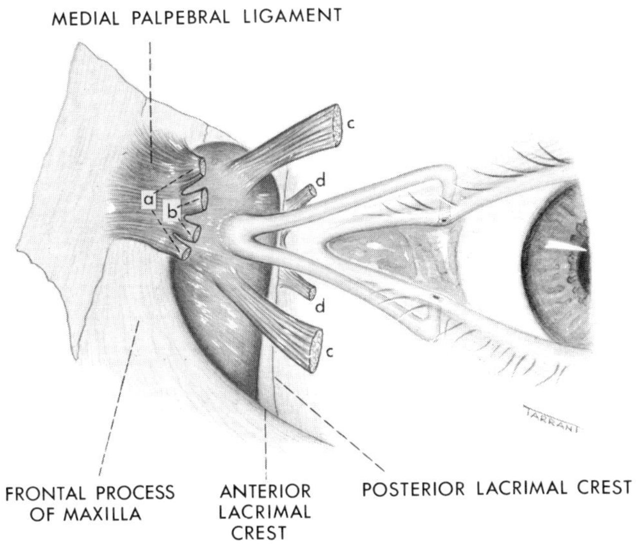

Fig. 3. The origin of the palpebral part of the orbicularis oculi muscle. a, superficial heads of preseptal orbicularis muscle; b, superficial heads of pretarsal orbicularis muscle; c, deep heads of preseptal orbicularis muscle; d, deep heads of pretarsal orbicularis muscle.

The upper and lower canaliculi usually unite to form a common canaliculus or sinus of Mair before entering the sac. The relationship of the canaliculi to the origin of the orbicularis oculi and the medial palpebral ligament are important to understanding the mechanism of the lacrimal pump.[10]

The medial palpebral ligament consists of a superficial part which arises near the fronto-maxillary suture. As it passes laterally, a deep or reflected part sweeps posteriorly to encircle the common canaliculus to be inserted into the posterior lacrimal crest. The palpebral orbicularis oculi muscle consists of a pretarsal and preseptal part (*Fig.* 3). The pretarsal part arises by two heads in both upper and lower lids; the anterior head from the superficial part of the medial palpebral ligament and the posterior one from the posterior lacrimal crest. A portion of this (Horner's muscle) is inserted around the canaliculus. The preseptal muscle also has a superficial head arising from the anterior part of the medial palpebral ligament and a deep one from the lacrimal fascia.

The canaliculi are lined by stratified squamous epithelium. The vertical component where the punctum widens into the ampulla is about 2 mm in length and the horizontal component about 8 mm. Having united to form the common canaliculus, this passes through the reflected part of the medial palpebral ligament to enter the sac some 5 mm from its fundus. The common canaliculus is some 3–4 mm in length. Its entrance into the sac is surrounded by folds of mucosa (valve of Rosenmüller).

The Lacrimal Sac and Nasolacrimal Duct

The sac occupies the lacrimal fossa where its fundus is covered by the superficial part of the medial palpebral ligament and the lacrimal duct with which it is continuous, passes through the bony nasolacrimal duct to open after a short intrameatal course into the inferior meatus of the nose some 35 mm from the anterior nares. The lower end of the duct is usually protected by a fold of mucosa – Hasner's valve.

Normal Tear Drainage and the Lacrimal Pump

The exact mechanism by which those tears not lost by evaporation reach the nose via the lacrimal drainage apparatus has been a source of controversy over the years. During blinking the lids close from lateral to medial. The marginal tear strip is moved towards the inner canthus. Tears enter the puncta and this may be aided by capillarity, although patients who have had their puncta mutilated surgically may still drain tears, suggesting that a negative pressure exists in the canaliculi. As the lids close, the puncta are occluded and the ampulla and individual canaliculi are compressed, pushing tears towards the sac. Reflux of tears from the sac tends to be prevented by the valves that surround the internal opening of the canaliculi.

According to Jones,[10] the contraction of the preseptal muscle pulls the lacrimal fascia laterally, producing a negative pressure within the sac and thus drawing the tears onwards. Relaxation of this muscle after blinking allows the lacrimal diaphragm to recoil, which would propel the fluid through the nasolacrimal duct to the nose. Others have found that there is an increase in pressure within the sac during blinking.[11,12] Integrity of the valves both at the internal opening and within the nasolacrimal duct is not, however, universal.

Most authors agree on the importance of the pumping action of the orbicularis on the canaliculi but many consider the sac's role to be entirely passive, acting only as a reservoir and draining by gravity. Indeed, there is evidence that resistance to tear flow is normally present in the nasolacrimal duct. Such a theory would anticipate that tear drainage would be enhanced by dacryocystorhinostomy.[13]

The progress of tears through the normal drainage apparatus is surprisingly rapid. Artificial tears labelled with gamma-emitting ^{99c}Tc sulphur colloid instilled in the conjunctival sac enter the tear sac in 5–10 s and can be identified in the nose in a minute.[14] The assumption that tears drain in a linear fashion from compartment to compartment has recently been questioned.[15] These authors showed that tear drainage was complex with variable flow and reflux between the various compartments of the system being possible.

Symptoms

Consisting as it does of canaliculi, tear sac and nasolacrimal duct, the lacrimal drainage apparatus may be involved in a variety of congenital malformations or acquired diseases. These pathological processes may have their origins within the system itself or encroach upon it from the surrounding structures. In the presence of a normal secretory apparatus such lesions may cause embarrassment to tear drainage and produce the troublesome symptom of epiphora.

Epiphora is not, however, the only symptom of lacrimal drainage disease, and patients may also be troubled by pain, swelling or discharge and occasionally by the presence of a fistula.

An overful tear film can interfere with vision and constant wiping of infected tears from the lower lid causes a troublesome dermatitis.

Diagnosis

Investigation of the tear drainage apparatus is directed towards identifying those patients with normal excretory passages whose symptoms are the result of excessive tear production (lacrimation) and treating the provoking agent. Such treatment is usually medical. In those patients where the symptoms are due to an obstructive cause, the object is to localize the level of the obstruction accurately and, if possible, identify its cause. When this information is available such patients can usually be completely relieved of their symptoms by appropriate surgery.

Assessment of Tear Drainage Apparatus

An accurate history from the patient about the duration and mode of onset of his symptoms can reveal important diagnostic information. In the case of watering it is helpful to know whether the condition was preceded by any conjunctival inflammation or discharge. A history of trauma should be specifically sought. Inquiry should also be made concerning any previous nasal or paranasal disease. Occasionally, the tear passages are involved in systemic disease and inquiry should be made concerning the patient's general health and whether or not he is receiving or has received any ocular or systemic medication.

Toxic effects on the conjunctival or canalicular mucosae may be produced by such drugs as IDU or miotics and systemic therapy with nicotinic acid, fluorouracil or bromhexine may be associated with increased tear production.

The Lids and Conjunctiva

Having obtained an accurate history, attention should then be directed to the lids. Is there any evidence of facial muscle weakness? And what is the state of tone of the lids? The presence or absence of fistulas should be specifically sought, as these are readily overlooked. Gentle palpation over the lacrimal fossa will reveal the presence of a mucocele and whether or not such pressure produces any regurgitation.

The conjunctiva should be examined with the slit lamp on both its bulbar and tarsal aspects for any evidence of inflammation or scarring disease, e.g. trachoma.

The Puncta

The position of the puncta and their relation to the marginal tear strip should always be determined. This examination is facilitated by the instillation of a drop of fluorescein. Minor degrees of ectropion are easily overlooked; they can be corrected by retropunctal cautery[16] or the excision of a diamond-shaped piece of conjunctiva from behind the punctum.[10]

When the ectropion is more extensive, a more formal plastic procedure may be required to correct it. Stenosis of the punctum is usually secondary to its occupying an ectopic position, where it becomes dry and keratinized. It usually resolves on repositioning of the punctum in contact with the marginal tear strip.

Stenosis of the lacrimal punctum, whether primary or secondary to conjunctival scarring disease, may be dealt with by a one- or three-snip procedure or using a specially designed punch to remove the posterior margin of the punctum.[17]

Tests for the Functional Patency of the Lacrimal Drainage Apparatus

These tests of lacrimal drainage function depend on the recovery from the pharynx of substances introduced into the palpebral aperture. They are sometimes referred to as 'primary' or 'physiological tests' because nothing is done to interfere with the normal flow of tears. They are of several types: taste, dye, radiological and radionucleotide tests.

TASTE TESTS

Various substances have been used, of which quinine[18] and saccharin[19] are examples. These tests are interpreted as positive if the substance can be tasted after its introduction into the eye.

DYE TESTS

Functional patency is verified by the detection of coloured fluid in the nose after its introduction into the conjunctival sac. Fluorescein is the most popular substance,[20] but recognition of the dye in the nose can be difficult and is possible in only 77 per cent of normals.[21] This test also depends on the tear flow rate. Recognition of the dye in the nose may be facilitated by its examination with a Wood's light.[22] The usual method is to pass a small pledget of cotton-wool under the inferior turbinate.

Because of the difficulties encountered, others have preferred to measure the rate of disappearance of the dye from the conjunctival sac.[23]

RADIOLOGICAL TESTS

Although used for many years to demonstrate anatomical defects in the drainage apparatus, radio-opaque material can be used to make functional assessments. The progress of Lipiodol ultra fluid or Angiografin instilled in the conjunctival sac through the system can be observed radiologically. The times taken for these substances to reach various levels have been determined for normal individuals, and patients with abnormalities of tear conduction through the upper part of the system (puncta and canaliculi) can be separated from those with more distally located lesions (sac, nasolacrimal duct).[24]

RADIONUCLEOTIDE TESTS

The progress of tears labelled with radioactive tracers can be monitored using a suitably modified gamma camera.[25] Valuable quantitative as well as qualitative information can be obtained, particularly if the system incorporates a digital computer, as in the technique of quantitative lacrimal scintillography.[14]

This test is particularly useful in assessing the efficiency of the canalicular pump mechanism but must be interpreted cautiously with regard to nasolacrimal duct function (where delayed emptying may have a physiological basis).[13]

Determination of the Anatomical State of Lacrimal Drainage Passages

Although the aetiology of lacrimal obstruction frequently remains obscure, the vast majority of such afflicted patients can be permanently relieved of their symptoms by appropriate surgery.

The nature of that surgery depends on the accurate preoperative localization of the level of obstruction within the system. Abnormalities in the canalicular system frequently co-exist with more distal lesions and preoperative knowledge of this is mandatory if all abnormalities are to be dealt with at the time of surgery and disappointing results avoided.[26]

DIAGNOSTIC SYRINGEING AND PROBING

The lacrimal syringe and cannula, introduced by Anel in 1713,[27] is the most commonly used instrument for assessing the patency or otherwise of the tear drainage system. A drop of local anaesthetic is instilled into the eye and the punctum gently dilated with a Nettleship's dilator. The tip of the cannula is then introduced through the punctum into the ampulla at right angles to the lid margin. Having drawn the lid laterally with a finger of the other hand to straighten out the canaliculus, the syringe is rotated laterally until the canula is parallel with it and its tip then advanced some 5 mm towards the sac, depending on the particular circumstances. The passages are then gently irrigated with saline. Great caution is required as it is possible to generate high pressures with the syringe and this may damage the membranous passages or produce artefacts. The statement recorded in the patient's notes that the passages were patent with pressure is of no use. Having said that, an experienced observer will be able to judge whether or not there is any undue resistance to the irrigation.

In addition to establishing whether or not patency is present, the syringeing reveals other important information. Should saline regurgitate from the opposite punctum, this confirms the patency of the canaliculi at least as far as the common canaliculus. If mucus or mucopus regurgitates, this usually implies that there is an obstruction located within the sac.

In addition to the information obtained from the syringeing, the canula may be introduced further into the system and an appraisal made of the individual and common canaliculus and whether or not the sac can be entered. Such a diagnostic probing is more usually performed using a fine lacrimal probe, such as those designed by Liebreich.

Although available in various gauges, it is recommended that only the fine ones are used. Those larger than 1/0 and designed by Bowman may damage the punctum. Fine probes are particularly useful for localizing obstructions in the individual canaliculi accurately and delineating fistula tracts.

Dacryocystography

Some 20 per cent of patients with epiphora have obstruction of the lacrimal drainage apparatus involving the upper part of the sac or canalicular system.[28] Accurate preoperative localization of the site of obstruction is essential if appropriate surgery is to be performed. Some authors have maintained that the information gained from syringeing and probing is sufficient in itself,[29] while others have emphasized the useful information that can be obtained by preoperative contrast radiology.[30,31] This information not only includes the accurate delineation of the level of obstructions and stenoses, but may also reveal the presence of diverticuli, filling defects associated with tumours or stones and outline fistula tracts.

In the case of streptothrix infections, the appearances are diagnostic.

The conventional method of dacryocystography introduced by Ewing in 1909[32] consists of the canalization of the inferior or superior canaliculus, and injection of contrast medium into the duct system followed by postero-anterior and lateral X-ray films taken after the removal of the cannula. This method was superseded in the mid 1950s[33] by an intubation technique introduced by Professor Barrie Jones in which the upper or lower canaliculus was intubated with a fine nylon catheter. By injecting non-viscous Lipiodol, a continuous stream of contrast medium distends the duct system and films are taken during the injection.

In 1964 Campbell[34] described a system of macroradiography for dacryocystograms and in 1972 intubation macrodacryocystography was described,[35] in which the advantages of the two above methods were combined. In particular patients, by taking a control film before the injection is made and ensuring that the patient's head remains motionless throughout the procedure, bone-free pictures may be obtained.

This technique of subtraction macrodacryocystography[36] is particularly useful in demonstrating lesions of the common canaliculus.

Nasal Examination

No assessment of the lacrimal drainage apparatus is complete without examination of the nose. This should exclude any obvious nasal pathology embarrassing the duct system and also include an appraisal of the position of the septum and the anterior end of the middle turbinate, both of which may be relevant to any planned surgery.

Other Investigations

From the practical point of view the information obtained from the above investigations will usually be sufficient for the surgeon to make an accurate anatomical diagnosis and plan his surgery accordingly. On occasions it may be helpful to carry out more sophisticated investigations, such as fluoroscopic examination of the duct system. CAT scanning or hypocycloidal tomography after injecting the duct system with contrast medium have proved extremely useful in traumatic cases where preoperative knowledge of its relationship to the damaged orbital and paranasal structures is desirable.

In the past few years a technique for directly viewing the interior of the tear passages through a miniature endoscope has been developed.[37] This may well prove useful clinically, while it is doubtful whether the techniques of thermography and chemiluminescence,[38] despite the spectacular appearances of the displays, will prove to have any widespread clinical application.

Functional Block

This term, together with 'lacrimal insufficiency', is used to describe those patients who, despite patent passages, fail to transmit tears to the nose. The term was introduced to distinguish these cases from those with complete obstructions. When assessed by the techniques described above, many will be found to have demonstrable pathology to account for their symptoms. For example, stenosis of the common canaliculus or nasolacrimal duct; the presence of a dacryolith or streptothrix or an infected sac diverticulum could all account for persistent epiphora in an otherwise patent system. Such patients should not be labelled as having a functional block as they all have a pathological basis for their symptoms. When these cases have been excluded, there remains a group of patients whose tear passages are normal radiologically but who fail to transmit tears as demonstrated by the scintillography technique. These patients usually have a failure in the tear pump mechanism, either as a result of neurogenic weakness of their orbicularis muscle or simply loss of tone in that muscle from the ageing process. Such patients are difficult to manage and may require bypass surgery to control their symptoms. They may legitimately be described as having a functional obstruction.

MANAGEMENT OF DISORDERS OF THE LACRIMAL DRAINAGE APPARATUS

Congenital Abnormalities

Normal Development

The nasolacrimal drainage system arises from a thickening in the surface ectoderm of the naso-optic fissure in the 7 mm or 32-day embryo. This thickened epithelium becomes buried in the mesenchyme between the lateral nasal and maxillary processes at the 12 mm or 42-day embryo, and separates from the surface. Caudal and cephalic extension of the cord then occurs forming the nasolacrimal duct and canaliculi. Segmental canalization of the solid cord begins at the 32–36 mm or 62-day embryo. The puncta are patent by the seventh fetal month.

At birth or soon thereafter the nasolacrimal duct opens into the nose.

The process whereby the cord of cells – 'the lacrimal anlage' as it is sometimes referred to – separates from the surface, canalizes and eventually opens to the lids and nose, may go awry in one of several ways: first, there may be a total or partial failure of the anlage to develop or canalize, giving rise to agenesis of the sac or canaliculi. Accessory budding may produce fistulas or multiple puncta. There may be non-perforation of the passages to the surface ectoderm, either at the lids or in the nose.

Finally, the tear passages may be ectatic. This occurs in association with facial clefts which themselves may be typical, due to the malunion of the facial processes, or atypical where they are considered to be due to amniotic bands. Surgical correction of these clefts may itself further interfere with the tear drainage mechanism.

Congenital Nasolacrimal Duct Obstruction

This, the most common congenital lacrimal anomaly, is due to the non-perforation of a membrane at the lower end of the nasolacrimal duct. Occasionally, however, a more extensive agenesis of the duct or abnormality of the bony canal is responsible. Its incidence varies according to different series between 6 per cent[39] and 54 per cent.[40]

The outcome of this non-perforation is that the child will be noted by its mother to have a watering eye usually within the first few days of birth. If patency does not occur spontaneously the child may develop a mucocoele or chronic dacryocystitis. Uncommonly, the obstructed system is invaded with pyogenic organisms and the child develops acute dacryocystitis. This itself may be complicated by spontaneous fistula formation.

Two schools of thought exist as to how these patients should be managed. The early interventionists argue that should spontaneous resolution not have occurred within 2 weeks of the child being presented, the tear passages should be irrigated and if necessary probed forthwith. By acting promptly they argue that the possibility of chronic inflammation scarring the sac and duct is reduced and the prognosis for a favourable outcome improved. In addition, they will have pre-empted the possible complication of dacryocystitis referred to above.

Alternatively, the late interventionists argue that if congenital nasolacrimal duct obstruction is so common, so also is the rate of spontaneous remission. The spontaneous cure rate using a conservative regime of antibiotic drops and instructing the parents how to evacuate the sac by gentle pressure over the lacrimal fossa is very similar – about 90 per cent up to the age of six months[41] – to that achieved by the interventionists. In fact, spontaneous resolution may occur after this but becomes much less likely after the age of 1 year.

These patients all have a normal canalicular system and since there is a small but real morbidity to these structures from the manipulations involved, a conservative approach is probably correct in the first instance. It also has the advantage that it defers the necessity for an anaesthetic until the child is older.

If spontaneous resolution has not occurred by the age of 6 months, arrangements should be made to examine the child under an anaesthetic. Ketamine is a convenient agent for this purpose.

After gently dilating the punctum with a Nettleship's dilator, the canaliculus is gently irrigated with saline. Whether the upper or lower is used for the purpose is of no importance. It is the common canaliculus which is the structure most at risk and this can be damaged just as readily through the upper as through the lower route.

If patency is not present, the lacrimal canula is advanced cautiously into the sac. This is facilitated by pulling the lid laterally and 'straightening out', the canaliculi. Having reached the lumen of the sac, the tip of the canula can be slipped down its medial wall to the nasolacrimal duct. Great care must be taken to ensure that the sac has been entered before rotating the canula downwards for it is at this point that the common canaliculus or the valves surrounding its internal opening may be traumatized.

Once the examiner is satisfied that he is in the nasolacrimal duct he may irrigate again, this time with a moderate pressure. In many cases this pressure will be sufficient to break down the membrane and establish patency, in which case the syringe and canula may be withdrawn. If patency is not established, then either the tip of the canula may be used to probe the nasolacrimal duct or the instrument may be withdrawn and a fine Liebreich's probe used for the purpose. That the membrane has been breached can be confirmed either by observing the tip of the probe in the nose or by a subsequent syringeing. The child is then prescribed antibiotic drops or ointment and seen again after an interval of about a month. Should the symptoms persist then the procedure may be repeated.

On this occasion it is useful to obtain a dacryocystogram before repeating the probing to establish the normality of the canaliculi and accurately delineate the level of the block in the sac or nasolacrimal duct.

If it proves impossible to negotiate the nasolacrimal duct, which may occur in association with its complete atresia or bony defects of the canal, then a dacryocystorhinostomy is mandatory.

Should a second probing properly effected not bring about relief of the symptoms, then it is unlikely that one is dealing with a simple membranous obstruction, but rather with a more extensive abnormality. It is unlikely that further probing will effect a cure and further attempts to do so should be resisted.

These children are all curable by a dacryocystorhinostomy. The timing of this procedure presents some problems, as although it is not difficult to perform such an operation even in quite small babies, a better cosmetic scar can be obtained and there is obviously an advantage from the anaesthetic point of view by deferring the operation until about the age of 4 years, before the child goes to school. The parents should have the advantages of this delay explained to them and they usually readily accept this advice.

If insurmountable problems arise and the parents are unable to keep the eye acceptably clean by regular expression of the sac and antibiotic drops, the plan can be altered and the date of surgery advanced. During this waiting period a significant number of cases will resolve spontaneously.

Vertical intubation of the nasolacrimal duct, using fine nylon or silicone tubing, has been widely recommended for children who have had unsuccessful probings as an alternative to carrying out a dacryocystorhinostomy. These tubes may be introduced from above[42] using a special introducer or the tubes may be swaged on to a metal introducer.[43] Alternatively, the nasolacrimal duct may be intubated from below, as in the technique described by Nagashima.[44] These tubes are left in position for some months. There is no doubt that their use may be attended by success, but the manipulations necessary for their introduction and the presence of tubing in the canaliculi represent a real hazard to the integrity of these structures.

Some of these children harbour bony abnormalities of the nasolacrimal duct, which are unlikely to be helped by the technique. Since all these patients are completely curable by a properly constructed dacryocystorhinostomy and since trauma to the canaliculi may condemn the patient to the lifetime use of a bypass tube, their use is best avoided except in exceptional circumstances and in expert hands.

Amniotocoele

Occasionally newborn babies may be seen with a tense swelling of the lacrimal sac which is distended with amniotic fluid. This is prevented from regurgitating by the valves around the internal opening of the common canaliculus and its presence implies the non-perforation of the nasolacrimal duct. Gentle pressure over the sac will usually effect a cure. If not, a probing may well be necessary.

Acute Dacryocystitis in Children

Invasion of the congenitally obstructed tear passages by pyogenic organisms may result in acute inflammation of the tear sac and its surrounding structures (pericystitis). If an abscess forms, this may lead to external fistulization. After 24 hours' treatment with appropriate systemic antibiotics a complete resolution of the condition can nearly always be achieved by probing the nasolacrimal duct. The antibiotics are continued to cover the immediate postoperative period.

Should the dacryocystitis not respond to probing or recur, then it may be necessary to carry out a dacryocystorhinostomy under antibiotic cover.

Chronic Dacryocystitis

This is the more common outcome than the acute variety, with persistent watering and mucopurulent discharge. If it does not respond to probing, resort will have to be made to dacryocystorhinostomy.

Not all dacryocystitis in children is secondary to membranous nasolacrimal duct obstruction. In addition to obstructions associated with craniofacial defects, a significant number of children have secondary obstructions associated with trauma, cystic fibrosis or retained foreign bodies in the nose. Such a possibility should always be borne in mind.

Punctal and Canalicular Agenesis

Non-perforation of the surface epithelium at the punctum may occur. In such patients examination of the lid margins with the aid of the microscope will usually reveal the site of the papilla. The occluding membrane can be perforated by a punctum seeker and then gently dilated. No other treatment is necessary.

Complete absence of either one or both canaliculi is less common.

In patients with one punctum, a dacryocystogram will invariably demonstrate the presence of an associated obstruction of the nasolacrimal duct. If this obstruction is not relieved by probing, than a dacryocystorhinostomy (DCR) will usually render such a patient symptom-free. Had the patients not had obstruction in the nasolacrimal duct, of course, they would not have developed symptoms and presented in the first place. A single canaliculus, be it upper or lower, provided the distal system is normal, is usually sufficient to keep a patient free from symptoms in normal circumstances.

When both puncta are absent there is unlikely to be any underlying canalicular tissue. Blind intubations and exploratory operations of the lids are unlikely to prove rewarding. These patients require a bypass tube to control their symptoms, which will become more pressing in their 'teens. An exploratory DCR is then performed at which time a search is retrogradely made for canalicular remnants. If they exist, it is occasionally possible to marsupialize them on to the lid margin. Such a retrograde canaliculostomy may prove functional even if its opening lies medial to the caruncle. As is more commonly the case, no such remnants exist; then, if the symptoms warrant it, a bypass tube may be inserted.

At such an exploratory operation it may occasionally be found that the sac itself is absent, either totally or partially. This does not preclude the creation of a rhinostomy or the insertion of a bypass tube, but some difficulty may be encountered with herniation of orbital fat.

Supernumerary Puncta

The presence of more than one punctum on the lid margin may be associated with watering. Presumably this occurs because the additional punctum is incompetent during blinking and it is easier for tears to emerge from this site than be propelled towards the nose. Occasionally one sees patients where the roof of the canaliculus, though not perforate, is obviously defective. Attempts to close such defects are unrewarding and the logical treatment, providing the other canaliculus appears normal, is to obliterate the offending canaliculus and accessory punctum with cautery (*Fig. 4*).

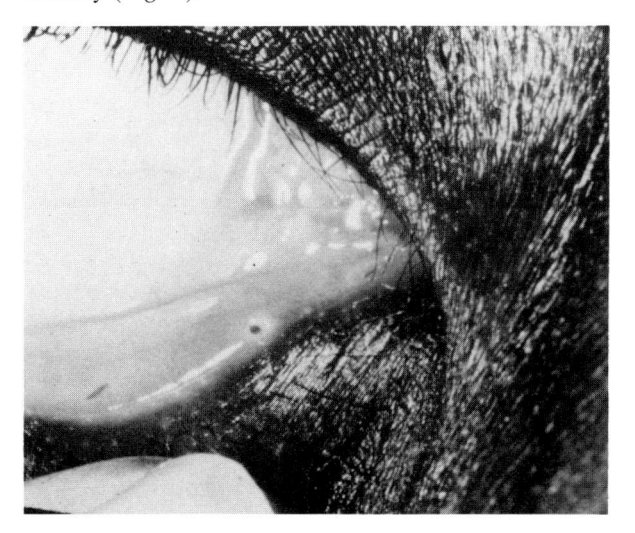

Fig. 4. Supernumerary punctum of lower canaliculus.

Congenital Lacrimal Fistula

This not uncommon congenital anomaly is considered by some to represent a persistence of the lacrimal anlage.[45] Although this may occasionally be the case, with the fistula communicating with the lacrimal sac, in the majority of patients the fistula represents an abnormal branching of the developing canalicular system. Histologically these fistulas are identical with canaliculi and usually communicate with the common canaliculus. Their external openings are most commonly found just below the superficial part of the medial palpebral ligament (*Fig. 5*).

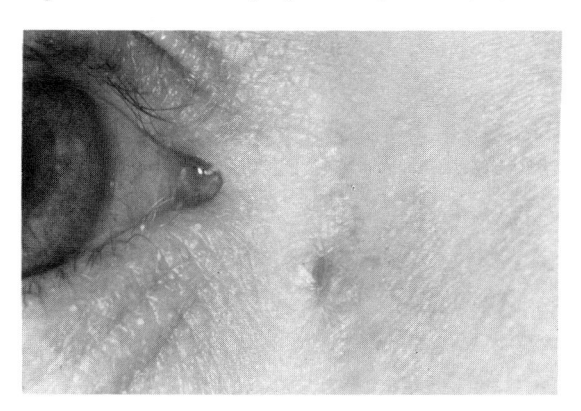

Fig. 5. Congenital lacrimal fistula.

Such fistulas only require treatment when symptoms arise. These usually consist of tears escaping from the fistula but the tract may become infected or a troublesome irritation of the skin develop about its opening.

The majority of patients have an associated, more distally located, obstruction in the sac or nasolacrimal duct. Although some authors have recommended simple excision or cautery to the tract, a less hazardous approach is to explore the common canaliculus and excise the fistula in its entirety, combining this with a dacryocystorhinostomy and leaving the canalicular system temporarily intubated.[46]

Other Congenital Abnormalities

The lacrimal passages are frequently involved in craniofacial abnormalities, either as a result of the defect itself or surgery invoked to correct it. The resultant chronic dacryocystitis is often amenable to treatment by dacryocystorhinostomy and its completion greatly facilitates the manoeuvres of the plastic surgeon to correct the cosmetic defect.

Acquired Lacrimal Disease

Dacryocystitis

Inflammation of the tear sac and duct is a common occurrence. It shows little tendency to resolve spontaneously and the symptoms it causes are unpleasant.

In adults the aetiology of the underlying obstruction remains obscure in the vast majority of patients. It is known that excluding the congenital cases, the condition becomes more prevalent with age and is much more common in women than men.

The affliction is said to be rare in Negroes and there is a familial and hereditary tendency. Sufferers frequently have a history or signs of nasal and paranasal sinus disease. Presumably all these factors exercise their effects by a tendency to impair the outflow of tears from the sac and the stasis eventually becomes associated with secondary changes in the sac and duct mucosa that are irreversible. The com-

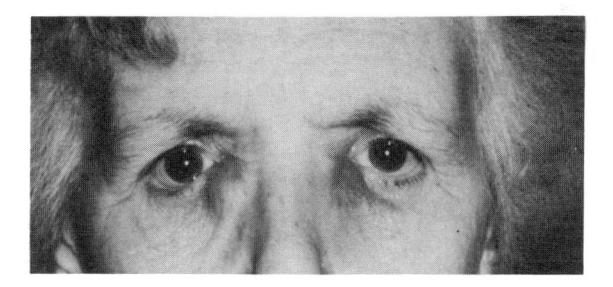

Fig. 6. Chronic dacryocystitis with bilateral mucocoeles.

bination of stasis and secondary infection eventually leads to complete closure of the passages.

The obstructed sac then becomes a reservoir for tears and mucous (*Fig. 6*).

Depending on the state of the sac wall, it may dilate to form a mucocele or, if invaded by more virulent organisms, a purulent discharge may ensue. Further inflammatory change in the sac wall may cause it to shrink or the exudate may become deposited around the opening of the common canaliculus and contribute to its obstruction. Debris within the sac may form dacryoliths which are commonly found at the time of surgery.

Whether such 'stones' are the cause or consequence of the obstruction is not clear. This debris – particularly in younger adults – may occasionally form a 'cast' of the tear sac and protrude through the nasolacrimal duct into the nose from whence material detaches itself from time to time.

Acute Dacryocystitis

This may arise *de novo* or more commonly in a patient with a known history of lacrimal obstruction. Pyogenic organisms invade the sac mucosa. The condition is extremely painful, with swelling, tenderness and general malaise. Prompt treatment with systemic antibiotics may bring about resolution but if the surrounding structures become involved (peridacryocystitis) abscess formation can occur and this can break through the skin to give rise to an external lacrimal fistula.

Occasionally, the abscess may burst into the nose to produce an internal lacrimal fistula.

The pain from acute dacryocystitis is severe and can be relieved by incising the sac. Such a procedure inevitably leads to a persistent fistula. Large doses of systemic antibiotics will usually bring about control of the pain and after a few days, partial resolution of the inflammation. Complete resolution may be effected by performing a dacryocystorhinostomy. Care should be taken to ensure that any perisac abscess is also marsupialized to the nose.

Acute Intermittent Dacryocystitis

From time to time one encounters a young adult with a history of recurrent attacks of epiphora, associated with severe pain over the lacrimal sac, often with swelling, but never with inflammatory signs. These episodes can last several days to resolve spontaneously and completely for several months or years. Between the attacks a dacryocystogram may be quite normal, although in the immediate period following such an attack it may be abnormally dilated. This condition has been labelled 'acute dacryocystitic retention'.[47] If the attacks are frequent and troublesome, they can be prevented by a dacryocystorhinostomy.

Secondary Dacryocystitis

Although in the vast majority of patients suffering from dacryocystitis the aetiology of the obstruction is obscure, the practitioner must always be aware that a specific cause for the obstruction may be present. Such an obstruction may arise within the lumen of the tear passages. Dacryoliths have already been mentioned, but occasionally foreign bodies may be present, possibly the result of trauma, but occasionally left behind following the attentions of another surgeon.

Rarely a primary transitional cell carcinoma may arise from the mucosa of the tear passages or, less rarely, the tear passages are invaded by secondary tumours, particularly from the adjacent paranasal sinuses.

Other afflictions of the adjacent nasal structures such as sacroid or Wagener's granulamotosis can also involve the tear passages and cause dacryocystitis.

Specific Types of Dacryocystitis

Although the organisms that invade the obstructed tear passages are protean and of the nasal, rather than the conjunctival type, specific types of dacryocystitis have been described in trachoma, tuberculosis, syphilis and certain other chronic infectious diseases. Their interest is largely academic.

Indications for Lacrimal Surgery (Table I)

The presence of tears spilling over the lid margin represents a source of irritation and embarrassment to the sufferer. Not only is it a cosmetic blemish, but the over-full tear film interferes with vision.

Table I. Indications for lacrimal surgery

Epiphora	Cosmetic / Optical
Dacryocytitis	Chronic – discharge, swelling / Acute – pain, fistula formation
Proposed intraocular surgery	
Skin excoration	
Malignant disease	

In women the use of cosmetics is precluded. Constant wiping of the eye may lead to stretching of the lower lid, producing ectropion, which compounds the problem. In chronic dacryocystitis the mucopurulent discharge, together with the trauma of constant wiping, may produce an unpleasant irritation of the skin of the lower lid. The mucopurulent discharge in the tear film also interferes with vision. The reservoir of potentially infective material represents a hazard should intraocular surgery be contemplated.

The onset of pain and the possible development of a fistula with acute dacryocystitis are all symptoms that may justify lacrimal surgery. Surgical intervention may also be indicated in suspected or proved malignant disease of the tear passages.

Notwithstanding that the cause for obstruction in the tear passages usually remains obscure, most patients whose symptoms can be attributed to an obstruction can be totally and permanently relieved by properly executed surgery.

Anaesthesia for Lacrimal Surgery

Lacrimal surgery may be performed under either general or local anaesthesia. General anaesthetics offer the advantages that the airway can be protected with an endotracheal tube.[48]

The face and nose are richly endowed with blood vessels and control of bleeding is an important factor in allowing the surgeon successfully to execute his task. It is particularly important when carrying out procedures on the canaliculi using the operating microscope.

Physiologically, bleeding can occur only from a cut vessel when the intraluminal pressure is greater than the elastic recoil and the muscular contraction of the walls of the vessel. Both these factors can be influenced pharmacologically. Vasoconstriction is usually produced by infiltrating the canthal area with diluted adrenaline and packing the nose with a mixture of cocaine and adrenaline.

Anaesthetists have grown accustomed to restricting the free use of adrenaline in effective concentrates because of the danger of death from ventricular fibrillation when used in the presence of halothane. Beta-adrenergic blocking agents such as propranalol obviate this risk or alternatively a vasoconstrictor with a pure alpha effect, such as methoxamine (Vasoxine) may be used.

Except in small children or patients with cerebrovascular disease, a controlled hypotensive anaesthetic provides the best operating conditions. This may be achieved in different ways, but the most commonly employed consists of a 'head-up tilt' of the patient. Halothane in a concentration of about 1 per cent is given with intermittent positive pressure ventilation, sometimes with positive pressure in the expiratory phase, autonomic blockage with pentolinium tartrate (Ansolysen) and control of the tachycardia with propranolol. The patient should be continuously monitored throughout the procedure.

If the services of a skilled anaesthetist are not available, or if general medical considerations preclude a general anaesthetic, then adequate local anaesthesia can be obtained by packing the nose with cocaine and blocking the supra-trochlear and intra-orbital nerves with a long acting local anaesthetic agent.

In addition to the above measures, the amount of haemorrhage encountered can be significantly limited by the technique of the surgeon. The angular vein should be avoided, and tissue planes adhered to. The liberal use of traction sutures improves access and limits bleeding. The divided lacrimal or nasal mucosa should be carefully sutured into its new desired position.

Finally, the careful use of the sucker passed up the nostril, removing any ooze from behind the operation site, greatly facilitates the surgery. Its careless use can severely traumatize the nasal mucosa and contribute to considerable haemorrhage.

Obstructive Lacrimal Disease

The treatment of obstructive lesions in the lacrimal drainage apparatus has a history dating back to antiquity. Galen himself is said to have advocated breaking through the lacrimal bone and introducing a caustic substance to inhibit closure of the newly formed passageway.

Following the description of the lacrimal syringe by Anel in 1713[27] and the introduction of graded lacrimal probes by Bowman in 1857,[49] syringeing and probing became the conventional methods of treatment. Patients with persistent infection were treated by extirpation of the lacrimal sac. This invariably left the patient with a watering eye. Although the use of therapeutic syringeing and probing still has its advocates, except in the case of congenital nasolacrimal duct obstruction, such manoeuvres are largely useless and not infrequently make the situation worse.[50]

In 1904 Adeo Toti,[51] a French ophthalmologist working in Florence, revolutionized the treatment of obstructive epiphora. He suggested that having made an external approach to the tear sac, that part of it adjacent to the canaliculi should be preserved and absorbed into the nose, from which part of the lateral wall had been removed. He called his operation 'dacryocystorhinostomy'.

Although good initial results were obtained, late failures were not infrequent. In 1921 Dupey-Dutemps and Bourguet[52] concluded that these failures could be avoided by suturing the divided nasal and sac mucosal edges over the bony margins of the osteotomy. The operation, as they described it, is highly successful in patients whose site of obstruction lies beyond the internal opening of the common canaliculus, in which a success rate approaching 100 per cent may be anticipated.

For more proximally sited lesions, different techniques are appropriate, depending on the level of obstruction. Such obstructions may be located at the level of the common canaliculus or involve the individual canaliculi.

Dacryocystorhinostomy

This operation is indicated where the patient's symptoms can be attributed to an obstruction located distal to the internal opening of the common canaliculus. The aim of the operation is to make that part of the sac which harbours the opening of the canaliculi an integral part of the nose. Following the operation, the sac should cease to exist and be marsupialized to the nose.

The Incision

The incision (*Fig. 7*) should be straight to avoid the possible disfigurement of a bowstring scar and made some 8 mm medial to the inner canthus on the side of the nose. It extends downwards and slightly laterally for some 20 mm from a point roughly 2 mm above the lower border of the medial palpebral tendon. The skin edges and subcutaneous tissue should be separated carefully as the angular vein lies immediately

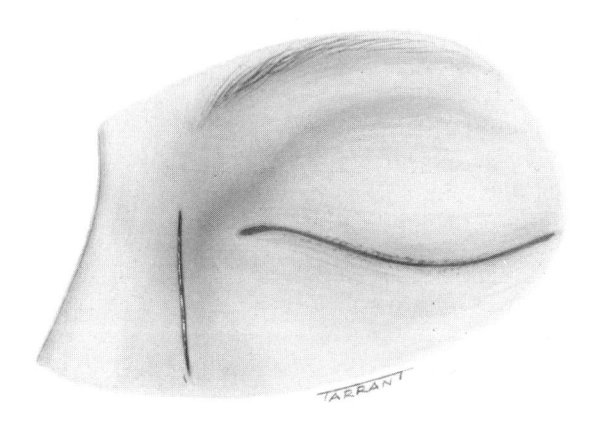

Fig. 7. Dacryocystorhinostomy – the incision.

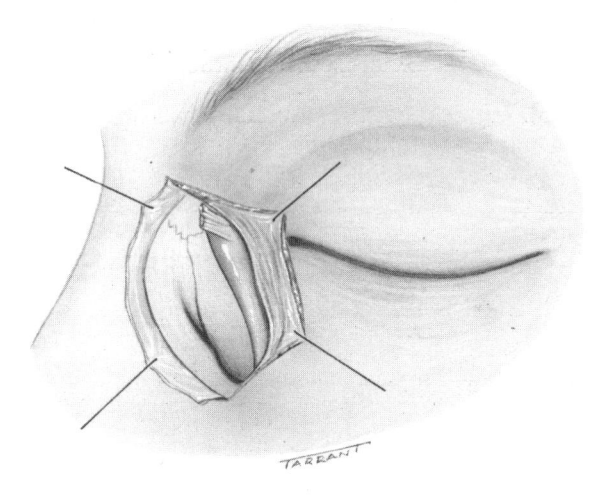

Fig. 8. Dacryocystorhinostomy – exposure of the lacrimal fossa.

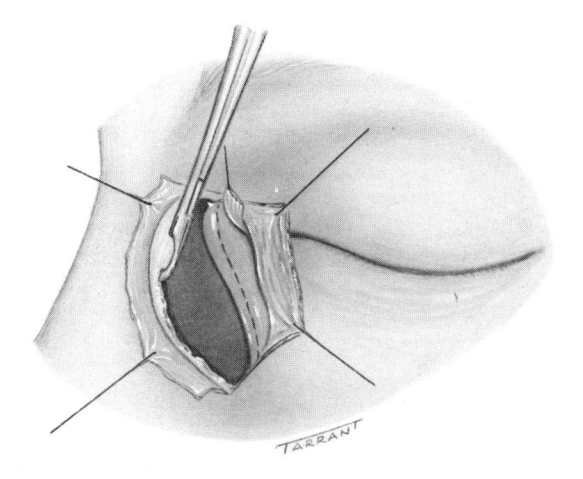

Fig. 9. Dacryocystorhinostomy – the rhinostomy.

under the incision on the orbital part of the orbicularis muscle.

The periosteum over the anterior lacrimal crest is then exposed by separating the orbital and palpebral parts of the orbicularis. Traction sutures are inserted to the subcutaneous tissue of the skin margins to give exposure, with two or three sutures around the orbital part of the orbicularis muscle and its overlying vein to draw them out of the way.

The periosteum is divided using a sharp rugine just anterior to the anterior lacrimal crest, from a spine which usually lies in front of the exit of the nasolacrimal duct upwards beyond the sharp part of the crest, to include the insertion to the periosteum of the superficial part of the medial palpebral ligament. The periosteum is reflected forwards to expose the bone for about 5 mm. This periosteal edge is also secured with traction stitches (*Fig.* 8).

Using the rugine, the sac is reflected laterally to expose the whole lacrimal fossa. This implies that all the bone medial to the sac from its fundus to the nasolacrimal duct and backwards to a line just anterior to the posterior lacrimal crest has been exposed.

Having thus cleared the area of periosteum, sufficient bone must be removed to allow the surgeon to incorporate the sac in the nose. If this bony opening is only large enough to allow a small anastomotic bridge between the nasal mucosa and a part of the sac, then a proportion of failures can be anticipated.[53] In practice, the ideal bony window extends backwards to just short of the posterior lacrimal crest, which should not be disturbed. Above, the opening should extend to the fundus of the sac, i.e., about 5 mm above the internal opening of the common canaliculus. Below, it should extend down the bony nasolacrimal canal – some 8 mm – removing that bone between the duct and the nose and also some of the bone from in front of it. Anteriorly, the osteotomy should include the lacrimal crest and extend forwards about half way from that structure to the nasal bone.

How far the osteotomy is enlarged forwards depends partly on how much nasal mucosa is required to fashion the flaps. It matters little how this osteotomy is created provided care is taken not to damage the underlying mucosa.

Some surgeons use a hand trephine, while others favour the use of a motorized burr or a gouge and hammer. I personally perforate the thin bone at a convenient suture in the floor of the fossa using a Traquair's periosteal elevator.

Whichever method is employed, the bony opening is enlarged using bone punches such as those designed by Citelli. A pair of Jensen's bone forceps is very useful for removing the bone of the upper part of the nasolacrimal duct (*Fig.* 9).

While removing the bone from the floor of the lacrimal fossa, the operator will frequently encounter either an ethmoid air cell or bone which is part of

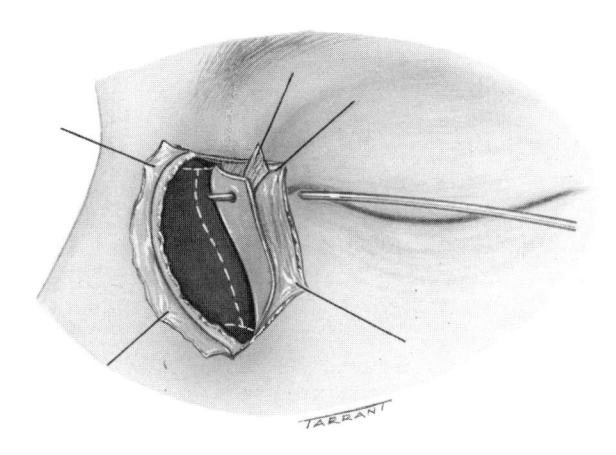

Fig. 10. Dacryocystorhinostomy – the opened sac.

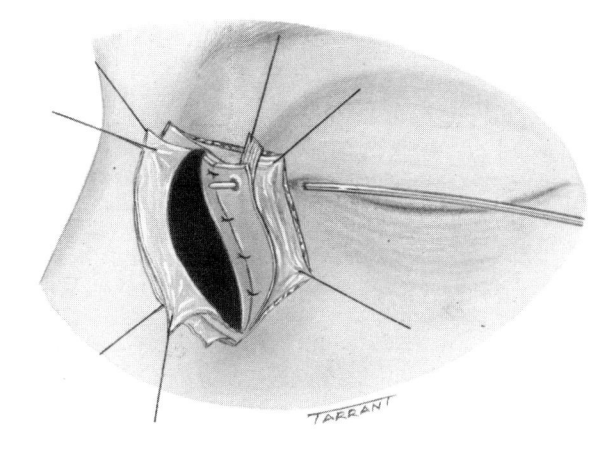

Fig. 11. Dacryocystorhinostomy – the sutured posterior mucosal flaps.

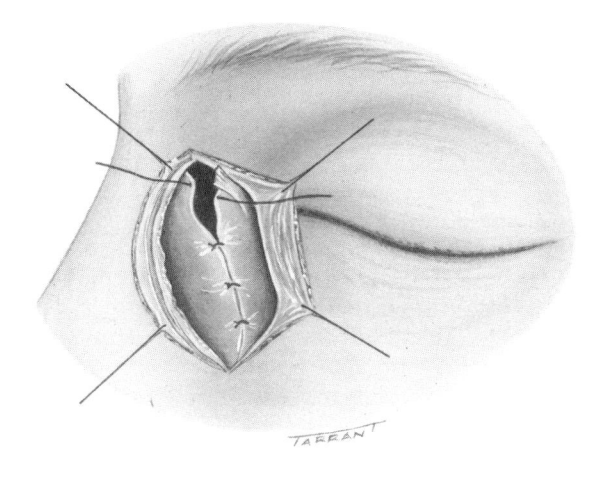

Fig. 12. Dacryocystorhinostomy – completion of the anterior mucosal anastomosis.

the skeleton of the middle turbinate. If the presence of these structures interferes with the construction of the rhinostomy, they should be removed.

Preparation of the Mucosal Flaps

After the introduction of a probe via a canaliculus to identify the lumen of the sac, a vertical incision is made in its medial wall. This is conveniently performed by making the initial incision with a sac knife and extending it with Werb's angled scissors.

The anterior and posterior flaps should be roughly of equal size. By extending the incision from well down in the nasolacrimal duct to the fundus, it will be found that the sac splays open like the opened leaves of a book (*Fig. 10*).

It is convenient at this point, with the lacrimal probe in position, to confirm the normality of the internal common opening. If it is compromised by adhesions or debris, these should be carefully removed, and if there is any doubt about its normality, the canaliculi should be intubated.

It may be necessary to separate or divide adhesions to allow the sac to be opened fully. Attention is then directed to fashioning the anterior and posterior nasal mucosal flaps. A vertical incision with the sac knife is made to divide the nasal mucosa roughly into an anterior two-thirds and posterior one-third. A small horizontal relieving incision may facilitate the forward hinging of the anterior flap.

SUTURING THE MUCOSAL FLAPS

The posterior flap of the sac is sutured to that of the posterior nasal mucosa using three or four absorbable 6/0 Dexon or collagen sutures (*Fig. 11*).

This manoeuvre is not universally undertaken, but such posteriorly placed sutures do have several important advantages. Their presence rapidly controls any bleeding coming from that source; the mucosa-to-mucosa anastomosis precludes the development of granulation tissue, presence of which may be associated with scarring or secondary haemorrhage. The fixation of the flap obviates its chance adhesion to the anterior part of the anastomosis and precludes the requirement for leaving a foreign body, such as a rubber catheter, in the rhinostomy to prevent this eventuality.

The placement of posterior sutures is not particularly difficult, provided that a large enough osteotomy has been prepared and the posterior nasal mucosal flap made sufficiently substantial. A source of axial illumination, i.e. 'a headlight', may be helpful. Haemorrhage is a reason for the insertion rather than the omission of posterior flap sutures.

Closure

The anterior flaps are similarly joined with absorbable sutures. This holds the anterior leaf of the sac well forward. What used to be the lumen of the sac should now have ceased to exist (*Fig. 12*).

If the operation has been performed in the plane between the orbital and palpebral parts of the orbicularis muscle, it is not usually necessary to place subcutaneous sutures, neither is it necessary to attach the divided superficial part of the medial palpebral ligament. All these structures normally fall back into place. The skin is closed either by interrupted fine nylon sutures or using a subcuticular stitch.

Complications of Lacrimal Surgery

Primary or secondary haemorrhage are the most feared complications of lacrimal surgery. Primary haemorrhage is extremely rare if the surgeon concerned operates in tissue planes and always sutures the anterior and posterior mucosal flaps as described above. It usually responds to sedation, blood transfusion and packing the nose.

Secondary haemorrhage is more common, particularly in patients who have been fitted with a bypass tube. It occurs from days 4 to 7 when infection of the mucosa, presumably in relation to a suture or the prosthesis, involves an adjacent blood vessel. It responds to treatment with systemic antibiotics. Transfusion and nasal packing may be required while the antibiotics take effect. Torrential haemorrhage is occasionally said to require the clipping of the anterior ethmoidal artery.

Secondary infection is uncommon in this vascular area. The occasional stitch abscess responds to the removal of the offending suture. Infection of the deeper structures can occur in patients whose tissues have been compromised by previous radiotherapy. Such patients require systemic antibiotics.

Unsightly scars following lacrimal surgery are best avoided by placing a linear skin incision at least 8 mm medial to the inner canthus. An unsightly bowed scar is usually the sequela of a more laterally placed curved incision. Should this unfortunate outcome ensue, it can be corrected by an appropriate Z-plasty. Keloids are uncommon on the inner canthus but should the scar be unduly thickened, a long-acting corticosteroid may be injected adjacent to the scar.

Failure to achieve the objective of a dry-eyed patient with tears draining freely to the nose can occur for two reasons. The first is that the surgeon concerned has carried out an inappropriate procedure. This usually stems from an error in diagnosis. In the absence of a regurgitating mucocoele it is always prudent to perform preoperative contrast studies. Failure to recognize a common canaliculus obstruction is a common reason for the unsuccessful outcome of a dacryocystorhinostomy.

Secondly, failure may be the result of errors in the technique of the surgeon concerned. This usually consists of not adequately marsupializing the sac to the nose, either as a result of not creating a large enough rhinostomy or, having done so, not suturing the anterior and posterior mucosal flaps over the bony margins, thus reducing the chances of haemorrhage, secondary infection and fibrosis. The anastomosis of the sac to the antrum or an ethmoid air cell is uncommon but does occur.

Re-operation for Failed Lacrimal Surgery

Provided there is still 8 mm or more of healthy canalicular tissue remaining, the prognosis for achieving a functional result by further surgery and without recourse to a bypass tube, is extremely high.[53] All such patients should be assessed with intubation dacryocystography to establish how much sac and canalicular tissue remains.

At operation, unless there is a large sac remnant still present, the common canaliculus should first be identified by careful dissection in what should be relatively normal tissue in the plane lateral to the sac. Only then should the anterior edge of the previous rhinostomy be identified and enlarged above anteriorly and below to expose normal nasal mucosa. This manoeuvre inevitably provokes some bleeding. The nose should then be entered by making a vertical incision in the nasal mucosa close to the common canaliculus and a large anterior flap of nasal mucosa fashioned. A large amount of scar tissue from the previous operation may need to be dissected from it. Fine probes passed along the canaliculi can then be cut down on to, and small anterior and posterior flaps of either sac or canaliculus created. The canaliculi should then be intubated and the posterior flap sutured to the adjacent nasal mucosa. If there is still bone or scar tissue compromising the posterior part of the rhinostomy it can be removed and a fresh posterior nasal mucosal flap fashioned. The canalicular tubing is passed through the rhinostomy and the anterior flaps sutured in place. Should there still be a large sac remnant, dissection of the canaliculi is not essential before enlarging the original rhinostomy. However, if there is the slightest doubt always identify the canaliculi first. This dissection greatly facilitates the identification of the sac lumen, which can be extremely difficult following previous surgery.

Having opened the nose, a large anterior nasal mucosal flap should be turned forwards and then the sac opened and the normality of the internal common canalicular opening checked before re-suturing the mucosal flaps in position.

Intubation of the canaliculi is not necessary unless the line of the anastomosis encroaches on the internal opening. It is desirable at the end of these reoperations to be satisfied that the anterior and posterior flaps, while not under any tension, are fixed fairly firmly in a position that ensures that the internal opening is held wide open.

Canalicular Obstructions

The Common Canaliculus

This structure may be obstructed throughout its length or at its junction with the lumen of the sac.

The former situation pertains in about one-third of patients presenting with common canalicular obstruction in the United Kingdom[54] and in these cases the sac is commonly normal and the obstruction appears to be due to a pericanalicular fibrosis. Occasionally patients show evidence of previous trachomatous infection but usually the aetiology is not known. This type of obstruction is referred to as a 'lateral' or 'fibrous' type of obstruction, to distinguish it from the medial or mucosal type which affects the remaining two-thirds of cases. In these patients the common canaliculus is obstructed by a membrane which forms over the internal common opening of the canaliculi and which is invariably a complication of chronic inflammatory disease within the sac (*Fig.* 13).

the sac as a bridge, having excised the obstructed canalicular tissue. It is important to remember that approximately 30 per cent of tears pass via the upper canaliculus and most patients with only one functional canaliculus – be it upper or lower – do not develop watering under normal conditions.

The technique for such a canaliculodacryocystorhinostomy (CDCR) was described by Professor B. Jones in 1960[55] and is as follows.

Having made a routine dacryocystorhinostomy incision, the superficial part of the medial palpebral ligament is reflected laterally and with probes in the individual canaliculi the common canaliculus is identified. The dissection is carried laterally into the lid to expose the site of obstruction. This dissection is

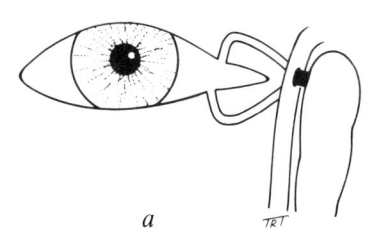

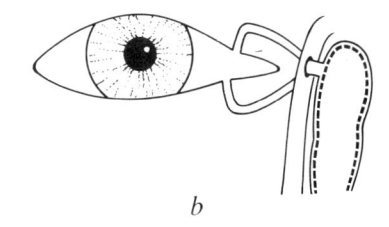

Fig. 13. Obstruction of the common canaliculus. *a*, Lateral; *b*, Mucosal.

Mucosal Type of Common Canaliculus Obstruction

Since the membranous obstruction is itself a complication of chronic sac infection, relief of the latter condition by a dacryocystorhinostomy combined with careful separation of the membranous adhesions about the internal common opening will usually effect a cure.

This dissection should be carried out with extreme caution from its sac aspect, having passed a fine probe through the canaliculus to delineate the obstruction and tent it up. It is extremely easy to create a false passage or damage the adjacent valves and mucosa. Having separated or divided the membranous obstruction, it is customary to intubate the upper and lower canaliculus with fine silicone or polyethylene tubing (No. 10 Portex). This tubing separates the margins of the recently traumatized mucosa and prevents re-adhesion while the surfaces re-epithelize. The ends of the tubing are passed through the rhinostomy and joined at the external nares. The tubes are left in position for about 3 months when they can then easily be removed by dividing the loop between the two puncta and pulling on the nasal ends.

Lateral Type of Common Canaliculus Obstruction

For patients whose common canaliculus is obstructed lateral to the sac, or for those who have obstruction of the individual canaliculi, provided there is at least 8 mm of either canaliculus present, it is usually possible to secure a functional mucosal anastomosis between the patent canaliculus and the nose, using

greatly facilitated by the use of an operating microscope, and fastidious haemostasis is mandatory. It is also essential that this dissection is carried out before the sac itself is mobilized from its position in the lacrimal fossa (*Fig.* 14).

Having located the site of obstruction, a large rhinostomy is performed. The obstructed canalicular tissue is excised and healthy canalicular tissue, having been intubated, is then anastomosed to a newly prepared opening in the opened sac. The dacryocystorhinostomy is completed in the normal manner having passed the tubing through the rhinostomy to the external nares. This tubing is left in situ for 3 months (*Fig.* 15).

A simpler method of carrying out a CDCR, and one that has the advantage that the deep attachments of the medial palpebral ligament are not disturbed, which has important implications should a bypass tube subsequently be required, is as follows.

Having reflected the superficial part of the medial palpebral ligament and exposed the common canaliculus, only its anterior aspect and upper and lower borders are dissected to identify the level of obstruction. The canaliculi are then divided and intubated.

Having completed a large rhinostomy, instead of incising the sac along its medial aspect, the sac is opened along its anterior border. This allows the sac to be opened backwards and entirely incorporated in the posterior anastomosis by suturing its lateral aspect to the posterior edge of the divided canaliculi and what was its medial edge well back in the nose to a short posterior nasal flap. The tubing is then passed through the rhinostomy and the large anterior nasal flap sutured directly to the front edges of the canaliculi (*Fig.* 16).

Using the above described techniques, a functional success rate in the order of 85 per cent can be anticipated in dealing with canalicular obstructions.

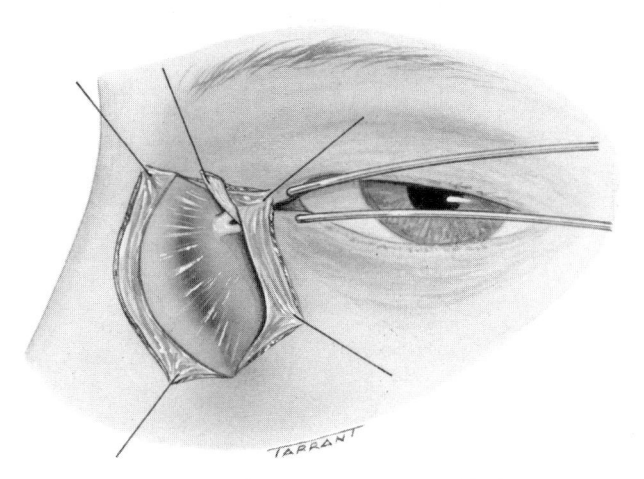

Bypass Surgery

Where there is less than 8 mm of healthy patent canaliculus present, canaliculodacryocystorhinostomy gives disappointing results. The creation of an alternative passageway for the drainage of tears then offers the best prospect for symptomatic relief. Vein grafts have not proved a satisfactory substitute for canaliculi,[56] and although the fistula created by the operation of conjuntivodacryocystorhinostomy described by Stallard,[57] in which the fundus of the sac is anastomosed to the lacus lacrimalis with or without a rhinostomy, usually remains patent, such an arrangement is seldom functional.

In 1961 Lester Jones[58] suggested that a thin glass capillary tube inserted between the inner canthus and nose would attract tears by its capillarity and that the negative phase of respiration allow drainage of tears to the nose. The indication for the use of such a prosthesis is the presence of epiphora in a patient with less than 8 mm of either canaliculus present or canaliculi which are non-functional.

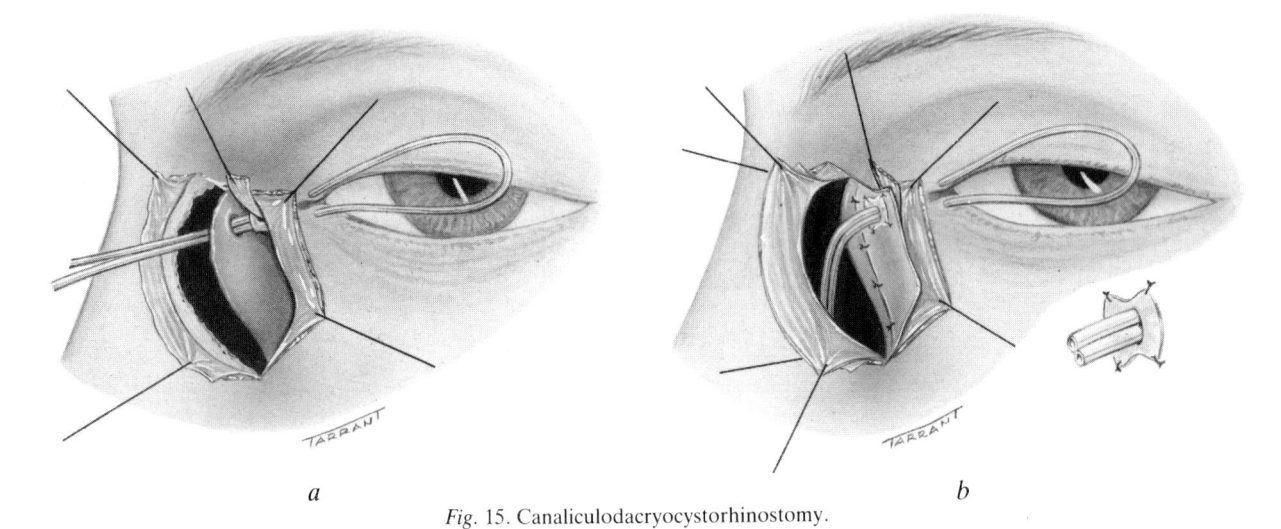

Fig. 14. Exposure of the common canaliculus.

Fig. 15. Canaliculodacryocystorhinostomy.

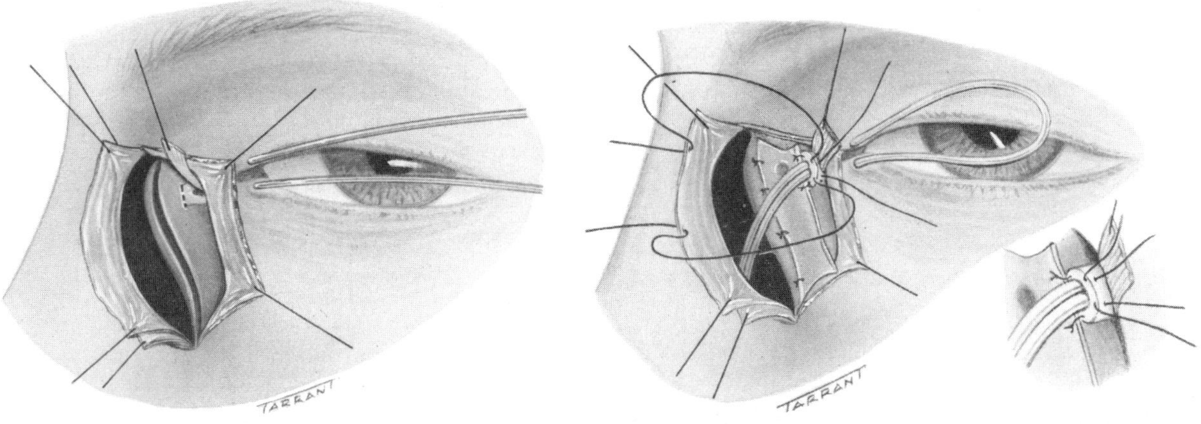

Fig. 16. Modified canaliculodacryocystorhinostomy.

Unlike elsewhere in the lacrimal drainage apparatus the causes of obstruction of the individual canaliculi are usually obvious.

The aetiology of canalicular obstruction in a series of 204 patients undergoing bypass surgery is given in *Table* II.

Table II. Aetiology of canalicular obstruction

Cause of canalicular obstruction	%
Herpex simplex canaliculitis	28
Trauma	22
Irradiation of rodent ulcers	13
Previously unsuccessful lacrimal surgery	13
Congenital absence of canaliculi	8
Stevens–Johnson syndrome	4
Facial palsy	1
Other	11

The technique for the insertion of a bypass tube is simple. A dacryocystorhinostomy is performed in the normal manner. When the posterior mucosal flaps have been sutured, attention is directed to the inner canthus. The track to embody the prosthesis is then prepared. The caruncle is excised and a needle inserted inwards and downwards to emerge within the sac in the region of the internal common opening. This track is then enlarged using a Graefe knife or a trephine as suggested by Henderson[59] and a No. 240 polythene tube inserted. This tube is about 18 mm long and its medial end is trimmed short of the nasal septum and its expanded lateral end sutured at the inner canthus. The DCR is then completed and about a week later this tube is replaced by a 2 mm glass capillary tube some 10–16 mm in length. The lateral end of this tube has a cuff 3–4 mm in diameter and its medial end is expanded to 2·25 mm (*Fig.* 17 and 18).

It is not always necessary to excise the whole of the caruncle for the insertion of the tube and occasionally when the first part of the canaliculus is normal a more satisfactory alternative is for the surgeon to remove the posterior wall of the ampulla and insert the prosthesis via the lid.

Complications

The insertion of a bypass tube has proved to be an effective method of controlling epiphora in over 90 per cent of patients so managed.

The prosthesis once inserted must remain in use indefinitely. Its removal, even after many years' usage, is attended by the prompt return of watering in all but a handful of patients (less than 5 per cent). Loss or temporary blockage of the tube is not infrequent and repositioning usually requires a general anaesthetic.

Other problems encountered include the formation of granulation tissue beneath the tube and embarrassment of its lumen by hypertrophy of the plica. No recurrence of the granulation tissue has followed its local excision and cauterization of the area with silver nitrate. Hypertrophy of the plica appears to be a response to its irritation by the cuff of the tube and usually responds well to a change in the shape of the one used.

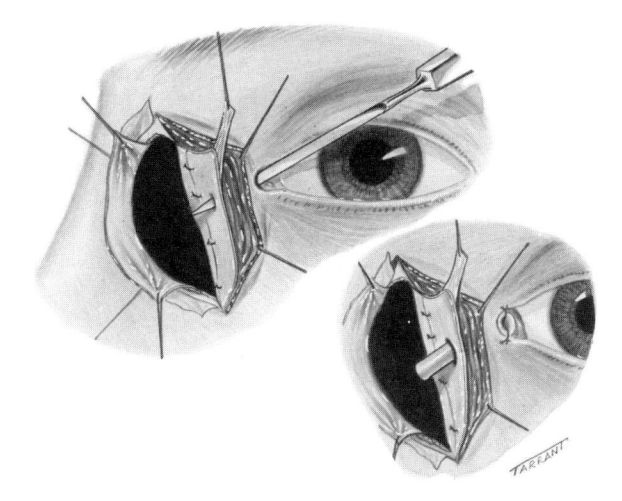

Fig. 17. Technique for insertion of bypass tube.

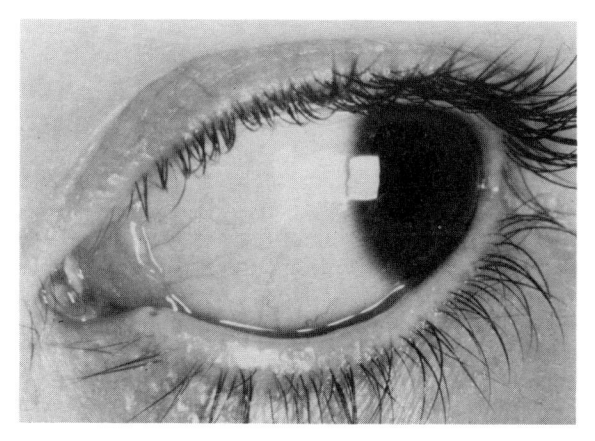

Fig. 18. Bypass tube inserted after removal of caruncle.

Cosmetically the appearance of the tube is quite acceptable and its presence usually passes unnoticed. Occasionally migration gives rise to problems.

In patients who have had extensive dissection of the deep part of the medial palpebral ligament during previously unsuccessful canalicular surgery, the presence of the tube may cause a somewhat unsightly deepening of the inner canthus. Forward migration has been troublesome in occasional patients who have scarring of the conjunctiva either as a result of previous trauma or who have sustained damage to the adjacent conjunctiva at the time of removing the caruncle.

If a Pyrex tube with a small diameter lip is inserted as a primary procedure or as a replacement for the polyethylene one it may become buried beneath the surface of the inner canthus and even be wedged between canthus and septum of the nose. Watering promptly returns. It is usually not possible to recover or re-position these tubes under local anaesthesia and should any difficulties be encountered the rhinostomy should be reopened under a general anaesthetic and the tube adjusted under direct vision.

Canaliculitis

Worldwide the most common cause of canaliculitis is trachoma. Its presence has been observed in some 37 per cent of cases.[62] This inflammation spreads to the canaliculi from the conjunctiva and frequently leads to canalicular stricture or complete obstruction often at the level of the common canaliculus. Secondary infection may lead to purulent canaliculitis. Such obstructions are amenable to cure by the operation of canaliculodacryocystorhinostomy. Other specific types of canaliculitis do occur and can cause canalicular obstruction. Thus the viruses of herpes simplex, herpes zoster, vaccinia and chickenpox may all be responsible. The obstruction caused by herpes simplex leads to a mid-canalicular block and usually requires a bypass tube to control the ensuing epiphora.[63]

Actinomycosis or Streptothrix of the Canaliculus

The presence of epiphora in a patient whose tear passages are patent to syringeing should always alert the ophthalmologist to the possibility of a fungal infection of the canaliculus. The condition is usually chronic and often the patient has been seen by a number of oculists with a history of watering and inflammation that has failed to respond to a variety of different antibiotic drops. Characteristically, the condition is unilateral and affects the lower canaliculus more frequently than the upper. The affected lid is swollen with pouting of the punctum from which may be expressed purulent discharge or particulate matter. The adjacent plica and conjunctiva are often swollen and congested. Dacryocystography will reveal a grossly dilated and ragged appearance of the canaliculus due to the presence of stones (*Fig.* 19). Although this condition is referred to as a streptothrix or actinomycosis of the canaliculus, this organism is not universally present. The exact aetiology of these stones and their associated canaliculitis is not entirely clear. Von Graefe in 1854 recognized actinomyces as a causative organism but cases may be associated with organisms other than *Actinomyces israelii*. These include Fusarium spp. and *Arachnia propionica*.[64]

Whatever the cause, once recognized the condition is easy to treat. The affected canaliculus is split open using either a specially designed canaliculostomy knife or a pair of sharp pointed scissors. The stones and concretions are curetted from the dilated canaliculus, which may show gross follicular hyperplasia, and are sent for bacteriology. Removal of all the stones is probably all that is necessary to effect a cure but traditionally the exposed mucosa is painted with an iodine solution or touched with a silver nitrate stick.

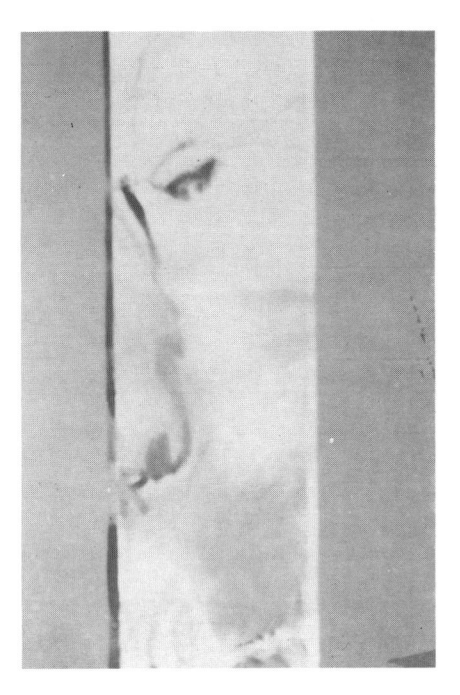

Fig. 19. Subtraction dacryocystogram of a patient with streptothrix showing a grossly dilate lower canaliculus.

Removal of the stones, which may be multiple, brings about an immediate resolution of the symptoms. The use of antibiotics is not necessary. Failure, should it occur, is due to a stone being overlooked or its not having been recognized that both canaliculi were involved in the condition.

Trauma to the Lacrimal Passages

Damage to the membranous tear passages may result from direct or indirect trauma to the region of the inner canthus of the eye. Such injuries are usually the result of road traffic accidents, criminal or domestic assaults, or animal bites. Incorrect management may condemn the patient to a lifetime of a watering eye.

Infection is seldom a problem in this vascular region but such injuries may be contaminated and patients should receive appropriate tetanus prophylaxis and systemic antibiotics.

These patients frequently arrive in the eye department late in the evening or in the early hours of the morning. Unless there is a major problem with uncontrolled haemorrhage the best results will be obtained by carrying out a planned surgical procedure the following day. A clear understanding of the normal anatomy and physiology of the tear drainage mechanism is essential before undertaking any surgery. Significant tissue loss is uncommon and a careful search will usually identify the individual tissues even though they may be disorganized.

As stated previously, tears are normally pumped to the tear sac via the canaliculi. Approximately 30 per cent of this volume is transmitted through the upper canaliculus and 70 per cent by the lower. The tear sac drains by gravity and the maximal resistance to tear flow is located in the nasolacrimal duct.

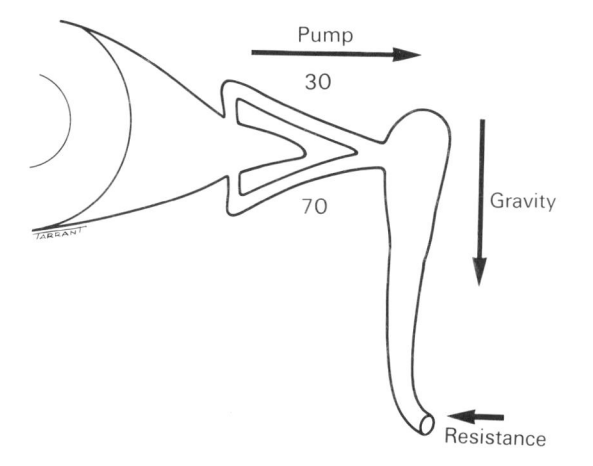

Fig. 20. Normal tear drainage.

Whether an eye waters or not depends on the efficiency with which this system copes with the volume of tears produced. This varies under different physiological conditions. Most eyes with an obstructed lower canaliculus do not water under ordinary circumstances and the few that do can often be rendered symptom-free by carrying out a dacryocystorhinostomy which has the effect of enhancing the flow along the upper canaliculus (*Fig.* 20).

Neither canaliculus can function if the position of the lid margin precludes entry of tears into the system. These facts must be kept clearly in mind when contemplating the management of patients with lacerations of the individual canaliculi. It is of paramount importance that the surgeon does nothing to prejudice the patency of the uninjured canaliculus, be it upper or lower.

Two retrospective studies on the attempted repair of such injuries using the pigtail probe method[60,61] have demonstrated how uncommon it is to get epiphora unless both canaliculi are obstructed. The studies also reveal a low level of patency achieved from such attempted repairs. Temporary intubation of the lacerated canaliculus without direct suturing of the mucosa is unlikely to remain patent and in view of the known lack of symptoms with or without patency it seems a much more reasonable approach to repair the lid margin as accurately as possible.

If the canaliculus medial to the laceration can be marsupialized to the conjunctiva in the lacus, this should be done by a three-snip type of procedure. Leaving a stent in the lower canaliculus tends to distort the lid margin and cause ectropion and is best avoided, as is also the passing of a pigtail probe and leaving both canaliculi intubated. This manoeuvre or the presence of the tubes may prejudice the non-traumatized canaliculus. Such an outcome will almost certainly condemn the patient to the lifetime use of a bypass tube to control his or her epiphora, which in the absence of surgical interference may well have never occurred.

Common canalicular lacerations, unless repaired, inevitably lead to watering in a normal individual. Such a repair may be effected using the technique of canaliculodacryocystorhinostomy. Absorbable mucosa to mucosa sutures should be used and the system left intubated for at least 3 months. The modification to the technique, whereby the whole of the sac is incorporated in the posterior anastomoses and the anterior edge of the divided canaliculus is sutured to a large anterior nasal mucosal flap, is particularly appropriate in these circumstances.

Tear sac lacerations are best managed by carrying out an immediate dacryocystorhinostomy. Although this might appear drastic, the outcome is much more predictable than a repair limited to suturing the wall alone.

Where there is extensive destruction of the lacrimal drainage system, surgery should be restricted to obtaining the best possible repair of the lids and face.

There is no place for the insertion of the bypass tubes as a primary procedure, though this may be necessary subsequently. Medial canthoplasty with or without transnasal wiring may be required as a secondary procedure in some cases of extensive medial canthal trauma, and this may be combined with the insertion of a bypass tube.

Lesions of the Punctum

The lacrimal puncta may be the site of a variety of skin tumours. Although such lesions are usually benign, a biopsy excision is desirable to exclude the possibility of malignancy. This can be effected by passing the pigtail probe from the opposite punctum and removing a cone of tissue from around its tip and then leaving the system temporarily intubated.

REFERENCES

1. Foster J. Evaluation of current treatment of stricture of the valve of Krause. *Ann. R. Coll. Surg. Engl.* 1956; **18,** 143–63.
2. Mishima S., Gasset A., Klyce S. D. et al. Determination of tear volume and tear flow. *Invest. Ophthalmol.* 1966; **5,** 264.
3. Pel P. K. Augenkrisen bei tabes dorsalis (crises ophthalmiques). *Berl. Klin. Wochenschr.* 1898, pp. 25–7.

4. de Roeth A. Lacrimation in normal eyes. *Arch. Ophthalmol.* 1953; **49**, 185–9.
5. Rycroft B. Problems of lacrimal obstruction. *Trans. Ophthalmol. Soc. UK* 1956; **36**, 395–7.
6. Jameson P. C. Subconjuctival section of the ductules of the lacrimal gland as a cure for epiphora. *Arch. Ophthalmol.* 1937; **17**, 206–8.
7. Whitwell J. Denervation of the lacrimal gland. *Br. J. Ophthalmol.* 1958; **42**, 518–25.
8. Golding-Wood P. Observations on petrosal and Vidian neurectomy in chronic vasomotor rhinitis. *J. Laryngol. Otol.* 1961; **75**, 232–47.
9. Antonelli A. Anomolie fonctionnelle congénitale de la glande lacrymale du côte droit. *Clin. Ophthal. (Fr.)* 1902; **8**, 35–6.
10. Jones L. T. An anatomical approach to problems of the eyelids and lacrimal apparatus. *Arch. Ophthalmol.* 1961; **66**, 111–24.
11. Rosengren B. On lacrimal drainage. *Ophthalmologica* 1972; **164**, 409–21.
12. Maurice D. M. The dynamics and drainage of tears. *Int. Ophthalmol. Clin.* 1973; **13**, 103.
13. Chavis R. M., Welham R. A. N. and Maisey M. N. Quantitative lacrimal scintillography. *Arch. Ophthalmol.* 1978; **96**, 2066–8.
14. Hurwitz J. J., Maisey M. N. and Welham R. A. N. Quantitative lacrimal scintillography. *Br. J. Ophthalmol.* 1975; **59**, 308–22.
15. Hildditch T. E., Kwok C. S. and Amananat L. A. Lacrimal scintigraphy. 1. Compartmental analysis of data. *Br. J. Ophthalmol.* 1983; **67**, 713–19.
16. Jones B. R. Cautery to cure epiphora from punctal eversion. *Trans. Ophthalmol. Soc. UK* 1973; **93**, 597–9.
17. Hughes W. L. and Maris C. S. G. A clip procedure for stenosis and eversion of the lacrimal punctum. *Trans. Am. Acad. Ophthalmol.* 1967; **71**, 653–5.
18. Lipsius E. I. Sodium saccharine for testing the patency of the lacrimal passages. *Am. J. Ophthalmol.* 1956; **41**, 320.
19. Hornblass A. A simple taste test for lacrimal obstruction. *Arch. Ophthalmol.* 1973; **90**, 435.
20. Linn M. L. and Jones L. T. Rate of lacrimal excretion of ophthalmic vehicles. *Am. J. Ophthalmol.* 1969; **65**, 76–8.
21. Zappia R. J. and Milder B. Lacrimal drainage function. 1. The Jones fluorescein test. *Am. J. Ophthalmol.* 1972; **74**, 154–9.
22. Vergez A. Contribution au diagnostic et au traitment non-opératoire des affections des voies lacrymales. *Ann Oculistique* 1961; **194**, 193–215.
23. Zappia R. J. and Milder B. Lacrimal drainage function. 2. The fluorescein dye disappearance test. *Am. J. Ophthalmol.* 1972; **74**, 160–2.
24. Hurwitz J. J. and Welham R. A. N. Radiology in functional lacrimal testing. *Br. J. Ophthalmol.* 1975; **59**, 323–31.
25. Rossomondo R. M., Carlton W. H., Trueblood J. H. et al. A new method of evaluating lacrimal drainage. *Arch. Ophthalmol.* 1972; **88**, 523–5.
26. Welham R. A. N. Canilicular obstructions and the Lester Jones tube, what to do when all else fails. *Trans. Ophthalmol. Soc. UK* 1973; **93**, 623–32.
27. Anel D. *Observations Singuliere sur la Fistule Lacrimale*. Gennes, Cionoco, 1713.
28. Campbell W. Radiology of the lacrimal system. *Int. Ophth. Clin.* 1964; **4**, 399–441.
29. Lyle T. K. Problems of lacrimal obstruction. *Trans. Ophthalmol. Soc. UK* 1956; **76**, 369–84.
30. Campbell D. M., Carter J. M. and Doub H. P. Roentgen ray studies of the naso-lacrimal passages. *Arch. Ophthalmol.* 1922; **51**, 462–70.
31. Rycroft B. W. Observations on corneo-plastic surgery. *Proc. R. Soc. Med.* 1960; **53**, 303–10.
32. Ewing A. E. Roentgen ray demonstration of the lacrimal abscess cavity. *Am. J. Ophthalmol.* 1909; **26**, 1–4.
33. Jones B. R. Personnal communication, 1959.
34. Campbell W. The radiology of the lacrimal system. *Br. J. Radiol.* 1964; **37**, 1.
35. Lloyd G. A. S., Jones B. R. and Welham R. A. N. Intubation macrodacryocystography. *Br. J. Ophthalmol.* 1972; **56**, 600–3.
36. Lloyd G. A. S. and Welham R. A. N. Subtraction macrodacryocystography. *Br. J. Radiol.* 1972; **47**, 379–82.
37. Cohen S. W., Prescott R., Sherman M. et al. Dacryoscopy. *Ophthalmic. Surg.* 1979; **10**, 57–63.
38. Raflo G. T. and Hurwitz J. J. Assessment of the efficiency of chemiluminescent evaluation of the human lacrimal drainage system. *Ophthalmic. Surg.* 1982; **13**, 36–46.
39. Guerry D. and Kendig E. L. Congenital impatency of the naso-lacrimal duct. *Arch. Ophthalmol.* 1948; **39**, 193–201.
40. Korchmaros I., Szalay E., Fodor M. et al. Spontaneous opening rate of the congenitally blocked nasolacrimal ducts. In: *Recent Advances in the Lacrimal System*. Tokyo, Ashai Press, 1980.
41. Evans P. J. Problems of lacrimal obstruction. *Trans. Ophthalmol. Soc. UK* 1956; **76**, 343–53.
42. Keith G. C. Lacrimal obstruction. *Trans. Ophthalmol. Soc. UK* 1968; **88**, 519–22.
43. Guibor R. P. Canaliculus intubation set. *Trans. Am. Acad. Ophthalmol. Otolaryngol.* 1975; **79**, 419–20.
44. Nagashima K. Retrograde silicon intubation of the nasolacrimal duct in children. In: *Recent Advances in the Lacrimal System*. Tokyo, Ashai Press, 1980, pp. 163–9.
45. Jones L. T. and Wobig J. L. *Surgery of the Eyelids and Lacrimal System*. Birmingham Ala, Aesculapius, 1976; 167–73.
46. Welham R. A. N. and Bergin D. J. Congenital lacrimal fistulae. *Arch. Ophthalmol.* 1985; **103**, 545–8.
47. Smith B., Tenzel R. R., Buffam F. V. et al. Acute dacryocystic retention. *Arch. Ophthalmol.* 1976; **94**, 1903–4.
48. Smith B. Anaesthesia for lacrimal surgery. *Trans. Ophthalmol. Soc. UK* 1973; **93**, 619–21.
49. Bowman W. On the treatment of lacrymal obstructions. *Ophthal. Hosp. Rep.* 1857; **1**, 10–20.

50. Foster J. Evaluation of the current treatment of stricture of the valve of Krause. *Ann. R. Coll. Surg. Engl.* 1956; **18,** 143–63.
51. Toti A. Nuovo metodo conservatore di cura radicale delle supperatzioni croniche del sacco lacrimale. *Clin. Mod. Firenze* 1904; **10,** 385.
52. Dupey-Dutemps L. and Bourguet J. Procede plastique de dacryocysto-rhinostomie et ses resultats. *Ann. Ocul.* 1921; **158,** 241–61.
53. Welham R. A. N. and Henderson P. Results of dacryocystorhinostomy: Analysis of causes for failure. *Trans. Ophthalmol. Soc. UK* 1973; **93,** 601–9.
54. Welham R. A. N. Canalicular obstructions and the Lester Jones tube. What to do when all else fails. *Trans. Ophthalmol. Soc. UK* 1973; **93,** 623–32.
55. Jones B. R. The surgical cure of obstruction in the common canaliculus. *Trans. Ophthalmol. Soc. UK* 1960; **80,** 343.
56. Jones B. R. and Corrigan M. J. *Obstruction of the Lacrimal Canaliculi.* (Proceedings of 2nd Corneoplastic Conference.) Oxford, Pergamon Press, 1969, pp. 101–11.
57. Stallard H. B. An operation for epiphora. *Lancet* 1940; **2,** 743.
58. Jones L. T. An anatomical approach to problems of the eyelids and lacrimal apparatus. *Arch. Ophthalmol.* 1961; **66,** 111–23.
59. Henderson P. N. A trephining technique for the insertion of Lester Jones tubes. *Arch. Ophthalmol.* 1971; **85,** 448–50.
60. Saunders D. H., Shannon G. H. and Flanagan J. C. The effectiveness of the pigtail probe method of repairing canalicular lacerations. *Ophthal. Surg.* 1978; **9,** 33–9.
61. Canavan Y. M. and Archer D. B. Long term review of injuries to the lacrimal drainage apparatus. *Trans. Ophthalmol. Soc. UK* 1979; **63,** 201–4.
62. Djacos C. La contamination trachomateuse des canalicules lacrimaux. *Ann. Ocul.* 1950; **183,** 135–41.
63. Coster D. J. and Welham R. A. N. Herpetic canalicular obstruction. *Br. J. Ophthalmol.* 1979; **60,** 259–62.
64. Berlin A. J., Rath R. and Rich L. Lacrimal system dacryoliths. *Ophthal. Surg.* 1980; **11,** 435–6.

Chapter 17

Concomitant and Incomitant Squint

Strabismus

Peter Fells

VISUAL SCREENING AND SQUINT DETECTION

Adults and older children whose eyes cease moving together complain of double vision and visit their doctor. In young children and infants the parents first notice the misalignment of the eyes, which is often intermittent, and then seek advice.

The consequences of strabismus for the development of high visual acuity are profound and early treatment is necessary to avoid poor visual acuity – amblyopia – in the deviating eye. Unfortunately, serious amblyopia can result from unequal focusing – anisometropia – of the two eyes with no strabismus. Therefore, visual screening is necessary and must be earlier and more effective than the present screening by health visitors, well baby clinics and general practitioners. Ideally, all children should be checked at 9 months of age and at 3 years old by orthoptists, and any child with a squint or amblyopia, or a suspicion of these, should be referred on to the ophthalmologist.

Amblyopia (Blunt Vision)

Three main types of amblyopia are recognized:
1. Stimulus deprivation amblyopia, where a formed image cannot reach the retina because the optical path is blocked by ptosis, corneal or lenticular opacity.
2. Strabismic amblyopia, in association with a constant deviation of one eye.
3. Anisometropic amblyopia, where the eyes have unequal refractive powers.

Neurophysiology

In types 2 and 3 ophthalmic examination shows clear ocular media and normal fundi. The problem must arise in the pathways to the visual cortex. A series of brilliant neurophysiological experiments in kittens by Hubel and Wiesel beginning in 1962 has elucidated the mechanisms involved and provided the rationale behind the empirical therapy of human amblyopia.

The striate cortical cells responded to bars or edges in the field of vision, either light or dark, at a particular orientation which were being moved at right angles to their long axis. The cortical cells were classified separately in relation to ocular dominance. Cells driven only by the contralateral eye were group 1, those driven only by the ipsilateral eye, group 7, with five intermediate groups, the group 4 cells being driven equally by either eye. These cortical cells were arranged in columns containing cells that had the same ocular dominance and orientation responses and differed only slightly from adjacent columns (*Fig.* 1).

Interruption of visual input from one eye in the kitten resulted in cortical cells being driven solely by the undeprived eye. The cortical columns from the stimulated eye enlarged as those from the deprived eye shrank and it was proposed that the optic radiations competed for synaptic space on the cortical cell bodies. Visual deprivation in the kitten had these effects from 3 weeks to 3 months of life: this is known as the sensitive period. Experiments with juvenile monkeys show a similar sensitive period.

Work along different lines has shown that there are three different types (W, X and Y) of retinal ganglion cells in cats. Type X cells predominate in the area centralis, have small receptive fields with well developed inhibitional surrounds and respond well to accurately focused targets. As the refractive error and hence the blur increases, the X cell response falls. If one eye is defocused, e.g. by atropinization, or surgical removal of the lens, or surgically induced strabismus in the kitten, this causes inadequate X cell stimulation with poor spatial resolution and amblyopia. Ikeda, Wright and Tremain, who have carried out these experiments, propose that amblyopia is a consequence of retinal blur (*Fig.* 2). Experiments with bilateral atropinization in kittens have reduced spatial resolution in each eye but the ocular dominance histogram remains normal. Alternating strabismus produced surgically preserves normal visual acuity but binocularity is lost. It is important in experiments to distinguish between loss of spatial resolution of retinal ganglion cells and of binocularity in the cortical cells.

The clinical implications of this new neurophysiology are significant. Inequalities of refractive error between the two eyes and high, equal refractive errors must be corrected early in life. Occlusion therapy must be carried out for as short a period as may be expected to give improvement in the acuity of the amblyopic eye and yet avoid the risk of the occluded eye itself becoming amblyopic from lack of visual input. A sensitive period has been identified in children who have responded to occlusion therapy by a temporary switching of amblyopia to the occluded eye. Children show the highest sensitivity during the first 2 years of life, and a decreasing response to occlusion up to 7 years of age.

Management of a Possibly Squinting Infant Child

Parents may notice that their infant's eyes do not move together, either intermittently or constantly. A constant deviation at any age needs ophthalmic examination. An intermittent deviation persisting beyond 4 months of age also demands investigation. Significant facts in the history may be pre-natal, e.g. maternal illness or medication during early pregnancy, premature birth, any instrumentation to assist delivery, any special care, e.g. O_2 therapy immediately after birth. Family history of strabismus or lazy eye in siblings, parents or close relatives is relevant. Siblings of a strabismic child should all be screened. Epicanthic lid folds may present as an apparent squint. Remember that epicanthic folds may coexist with a true esotropia (convergent squint), which is by far the most common deviation. Check that each eye can take up fixation and that temporary occlusion of each eye is acceptable. Avoidance of occlusion of

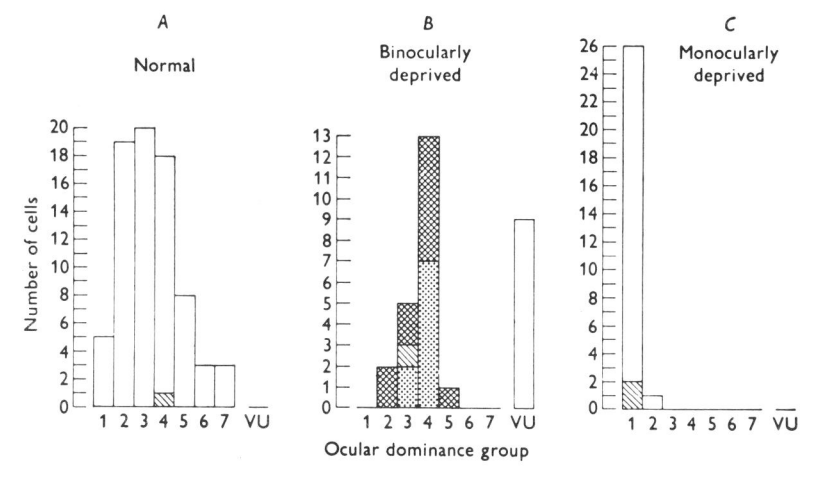

Fig. 1. Ocular dominance histograms of visual cortical cells in kittens showing : *A*, the normal distribution of the seven cell groups; *B*, the similar shape of the histogram when the kitten has been binocularly deprived, indicating that binocular potential has been preserved but there has been a big increase in the number of visually unresponsive (VU) cells. *C*, the monocularly deprived kitten has a completely altered histogram with the cortical cells responding to the experienced eye alone.

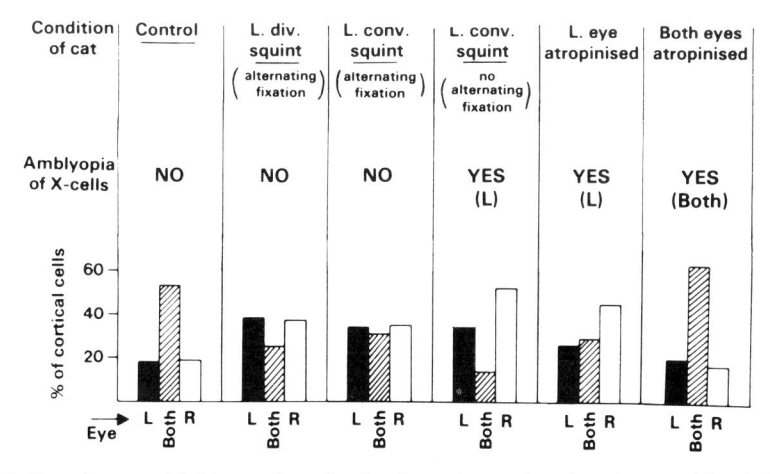

Fig. 2. Experiments with kittens show that in alternating squints there is no amblyopia but a decrease in the cortical cells that can respond to both eyes. Unilateral left strabismus or left defocusing produces left amblyopia and a reduction in cortical cells responding to left ocular stimulation. Bilateral atropinization caused bilateral amblyopia but the cortical cells maintained binocularity.

one eye is good evidence that that eye is the preferred one and that the squinting eye is amblyopic. No objection to occlusion of either eye in a seeing child suggests each eye can fixate adequately.

The esotropic infant may not abduct either eye fully but uses the in-turned eye to cross-fixate objects on its opposite side. This strategy appears to be in the interests of economy of ocular movements, the infant merely switching attention from one eye to the more deviant one without any change in ocular position. If the infant will not follow a target to demonstrate abduction then doll's head rotation should be used, where the infant fixates on the examiner's face as the head is rotated to either side. If necessary the eye on the side of the direction of rotation may be temporarily occluded by the examiner's hand to make the other eye abduct. Full abduction only needs to be elicited once to know that the lateral rectus and its nerve are intact. Whole body rotation with the infant held at arm's length and rotated around the doctor induces nystagmus with the fast phase in the direction of the infant's rotation. If quick phase nystagmus can be induced by rotation to either side by the vestibular input, there cannot be bilateral VIth nerve palsies. When infant rotation ceases, the induced nystagmus should stop with no more than one or at most two beats post-rotation showing good visual inhibition of the vestibulo-ocular reflex.

Next the ocular media, fundi and refraction must be checked. With most children cycloplegia with cylopentolate 1 per cent drops, one to each eye and repeated after 5 min, with examination after 20 min, is usually adequate. (Some doctors always use Oc. atropine 1 per cent twice daily for 4 days immediately before seeing the child for the first refraction in any child up to 3 years of age. Others reserve atropine for uncooperative patients or those with high degrees of hypermetropia or who give inconsistent results with cyclopentolate.) When refracting the young child it is helpful if one parent goes to the 6 metre position to act as fixation target. Whichever cycloplegic is used, allowance is made for the working distance only, usually $\frac{2}{3}$ metre for children, often $\frac{1}{2}$ metre for infants. No allowance is made for any cycloplegic used as residual ciliary muscle tonus is a myth.

Spectacles are rarely used before one year of age unless there are more than two dioptres of anisometropia. If astigmatism is present but equal in the two eyes, glasses are not used before 2 years old. Myopia, unless greater than two dioptres, is not corrected before 2 years old. Hypermetropia of more than two dioptres is corrected after one year of age in esotropic patients as it reduces the deviation. Glasses should have plastic lenses, and fit comfortably or they will not be worn.

Transparency of the ocular media must be assessed and developmental lens opacities looked for. Equal size and colouring of the optic discs is important and optic disc hypoplasia recognized when present. The degree of retinal pigmentation and macular development should be noted.

Equal use of the eyes must be established by repeated examination and use of part-time occlusion therapy. Up to 1 year of age occlusion of 15 min daily is used, with glasses worn if indicated. During the first 4 years any occlusion is best carried out using a patch which adheres over the preferred eye and glasses are worn over this. Light-tight patches eliminating both light and form vision are most effective.

A few children seem quite unable to tolerate facial occlusion despite repeated explanations to parents of its importance. In such cases 'penalization' methods may be used. (The word has overtones of punishment which is unfortunate since it has been transliterated from the French which means 'hindrance'.) A child with dense unilateral amblyopia has G. Atropine 1 per cent used every morning to the fixating eye and glasses giving full refractive correction are worn. Furthermore, the lens for the atropinized, dominant eye is overcorrected by +3 dioptres so that this eye is used only for near and the amblyopic eye is in better focus for all other distances.

Supervision of occlusion therapy until alternation of fixation is achieved is best performed by orthoptists. Any manifest squint when glasses are worn is then dealt with surgically. Orthoptic checking must continue after surgery to ensure that amblyopia does not recur. In children of 5 years or older, once the amblyopic eye has corrected acuity of better than 6/18, spectacle occlusion using a double layer of Blenderm tape on the inside of the spectacle lens may be preferred.

Congenital Esotropia (Infantile Esotropia)

Esotropia which is known to have been present during the first six months of life is accepted as congenital esotropia provided that photographs show an unequivocal convergent squint or the infant has been seen to be esotropic by the ophthalmologist. Many, if not all, of these congenital esotropes will develop latent nystagmus and dissociated vertical divergence (DVD) by 2–3 years of age. When one eye is occluded the uncovered eye makes nystagmoid jerks with the fast phase towards the uncovered side. When the occluder is removed, the previously covered eye is seen to make recovery movements from its position of elevation and extorsion by downward rotation of the eye plus intorsion movements. There is no nystagmus with both eyes uncovered but in the older child the DVD may become apparent spontaneously in the non-dominant eye and present as a cosmetic defect.

There is still disagreement about the timing of surgical intervention in constant squints. Many ophthalmologists believe that if the eyes can be made straight by surgery before the second birthday, or at least to within ten prism dioptres of straight, there is the possibility of normal binocular single vision developing. Others claim that a residual microstrabismus of up to eight prism dioptres persists and that only a compromised form of binocular single vision with anomalous correspondence of the two eyes can be achieved. The problems of such early surgery, on a patient less than 2 years old, are gaining accurate examination and measurements of the eyes on which to base the operation. In addition, if more than one operation is necessary to straighten the eyes, then all the surgery must be performed before the second birthday.

Exotropia

In exotropia the treatment is usually less urgent because most divergent squints are intermittent, of exotropia recession of the lateral rectus and resection of the medial rectus of the divergent eye is advised. Surgery should aim to correct the squint exactly in the visually immature, that is, up to 6 years old. After that age a slight overcorrection of the exotropia by ten prism dioptres gives the best long term results as the resultant diplopia is a powerful stimulus to fusion in the immediate postoperative period.

A- and V-Patterns

Unfortunately, neither eso- nor exotropia are always of equal extent away from the primary position. When the horizontal separation of the eyes decreases on down gaze this is called a V-pattern (*Fig.* 3). Obviously a V-pattern of esotropia (V-ET) becomes

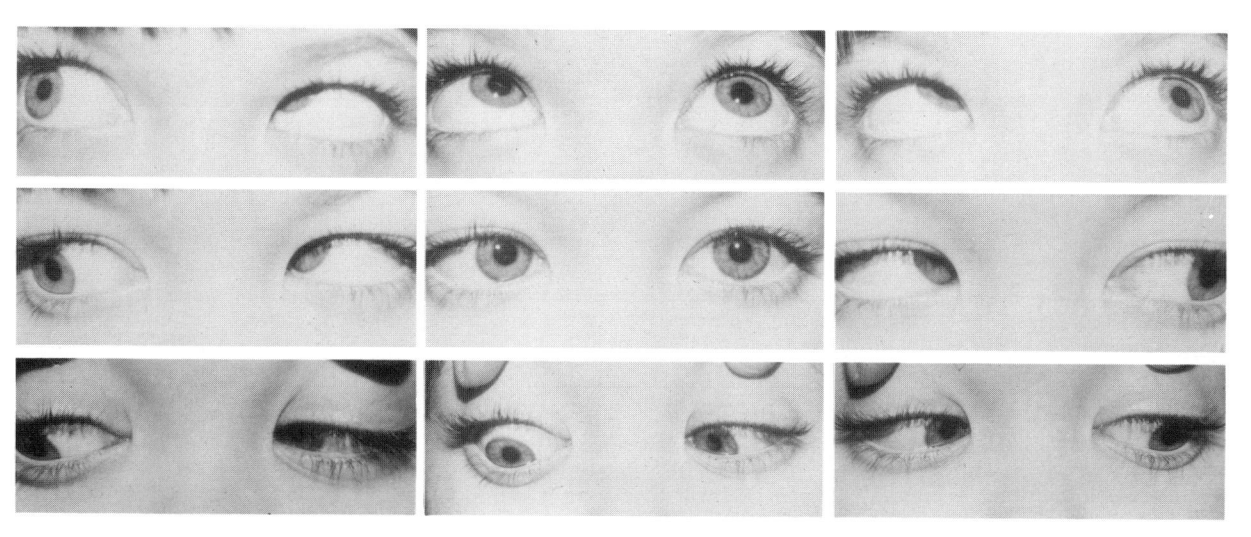

Fig. 3. V-pattern of esotropia. Note the overelevation of each eye on side gaze due to inferior oblique overactions.

being manifest for the distance, or far distance beyond 6 metres, but controlled for near. As long as the eyes are being used together for near work, normal binocular reflexes are being established and treatment is not urgent. If the distance exotropia is 30 prism dioptres or more it is highly likely that surgical treatment will prove necessary but first refraction must be corrected, and any tendency to suppression of the deviating eye overcome by part-time occlusion of the preferred eye. If the refraction shows low to moderate hypermetropia no glasses are necessary as the subject's focusing effort helps to control the deviation. If there are four dioptres or more of hypermetropia then glasses must be worn and the angle of exotropia manifest through the glasses corrected surgically. Any myopia when corrected with spectacles will help to control the divergent deviation. For true divergence excess, where the distance divergence is much larger than for near, and the near deviation is not increased when accommodative convergence is largely eliminated by the use of +3 dioptre lenses over each eye, bilateral recessions of the lateral rectus are carried out. For all other forms

worse on down gaze, whereas a V-pattern of exotropia (V-XT) shows better control of down gaze. If the horizontal separation of the eyes increases on down gaze this is an A-pattern of strabismus (*Fig.* 4). A-pattern of esotropia (A-ET) is better on down gaze, but A-pattern of exotropia (A-XT) is worse on down gaze.

The two important conditions are those that become worse on down gaze (V-ET and A-XT) since these patients may look good and even be straight in the primary position but have a manifest squint on down gaze. When the patient is examined looking down it may be necessary to hold up the lids to reveal any misalignment of the eyes in the important reading position. The vast majority of A- and V-patterns are due to abnormal insertions of the oblique muscles which commonly show considerable variation from the anatomically averaged positions that are quoted in textbooks as the standard. The line of muscle action of the superior oblique, from trochlea to insertion, is quoted as being at 54° to the vertical plane and at 51° for the inferior oblique. Measurements in 122 human cadavers by Fink showed that the variation for the superior oblique was between 20° and 71° with an average of 45°. The inferior oblique measurements ranged from 32° to 70° with an average of 45·5°. When the oblique muscle pair act along the same line they rotate the eyeball around an axis at right angles to their line of pull and lying in the horizontal plane (*Fig.* 5). If the inferior oblique is inserted very posteriorly, i.e. at an acute angle to the anteroposterior plane, and the superior oblique is inserted anteriorly at a wide angle to the anteroposterior direction, the plane containing their common axis around which the oblique pair work is tilted upwards at the medial end. Clinical confirmation of this fact is readily gained by observing the posterior pole of the fundus and seeing that the optic disc is higher than the fovea. Visual field testing in older patients shows that the blind spot is lower than normal. These features typify the V-pattern.

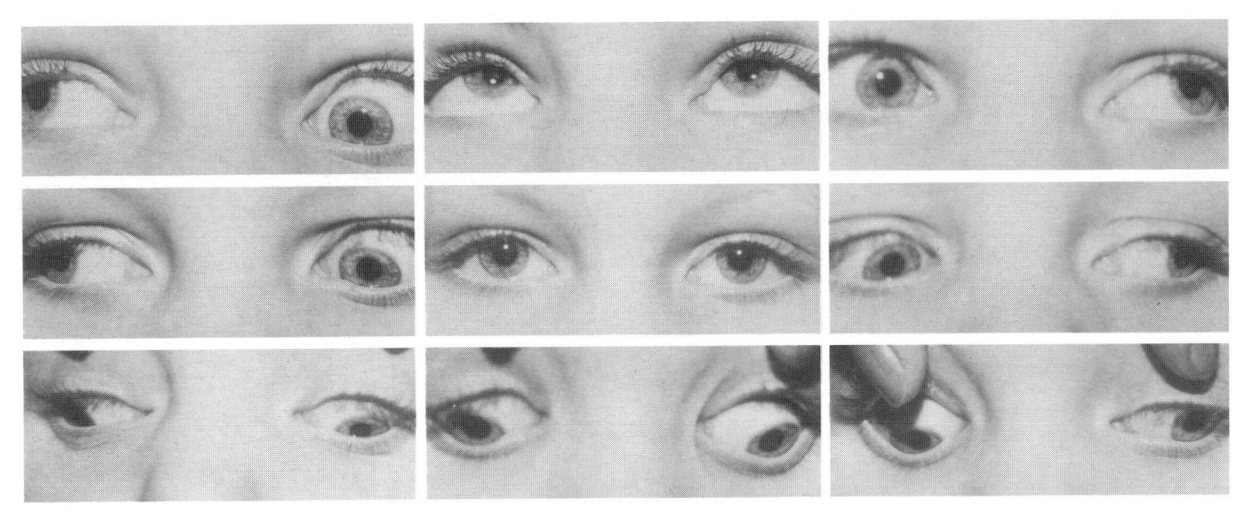

Exactly the reverse is found in A-patterns with the superior oblique attached very posteriorly and the plane containing the common oblique pair axis being tilted downwards at the medial end. Surgical correction of a V-pattern must include bilateral recessions of the overacting inferior obliques plus appropriate horizontal rectus surgery at the one operation. For A-patterns the superior obliques must be weakened either by disinsertion of the posterior three-quarters of the tendon, or for severe cases by superior oblique tenotomies nasal to the superior rectus plus the indicated horizontal rectus surgery. Up to 25 per cent of apparently concomitant horizontal squints have significant A- or V-patterns of ocular movement.

Accommodative Esotropia

Some children only begin to squint at 2½–3 years of age when they start to look more closely at small objects. The esotropia is brought about by accommodation but the overconvergence due to accommodation may begin at any age from 9 months to 7 years. Full (cycloplegic) correction of the hypermetropia will permit the eyes to be used binocularly at all distances. However, some children will have correction of the squint at distance by glasses for hypermetropia, but will still overconverge for near. These children have an abnormally high ratio of accommodative convergence to accommodation (AC/A ratio) so that the unusually high gearing of their near reflex produces excessive convergence for the usual 3 dioptres of accommodation for near. If the child is 5–6 years old he may be helped by the wearing of bifocal glasses. Although formulae using the near and distance esotropia measurements and the interpupillary distance allow calculation of the necessary near addition, in practice equal strength plus lenses are added to each side of the trial frame containing the distance correction until control of the deviation at near to an accommodative target is attained. It is rare for the addition to need to be as high as +3·00 dioptres each eye.

Because the child has an accommodative range of some 12 dioptres there is no incentive to use the bifocal part of the lens, as there is for a presbyopic adult. Consequently the glasses must be of the 'executive' type with the horizontal line separating near and distance correction being as high as the lower pupillary border with the eyes in the primary position. The glasses must stay in this position during normal activities and not slip down the nose. The ultimate test is to raise the child's book as he reads and note that his chin automatically elevates to maintain binocularity as he uses the bifocal addition. Over the next few years the child should be refracted every 6 months and checked to see if the bifocal addition can be made weaker. It is not worth reducing the addition by less than 0·5 dioptres each side. Every endeavour must be made to keep full hypermetropic correction in the distance segment as this, too, keeps the 'add' to a minimum.

If no reduction in the 'add' is possible by 8½ years of age then surgery of bimedial rectus recessions should be performed, since the aim is for full control of the esotropia with single focus glasses by 10 years old. The possibility of later surgery after several years of bifocals leads some surgeons to offer surgery as soon as it is apparent that the full hypermetropic correction does not eliminate esotropia for near. Either bimedial rectus recessions, or bilateral Faden operations to the medial recti (posterior fixation sutures), or a combination of both, may be recommended.

Phospholine iodide drops, 0.06 per cent, may be used every morning for a few weeks in a child whose esotropia seems to be almost controlled for near by the glasses for hypermetropia alone and are then 'tailed off' slowly over the next 3 weeks. Occasionally this will establish control of the esodeviation at all distances. Phospholine iodide drops are not used long term because of the risks of iris cyst formation and possibly of cataracts. These drops also cause a serious depletion of the pseudocholinesterases in the blood and if succinylcholine is used prior to intubation in general anaesthesia there may be prolonged depression of spontaneous respiration. Phospholine iodide drops may be helpful in the immediate postoperative period if there is a small residual esotropia for near despite medial rectus recessions.

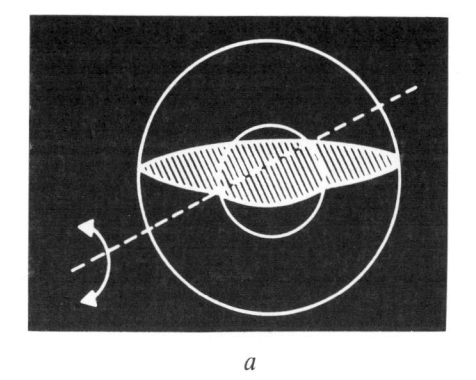

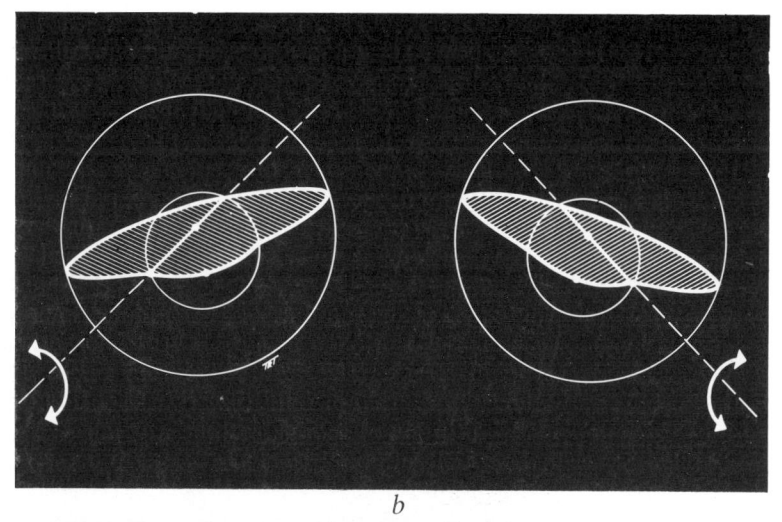

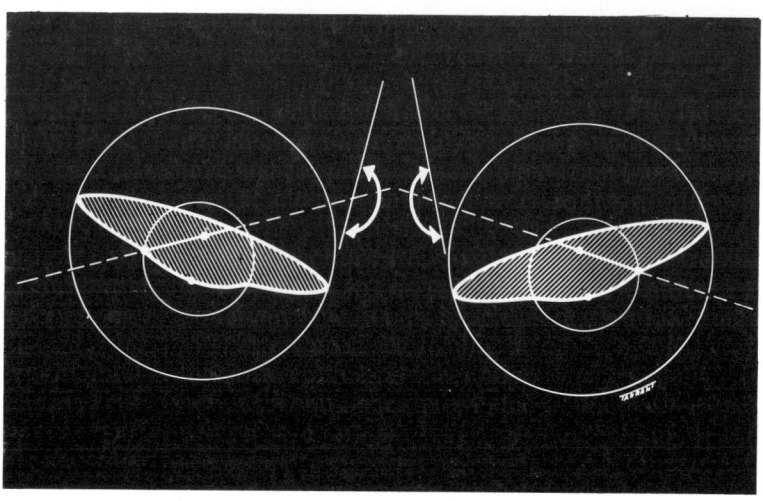

Fig. 5. *a*, Right eye from in front showing the horizontal plane (shaded) which contains the common axis around which the oblique muscle pair rotate the globe. *b*, When the plane containing the common axis is tilted upwards at its medial end the V-pattern of ocular movements results. *c*, If this plane is tilted downwards at its medial end A-pattern movements are seen.

Abnormal/Compensatory Head Postures

Some parents may notice that their child adopts an unusual position of the head whenever detailed vision is required. It is always worth observing the child's behaviour while the history is being taken as there may be a suggestion of an abnormal head posture when the child is unaware that he is under scrutiny. Many infants will not show an abnormal head posture (AHP) until they have been walking for some months. An AHP that appears immediately an infant sits up suggests cervical vertebral anomalies, such as hemi-vertebrae.

Although there are several other causes of AHP in children, such as unilateral deafness, enlarged or tender cervical lymph nodes, or rarely torticollis due to a tight sternomastoid muscle on one side, ocular movement abnormalities are by far the most common. These are best demonstrated by asking the child strives subconsciously to maintain binocular single vision by putting the eyes into their most advantageous position. Always describe an AHP in terms of face *turn*, head *tilt* and chin *tip*.

The older child of 8 or 9 years may have learned to keep the head straight at the cost of less satisfactory vision, e.g. a child with congenital nystagmus and highest acuity with a face turn to one side may appear to have a normal head posture until he is asked to read down the test chart at 6 metres. To obtain best vision the face turn has to be adopted to an increasing extent for the smaller optotypes. Ideally, surgery to the ocular muscles to reduce and occasionally abolish an AHP should be completed before the fifth birth-

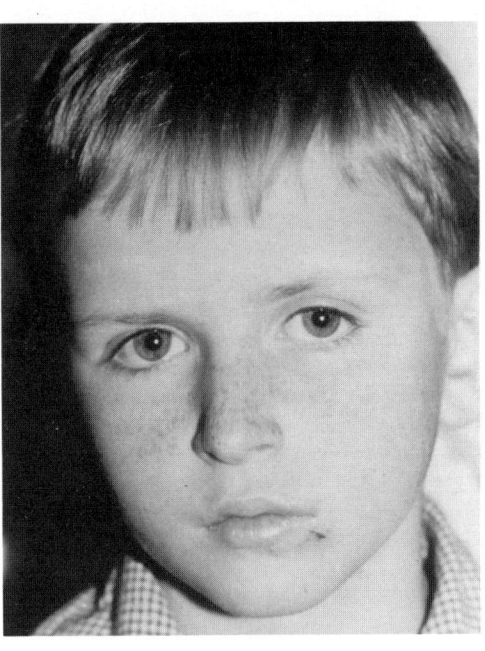

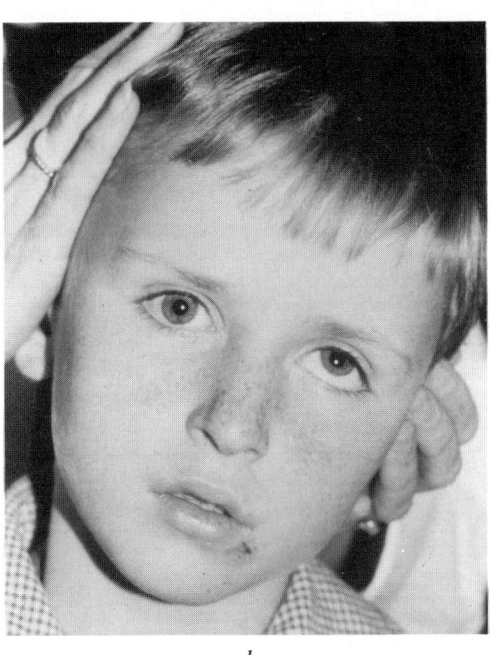

Fig. 6. *a*, Compensatory head tilt to the right with chin depression and slight face turn to the right in a child with left superior oblique palsy. *b*, When the head is forcibly tilted to the left the necessary left intorsion can be generated by the left superior rectus only as the other left intorter is palsied. As a result, unopposed overelevation of the left eye occurs. This is called the Bielschowsky head tilt test.

to stand up to attention, e.g. pretending to be a soldier, with feet together pointing towards the observer and arms by the side and certainly not reaching backwards to lean on mother. The observer is directly in front of the child and is kneeling or squatting so that his eyes are at the same level as the child's. This is the easiest and most repeatable way of disclosing an AHP. Perusal of the family photograph album often serves the same purpose of revealing a preferred head position. The child with an abducent palsy or typical Duane's syndrome will have a face turn towards the side of deficient abduction. A consistent tilt of the head towards one shoulder may give the clue to a developmental trochlear nerve palsy of the opposite side so that the head is tilted towards the lower, or hypotropic, eye (*Fig.* 6).

Depression of the chin in a V-pattern esotropia, or A-pattern exotropia may be seen as the child day if permanent cervical growth changes are to be avoided. An uncorrected AHP in childhood means painful cervical symptoms are more likely in early middle age.

OCULAR MUSCLE PALSIES

These may be present at birth or become apparent in the early years of life. Developmental palsy is a better name than the usual congenital palsy, which strictly means present at birth. These childhood palsies have no clear-cut beginning but parents may notice an intermittent squint, particularly when the child looks to one side, and also an AHP. When a developmental palsy begins to decompensate in middle life the patient may have diplopia whenever he looks in a particular direction and find that reading is easier with one eye closed. These features contrast sharply with the acquired ocular palsy, where sudden onset of diplopia with an easily noticeable squint sends the patient to seek urgent medical advice.

The aetiology of developmental ocular palsies is not understood but there is certainly a familial pattern in some cases. There are many causes of acquired ocular palsies and these may be classified in various ways, e.g. according to the pathological process involved, or with reference to the anatomical site, such as the nerve nucleus, or its nerve fibres, the neuromuscular junction or the muscle itself. The long course of the cranial ocular motor nerves makes them vulnerable at several sites, e.g. in the interpeduncular fossa by an aneurysm of the posterior communicating artery, or by basilar meningitis. Within the cavernous sinus the association of particular nerve involvements allows the sinus lesion to be placed posteriorly or anteriorly. At the orbital apex there is additional involvement of the optic nerve and sometimes proptosis.

The possible pathological headings to consider are:

1. Trauma, which typically causes disruption of the ocular motor nerve fibres as they leave the brain stem, but may also produce intraneural haemorrhage or direct ocular muscle haematoma and bruising.

2. Vascular, e.g. thrombosis, haemorrhage or aneurysm.

3. Inflammatory, which may be immunological or infective, e.g. multiple sclerosis, Gradenigo's syndrome where inflammation of the petrous part of the temporal bone involves the ipsilateral VIIth, VIth and Vth cranial nerves.

4. Metabolic, e.g. diabetes mellitus, thiamine deficiency.

5. Toxic, e.g. lead, botulinus toxin.

6. Neoplastic, e.g. glioma, pituitary tumour, orbital metastases.

7. Degenerative, e.g. progressive external ophthalmoplegia.

Mechanical Restriction

In addition to the above processes which may prevent normal muscle contraction, mechanical restrictions may reduce the range of ocular rotations. A fibrotic reaction in a muscle may tether the globe by stopping the normal relaxation and extension of the muscle as the other member of the muscle pair contracts. This is typically seen in thyroid ophthalmopathy where a tight inferior rectus prevents the expected elevation of the eye as the superior rectus muscle contracts. Alternatively, the fibrous connective tissue septa of the orbit may have become trapped, as in an orbital wall blow-out fracture, and limit the full movement of the globe.

Developmental Ocular Muscle Palsy

Duane's Retraction Syndrome

Classically these children have absent or severely limited abduction of the left eye with a compensatory face turn to the same side. The right eye may be similarly but less often affected, and bilateral involvement is rare. On attempted gaze to the affected side the palpebral aperture widens, while gaze to the opposite side produces narrowing of the palpebral fissure plus retraction of the globe (*Fig. 7*). Adduction of the affected eye may be reduced or normal. The visual acuity is often normal or only slightly reduced on the involved side with good quality fusion and stereopsis except on looking to the affected side where suppression usually prevents diplopia. A marked compensatory face turn leads to cervical symptoms in adult life and surgical correction is often advised to reduce this. The medial rectus has a

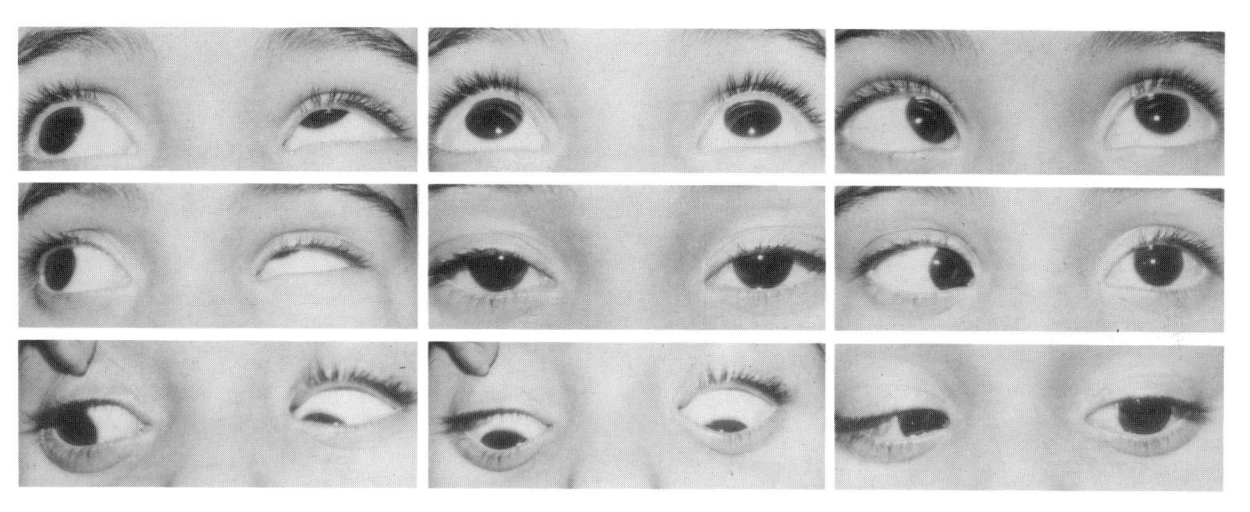

Fig. 7. Left Duane's retraction syndrome showing failure of left abduction with widening of the palpebral fissure on attempting to look left and narrowing of the palpebral fissure on right gaze. Note the abnormal vertical position of the left eye when looking up and right, and down and right, due to the tight lateral rectus.

3·5 mm recession combined with temporal transfer of the whole of the vertical recti, preferably by five years of age. Recent work suggests that in some cases the involved lateral rectus receives dual innervation by both the VIth and IIIrd nerves. There is an atypical Duane's syndrome where adduction is more limited than abduction and is associated with exotropia and a face turn towards the opposite side.

Developmental VIth Nerve Palsy

This is less common than Duane's syndrome although the condition is often erroneously suspected in congenital esotropia. In congenital esotropes abduction can usually be demonstrated by doll's head rotation of the infant, or by whole body rotation that induces nystagmus. Surgical treatment, after appropriate occlusion therapy for amblyopia, is the same three-muscle operation as for Duane's syndrome, but it is often carried out at an earlier age.

Developmental IVth Nerve Palsy

This may present as a face turn and tilt away from the affected side to allow the eyes to work together. Such patients may appear to have a V-pattern of esotropia but careful testing reveals truly unilateral inferior oblique overaction on the involved side. After correction of refractive error and amblyopia, surgery to the horizontal muscles plus unilateral inferior oblique recession is required.

When developmental trochlear palsy becomes decompensated in older patients, vertical surgery only may be needed. This would be ipsilateral inferior oblique recession plus inferior rectus recession of the opposite eye using an adjustable suture.

Developmental IIIrd Nerve Palsy

This may be complete or partial. If complete the ptotic lid needs opening by a sling to the frontalis muscle to prevent stimulus deprivation amblyopia. At a later stage, at about 3½ years of age, a definitive ptosis repair can be performed (*Fig.* 8). Because so many extraocular muscles are supplied by the oculomotor nerve the best that may be achieved is straight eyes in the primary position but there will be abduction, and intorsion with depression from continued action of lateral rectus and superior oblique muscles respectively.

If the palsy is only partial it may be possible to produce a small, central field of binocular fixation. Oculomotor palsy beginning during the first 2 years of life may produce the rare condition of IIIrd nerve palsy with cyclic spasms where the ptosis varies, being least when the pupil is miosed and becoming a complete ptosis that covers a dilated pupil with a cycle of approximately 2 min. This cyclic condition becomes less marked over the years and more like a total oculomotor palsy.

Brown's Syndrome

This was formerly called superior oblique tendon sheath syndrome. These children have failure of elevation in adduction of the right eye more often than the left, and sometimes bilaterally. Their parents may complain of the overelevation of the unaffected eye (*Fig.* 9). In severe cases an AHP of chin elevation is adopted. Study of the natural history of the condition shows that from 7 to 10 years of age the condition becomes painful with localized tenderness and 'clicking' over the involved trochlea. This phase appears to be part of the spontaneous recovery that occurs in most patients, with usually complete resolution by 15 years of age. A few children with severe forms of the syndrome and an AHP, or those with such downdrift of the affected eye on looking to the opposite side that fusion is impossible except down and to the same side, may require surgery at 4 or 5 years. A positive traction test confirms the diagnosis and the superior oblique tendon is severed at the nasal

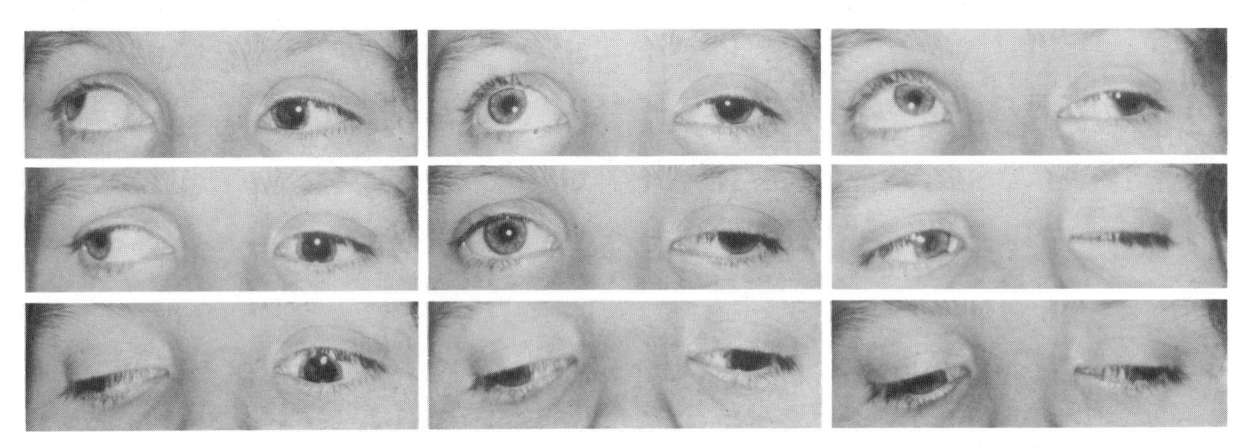

Fig. 8. Left IIIrd nerve palsy with very reduced vertical movements and only partial medial rectus action is preserved. The left ptosis becomes worse on left gaze but the left lid elevates on right gaze with maximal retraction appearing on dextro-depression. This indicates misdirection–regeneration of the IIIrd nerve. Note the dilated left pupil.

side of the superior rectus giving a normal traction test. In some of these patients a superior oblique palsy develops over the next 6 months, necessitating inferior oblique recession.

from a tight medial rectus and poor depression from superior rectus fibrosis are the next most often restricted rotations. Poor elevation and abduction have long been attributed erroneously to superior rectus

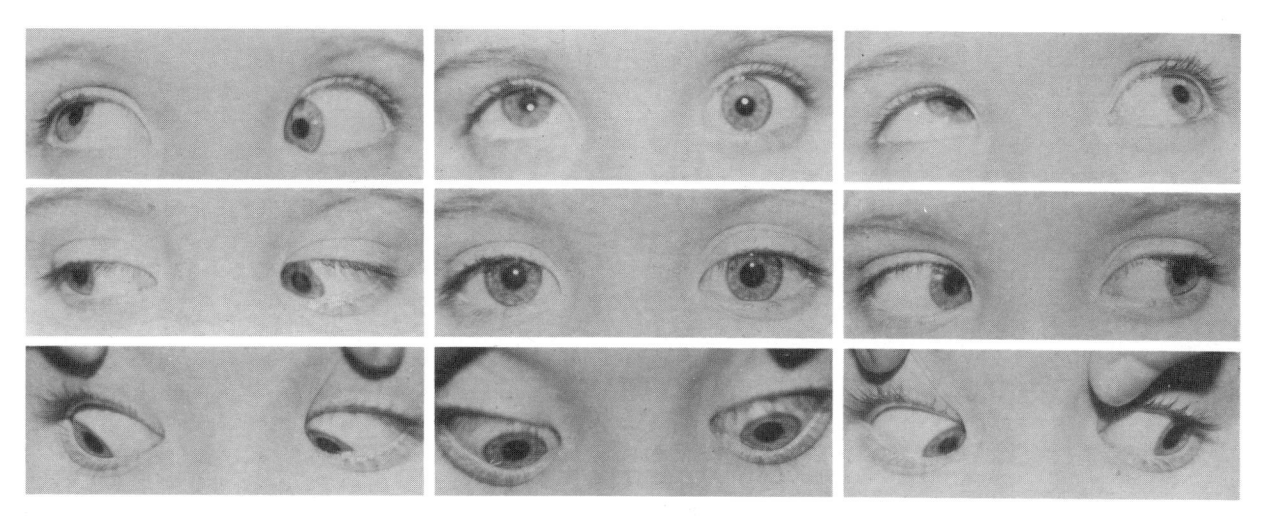

Fig. 9. Left Brown's syndrome. The left eye cannot elevate in adduction but has virtually full laevo-elevation. Note the downdrift of the left eye on dextroversion. The superior oblique produces normal depression in adduction.

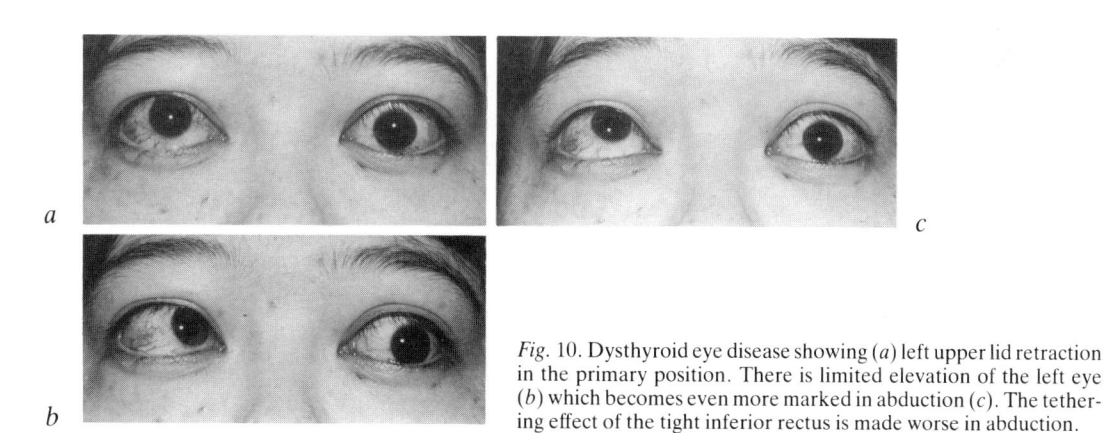

Fig. 10. Dysthyroid eye disease showing (*a*) left upper lid retraction in the primary position. There is limited elevation of the left eye (*b*) which becomes even more marked in abduction (*c*). The tethering effect of the tight inferior rectus is made worse in abduction.

Strabismus Fixus

This is a rare congenital condition with the eyes fixed in esotropia bilaterally. Surgery is difficult because disinsertion of the medial rectus has no effect but allows access to the deep, solid fibrous bands anchoring the eyes in adduction, which have to be severed.

Adult Mechanical Restriction of Ocular Rotations

Dysthyroid Eye Disease

Dysthyroid eye disease may present as diplopia of gradual onset, often with an AHP of chin elevation (*Fig.* 10). There may be associated hyperthyroidism, past or present, but not necessarily so, and there need never have been proptosis at any stage. Decreased elevation, due to inferior rectus tethering, is the most frequently affected movement. Reduced abduction

and lateral rectus weakness respectively. Surgical treatment at the right time is by recession of the fibrosed muscle(s), preferably using the adjustable suture technique, once any hyperthyroidism has been controlled and overtreatment into *hypo*thyroidism avoided.

Orbital Floor Fractures

In orbital floor fractures with an intact rim – blow out fractures – the failure of elevation is not due to a trapped inferior rectus but to tethering by radially running orbital fibrous tissue septa. The not infrequently reduced depression of the involved eye may be due to direct injury of the inferior rectus muscle or its nerve, but this is not yet proved (*Fig.* 11). Provided enophthalmos is less than 3 mm and the ocular rotations are showing objective improvement and there is no retraction of the affected globe on attempted up gaze, surgical intervention is not indicated. The patient is encouraged to make vertical ductions to keep orbital fibrosis and scarring to a minimum.

When there is retraction on attempted up gaze and no improvement of ocular movements, surgical exploration of the orbital floor via the skin of the lower lid is indicated and subperiosteal exposure of the fracture in the orbital floor. Herniated orbital contents are returned to the orbit and silicone sheeting is shaped to cover the whole orbital floor and inserted beneath the periosteum. Postoperative duction exercises are still necessary.

Acquired Brown's Syndrome

This condition results from broken windscreen injuries to the trochlea and superior oblique tendon

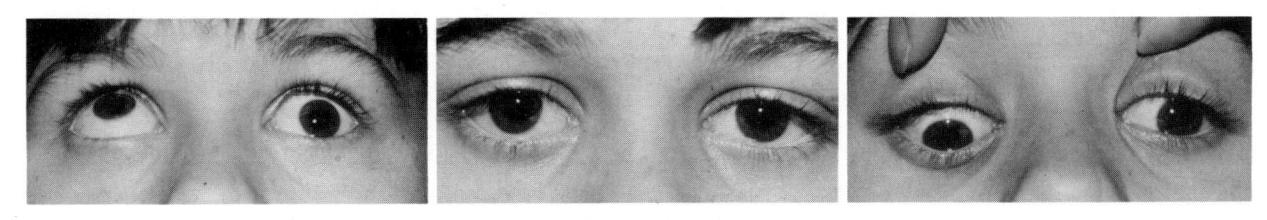

Fig. 11. Left orbital floor blow-out fracture with minimal enophthalmos but severely limited elevation and depression of that eye.

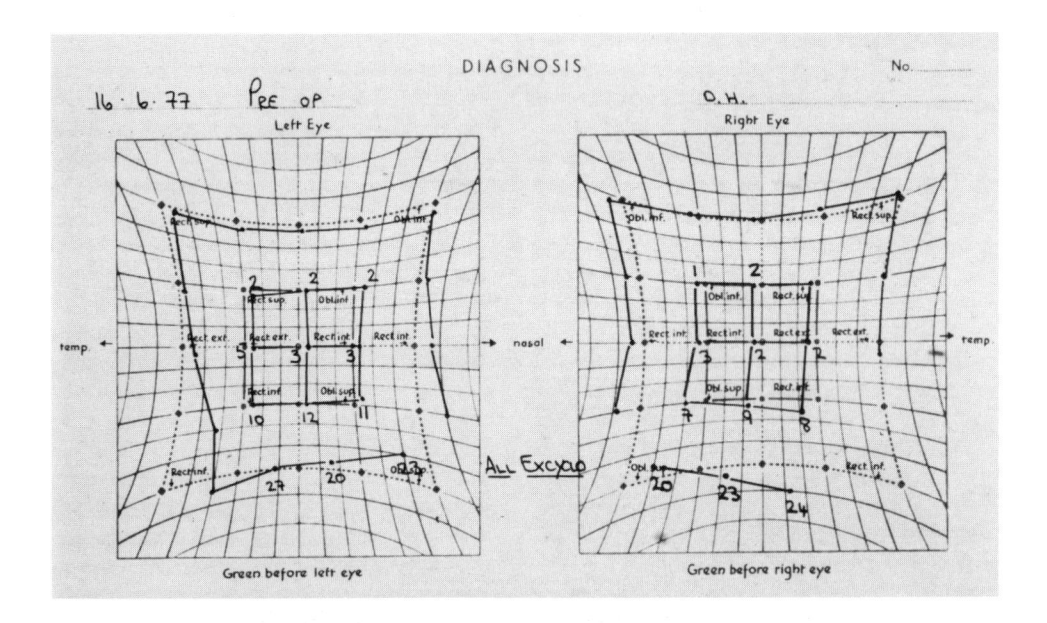

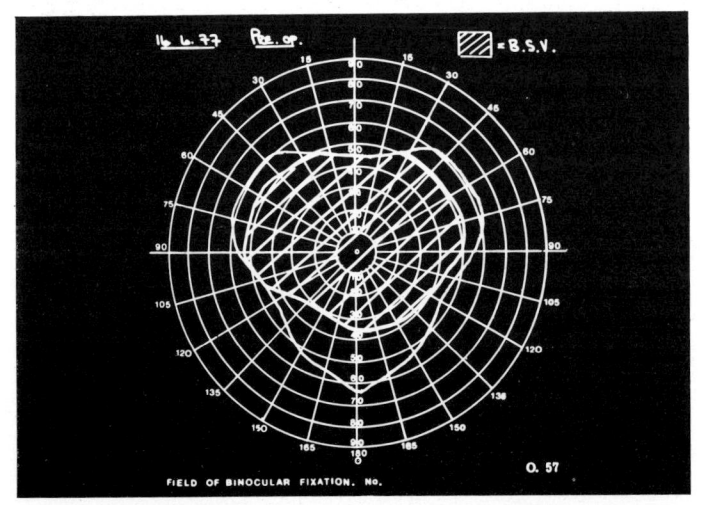

a

and, less often, from screwdriver or similar localized orbital trauma. Removal of glass foreign bodies from the trochlea rarely if ever improves elevation in adduction. Simultaneous superior oblique tenotomy and ipsilateral inferior oblique recession give the best hope of improvement.

Acquired Ocular Muscle Palsies

In addition to each of the ocular motor nerves being affected individually by various pathological processes, trauma may cause bilateral VIth nerve palsies or bilateral IVth nerve palsies, or even all four nerve palsies together. Surgical treatment of total VIth nerve palsies in patients over 20 years of age needs Jensen's procedure to avoid anterior segment ischaemia. Surgery to three rectus muscles of the same eye usually interferes with the blood supply unless the adjacent halves of longitudinally split superior and lateral recti are sutured together at the equator with similar surgery to adjacent halves of the split lateral and inferior recti. At the same time the medial rectus usually needs a small recession.

Traumatic Bilateral IVth Nerve Palsies

These are particularly disabling as torsional diplopia results, which may easily be misdiagnosed by a neurologist as 'functional' or 'compensitis'. Special orthoptic measurements of torsion are essential in diagnosing these cases (*Fig.* 12). Even though fusion may not always be demonstrable in such patients, surgical advancement of the anterior half of both superior oblique insertions gives very good results in the majority of cases.

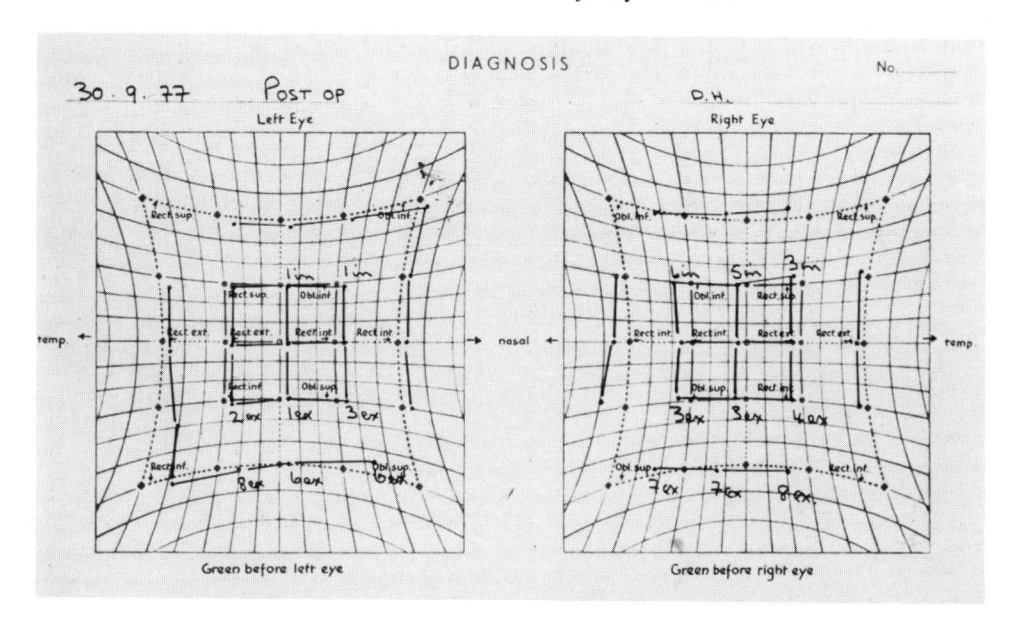

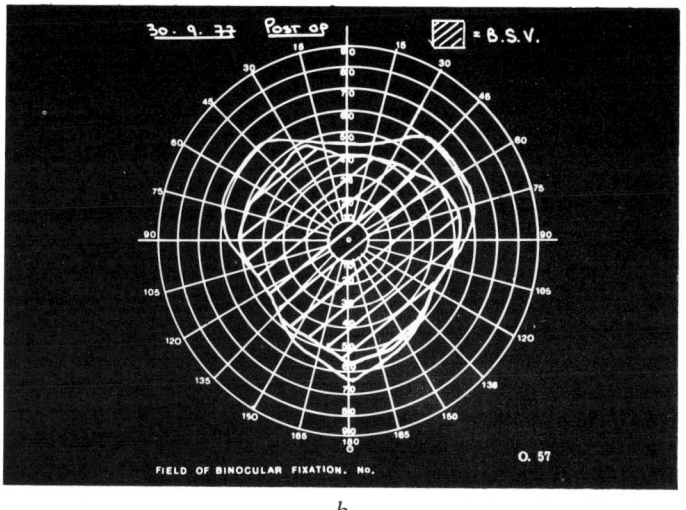

Fig. 12. *a*, Hess chart of a patient with bilateral IVth nerve pareses plotted at the Lees screen using the T-piece modification to the pointer to allow torsion to be measured as well. The field of binocular fixation is limited on down gaze by the severely disabling torsional diplopia. *b*, Hess chart and field of binocular fixation after surgery to the superior oblique muscles to restore intorsion on down gaze.

Orthoptics

Although every effort is made to try to establish the cause of acquired ocular motor palsies and give appropriate treatment to conditions such as hydrocephalus in children, or hypertension or diabetes in adults, it must be admitted that diagnoses are made in less than half of all cases. The role of the orthoptist is particularly important in their management because most ophthalmologists merely diagnose the involved ocular muscle(s). The orthoptist makes measurements of the size of the deviation and of any remaining fusion. Prism cover tests are useful in the primary position but synoptophore measurements in the nine gaze positions are most informative and can include torsional assessment. Even more helpful is the Hess or Lees screen showing the relative excursions of the two eyes, particularly when combined with the modified pointer to give very accurate torsional deviations too. At each visit the field of binocular fixation is plotted using an adapted Lister perimeter. These vital measurements give objective, numerical evidence of the ocular movements that can readily be repeated serially to show any recovery or other changes with time.

Many acquired palsies show improvement within 3 months which may continue over a total of 6 months. During this waiting period the orthoptist instructs the patient about the best head posture to adopt to relieve diplopia, aided when necessary by Fresnel prisms on glasses. If the deviation is too large for these methods, the affected eye is occluded. Once the orthoptic tests show that the ocular state has been stable for a minimum of 3 and usually 6 months muscle surgery may be offered. This will be first to the affected eye and later any residual diplopia may be reduced by operating on the overacting muscles of the fellow eye to give the maximum field of binocular cooperation.

REFERENCES

*Blakemore C. Maturation and modification in the developing visual pathway. In: Held R., Leibowitz H. W. and Teuber H. L. (ed.) *Handbook of Sensory Physiology*, vol. VIII: *Perception.* Springer-Verlag, Berlin 1978, p. 437–488.
Burian H. M. and von Noorden G. K. *Binocular Vision and Ocular Motility*, 2nd ed. St Louis, Mo, Mosby, 1980.
Fells P. The treatment of non-comitant strabismus. In: van Balen A. Th. M. and Houtman W. A. (ed.) *Documenta Ophthalmologica Proceedings Series 32*. The Hague, Junk Publishers, 1982, pp. 197–207.
*Vaegan, Arden G. B. and Fells P. Amblyopia: some possible relations between experimental models and clinical experience. In: Wybar K. C. and Taylor D. (ed.) *Paediatric Ophthalmology*. New York, Marcel Dekker, 1983, pp. 291–312.

* These chapters contain many references to the important work by Hubel and Wiesel, and by Ikeda, Wright and Tremaine.

The Ocular Motor System

M. D. Sanders and T. J. K. Leonard

Many neurological lesions produce abnormalities of eye movements, and clinical recognition of specific eye movement disorders may facilitate diagnosis. In addition, accurate examination may produce precise neurological localization.

INTRODUCTION

The perfect functioning of the binocular visual system of primates depends upon a complex anatomical framework and a number of finely tuned coordinating systems. The fovea of each eye must be directed at the object of regard to obtain optimum visual acuity and binocular single vision. Refixation of new targets by saccades or tracking of moving objects by pursuit movements require the two eyes to be moved harmoniously in the same direction. Binocular single vision of objects moving towards or away from the observer may require the eyes to move in opposite directions and result in convergence or divergence. Saccadic, pursuit and vergence systems are each served by sub-systems with different anatomical and physiological features.

In addition, during head or body movement, compensatory ocular movements are made to prevent slipping of the retinal image and visual blurring. Head movements prompt compensatory vestibular ocular movements. Sustained turns or tilts of the head do not disturb binocular vision since the optokinetic system produces compensatory ocular movements through the otolithic pathways.

ANATOMICAL AND PHYSIOLOGICAL SUBSTRATES OF OCULAR MOTOR CONTROL

History

Bender[1] reviewed the early history of clinicopathological correlation of eye movement disorders. In 1858 Foville[2] postulated the existence of a control centre in the pons for horizontal gaze. Thirty years later, Parinaud,[3] in a series of classic papers, correctly designated the quadrigeminal plate as the site of vertical gaze disorders associated with pupillary anomalies. Post-morten findings of tuberculomas in various locations supplied much information concerning the organization of eye movements. These lesions were gross yet produced specific eye movement anomalies. The evolution of computerized tomography and magnetic resonance imaging has enabled us to localize in the living patient cerebral lesions that may be correlated with clinical signs. Eye movement recordings calibrate clinical findings, anatomical tracer substances provide histological information and microelectric stimulation techniques provide useful neurophysiological information. Localization of long standing disease of the ocular motor systems remains difficult, however, even with sophisticated investigative techniques, because of the remarkable adaptive capability of the neural system and, in particular, the cerebellum.

Basic Mechanisms of Conjugate Ocular Movement

Our interpretation of ocular motor control mechanisms has been enhanced by biomedical engineers and neurophysiologists with original concepts of the mechanism of the generation and control of eye movements. This information, gained from experimental work in primates with computer analogues, shows that in the generation of saccades a 'pulse step' innervational pattern is necessary.

The *saccadic pulse* is an eye velocity command which generates a high frequency phasic change in innervation to move the eye rapidly from one position to another against orbital viscous forces. The *saccadic step* is an eye position command that generates the new level of innervation at the end of the saccade to hold the eye in its new position against restoring orbital elastic forces.

This concept of a coding for the eye velocity command (pulse) and the eye position command (step) is useful in the interpretation of disorders of the ocular motor system. There is sound neurophysiological evidence for this pulse–step coding of all conjugate ocular movement.[4]

The saccadic pulse is thought to be generated by 'burst cells' in the pontine and mesencephalic reticular formation. Burst neurones are so called since they produce high frequency discharge commencing just before a saccade. Burst cells therefore initiate a saccade, which moves the eyes rapidly to the desired position.

An appropriate innervation signal (step) is now required to hold the eyes in the new position. The step signal is produced from a second group of specialized cells in the pontine reticular formation – the tonic cells. In order for eye position and velocity movements to be closely coordinated, some form of integration is necessary.

A mathematical concept is useful to explain how the appropriate step signal is derived from the saccadic velocity or pulse signal. It is thought that a neural network, probably existing in the perihypoglossal nuclei of the rostral medulla,[5] acts as a neural integrator, though the flocculus of the cerebellum is also important.

The Ocular Motor Pathways

Horizontal and vertical ocular movements are generated in the brain stem and influenced by supranuclear pathways and the cerebellum.

Brain Stem Organization of Horizontal Eye Movement

On each side of the midline between the levels of the IVth and VIth nerve nuclei lie a collection of neurones termed the paramedian pontine reticular formation (PPRF), or pontine gaze centre. The PPRF contains specialized cells for the generation of the pulse and step components of conjugate ocular movement. Velocity commands from the burst cells

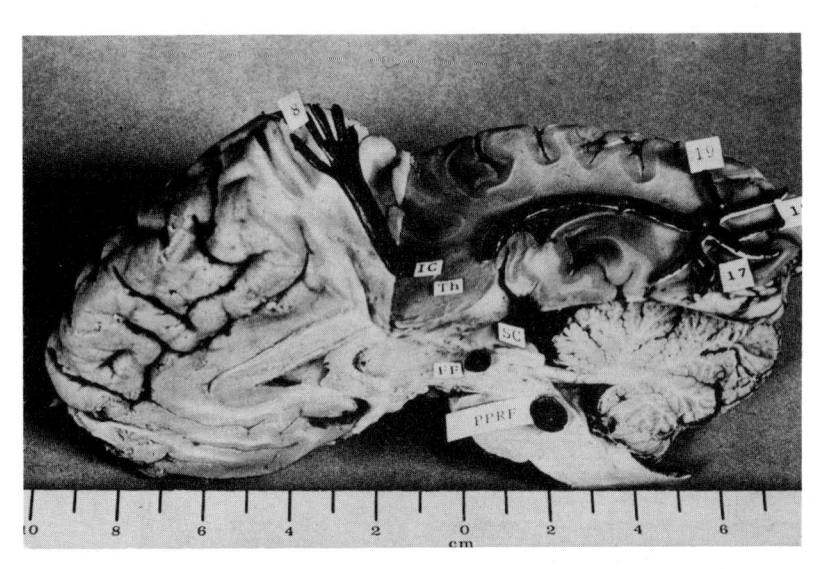

Fig. 1. The descending pathway from the frontal eye fields is seen passing to the anterior limb of the internal capsule (IC). The occipital pathway subserving visual pursuit passes round the posterior horn of the lateral ventricle into the posterior portion of the internal capsule. These two pathways descend under the thalamus (Th) to pass to the paramedian pontine reticular formation (PPRF) in the superior colliculus (SC).

A third class of neurone within the pontine reticular formation – the pause cell – is also concerned with saccadic eye movement. Pause cells are so called from their ability to arrest saccades by inhibiting burst cells. The relationship between burst cells, tonic cells and pause cells is shown in *Fig.* 1.

The generation of vergence movement is poorly understood. Recently Mays[6] has described cells lateral to the IIIrd nerve nuclear complex which discharge according to the angle of vergence. Buttner-Ennever[7] has demonstrated, with elegant tracer techniques, an accessory population of small motor neurones alongside the IIIrd nerve nucleus which may also be relevant to vergence movement.

In summary, conjugate eye movements require a pulse–step coding. The signals are generated in specialized cells in the brain stem. Disjunctive eye movements are generated differently and there is some evidence that neurones adjacent to the main IIIrd nerve nucleus may be responsible.

are projected to the ipsilateral VIth nerve nucleus which contains two types of neurones – abducens motor neurones and abducens internuclear neurones.

The abducens motor neurones supply the ipsilateral lateral rectus muscle. The internuclear neurones project through the medial longitudinal fasciculus (MLF) to the medial rectus division of the contralateral IIIrd nerve nucleus. The abducens nuclei, as Foville had suspected, contain the final common pathway for conjugate eye movements. VIth nerve nuclear lesions, not surprisingly, cause failure of ipsilateral conjugate gaze with loss of horizontal saccadic, pursuit and vestibular movement. Vergence, however, is unaffected.

Brain Stem Organization of Vertical Ocular Movements

Certain areas of the rostral midbrain are associated with the synthesis of upward and downward saccades.

Although termed nuclei, these areas should be considered as collections of neurones rather than as specific anatomical entities.

Burst neurones in the dorsal midbrain are important, particularly in the region of the posterior commissure, the interstitial nucleus of Cahal and the nucleus of Darkschewitsch. Descending neurones have been identified from the nucleus of Cahal to bilateral IIIrd and contralateral IVth nerve nuclei. Unilateral lesions in this region cause bilateral failure of upward saccades.

Failure of downward gaze in the monkey may be produced by bilateral lesions of the area known as the rostral interstitial nucleus of the MLF.[8] Bilateral collections of neurones are situated medially near the third ventricle in the prerubral field at the junction of the midbrain and thalamus. Projections from the RIMLF to the ipsilateral IIIrd and IVth nerve nuclei relay information for downward saccades.

Although burst neurones in these areas generate vertical saccadic movements, important ascending tracts from the PPRF may influence normal function. Bilateral pontine disease may therefore be associated with slow vertical saccades.

Vertical pursuit and vestibular movements are generated in the PPRF and ascend to the midbrain through the MLF. Vertical pursuit and vertical vestibular optic reflexes are thus affected by lesions in the PPRF and MLF.

In summary, the generation of horizontal and vertical eye movements is localized to the brain stem. Horizontal conjugate movements are synthesized in the PPRF and require an intact VIth nerve nucleus for normal function. While vertical pursuit and vestibular movements originate in the PPRF, vertical saccades are generated more rostrally in specialized groups of cells but are influenced by input from the PPRF. The bilateral integration of normal horizontal and vertical eye movements in the brain stem requires an intact medial longitudinal fasciculus.

Supranuclear and Vestibular Influences on Conjugate Ocular Movement

The inputs to the brain stem centres for generation of conjugate ocular movements are complicated and incompletely understood. Certain aspects are known, however, and have a clinical relevance.

Supranuclear Influence on Saccadic Eye Movement

More than one hundred years ago, Ferrier[9] had established the existence of frontal eye fields (FEF) in area 8 of the cerebral cortex. The ipsilateral FEF contain neurones which, when stimulated, cause contralateral horizontal saccades. Vertical saccadic movements require a bilateral output from the FEF.

For control of saccadic eye movement the important output from the FEF is a descending tract to the anterior limb of the internal capsule (see Fig. 1).

A diffuse ocular motor decussation of the descending tract occurs between the levels of the IVth and VIth nuclei with the principal component terminating in the PPRF. Subsidiary pathways may also be in existence.

For practical purposes, clinical evaluation of the supranuclear horizontal saccadic movement involves the pathway from the FEF of either side to the contralateral PPRF. Vertical saccadic deficits cannot be lateralized since the supranuclear input to the rostral brain stem premotor centres is bilateral.

Pursuit Movements

The pursuit system is phylogenetically recent and only assumes importance in primates. Damage to the parieto-occipital association cortex (area 7) impairs smooth pursuit to the ipsilateral side. Input to the ipsilateral area 7 is from the visual cortices of both sides, which contain neurones that respond to moving stimuli. A descending pathway gains the posterior limb of the internal capsule to reach the ipsilateral PPRF. Lesions of this pathway may affect the adjacent visual radiation in the parietal lobe, causing contralateral hemianopia with loss of ipsilateral pursuit movements.[10]

Pathways from area 7 project to the frontal eye fields, the deeper layers of the superior colliculi and the pretectal nuclei.[11] Supranuclear horizontal pursuit disorders suggest a lesion involving descending pathways from area 7 to the brain stem. Vertical pursuit requires a bilateral input and disorders cannot be localized by ocular motor examination.

Superior Collicular Influence on Ocular Movement[12]

The superior colliculus in primates is rather less important for eye movement control than in other species. Destruction of the superior colliculi in monkeys produces various ocular motor deficits including saccadic dysmetria, and reduced frequency of spontaneous saccades.

Vestibulo-ocular Reflex (VOR)

A normal VOR is essential for optimum visual function. Even transmitted resting cardiac pulsation requires small compensatory eye movements to prevent slip of the retinal image and visual blurring.

Fortunately, visual processing through the retina is slow ($\simeq 70$ msec) so the vestibulo-ocular reflex (<12 msec), mediated through the movement of endolymph in the semicircular canals, allows sufficiently prompt compensatory eye movements to occur. Signals from the canals are projected to the ipsilateral vestibular nuclei.

Vestibular eye movements, like saccades, are composed of both a velocity component (the pulse) and a tonic component to maintain eye position (the step). The velocity-coded component must be integrated with head movement velocity, a process which is incompletely understood. During pursuit movements of slow moving targets with the head also moving, the VOR must be cancelled. VOR cancellation is not yet fully understood but may represent a separate ocular motor control system.

The Cerebellum

In 1664 Thomas Willis suggested that the cerebellum might control involuntary movements. Sherrington[13] noted that the cerebellum related to posture and did not initiate movement, and therefore considered the cerebellum to be the most important 'ganglion' in the proprioceptive system. Currently, neurophysiologists and neuroanatomists are attempting to delineate specific control areas in the cerebellum for various eye movements.

The central lobe of the cerebellum or vermis is of major importance. A series of lobules is divisible into anterior, middle and posterior portions. The middle portion of the cerebellum, consisting of lobules V to VII, contains cells that help control eye movements concerned with non-visual feedback, such as auditory stimuli. The cells here fire during saccades and lesions cause specific dysmetria and flutter-like ocular movements. Some evidence suggests that midline lesions cause vertical dysmetria, while lateral lesions cause horizontal dysmetria. The more anterior the lesions, the more the dysmetria occurs on up gaze, while the more posterior lesions accentuate dysmetria in down gaze.

The posterior portion of the vermis is responsible for visual monitoring of ocular movement: that is, tracking a moving target, maintenance of accurate fixation on a target, optokinetic response, maintenance of eccentric gaze and VOR suppression. All these functions require visual input.

Lateral outpouchings of the vermis – the flocculi – contain cells that are activated by tracking movements. If only the flocculi are removed in monkeys, the clinical signs mimic those seen with posterior fossa lesions in humans.

EXAMINATION OF THE OCULAR MOTOR SYSTEM

Adequate clinical examination of the ocular motor system must always be preceded by the taking of a careful history, an examination of the visual system and a full neurological examination. Neurological signs may provide localizing or diagnostic information. Drug therapy, particularly anticonvulsants and tranquilizers, may also produce abnormal changes.

By testing the saccadic, pursuit, vestibular and vergence movements systematically, it may be possible to localize the site of the responsible lesion.

Saccadic Movements

The patient must be asked to fixate two targets alternately. A pen held in one hand and the raised finger of the other should suffice as targets. Horizontal and vertical saccades are evaluated by asking the patient to look from the finger to the pen on command (*Fig. 2a*).

The velocity and accuracy of saccades is important. The speed of initiation and any overshoot (dysmetria) must be considered. Apraxic movements of the head, to compensate for inadequate saccades, should be noted.

Smooth Pursuit Movements

A fixation target of approximately 2 cm in diameter, attached to a wand, should be used and held some 40 cm from the face. The patient should be instructed to follow the target smoothly in horizontal and vertical directions. The target should be moved slowly, and the speed of movement gradually increased, until the smooth pursuit movement is broken up, due to physiological intrusion of saccades (*Fig. 2b*).

Broken up pursuit, corrective compensatory saccades or any nystagmus should be noted. Accurate tracking of a moving target should occur in a normal individual with conjugate smooth pursuit movements.

Optokinetic Nystagmus (OKN)

The optokinetic tape or drum is useful, particularly when saccadic or pursuit abnormalities are mild. Care should be taken not to hold the drum or tape too close to the patient and thus induce convergence.

The target should be moved or rotated slowly and the patient asked to count the picture or stripes to ensure adequate concentration (*Fig. 2c*). A pictorial representation may produce a better response than stripes, particularly in children. Optokinetic responses do not give an accurate guide to visual acuity.

Vergence Movements

Convergence movements may be simply tested by asking the patient to approximate his own finger from arms length to just beyond his nose. Reading material may also be used. In addition the patient is asked to look from a distant fixation target to his own finger. Measurements of convergence are made possible by the use of prisms, lenses or the synoptophore.

Doll's Head Movements

With the patient fixating a target, the head is rotated and a slow pursuit movement should culminate in the eyes being in an extreme position of either horizontal or vertical gaze. This indicates the functioning of the vestibulo-ocular system (*Fig. 2d*).

Vestibulo-ocular Reflex

This reflex is tested by asking the patient to fixate a target which moves in harmony with the head.

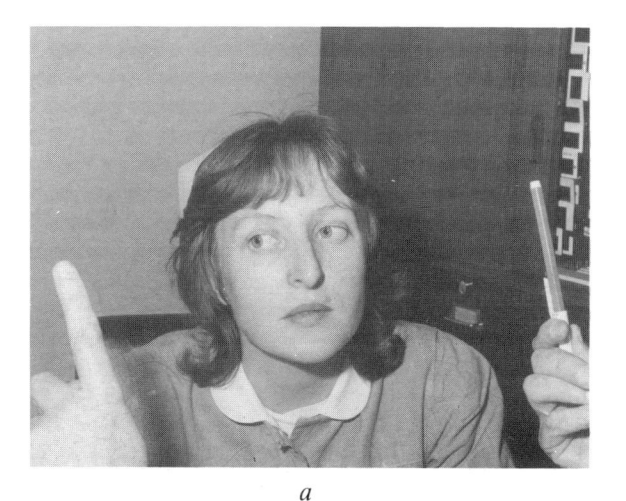

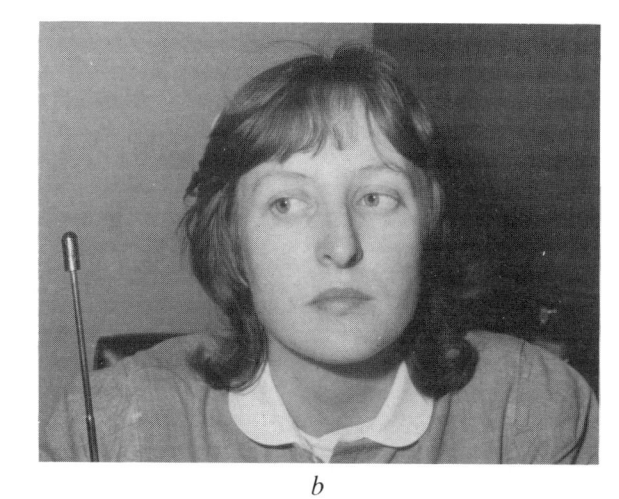

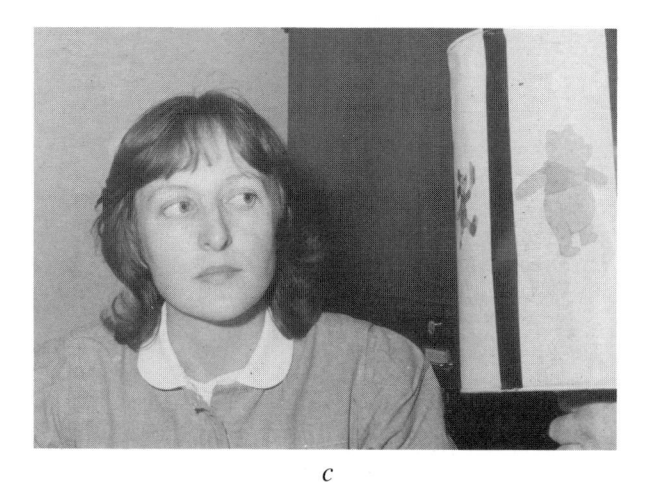

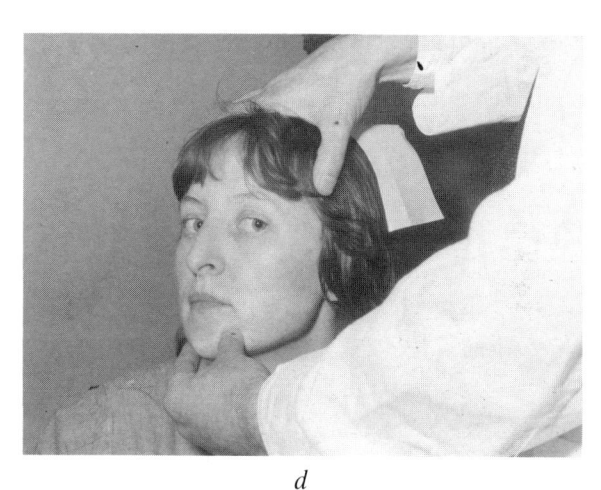

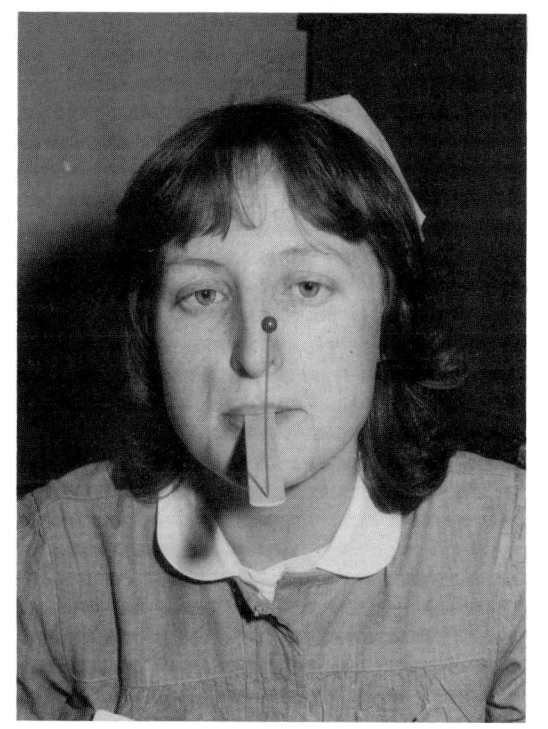

Fig. 2. Testing of saccadic eye movements. *a*, It is important to gain normal values for the velocity of eye movements from one point to another. This method can also be used in the vertical plane. *b*, Smooth pursuit. The eye should smoothly pursue a target up to about 40° per second. After this, voluntary saccadic movements are added. Within this range, however, jerky pursuit movements should be noted. *c*, Optokinetic nystagmus. The patient is asked to observe a rotating drum which initiates pursuit movement in the direction of the drum and a saccadic movement in the opposite direction. In the detection of cerebral lesions an abnormality is noted when the drum rotates towards the side of the lesion. *d*, Doll's head manoeuvre. Here the head is turned to the right with the eyes obtaining a full excursion to the left. *e*, Fixation of a target is obtained and when the head is straight the eyes should remain fixated on the target. Abnormal results occur when the eyes deviate and make microsaccadic movements.

Normally the eyes would deviate in the opposite direction, but with the fixation target the normal vestibular responses have to be inhibited. For practical purposes this can be done with a spatula gripped between the teeth with a fixation target on the end of the spatula (*Fig. 2e*).

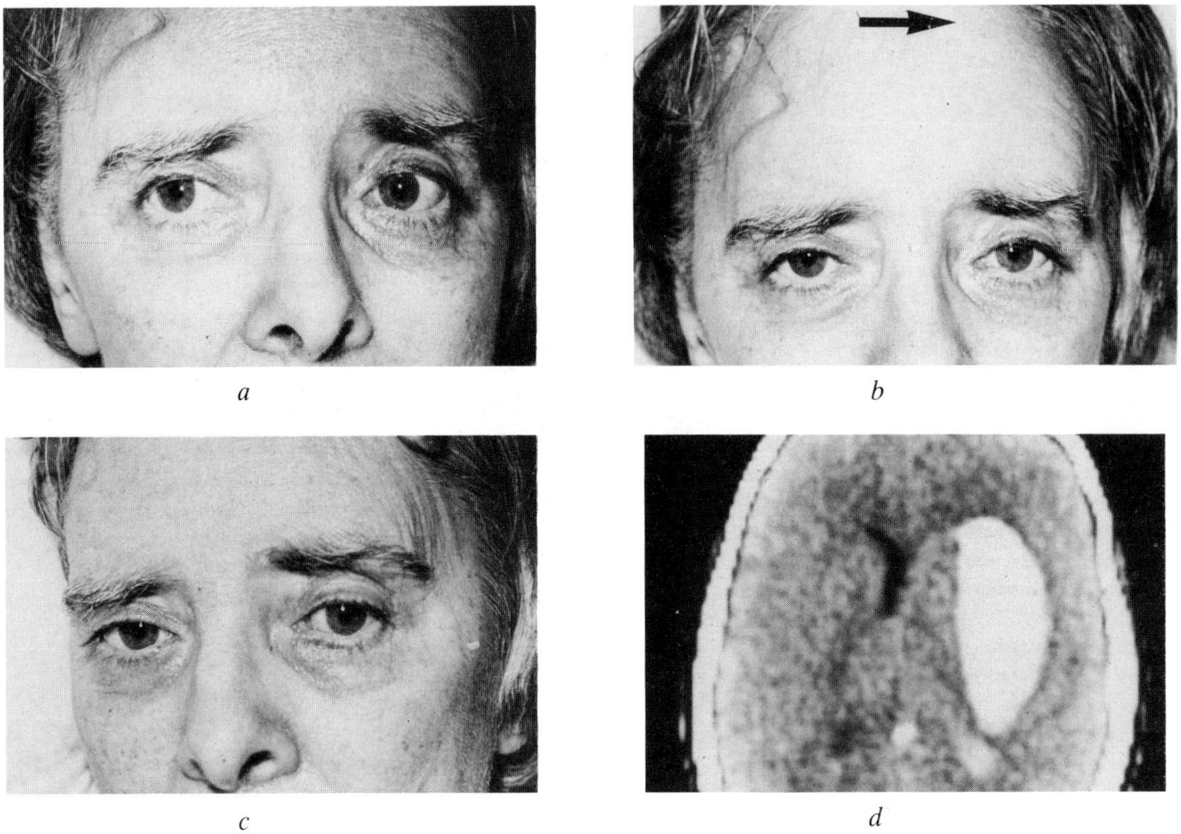

Horizontal Movements

Frontal Gaze Palsy (Supranuclear)

A frontal supranuclear gaze palsy is usually seen after an acute frontal insult such as frontal haematoma or infarct, often traumatic. The eyes are deviated

Fig. 3. Frontal gaze palsy. *a*, This elderly woman presented with eyes deviated to the right. Voluntary and command movements were unable to produce a movement to the left. Movements could not be elicited by voluntary suggestion (*b*). Doll's head manoeuvre, however, showed that a full range of gaze to the left could be elicited (*c*), indicating the supranuclear nature of the disorder. CT scan (*d*), shows a large haematoma in the right fronto-parietal region.

Abnormalities of saccadic, pursuit or vestibular movements indicate whether an ocular motor problem is supranuclear, internuclear or infranuclear.

DISORDERS OF THE OCULAR MOTOR SYSTEM

Disorders of Saccadic Eye Movement

Abnormalities of saccadic eye movements include (*a*) supranuclear gaze palsy; (*b*) total gaze palsy (pontine); (*c*) partial gaze palsy and/or slow saccades and (*d*) dysmetria. These may be analysed in terms of disorders of the saccadic pulse, saccadic step or a mismatch of pulse and step signals. For example, dysmetric saccades are caused by a change in amplitude of the saccadic pulse, reflecting disease in the dorsal vermis of the cerebellum.

to the side of the lesion, because of the inability to generate contralateral saccades. Contralateral gaze may, however, be induced by pursuit, Doll's head movements or caloric stimulation (*Fig. 3*). Chronic horizontal gaze palsy may be an early sign of conditions such as Huntington's chorea, Wilson's disease and adult Gaucher's disease.

Pontine Gaze Palsy

A pontine gaze palsy may be total or partial. A total pontine gaze palsy demonstrates ipsilateral loss of conjugate gaze to saccades, pursuit, OKN and vestibulo-ocular and caloric testing (*Fig. 4*). The chronic condition, which is precipitated acutely by infarcts, haemorrhages and, occasionally, demyelinating disease, may be seen with infiltrating conditions such as glioma and secondary tumours. Facial nerve involvement is usual, and the ophthalmologist should assess convergence, which is usually intact due to the integrity of the midbrain.

A partial gaze palsy may be due to any of the above causes but sufficient neural tissue remains to allow restricted movements. Thus saccades, though present, may be reduced in either amplitude or velocity. Saccades that are reduced in range may be of normal velocity, but may be associated with a slow gaze paretic type of nystagmus. Slow saccades may be interpreted as a disorder of the burst cells.

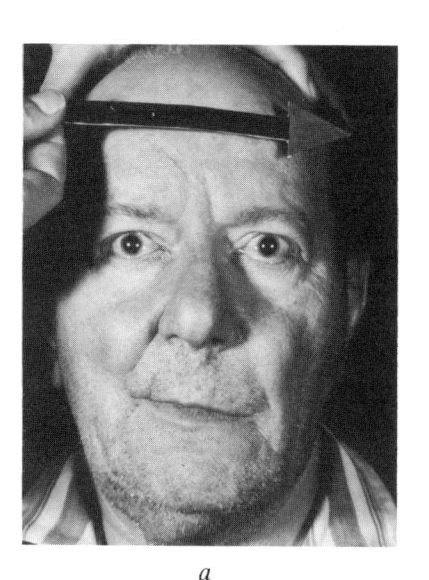

3. Refraction abnormalities due to a reduction in the amplitude of accommodation.
4. Pupillary light–near dissociation (*Fig. 5*).
5. Papilloedema due to obstruction of the aqueduct of Sylvius.

The lesions responsible for these signs are most frequently related to the pineal gland, and include teratomas or pinealomas. However, gliomas, vascular malformations, trauma and secondary tumours may all present in this manner.

The presumed mechanism for the signs is down-

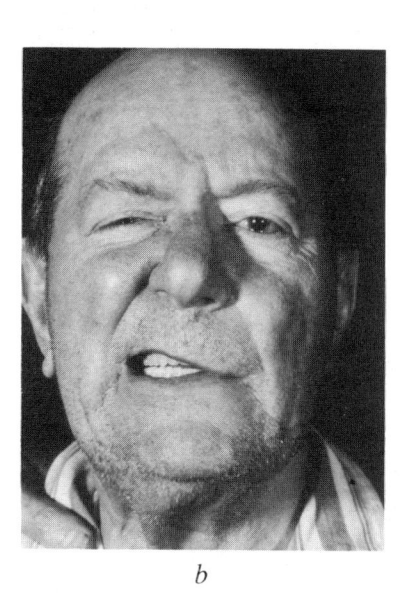

Fig. 4. Total pontine gaze palsy. *a*, This elderly man presented with an acute left pontine infarct. He was unable to move the eyes to the left by command, by pursuit, by Doll's head manoeuvre or by caloric measures. *b*, In addition, this was associated with the left facial palsy.

Vertical Movements

The absence, reduction in amplitude or in velocity of vertical saccades reflects disease in the rostral midbrain, and the ophthalmologist may play a crucial role in diagnosis.

Sylvian Aqueduct Syndrome, Parinaud's Syndrome, Dorsal Midbrain Syndrome or the Koerber–Salus–Elschnig Syndrome

The variety of eponyms and anatomical terms, though confusing, serves to emphasize the importance in recognizing this syndrome. Characteristically occurring in children and young adults, lesions in this region produce a variety of important neuro-ophthalmic signs, any of which may be the presenting feature. They include:

1. Loss of elevation to saccades, but later also pursuit and vestibular ocular responses.
2. Convergence retraction nystagmus on attempted elevation of the eyes (best demonstrated with a downward rotating OKN drum).

ward pressure on the posterior commissure area where the premotor centre for upward saccades and pupillary light–near fibres are in close proximity.

Progressive Supranuclear Palsy (PSP or Steele–Richardson–Olszewski Syndrome)

This is a degenerative condition of elderly patients with a poor prognosis and characteristic ocular motor findings. The patient cannot make downward saccades and finds difficulty in reading. Later upward and horizontal saccades are also involved before pursuit is affected (*Fig. 6*). Ocular vestibular responses remain intact, indicating the supranuclear nature of this disorder. Neurones in the basal ganglia and midbrain degenerate. Eventually, muscle rigidity sudden falls and dementia occurs.

Ophthalmoplegic Lipidosis

Similar ocular motor abnormalities to PSP are seen in ophthalmoplegic lipidosis, a progressive neurological disease of young children. Compensatory move-

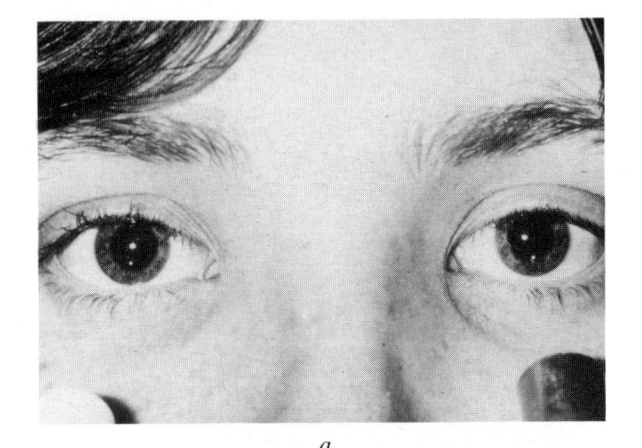

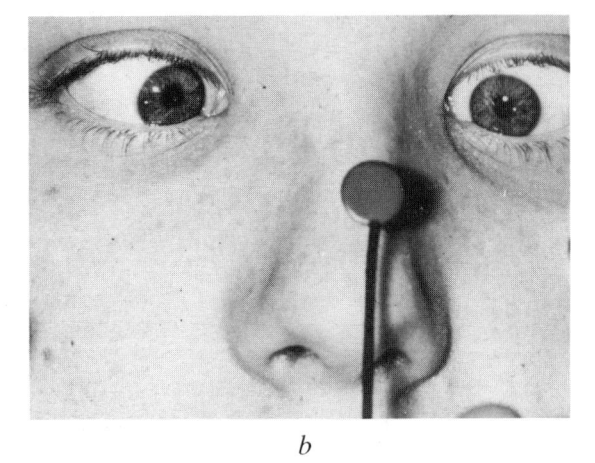

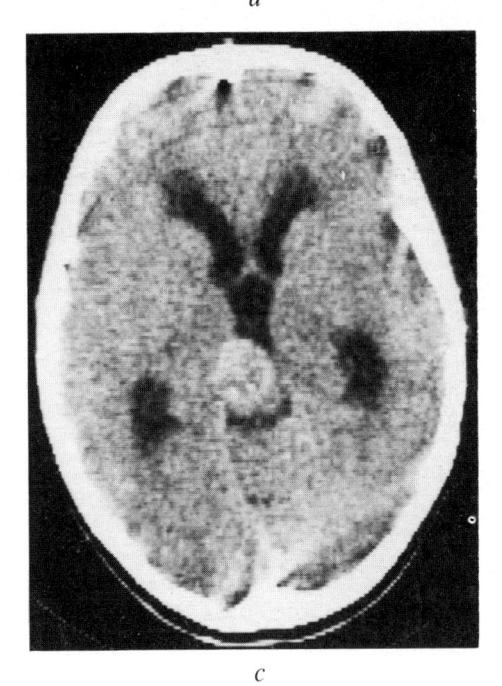

Fig. 5. Sylvian aqueduct syndrome. *a*, Light–near dissociation. The pupils are dilated and do not react to a light. *b*, A near response, however, produces pupillary constriction. *c*, CT scan showing a dysgerminoma of the pineal gland.

ments of the head may be substituted for absent vertical saccades. A lysosomal storage disease of unknown aetiology is the cause of this condition and there is no treatment.

Some saccadic disorders are accompanied by blinks or head movements (apraxic movements) which help initiate the saccade. This is particularly noticeable in ocular motor apraxia but is also seen in Huntington's chorea and Parkinsonism.

Further Abnormal Ocular Oscillations due to Disorders of Saccades

SQUARE WAVE JERKS

These are small amplitude horizontal saccades (<5 degrees) which may be seen on careful clinical evaluation but facilitated by the use of the slit lamp. A corrective saccade follows within 200 ms. They are associated with cerebellar disease, progressive supranuclear palsy and may be seen in elderly patients without established neurological disease.

MACRO SQUARE WAVE JERKS

These consist of large amplitude saccades, usually horizontal, and the saccadic amplitude is increased (to 10–40 degrees). They are found in multiple sclerosis and olivoponto cerebellar atrophy.

Ocular Flutter

Rapid conjugate horizontal ocular motor oscillations may be seen in two clinical situations. First, as a rapid onset cerebellar syndrome often suggestive of an inflammatory process. Secondly, flutter-like oscillations may be seen as part of a more generalized cerebellar and neurological disorder. Recordings show absence of the intersaccadic interval.

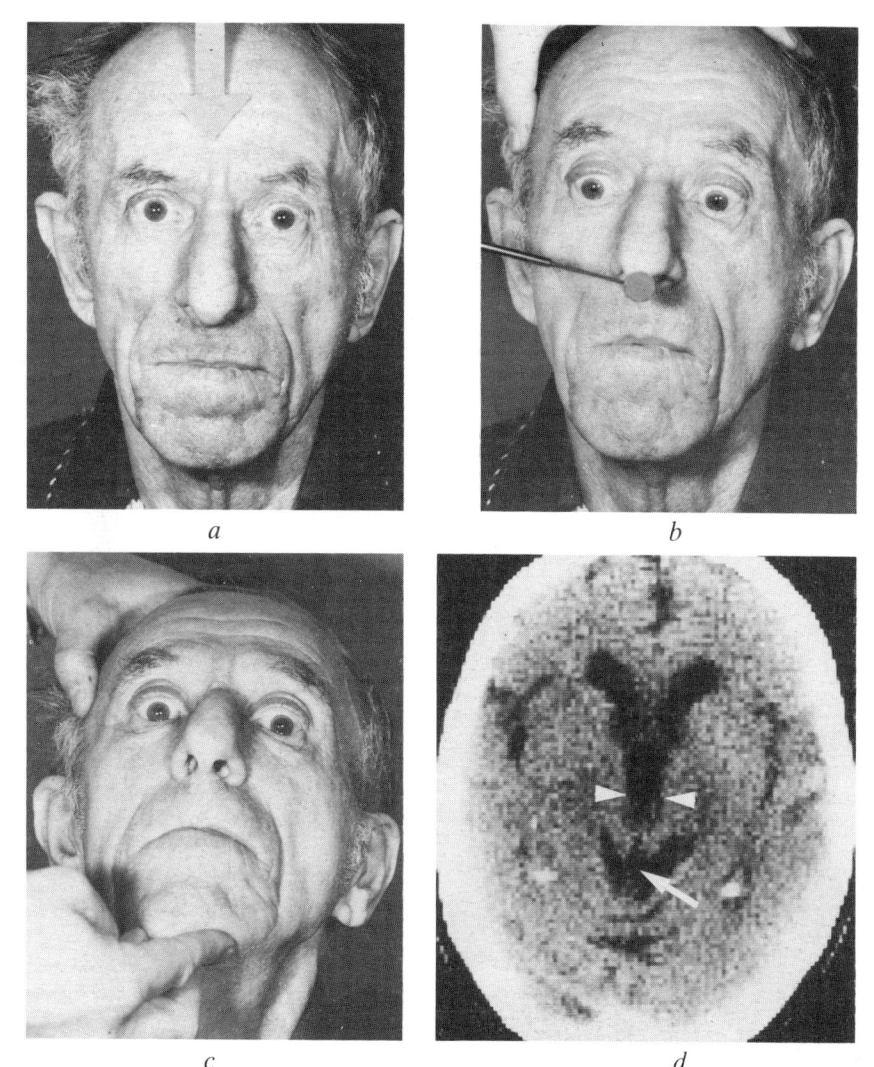

Fig. 6. Supranuclear palsy. An elderly man was admitted with a history of repeated falls and paucity of facial expression. He was unable to move his eyes downwards to command (*a*), to pursuit movements his down gaze was limited (*b*), but with Doll's head manoeuvres he had a full range of down gaze (*c*). These findings indicated a supranuclear palsy and CT scan showed dilatation of the ventricles with diffuse loss of cerebral tissue (*d*).

OPSOCLONUS

Rapid saccades in all planes (saccadomania)[14] are termed opsoclonus and associated with blinking and, often, movements of the limbs. Similar eye movements occur with (*a*) dancing eyes syndrome, (*b*) carcinoma – distant or proximal; and (*c*) neuroblastoma in children.

Ocular flutter and opsoclonus may represent a failure of the midline pause cells, which should fire continuously save during saccades. Saccadic movements occur in an uninhibited chaotic fashion.[15,16]

Disorders of Pursuit Movement

Broken up pursuit is seen in diffuse cerebral or cerebellar disease. Sedatives and anticonvulsants are a common cause. Recognition fails to provide diagnostic localization. In deep parietal lesions, despite normal saccades and smooth pursuit, OKN testing may be grossly abnormal.[17,18] This indicates the value of optokinetic nystagmus in the detection of cerebral lesions (*Fig. 7*).

Supranuclear failure of gaze may be diagnosed by the loss of saccadic or pursuit movements, but the preservation of vestibulo-ocular reflexes. Vergence movements are not involved with supranuclear disease. There are certain specific abnormalities of the saccadic system, which include; opsoclonus, ocular flutter, square wave jerks and macro-oscillations.

Internuclear Disorders

Internuclear Ophthalmoplegia (INO)

The medial longitudinal fasciculi (MLF) comprises two parallel tracts which are phylogenetically old, and appear at an early stage of embryological

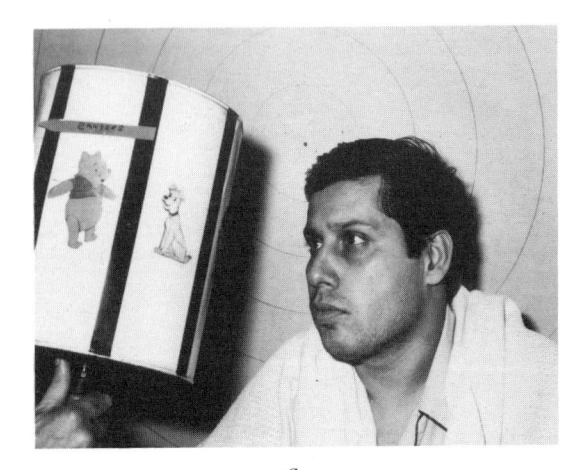

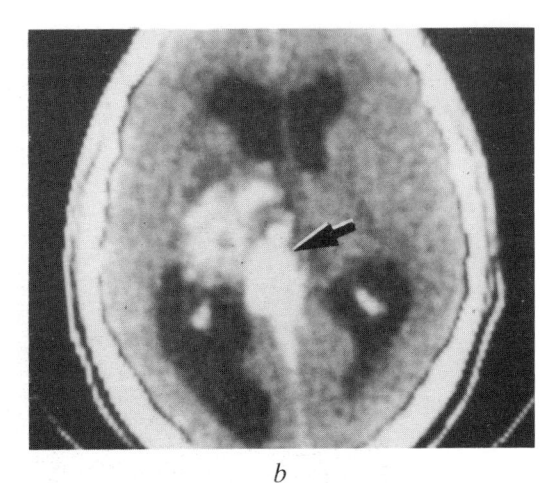

Fig. 7. Deep parietal lesion. *a*, Patient with normal saccadic and pursuit movements whose optokinetic nystagmus was grossly reduced with the drum rotating to the left. *b*, CT scan shows a deep left parietal lesion (arrow).

development and link the lower pons with the tegmentum. Inputs arise from the vestibular nuclei, afferents from cervical joints and muscles and fibres from the cerebellum.

Lesions of the MLF cause an internuclear ophthalmoplegia (INO) with impaired ipsilateral adduction and abduction nystagmus of the contralateral eye. The clinical signs may vary from a complete inability to adduct the ipsilateral eye (*Fig.* 8), to a subtle decrease in the speed of adducting saccades, often

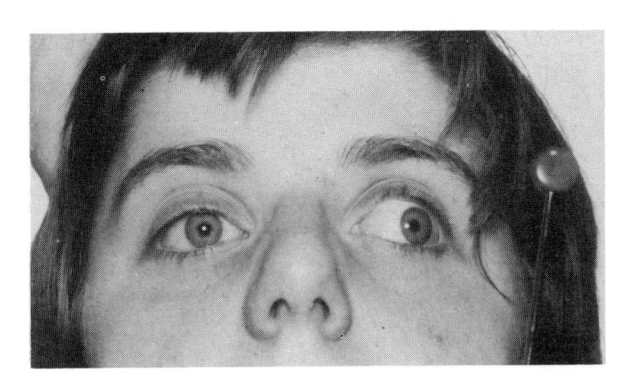

Fig. 8. Right internuclear ophthalmoplegia. The patient was unable to adduct the right eye and there was abduction nystagmus in the left eye. Convergence was normal and showed a greater amplitude than adduction. The diagnosis was demyelinating disease.

termed adduction lag. Subtle INO may be elicited by using the optokinetic drum, where the saccadic movements on the ipsilateral side become slower and smaller. The adduction paresis affects saccadic, pursuit and vestibular movements, but vergence is unchanged unless the IIIrd nerve nucleus is also involved. Certainty of diagnosis is only obtained when the range of vergence exceeds the range of adduction, and they may be difficult to assess in the elderly with convergence weakness. Other signs may suggest associated brain stem disease.

The mechanism of the abducting nystagmus is controversial. Theories include anomalies of convergence,[19] impaired inhibition of the contralateral medial rectus muscle,[20] and interruption of descending internuclear fibres which project to the abducens nucleus.[21] Other ideas noted have been a gaze evoked nystagmus[22] or the effect of adaptation to the contralateral medial rectus weakness.[23,24]

Skew deviation is a common associated finding in INO with diplopia and the ipsilateral eye is usually hypertropic.

Patients with bilateral INO have bilateral adduction weakness, with bilateral abducting nystagmus. The vertical vestibular and vertical pursuit movements are also abnormal, with gaze evoked nystagmus on elevation and depression.

Oscillopsia is a frequent symptom in patients with INO. Horizontal oscillopsia is possibly due to the abduction nystagmus. Vertical oscillopsia is associated with head movements and is due to the deficient vertical vestibulo-ocular reflex.[25] The horizontal oscillopsia is usually most evident at the onset of INO but diminishes, probably due to central adaptive mechanisms.

The One and a Half Syndrome[26]

When lesions involve both the MLF and adjacent PPRF or the descending cortico-spinal tract on one side of the brain stem, the result is an ipsilateral horizontal gaze palsy and ipsilateral INO. The only intact horizontal movement is contralateral abduction, which may be associated with nystagmus. Convergence is usually intact. The term paralytic exotropia is used to describe the ocular posture of patients with the 'one and a half' syndrome when attempting to look straight ahead (*Fig.* 9).

The ipsilateral horizontal gaze palsy is due to the PPRF lesion. This may be complete for all versional movements, but if the lesion is situated rostrally in the PPRF, then vestibular movements are preserved.

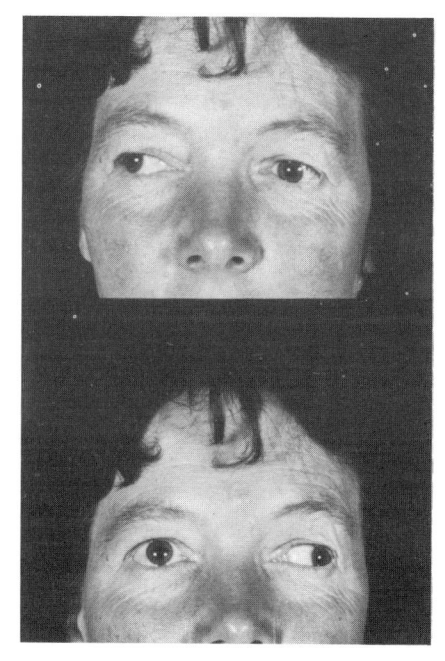

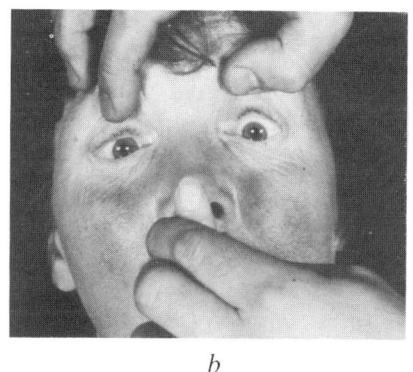

Fig. 9. 'One and a half' syndrome. *a*, This patient presented acutely with a bilateral internuclear ophthalmoplegia. She demonstrates paralytic pontine exotropia. Convergence, however (*b*), showed a full range.

The ipsilateral failure of adduction and contralateral abducting nystagmus is due to the INO.

Causes of INO

Multiple sclerosis (usually bilateral).
Infarction (usually unilateral).
Tumour.
Syringobulbia[27] with Arnold–Chiari malformation.
Infection: usually with encephalitis.
Metabolic, e.g. hepatic encephalopathy.
Drug intoxication (tricyclics,[28] phenothiazines.[29])
Trauma.
Syphilis.

Pseudo-INO

Myasthenia gravis, Fisher's syndrome,[30] thyroid and orbital myosistis may exactly mimic an internuclear ophthalmoplegia. However, other clinical signs will suggest the correct diagnosis.

Disorders of Vestibular Eye Movement

Acute unilateral destructive lesions of the vestibular labyrinth or nerve produce a tonic imbalance between resting discharge rates of the left and right vestibular nuclei. Initially, the eyes drift ipsilaterally towards the side of the lesion accompanied by contralateral nystagmus (fast phase away from the side of the lesion).

Acute unilateral vestibular disturbances cause symptoms for a few days or weeks before central adaptation takes place. The aetiology is usually demyelination or vascular disease but the cause of acute labyrinthitis often remains unestablished.

If bilateral failure of the labyrinths occurs, head movements cause oscillopsia since the vestibulo-ocular reflex is abolished. Symptoms include blurring of vision on walking, which may be misinterpreted as Uhthoff's phenomenon.

Examination of the patient should include checking the visual acuity while shaking the head. The acuity will deteriorate since the absent VOR no longer stabilizes the eyes during head movement. Central adaptation to peripheral vestibular disease, however, is remarkable, with compensation for bilateral deficits frequently occurring.

Use of Vestibulo-ocular Reflex in the Unconscious Patient

In the unconscious patient caloric stimulation may give useful clues to the severity of the injury or coma. Quick phases of nystagmus will be abolished in severe coma but stimulation of semicircular canals by warm or cold water will produce deviation of the eyes towards (warm) or away from (cold) the examined side. A useful mnemonic, COWS (cold opposite warm same) has been introduced and relates to the fast phase of the nystagmus. Loss of these VOR induced movements indicates structural damage to the brain stem.

Infranuclear Disorders

The onset of diplopia reflecting ocular motor dysfunction is sudden and indicates nuclear or more commonly infranuclear disease. Present understanding of the mechanics of diplopia is still derived from Ewald Hering's[31] observations of 1864! Diplopia, due to an infranuclear lesion, may be defined as the simultaneous appreciation of two images of the same object due to misalignment of the visual axes.

Diplopia

Two visual problems are produced by misaligned ocular axes. Appreciation of two separate images of the same object is due to stimulation of non-corresponding retinal points, and results in diplopia. The foveae, however, are able to appreciate two different objects in space. One fovea – in the correctly aligned eye – will receive the true image of the object of regard, but the misaligned fovea will receive a different image of the object. This causes confusion rather than diplopia with an accompanying set of symptoms including oscillopsia, unsteadiness and visual blurring. Oscillopsia and unsteadiness are probably caused by inadequate compensatory movement of the eyes during head and body movement.

Patients with misaligned visual axes who do not appreciate diplopia have usually had this problem from childhood and have never developed binocular vision.

Constant diplopia, with no other symptoms, suggests ocular motor nerve paresis. If, however, other symptoms are present, examination may indicate the precise anatomical site of the lesion, which may be in the cavernous sinus, orbital fissure, orbit, or the ocular muscle. The patient with diplopia may often indicate the area of maximal separation, and the orientation of the false image, indicating the probable affected muscle. Patients who complain of horizontal diplopia worse for distance may have complete or partial VIth nerve palsies. Patients with vertical diplopia greater for near are likely to have an oblique palsy (usually superior), whereas those with distance diplopia are more likely to have a vertical rectus weakness.

Intermittent Diplopia

This is a relatively uncommon symptom and must be distinguished from the variability in degree of diplopia suggestive of myasthenia.

Inquiry should be directed to the possibility of a childhood squint managed by patching, glasses or surgery, all of which suggest a long standing problem. Patients who develop some degree of binocular vision early in life despite abnormal ocular motility sometimes lose their ability to fuse two images all the time and diplopia results. The symptoms either for distance or near are intermittent, often being worse when tired.

Examination of Diplopia

The examination for diplopia consists of eliciting the site of maximum disparity, determining the eye producing the most peripheral or false image and confirming these findings by further documentation.

OBJECTIVE DIPLOPIA TEST

Several objective methods for assessing diplopia are available. Gross misalignment of the visual axes in children may be detected by examination of the corneal reflections of a bright torch light held in front of the patient and then in positions of extreme gaze.

Examination of the adult with diplopia may be performed with a wand or Lancaster red–green goggles.

Use of the wand may provide the true diagnosis, and is preferable to a small torch because it provides evidence of torsion. The aim is to determine the site of maximal separation, and then to cover alternate eyes until the false or peripheral image, which comes from the paretic eye, is appreciated. In vertical diplopia torsion must be assessed and in a superior oblique palsy if the wand appears double the apex of the two images points to the responsible eye. The cover test may also be performed in different positions of gaze.

Measurement of diplopia may also be performed by the Lancaster red–green test. A red glass is placed in front of the right eye and a green glass before the left. The patient is given a torch which carries a red filter allowing him to project a thin pencil of light on to a screen. The examiner holds a similar torch but with a green filter. The goggles ensure the patient can only see the red pencil of light with his right eye and the green pencil of light with the left. The examiner moves his green torch to project targets in the nine positions of gaze. The patient is asked to cover the green pencil of light with his red one. Any discrepancy between the two pencils can be noted and will immediately resolve the nature of the diplopia. Horizontal diplopia is best investigated by using a vertical beam while vertical diplopia is most easily elicited if the beam is projected horizontally.

A forced duction test is another possibility, although it is surrounded by confusion and difficulty. The anaesthetized eye may be moved into the paretic field by a cotton-wool bud, a pair of forceps or a contact lens.

If the eye can be passively moved into the paretic field by pressure from the applicator, there is no mechanical restriction. If there is resistance to this manoeuvre, then mechanical restriction may be responsible for the diplopia and this constitutes a positive forced duction test. The test is difficult to interpret and meaningful results are often obtained only under general anaesthetic.

VERTICAL DEVIATION AND HEAD TILT TEST
(BIELSCHOWSKY HEAD TILT TEST)

To determine which extraocular muscle is responsible for a vertical strabismus, a four-stage procedure is required:
1. A cover test determines the hypertropic eye.
2. The patient looks horizontally left and right. The hypertropia will increase in one or other direction.
3. The patient is asked to look up and down. The hypertropia will increase in either up or down gaze.
4. Finally, the head is tilted to each shoulder alternately and any change in the size of deviation noted.

The probable physiological basis of the Bielschowsky test is interesting. During a lateral head tilt the vertical eye muscles are no longer working in pairs as 'yoked' muscles. The vestibular otoliths produce a compensatory cyclorotation of the eyes by co-innervation of the ipsilateral (ipsilateral to the direction of head tilt) superior rectus and superior oblique muscles. The result is ipsilateral intorsion. At the same time there is contralateral extorsion due to the induced action of the contralateral inferior oblique and inferior rectus muscles.

Head tilt tests usually remain useful, even in long standing oblique muscle paresis.

Primary and Secondary Deviations in Strabismus

In paralytic strabismus primary deviation refers to the angle between the visual axes when the normal eye fixes the target. The angle between the visual axes when the paretic eye fixates the target is referred to as the secondary deviation.

A relatively greater effort is required to move the paretic eye in the direction of action of the paretic muscle than is necessary to move the normal eye in that same direction. This is reflected by a greater deviation of the normal eye due to the co-innervation of the yoke muscle. The secondary deviation is thus greater than the primary deviation.

Head Postures

Patients with strabismus often turn or tilt their heads to alleviate the diplopia. Horizontal muscle weakness – usually from VIth nerve palsy – is compensated by turning the head into the direction of action of the muscle. Paresis of depression requires depression and paresis of elevation requires elevation of the head. Torsional paresis, usually from oblique muscle involvement, requires a head tilt. A right superior oblique palsy would include loss of intorsion of the right eye. The head is then 'intorted' instead to compensate, so is thus inclined towards the opposite shoulder. The accompanying loss of normal ocular depression requires depression of the chin. While most patients with ocular muscle paresis move their heads to lessen the diplopia, occasionally the head is moved in the opposite direction, increasing the deviation. This probably facilitates suppression of the image from the paretic eye with alleviation of the diplopia.

Differentiation of Concomitant and Incomitant Strabismus causing Diplopia

Concomitant strabismus is characterized by a constant angle of deviation in all directions of gaze, whichever eye is fixating. Incomitant strabismus is accompanied by different angles of deviation depending on the direction of gaze. Many people have some degree of concomitant heterophoria which may be elicited on breaking fusion by covering one eye. With both eyes open under normal conditions fusional mechanisms compensate for the small phoria and prevent diplopia.

Refractive or accommodative factors change the fusional mechanism, producing decompensation and intermittent diplopia.

Ocular Motor Nerve Palsies (Abducens Palsy)

Paralysis of the abducens nerve is the most common ocular motor paralysis. Several large retrospective studies have analysed the causes and indicate a predominantly idiopathic group in adults, whereas in children the aetiology is usually malignant (*Table* I).[36]

Table I. Reported causes of paralysis of the abducens nerve

Aetiology (%)	Rucker, 1958[32] (n = 545)	and Schlezinger, 1960[33] (n = 104)	Rucker, 1966[34] (n = 607)	Johnston, 1968[35] (n = 158)	Robertson et al., 1970[36] (n = 133)
Undetermined	30	24	20	8	9
Trauma	16	3	12	32	20
Neoplasm	21	7	33	13	9
Ischaemia	11	36	8	16	0
Aneurysm	6	0	3	1	3
Miscellaneous	16	30	24	30	29

The aetiology may be examined in a logical manner by considering the course of the VIth nerve from nucleus to orbit.

Nuclear VIth Nerve Palsy

Nuclear VIth nerve palsies are unusual and are commonly associated with disorders involving the adjacent VIIth nerve nucleus. Nuclear VIth nerve palsies cause disturbance of ipsilateral horizontal gaze since neurones to the ipsilateral lateral rectus and contralateral medial rectus are involved.

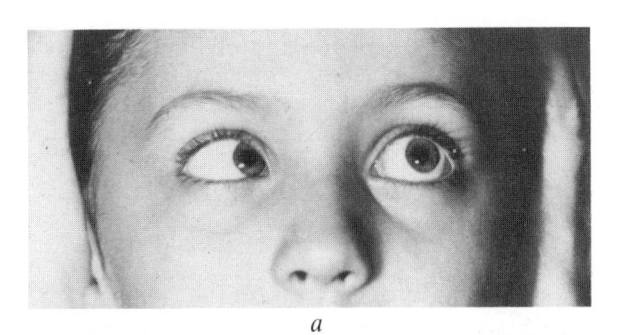

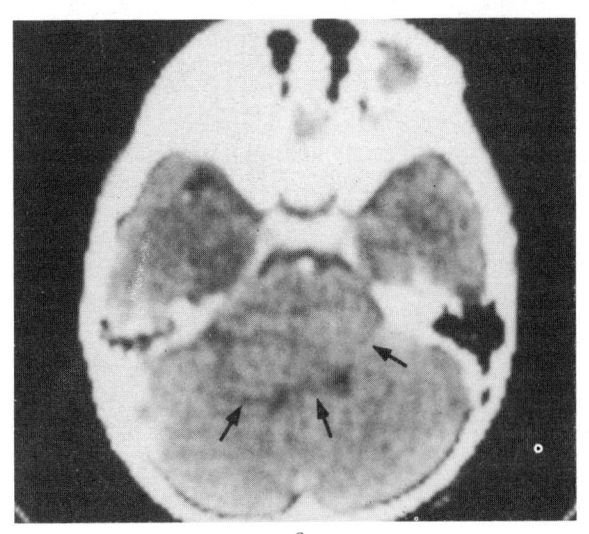

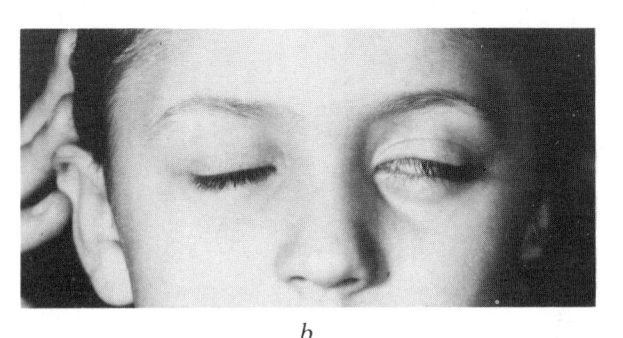

Fig. 10. Left VIth nerve palsy. *a*, All horizontal eye movements were extremely slow on testing, though the integrity of R adduction demonstrates the fascicular nature of this left VIth nerve palsy. *b*, There is a left facial palsy, indicating extensive pontine involvement. *c*, CT scan shows a fat pons due to a glioma with greater extension on the left (arrows).

Isolated nuclear VIth nerve palsies are excessively rare, but may occur from congenital absence of the nucleus. Two important syndromes should be considered in this context.

Moebius Syndrome

This is a combination of bilateral congenital hypoplasia of the VIth and VIIth nerve nuclei leading to a horizontal gaze palsy with bilateral facial weakness. Mental retardation, bulbar lesions and limb abnormalities are found.

Duane's Retraction Syndrome[37,38]

This interesting condition is detailed elsewhere (pp. 419–20). Recent clinicopathological information[44] has confirmed abnormalities of the abducens nuclei and nerves.[37]

Fascicular VIth Nerve Lesions

As the fascicles emerge from the nucleus to the ventral brain stem they pass near the pyramidal tract. Infarction, tumour (*Fig.* 10) or demyelination here will cause the Millard–Grubler syndrome – abducens palsy, ipsilateral facial weakness and contralateral hemiplegia.

Within the subarachnoid space, meningitis, compression and displacement of the brain stem (from raised intracranial pressure) may involve the VIth nerve, often causing bilateral lesions. VIth nerve palsy occasionally occurs after lumbar puncture,[39] especially if there is injection of contrast fluid via a cisternal puncture.

The VIth nerve is closely apposed to bone over the petrous crest, where infections (mastoiditis) may occur. A combination of pain, diplopia and deafness (Gradenigo's syndrome) is seen in patients with chronic ear disease or sometimes with invasive nasopharyngeal carcinoma.

Once the VIth nerve has entered the cavernous sinus, it may be involved along with the other oculomotor nerves and the trigeminal nerve in inflammatory or neoplastic processes; compression from intracavernous carotid aneurysms may also occur.

More anteriorly, the VIth nerve passes through the orbital fissure, and lesions at the orbital apex may cause a combination of ocular motility disturbance, proptosis and visual loss.

VIth Nerve Palsy in Children

Abducens palsy in childhood should be regarded with suspicion. Pontine gliomas may cause bilateral VIth nerve palsies with horizontal gaze failure. Usually there is an associated facial weakness. A 'fat' pons may be seen on CT scan. Posterior fossa tumours, including medulloblastoma, also cause abducens weakness. However, benign VIth nerve palsy[40] in childhood may accompany viral illness with an excellent prognosis for a return of normal motility.

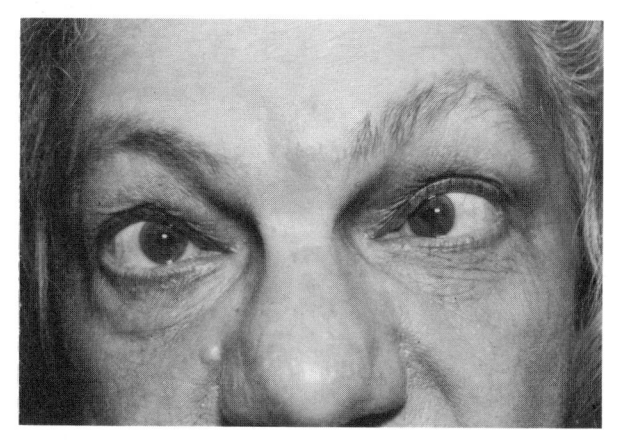

Fig. 11. Bilateral VIth nerve palsy of unknown aetiology.

Bilateral VIth Nerve Weakness

Many of these causes of unilateral VIth nerve palsy may also affect the opposite nerve, giving bilateral abduction weakness. This especially applies to raised intracranial pressure from tumours or benign intracranial hypertension, where there is downward displacement of the brain stem[41] (*Fig.* 11).

Trochlear (IVth) Nerve Palsy

Head trauma, usually blunt frontal injury, is the most frequent cause of IVth nerve palsy. Bilateral involvement is more common; the probable site of the lesion is the anterior medullary velum where the trochlear nerves decussate.

Patients with IVth nerve paresis complain of vertical and torsional diplopia on down gaze (*Fig.* 12). Thus they often have difficulty in reading. Bilateral IVth nerve palsies show alternating vertical diplopia depending on the position of gaze. Both unilateral and bilateral IVth nerve palsies tend to make the patient adopt a characteristic head posture to alleviate the problem.

The chin is depressed, the face turned away from the affected side and the head tilted to the opposite shoulder. Thus the loss of depression, abduction and intorsion are compensated by an abnormal head posture.

Cover testing will demonstrate a vertical tropia which is accentuated on adduction of the affected eye, where the oblique muscles should be acting at the best mechanical advantage. The eye movements typically show a reduction in ipsilateral depression, again most obvious when the affected eye is in adduction. The Lancaster red–green test is often helpful in subtle IVth nerve palsies, especially with bilateral involvement.

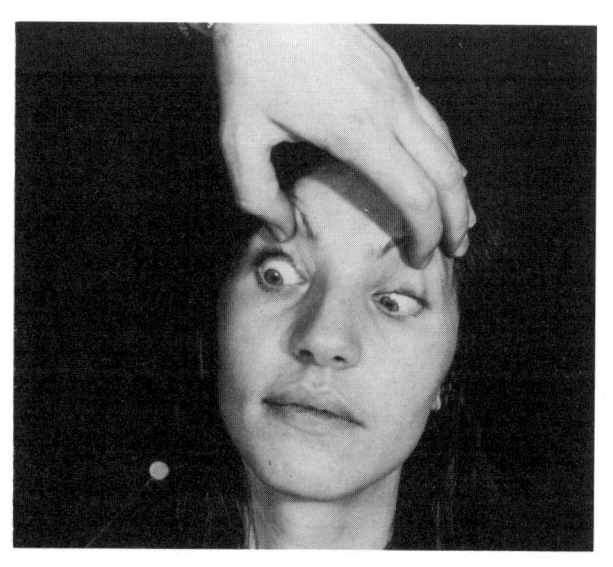

Fig. 12. Trochlear nerve palsy. This patient had a right IVth nerve palsy with characteristic head tilt. Unusually the lesion was due to a petrous tumour.

Confusion may occur with skew deviation in the differential diagnosis of trochlear paresis, because a long standing trochlear palsy may become comitant. Skew deviation refers to a vertical misalignment of the visual axes due to abnormal prenuclear input. Usually the hypertropia is constant for all positions of gaze but may alternate, resembling bilateral IVth nerve palsies. Isolated skew deviation occurs but generally it is associated with other neurological signs which aid the clinician in making a diagnosis.

A number of conditions are associated with skew deviation, especially unilateral internuclear ophthalmoplegia where an ipsilateral hypertropia is found. Ascending otolithic pathways are most likely involved in the ipsilateral medial longitudinal fasciculus.

Oculomotor (IIIrd) Nerve Palsies

The oculomotor nerve supplies not only four extraocular muscles but also the levator palpebrae superioris and the pupil. Consequently IIIrd nerve paresis may be complicated by several different presentations. The aetiologies for oculomotor palsy are similar to those for abducens and trochlear disease.

IIIrd Nerve Palsies in Children

Oculomotor palsy in childhood is most often congenital. The signs are usually unilateral and incomplete, with aberrant regeneration a common finding.[42] Cyclic oculomotor[43] palsy is a rare anomaly where cycles of complete or incomplete palsy of the IIIrd nerve on one side alternate with periods of normal function. No cause has been established.

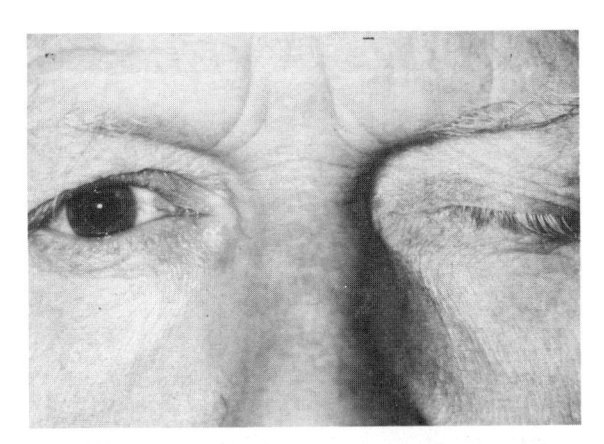

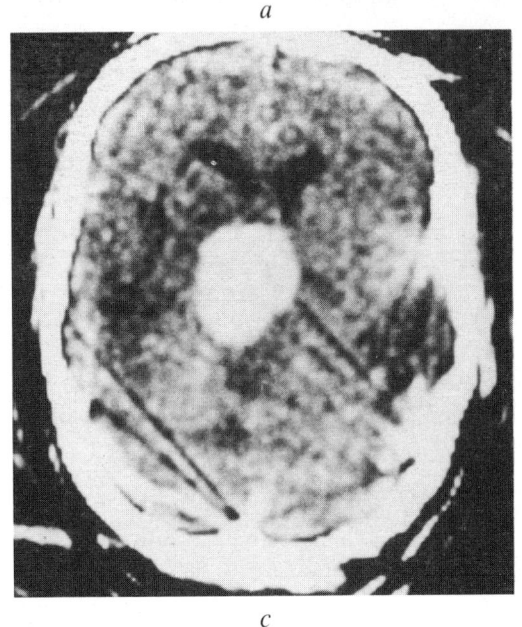

Ophthalmoplegic migraine is also found in children who develop a sudden complete IIIrd nerve palsy during a severe headache. Recurrent episodes may occur and it may even be bilateral, and though no cause is found, an angiogram is often indicated. Aberrant regeneration has been reported with ophthalmoplegic migraine.[44]

Nuclear IIIrd Nerve Lesions

The clinical signs include bilateral ptosis (from involvement of the paired levator nucleus) and contralateral superior rectus weakness (the superior rectus nuclear representation is crossed). The IIIrd nerve nucleus may be infiltrated by local lesions and it is impossible clinically to differentiate nuclear from fascicular involvement.

Fascicular IIIrd Nerve Syndromes

As the fascicles of the IIIrd nerve pass down through the midbrain, they traverse the red nucleus and the pyramidal tracts so that lesions at different levels may

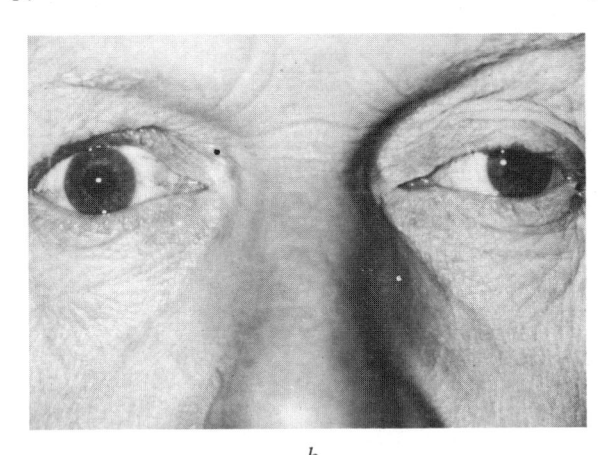

Fig. 13. *a* and *b*, This patient presented acutely with a left-sided ptosis, divergence of the visual axes and a large pupil. *c*, CT scan showed a large midbrain glioma.

be localized by recognition of pattern of physical signs (*Fig. 13*).

Posterior Communicating Artery Aneurysms

Aneurysms of the posterior communicating artery may affect the IIIrd nerve with a characteristic syndrome of ophthalmoplegia, ptosis and an efferent pupil defect with jaw or orbital pain. Pain is not always present, however, but pupillary involvement tends to confirm a compressive aetiology. Pupillary involvement is seen predominantly with aneurysms because of the peripheral location of the pupillary fibres in the IIIrd nerve. Aneurysms may, however, occur with pupil sparing, so in the non-diabetic patient, angiographic examination may still be indicated.

Multiple Ocular Motor Nerve Palsies

Combined IIIrd, IVth and VIth nerve palsy occurs in lesions of the cavernous sinus and orbital fissure. Trauma, infiltrations and granulomas are usually responsible. The involvement of branches of the Vth nerve facilitates localization.

Multiple cranial nerve palsies may occur with the Guillain–Barré syndrome but the Miller–Fisher variant may show signs confined to the ocular motor nerves. Controversy exists as to whether there is both central and peripheral involvement in the Miller–Fisher syndrome.

Recommended Investigation of Ocular Motor Nerve Palsy

Blood pressure.
Full blood count and differential ESR.
VDRL and FTA-antibodies.
Fasting glucose and lipids.
Antinuclear factor.
Radiology: plain skull X-ray.

Management

If the palsy is isolated – perform above investigations and follow up for 3 months; if no recovery – CT scan.

If negative – continue follow-up for 1 year. If signs of aberrant regeneration occur, angiography should be undertaken.

MYASTHENIA GRAVIS[45,46]

Ophthalmologists should always consider this rare disease in any patient with ptosis and an ocular motor disorder.

Ocular features are seen at presentation in half the patients and 90 per cent develop them at a later stage. Women are more frequently affected than men. However, a small group of patients have myasthenia that is clinically confined to the extraocular muscles and eyelids, and clinical features may be localized for many years.

Pathogenesis

The condition is a prime example of an autoimmune disease, with antibodies to motor end plates with increased degradation of postsynaptic acetylcholine receptors and destructive changes in the postsynaptic membrane.

About 87 per cent of patients with myasthenia gravis have circulating anticholinergic receptor antibodies. Patients who clinically have ocular involvement alone, have both a lower incidence and lower serum titre of receptor antibodies. The level of antibody does not indicate the activity of the disease.

Ocular Myasthenia

The extraocular muscle weakness is often asymmetrical and can mimic any brain stem disorder. A variability in symptoms combined with fatiguability demonstrable on clinical examination should make the diagnosis clear. Ptosis and orbicularis weakness are common and levator fatigue can be demonstrated by the Cogan lid twitch.[46]

After levator fatigue, the patient is asked to follow a target moving into down gaze. The target is then jerked rapidly upwards. On changing from down gaze to up gaze the levator palpebrae superioris makes rapid upward twitching movements and then descends slowly. Another useful clinical sign is to ask the patient to sustain up gaze for several minutes, which normal patients find easy; myasthenic patients rapidly fatigue.

Laboratory evaluation of ocular myasthenia has demonstrated characteristic changes[47] in normal saccades fixation. During large saccades eye movements slow down, especially after repeated fixations. Nystagmus increases during any sustained position of eccentric gaze and saccadic dysmetria is often found.

Peripheral mechanisms explain most, but not all, of the findings in ocular myasthenia. Failure of normal neuromuscular transmission affects the tonic extraocular muscle fibres rendering them vulnerable to fatigue as there are simply less postsynaptic acetylcholine receptors available.

The inability to sustain a saccade (lack of sustained pulse phase) allows the eye to drift backwards since the tonic fibres are also fatigued and eye position is not maintained. The drift backwards may be rapid, causing the whole attempted, ill-sustained saccade to resemble a 'quiver' movement. More detailed accounts of the ocular movements in myasthena gravis may be found elsewhere.[48,49]

The diagnosis of ocular myasthenia depends on a clinical suspicion, corroborative testing and pharmacological confirmation. The edrophonium test is useful but should not be attempted by the ophthalmologist in clinics without access to resuscitation facilities.

Treatment of ocular myasthenia is traditionally undertaken by neurologists, and thymectomy and immunosuppression is the treatment of choice in selected patients. Ophthalmologists may see the side effects of long term treatment with steroids or immunosuppression. CT scan of the anterior mediastinum is mandatory for the detection of a thymoma. Rarely, drugs precipitate myasthenia, penicillamine being the most frequent offender.

Chronic Progressive External Ophthalmoplegia (CPEO)

Several distinct neuromuscular diseases may present with slowly progressive ptosis and external ophthalmoplegia. Attempts to delineate these disorders have been limited by the lack of specific pathogenic mechanisms, but several clinical groups of disease have been classified recently.[50]

The different clinical categories of CPEO have similar ocular symptoms and signs. There is progressive limitation of ocular motility, to produce total ophthalmoplegia and progressive ptosis. Diplopia may be a problem, particularly for close work, and ocular muscle surgery may correct the progressive exotropia. Ptosis surgery should be discouraged since the ophthalmoplegia and absent Bell's sign may render the globe more vulnerable to exposure. Ptosis is therefore best managed by ptosis props on spectacles or contact lenses, with shelves to support the drooping lid.

The ophthalmologist may contribute diagnostically by the recognition of retinal pigmentary changes in 36 per cent of cases, and in some the condition may be severe and progressive.[51] The retinal changes may be due to enlarged mitochondria in the retinal pigment epithelial cells.[52]

General Features

Current biochemical studies on muscle biopsy specimens have isolated specific enzyme abnormalities, e.g. carnitine deficiency. Histological features show ragged red fibres, which are seen on electron microscopy to be due to mitochondrial abnormalities. The Kearns–Sayre syndrome merits recognition because of the associated endocrine and cardiac abnormalities.

DYSTHYROID DISEASE AND OPHTHALMOPLEGIA[53]

The ophthalmologist has an important role in the recognition, diagnosis and management of thyroid disease. Visual loss may be the most devastating effect of the disease. Ophthalmoplegia may occur with any form of dysthyroid disease, but is most common with hyperthyroidism, though this may only become detectable later in the course of the disease and especially with T3 toxicosis. The investigations currently available usually detect the underlying thyroid disease and include: (*a*) T4 estimation; (*b*) T3 estimation; (*c*) TRH test; (*d*) thyroid autoantibodies.

Ocular features include lid retraction, particularly on elevation, and lid lag on down gaze in combination with proptosis and ophthalmoplegia. Involvement may be asymmetrical, although the second eye is generally involved within 2 years.

The management of patients with dysthyroid ophthalmoplegia is difficult. The thyroid status of the patient needs stabilization with carbimazole, radioactive iodine and supported by beta-blockers. Surgery is advisable in young patients with severe thyrotoxicosis, and focal thyroid hyperplasia. Patients with tense orbits and threatened vision require urgent treatment, with large doses of systemic steroids. Visual loss is due to optic nerve compression at the orbital apex where the muscle swelling tends to be most marked on CT examination. Orbital decompression, therefore, if necessary, is aimed at improving space at the orbital apex.

Acute dysthyroid disease[54] may occasionally present with ophthalmoplegia, ptosis, visual loss and pain, mimicking orbital cellulitis. The diagnosis of dysthyroid disease can be made on orbital CT scan, where enlarged extraocular muscles are apparent. Large doses of systemic steroid effect rapid resolution of symptoms and signs.

The ophthalmoplegia in dysthyroid disease may affect solitary muscles, though more frequently all muscles are involved. Vertical diplopia may be the presenting symptom, presumably because of the special relationship between the inferior rectus and oblique muscles. Other muscles become involved, particularly the medial rectus, so that the eye becomes tethered in a downward and inward position.

The ophthalmoplegia is due to inflammatory changes in the orbit with replacement fibrosis causing tethering of the extraocular muscles. The immunology of dysthyroid ophthalmoplegia is complex and poorly understood. TSH receptors are found in orbital fat cells but not on the extraocular muscles. Thyroid stimulating immunoglobulin is present in 60 per cent of patients with euthyroid Graves's disease,[61] but circulating antibody levels have not been useful in assessing the activity or prognosis of the ocular complications. A circulating autoantibody against soluble ocular muscle antigen in patients with ophthalmic Graves's disease, but not in patients with thyrotoxicosis or goitre has been identified[55] more recently an ophthalmopathic immunoglobulin (IgG) has been detected.[56]

The management of mild dysthyroid ophthalmoplegia is conservative, with observation and serial Hess charts. Prisms or occlusion may relieve the immediate symptoms, especially vertical diplopia. If after 6 months the diplopia is stable, surgery may be considered.

Usually there is a vertical diplopia caused by tethering of the inferior recti (*Fig.* 14). Inferior rectus recession of the hypotropic eye may relieve the symptoms considerably, though the surgery may be difficult, and the use of adjustable sutures and local anaesthetic should be restricted to experienced surgeons. Prisms may still be required to achieve binocular single vision.

In summary, the ocular myopathies are a rare but important group of diseases. The initial presentation, with either diplopia or ptosis, is often in an ophthalmology clinic. If the possibility of a myopathy is considered, the diagnosis will not be missed.

OTHER CAUSES OF EXTRAOCULAR MUSCLE DYSFUNCTION

Orbital pseudotumour with ocular myositis may present with diplopia and pain on eye movement. The

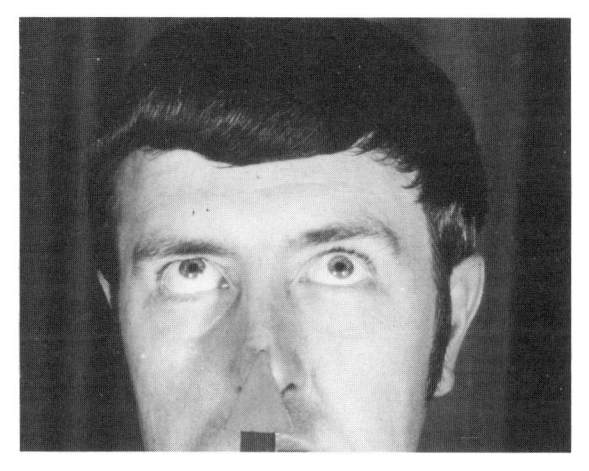

Fig. 14. Monocular elevator palsy. This patient presented with a monocular elevator palsy on the left which was due to a tumour at the base of the brain. The differential diagnosis of monocular elevator palsy is thyroid eye disease or a blow out fracture.

eye may be red and, rarely, there is associated uveitis. An orbital CT scan helps to distinguish this condition from dysthyroid ophthalmoplegia. Mosely and Sanders[57] have emphasized that ocular muscle enlargement in pseudotumour is mainly at the insertions while in dysthyroid disease the muscle body and orbital apex region are involved.

A dural fistula in the cavernous sinus may produce orbital hypoxia with swollen extraocular muscles and ophthalmoplegia. The differential diagnosis for thyroid may be difficult and continued examination necessary.

Nystagmus

Nystagmus is an important clinical sign indicating central nervous system disease. The term 'nystagmus' is derived from the Greek word for 'nodding in one's sleep'. The derivation is apt: the slow movements of the head towards one shoulder are followed by a rapid corrective movement as the subject almost awakens before the cycle is repeated.

Nystagmus is used to describe ocular movements which, by definition, should be rhythmic, involuntary and consist of to and fro oscillations of the eyes. The term embraces pendular nystagmus (smooth sinusoidal oscillations) and also jerk nystagmus (alternating oscillation of slow drifts and rapid corrective movements).

There is a conventional terminology in nystagmus. The direction is, by definition, the direction of the fast component. Appreciation of amplitude and rate are inaccurate clinically but are useful when measured by eye movement recordings. The form of the nystagmus may be horizontal, vertical, rotatory, circular or elliptical. Usually both eyes move in harmony; dissociated nystagmus is a term describing different movements in the two eyes.

Although the fast phase is, by convention, used to define the direction of the nystagmus, the clinician's attention should be focused on the slow phase. The slow phase is due to failure of the mechanisms to hold fixation steady. Eccentric gaze requires a balance of vestibular, optokinetic and pursuit systems. Disease of these systems leads to nystagmus.

No precise classification of nystagmus exists but, for practical purposes, it is enough to recognize certain oscillations as carrying clinical significance. It is important to identify an ocular oscillation as being congenital or acquired and to establish any localizing features which require further investigation.

Clinical Classification of Nystagmus

1. Physiological nystagmus
2. Voluntary nystagmus
3. Congenital nystagmus
4. Specific recognizable nystagmus with localizing value
5. Non-specific non-localizing nystagmus
6. Other ocular oscillations

Symptoms may include oscillopsia – a term used to describe movement of the visual environment – dizziness, unsteadiness, intermittent blurred vision or diplopia. The symptoms may only occur in certain positions of gaze, or with certain positions of the head, or at a specific time interval.

Physiological Nystagmus

Normal eyes wobble when held in extreme positions of gaze and the inexperienced examiner may derive spurious information from testing the eye movement excursions beyond the patient's field of binocular vision. Physiological nystagmus is also a normal response to certain stimuli. Cold or warm water, when introduced into the external auditory canal, will stimulate movement of endolymph in the semicircular canals. The imbalance in vestibular stimulation creates a physiological response of nystagmus. Cold water produces the fast phase of the nystagmus in the opposite or contralateral direction, while warm water induces movement in the same direction (COWS).

Physiological nystagmus is also seen in response to a rotating optokinetic (OKN) drum. A slow pursuit movement follows the stripe in the direction of drum rotations to its extreme before a corrective contralateral saccade effects refixation of the next stripe.

The OKN response has some useful clinical applications. Patients with homonymous hemianopias due to occipital lobe infarction generally retain normal OKN. However, Cogan[58] noted that tumours in the parieto-occipital area often caused loss of ipsilateral pursuit and a homonymous hemianopia since the pursuit pathways pass close to the posterior optic radiation.

Hysterical patients who allege no light perception but have an OKN response can be easily identified.

OKN is also useful to enhance signs of suspected disease of the ocular motor pathways. For example, fatiguing of saccades can accentuate the slow ipsilateral adduction of subtle internuclear ophthalmoplegia. OKN in myasthenia may be quite variable and bizarre.

Voluntary Nystagmus[59]

Some patients can sustain a series of saccades for short periods (e.g. 30 s), which resembles a pendular nystagmus. Clues as to the voluntary effort required may be offered by the accompanying facial grimacing.

Convergence spasm is another voluntary eye movement that confuses the clinical picture. Convergence spasm may accompany voluntary nystagmus, one set of bizarre symptoms and signs alternating with the other. The most common misdiagnosis is bilateral VIth nerve palsy or myasthenia. The pupils are usually small in convergence spasm as they too are incorporated in the synkinetic reflex. Patients with convergence spasm often complain of eye pain. The symptoms are usually relieved by atropinization.

Congenital Nystagmus

The history is extremely important and it is often difficult to be certain of the exact onset of the nystagmus. The eyes and ocular movements therefore need careful examination, for true congenital nystagmus has certain characteristics (Table II).

Table II. Characteristics of congenital nystagmus*

> Binocular
> Similar amplitude in both eyes
> Uniplanar, usually horizontal
> Distinctive waveforms
> Diminished (dampened) by convergence
> Increased by fixation attempt
> Superimposition of latent component
> Inversion of optokinetic reflex
> Associated head oscillation
> No oscillopsia
> Abolished in sleep

* After Daroff et al.[60]

There is some logic in dividing children with congenital nystagmus into two groups depending on the presence of associated disease of the anterior visual pathways.

Patients with congenital cataract, ocular albinism, aniridia or dyschromatopsia fail to develop normal fixation and may exhibit nystagmus in the first 6 months of life. Nystagmus in these patients is not often present at birth. Although the nystagmus is usually of the pendular type, prominent jerk nystagmus is also occasionally seen.

Patients without disease of the anterior visual pathway may show a pendular or jerk nystagmus from birth. The features detailed above may be present and it is especially important to be sure of the history in these patients regarding progressive visual loss. Rather than occlusion of the non-tested eye, a polarizing lens or strong spherical correction is more useful to lessen the effect of any latent nystagmus. The 'occluded' eye is defocused rather than completely covered, allowing uniocular visual acuity to be measured.

Spasmus Nutans

Spasmus nutans describes a clinical triad of ocular oscillations, head nodding and torticollis. The relevance of discussing spasmus nutans with congenital nystagmus is that spasmus nutans usually commences within the first 2 years of life.

Although the nystagmus is usually bilateral, it may be monocular in any direction. The nystagmus is often asymmetrical and varies in different positions of gaze. Head nodding is not always present, but occasionally precedes the nystagmus.

Spasmus nutans spontaneously disappears during the third or fourth year, although occasionally persists until 6 years of age.

Specific Recognizable Nystagmus with Localizing Value

Dissociated Nystagmus

The ocular movements of the two eyes are asymmetrical in dissociated nystagmus. Unilateral lesions of the medial longitudinal fasciculus produce ipsilateral adduction paresis on contralateral gaze. The abducting fellow eye moves more quickly but with characteristic jerky oscillations, resembling nystagmus. The mechanism for this abduction nystagmus is controversial, as has been discussed earlier.

More bizarre vertical and torsional dissociated movements are seen with posterior fossa lesions, usually demyelination or tumours.[60]

Dissociated vertical or oblique nystagmus should prompt a careful study of the posterior fossa, while the abduction nystagmus of the internuclear ophthalmoplegia is usually accompanied by other obvious signs.

See-Saw Nystagmus[61]

See-saw nystagmus is characterized by a curious extorting movement of one eye as it moves down while the fellow eye intorts as it rises. The movement alternates in a see-saw fashion. See-saw nystagmus is associated, particularly in children, with chiasmatic tumours. There is usually a bitemporal field defect.

Convergence Retraction Nystagmus

Convergence retraction nystagmus refers to the characteristic ocular motor disturbance found in the dorsal midbrain syndrome. On attempted elevation both eyes make adducting jerk movements accompanied by retraction of the globes. This can be detected by observing a rapidly elevated wand or a downward rotating drum. This unusual abnormality is due to co-firing of all ocular motor neurones on attempted elevation. Eye movement recordings have demonstrated that these movements are saccadic.[62]

Nystagmus of Cerebello-pontine Angle Disease

Tumours – usually acoustic neuromas or meningiomas – of the cerebello-pontine angle are associated with an unusual combination of peripheral vestibular nystagmus and gaze evoked nystagmus.

There is, therefore, a combination of a small amplitude rapid primary position nystagmus which beats away from the side of the lesion and a slow gaze evoked or gaze paretic type of nystagmus towards the side of the lesion.

Vestibular Nystagmus

Vestibular disease may be peripheral or central. There is a characteristic jerk nystagmus with the fast phase beating away from the side of the lesion. The form of the nystagmus may be horizontal or rotatory. There may be associated symptoms of tinnitus, deafness and vertigo, all of which are more prominent with peripheral vestibular disease. Peripheral vestibular nystagmus is usually more obvious without a fixation stimulus and is increased if the eyes are turned in the direction of the quick phase (Alexander's law).[63]

Central vestibular nystagmus may be purely torsional or vertical – either downbeating or upbeating. Removal of a fixation target does not usually alter the slow phase velocity of central vestibular nystagmus.

Downbeat Nystagmus

Downbeat nystagmus describes nystagmus with the fast phase in a downward direction while the eye is in the primary position, and thus the feature is accentuated on lateral gaze. Oscillopsia is particularly disabling, especially when going downstairs, and other neurological features are usually absent. The two most common causes are cerebellar ectopia (25 per cent) and cerebellar degeneration (25 per cent).[64] In 40 per cent of cases no cause is established and in the remainder a wide variety of conditions, including tumours, drugs and metabolic (cherry red spot myoclonus syndrome) are seen. Rarely, patients suffer from downbeat nystagmus after apparently uncomplicated general anaesthesia.

The pathogenesis of downbeat nystagmus is controversial. Upward slow phase drifts may be due to unopposed tonic input from the anterior semicircular canals. The central projections from the posterior canals cross the floor of the IVth ventricle and experimentally lesions in this area produce downbeat nystagmus. Other mechanisms postulated relate to decreased inhibition of the central vestibular connections of the anterior canals.

Although there are many causes of downbeat nystagmus, a careful search must always be made for a treatable lesion. In addition to routine CT, metrizamide CT scanning may be required, and MRI (magnetic resonance imaging) is becoming the investigation of choice in patients with the Arnold–Chiari malformation.

Upbeat Nystagmus

Upbeat nystagmus represents upbeating nystagmus in the primary position. Occurring mainly with intra-axial lesions, there are some reports with cerebellar lesions. The nystagmus is altered by head tilt and thus an otolith related component is responsible. Upbeat nystagmus is also found with Wernicke's encephalopathy and drug intoxication.

Periodic Alternating Nystagmus[65]

Periodic alternating nystagmus (PAN) describes an eye movement disorder in which the fast phase of the nystagmus regularly shifts its horizontal direction every 60–120 s. Smooth pursuit is usually impaired and there may be associated downbeat nystagmus.

The localizing value of PAN is limited but the syndrome is most often seen with lesions in the posterior fossa, including tumours and the Arnold–Chiari malformation. It is also found with multiple sclerosis, blind patients and anticonvulsant intoxication.

The diagnosis is usually missed because the examiner fails to observe the nystagmus for long enough.

Windmill nystagmus may be a variation of PAN, with excursions in horizontal, vertical and oblique planes.

Oculopalatal Myoclonus

Oculopalatal myoclonus was described in 1938.[66] The abnormal ocular movements usually commence several months after infarction of the brain stem. Characteristic vertical pendular oscillations (the term myoclonus is in fact misleading) are seen often with torsional or horizontal components. Synchronous movements of the soft palate, larynx and diaphragm may be found. The eye movements may disappear in sleep, but the palatal oscillations usually continue.

Histopathological findings of hypertrophy of the inferior olivary nucleus are characteristic of oculopalatal myoclonus. The hypertrophic neurones contain an increase in the products of the normal acetylcholinesterase reaction.

Abnormalities in the red nucleus and contralateral dentate nucleus are also found. Intravenous scopolamine has been found to abolish the ocular oscillations that cause severe oscillopsia.

Non-localizing Nystagmus, Gaze Evoked Nystagmus

Unlike the localizing forms of nystagmus, gaze evoked nystagmus is not present with the eyes held in the primary position. The mechanism is probably due to faulty neural integration with an inability to sustain eccentric eye positions. There is often, but not always, an associated gaze paresis.

Normal subjects may have a gaze evoked nystagmus on eccentric gaze as the physiological end point of gaze is exceeded for that individual. Physiological end point nystagmus is usually symmetrical and has a slower drift than gaze evoked nystagmus due to disease.

Cerebellar disease, drug intoxication especially anticonvulsants, and myasthenia may all cause gaze evoked nystagmus. It has no localizing value.

Rebound Nystagmus

In some patients with gaze evoked nystagmus rebound nystagmus occurs. After directing the eyes to an eccentric position to evoke nystagmus, the eyes are returned to the primary position. A brief nystagmus with the slow drifts in the direction of the previous gaze evoked nystagmus is seen – rebound nystagmus. Rebound nystagmus possibly represents central adaptive mechanisms.

Other Ocular Oscillations

A number of saccadic abnormalities produce abnormal patterns of ocular movement resembling nystagmus. 'Convergence–retraction nystagmus' – a disorder with abnormal adducting saccades – has been included already because of the associated localizing value. Often eye movement recordings are required to be certain of the exact nature of an unusual ocular oscillation.

Ocular Bobbing[67]

Ocular bobbing is usually seen in comatose patients with massive pontine haemorrhage or infarction. Glioblastoma multiforme or metabolic encephalopathy also produce this syndrome.

The term 'bobbing' is apt. A fast conjugate downward movement of the eyes is followed by a slow updrift to the primary position. Unlike downbeat nystagmus, the updrift is staggered such that the eyes appear to bob like a fisherman's float after the fish has taken the bait. Associated features are an absence of spontaneous or reflex (Doll's head) eye movements.

Superior Oblique Myokymia[68]

Superior oblique myokymia represents one of the most bizarre ocular oscillations. Symptoms usually include sudden monocular torsional diplopia with oscillopsia. A fast small amplitude torsional monocular movement may be seen on slit lamp examination, and is associated with a synchronous bruit over the orbit. Carbamizepine therapy occasionally provides relief.

ACKNOWLEDGEMENT

Figures 1, 2, 3, 5, 6, 7, 10 and 13 first appeared in *Computerized Tomography in Neuro-Ophthalmology*, by I. F. Moseley and M. D. Sanders, 1982. They are published here by kind permission of Chapman & Hall.

REFERENCES

1. Bender M. B. Brain control of conjugate horizontal and vertical eye movement A survey of the structural and functional correlations. *Brain* 1980; **103**, 23–69.
2. Foville A. L. Note sur une paralysie peu connue de certains muscles de l'oeil et sa liaison avec quelques ponts de l'anatomie de la pretuberenie annulaire. *Bull. Soc. Anat. Paris* 1858; **33**, 373–405.
3. Parinaud H. Paralysie des mouvements associes des yeux. *Arch. Neurol.* 1883; **5**, 145–72.
4. Robinson D. A. Ocular motor unit behaviour in the monkey. *J. Neurophysiol.* 1970; **33**, 393–404.
5. McCree R. H., Baker R. and Delgado-Garcia J. Afferent and efferent organisation of the prepositive hypoglossi nucleus. *Prog. Brain. Res.* 1979; **50**, 653–65.
6. Mays L. E. Neuronal correlates of vergence eye movements. *Soc. Neurosci. Abstr.* 1981; **7**, 133.
7. Bütner-Ennever J. A. and Akert A. Medial rectus subgroups of the ocular motor nucleus and their abducens internuclear input in the monkey. *J. Comp. Neurol.* 1981; **197**, 17–27.
8. Bütner-Ennever J. A., Buttner U., Cohen B. et al. Vertical paralysis and the rostral interstitial nucleus of the median longitudinal fasciculus. *Brain* 1982; **105**, 125–49.
9. Ferrier D. Experiments on the brain of monkeys. *Proc. R. Soc. Lond.* 1875; **23**, 409–32.
10. Goldberg M. E. and Bushnell H. C. Behavioural enhancement of visual responses in monkey cerebral cortex. Modulation in frontal eye fields specifically related to saccades. *J. Neurophysiol.* 1981; **46**, 773–87.
11. Lynch J. C. and McLarin J. W. The contribution of parieto-occipital association cortex to the control of slow eye movements. In: Lennerstrand G., Zee D. S. and Keller E. L. (ed.) *Functional Basis of Ocular Motility Disorders.* Oxford, Pergamon Press, 1982.
12. Wurtz R. H. and Albano J. E. Visual-motor function of the primate superior colliculus. *Ann. Rev. Neurosci.* 1980; **3**, 189–226.
13. Sherrington C. S. *The Integrative Action of the Nervous System.* London, 1908.
14. King W. M., Lisberger S. G. and Fuchs A. F. Response of fibres in the medial longitudinal fasciculus of alert

monkeys during horizontal and vertical conjugate eye movements evoked by visual or vestibular stimuli. *J. Neurophysiol.* 1976; **39**, 1135–49.
15. Pola J. and Robinson D. A. Oculomotor signals in the medial longitudinal fasciculus of the monkey. *J. Neurophysiol.* 1978; **41**, 245–59.
16. Zee D. S. and Robinson D. A. A hypothetical explanation of saccadic oscillations. *Ann. Neurol.* 1979; **5**, 504–14
17. Halmagyi G. M., Gresty M. A. and Leech J. Reversal optokinetic nystagmus (OKN) mechanisms and clinical significance. *Ann. Neurol.* 1980; **7**, 429–35.
18. Collewijm H., Winterson B. J. and Dubois M. F. W. Optokinetic eye movements in albino rabbits. Inversion in the anterior visual field. *Science* 1978; **199**, 1351–5.
19. Daroff R. B. and Hoyt W. F. Supranuclear disorders of ocular control systems in men: Clinical, anatomical and physiological correlations. In: Bach-y-Rita P., Collins C. S. and Hyde J. E. (ed.) *The Control of Eye Movements*. New York, Academic Press, 1971; pp. 75–235.
20. Stroud M. M., Newman N. M., Keltner J. L. et al. Abducting nystagmus in the medial longitudinal fasciculus syndrome – internuclear ophthalmoplegia. *Arch. Ophthalmol.* 1974; **82**, 2.
21. Pola J. and Robinson D. A. An explanation of eye movements seen in internuclear ophthalmoplegia. *Arch. Neurol.* 1976; **33**, 447.
22. Pierrot-Descilligny C. and Chain F. L'ophthalmoplegie internucleare. *Rev. Neurol (Paris)* 1979; **135**, 485.
23. Bender M. B. and Winstein E. A. Dissociated monocular nystagmus with paresis of the horizontal eye movements. *Arch. Ophthalmol.* 1939; **21**, 266.
24. Barloh R. W., Yee, R. D. and Homrubia, V. Internuclear ophthalmoplegia I. Saccades and dissociated nystagmus *Arch. Neurol.* 1978; **35**, 484.
25. Gresty M. A., Hess K. and Leech J. Disorders of the vestibulo-ocular reflex producing oscillopsia and mechanisms compensating for loss of labyrinthine function. *Brain* 1977; **100**, 693.
26. Pierrot-Descilligny C. H., Chain F., Serdaru M. et al. The 'one and a half' syndrome. Electro-oculographic analysis of five cases with deductions about the physiological mechanisms of lateral gaze. *Brain* 1981; **104**, 665.
27. Thrush D. C. and Foster J. B. An analysis of nystagmus in 100 consecutive patients with communicating syringomyelia. *J. Neurol. Sci.* 1973; **20**, 381.
28. Snyder B. D., Blonde L. and McWhinter W. R. Reversal of amitryptiline intoxication by physostigmine. *JAMA* 1974; **230**, 1433.
29. Cook F. F., Davis R. G. and Russol S. Internuclear ophthalmoplegia caused by phenothiazine intoxication. *Arch. Neurol.* 1981; **38**, 465.
30. Swick M. M. Pseudointernuclear ophthalmoplegia in acute idiopathic polyneuritis (Fisher's syndrome). *Am. J. Ophthalmol.* 1974; **77**, 725.
31. Hering E. *Beitr. Physiol. (Leipzig)*, 1864.
32. Rucker C. W. Paralysis of the third, fourth and sixth cranial nerves. *Am. J. Ophthalmol.* 1958; **46**, 787.
33. Shrader C. C. and Schlezinger N. D. Neuro-ophthalmologic evaluation of abducens nerve paralysis. *Arch. Ophthalmol.* 1970; **64**, 108.
34. Rucker C. W. The causes of paralysis of the third, fourth and sixth cranial nerves. *Am. J. Ophthalmol.* 1966; **61**, 1293.
35. Johnston A. C. Aetiology and treatment of abducens palsy. *Trans. Pacif. Coast Ophthalmol. Soc.* 1968; **49**, 259.
36. Robertson D. M., Hines J. D. and Ruke C. W. Acquired VI nerve paresis in children. *Arch. Ophthalmol.* 1970; **83**, 574.
37. Mario T., Kubota N., Akimoto H. et al. Duane's syndrome. *Jap J. Ophthalmol.* 1979; **23**, 453.
38. Hotchkiss M. G., Miller N. R., Clark A. W. et al. Bilateral Duane's retraction syndrome. A clinical pathologic case report. *Arch. Ophthalmol.* 1980; **98**, 876.
39. Bryce-Smith R. and MacIntosh R. R. Sixth nerve palsy after lumbar puncture and spinal analgesia. *Br. Med. J.* 1951; **1**, 275.
40. Knox D. L., Clerk, D. B. and Shuster F. F. Benign VI nerve palsies in childhood. *Paediatrics* 1967; **40**, 560.
41. Keane J. Bilateral VI nerve palsy. Analysis of 125 cases. *Arch. Neurol.* 1976; **33**, 681.
42. Burier K. M., van Allen M. C. O., Seaton R. R. et al. Substitution phenomenon in congenital and acquired supranuclear disorders of eye movement. *Trans. Am. Acad. Ophthalmol. Otolaryngol.* 1965; **69**, 1106.
43. Lowenfeld I. E. and Thompson H. S. Oculomotor paresis with cyclic spasms. A critical review of the literature and a new case. *Surv. Ophthalmol.* 1975; **20**, 81.
44. O'Day J., Billson F. and King J. Ophthalmoplegic migraine and aberrant regeneration of the third nerve. *Br. J. Ophthalmol.* 1980; **64**, 534.
45. Scadding G. K. and Havard C. W. K. Pathogenesis and treatment of myasthenia gravis. *Br. J. Med.* 1981; **283**, 1008.
46. Cogan D. G. Myasthenia gravis: A review of the disease and a description of lid twitch as a characteristic sign. *Arch. Ophthalmol.* 1965; **74**, 211.
47. Cogan D. G., Yee R. D. and Gitinger J. Rapid eye movements in myasthenia gravis. I: Clinical observations. *Arch. Ophthamol.* 1976; **94**, 1083.
48. Yee R. D., Cogan D. G., Zee D. S. et al. Rapid eye movements in myasthenia gravis. II: Electro-oculographic analysis *Arch. Ophthamol.* 1976; **95**, 1465.
49. Spooner J. W. and Baloh R. W. Eye movement fatigue in myasthenia gravis. *Neurology* 1979; **29**, 29.
50. Morgan Hughes J. A. Mitochondrial myopathies. In: Nastaglia F. L. and Walton J. H. (ed.) *Skeletal Muscle Pathology*. Edinburgh, Churchill Livingstone, 1982, pp. 309–39.

51. Mullie M. A., Harding A. E., Petty R. K. H. et al. Retinal manifestations of mitochondrial myopathy. *Arch. Ophthalmol.* 1985; **103,** 1825–30.
52. McKechnie N. M., King M. and Lee W. R. Retinal pathology in Kearns Sayre syndrome. *Br. J. Ophthalmol.* 1985; **69,** 63–75.
53. Winstanley J. The eye signs of Graves's disease. In: Clifford Rose F. (ed.) *The Eye in General Medicine.* London, Chapman and Hall, 1983, p. 428.
54. Leonard T. J. K., Graham E. M., Standford M. R. et al. A new presentation of Graves's disease. Bilateral acute painful proptosis, ptosis, ophthalmoplegia and visual loss. *Lancet* 1984; **2,** 431–3.
55. Atkinson S., Holcombe M., Kendall-Taylor P. Ophthalmopathic immunoglobulin in patients with Graves's ophthalmopathy. *Lancet* 1984; **2,** 374–6.
56. Kodarma K., Sikorsk A. H. and Bandy Defoc P. Demonstration of circulating autoantibody against soluble eye muscle antigens in Graves's ophthalmopathy. *Lancet* 1982; **2,** 1353–6.
57. Moseley I. F. and Sanders M. D. *Computerised Tomography in Neuro-Ophthalmology.* London, Chapman and Hall, 1982, pp. 21–30.
58. Cogan D. G. and Loeb D. R. Optokinetic spasm and intracranial lesions. *Arch. Neurol. Psychiatr. (Chicago)* 1949; **61,** 183.
59. Shultz W. T., Stral L., Hoyt W. F. et al. Normal saccadic structure of voluntary nystagmus. *Arch. Ophthalmol.* 1977; **95,** 1399.
60. Daroff R. B., Troost B. T. and Dell'Osso L. F. In: Glaser J. S. (ed.) *Neuro-Ophthalmology.* Hagerstown, Md, Harper and Row, 1978, p. 219.
61. Daroff R. B. See-saw nystagmus. *Neurology* 1965; **15,** 874–7.
62. Ocusa L., Stark L., Hoyt W. F. et al. Opposed adducting saccades in convergence–retraction nystagmus. A patient with sylvian aqueduct syndrome. *Brain* 1979; **102,** 497-508.
63. Alexander G. In: Pfaundler M. and Schlossman A. (ed.) *Handbuch der Kinder Heilkunde.* Leipzig, Vogel, 1912, pp. 84–96.
64. Halmagyi C. M., Rudge P., Gresty M. A. et al. Downbeating nystagmus. Review of 62 cases. *Arch. Neurol.* 1983; **90,** 777.
65. Davis D. G. and Smith J. L. Periodic alternating nystagmus. *Am. J. Ophthalmol.* 1971; **72,** 757–62.
66. Guillain G. The syndrome of synchronous rhythmic palato-pharyngo-laryngo-oculodiaphragmatic myoclonus. *Proc. R. Soc. Med.* 1938; **31,** 1031.
67. Susac J. O., Hoyt W. F. and Daroff R. B. Clinical spectrum of ocular bobbing. *J. Neurol. Neurosurg. Psychiatr.* 1970; **33,** 771–5.
68. Susac J. O., Smith J. L. and Schatz N. J. Superior oblique myokymia. *Arch. Neurol.* 1973; **29,** 432.

Chapter 18

Paediatric Ophthalmology

Françoise Cuendet and David Taylor

We intend first to describe the assessment of vision in childhood and outline the impact of visual handicap on the development of the child, concentrating on the first year of life (infancy). We will integrate this with aspects of general development and see how they interact in the child who has multiple handicaps.

In the second part of the chapter we will deal with some of the more common problems that present to an ophthalmologist who looks after children. Naturally, this review is not comprehensive, and for details on other topics in paediatric ophthalmology the reader is referred to more comprehensive works.[1-3]

INFANT DEVELOPMENT

Clinical Visual Assessment

Neurophysiological studies have increased the awareness of a critical period for the development of vision in infancy, and it is increasingly valuable to be able to assess visual function as early as possible. Advances in technology have allowed us to become more objective and to quantify visual functions in infancy. We should co-operate with the child, play with him, observe how he plays and how vision helps him.

History Taking

A paediatric ophthalmologist pays a great deal of attention to the prenatal, birth and perinatal history and discusses with the mother the pregnancy, the length of gestation, birth weight, the nature of the delivery, whether there were any problems in the neonatal period and then discusses the child's motor, social and speech milestones, together with his ability to hear, his general health and any treatment that he may have had. A family history with direct questions about squints, poor vision and consanguinity should be taken before a history of the visual problem itself.

The opinion of the mother, especially if she has had previous children, is very valuable, but should be interpreted carefully in the light of the mother's social and educational background. Direct questioning may be necessary about the baby's response to a silent smile and his ability to maintain eye to eye contact, especially during feeding. There is something unique about the communication that a mother and baby may have; when the baby sees, the communication is many times greater than that obtained when the eyes just happen to be looking at the mother but not seeing, as in a blind baby. Direct questions about visual interest, following, grasping of objects and facial expressiveness, together with questions about the presence and nature of any squint are important.

Where there is a suspicion of visual handicap, specific questions about the detection of toys by vision or by feel, or about whether the baby looks at immobile or only mobile objects, are necessary. The mother should also be asked whether the baby turns his head towards a window or a light, or is photophobic, or whether he has watering or unsteady eyes; whether the child tends to poke or rub his eyes; whether he bumps into furniture; whether he has head thrusts or whether there is abnormal behaviour, especially when he is left alone – for instance rhythmic, stereotyped movements with his body.

Observational Techniques in Visual Assessment

A most important variable when testing an infant's vision is his level of alertness and interest. The examination must be quick and every investigation should be planned to be carried out only once, although it may need to be repeated when the child is in a suitably cooperative and relaxed state. The best time is usually 1–2 h after feeding, but there is a great variation from one child to another and one must bear in mind that a negative response to subjective tests does not necessarily mean a visual handicap if the baby is sleepy or tired.

Direct Signs

PUPILLARY REACTIONS

Pupillary reactions are not a test of vision but they are a useful sign of the patency of the anterior visual pathways. They are reliably present in a premature child of at least 31 weeks' gestation, but absent at

29 weeks or less.[4] Because the pupils of a neonate are small and constrict and dilate slowly, a bright light is needed, and magnification may help. Because it is difficult to make an infant look at a distant object, the differentiation of the near reflex from the light reflexes is difficult. The amplitude and velocity of pupil reactions should be noted, as well as the presence or absence of a relative afferent pupillary defect, which occurs when there is a conduction defect in one eye that is greater than that in the other. This test, also known as the 'swinging flashlight' test, is elicited by moving the light from the 'good' eye quickly to the 'bad' eye. If there is a relative afferent defect when the light is moved to the 'bad' eye, the pupils will dilate, since the input to the pupillary system is less through the eye with the damaged conduction system. Paradoxical pupil reactions in which the pupils dilate in the light and constrict in the dark should be tested for in cases of suspected poor vision due to a retinal defect.

FIXATION AND FOLLOWING

This is the most reliable clinical test. Fixation is present at birth. A recent study[5] of visual behaviour in 70 newborns tested from 2 to 10 days after birth showed that 83 per cent followed a face, but not one followed a white light. One should note whether the fixation is central or eccentric, steady or unsteady, as well as the speed and the length of fixation.

Three-dimensional and colourful objects have greater interest to infants; in the first 3 weeks of life infants prefer to fixate simple targets (e.g. a four-checked square), but they prefer to look at more complex patterns as they get older.[6] There is a preference for the human face, therefore the quickest and easiest way to elicit fixing and following[7] is to hold the infant upright and move one's face slowly in front of him. If the examiner is unsuccessful he can ask the mother to try the same thing, warning her not to make any noise. While performing this test care must be taken not to rotate the infant, since this would induce a confusing vestibulo-ocular reflex. If a child responds to a silent smile, or if his face becomes alert when he looks at objects of interest to him, this is a very good sign of central vision. One should also notice the quality of refixations, how quickly and accurately an object in the peripheral field is brought into focus by the child.

VISUALLY DIRECTED REACHING

Visually directed reaching may start at less than 3 months of age. Hoyt et al.[7] have found that, in a clinical setting, this type of testing is not useful until the infant has developed a good postural tone and reflexes, which is usually at 6 months or even later. Very tiny cake decorations ('hundreds and thousands') – which are about 2 mm in diameter – put on to a sheet of paper are a test of both manual and visual skills. (*Fig.* 1). If the child does not want to reach for these one can try with any other kind of sweet of a larger size, the most popular of which are 'Smarties'. If possible, the child should be tested binocularly and then monocularly.

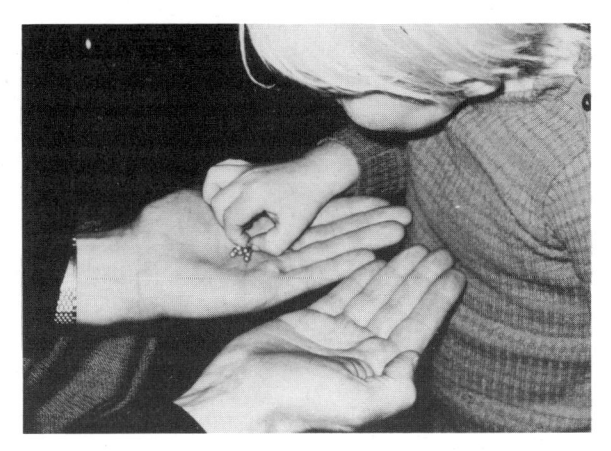

Fig. 1. *Vision testing.* The child who is suspected of having a visual handicap is presented with small objects (in this case tiny silver sweets) in the palm of one hand, with the other hand being held out simultaneously so that he can choose which hand has the sweets on it. Although a very crude test of visual ability, the use of different sized sweets can add depth to the examination.

Stycar mounted (*Fig.* 2) or rolling balls are a valuable test, but they only test visibility and not the power of resolution. They can, therefore, give an overestimation of acuity, especially if the child is alert. The rolling balls test was based on a technique described by Claud Worth in 1903. He observed the

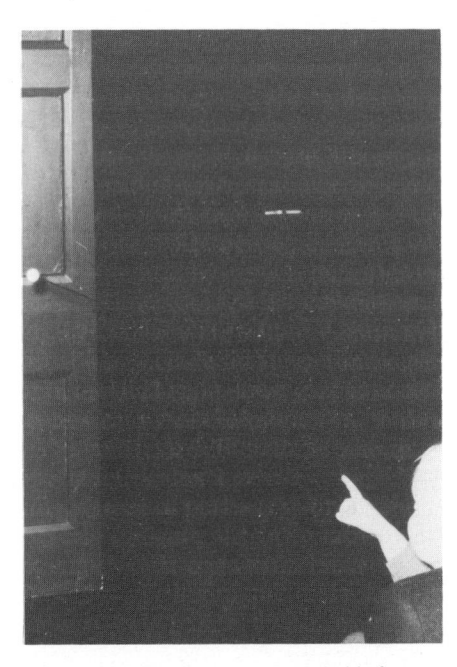

Fig. 2. *Vision testing.* The examiner hides behind a screen observing the child through a small slit. He then shows the child a ball mounted on the end of a stick and the child is encouraged to 'spot' it. This test gains some impression of the child's vision, including the visual field.

fixation of children who were being encouraged to follow specially graded ivory balls which he flicked with great dexterity while watching the child. Today the balls are made of polystyrene, but the observations are just as useful provided the examiner is aware of the test's limitations.

The standard tests for squint, especially the cover--uncover test and the alternate cover test and prism testing, will be helpful in determining whether the child has basic visual reflexes. Blinking to a bright light occurs in premature babies, even of 30 weeks' gestation.[4] The source of light should be bright and noiseless and the baby should be observed carefully, since the response may be transient. A positive test only indicates a bare minimum of function of the afferent and efferent pathways as far as the geniculate body.

Blinking to threat only appears at about 5 to 6 months and is an acquired response, it is therefore difficult to interpret in very young infants. Care must be taken to use a large threatening target and to move it in such a way that a cutaneous blink reflex is avoided.

Visual field testing in preverbal children is possible, at least to a crude extent (*Fig.* 3). The examiner holds the child's attention while he watches for refixation eye movements towards an object which is introduced into the peripheral field; the four quadrants can be evaluated in each eye.

Indirect Signs

Abnormal eye movements are the most common sign of poor vision: the more gross and less coordinated these wandering eye movements, the poorer the vision. The nystagmus of poor vision in infancy is usually 'pendular', with horizontal, vertical and rotary components.

Many young infants with severe visual defects use their fist or a finger to rub or poke the eye; the reasons for this are not fully understood, but are at least in part habitual. The action may be quite violent.

After a few months of age most infants are very expressive, but in blind children there is a striking lack of facial mobility and after 1 or 2 years they sometimes develop characteristic tics, which may also be found in sighted, but severely mentally retarded or autistic children.

OBJECTIVE TESTS

Visually evoked cortical responses (VER), electro-retinogram (ERG) and electro-encephalogram (EEG) are now frequently used in children's clinics. All can be carried out without the use of sedation. Electroretinography comes into its own in infancy to diagnose congenital retinal dystrophy, in which the eye may be normal[8] despite a severe visual handicap. ERGs are also useful in the assessment of the child with a visual handicap of other cause, for instance congenital cataract, to exclude the possibility of an associated retinal abnormality. VERs to a flash stimulus[9] are a very useful way of assessing the electrophysiological integrity of the visual pathway, without giving any estimate of visual acuity, but the presence of a normal response can be taken as an encouraging sign for the development of normal vision. Pattern visually evoked responses in infancy have been used to determine acuity,[10] but the technique is expensive and the results have yet to be confirmed. It does have the advantage of being an objective test.

Optokinetic nystagmus may be present in full term infants but it is reliably absent in blind and in many brain damaged infants (*Fig.* 4). One cannot be sure that optokinetic nystagmus is a purely cortical function and there is increasing evidence that there may be subcortical pathways which subserve optokinetic

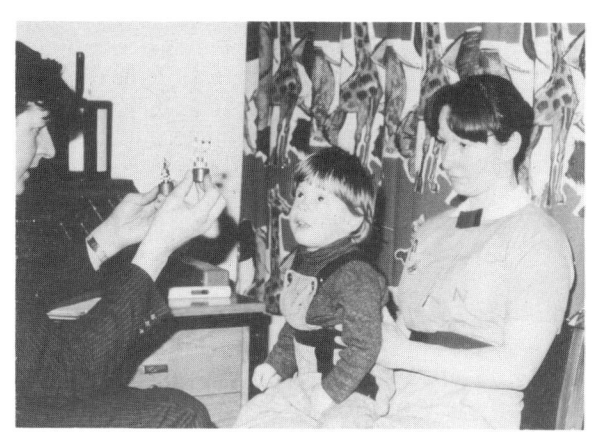

Fig. 3. Visual field testing. Visual field testing in an infant or small child is possible, although the evaluation is crude. Despite the crudeness of this test, it is still extremely useful to know whether a child will have a total homonymous hemianopia during his development and education. In this test the child's attention is attracted to one toy while another is brought in silently from one side and the child's refixation is observed.

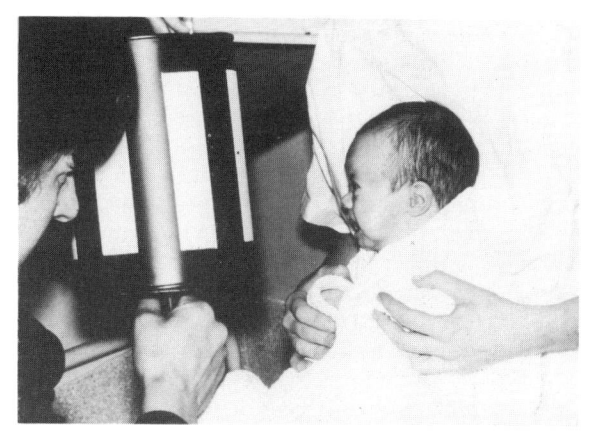

Fig. 4. Optokinetic nystagmus. Optokinetic nystagmus should not be thought of as a specific test for visual acuity, but as a test for vision and the integrity of the central nervous system. A positive test in a small child implies not only at least useful vision, but an intact central pathway for optokinetic movements.

nystagmus. Acuities estimated by optokinetic techniques are of less relevance than previously thought, being highly dependent on attention, interest and motor responses. The test is one of minimum visible and not minimum resolvable and in clinical practice simple techniques using a very large drum or a bright scarf with stripes on it, are used. Failure to elicit OKN by these techniques in very young children should never be relied on as the only evidence of visual impairment.

A device known as the Catford drum has been introduced to measure vision in infancy; it measures more the ability of the child to follow a small object than his acuity, and therefore measurements may be somewhat misleading, especially if the child has reduced acuity.

Spinning the child is a useful technique to elicit both vestibulo-ocular reflexes and optokinetic nystagmus. With smaller children this can be done by the examiner holding the child up in front of him, but with heavier infants it is more comfortable to perform the test while sitting on a rotating chair with the axis of rotation running through the crown/rump axis of the child.

Providing there are no oculomotor abnormalities, the only true indication of visual awareness is the ability to suppress nystagmus in two situations:

1. When the rotation is stopped suddenly, a normal child will show only one or two afterbeats, but a blind infant will continue to have nystagmus for several beats. This test is normal in a child with one blind eye and one sighted eye, unless the sighted eye is covered.

2. During rotation, a child from 3 months old may be able to suppress nystagmus while transiently looking at the examiner.

Tonic deviation of the eyes in the direction opposite to the rotation also occurs in infants with neurological disorders which give rise to a saccade (rapid eye movement) palsy. Blindness can be misdiagnosed in a child with oculomotor apraxia or one with cerebral palsy with a saccade palsy who cannot generate saccades and therefore may not appear to see.

Refraction is all too often overlooked. Ingram et al.[11] have shown that if a 1-year-old child has 2·5 dioptres of hypermetropia in any one meridian, he has a significant chance of developing a squint or becoming amblyopic. Bilateral hypermetropia, astigmatism or anisometropia are also significantly associated with squint and amblyopia. Visually impaired children have a higher incidence of refractive error, but these may be difficult to assess because of opacities in the refractive media.[12] Photo refraction, a simple technique for screening for refractive errors, has recently been introduced; the difference in the brightness of the light reflected through the pupil from the fundi indicates the amount of refractive error and the presence of anisometropia.[13]

In the forced-choice (for the observer) preferential looking method (FPL), the child is presented with one blank screen and one patterned screen of matching luminance which are randomly changed from one side to the other. If the child looks more consistently at the pattern he can detect it. The optimal age for testing by this method is between 1 and 6 months (or later in patients with mental retardation). Visual acuity can be estimated by the stripe width (spatial frequency) and the technique can also be used for testing for colour vision or contrast sensitivity. The information given by FPL is nearer to the clinical examination of vision,[14] but is less objective than VERs.

Visual Development

The infant eye undergoes phenomenal anatomical and neurophysiological development in the first year of life. There is an increase in the diameter of the globe which is 16·5 mm at birth and becomes 24·5 mm by adulthood; most of this growth occurs in the first year of life, which demands profound changes in refraction, accommodation and depth of focus.

Development of Eye Position and Motility

The position of the eyes of a premature baby during sleep gradually changes from the straight ahead to the sleep position of the adult. This usually occurs by 3 weeks for a full term baby. Spontaneous opening of the lids is rare in the very premature infant, but is normal in a full term neonate.

Saccadic horizontal movements are present from birth, but are very hypometric.[7,15] The baby may produce multiple small rapid movements (saccades) which are of low amplitude to reach a target. It is often impossible to elicit any vertical saccades until at least 4–6 weeks of age. Between 6 weeks and 3 months smooth pursuit movements may first be observed. The vestibular system is well developed in most neonates and provides a consistent way of evaluating the range of ocular movements.

Accommodation, Vergences and Binocular Single Vision

In neonates, a limited power of accommodation produces a relatively fixed focal length for the eye, up to about 20–30 cm from the baby; at around 3 months children adjust their accommodation for targets as far as 75 cm.[16] It is usually not before 6 months that an infant can accommodate to a target over the entire working range from near to infinity.[7,13] Convergence to moving targets occurs in 1-month-old babies but a normal infant with normal binocular vision will not usually overcome a base-out prism employed to induce convergence until he is 6 months old.

There is not yet a precise estimate of stereo acuity as a function of age in infancy, but Braddick and Atkinson[17] showed that at around 3 months of age there was binocular enhancement of the uniocular response.

While the eyes are less often 'straight' in the newborn than in adults, or older children, the great majority of eye movements are conjugate. Most infants establish constant ocular alignment within 3–4 weeks of life.[7]

Fixation and Development of Visual Acuity

The anatomical substrate for visual development is present even after 33 weeks' gestation. The 1-month-old's acuity allows him to distinguish the principal features of a face at less than one metre. At 2–3 months old an infant resolves objects of a few millimetres at 1 m. Progressively his eyes fix a target more accurately, more quickly and for a longer time.

There are marked individual differences in the rates of increase in infant acuity and great variations between the different ways of testing (VEP, FPL, OKN). By VEP methods acuity values equal to those of an adult $(1.0 = 20/20 = 6/6)$ are reached at 6 months, but only by 2 years if a forced preferential looking method is used.[14] By OKN testing 6/6 acuity is achieved at around 20–30 months.[6] Thresholds for gratings are higher for amblyopes and children with ocular anomalies than with standard methods of testing, even with isolated letter testing. The surrounded single letter (or letters) read in a row shows poor initial acuity with greater development later on; thus the best test is the surrounded letter (e.g., contour interaction with bar format ((E)) is the best test because it is less confusing for a child than the Landolt 'C' or illiterate 'E' with pseudo-optotypes).[18] Single letter studies show high levels of visual acuity at early ages and little development thereafter. In a 3-year-old the contrast sensitivity is similar to the adult's.[12]

Perceptual Abilities

In the first months of life an infant can pick up some of the clues which give a three-dimensional impression, although without a complete sense of space. Infants gradually learn orientation and movement and acquire recognition of objects. At 5–7 weeks infants can usually differentiate between the face pictures of different individuals. However, under 2 months, infants usually ignore the inert features of objects, therefore, recognition of a face is made on the outlines rather than the eyes and mouth.[13]

Colour Vision

The spectral sensitivity of a 2-month-old infant resembles the adult. The most rapid period of maturation in all visual capabilities seems to be early in the first 6 months of life.

General Developmental Milestones

The factor that affects the rate of a child's development more than any other is his intelligence;[19] however, prematurity, environment, family, sex (girls quicker, at least initially!), personality, general health, sensory deprivation, autism, lack of stimulation, lack of love, may explain the range of variations in normal developmental milestones.

No child is thought of as mentally retarded if backward in a single field of development and normal in all other fields. The mentally retarded child is backward in his social behaviour, in his speech and in his manipulation, though he can sometimes sit or walk at the average age, and perform well in a circumscribed area. The age at which main milestones in the three most important fields of development should be obtained is shown in *Table I*.

Table I. Milestones in child development

| Age | Motor | | Social | Speech |
	Gross	Fine		
4 wk	(Postures and movements of limbs and trunk dominated by primary reflexes).			
6 wk			*Social smile:*	
2 mth	*Gross head control:* no head control when pulled to sit (3 mth)	Holding of toys but no hand/eye coordination (3 mth)	Turns head to sounds Laughing	Cooing
			Still friendly to foreigner	
6 mth	*Sits* unaided	Palmar grasp and transfer		*Babbling* (change in intonation)
9 mth	Attempts to crawl: stands holding on	Picks up a pellet scissor fashion, grasping	Delighted imitation Understands 'no'	Recognizable syllables
1 yr	*Walks* with hand held *Walks* alone but tumbles	*Pincer grasp*	Situational understanding and imitation by 9 mth to 1 yr. Wave goodbye Looks for fallen objects	*Single words* 'mama, dada'
1½ yr	Walks well	Builds tower of three bricks	Enjoys picture books	Words – vocabulary rapidly increasing
2 yrs	Runs well			Word combination

A smile as an answer to a smile should be obtained at 6 weeks in a full term baby. A delay of motor development, a lateralization appearing before 1 year or other neurological dysfunction may be a sign of cerebral palsy.

With a little practice the ophthalmologist can take a very useful history which will alert him to the presence of any significant developmental problems. In addition to the service to the patient, this concern for the child's general development is often reassuring and confidence-inspiring to the mother. There are several useful books on child development to which the clinician can refer.[20,21,22]

The Effect of a Visual Defect on General Development

Development depends on the maturation of the nervous system, and until that has occurred, no amount of practice will help a child to learn a skill. But when practice is denied, or when there is a lack of stimulus due to a visual handicap, the ability may lie dormant. The sequence of development is the same for all children, but the rate of development varies and is considerably slowed by sensory handicaps. Early stimulation by alternative means to vision achieves the best developmental results.[23,24]

In a blind child there is no eye-to-eye contact with his mother and therefore a less intense communication. A baby who can't communicate and 'bond' through sight and who lacks facial mobility and expression is less rewarding for the mother and has less contact. He is at risk of remaining without a clear concept of his surroundings. The blind child cannot build a stable image of himself or his parents, and it is hard for him to understand finally who's who, and what's what. He cannot make himself understood because he has less facial expression; he cannot point, and cannot bring the interest of people to the thing that interests him. Not only is the world difficult for him to understand, but it is as difficult for him to make himself understood. Location of touch and sound is normally done through visual associations, and must be replaced by auditory–tactile associations (e.g. guidance of a baby's hands towards the sound). Because he does not see his hands and feet, a blind baby should be made aware of them and encouraged to explore and play with them and to find their use in exploration. Fraiberg found that sitting or standing are not greatly delayed in blind babies whereas mobility milestones are.[25,26] The language of a blind child may appear satisfactorily developed, but it frequently hides an imprecise linguistic understanding, because his words remain without 'concrete' meanings. Some blind children remain very silent in their first year, unable perhaps to mimic mother's lip movements. Apart from the difficulty of understanding the permanence of objects, there is the difficulty of grasping the relationship between them.

Since vision is the prime coordinating sense in the early stage of development, and because of the lack of curiosity induced by sight, visually impaired children are at a high risk of withdrawal behaviour, with stereotyped rocking body movements. They often pass through an echolalic phase and should ideally be carefully followed up by a competent and interested paediatrician to avoid secondary handicaps. Of course the less severe the visual handicap, the nearer to normal will be the acquisition of skills.

The Multiply Handicapped Infant and Young Child

The risk of visual defect is a hundred times higher in multiply handicapped children[12] and there is a need for special management.

The best assessment is gained in the child's own surroundings, ideally with the help of a multi-disciplinary team to assist in communication, selection and training for the best test corresponding to the child's capabilities. The test should first be performed for near, then at greater distances. In very severely affected children only indirect observations of reactions to visual stimuli can be used, such as irregularity in breathing, decrease in motor activity while fixing, emotional reaction with widening of palpebral fissures, or expressions of joy or fear. In mentally retarded children a lack of visual interest may be interpreted as poor vision.

For older children, before using an illiterate 'E' test or a single letter matching test, one must be sure that the child has a good spatial orientation. 'Perceptual disorders', like hand–eye co-ordination, right–left motion, or the 'crowding' phenomenon are seen in cerebral palsy, minimal brain dysfunction and in mentally retarded children.[12]

Visual field testing is often very difficult and one must rely on behavioural observation. Hemianopsia is common and easily overlooked in cerebral palsy, when it may be a serious additional visual problem. The 'two targets' method is very useful in eliciting a gross (but developmentally significant) homonymous defect in a very young child (see Fig. 3).

Refractive errors, squint and amblyopia are more common in the multiply handicapped child and should be managed much as in other children; it is a mistake not to treat a refractive error or squint because of misplaced kindness. An atropine refraction is often better than cycloplegia with a short acting drug because the examination may be much quicker and the child more easily distracted by the 'game' of the test. In premature children myopia is common. The correction of the refractive error must be proportionate to the child's needs and to his corrected vision. Glasses are sometimes reluctantly accepted by retarded children and they require plastic or toughened glass lenses, strong and comfortable frames, sometimes needing to be tied on. Elbow restraints may be helpful; this is not a cruel procedure and, once started, often becomes unnecessary because of increased compliance.

Emotionally immature children often resent the occlusion of one eye, therefore it may be helpful to use atropine to defocus the fixing eye instead. The treatment of amblyopia lessens at least one of their handicaps, but the proportion of the visual defect accounted for by organic disease should be evaluated before starting on treatment. Even if there is mild asymmetry in optic disc colour with a relative afferent pupillary defect, occlusion therapy is worthwhile as amblyopia may cause part of the defect.

Squint occurs in children with cerebral palsy more than ten times as frequently as in the general population, the figures varying from 37 to 60 per cent, the higher incidence being in the more handicapped children. In addition, these squints are much more frequently incomitant, paralytic and complicated by nystagmus, gaze palsies or uncoordinated eye movements. A concomitant squint may result from an initially incomitant deviation or be due to poor vision in one or both eyes, poor fusion or significant refractive errors.[27] A squint in the multiply handicapped child should be dealt with as in any other child, but any pathological causes, and especially raised intracranial pressure, should be excluded. The angle of deviation should be measured so that an increase can be detected. Especially if associated with papilloedema, a squint can be the first sign of a blocked valve in shunted hydrocephalus and it should be treated as a matter of urgency. An atrophic disc, because of the lack of nerve fibres which normally become swollen in papilloedema, may no longer show swelling. If the shunt blockage is acute, there may be insufficient time for the development of papilloedema. The parents should be warned to report any sudden deterioration.

VIth nerve palsy is more frequent and the differential diagnosis between esotropia, with pseudo-limitation of both lateral recti, and a real paresis of the VIth nerve is important. Care should be taken that 'A' or 'V' phenomena (an increase or decrease in the angle of a squint in up or down gaze) are not overlooked.

Before planning surgery, any causative conditions should be stable. The problem of recurrent admissions to hospital and the risks of a general anaesthetic in these vulnerable children must be weighed carefully against the benefits directly to the child himself or indirectly to the child through his family. The choice of early or late surgery depends substantially on the parent's wishes and the most convenient time for the child's development. The long term result of surgery is unpredictable, especially when the angle of squint is variable or the squint associated with uncoordinated movements. The frequency of consecutive divergence should make the surgeon undercorrect a convergent squint in retarded children. Few multiply handicapped children will develop binocular vision and therefore a squint operation has often a largely cosmetic aim.

Vision can also be trained; for instance, the infant can be surrounded by objects with clearly visible visual surfaces coinciding with clearly felt tactile surfaces (e.g. dark materials of smooth surface and light coloured materials of rough texture). Parents can wear bright colours to help the child recognize them at a distance. All objects with which the toddler is in daily contact should be made attractive and colourful. Balls and other toys can be used to train fixation and visuo-motor coordination. When different echo-surfaces, like a mirror, are added to the child's environment, he can use them to experiment with different auditory and visual stimuli.[23] The best stimulation is the child's mother's face and body games where parents help the child progressively to take notice of his midline by bringing his hands together. An important part of the management of the multiply handicapped child is support for the parents and the whole family. A clear explanation should be given about the diagnosis and the amount the child can see, perhaps with the help of a drawing. Parents may be relieved by contact with other parents who have a child affected like their own, but who cope well in life.

A recommended book[28] or association (the Royal National Institute for the Blind), or a visit to a low visual aid clinic, can bring great comfort. The discussion regarding an eventual school placement must not be done too early because it can alarm parents. In order to determine the best education, it is necessary to separate the role of mental deficit from the role of visual deficit. Deaf children are very vulnerable and should be handled with special care. Deafness added to blindness does not mean an addition of two sensory defects, but a multiplication of the sensory defect, therefore children at risk, like rubella children and infants with Norrie's disease, should be particularly watched and helped.

SOME EYE PROBLEMS IN INFANCY

The Baby who Does Not See

The history and examination of the infant with suspected poor vision are taken as detailed earlier. This is followed by a close inspection of the external features, including the orbits and lids. If necessary, slit lamp examination can be carried out on a child of any age, and direct and indirect ophthalmoscopy and refraction very rarely require an anaesthetic or sedation in infancy. The most important thing is to be prepared to spend a substantial amount of time on the examination.

It is most important to look thoroughly for the treatable bilateral causes of poor vision in infancy (*Table* II). In particular:
Congenital cataracts
Congenital glaucoma
Retinoblastoma
High refractive error

Table II. Stages to diagnosis of a blind infant

Look for the obvious
    refractive error
    opaque media
    macular disorder
    optic disc abnormalities
Think again of the treatable
    glaucoma
    cataract
    retinoblastoma
    refractive error
If examination of the eye normal, think of
    Leber's amaurosis
    Cerebral blindness
    Optic disc hypoplasia
    Albinism
    Optic atrophy
    Delayed visual development
Investigate non-invasively
    If ERG abnormal do investigations for Leber's congenital amaurosis (urine concentration, liver function) or other retinal dystrophies/dysplasia, in conjunction with paediatrician.
    If ERG and VER normal, wait and repeat the examinations soon
    If ERG normal and VER abnormal, go to next stage
Invasive investigation (in this age group), CT scan in conjunction with neurologist

If there is no obvious cause on examination, it is best to pause and then go back through an anatomical approach to the possible causes, looking at the anterior segment, in particular at the cornea, considering whether there are diffuse corneal opacities that may not be immediately obvious but which may disrupt vision substantially; or whether there is a subtle congenital cataract which allows a good red reflex but no focused image on the retina. Many other causes of poor vision in infancy will be found in the posterior segment. The retinopathy of prematurity and retinal abnormalities are the largest cause, but one must not forget that retinal infections may occur, albeit rarely. Albinism can be an obvious cause of poor vision, but in its more subtle manifestations may easily be overlooked, unless specifically sought. Similarly optic atrophy or subtle manifestations of colobomas (*Fig.* 5) may well be missed in a child with a pale fundus background. One should never forget that the apparently blind child may have normal eyes, but a brain abnormality or delayed visual development.

The Blind Baby with No Obvious Cause

If one does not find an abnormality at the initial examination, the main causes of blindness to look for are (*Table* III):

Leber's Amaurosis and other Retinal Disorders (*Fig.* 6)

In this condition the child presents with a poor visual response, usually with nystagmus, sluggishly reacting pupils and a fundus abnormality, which is often extremely mild and sometimes described as normal.[8,29]

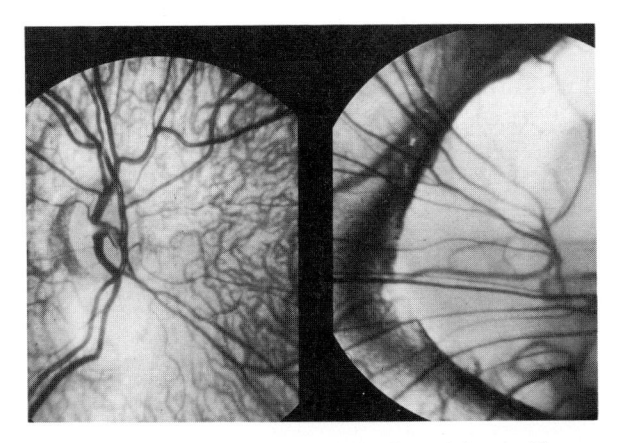

Fig. 5. Coloboma. Right, severe optic disc coloboma. The eye has no useful vision. *Left,* a small defect in the choroid over which retinal vessels dip. This is a small coloboma, and although it has no functional significance, it may have great diagnostic significance.

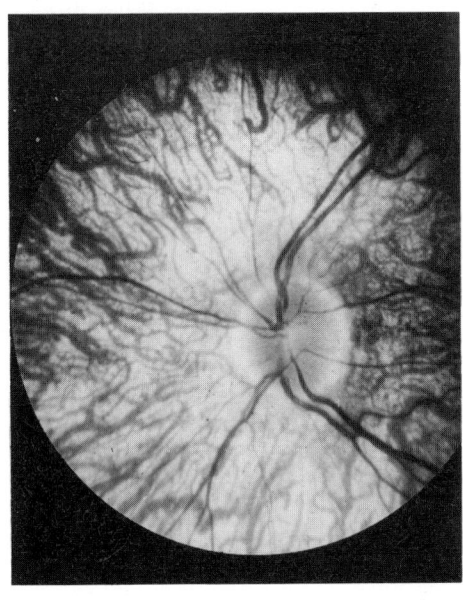

Fig. 6. Leber's amaurosis. This child presented with unsteady eyes in infancy and by the age of 4 months was thought to have extremely poor vision. The retinal pigment epithelium is very thin and there is some attenuation of the arterioles. The ERG was absent, confirming the diagnosis of Leber's amaurosis, which is a heterogeneous group of conditions which have a congenital retinal dystrophy.

Particular attention should be paid to the retinal arterioles, since arteriolar thinning is a very subtle sign in Leber's amaurosis. An electroretinogram will confirm the defect.

Optic Disc Hypoplasia (*Fig.* 7)

This condition is often missed if the clinician uses only an indirect ophthalmoscope, and therefore an

Table III. Main causes of blindness in cases with no obvious abnormality

	Leber's amaurosis	Optic disc hypoplasia	Cerebral blindness	Albinism	Optic atrophy	Cone dystrophy (Achromatopsia)	Delayed visual development	'Apparent blindness' secondary to severe developmental delay
Pupillary reflex	Usually sluggish, sometimes normal or absent	Often sluggish	Brisk	Normal	Depending on severity	Normal or paradoxical	Normal	Brisk
Nystagmus	Very frequent	Frequent	Not marked	Almost always	Depends on severity and age of onset	Constant – lessening with time	No	No
Photophobia	Frequent	No	No	Sometimes present	No	Marked	No	No
Optic disc	Normal, some swelling, or pallor	Small, double ring, mis-shapen	Normal	Normal	Pallor and diminution of arterioles on disc, thinning of NFL	Normal	Normal	Normal
VER	Low amplitude or absent, occasionally relatively normal	Latencies near normal, but waveform and amplitudes abnormal	Diminished or absent	Flash normal Pattern VER may reflect abnormal crossover at chiasm	Variably reduced	Normal to flash Abnormal pattern response	Usually normal	Normal, unless associated with cerebral defect
ERG	Unrecordable or severely depressed	Normal	Normal	Flash ERG normal	Normal	Photopic: abnormal to unrecordable Scotopic: may be sub-normal Low flicker fusion frequency	Normal	Normal
EEG	Normal	Normal, unless severe cerebral malformation	Abnormal	Normal	Normal, unless severe cerebral disorder associated	Normal	Normal	Abnormal
Inheritance	Probably autosomal recessive Heterogeneity	Sporadic	Secondary to intracranial disease, therefore, any inheritance is that of the primary condition	Autosomal dominant/recessive X-linked recessive	AR congenital type very rare usually secondary to ocular, orbital or intracranial disease	AR (AR or X-linked for incomplete form)	Sporadic in prematures or small-for-dates infants	Depending on the aetiology of the mental retardation. Cerebral development abnormal

examination with the direct ophthalmoscope is helpful, in order to distinguish it from optic atrophy by the identification of a white ring of choroidal and pigment epithelial atrophy around the tiny hypoplastic disc.

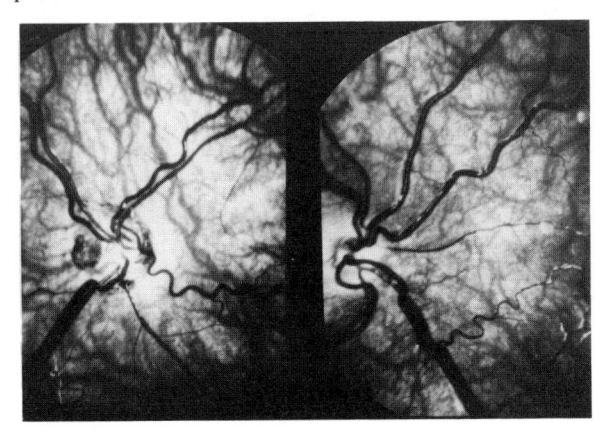

Fig. 7. Optic disc hypoplasia. This blind baby began to fail to thrive when he was about 3 years old, because the optic disc hypoplasia was associated with developmental brain abnormalities. The optic discs are minute, in this case being surrounded by a pigmented halo in the right eye and by a pale halo in the left eye.

Cerebral blindness (Fig. 8)

This should be suspected, especially if the child's general development is delayed, if there are midline defects, such as a cleft lip, or palate or nose, other dysmorphism, or any suggestion of seizures.

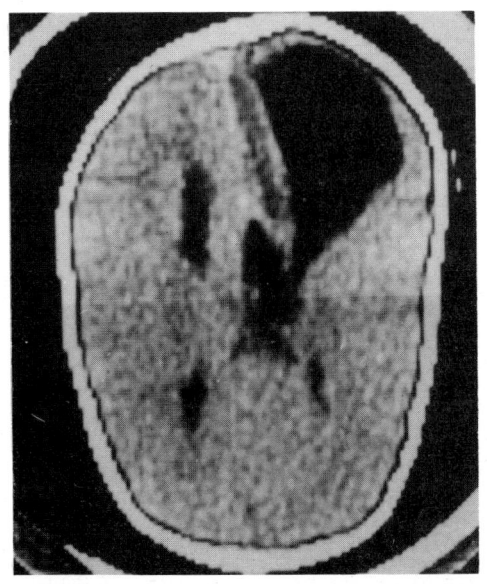

Fig. 8. Cerebral blindness. This child has a porencephalic cyst of the left occipital pole and has a total right homonymous hemianopia.

Albinism

This should be suspected in any child with a relatively poor visual response and photophobia, even if they are not particularly fair haired, when there is a 'compound' type of nystagmus. Iris transilluminence is diagnosed by slit lamp examination with retro-illumination of the iris or transillumination through the lower lid. A positive transillumination is only pathognomonic in brown irides, unless it is marked.

Optic Atrophy (Fig. 9)

This is the end result of many different causes, the most common of which is perinatal anoxia. It is particularly easily missed if the child is fair skinned and has a lightly pigmented fundus. The distinction between a normal and a pale optic disc in infancy is not easy, but one should rely not only on the colour

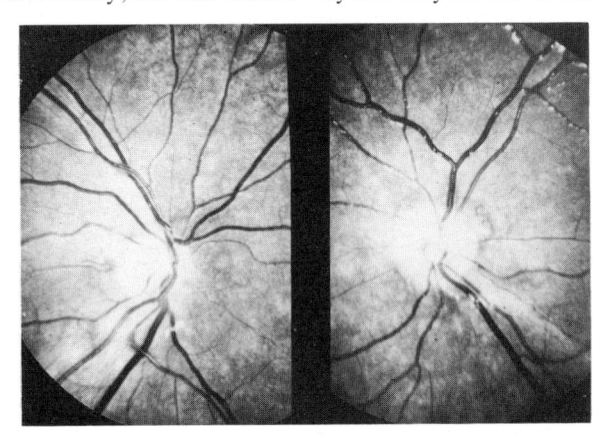

Fig. 9. Optic atrophy. Optic atrophy in infancy may be difficult to determine because of the colour of the background of the fundus, which is often rather pale in appearance. Other clues to the diagnosis are the way in which, because of the thinning of the nerve fibre layer, the vessels stand out against the internal limiting membrane of the retina, especially well seen in parallax. In this case the baby suffered from late prenatal damage, was premature and suffered hypoxia. The optic atrophy was associated with brain defects.

per se but its colour in relation to the background colour of the fundus. The small vessels on the disc itself and the state of the nerve fibre layer should also be examined by both direct and indirect ophthalmoscopy. Unless there is an obvious ophthalmological cause, optic atrophy should be investigated in conjunction with a neurologist.

Cone dystrophy

Cone dystrophy is a rare, usually autosomal recessive, disorder of central vision. Children present because of poor acuity, nystagmus, photophobia, or poor colour vision. They have characteristic abnormalities of the photopic ERG and the fundus may show a macular pigmentary disturbance or a bull's-eye maculopathy.

Delayed Visual Development

This occurs in two different settings: in a normal child, and secondly in a child who is developmentally delayed. In a normal child it is unusual for apparently poor vision to occur without there being an organic basis for it after 4 months of age. There are some children who have a specific delay in their visual development for no apparent cause and who make a full and complete recovery. In these circumstances electrodiagnostic tests may be very helpful, in particular a VER, and ERG, and an EEG will exclude major organic disease. If these are normal, a more confident prognosis can be given, but the child must be kept carefully under review. In the second situation the child will show other aspects of developmental delay and his apparently poor vision is to be thought of more as a result of poor visual attention than of purely poor visual responses. In these patients there is often a severely abnormal EEG, although the visually evoked cortical responses are normal, or not severely abnormal, and the ERG is also normal. Since the child's visual development will appear to improve as his general development and level of attention improve, a cautiously optimistic line is taken with the parents.

While diagnosis is very important, one should not forget that the parents are most concerned with the visual prognosis, the genetic implications and whether or not the visual problems are associated with any other disorders, and the child should be looked at as a whole rather than as a specifically ophthalmological problem. The occurrence of a possible visual handicap in a small baby raises frightening questions with the parents and it is best to have an honest, but sympathetic approach to them even if it is difficult to be accurate about a prognosis.

The Child with Epileptic Fits

Some 5·7 per cent of the population under 5 years old suffer from convulsions, and the paediatrician may refer a child with fits to the ophthalmologist in the hope of some diagnostic clues.

Neonatal convulsions frequently have an organic basis, often with a grave prognosis; about half the children die or are severely retarded.

Patients with congenital toxoplasmosis, apart from many intracerebral calcifications, mental retardation, microcephaly or hydrocephalus, often present with fits and ocular paresis. The typical lesions of retinochoroiditis can be present at birth or later (*Fig. 10*). They are frequently in the macular region, where they could be confused with macular coloboma, but they have less clearly defined edges, with considerable chorioretinal scarring and vitreous involvement.

A common presentation of tuberous sclerosis (Bourneville's disease) is infantile spasms with mental regression that can lead to an appearance of blindness. In this dominantly inherited disorder the best known manifestations are adenoma sebaceum of the cheeks and nasolabial folds, areas of depigmentation on the skin (ash leaf spots) and in the iris or fundus.[30] In about 50 per cent of cases astrocytic hamartomas of the retina occur.[31] They are of two basic types.

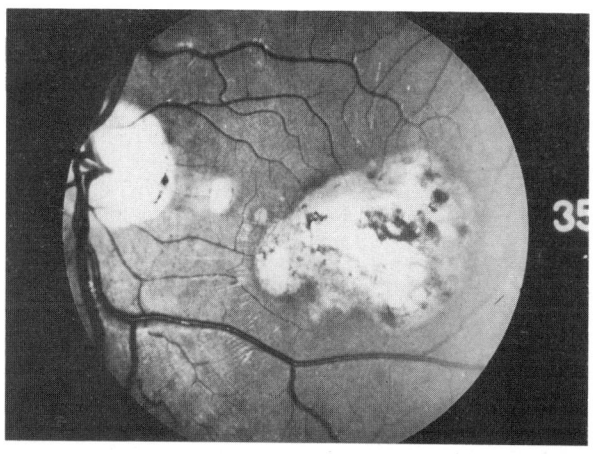

Fig. 10. Toxoplasmosis. A typical toxoplasmosis macular scar destroying fine vision. The patient presented with poor vision in infancy and unsteady eye movements and this well-demarcated macular scar with hyperpigmentation was found on examination.

The first is the flat, semitranslucent lesions superficial to the retinal vessels, with poorly defined boundaries (*Fig. 11*), which become elevated with time (*Fig. 12*). Secondly, there are the elevated, solid, 'mulberry' lesions more frequently found at the optic disc and containing calcium (*Fig. 13*). The relatively small, flat lesions seem to be the first stage of the elevated nodular lesions and can easily be overlooked if careful ophthalmoscopy is not used. The discovery of these lesions is very important, because they are often the first specific sign of tuberous sclerosis in a fitting child before the appearance of adenoma sebaceum and intracerebral calcifications.[32] These patients may also show papilloedema, owing to raised intracranial pressure.

The Sturge Weber syndrome (encephalotrigeminal angiomatosis) may present with convulsions and often these children develop hemiplegia, sometimes with an homonymous field defect. The characteristic feature is a 'port wine stain' of the face, in the territory of V1 and V2 cranial nerves, usually unilateral, with an ipsilateral angiomatous malformation of the meninges and brain with intracranial calcifications and contralateral seizures. An ipsilateral choroidal haemangioma, localized or diffuse, occurs giving a 'ketchup' like appearance to the fundus with masking of the normal choroidal pattern, and finally an ipsilateral glaucoma, which is usually congenital but which can appear later on in life. Sometimes a localized haemangioma can lead to serous detachment of the retina. Dilated episcleral vessels are quite common and heterochromia of the iris can occur. This is the only phakomatosis which is not autosomal dominant and which is probably not heredofamilial.

Neurofibromatosis (von Recklinghausen's disease) only occasionally presents with epilepsy; these children have eye signs including pigmented spots on the skin ('cafe-au-lait'), iris nodules or naevi, cutaneous lid fibroma as well as an orbital or lid plexiform neuroma ('bag of worms') which may be accompanied by congenital glaucoma. Thickened corneal nerves, optic atrophy secondary to glioma of the optic nerve, choroidal and retinal neurofibromas also occur and enophthalmos due to sphenoid dysplasia is described.

Neurometabolic diseases may present with seizures. Among the neurolipidoses, Batten's disease of the infantile type (onset 6–18 months), or in the late infantile form (onset 18 months–4 years), presents with developmental regression, behavioural problems, myoclonic jerks, visual impairment and dementia, the final outcome being death at around 4–10 years. In the juvenile type (onset 6–8 years), central visual loss usually precedes behaviour changes and grand mal fits.[33] Fundus changes occur early, with epithelial defects that can give a 'bull's eye' appearance, the arterioles become thinned and pigment epithelial changes may occur. All types of Batten's disease are autosomal recessive neuronal storage disorders which show early modification of ERG and later of the VER. The diagnosis can be initially established by finding vacuolated lymphocytes in a blood smear and confirmed by rectal biopsy which shows characteristic ultramicroscopic inclusions. In older children ophthalmoplegic lipidosis (Niemann Pick type C) may present with ataxia, dementia and onset of fits. The degree of hepatosplenomegaly is variable. Vertical supranuclear ophthalmoplegia, affecting mainly the downwards saccades, is an important diagnostic clue. Among the gangliosidoses, Tay–Sach's disease may present with seizures in the first months of life. The most common initial symptom is a startled reaction to sound. Vision is affected early, with the storage of white gangliosides in the ganglion cells, giving the classic appearance of cherry red spot (*Fig.* 14) due to the absence of ganglion cells at the fovea with multilayered white ganglion cells around it. Death usually occurs before

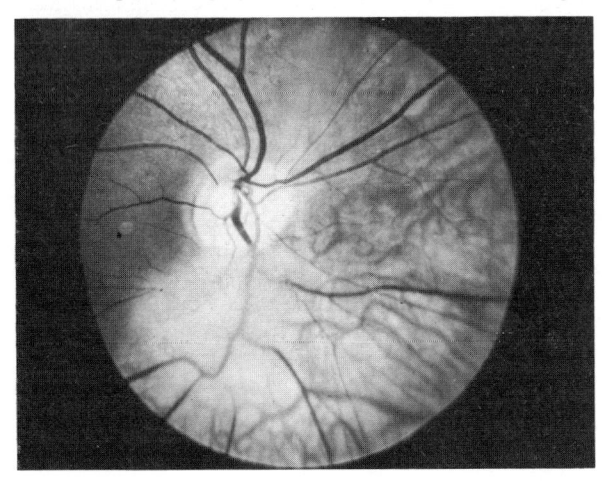

Fig. 11. Tuberous sclerosis. Above and below the disc there are opalescent areas partially obscuring the underlying retina. These are phacomas in the retina.

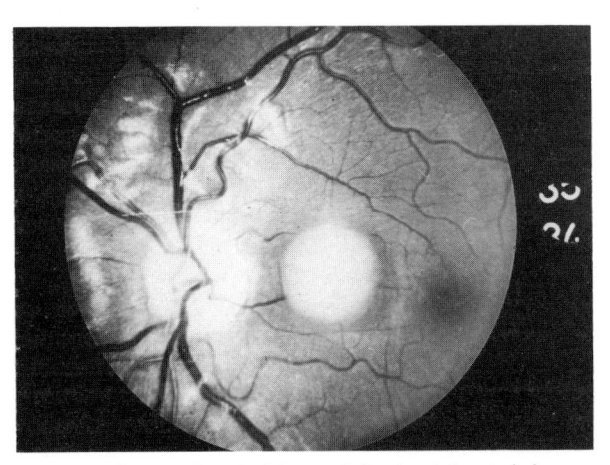

Fig. 12. Tuberous sclerosis. A better defined and elevated phacoma between the fovea and the optic disc.

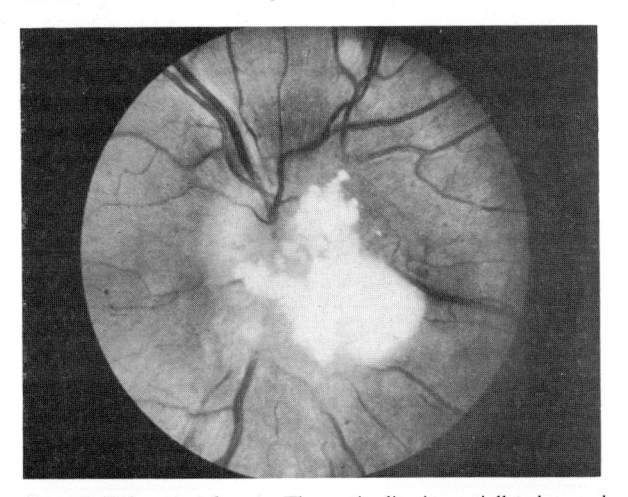

Fig. 13. Tuberous sclerosis. The optic disc is partially obscured by a so-called 'mulberry tumour'. This is a white knobbly excrescence which contains calcium, which may be sometimes seen on a CT scan. This child presented with intractable fits in infancy.

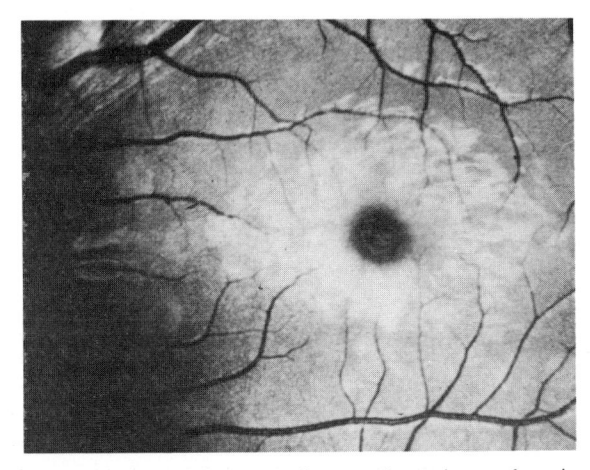

Fig. 14. A cherry red spot. A cherry red spot is seen here in a patient with Tay–Sach's disease, because the ganglion cells become filled by the abnormal accumulation of gangliosides. The area around the fovea becomes opalescent; since there are no ganglion cells at the fovea, this shines out as a bright red spot in contrast to the white surroundings. The red spot itself is normal, it is the white surround that is the abnormal feature. As the ganglion cells die, the cherry red spot appearance fades.

3 years of age. The disorder is autosomal recessive with a very frequent carrier state in Ashkenazic Jews. Unlike in Batten's disease, the ERG is normal while the VER is abnormal. Sandhoff's disease and juvenile GM2 gangliosidosis present the same type of features.

Infantile spasms with severe retardation are also seen in Aicardi's syndrome. Only girls are affected, with agenesis of the corpus callosum and ectopic grey matter seen on CT scan and very characteristic fundi[32] (*Fig.* 15). This pathognomonic fundus appearance establishes the diagnosis and enables the doctor to give reassurance of the lack of familial incidence.

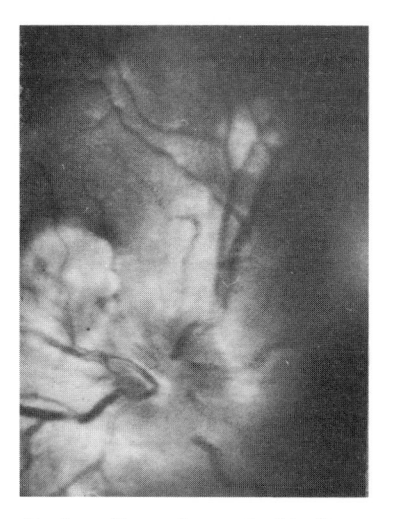

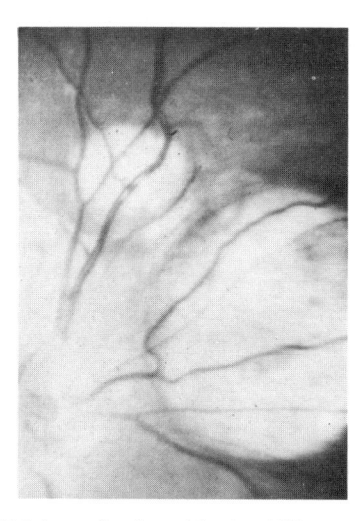

Fig. 15. Aicardi's syndrome. In this disease, which is confined to girls, the children present with infantile spasms and have cerebral malformations, including agenesis of the corpus callosum and ectopic grey matter. There are characteristic fundus findings which consist of punched-out areas in the retina without pigment hyperplasia and sometimes dysplastic optic discs.

Pre-retinal and retinal haemorrhages are a common feature of non-accidental injury (NAI), which should be remembered, especially in children under 2 years of age presenting with a disproportionate degree of soft tissue injuries in different stages of resolution, with fits and often subdural haematomas leading to hydrocephalus (*Fig.* 16). NAI can lead to dramatic loss of vision with optic atrophy, macular scarring and patchy atrophy of the choroid. In the fundus, haemorrhages at different stages of resolution can be a useful clinical clue.

The ophthalmologist might also help in the diagnosis between hyperpyrexic convulsions and those associated with meningoencephalitis, and occasionally in cases of fits due to acute nephropathies, arterial hypertension and some intoxications.

In the rare cases of epilepsy due to intracranial tumours in children, papilloedema may be present and cataracts are occasionally clinical clues in fits due to hypoglycaemia or hypocalcaemia. In hypoglycaemic fits one should exclude optic disc hypoplasia, with its associated hypothalamic abnormalities.

Hoyt's study[32] suggested that a careful examination of the fundus of children with infantile spasms will help to establish diagnosis in 20 per cent of cases.

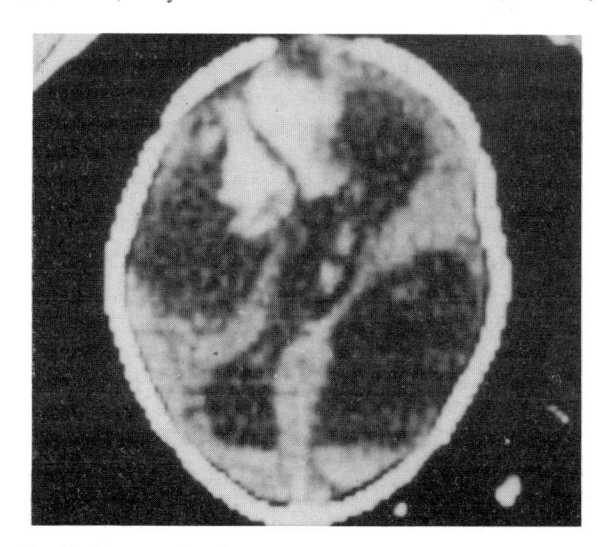

The Eye of the Infant who Fails to Thrive

The paediatric ophthalmologist is asked to provide diagnostic clues to the infant who is failing to grow or develop normally. An investigation of these patients may follow the guidelines described previously. There are certain specific diagnoses in which the ophthalmologist particularly may help.

Congenital Infection – Toxoplasmosis

These children present with a chronic encephalitis, hydrocephalus or microcephaly. They have intracerebral calcification and their fundus may show signs of toxoplasmosis (*see Fig.* 10). Rubella babies are small, often have a rash after birth, they may have cataracts, may be deaf and have heart defects. They

Fig. 16. Non-accidental injury. This child, who suffered a severe non-accidental injury in early infancy, has hydrocephalus, extensive brain atrophy and areas of organized intracerebral haemorrhage.

thrive poorly in the first year of life. The most common eye abnormality is a retinopathy, with a diffuse pigment epithelial disturbance which usually has only a mild functional significance.

Miliary tuberculosis is found most frequently in the United Kingdom in sick children of lower socio-economic groups and the commonest ocular manifestation is multiple choroidal tubercles; many develop optic atrophy.

Metabolic Disorders

Mucopolysaccharides, mucolipidosis and neurolipidoses may have corneal and retinal abnormalities, the latter being either a retinitis pigmentosa-like disorder or cherry red spots. Cystinosis presents as a child who fails to thrive, is usually fair haired, and who may have a prolific production of urine; corneal and conjunctival crystals may be found only on slit lamp examination.

Other Renal Disorders

These include Alport's syndrome, in which the commonest abnormality is a posterior lenticonus most easily seen on retinoscopy as a reflex similar to that obtained in keratoconus; retinal abnormalities also occur. Medullary cystic disease of the kidney occurs in association with a retinal dystrophy in Leber's amaurosis and Laurence–Moon–Biedl syndrome, or in Senior's syndrome.

Associated Hepatic Disease

Possibilities are Wilson's disease or Zellweger's syndrome. In the latter, brain malformations occur with renal and liver disorders, and a retinal dystrophy. Leigh's subacute necrotizing encephalopathy may present, with optic atrophy, ophthalmoplegia, mental retardation and spasticity. Treatment with large doses of thiamine has been successful.

Chromosomal Abnormalities

A variety of chromosomal disorders[34] are associated with delayed development and failure to thrive, many with dysmorphic features and eye abnormalities.

Syndromes Associated with Failure to Thrive

de Morsier's Syndrome (Septo-optic Dysplasia) (Fig. 17)

Optic disc hypoplasia may be associated with a variety of developmental brain disorders, the most common of which is an absence of the septum pellucidum. Although growth defects do not usually occur until the child is over 3 years old, the child may have diabetes insipidus or a generalized failure to thrive. The detection of optic disc hypoplasia is a vital clue to the diagnosis (see Fig. 7).

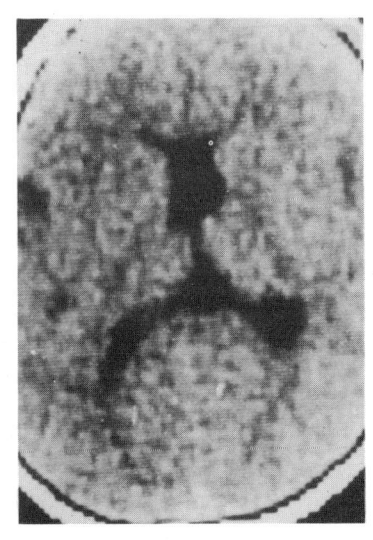

Fig. 17. Septo-optic dysplasia. This CT scan shows the absence of the septum pellucidum, which is normally seen as a thin white line between the anterior horns of the ventricles.

Bone Defects and Dysplasias

In patients with bony defects and dysplasia there are frequently eye abnormalities. In Marfan's syndrome there is often a refractive error and a very high incidence of dislocated lenses. In osteopetrosis the optic canals may be small and optic nerve compression may occur. In some cases there is also an associated retinal dystrophy and ERG in these patients is essential. Diagnosis is radiological and treatment is now available by bone-marrow transplantation in selected cases. In the craniofacial dysostoses there is a skull malformation and a very high incidence of squint is found, together with papilloedema, which may decompensate and cause optic atrophy.

Coloboma Associations

One of the commonest coloboma syndromes is the CHARGE association. A mild mental defect occurs with a variety of heart defects, coloboma of the uvea, ear abnormalities, deafness, a VIIth nerve palsy and choanal atresia or tracheo-oesophageal fistula.

Other associations are the Golz syndrome, Lenz microphthalmos syndrome and Meckel's syndrome. For a more detailed description the reader is referred to a textbook on dysmorphism.[34]

Suprasellar Gliomas and Craniopharyngiomas

The presentation is one of failure to thrive, diabetes insipidus or hydrocephalus (Fig. 18), and they may have optic atrophy (Fig. 19), developmental optic nerve defects, nystagmus or strabismus.

Other Tumours

A patient with a neuroblastoma may fail to thrive and among the ophthalmological abnormalities are opsoclonus (a wildly multidirectional nystagmus),

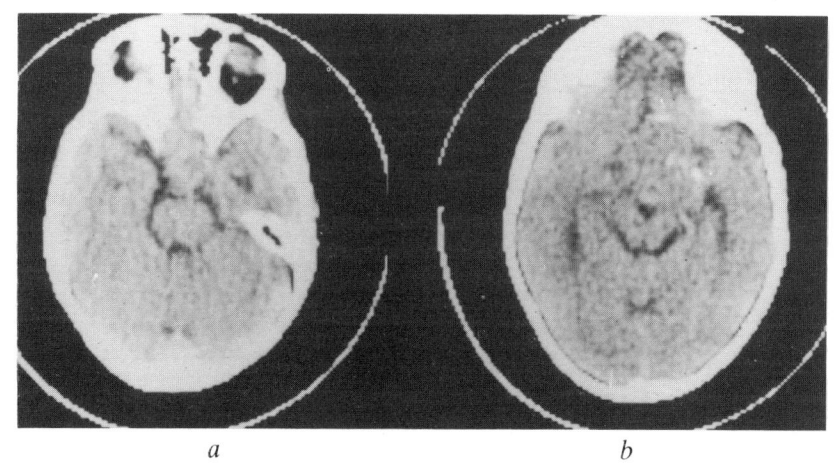

Fig. 18. Chiasmal glioma. This child presented in infancy with poor vision secondary to optic atrophy and unsteady eye movements. The CT scan (*a*) shows a small tumour in the suprasellar cystern and this extends up into the third ventricle (*b*). The child had von Recklinghausen's disease, which is associated with chiasmal gliomas.

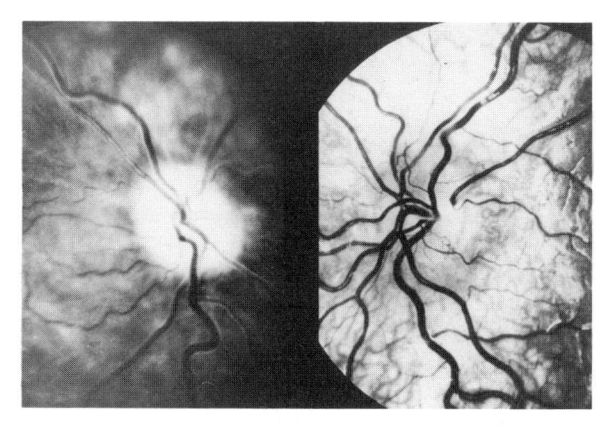

Fig. 19. Chiasmal glioma. This teenage child had been blind in the right eye for very many years and the optic atrophy is evident. There was a total left homonymous hemianopia from the glioma which extended from the right optic nerve into the chiasm. As the tumour grew, it occluded the foramen of Monro and caused hydrocephalus. The swelling of the left optic disc is most marked in the superior and inferior poles which are the areas which carry the nerve fibres from the intact nasal field. This bilobed papilloedema, also known as 'twin-peaks' papilloedema, reflects the visual field defect.

periorbital ecchymosis and proptosis, which may lead to blindness.

Patients with histiocytosis X may have orbital involvement and sometimes lid lesions, and some patients with Wilm's tumour may have aniridia, and those with IIp− syndrome have genital anomalies and mental retardation.

Developmental Abnormalities

Certain developmental central nervous system and face malformations may be associated with developmental delay and failure to thrive as a result of hypothalamic disturbances. These include craniofacial dysostoses, patients with porencephaly and those with a variety of causes of cerebral palsy.

Others

One must remember that children with non-accidental injury may present as failure to thrive (*see Fig. 16*) and in Lowe's syndrome infants who are floppy from birth and fail to thrive have congenital cataract and glaucoma.

Refractive Errors in Infancy

In the first year of life the only indication for the prescription of spectacles or contact lenses is the prevention of amblyopia. Even patients with very high refractive errors probably do not require optical correction for the purpose of providing a sharp image alone, unless this is part of the treatment or prevention of amblyopia.

Bilateral hypermetropia, whatever its degree, does not require treatment unless as part of the management of a squint. However, patients with over +2·50 dioptres of hypermetropia should be regarded as at risk both for squint and amblyopia and should be reviewed at least at yearly intervals, and the prescription of spectacles may be reconsidered when the child comes of school age, even if a squint has not developed.

In infancy, bilateral myopia does not usually require treatment whatever the degree, although one must be cautious in patients with over −15·00 dioptres since these children may develop amblyopia, preventable by the early prescription of contact lenses. If a decision is made to correct high degrees of myopia, the full, or very nearly full, prescription should be given. If there is any contraindication for contact lenses, or if they are not available, tie on spectacles can always be tried, though they are very heavy for that age group.

For anisometropia in infancy it is not usually necessary to prescribe spectacles or contact lenses unless the difference is over 2·00 dioptres, when the child is at risk from amblyopia in which case the use of a contact lens may be considered, together with occlusion therapy where appropriate.

Astigmatism is a normal finding in infancy and even astigmatic errors of 1·50 or 2·00 dioptres need not be corrected in the first year of life, although the patient should be kept under review. Even very high degrees of astigmatism, if symmetrical and bilateral, need not necessarily be treated with spectacles at an early stage, but the patient should be kept under review.

Contact lenses should be reserved only for those infants who are likely to become amblyopic, either because of anisometropia or very high refractive errors, such as in those patients who have had surgery for congenital cataract. There is a substantial risk to the use of continuous wear contact lenses that is only worth taking if the benefits are sufficiently high.

Eye Movement Disorders in Infancy

The parents of an infant with an eye movement disorder often have little concern for some months, because they are unsure whether or not it is normal. The taking of a detailed history is important in order to get some impression of the early stages of the disorder, in particular the time of onset and its progression, changes in direction of any nystagmus, its relationship to startle, whether or not there is a family history, the presence of a head shake or abnormal head position. In addition, direct questions about visual development and general development, and the relationship of the onset to any fever, are important.

Examination of the infant does not require special equipment and diagnosis is still made at a clinical level in virtually every case.[35] An assessment of the child's vision is important, and nystagmus directions, whether or not the eye movement defects are horizontal, vertical, rotary or circum-rotary, can be charted as in *Fig.* 20. The presence of squint should not be overlooked and a detailed general eye examination is mandatory, together with the specific search for episodes of head shaking on fixation, or head shaking when the child is not concentrating. The presence of the vestibulo-ocular reflexes may be elicited by spinning a small infant or by moving his head from side to side while he is lying in a cot or with his head on a pillow. A brief general examination should also be carried out.

Specific Patterns of Nystagmus

Congenital Idiopathic Nystagmus

This should be thought of as being horizontal in all positions of gaze, but in any case the clinician should beware of making the diagnosis except as one of exclusion. The nystagmus may be associated with an abnormal head posture or shake, and it may be 'pendular' or 'jerk'. Either of these patterns may have amplification on lateral gaze. There is a high inci-

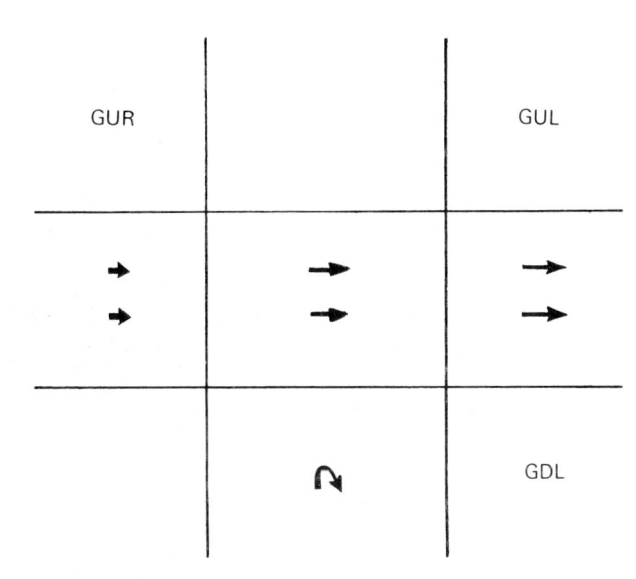

GUR Gaze up and right
GUL Gaze up and left
GDL Gaze down and left
Arrow refers to direction of fast phase
Number of arrows refers to frequency
Length of arrow refers to amplitude
Curved arrow refers to rotary nystagmus

Fig. 20. Method of charting the features of nystagmus.

dence of squint and astigmatic refractive errors and the acuity in older children is relatively good, especially for near. These children always have normal visual fields, colour vision and electrodiagnostic studies, and their general development is normal. If any of these factors is not normal, they should be investigated further, preferably in conjunction with a paediatric neurologist. There is sometimes a positive family history.

Secondary Nystagmoid Eye Movements

POOR VISION

The eye movement abnormality is a severe visual defect in infancy. It usually takes the form of 'roving eye movements' with random, large amplitude, purposeless eye movements which are not just horizontal or vertical, but are also circum-rotary. This is frequently the presenting feature of poor vision in infancy, often associated with squint. Since the cause usually lies in the anterior visual pathways (cortical blindness does not typically present with quite such marked roving eye movements) the pupil reactions are often abnormal and other ocular abnormalities common on examination. Patients with anything other than purely horizontal nystagmus in all positions of gaze should be suspected of having an underlying visual defect.

MOTOR DEFECTS

Acute Cerebellar Syndromes: These most frequently occur after non-specific acute infections in childhood, but they also occur with neuroblastoma and in older children with other tumours.

Opsoclonus consists of bursts of large amplitude, high velocity, horizontal, vertical and circum-rotary movements which occur usually on attempted fixation in patients who have a severe truncal ataxia.

Ocular flutter is a purely horizontal eye movement defect which may occur by itself, as part of a para-infectious encephalitis, or following opsoclonus. The bursts of high amplitude, high frequency, horizontal oscillations occur usually on attempted fixation, but may be spontaneous. The prognosis is good, with resolution occurring after some days or weeks.

Hydrocephalus: This may cause an up gaze palsy together with lid retraction; the combination of these two signs gives rise to the 'setting sun' sign which resolves immediately when the intracranial pressure is lowered.

Convergence–Retraction Nystagmus: This occurs as a result of space occupying lesions around the Sylvian aqueduct. These are high velocity, bilateral adducting eye movements which occur when the patient makes upward saccades, such as those generated by downward optokinetic nystagmus. As well as adducting, the eye appears to retract; it is often associated with light–near dissociation of the pupil reflexes and sometimes with vertical gaze palsies or nystagmus.

Vertical Nystagmus: Upbeat nystagmus occurs most frequently in patients on relatively high doses of anti-epileptic drugs. The nystagmus may be upbeat in all positions of gaze, but is most frequently elicited by getting the patient to look upwards. It may also be found as a non-specific sign in patients with a variety of posterior fossa disorders.

Downbeat nystagmus that increases in amplitude on down gaze is a non-specific sign of a posterior fossa disorder or drug ingestion, but there is a specific down beat nystagmus that becomes of much greater amplitude on looking downwards and laterally to either side. It is associated with lower brain stem defects, and the commonest abnormality which gives rise to this in childhood is a form of Arnold–Chiari malformation.

Periodic Alternating Nystagmus: Although usually detected only in older children, this condition, which is associated with a variety of cerebral defects, should be suspected when a variable pattern of nystagmus appears at different times. A change of direction of nystagmus, and sometimes a change in the compensatory head posture, may occur with a frequency that is usually around $1\frac{1}{2}$–2 min. There are often associated cerebellar signs.

Other Cerebellar Defects: These may be detected in the infant, but they are less prominent than in older children. They include nystagmus, with the fast phase beating in the direction of gaze, rebound nystagmus (nystagmus which occurs on gaze in one direction and then decreases in amplitude and on return to the primary position beats in the opposite direction), overshoot and undershoot dysmetria, and failure of suppression of the vestibulo-ocular reflexes.

Nystagmus with Head Shake: Head shaking with nystagmus may occur because both the nystagmus and the head shake are the result of the same underlying tremor. The head shake and nystagmus in this situation are usually not influenced by attempts to fixate.

There are several adaptive mechanisms that improve vision. The head shake is brought about at a time when the patient is trying to concentrate on an object; only older infants, who have the ability to control the head movements, will exhibit such head shakes.

In compensatory head shaking the head shake is opposite and equal to the nystagmus and therefore the eye in space becomes steady. This is not usually a clear-cut relationship, but more a mechanism whereby transient plateaux of steadiness are brought about. During these plateaux of steadiness a high level of acuity may be achieved.

Head shaking also induces the vestibulo-ocular reflex, which is a powerful primitive reflex for stabilization of the eye. By shaking the head some patients appear to 'switch off' or override their nystagmus.

In oculo-motor apraxia there is a relative and sometimes intermittent defect in the ability to generate rapid, horizontal eye movements. The only way in which the eyes can be moved from one position to another is for the patient to make large amplitude head thrusts, which bring the eyes into extremes of version from which position they are dragged to the position of fixation, at which time the head returns to the straight ahead position, giving rise to the sequence of a rapid head thrust with a relatively slow return movement. It usually is unassociated with any neurological disorder, but several cases have been described, with a variety of brain defects and also in association with retinal dystrophies.

Ocular myoclonus may occur with generalized myoclonic syndromes and acute cerebellar syndromes may also be associated with head tremors and unsteadiness, with or without an intact vestibulo-ocular reflex.

ACKNOWLEDGEMENTS

We would like to thank Miss Josephine Lace and Miss Yvonne Robinson who produced the drafts and the final manuscript.

REFERENCES

1. Wybar K. C. and Taylor D. S. I. (ed.) *Pediatric Ophthalmology – Current Aspects.* New York, Marcel Dekker, 1983.
2. Crawford J. D. and Morin J. D. (ed.) *The Eye in Childhood.* New York, Grune and Stratton, 1983.
3. Harley R. D. (ed.) *Pediatric Ophthalmology* Philadelphia, Saunders, 1982.
4. Robinson R. J. Assessment of gestational age by neurological examination. *Arch. Dis. Childh.* 1966; **41,** 437–41.
5. La Roche G. R., Anderson D. P. and Allen A. C. Visual behaviour in newborn infants. Ravault A. P. and Lenk M. (ed.) *Transactions of the Vth International Orthoptic Congress, Cannes, France, 10–13 October 1983.* Lyons, Lips, pp. 23–31.
6. Brennon W. M., Ames E. W. and Moore R. W. Age differences in infants' attention to patterns of different complexities. *Science* 1966; **151,** 354–6.
7. Hoyt C. S., Nickel B. L. and Billson F. A. Ophthalmological examination of the infant. *Surv. Ophthalmol.* 1982; **26,** 177–89.
8. Keast-Butler J. Congenital retinal blindness. In: Wybar K. and Taylor D. (ed.) *Pediatric Ophthalmology – Current Aspects.* New York, Marcel Dekker, 1983, pp. 209–17.
9. Harden A. Electrodiagnostic assessment in infancy. In: Wybar K. and Taylor D. (ed.) *Pediatric Ophthalmology – Current Aspects.* New York, Marcel Dekker, 1983, pp. 11–18.
10. Marg E., Freeman D. N., Peltzman P. et al. Visual acuity development in human infants: Evoked potential measurements. *Invest. Ophthalmol. Vis. Sci.* 1976; **15,** 150–3.
11. Ingram R. M., Traynar M. J., Walker C. et al. Screening for refractive errors at age 1 year: a pilot study. *Br. J. Ophthalmol.* 1979; **63,** 143–250.
12. Hyvarinen L. and Lindstedt E. *Assessment of Vision in Children.* Stockholm, SRF Tal & Punkt, 1981.
13. Atkinson J. and Braddick O. The development of visual function. In: Davis J. A. and Dobbling J. (ed.) *Scientific Foundations of Paediatrics,* 2nd ed. London, Heinemann, 1981, pp. 865–77.
14. Fulton A. B., Hansen R. M. and Manning K. A. Measuring visual acuity in infants. *Surv. Ophthalmol.* 1981; **25,** 325–32.
15. Aslin R. N. and Salapatek P. Saccadic localization of peripheral targets by the very young human infant. *Percept. Psychophys.* 1975; **17,** 293–302.
16. Sheridan M. D. *Children's Developmental Progress from Birth to Five Years: The Stycar Sequences.* Windsor, NFER Publishing, 1975.
17. Braddick O. and Atkinson J. The development of binocular function in infancy. (Symposium on early visual development March 1982, Solna, Sweden.) *Acta Ophthalmol. (Kbh.)* 1983; Suppl. 157, 27–35.
18. Simons K. Visual acuity norms in young children. *Surv. Ophthalmol.* 1983; **28,** 84–92.
19. Illingworth R. S. *The Normal Child: Some Problems of the Early Years and their Treatment,* 7th ed. Edinburgh, Churchill Livingstone, 1979.
20. Egan B., Illingworth R. S. and McKeith R. C. Developmental screening 0–5 years. *Clinics in Developmental Medicine,* no. 30. London, Heinemann, 1969.
21. Illingworth R. S. *The Development of the Infant and Young Child; Normal and Abnormal,* 7th ed. Edinburgh, Churchill Livingstone, 1980.
22. Sheridan M. D. *From Birth to Five Years: Children's Developmental Progress,* 3rd ed. Windsor, NFER-Nelson Publishing, 1975, reprinted 1982.
23. Hyvarinen L. Early stimulation of visually impaired infants. *Ophthalmic Paediatr. Genet.,* 1983; **2,** 129–33.
24. Sonksen P. N. Vision and early development. In: Wybar K. and Taylor D. (ed.) *Pediatric Ophthalmology – Current Aspects.* New York, Marcel Dekker, 1983; pp. 85–94.
25. Fraiberg S. *Insights from the Blind.* London, Souvenir Press (Horizon Series), 1977.
26. Reynell J. *Manual for the Reynell–Zinkin Scales.* (Developmental Scales for Young Visually Handicapped Children – Part I: Mental Development.) Windsor, NFER, 1979.
27. Harcourt B. Strabismus affecting children with multiple handicaps. *Br. J. Ophthalmol.* 1974; **58,** 272–80.
28. Scott E. P., Jan S. E. and Freeman R. D. *Can't your Child See?* Baltimore and London, University Park Press, 1977.
29. Stanley J. H., MacDonald J. and Flynn J. T. Leber's congenital amaurosis: A clinical study. In: Lawton Smith J. (ed.) *Neuro-Ophthalmology Update.* New York, Masson, 1977, pp. 91–7.
30. Lucchese N. J. and Goldberg M. F. Iris and fundus pigmentary changes in tuberous sclerosis. *J. Pediatr. Ophthalmol. Strabismus* 1981; **18,** 45–6.
31. Nyboer J. H., Robertson D. M. and Camey M. R. Retinal lesions in tuberous sclerosis. *Arch. Ophthalmol.* 1976; **94,** 1277–80.
32. Hoyt C. S. The ocular findings in infantile spasm. *Ophthalmology* 1979; **86,** 1994–2802.
33. Spalton D. J., Taylor D. S. I. and Sanders M. D. Juvenile Batten's disease: An ophthalmological assessment of 26 patients. *Br. J. Ophthalmol.* 1980; **64,** 726–32.
34. Smith D. W. *Recognisable Patterns of Human Malformation,* 3rd ed. Philadelphia, Saunders, 1982.
35. Taylor D. Disorders of head and eye movements in children. *Trans. Ophthalmol. Soc. UK* 1980; **100,** 489–94.

Chapter 19

Hereditary Diseases

Barrie Jay

Since the beginning of this century, ophthalmologists have made significant contributions to human genetics, at least in part because a number of the more common causes of visual impairment, and many of the rarer causes, have a genetic component in their aetiology. In this chapter the principles of human genetics will be presented, and these principles will be illustrated by disorders that involve the eye, and thus interest the ophthalmologist. In no way is this intended to be a complete list of those genetically determined disorders of ophthalmic interest; appropriate references will be found to more comprehensive texts at the end of the chapter.

CHROMOSOMES AND THEIR ABERRATIONS

Inherited human characteristics, both normal and abnormal, are determined by genes carried on chromosomes. Man has 23 pairs of chromosomes in each somatic cell, 22 pairs of autosomes and one pair of sex chromosomes – a pair of X in the female and an X and a Y chromosome in the male. The sex cells each have a single set of 22 autosomes and one X or one Y chromosome.

Various errors can occur at mitosis or meiosis that can lead to an anomaly of chromosome number, resulting in aneuploidy or polyploidy. Aneuploidy is the result of the gain or loss of a chromosome. Polyploidy is where there is a multiple of the normal haploid number of chromosomes (23), as in triploidy (69 chromosomes) or tetraploidy (92 chromosomes). An individual with an extra chromosome is *trisomic* for that chromosome (*see* trisomies 13 and 21, below), one with the loss of a chromosome is *monosomic* for that chromosome. Autosomal trisomies and monosomies are seldom compatible with life, at best they produce major abnormalities of many systems of the body. The most common trisomies compatible with life are trisomy 21 (Down's syndrome) and the triple X syndrome (women with 47 chromosomes, including 3 X chromosomes); others are trisomy 13 (Patau's syndrome) and trisomy 18 (Edward's syndrome). The only monosomies compatible with life are Turner's syndrome (women with 45 chromosomes, including only one X) and monosomy 21. Two of these aneuploidies have interesting ocular manifestations.

Trisomy 13 (Patau's Syndrome)

This trisomy, which usually results in death within a few months, is of particular interest to ophthalmologists. It is characterized by microcephaly with scalp defects, cleft lip and palate, malformed ears, polydactyly, 'rocker-bottom' feet, undescended testes and hernias. In addition, there are malformations of the central nervous system, and cardiac and genitourinary defects. The most common ocular abnormalities are microphthalmos, coloboma, cataract and retinal dysplasia, the last being characteristic of trisomy 13 (although it does occur in other conditions). The retina is often infolded and detached, and the folds, when cut transversely, result in the appearance of rosettes.

Trisomy 21 (Down's Syndrome, Mongolism)

The clinical picture of trisomy 21 is well known. Mental deficiency, small stature, brachycephaly and cardiac anomalies are just a few of the characteristic abnormalities. The typical facies result in part from the epicanthic folds and the short rounded palpebral apertures which slant upwards and outwards. The ocular manifestations include cataract, nodules on the iris and keratoconus. The lens opacities, which are usually apparent from puberty, are very common and may be of several different types: arcuate opacities radiating anteriorly and posteriorly within the fetal nucleus; sutural opacities along the Y sutures of the fetal nucleus; and flakey opacities, often in large numbers, usually within the infantile and adult nuclei. The iris nodules (Brushfield's spots) – areas of increased density in the iris stroma – are seen as white or yellowish elevated spots around the periphery of the iris in the majority of patients with trisomy 21; they also occur in about 20 per cent of normal individuals. Keratoconus, and particularly the acute form, is much more common in trisomy 21 than in the normal population.

In addition to the anomalies of chromosome number (aneuploidy and polyploidy), chromosomes may undergo structural changes which result in part of a chromosome being deleted or duplicated (deletion or partial trisomy), in a rearrangement of genetic material within a chromosome (inversion), in a transfer of a chromosome segment from its normal position to another position either in the same chromosome (shift) or in another (insertion), or the exchange of segments between two different chromosomes (reciprocal translocation) (*Fig.* 1). Two deletions are of particular importance to ophthalmologists, the 11p13 and the 13q14 deletions. (In current terminology the first number indicates the chromosome involved, the letter indicates the short arm (p) or the long arm (q), while the second pair of digits indicates the band that is involved.)

patients have an interstitial deletion of band 13 on the short arm of chromosome 11. All babies with sporadic aniridia should be regularly examined to exclude a Wilms's tumour. Clinical examination of the abdomen is not sufficient; ultrasonic examinations should be performed periodically until puberty, although most children develop the tumour before 3 years of age.

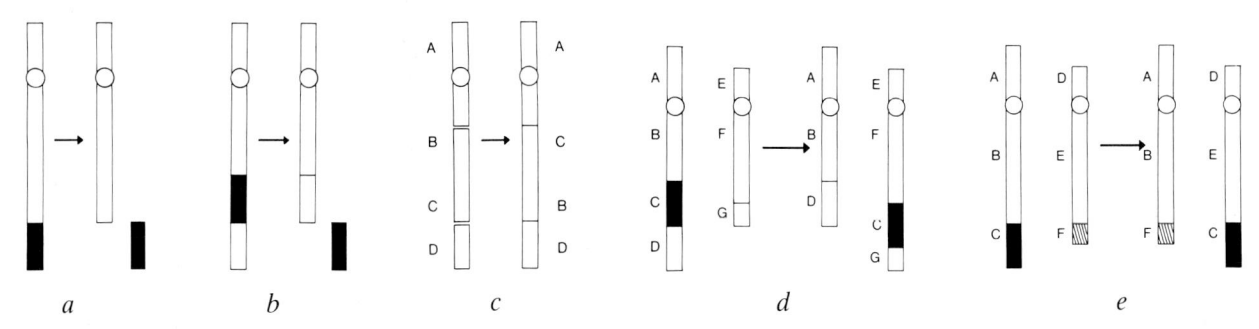

Fig. 1. Structural changes in chromosomes. *a*, Terminal deletion. Loss of the terminal part of a chromosome. *b*, Interstitial deletion. Loss of a segment of chromosome between its centromere and one of its ends. *c*, Paracentric inversion. Rearrangement of the genetic material within a chromosome. *d*, Insertion. Transfer of a chromosome segment from one chromosome to another (in this case a segment was transferred from the longer to the shorter chromosome). *e*, Reciprocal translocation. Exchange of chromosome segments between two different chromosomes.

Aniridia

Until recently, two types of congenital aniridia have been distinguished – a hereditary autosomal dominant type and a sporadic type. The clinical picture of aniridia is variable. Most patients have a clinically absent iris, although on gonioscopy a small fringe of iris becomes visible. A smaller number have a clinically visible fringe of iris, while a few members of affected families have an appreciable, though reduced, amount of iris present. Ocular complications are common: cataract and nystagmus occur in about 80 per cent, glaucoma in some 50 per cent and subluxated lenses in about 25 per cent. The majority of children with aniridia have reduced vision, 6/18 or worse, while the long term visual prognosis is very poor. A few families have appreciably better vision, with fewer long term complications, and these may indicate a separate and milder form of the disorder. The hereditary form is seldom associated with other abnormalities, in contrast to the sporadic form.

11p13 Deletion (Deletion of the Short Arm of Chromosome 11)

The sporadic type of aniridia is sometimes associated with mental retardation and with numerous other anomalies such as micro- or macrocephaly, genito-urinary anomalies and skeletal malformations. Many of these patients also develop a Wilms's tumour. Chromosome studies have indicated that these

Retinoblastoma

There have recently been interesting advances in our understanding of retinoblastoma and of its genetics. About 40 per cent of cases are bilateral, and these are now all assumed to be hereditary.

Cases of retinoblastoma can be divided into three groups (the percentages mentioned are approximate, and vary considerably between different series):

1. *Somatic mutation*: About 75 per cent of all cases of retinoblastoma are sporadic (no family history) and, of these, about one-third are thought to result from a new dominant mutation, while the remainder result from a somatic mutation. These latter cases would, of necessity, be non-hereditary, and have unilateral and solitary tumours (but not all unilateral cases are necessarily the result of a somatic mutation – *see below*). The non-hereditary cases have a higher age of onset of their tumour (average 26 months) than do the hereditary cases (average 8 months), and if the age of onset of a unilateral case exceeds 4 years, it can be assumed to be non-hereditary.

2. *Autosomal dominant retinoblastoma*: About 20 per cent of cases of retinoblastoma have a family history of the tumour, and a certain additional number are the result of a new autosomal dominant mutation. Carriers of the gene for retinoblastoma are usually affected and, of these, 60 per cent have bilateral and 40 per cent unilateral tumours. A small number of these carriers are unaffected, or have evidence of a stationary lesion in the retina (originally thought to be a 'spontaneous regression', now called a retinoma). A retinoma, which is a benign manifestation of the retinoblastoma gene, has a characteristic appearance. It is a stationary, translucent, greyish retinal mass protruding into the vitreous, which

usually contains calcification and is frequently associated with migration and proliferation of the retinal pigment epithelium. The retinoma has an intact blood supply, as demonstrated on fluorescein angiography, in contrast to a retinoblastoma, which frequently undergoes ischaemic necrosis. The presence of a retinoma indicates that the patient has the retinoblastoma gene which can be transmitted to half his/her children.

Recent studies have indicated that there is linkage between the retinoblastoma gene and that for esterase D. The gene for esterase D (an enzyme with no known biological action) has been assigned to chromosome band 13q14, thus indicating that the gene for retinoblastoma is also on this band. In addition to the very high risk of developing retinoblastoma, carriers of the gene also have a 15–30 per cent chance of developing a second non-ocular malignancy (usually an osteogenic sarcoma) in their second or third decade of life.

3. *13q14 deletion*: Probably about 5 per cent of all cases of retinoblastoma result from the loss of a small segment of the long arm of chromosome 13.

Genetic counselling in retinoblastoma is an important aspect of the management of families in which this tumour has occurred. All bilateral cases must be assumed to result from the presence of an autosomal dominant gene, so their offspring have a 50 per cent chance of inheriting the gene. Unilateral cases that are known to be hereditary have a 45 per cent chance of producing affected children, while unilateral cases with no family history have a 5–10 per cent chance of producing affected children. If unaffected parents with no other family history of the disease have produced one affected child, their chances of producing a second affected child are small, probably in the region of 1–2 per cent.

13q14 Deletion (Deletion of the Long Arm of Chromosome 13)

The uncommon occurrence of sporadic retinoblastoma in association with mental retardation is now known to result from an interstitial deletion of band 14 of the long arm of chromosome 13 (*Fig.* 2). As the gene for esterase D has been assigned to this band, an assay of this enzyme could indicate the presence of a small deletion, useful in the diagnosis of retinoblastoma and in genetic counselling.

MENDELIAN INHERITANCE

The foundation of modern genetics resulted from experiments conducted by Gregor Mendel, an Augustinian monk, on the garden pea in the middle of the nineteenth century. Although this work was largely neglected for some 40 years, its rediscovery at the beginning of this century led to the appreciation of the importance of the particulate nature of many inherited characteristics and disorders. The 22 auto-

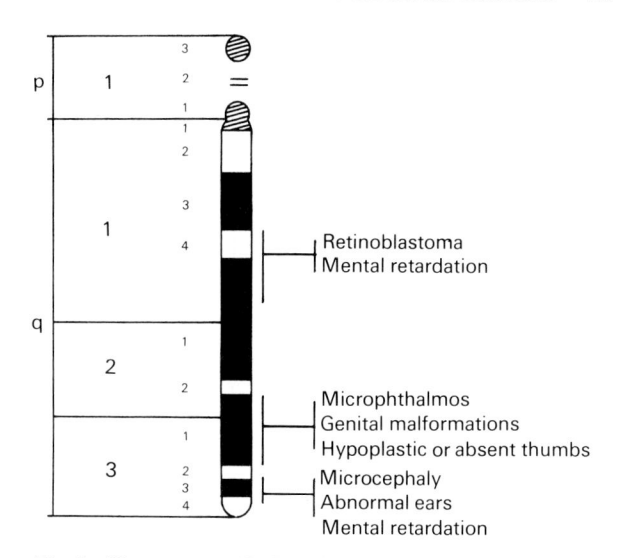

Fig. 2. Chromosome 13. Deletion of different segments of this chromosome produces different syndromes. The retinoblastoma gene (and also that for esterase D) is on band 14 of the long arm, and a deletion of this segment of the chromosome occurs in about 5 per cent of cases of retinoblastoma.

somes, and the X chromosome in the female, occur in pairs, and genes that are at the same locus on a pair of chromosomes are called alleles. If two allelic genes are identical, the person is said to be homozygous; if they are different, he or she is said to be heterozygous. In the male, who has only one X chromosome, he is said to be hemizygous for genes on that chromosome.

Characteristics or disorders transmitted as classic Mendelian traits result from the presence of a particular gene either in a single dose (the heterozygous state seen in dominant conditions) or in a double dose (the homozygous state seen in recessive conditions). Most traits are determined by genes on one of the autosomal chromosomes (autosomal traits); a few are determined by genes on the X chromosome (X-linked traits). The small Y chromosome appears to be responsible for little other than maleness; Y-linked traits, if they occur, appear not to be important in clinical genetics.

Autosomal Dominant Inheritance

The typical pedigree of an autosomal dominant trait is one where there are affected individuals in three or more generations. An affected person, who must be heterozygous for the responsible gene, will have, on average, half his or her children affected (*Fig.* 3). As the gene is on an autosome, males and females will be equally affected and, unlike X-linked inheritance, there will be male-to-male transmission. In many families the above conditions will not be met, partly because some patients with an autosomal dominant trait will have resulted from a new mutation and, in this instance, there will be no previous family history (the finding of an elevated mean paternal age supports the possibility that a condition is the result of new dominant mutation). In some families it may not be possible to confirm the diagnosis in previous generations who may not be available for examination. In others, the condition may have been so mild in previous generations that the condition may not have been suspected (*see* discussion of Penetrance and Expressivity below). If an accurate diagnosis has been made, and if the condition is always inherited as an autosomal dominant trait, a pedigree demonstrating all the characteristics of this form of inheritance is not essential.

Fig. 3. Autosomal dominant inheritance. An affected heterozygote (with one abnormal gene) transmits the abnormal gene to half his or her children.

Stickler's Syndrome (Hereditary Progressive Arthro-ophthalmopathy)

The major features of this autosomal dominant trait have been grouped into ocular and non-ocular abnormalities, the ocular abnormalities being the more common. The chief ocular signs are progressive myopia, open angle glaucoma, cataract, vitreo-retinal degeneration, perivascular pigmentary retinopathy and retinal detachment, frequently resulting in blindness. The most notable of the non-ocular findings are hearing loss and subtle facial abnormalities, including maxillary hypoplasia, depressed bridge of nose, small chin and cleft palate. Major generalized skeletal abnormalities include joint hyperextensibility and enlargement, arthritis and mild spondyloepiphyseal dysplasia.

This is a common connective tissue dysplasia, usually presenting to the ophthalmologist, in which the systemic manifestations are frequently unrecognized. Early diagnosis of Stickler's syndrome is important. Blindness may be prevented by regular ophthalmic examination and, where appropriate, by prophylactic treatment of retinal breaks and appropriate glaucoma therapy. In view of the serious nature of the complications, appropriate genetic counselling is desirable.

The ocular manifestations of Stickler's syndrome are similar to those described as Wagner's hyaloideoretinal degeneration, except that in Wagner's original large family there were no reported cases of retinal detachment, and no description of non-ocular manifestations. Some believe that the two conditions are identical; others consider that the family reported by Wagner is a separate, but very rare, entity.

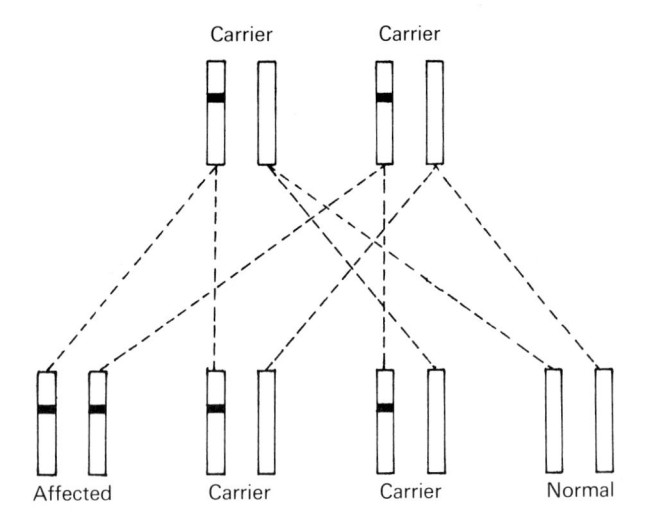

Fig. 4. Autosomal recessive inheritance. The carrier parents, each with one abnormal gene (heterozygote), transmit two abnormal genes to one-quarter of their children (who will be homozygous and affected), and one abnormal gene to half their children (who will be heterozygotes like their parents).

Autosomal Recessive Inheritance

When two individuals, each heterozygous for the same recessive gene, have children, one in four of the children will inherit two abnormal genes and will be homozygous and affected (*Fig.* 4). In communities where consanguineous marriages are common, autosomal recessive traits are prevalent, as the most likely way in which two individuals will have the same recessive gene is if they are related. This is particularly true for very rare traits, where the chances of two unrelated individuals having the same rare gene are extremely small. It is a good working rule that if a rare abnormality results from a consanguineous marriage, it should be considered to be an autosomal recessive trait until proved otherwise. In many instances, however, autosomal recessive traits occur by chance; they appear in one generation of a pedigree and then disappear, because the offspring of a homozygous (affected) individual with an autosomal recessive trait will inherit only one of the parent's abnormal genes and will, therefore, be unaffected. As with autosomal dominant transmission, as the genes are on autosomes, males and females will be equally affected.

If an abnormality has been shown to result from an enzyme deficiency, and if both parents show a partial deficiency for that enzyme, autosomal recessive inheritance is almost certain. It is a useful generalization to consider that autosomal recessive traits result from an enzyme deficiency, while autosomal dominant traits result from an abnormality of a structural protein, such as collagen.

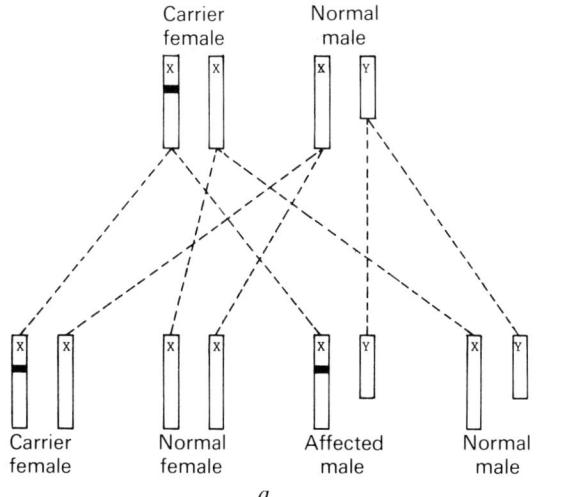

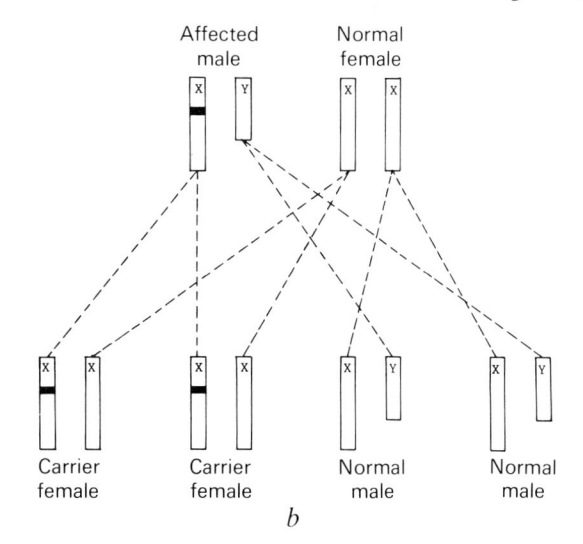

Fig. 5. X-linked inheritance. *a*, A heterozygous (carrier) female, with an abnormal gene on one of her X chromosomes, will transmit the abnormal gene to half her daughters (who will be heterozygous and carriers), and to half her sons (who will be hemizygous and affected). *b*, A hemizygous (affected) male will transmit the abnormal gene to all his daughters (who will be heterozygous and carriers), but to none of his sons (who inherit their Y chromosome from their father).

Gyrate Atrophy (Hyperornithinaemia)

Gyrate atrophy of the retina and choroid, one of the tapetoretinal dystrophies, and a very uncommon autosomal recessive trait, was recently shown to be associated with hyperornithinaemia, and to be the result of deficiency of the enzyme ornithine ketoacid aminotransferase. It presents in the first decade of life with gradually enlarging sharply defined areas of atrophy of the pigment epithelium, the retina and choroid, starting in the midperiphery, which gradually spread towards the posterior pole. It is followed by constriction of the visual fields, night blindness and cataract.

The concentration of ornithine in the plasma can be lowered towards normal with low protein, low arginine diets in all cases so far studied, and with vitamin B_6 (pyridoxine) in some cases. The responsiveness of some patients to vitamin B_6 suggests genetic heterogeneity (*see below*). It is too early to say whether treatment will influence the course of the ocular changes.

X-linked Inheritance

When a pedigree consists of affected males in two or more sibships connected through unaffected, or mildly affected, females, X-linked inheritance should be suspected. There must be no father-to-son transmission, for a son inherits his Y chromosome from his father, his X chromosome coming from his mother. If an abnormality has been shown to result from an enzyme deficiency, and if the mother (but not the father) shows an intermediate level of that enzyme activity, X-linked inheritance is almost certain.

In an X-linked trait, a hemizygous (affected) male will transmit his X chromosome to all his daughters, who will be heterozygotes (carriers), but to none of his sons. A heterozygous female will transmit the X chromosome with the abnormal gene to half her daughters, who will be carriers like their mother, and to half her sons, who will be affected (*Fig.* 5).

X-linked Retinoschisis

This is a fairly common, but frequently undiagnosed, X-linked vitreo-retinal dystrophy. It occurs virtually only in males, who inherit their abnormal gene from their mothers who themselves show no abnormalities, either ophthalmoscopically or electrophysiologically. The gene is highly penetrant, but the expressivity is variable (*see* Penetrance and Expressivity below).

The condition frequently presents in childhood, usually with reduced vision, but occasionally with vitreous haemorrhage. The pathognomonic sign, present in every case, is foveal retinoschisis, and this is the only sign of the disease in about 50 per cent of cases. At the fovea there is an optically empty zone delimited by two retinal layers of which the more superficial one is very thin and shows characteristic radial folds (*Plate* XV*a*). Silver-grey glistening spots can be found scattered over the retina, lattice-like changes may be seen, particularly in the lower temporal periphery, where true retinoschisis may be found in about half the cases. When the retinal changes are marked, there are accompanying vitreous changes. The electroretinogram shows a subnormal b-wave. True retinal detachment, when holes are present in both inner and outer layers of the retina, is uncommon.

In some patients the visual acuity remains remarkably good for many years; in others it is considerably reduced in childhood. The disease is slowly progressive throughout life.

Heterogeneity

> ... when a genetic disorder is examined closely, what at first is thought to be one entity is found in fact to be several clinically (that is, phenotypically) similar but fundamentally (genotypically) distinct disorders.
> V. A. McKusick

The importance of an accurate diagnosis in assessing genetic risk, and in determining the fundamental defect, in any particular genetically determined condition cannot be overemphasized. It has become apparent that in many instances more than one genetic cause leads to the same or similar clinical appearance (heterogeneity), and what was once thought to be a single entity has proved on close study to consist of several distinct disorders. Several examples of heterogeneity will be used to illustrate this point, the first (retinitis pigmentosa) also illustrating the three classic modes of Mendelian inheritance.

Retinitis Pigmentosa

A classic example of genetic heterogeneity is retinitis pigmentosa, a group of hereditary disorders of unknown aetiology characterized by a progressive deterioration in the function of the retinal receptors, leading most frequently to blindness in adult life or old age. For many years it has been recognized that isolated retinitis pigmentosa can be transmitted as an autosomal dominant (*Fig. 6*), an autosomal recessive (*Fig. 7*), or an X-linked trait (*Fig. 8*), and that an appreciable percentage of patients have no family history of the disease ('simplex' cases – not all of which are autosomal recessive). It would appear that in Britain about 25 per cent of all cases of retinitis pigmentosa are autosomal dominant, 40 per cent are autosomal recessive and 20 per cent are X-linked. The genetic status of the remainder is uncertain.

Although the majority of patients with retinitis pigmentosa have night blindness as their first symptom, followed by constriction of their visual fields, and all have characteristic ophthalmoscopic changes, the rate of progression and severity of the disease differs in the different genetic forms. The autosomal dominant form is the mildest; most patients keeping useful central vision into their 60s or later, although their visual fields are grossly constricted by middle age. The autosomal recessive and X-linked forms are much more severe, with gross constriction of their fields by the 20s and loss of useful central vision usually by the age of 40 years. It is therefore relevant to determine the correct genetic form, not only for genetic counselling, but also to give an accurate prognosis for vision. As it is almost certain that each of the different genetic forms has a different aetiology, it is necessary to make an accurate genetic diagnosis in order to study each disease meaningfully with the aim of determining the basic aetiological defect.

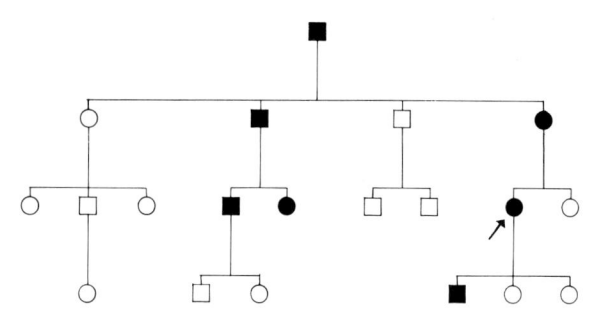

Fig. 6. Pedigree of autosomal dominant retinitis pigmentosa. In this family the disorder is transmitted through four generations. Males and females are equally affected, each affected person transmits the disorder to half the children, and there is father-to-son transmission (which excludes X-linked inheritance).

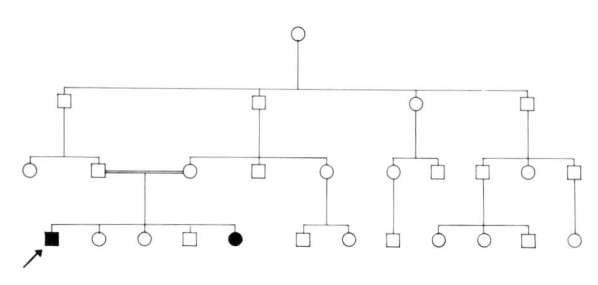

Fig. 7. Pedigree of autosomal recessive retinitis pigmentosa. In this family two first cousins, who must each have been heterozygous for the abnormal gene, married and had five children, two of whom were affected.

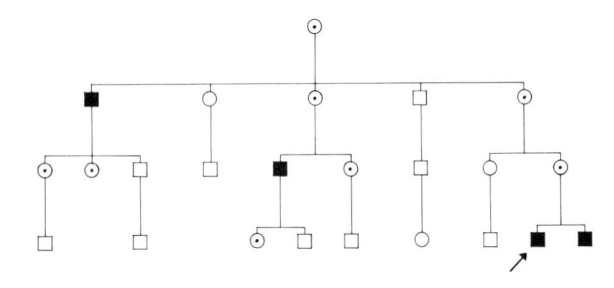

Fig. 8. Pedigree of X-linked retinitis pigmentosa. In this family only males are affected, and they have inherited their abnormal gene from their mothers. The heterozygous (carrier) females are shown on this pedigree by a dot in the circles, indicating female members.

X-linked retinitis pigmentosa merits further comment. As has already been stated, the hemizygous males are severely affected. The heterozygous (carrier) females usually show changes in their fundi; a few have a glistening tapetal reflex, and a number have a characteristic granular retinal periphery with small white spots scattered over it. The most characteristic changes are segmental areas of atrophy of the pigment epithelium with pigmentary migration into the retina. A few fundi show segmental retinitis pigmentosa or even frank generalized retinitis pigmentosa. Small defects in the visual fields are usually demonstrable, corresponding to the areas of greatest retinal involvement. In those heterozygous females with gross retinal changes, the field changes are correspondingly gross, but never as extensive as the changes found in affected males of similar age. The significance of these changes will be discussed later (Lyon hypothesis).

Several systemic disorders initially present with a retinal dystrophy that is similar to, or misdiagnosed as, retinitis pigmentosa. Three are worth mentioning: Batten's disease, abetalipoproteinaemia and Refsum's syndrome.

Batten's Disease (Neuronal Ceroid-lipofuscinosis)

Batten's disease is the preferred name for a group of uncommon neurolipidoses, each transmitted as an autosomal recessive trait. The three disorders in the group are: the infantile form (Haltia–Santavouri), the late infantile form (Jansky–Bielschowsky) and the juvenile form (Spielmeyer–Vogt, Batten–Mayou), but it is only in the last named that visual disturbance is the presenting symptom.

Juvenile Batten's Disease

This presents between 5 and 8 years of age, usually with loss of central vision, night blindness and central pigment epithelial defects. There is narrowing of the retinal vessels and mild peripheral pigment epithelial thinning and granularity, followed by progressive neuroepithelial degeneration and optic atrophy. Seizures and behavioural changes usually follow visual deterioration by several years, and death occurs at between 15 and 20 years of age, preceded by dementia and blindness. Diagnosis is confirmed by the finding of autofluorescent inclusions with characteristic staining in the neurones in a rectal biopsy.

Abetalipoproteinaemia (Bassen–Kornzweig Syndrome)

This uncommon and interesting autosomal recessive trait presents in infancy with steatorrhoea and retarded growth. Diminished tendon reflexes, proprioceptive defects and cerebellar signs develop in childhood. Acanthocytosis (crenated red blood cells with spiny excrescences) is an integral part of the syndrome, as is absence of low density plasma lipoproteins; both are probably present at a very early age.

The retinae show multiple areas of pigment epithelial atrophy with white spots and some pigment migration. The retinal changes are progressive, and pallor of the optic discs and narrowing of the retinal vessels develop. The dark adaptation threshold is raised and the electroretinogram extinguished.

Parenteral vitamin A, particularly if given early enough, results in dark adaptation and the electroretinogram returning to normal. This is the only retinal dystrophy for which vitamin A is indicated.

Refsum's Syndrome

In this rare autosomal recessive disorder, due to a deficiency of the enzyme phytanic acid alpha hydroxylase, a diffuse retinal dystrophy resembling retinitis pigmentosa is associated with polyneuritis, ataxia, deafness and tetraplegia. The neurological abnormalities are arrested by a low phytanic acid diet.

Albinism

Albinism may be defined as congenital heritable hypomelanosis involving the eye, skin and hair (oculocutaneous albinism – OCA), or apparently limited to the eye (ocular albinism – OA). Nystagmus, photophobia and reduced visual acuity occur in all forms of albinism; in their absence hypomelanosis should be termed albinoidism or cutaneous hypopigmentation. Both oculocutaneous and ocular albinism are heterogeneous groups of disorders which may be subdivided on anatomical, genetic or biochemical grounds. All forms of oculocutaneous albinism are transmitted as autosomal recessive traits, while ocular albinism may be autosomal recessive (AROA) or X-linked (XOA).

Oculocutaneous albinism has been divided into tyrosinase-negative (ty-neg) and tyrosinase-positive (ty-pos) forms on the basis of the hair bulb incubation test. This test, which consists of incubating a hair bulb with tyrosine, demonstrates the presence of the enzyme tyrosinase by the appearance of the pigment melanin. Unfortunately, the test is unreliable in the first 2 or 3 years of life. These two forms of OCA are non-allelic, that is, the genes responsible for each disorder are not at the same loci. This has been determined by finding several couples, each with one of these forms of OCA, whose children are not albinos. There are several other less common forms of OCA which will not be discussed here.

Tyrosinase-negative OCA

In this, the most extreme form of albinism, there is an absence of pigment in the skin, hair and eyes, and this does not change with age. The skin is pink and the hair white. The colour of the iris, which is grossly translucent, varies from grey to blue, and the pupil is red. There is no visible pigment in the fundi. Severe nystagmus and photophobia occur, strabismus is common and the visual acuity is greatly reduced, usually being in the region of 6/60. Many children with this form of OCA require special schooling because of their reduced visual acuity.

Tyrosinase-positive OCA

In this form of albinism, although pigment is usually absent in Caucasian and Negro infants, and in some Caucasian adults, it tends to vary with race and increase with age. The hair is white in infancy but may change to flaxen or yellow with age. The skin is pink but freckles and pigmented naevi are common. Negroes often have a darker skin colour than blond Caucasians. The colour of the iris, which is moderately to markedly translucent, frequently changes from blue to hazel, or even to light brown.

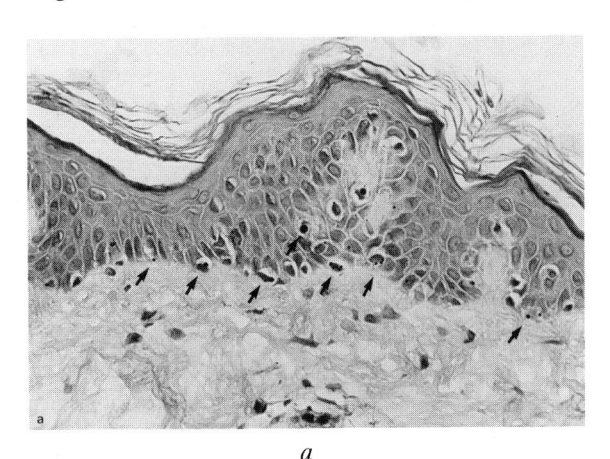

X-linked Ocular Albinism

The classic form of X-linked OA was first described by Nettleship at the beginning of this century. Affected males have nystagmus, reduced visual acuity, photophobia, translucent irides and albinotic fundi. Heterozygous (carrier) females frequently show some degree of translucency of their irides, and almost always have characteristic fundus changes consisting of areas of hypopigmentation interspersed between areas of normal or hyperpigmented retina (*Plate* XV*b,c*), despite normal visual functions.

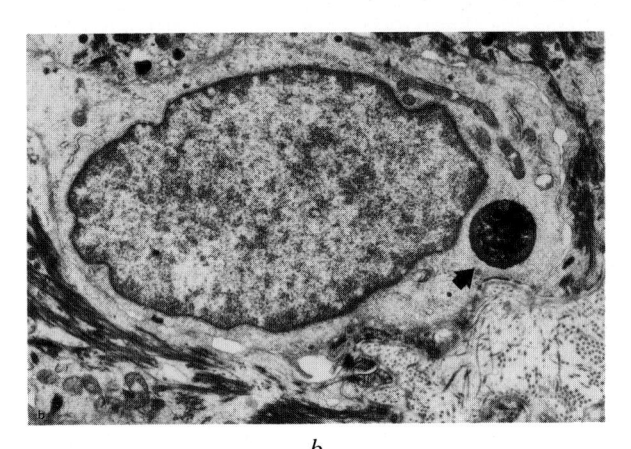

Fig. 9. Giant melanosomes in X-linked ocular albinism. *a*, Light micrograph of skin, showing giant melanosomes (arrows) in the epidermis, mainly within melanocytes in the basal layer of the epidermis. *b*, Electron micrograph of a melanocyte from the basal layer of the epidermis, showing a giant melanosome (arrow).

A red pupillary reflex is common in infancy. There is no visible pigment in the infant's fundus, but choroidal pigment gradually accumulates with age, particularly in Negroes. Nystagmus and photophobia are usually marked, but less so than in the ty-neg form, and visual acuity, which is greatly reduced in infants, may improve with age, being 6/18 to 6/36 in the majority of adults. The majority of children with ty-pos OCA can manage at normal schools.

Autosomal Recessive Ocular Albinism

In this form of albinism all patients are lightly pigmented at birth with blond or platinum-coloured hair which gradually darkens shortly after birth. Most patients tan slightly and all have freckles and pigmented naevi. The colour of the iris, which is moderately translucent, often changes from blue to hazel or brown. There is usually a little pigment in the infant's fundus; this increases with age. Nystagmus and photophobia are always present, but are not usually as marked as in OCA. Strabismus is common, and the visual acuity is usually 6/18 to 6/24. Autosomal recessive ocular albinism, which is not rare, is often misdiagnosed as ocular nystagmus. Although the distinction between ty-post OCA and AROA is useful clinically, it may be that this division is artificial.

Of particular interest is the recent observation of giant melanosomes in the skin and eyes both of Caucasian and Negro affected males and of heterozygous females with X-linked ocular albinism (*Fig.* 9). This indicates the widespread nature of the disturbance in the structure of melanosomes.

Higher Visual Pathways

In recent years a considerable body of evidence has accumulated indicating that, in all the albino animals so far studied, there is an increase in the number of fibres that cross in the optic chiasm (*Plate* XV*d*). Visual evoked potentials have been studied in human oculocutaneous and ocular albinos and these confirm that in man each occipital cortex receives a predominantly monocular input from the contralateral eye. An anatomical study of the dorsal lateral geniculate nucleus in human albinos has confirmed that the retinogeniculate pathways are abnormal, the abnormality in the nucleus being consistent with its being innervated by one eye.

Marfan's Syndrome

This, one of the 'heritable disorders of connective tissue', commonly presents to the ophthalmologist in childhood because of the ocular manifestations of the syndrome. Marfan's syndrome involves mainly the eye and the skeletal and cardiovascular systems and is transmitted as an autosomal dominant trait, due to the presence of a *pleiotropic* gene, a single gene responsible for multiple manifestations. In common with many other autosomal dominant traits, there is wide variation in the clinical picture from case to case, and this is true even for affected members of the same family. This wide spectrum of clinical picture accounts for the apparently large number of sporadic cases of Marfan's syndrome; in the majority of these apparently sporadic cases, careful clinical examination of other members of the family will bring to light mildly affected members.

Ectopia lentis, which is bilateral and symmetrical, is the most characteristic ocular manifestation of this syndrome, present in about 80 per cent of cases. It may be demonstrable at birth; it frequently develops during childhood. Characteristically, the lens, which is often small and spherical, is displaced upwards and outwards, in contrast to homocystinuria, where the lens is typically displaced downwards (*see below*). When the lens is subluxated, iridodonesis is almost invariably present. Other common ocular manifestations include high myopia and spontaneous retinal detachment; blue sclerae, megalocornea and developmental anomalies of the angle of the anterior chamber also occur.

The typical skeletal abnormalities include long extremities, characteristic facies and pectus excavatum ('funnel chest'). The excessive length of the limbs can often be shown by the pubis-to-sole being greater than that of the pubis-to-vertex measurement, and the arm span being greater than the height. The more distal bones of the extremities are particularly involved, resulting in arachnodactyly (spider fingers). The characteristic facies include a long narrow face, high arched palate and prominent lower jaw. A kyphoscoliosis is very common, as is hyperextensibility of the joints.

The cardiovascular manifestations result from a weakness of the tunica media of the aorta and main pulmonary artery, resulting particularly in diffuse dilatation and/or dissecting aneurysms of the aorta. Mitral regurgitation, due to a 'floppy mitral valve', is also common. These cardiovascular complications account for about 95 per cent of deaths in Marfan's syndrome, the average age of death being about 30 years.

An accurate diagnosis of Marfan's syndrome is becoming increasingly important now that treatment for the cardiovascular complications is feasible. Aortic dilatation is now being managed by prophylactic propranolol, and such patients need counselling about sports and pregnancy (where there is an increased risk of vascular rupture). Certain patients are suitable candidates for prophylactic cardiovascular surgery.

It must be remembered that, in addition to homocystinuria (*see below*), there are a number of other causes of subluxated lenses (*Table* I). A number of conditions also mimic the increased height and long limbs of Marfan's syndrome: certain Negro tribes, eunuchs, Klinefelter's syndrome (a male with a 47,XXY karyotype – his cells containing an extra X chromosome) and sickle cell anaemia.

Homocystinuria

Before its description in 1962, this inborn error of metabolism, due to a deficiency of the enzyme cystathionine synthase, was frequently misdiagnosed as Marfan's syndrome. Like Marfan's syndrome, it has ocular, skeletal and cardiovascular manifestations, but unlike Marfan's syndrome mental subnormality occurs in about 70 per cent of cases. It is inherited as an autosomal recessive trait.

Ectopia lentis, which is bilateral and symmetrical, occurs in about 90 per cent of cases of homocystinuria, the lens being most frequently displaced downwards and inwards, in contrast to Marfan's syndrome where it is displaced upwards and outwards. The subluxation is progressive, and dislocation into the anterior chamber is more frequent than in Marfan's syndrome.

The skeletal manifestations include excessive height, generalized osteoporosis, scoliosis, widened epiphyses and vertebral collapse. The cardiovascular complications result from thromboses in medium sized arteries; intracranial venous and arterial thromboses, thrombophlebitis with pulmonary embolism, coronary artery occlusion and renal artery stenosis all occur. Patients with homocystinuria are liable to develop thrombotic episodes during or after general anaesthesia.

The diagnosis should be suspected in any patient with spontaneous subluxation of the lens. The cyanide nitroprusside test on urine is a simple and useful screening measure; if positive, it should be followed by high voltage paper electrophoresis.

Genetic heterogeneity is illustrated by the separation of homocystinuria from Marfan's syndrome. In addition, there appear to be at least two forms of homocystinuria: one which responds to vitamin B_6, and one which does not. The former is often associated with normal mentality and responds to treatment by pyridoxine (vitamin B_6), particularly if treatment is started early enough.

Penetrance and Expressivity

We have already seen in retinoblastoma that not all individuals who are heterozygous for the relevant gene manifest the disease. When this occurs, the condition may skip a generation. The degree of penetrance is a measure of the percentage of individuals of the relevant genotype who manifest the disease. In retinoblastoma, for example, a parent with retinoblastoma will transmit the abnormal gene to 50 per cent of his or her children, but only 90 per cent of the children who inherit the abnormal gene will

Table I. Causes of ectopia lentis

	Inheritance	McKusick no.*
Without systemic manifestations		
Simple ectopia lentis	AD	12960
Late spontaneous ectopia lentis	AD	18545
Ectopia lentis et pupillae	AR	22520
Systemic disorders associated with ectopia lentis		
Marfan's syndrome	AD	15470
Homocystinuria	AR	23620
Weill–Marchesani syndrome	AR	27760
Hyperlysinaemia	AR	23870
Molybdenum cofactor deficiency	AR	25215
Sulphite oxidase deficiency	AR	27230
Ocular disorders with ectopia lentis		
Trauma		
Aniridia	AD	10620
High myopia		
Blepharoptosis, myopia, ectopia lentis	AD	11015
Cornea plana		
Eales's disease		
Congenital glaucoma		
Megalocornea		
Microphthalmos		
Persistent pupillary membrane		
Persistent hyperplastic primary vitreous		
Retinitis pigmentosa		
Rieger syndrome	AD	18050
Uveal coloboma		
Systemic disorders rarely associated with ectopia lentis		
Crouzon's disease	AD	12350
Ehlers–Danlos syndrome		
Kniest disease	AD	15655
Mandibulofacial dysostosis	AD	15450
Refsum syndrome	AR	26650
Scleroderma		
Sturge–Weber syndrome	—	18530
Syphilis		

Some of the above ocular disorders with ectopia lentis, and systemic disorders rarely associated with ectopia lentis, may be fortuitous associations.
AD, Autosomal Dominant; AR, autosomal recessive.
* McKusick V. A. *Mendelian Inheritance in Man*, 6th ed. Baltimore, Md, Johns Hopkins University Press, 1983.

manifest the disease (i.e., 45 per cent of all his or her children will manifest the disease – 90 per cent penetrance).

We have also seen, in Marfan's syndrome for example, that there can be considerable variation in the clinical picture from case to case, some individuals being so mildly affected that they (and their family) may be unaware of their having the disease. Marfan's syndrome is therefore said to have variable expressivity.

Variable expressivity can create diagnostic problems, and, with reduced penetrance, can complicate accurate genetic counselling. The phakomatoses are a group of disorders characterized by neural and vascular tumours involving the skin, eye and nervous system. The group comprises neurofibromatosis, tuberous sclerosis and the von Hippel–Lindau syndrome, and each demonstrates variable expressivity.

The Sturge–Weber syndrome is another member of the group, but it is not genetically determined.

Neurofibromatosis (von Recklinghausen's Disease)

The consistent features of neurofibromatosis are cafe-au-lait spots and fibromatous skin tumours which arise from cutaneous nerves. The cafe-au-lait spots are flat, light brown patches on the skin and the presence of at least six, each more than 1·5 cm in diameter, is necessary to confirm the diagnosis. The disease, which is transmitted as an autosomal dominant trait, varies widely in its severity. Some patients have a few cafe-au-lait spots and the occasional fibroma, others are grotesquely affected with multiple skin tumours, neurofibromas on numerous peripheral and central nerves, and deformities and cystic rarefactions of bones (Quasimodo, in Victor

Hugo's *Notre Dame de Paris*, probably suffered from this disease.)

Almost every tissue in and around the eye can be involved, but the more important ocular manifestations are plexiform neuroma of the eyelid, congenital or infantile glaucoma, orbital neuromas and gliomas of the optic nerve and chiasm. Glaucoma is usually associated with a plexiform neuroma of the upper lid (and sometimes with hemihypertrophy of the face), so all patients with this neuroma should be periodically examined to exclude glaucoma, which results from infiltration by neurofibroma of the angle of the anterior chamber. The orbital tumours may be solitary neurofibromas or plexiform neuromas; they are often associated with an enlarged orbit and bony defects in the orbital walls. About 15 per cent of primary optic nerve tumours are associated with neurofibromatosis.

Tuberous Sclerosis (Bourneville's Disease, Epiloia)

This autosomal dominant trait with variable expressivity is characterized, in its complete form, by epilepsy, mental deficiency and 'adenoma sebaceum' of the face (more correctly facial angiofibroma). Multiple fibro-angiomatous or glio-angiomatous tumours occur in the brain, kidneys, heart and other organs. In the eye mulberry-like tumours occur in the retina or project from the optic nerve head. The presence of white leaf-shaped skin lesions is a useful diagnostic aid.

von Hippel–Lindau Syndrome

The cardinal features of this autosomal dominant disease with variable expressivity and low penetrance are angiomas of the retina and haemangioblastomas of the cerebellum. Tumours also occur in other organs. The retinal angiomas, which are treatable, are frequently associated with dilated and tortuous retinal vessels. Secondary polycythaemia, due to cerebellar haemangioblastoma or to phaeochromocytoma, occurs in some patients.

Sturge–Weber Syndrome

This non-genetic disease is included here for completeness. It is characterized by a capillary angioma of the face (naevus flammeus) associated with a meningeal angioma. The latter tumour may cause epilepsy or mental subnormality, and is frequently associated with 'tram-line' calcification in the underlying cerebral cortex. Congenital or infantile glaucoma may occur, particularly if the facial angioma involves the upper lid, and choroidal angiomas may be present.

Lyon Hypothesis

From a study of sex chromosome abnormalities it has become apparent that the presence of a Y chromosome determines male development, irrespective of the number of X chromosomes that are present, while the absence of a Y chromosome results in female development. For example, the karyotype of a normal male is 46,XY, while that of a male with Klinefelter's syndrome is 47,XXY. The karyotype of females with Turner's syndrome is 45,X, that of a normal female is 46,XX, while that of a triple X female is 47,XXX.

As the Y chromosome is small, it would appear at first sight that the female has considerably more DNA than the male. If a considerable excess or deficiency of DNA were to occur in autosomes, the effect would probably be lethal. It would appear necessary, therefore, for some sort of gene dosage compensation to operate, and Mary Lyon has produced an acceptable explanation for this.

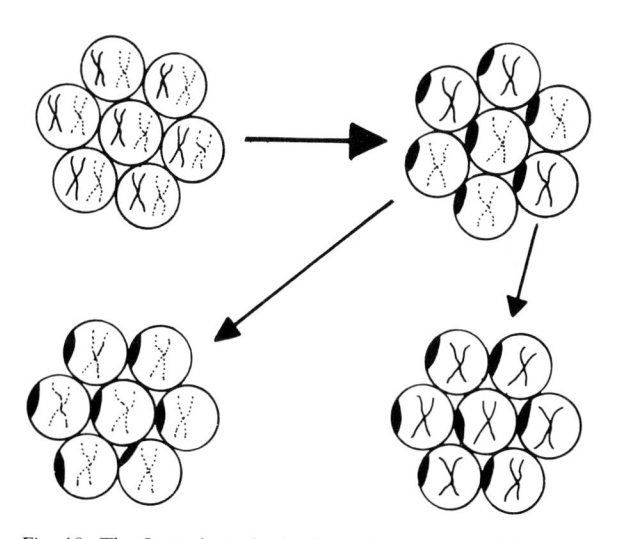

Fig. 10. The Lyon hypothesis. Early in embryonic life, in each somatic cell of a female embryo, one of the X chromosomes becomes inactivated and forms the Barr body. Descendants of these somatic cells contain the same active X chromosome as their ancestor cell. The female somatic cells, therefore, contain one active X chromosome; in some cells these are paternally derived, in the remainder they are maternally derived.

The Lyon hypothesis states that early in embryonic life, however many X chromosomes are present in a somatic cell, only one remains active. This process of inactivation occurs at random, so that paternal and maternal X chromosomes have an equal chance of being inactivated. Once inactivation has occurred, the same X chromosome will be inactivated in the descendants of any one cell (*Fig.* 10). We now know that the inactivated X chromosomes produce the Barr bodies, so that a normal male (46,XY) and a female with Turner's syndrome (45,X) have no Barr bodies, a normal female (46,XX) and a male with Klinefelter's syndrome (47,XXY) have one Barr body, and a triple X female (47,XXX) has 2 Barr bodies.

One implication of the Lyon hypothesis is that females are mosaics; they have, as far as their X chromosome is concerned, two cell lines, one where the active X chromosome is paternally derived, and the other where it is maternally derived. Evidence of this mosaicism can be seen in the fundi of heterozygotes for several X-linked diseases. In heterozygotes for X-linked ocular albinism the fundus has small areas of non-pigmented (albino) fundus interspersed in a random fashion with areas of pigmented fundus; this is what could be expected if the Lyon hypothesis applied to retinal cells early in their development. In heterozygotes for X-linked retinitis pigmentosa the result appears to be somewhat different, the fundus appearing midway between that of the hemizygous (affected) male and that of the normal individual. This may indicate that the gene action in this case is more distant from the retina. If inactivation of the X chromosome occurs early enough in development, it will only involve a few cells destined to become the target organ. It is not surprising, therefore, that the clinical appearance of these heterozygotes varies from normal to that of the affected male, the majority of heterozygotes having an appearance midway in severity between the two. Occasional severely affected heterozygotes (manifesting heterozygotes) are seen in X-linked retinitis pigmentosa, in X-linked ocular albinism and in choroideremia.

Choroideremia

In addition to retinitis pigmentosa, the generalized receptor dystrophies include choroideremia, an uncommon X-linked disorder that is frequently misdiagnosed. The first symptoms are night blindness in childhood, followed by constriction of the visual fields, usually first noticed in the 'teens. Central vision is retained longer than in X-linked retinitis pigmentosa; most hemizygous males keep useful central vision at least into their 50s. In childhood, the fundi show fine pigment stippling of the entire retina followed, over many years, by a gradual atrophy of the choriocapillaris. Pigment migration is not a prominent feature; it tends to be maximal in the midperiphery of the fundus. Eventually the retina and choroid almost completely disappear; all that remains are the larger retinal vessels which are narrowed, and scattered clumps of pigment, particularly around the posterior pole. As in retinitis pigmentosa, the optic disc becomes atrophic.

In choroideremia, the heterozygous females show minimal pigment stippling at the posterior pole, but in the midperiphery and beyond there is spotty pigmentation, often in a linear configuration, with focal areas of pigment epithelial atrophy (*Plate* XV*e,f*). Some heterozygotes have small peripheral areas of atrophy of the choriocapillaris, and occasional heterozygotes (manifesting heterozygotes) have a degree of severity approaching that of hemizygous males. Most heterozygous females have only slight involvement of their visual functions; not surprisingly, manifesting heterozygotes can be severely affected.

Phenocopy

A phenocopy is a condition due to environmental factors which mimics one that is genetically determined. Phenocopies are commonly encountered in ophthalmology and raise problems in diagnosis and, therefore, for genetic counselling. In two groups of disorders, congenital cataract and optic atrophy, they are numerically of considerable importance.

Congenital Cataract

Cataracts that are present at birth or become apparent in the first year of life are an important cause of visual handicap in childhood, accounting for just under 20 per cent of all causes in children under the age of 15 years registered as blind in England and Wales. About half the cases are genetically determined, and an appreciable percentage of the remainder are associated with prematurity or perinatal difficulties. A small but important group, important because they are preventable, are caused by the rubella syndrome.

Genetically determined cataracts are a heterogeneous group of disorders. Most commonly they are an isolated finding, often they are associated with other ocular abnormalities, such as microphthalmos or coloboma. A small number are part of a systemic syndrome, of which there are a large number, most being uncommon or rare (*Table* II).

Genetically Determined Isolated Cataract

Isolated hereditary cataract may be transmitted as autosomal dominant, autosomal recessive, or X-linked traits, the autosomal dominant being by far the most common.

Autosomal dominant cataracts are most commonly lamellar, although not all lamellar cataracts are genetically determined.

Autosomal recessive cataracts are uncommon in Britain, although they occur more frequently in communities where consanguinity is common. If a cataract occurs in a consanguineous marriage, it is important to exclude the autosomal recessive systemic disorders with which cataract may be associated and, in particular, galactosaemia and galactokinase deficiency.

X-linked isolated cataracts are rare. The hemizygous (affected) males tend to have nuclear cataracts which may progress to maturation in early adult life. The heterozygous (carrier) females have characteristic posterior Y-sutural opacities (*Fig.* 11); these are difficult to see without a slit lamp microscope and seldom affect vision. X-linked isolated cataract is a distinct entity and should not be confused with the Lowe oculocerebrorenal syndrome which is also transmitted as an X-linked trait.

Table II. Aetiology of cataract within the first year of life

	McKusick no*
Chromosomal anomalies	
Deletion of short arm of chromosome 4 (Wolf–Hirschhorn syndrome)	
Trisomy 13 (Patau syndrome)	
Trisomy 18 (Edwards' syndrome)	
Trisomy 21 (Down's syndrome)	
Genetically determined	
Autosomal dominant cataract (several genetically distinct forms)	11570–11680
Autosomal recessive cataract	
X-linked cataract	30220
Intrauterine infections	
Cytomegalovirus	
Rubella	
Varicella-zoster	
Prematurity or perinatal difficulties	
Associated with ocular disorders	
Aniridia	
Anterior chamber cleavage syndromes	
Coloboma	
Microphthalmos	
Retinoblastoma	
Retrolental fibroplasia	
Central nervous system disorders	
Cataract–mental retardation–hypogonadism	21272
Crome syndrome	21890
Marinesco–Sjögren syndrome	24880
Meckel syndrome	24900
Cerebrohepatorenal syndrome (Zellweger syndrome)	21410
Craniofacial and facial syndromes	
Hallerman–Streiff syndrome	23410
Pierre Robin syndrome	
Rubinstein–Taybi syndrome	26860
Smith–Lemli–Opitz syndrome	27040
Mandibulofacial dysostosis (Treacher Collins syndrome)	15450
Dermatological disorders	
Anhidrotic ectodermal dysplasia	30510
Gorlin syndrome	23350
Congenital ichthyosis	21240
Incontinentia pigmenti	30830
Rothmund–Thomson syndrome (Poikiloderma atrophicans)	26840
Metabolic disorders	
Alport syndrome	10420
Galactosaemia	23040
Galactokinase deficiency	23020
Hypocalcaemia	
Hypoglycaemia	
Lowe syndrome	30900
Muscular disorders	
Cataract and cardiomyopathy	21235
Skeletal disorders	
Cataract, microcephaly, arthrogryposis, kyphosis syndrome	21253
Cataract, microcephaly, failure to thrive, kyphoscoliosis syndrome	21254
Chondrodysplasia punctata (Conradi syndrome)	21510
Absence deformity of leg	24600
Marfan's syndrome	15470
Meckel syndrome	24900
Oculodentodigital dysplasia	16420
Osteogenesis imperfecta congenita, microcephaly and cataracts	25941
Rubinstein–Taybi syndrome	26860
Trauma	
Accidental injury	
Non-accidental injury	
Radiotherapy	

* McKusick V. A. *Mendelian Inheritance in Man*, 6th ed. Baltimore, Md, Johns Hopkins University Press, 1983.

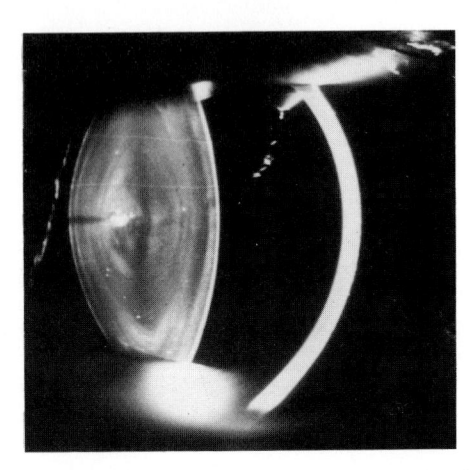

Fig. 11. Lens of a heterozygote for X-linked cataract showing fine central opacities in the region of the Y sutures.

Genetically Determined Cataract associated with Systemic Disorders

Of the many genetically determined systemic disorders that are associated with cataract, three deserve brief mention.

Galactosaemia

An autosomal recessive trait due to a deficiency of the enzyme galactose-1-phosphate uridyltransferase, galactosaemia presents in early infancy as a failure to thrive, with mental retardation, hepatomegaly and galactose in serum and urine. Slit lamp examination reveals 'oil-droplet' cataracts. By excluding galactose from the diet, the condition may be reversed. Heterozygotes for galactosaemia may be identified by measuring the activity of uridyltransferase in their red and white blood cells; it is about 50 per cent of normal.

Galactokinase deficiency

Another autosomal recessive trait, galactokinase deficiency results in cataracts in childhood associated with galactose in the serum and urine, but without the other systemic features of galactosaemia. Cataract formation can be prevented by excluding milk from the diet at an early age. All children with cataracts should have their urine examined for galactose, as both galactokinase deficiency and galactosaemia are treatable if diagnosed early enough.

The Lowe Oculocerebrorenal Syndrome

This syndrome is transmitted as an X-linked trait. It is characterized by cataract, marginal corneal opacity, congenital glaucoma, mental retardation, vitamin D-resistant rickets, aminoaciduria and reduced ammonia production by the kidneys. Babies with this syndrome present with failure to thrive, nystagmus and visual handicap, and mental retardation.

Non-hereditary Cataract

Having described some of the more common types of genetically determined cataract, mention must now be made of two groups of *phenocopies*: those associated with perinatal problems, and those resulting from rubella infection in the first trimester of pregnancy.

Perinatal Problems

Congenital cataract is frequently seen in children who were of low birth weight or who had perinatal problems. These children have a high incidence of neurological defects, mental retardation and epilepsy, and these associations make it important for all visually handicapped children, whatever the apparent cause of the handicap, to be examined by a paediatrician.

Rubella Syndrome

Fetal infection and damage may occur when a primary rubella infection occurs during the first 20 weeks of pregnancy; infection after 10 weeks of gestation usually results in a single defect, almost always deafness. The rubella syndrome comprises multiple congenital abnormalities, the most common being retardation of growth and mental development, microcephaly, cataracts, deafness and congenital heart defects. In addition to cataracts, other common ocular disorders are retinopathy, strabismus, nystagmus, microphthalmos, optic atrophy, corneal haze and glaucoma. The retinopathy, which may mimic retinitis pigmentosa, consists most commonly of a widespread pigmentary disturbance which is non-progressive and has little effect on visual function.

Optic Atrophy

Optic atrophy accounts for 30 per cent of all those under the age of 15 years registered as blind in England and Wales. Just over half these cases are congenital or hereditary, the remainder are acquired. The congenital and hereditary group consists of a minority of cases of hereditary optic atrophy and a majority where the optic atrophy is associated with perinatal difficulties. The acquired group must contain many cases that result from compressive lesions.

Genetically Determined Optic Atrophy

Autosomal Dominant Optic Atrophy

This is the most common genetically determined type. The onset of visual difficulty is in childhood, the visual acuity seldom falls below 6/60 and nystagmus is not present. There is temporal pallor of the optic discs and an acquired blue–yellow dyschromatopsia.

Autosomal Recessive Optic Atrophy

This is very rare, with an onset in early childhood. There is severe visual impairment with nystagmus, and the optic discs are very pale with attenuated retinal vessels. The condition must be distinguished from Leber's amaurosis (retinal aplasia); in autosomal recessive optic atrophy the electroretinogram is present, while in Leber's amaurosis it is extinguished.

Behr's Syndrome

Behr's syndrome is another autosomal recessive trait with onset in childhood. Bilateral optic atrophy is associated with nystagmus, spasticity, hypertonia, ataxia and mild mental retardation.

Diabetes Mellitus and Insipidus with Optic Atrophy and Deafness

DIDMOAD syndrome or Wolfram's syndrome has an onset in childhood, the juvenile diabetes mellitus preceding the optic atrophy, both of which are prominent signs. Diabetes insipidus and mild deafness may be missed.

Leber's Optic Atrophy

This results in the sudden onset of visual loss in the second and third decades, the second eye usually becoming involved within a few days of the first. In the acute phase the optic disc shows circumpapillary telangiectatic microangiopathy with swelling of the nerve fibre layer around the disc. In the late phase of the disease both optic discs become pale and flat, there is marked loss of nerve fibres temporal to the disc, and there is loss of capillaries both on and around the disc. The majority of cases show no recovery of vision, which remains at 6/60 or worse. Pyramidal and cerebellar symptoms and peripheral nerve involvement may occur.

The mode of inheritance in Leber's optic atrophy is still uncertain. The disease involves mainly males, but males never transmit the disease to their descendants. Heterozygous females, who may be affected or unaffected, transmit the disease to about half their sons and to most (? all) of their daughters. In addition to a genetic component (which might be autosomal), it has been suggested that an environmental factor, possibly cyanide intoxication or a slow virus, may play a part in the aetiology, although the present view is that the disorder results from mitochondrial inheritance.

Non-hereditary Optic Atrophy

The majority of cases of congenital optic atrophy are non-hereditary; many have a history of perinatal difficulties and are associated with other signs of damage to the central nervous system. It is important to distinguish optic nerve hypoplasia from optic atrophy; the two conditions can look superficially similar. The acquired causes of optic atrophy are important; in childhood they most commonly result from compression of the anterior visual pathways in hydrocephalus, glioma and craniopharyngioma.

MULTIFACTORIAL INHERITANCE

The diseases so far discussed in this chapter have been transmitted by the various classic modes of Mendelian inheritance. These modes account for the transmission of many genetically determined diseases and, in particular, the uncommon diseases whose patterns of inheritance have, in many cases, been understood since the early part of this century.

It has been recognized for many years that there are a number of common disorders that have a hereditary predisposition, but the patterns of inheritance cannot be adequately explained in terms of Mendelian inheritance. Two such ocular disorders are chronic simple glaucoma and strabismus. In recent years there has accumulated statistical evidence to suggest that these common disorders are examples of multifactorial inheritance, that is, inheritance resulting from a number of factors, some genetic and others environmental. It is not the intention to discuss here the theoretical basis for this statement; only its implications will be considered.

Implicit in the concept of multifactorial inheritance is the threshold effect, in which independently inherited genes have an additive effect; only when a threshold has been exceeded does their combined effect produce the disorder. It can be shown mathematically that such a model will result in the frequency of affected members in a family decreasing very rapidly as the relationship becomes more remote. In an autosomal dominant trait, the incidence of the disorder in first degree relatives (parents, sibs, children) is 0·5, in second degree relatives (grandparents, grandchildren, aunts, uncles, nieces, nephews) it is 0·25, while in third degree relatives (cousins, great-grandchildren, great-uncles, etc) it is 0·125 (i.e. 1 in 8 will be affected). In multifactorial inheritance, on the other hand, the incidence of the disease decreases markedly between first and second degree relatives. In harelip and cleft palate, an example of multifactorial inheritance, where the incidence in different relatives has been ascertained, the results are as follows: in first degree relatives of an affected person the incidence of the disease is 30 to 40 times higher than in the general population; in second degree relatives it is seven times higher; while in third degree relatives the incidence is only two to three times higher than in the general population.

This pattern of disease within a family becomes relevant when the prevention of these common diseases is considered. In chronic simple glaucoma, for example, first degree relatives have about ten times more chance of developing the disease than do people without a family history of glaucoma; they must therefore be screened regularly for the disease, particularly if screening the whole population is unrealistic or uneconomical.

The implications of multifactorial inheritance are that a search for a single abnormality, whether it be a deficient enzyme or an abnormal structural gene, underlying each of these conditions is unlikely to be profitable and that there is a need to discover the individual genes involved and the nature of any additional environmental factors contributing to their aetiology. It should also be remembered that in multifactorial inheritance the risk to relatives will vary from family to family, will increase if two or more members are already affected, and will also be increased if the index patient is severely affected.

FURTHER READING

Bergsma D., Bron A. J. and Cotlier E. (ed.) *The Eye and Inborn Errors of Metabolism*. New York, Liss, 1976.
Cotlier E., Maumenee I. H. and Berman E. R. (ed.) *Genetic Eye Diseases. Retinitis Pigmentosa and Other Inherited Eye Disorders*. New York, Liss, 1982.
Duke-Elder S. *System of Ophthalmology. Vol. III: Normal and Abnormal Development – Part 2 Congenital Deformities*. London, Kimpton, 1964.
François J. *Heredity in Ophthalmology*. St Louis, Mo, Mosby, 1961.
Goldberg M. F. (ed.) *Genetic and Metabolic Eye Disease*. Boston, Mass, Little Brown, 1974.
Keith C. G. *Genetics and Ophthalmology*. Edinburgh, Churchill Livingstone, 1978.
Krill A. E. *Hereditary Retinal and Choroidal Diseases. Vol. I: Evaluation*. Hagerstown, Md, Harper and Row, 1972.
Krill A. E. and Archer D. B. *Krill's Hereditary Retinal and Choroidal Diseases. Vol. II: Clinical Characteristics*. Hagerstown, Md, Harper and Row, 1977.
McKusick V. A. *Mendelian Inheritance in Man. Catalogs of Autosomal Dominant, Autosomal Recessive, and X-linked Phenotypes*, 6th ed. Baltimore, Md, Johns Hopkins University Press, 1983.
Sorsby A. *Ophthalmic Genetics*, 2nd ed. London, Butterworths, 1970.
Waardenburg P. J. Franceschetti A. and Klein D. *Genetics and Ophthalmology*. Assen, Royal VanGorcum, 1961.
Waardenburg P. J. *Genetics and Ophthalmology*, vol. II (Neuro-Opthalmology Section) Assen, Royal VanGorcum, 1963.

Chapter 20

Immunology and the Eye

Immunopathology

Amjad H. S. Rahi

BASIC IMMUNE MECHANISMS

The survival of the human race in the face of constant microbial invasion and frequent neoplastic revolution depends upon a combination of *non-specific protective mechanisms* common to most vertebrates and a highly evolved and elaborate *specific mechanism* consisting of antibodies and a heterogeneous population of thymus derived T-lymphocytes.

The Lymphoid System

The precursors of lymphocytes are derived from mesenchymal cells in the yolk sac, which during intrauterine development migrate to organs involved in haemopoiesis. In the postnatal life they are confined to the bone-marrow. The lymphoid system has a central and peripheral component; the central lymphoid organs act as a training ground and consist of the thymus and the bone-marrow. It is here that lymphocytes mature and become antigen sensitive. The mature lymphocytes then enter the circulation and disseminate to various structures, including the lymph nodes, spleen, Peyer's patches, tonsils, the conjunctival submucosae and the lacrimal glands to form the peripheral lymphoid tissues (*Fig.* 1). Human lymphocytes thus consist of a mixture of several classes, each of which has separate surface characteristics and separate functions.

Thymus Derived (T) Lymphocytes

A population of prelymphocytes from the bone-marrow migrates to the thymus where under the influence of thymic hormones and the microenvironment of epithelial cells, they proliferate and differentiate into mature T-lymphocytes. These cells then migrate to the paracortical areas of the lymph node, the periarteriolar sheath in the spleen and the interfollicular zone of the conjunctival and other submucous lymphoid aggregates. These areas are therefore called thymus dependent areas which gradually expand to take part in the cell mediated immune response to infective agents, contact allergens, malignant tumours and homologous grafts. In adult life the precursors of T-lymphocytes continue to migrate from bone-marrow to the thymus and mature T-cells continue to feed the peripheral lymphoid organs, but at a much reduced rate. Although T-lymphocytes are morphologically indistinguishable from bone-marrow derived B-lymphocytes, they possess certain unique cell membrane proteins and have characteristic physical, histochemical and biochemical qualities by which

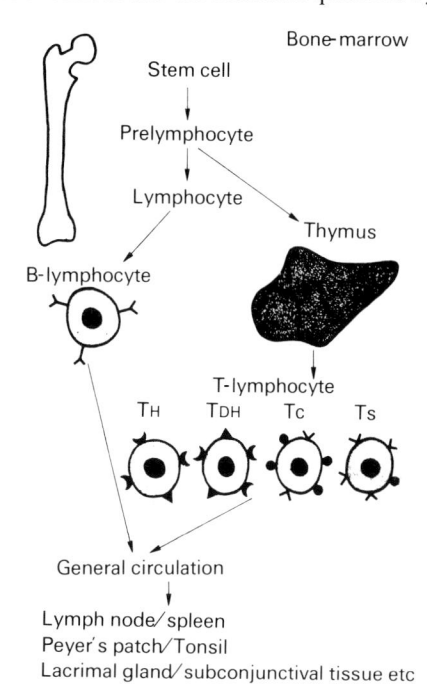

Fig. 1. The origin, development, distribution and function of B- and T-lymphocytes.

they can be recognized. The T-lymphocytes form spontaneous rosettes when mixed with sheep red blood cells (E-rosette) and react selectively with commercially available monoclonal antibodies. Human T-cells have been conveniently divided into four subclasses according to their function and surface characteristics:

1. Helper T-cells (T_H) react with antigens taken up by macrophages and secrete lymphocyte growth factors (interleukin).
2. Cells involved in delayed hypersensitivity (T_{DH}) produce inflammatory lymphokine.

3. Cytotoxic T-cells (Tc) destroy virus infected cells and grafted tissue.
4. Suppressor T-cells (Ts) modulate immune response.

It has been estimated that about 15 per cent of the peripheral blood lymphocytes are B-cells, 70 per cent are T-lymphocytes and the remaining 15 per cent, having the characteristics of neither B- nor T-lymphocytes, are known as null cells.

B-lymphocytes

These cells originate and mature in the bone-marrow. Pre-B-lymphocytes contain small amounts of cytoplasmic immunoglobulin but they are not expressed as receptors on the surface membrane until these cells become mature. First IgM bearing lymphocytes appear followed by IgD, IgG and others. Immunoglobulins are synthesized in the cytoplasm of B-lymphocytes and are then transported to the cell surface where they act as receptors for a variety of antigens. The lymphocytes that initially express a particular immunoglobulin on their surface may transform following antigenic stimulus into IgG, IgA, IgM, IgD or IgE producing plasma cells. HLA-DR, a histocompatibility antigen, is expressed on all B-lymphocytes, antigen binding macrophages and Langerhans cells, but only on a small number of activated T-lymphocytes. Monoclonal antibodies against surface immunoglobulin and HLA-DR are thus conveniently employed to differentiate between B- and T-lymphocytes in peripheral blood and tissue biopsies. This has greatly improved our understanding of chronic inflammatory diseases of unknown aetiology and the histogenesis of lymphocytic tumours of the lymph nodes, orbit and the central nervous system.

Null Cells, K-Cells and NK-Cells

Null lymphocytes are unclassified mononuclear cells. They do not form rosettes with sheep RBCs and do not have surface immunoglobulins. Null cells are increased and T-cells are reduced in active SLE and the ratio returns to normal following treatment. It is therefore thought that null cells are immature T-lymphocytes.

K-cells, a subclass of null cells, can kill IgG coated target cells through an extracellular non-phagocytic mechanism – known as antibody dependent cellular cytotoxicity (ADCC). K-cells play an important role in type II hypersensitivity and are of importance in corneal and other graft rejection and in circumstances where the target is too large for phagocytosis.

The natural killer (NK)-cells are also uncategorized lymphoid cells but they kill in the absence of immunoglobulin. The mechanism involved is similar, however, leading to changes in the target cell membrane permeability, osmotic swelling and membrane disruption. NK-cells appear to play an important role in anti-tumour surveillance. Patients with immunodeficiency states such as Chédiak–Higashi syndrome lack NK-cell activity and thus develop lymphoma-like lesions. NK-cell activity is also depressed in Wiskott–Aldrich syndrome, ataxia–telengiectasia and in patients on immunosuppressive therapy. In these types of patient there is a high risk of malignancy.

Antigens and Adjuvants

A substance that specifically stimulates the immune system is called an antigen (*anti*body *gen*erating); when it leads to a positive response in the form of antibody or sensitized T-cell, it is more appropriately designated as an immunogen. A tolerogen produces a negative response in the form of immunological tolerance or unresponsiveness. Most antigens are proteins, lipoproteins or glycoproteins. Lipids on their own are non-antigenic but high molecular weight polysaccharides can stimulate an immune response. Many non-immunogenic substances may combine, however, with tissue proteins or other compounds, to become antigenic. Such substances are called haptens. Drugs and various chemicals, such as preservatives in eye drops, may cause a hypersensitivity reaction acting as haptens.

Adjuvants are immune potentiators or immune accelerators. Freund's complete adjuvant contains paraffin oil, an emulsifier, and killed mycobacteria. Adjuvants increase antibody response to thymus dependent antigens and stimulate delayed hypersensitivity responses. They also produce a granuloma at the site of injection, thus acting as a depot for the slow release of the injected antigens. Macrophages are activated by adjuvants. Tissue antigens, when incorporated with adjuvant, produce autoimmunity in experimental animals.

Immunoglobulins

Antibodies, which are also called immunoglobulins, are divided into five major groups, known as IgG, IgA, IgM, IgD and IgE. They differ from one another in their physicochemical and biological properties (*Table* I). IgG consist of four polypeptide chains, joined together by disulphide bonds.

IgG is the smallest and most common immunoglobulin in the blood, the normal serum concentration being 1500 mg/100 ml. It perfuses through blood vessel walls and is present in tissue fluids. Its concentration in physiological tears is about 5 mg/100 ml and slightly less in the normal aqueous humour. IgG is responsible for humoral immunity against bacterial and virus infections. Four subclasses are known: ($IgG_1 \ldots IgG_4$). IgG_1 and IgG_3 bind to monocytes, macrophages and K-cells and predominantly activate complement. Polymorphs have receptors for all the four subclasses of IgG.

IgA occurs in the plasma as a single molecule (i.e. as a monomer), but is present, due to a joining (i.e. J) piece, in dimeric form (i.e. Ig[A]2) in tears and other seromucous secretions where it plays an impor-

Table I. Physical and biological properties of human immunoglobulins

	IgG	IgA	IgM	IgD	IgE
Molecular weight	150 000	160 000 (secretory 370 000)	900 000	186 000	200 000
Molecular composition					
Heavy chains	$\gamma_1, \gamma_2, \gamma_3, \gamma_4$	α_1, α_2	μ	δ	ε
Light chains	κ or λ	κ or λ	κ or λ	κ or λ	κ or λ
J chain	−	+	+	−	−
Secretory piece	−	+	−	−	−
Subtypes	$IgG_1, IgG_2, IgG_3, IgG_4$	IgA_1, IgA_2	?	?	?
Serum concentration (mg/100 ml)	800–1600	150–400	60–200	0·3–3	<100 i.u./ml
Concentration in tears (mg/100 ml)	5	20	Undetectable	Undetectable	<3 i.u./ml
Concentration in aqueous humour (mg/100 ml)	2–4	<1	Undetectable	Undetectable	Undetectable
Biological function:					
Binding to macrophages	+ (IgG_1, IgG_3)	? Aggregate IgA	−	−	? Antimetazoan IgE
Complement fixation	++ (IgG_1, IgG_2, IgG_3)	Alternative pathway	+++	?	? Alternative pathway
Placental transfer	+	−	−	−	−
Binding to mast cells	+	−	−	−	+++
Principal site of action	Tissue fluids	Seromucous membranes	Bloodstream	?	Seromucous membranes

tant role in maintaining local immunity. The IgA in secretions is therefore called secretory IgA (SIgA); it is stabilized against enzymatic degradation by the presence of another protein, called the secretory component. The dimeric IgA, in the case of tears, is produced by the plasma cells present in the lacrimal gland and to some extent by the conjunctival lymphoid tissue. The antibodies are then pinocytosed by the secretory duct epithelium of the lacrimal gland and the conjunctival epithelium, which synthesize the secretory component and attach it to the IgA before releasing it into the lacrimal fluid. SIgA may function either by coating the microorganism (or the exposed surfaces of the conjunctival and the corneal epithelium) and thus preventing their adherence to the surface of these cells. Aggregated IgA binds to neutrophils and can activate complement through the alternative pathway. IgA also acts in synergism with lysozyme in killing Gram-negative bacteria in the conjunctival sac and other mucosal surfaces. The mean concentration of IgA in blood is 300 mg/100 ml; its concentration in tears is variable, the mean being 20 mg/100 ml and most of which represents locally formed secretory IgA. In the normal aqueous humour, the concentration of IgA is very low, usually less than 1 mg/100 ml.

IgM is a very high molecular weight immunoglobulin because it occurs as a pentamer, in which five molecules of the antibody are joined together, and therefore it is largely restricted to intravascular compartments. It is absent in normal tear fluid and aqueous humour but becomes detectable in inflammation due to breakdown of the blood–ocular barrier. It does not cross placenta and it normally appears in the plasma 2–3 months after birth. The presence of IgM antibodies to toxoplasma and other organisms in infants' blood during the first few weeks after birth should therefore suggest intrauterine infection. In an immune response to a foreign antigen IgM production precedes IgG, and although of lower affinity, it appears to activate complement much more easily because of its pentameric nature.

IgE is responsible for acute allergic (i.e. anaphylactic) disorders such as drug and food allergies, hay fever, vernal disease and extrinsic asthma. High levels of IgE are also found in some cases of keratoconus, giant papillary conjunctivitis due to contact lens wear and in parasitic infections. Unlike other immunoglobulins IgE is heat labile. It remains firmly fixed to basophils and tissue mast cells in the skin, the uvea, the conjunctiva, the respiratory and gastrointestinal mucosa and the orbital tissues. Contact with allergens leads to mast cell degranulation with release of vasoactive amines and other inflammatory and chemotactic agents.

IgE, circulating freely in the blood or in tissue fluids, may interact with antigens, thus allowing the phagocytes to clear them from the system.

IgD is present in very small concentration in normal plasma and is raised in some cases of multiple myeloma, mycobacterial infections, Vogt–Koyanagi–Harada syndrome and chronic uveitis. IgD along with IgM act as receptors on B-lymphocytes and in experimental animals immunological tolerance can be induced only in those B-lymphocytes which lack IgD on their surface and are therefore immature.

Regulation of Immune Response

Antibodies are readily produced against soluble circulating antigens in contrast to cellular immunity which develops in response to particulate or fixed antigens such as homografts, solid tumours and contact allergens. The immune response has three distinct components: the *afferent arc*, whereby the antigen migrates to lymphoid tissues; the *central limb*, in which sensitized B- and T-lymphocytes differentiate, proliferate and secrete antibody and lymphokines; and the *efferent arc*, through which antigen specific T-lymphocytes or antibodies arrive at the site of antigen deposition and lead directly or indirectly to its elimination. An antigen is first taken up by the cells of the mononuclear phagocytic system, which after concentration and modification hand it over to helper T-cells. The helper T-cells secrete antigen specific helper factors which stimulate B-cells to form antibody producing plasma cells and encourage T-cells to expand the population of cytotoxic or lymphokine producing lymphocytes (*Fig.* 2). The various factors involved in the activation of lymphocytes and their growth have been named interleukins (e.g. interleukins I and II produced by macrophage and helper T-cell respectively). It has also been shown that for effective cellular interaction between macrophages and lymphocytes, or between lymphocytes and target cells, a double signal is essential; the helper T-cell thus reacts simultaneously with the foreign antigen (attached to the surface of a macrophage) and the HLA-DR, an immune associated transplantation antigen, present in the plasma membrane of the macrophage. Cytotoxic T-cells are similarly required to react with HLA-A and HLA-B transplantation antigens on the virus infected cells before mounting an effective cytolytic response. This HLA restriction of the immune response guards against harmful and irrelevant immune reactions and seems to be an important physiological function of transplantation antigens.

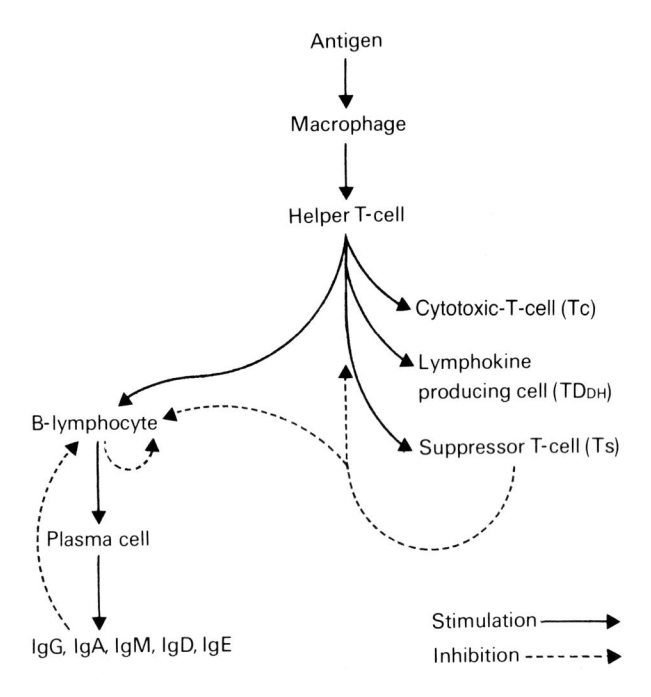

Fig. 2. Antigens are first taken up by macrophages and then handed over to helper T-cells which then induce B-lymphocytes and other subsets of T-cells to proliferate and differentiate. Some antigens do not require T-cell help, and can directly stimulate B-lymphocytes to produce plasma cells. During the immune response, however, suppressor T-cells are also generated which inhibit both B- and T-cell mediated responses.

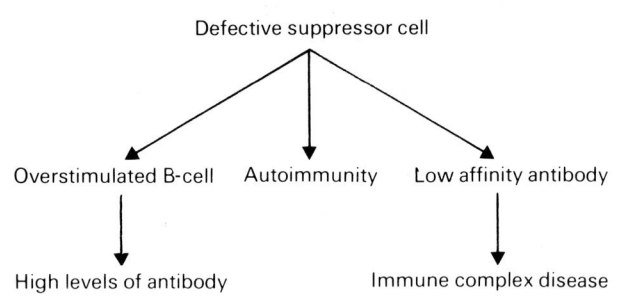

Fig. 3. The pathological effects as a result of aberrations in the regulatory mechanism.

Virus infections, which are believed to trigger autoimmune disorders, seem to encourage the target organs to commit suicide by expressing HLA-DR on their surface; the helper T-cells are thus tricked to interact and mount an immune response to the host tissue with resultant autodestruction.

After the first contact with an antigen, there is a latent period and then a primary (antibody) response. It is short lived and the production of IgM is followed by IgG and other immunoglobulins. Subsequent contact with the same antigen leads to an accelerated and prolonged response, consisting mainly of IgG. This enhanced secondary response is due to immunological memory, which resides mainly in the long lived helper T-cells. Antigen–antibody complexes produce a feedback inhibition of antibody production. In addition, suppressor T-cells produce regulatory factors which are inhibitory to both B- and T-lymphocytes. Apart from T cells, macrophages and tumours cells also produce immunosuppressive factors; similar factors are also produced during pregnancy, which protects the fetus against graft reaction and transplacental transfer of autoimmunity. Certain plasma cells produce a special class of autoantibody known as anti-idiotypic antibody; it is directed against antigen binding sites (i.e. receptors) on the surface of sensitized B- or T-lymphocytes and helps to switch off the immune response. It is therefore obvious that there exists a core regulatory mechanism which extends in a network fashion; not surprisingly, its failure leads to chronic inflammation and autoimmunity (*Fig.* 3).

PATHOLOGICAL IMMUNE MECHANISMS

There may be an overreaction (hyperergy), altered reaction (allergy) or no reaction (anergy) to a foreign antigen. The classic example of hyperergy is tuberculoid leprosy whereas anergy (of T-cells) is represented by lepromatous leprosy. A reaction to the host's own tissue components is autoallergy. An immune response beneficial to the host is known as immunity, whereas if it leads to tissue injury it is called allergy or hypersensitivity. The allergic reactions can be conveniently divided into two major categories: those mediated by B-lymphocytes and their products (i.e. antibodies), as distinct from those produced by T-lymphocytes and their products (i.e. lymphokines).

It is customary to divide antibody mediated allergic reactions into three types (type I ... type III); the T-cell mediated allergy is known as type IV reaction of Gell and Coombs.

IgE Mediated (Type I) Hypersensitivity

This reaction follows binding of an allergen to specific IgE on the surface of mast cells in the stroma as well as within the epithelial layer of the conjunctiva and other mucous membranes and on the basophils in blood. Changes occur in the mast cell and degranulation takes place. Apart from the release of preformed chemicals such as histamine, eosinophil and neutrophil chemotactic factors (ECF-A, NCFA) and kallikrein, the activated cell membrane of mast cells contributes to the production of platelet activation factor (PAF) and the slow-reacting substance of anaphylaxis (SRS-A). The latter is now called leukotriene C and D (LTC_4, D_4) (Fig. 4). Local examples of type I allergy include urticarial lid swelling, acute allergic conjunctivitis, hay fever conjunctivitis and vernal disease. A special class of IgG (e.g. IgG4) can occasionally cause mast cell degranulation. Non-IgE mediated mast cell degranulation can take place by physical trauma (rubbing, application of ice), anti-mast cell antibody, fragments of complement (C3a, C5a), known as anaphylatoxin, neutrophil basic protein, calcium ionophores and other chemical compounds. Thus features of acute allergy can be occasionally produced through non-IgE and even non-immune mechanisms.

Tissue Changes

The histological features of type I allergy are those of acute (but non-purulent) or subacute inflammation. There is dilatation and congestion of the microvasculature, which is followed by oedema (e.g. chemosis), exudation and infiltration by eosinophils. Mast cells are seen in various stages of degranulation. Eosinophils are involved in the synthesis of prostaglandins which inhibit further degranulation of mast cells (Fig. 5).

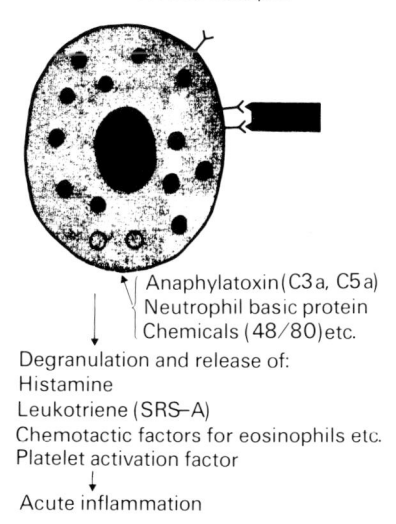

Fig. 4. Degranulation of mast cells following IgE and allergen interaction. Occasionally mast cells may also degranulate through non-IgE mediated immune and non-immune mechanisms.

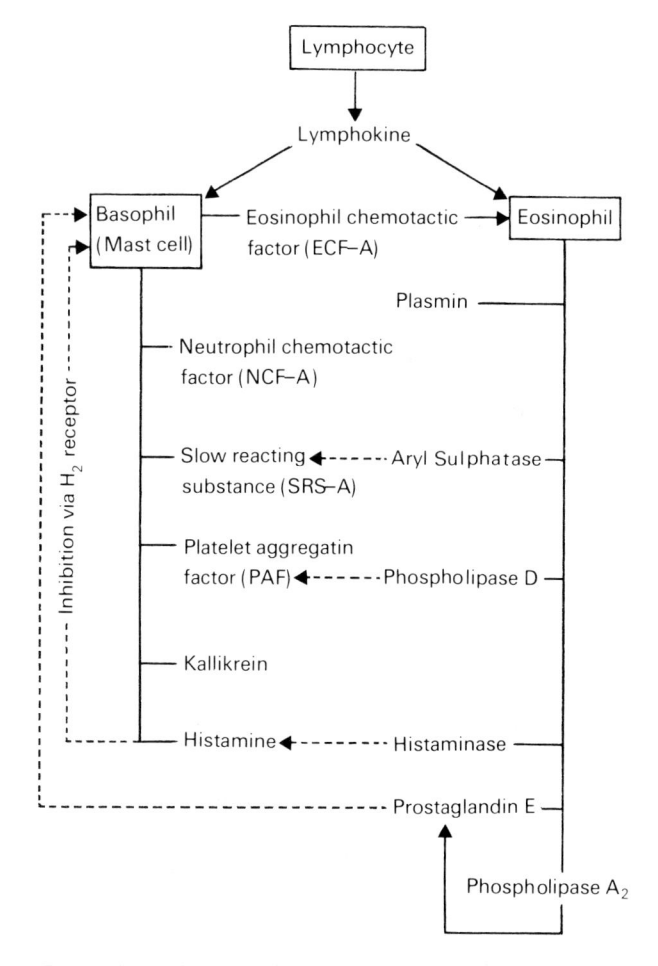

Fig. 5. The modulatory role of eosinophils in an allergic reaction. Apart from producing enzymes that destroy mast cell products, eosinophils seem to generate prostaglandin E, which is inhibitory to mast cells.

Atopy is a condition in which an individual makes IgE much more easily and (to a great extent) to irrelevant antigens. It seems to have a genetic basis and is related to histocompatibility antigens haplotypes A1:B8 and A3:B7. The suppressor T-cells appear to be abnormal in atopy and some patients have circulating antibodies to β-adrenergic receptors. Since adrenaline stabilizes mast cell and keeps the airways open, reduction of such receptors on smooth muscle and mast cells can lead to unstable bronchial physiology and mast cell degranulation.

Antibody, Complement and K-Cell Dependent (Type II) Reaction

The classic reaction depends upon IgG and IgM, which on combination with the target (e.g. bacteria, protozoa, parasite, tumour cells, graft tissue, vascular endothelium, corneal epithelium and the endothelium) activate a series of enzymes known collectively as the complement system. This leads to the creation of physiological and anatomical holes in the target cell membrane which allow osmotic swelling and lysis (*Fig. 6*).

Apart from the lytic effect of complement, there are at least four other mechanisms by which tissue damage is produced in a type II hypersensitivity. Neutrophils and macrophages possess receptors for IgG and C3, which facilitate phagocytosis of antibody coated (opsonization) and complement coated (immune adherence) target cells. IgG coated target cells can be further destroyed by K-cells and macrophages through a process of extracellular killing known as antibody dependent cellular cytotoxicity (ADCC). Monocytes and eosinophils also appear to react with IgG or IgE coated parasites, leading to their destruction. Examples of type II hypersensitivity include organ-specific autoimmune disorders, haemolytic anaemia, idiopathic thrombocytopenia, Goodpasture syndrome (in which the retinal pigment epithelium and Bruch's membrane may be involved), failed corneal and other grafts, Mooren's ulcer, pemphigus, pemphigoid and necrosis in choroidal melanoma and solid tumours. Apart from initiating cytolysis, antibodies can produce damage through other subtle mechanisms. It may thus combine with the basement membrane to produce physicochemical changes, thus altering its physiological task in vital organs such as the kidney. Sometimes the antibody may be directed against receptors for hormones such as TSH and insulin or neurotransmitters such as acetylcholine leading to stimulation, neutralization, modulation or destruction of receptors; this group includes hyperthyroidism, diabetes and myasthenia gravis.

Tissue Changes

There are no distinct histological features of type II hypersensitivity except necrosis of target cells and infiltration by neutrophils, monocytes, macrophages and K-cells. When antigen is adsorbed by vascular endothelium, it may be attacked by mononuclear cells to produce vasculitis. Damage to epithelial cells in mucous membrane and skin leads to bullous changes and ulceration.

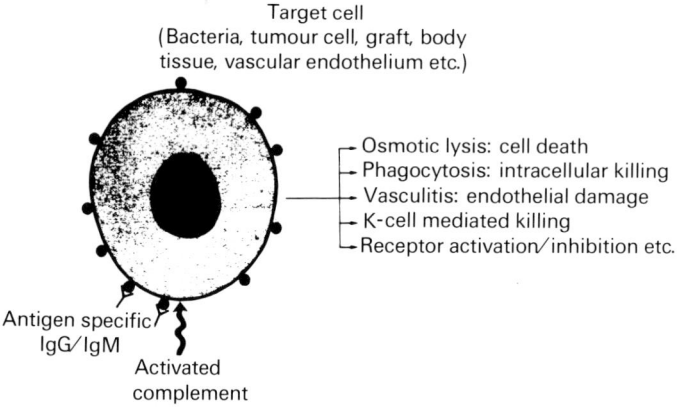

Fig. 6. Antibodies can induce target cell death by activating complement, thus leading to either osmotic lysis or intraocular and extracellular killing by leucocytes.

Immune Complex Mediated (Type III) Allergy

Antigen–antibody complexes are formed in the body all the time, particularly in response to antigens from food products and the bacterial flora in the gut. These complexes are removed regularly, however, by the cells of the mononuclear phagocytic system, particularly the Kupffer cells in the liver, mesangial cells in the kidney, littoral cells in the spleen and macrophages present in the bone-marrow and other tissues. Sometimes these aggregates, if small, cross the vascular endothelial barrier and, following deposition in and around blood vessels, activate complement as well as the clotting system leading to neutrophilic infiltration, thrombosis, haemorrhage, vasculitis and necrosis due to the release of lysosomal enzymes from inflammatory cells (*Fig.* 7). There is evidence that prostaglandins, leukotrienes, superoxide and singlet oxygen are also generated in immune complex initiated vasculitis, leading to further tissue injury. Examples of type III hypersensitivity include cutaneous vasculitis (erythema nodosum), Stevens–Johnson syndrome, serum sickness syndrome, connective tissue disorders, glomerulonephritis, endogenous uveitis, retinal vasculitis, some orbital pseudotumours, lens induced endophthalmitis and corneal immune ring in virus and mycotic infections and experimental Arthus reaction.

Fig. 7. Pathways of tissue damage in a type III allergic reaction.

Tissue Changes

The histological changes in type III hypersensitivity are wide and varied and depend to a large extent on the size of the immune complex; large antigen–antibody aggregates produced in antibody excess lead to granuloma formation. The affected tissue is infiltrated by monocytes, macrophages, epithelioid cells and multinucleate giant cells. Moderate size aggregates, formed when antigen and antibody are present in equivalent amounts, produce non-granulomatous inflammation in which the tissue is chiefly infiltrated by lymphocytes. In antigen excess, however, the Ag–Ab aggregates are very small (e.g. Arthus reaction) and often lead to acute vasculitis and infiltration of the tissue by neutrophils. There is also aggregation of platelets leading to thrombosis, necrosis and haemorrhage. Lens induced endophthalmitis may show all the three histological features mentioned above.

Cell Mediated (Type IV) Hypersensitivity

This reaction is also known as delayed hypersensitivity, delayed tissue allergy or cellular immunity. The reaction is mediated by cytotoxic and lymphokine producing T-lymphocytes. In the presence of active delayed hypersensitivity to bacterial or other products a granulomatous reaction may develop (e.g. tuberculoid leprosy). Apart from the direct cytotoxic effect of activated lymphoblasts, lymphokines can encourage tissue damage by producing a local inflammatory reaction. The macrophage inhibition (MIF) and activation (MAF) factors encourage intracellular killing of bacteria such as mycobacterium and extracellular killing of tumour cells and homografts (*Fig. 8*). T-cell mediated cytotoxicity in virus infection depends upon simultaneous recognition of HLA-A and B transplantation antigens and the virus coated antigen on the virus infected target cells. Granulomatous inflammation in tuberculosis, mycotic infection, sympathetic ophthalmitis and Vogt–Koyanagi–Harada syndrome are examples of type IV reaction. Contact hypersensitivity of the eyelid and the conjunctiva, viral keratitis and optic neuritis are further examples of type IV allergy, so are the ocular myopathies and the lacrimal gland involvement in Sjögren's syndrome.

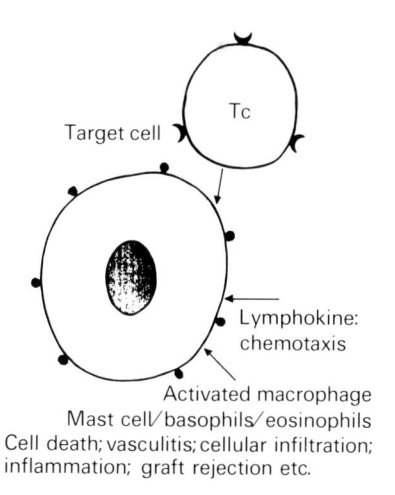

Fig. 8. The mechanism of tissue damage in a T-cell mediated allergic reaction.

Tissue changes

The earliest histological features of a classic type IV allergy consist of microvascular congestion and perivascular accumulation of lymphocytes and histiocytes. There is some oedema and swelling and there may be considerable deposition of fibrin, which is responsible for the induration seen in a positive Mantoux reaction. The morphological features may be modified by the injury inflicted by bacteria and their toxins. Granulomatous inflammation is a feature of delayed hypersensitivity and it involves epithelioid cells (derived from macrophages) and multinucleate giant cells which seem to develop following fusion of young and old macrophages or due to simultaneous phagocytosis of microorganism or particulate deposits. There are several varieties of type IV hypersensitivity; in contact allergy and cutaneous basophil hypersensitivity basophils are prominent at least in the early stages. Repeated injection of the same antigen (e.g. tuberculin) at the same site in a sensitized individual leads to tissue infiltration by eosinophils; this is known as retest phenomenon. Since vasculitis and eosinophilic infiltration are features of vernal disease, it is conceivable that vernal keratoconjunctivitis results from a combination of type I, III and IV allergic responses.

IMMUNOLOGICAL TOLERANCE AND AUTOIMMUNITY

Failure to produce antibody or cell mediated response following an antigenic challenge is called immunological tolerance or unresponsiveness. The factors that promote self tolerance include the maturity of the lymphoid tissue, the nature and dose of the antigen, the regulatory cells (e.g. suppressor T-cells) and various immunosuppressive factors in the serum. Autoimmunity results from type II, type III and type IV reactions in which structural and functional changes in the affected organs are produced by autoantibodies and autoreactive T-cells. It would seem that autoimmunity develops either from the emergence of autoreactive helper T-cells or inactivity of suppressor T-cells.

The ways in which tolerance to autoantigens may be bypassed include modification of autoantigens, emergence of cross-reacting antibodies as a result of virus and bacterial infection and release of sequestered autoantigen. It has been stated before that helper T-cells require a double signal for their activation; the antigen on the surface of a macrophage provides the first signal and the HLA-DR antigen normally present on macrophage (and B-lymphocytes) provides the second signal. HLA-DR is not normally present on parenchymal tissues such as thyrocytes and pancreatic islet cells, but following virus infection there seems to be a gene derepression which leads to the appearance of HLA-DR on these cells. The parenchymal cells may then behave as antigen presenting cells and lead to the activation of autoreactive helper T-cells which in turn may either lead to B-cell transformation (and autoantibody production) or activation of cytotoxic T-cells.

IMMUNOLOGICAL DISORDERS OF THE EYE

The eye is not spared the immunopathological processes which afflict other parts of the body. However, there are certain peculiarities of the ocular anatomy and physiology which tend to modify allergic inflammatory reactions. These aspects of ocular biology will be considered before embarking on a detailed discussion of specific immunological diseases of the eye.

Factors Modifying Ocular Immune Reactions

Avascularity of the Cornea and the Lens

In health, the cornea is completely avascular and meets its metabolic needs by diffusion from surrounding air, aqueous humour and the limbal circulation. The diffusion of macromolecules through the cornea is further impeded because of its unique structure, composed of collagen fibrils of uniform size laid in orderly fashion in a matrix of mucopolysaccharides. Thus obstruction to flow for molecules of about 0·5 nm diameter (such as sodium) is twofold and for albumin is eightfold. High molecular weight proteins such as IgM are completely obstructed and do not diffuse in the corneal stroma. This also means that antigenic substances present in the cornea, or those released following infection or trauma, will reach centres of lymphoid activity with great difficulty. Similarly, humoral antibodies and cytotoxic lymphocytes which may, ultimately, have been provoked, have restricted access to the source of antigen. The cornea, therefore, is a privileged site for successful graft. The disadvantage is that it takes some time for the cornea to recover from infection and associated inflammation. The avascular lens, surrounded by a thick capsulo-epithelial barrier, is completely isolated from the immune system. Liberation of lens protein following surgery or trauma may, therefore, lead to autoimmune intraocular inflammation.

Absence of Lymphatic Vessels

With the exception of the conjunctiva and the eyelids, the ocular tissues are devoid of lymphatic channels and therefore access of antigen to potentially reactive lymphoid tissue is further reduced. Avascularity and absence of lymphatics impede both the afferent and efferent arc of the immune response in the cornea. It is not surprising, therefore, that without the benefit of any tissue-matching about 90 per cent of corneal transplants are successful when the diseased cornea of the host is not vascularized. In contrast, corneal grafts will be rejected if vessels are brought to the site of the donor tissue, either by encouraging their growth by leaving a stitch, or transplanting the donor cornea into a vascularized bed. A further consequence of absence of lymphatic channels within the eye is that antigens gradually drain directly into the bloodstream, thus producing either immunological tolerance or a generalized and prolonged immune response.

Blood–Ocular Barriers

The concentration of serum proteins, including immunoglobulins, in the aqueous humour is not directly proportional to the composition of the circulating plasma. Thus, about 5–10 mg of IgG are present in 100 ml of aqueous humour, which also contains traces of IgA; IgM is not present in normal aqueous humour. Resistance to the transfer of immunoglobulins between blood and aqueous humour is provided by the size and shape of the molecule and the tight junctions between the vascular endothelium in the ciliary muscle and the non-pigmented epithelium of the ciliary body; in the iris it is provided by the blood vessels alone which are normally surrounded by a thick collar of collagen. Tissue grafted into the anterior chamber, therefore, survives for a prolonged period although it is ultimately rejected following invasion of blood capillaries from the iris.

Between the retina and its vascular supply there is a rather more effective barrier. The inner sensory retina is supplied by the branches of the central retinal artery and there the barrier is provided by a continuous endothelial lining which, because of tight junctions, is impervious to leucocytes and particulate antigen. The remainder of the retina is dependent on the choroidal circulation from which it is separated by Bruch's membrane and a layer of pigment epithelium, again bound by tight junctions.

Tissue Specific Antigens

The ocular tissues share most of the antigens with other organs in the body. Some of these antigens, however, show only limited cross-reactivity (e.g. retina contains antigens that cross-react with lymphocytes and brain tissue) and others are peculiar to the eye. Thus the lens, the retina and the cornea contain some cytoplasmic and membrane associated antigens which show strong organ specificity. The antigens of the lens are peculiar because of its anatomical relationship. Since the lens is segregated from the immune system during early embryogenesis, either there is no self tolerance to lens proteins or there is only a T-cell unresponsiveness. These antigens may, therefore, be treated as foreign should the lens capsule be damaged during operation or following perforating injury of the eye. This may result in autoimmune intraocular inflammation, most appropriately called phacoallergic endophthalmitis.

Depot Effect of Antigens Sequestered in the Vitreous

Intravitreal injection of foreign proteins in experimental animals delays its dispersion because the vitreous mucopolysaccharides not only act as a molecular sieve but also as an affinity column binding strongly to the foreign antigens. In clinical conditions, antigens entering the vitreous either as tissue breakdown products or derivatives of microbial agents may thus prolong any allergic inflammation.

Lymph Node-like Behaviour

The lymphocytes accumulating in the conjunctival tissue around the cornea (i.e. the limbal area) and in the uvea represent primary infection of these tissues but also indicate an immune response to antigenic stimuli originating in adjacent parts of the eye. This means that 'conjunctivitis' can be a reaction to corneal disease and the stimulus to uveitis can come from the vitreous, retina, lens and the sclera.

Mechanisms in Ocular Inflammation

Before considering specific allergic eye diseases, it will not be out of place to review the current concepts concerning initiation of ocular inflammation. The immune and non-immune mediators of inflammation which cause eye disease are essentially similar to those that are involved in the inflammatory disorders of other parts of the body. The eye is different, however, in having a highly labile vasomotor response. Evoked mainly as a protective phenomenon, it is mediated by a rich sensory and autonomic innervation and the biogenic lipids and amines elaborated by the uvea.

Experimental induction of inflammation in rats, guinea-pigs and rabbits has, in spite of its limitations, thrown much light on the nature of intraocular inflammation in man. As indicated in *Table* II, stimulation of the sensory nerves, irritation of ocular

Table II. Experimental induction of intraocular inflammation

Neurogenic Stimulus
   Stimulation of Vth Nerve

Physical agents
   Mechanical injury
   Laser/X-ray damage
   Contusion
   Paracentesis

Chemical irritants
   Nitrogen mustard
   Formaldehyde
   Acid/alkali burn

Endogenous inflammatory agents
   Histamine: bradykinin
   Prostaglandins: leukotrienes

Immunological insults
   Foreign proteins (e.g. BSA)
   Soluble retinal antigens

Bacterial products
   Endotoxin
   Freund's adjuvant

tissues by physical and chemical agents, intraocular injection of histamine, bradykinin, various biogenic lipids and foreign proteins and systemic injection of ocular antigens or bacterial products have been successfully used to produce features of intraocular inflammation. It is obvious, therefore, that the mechanism of ocular inflammation is rather complex and its evolution depends upon the intricate interactions of various neurogenic and immune and non-immune humoral and cellular factors.

Intraocular inflammation (*Fig.* 9) is like the three sides of a triangle and consists of (*a*) neurogenic components, (*b*) immune and non-immune humoral components and (*c*) immune and non-immune cellular components.

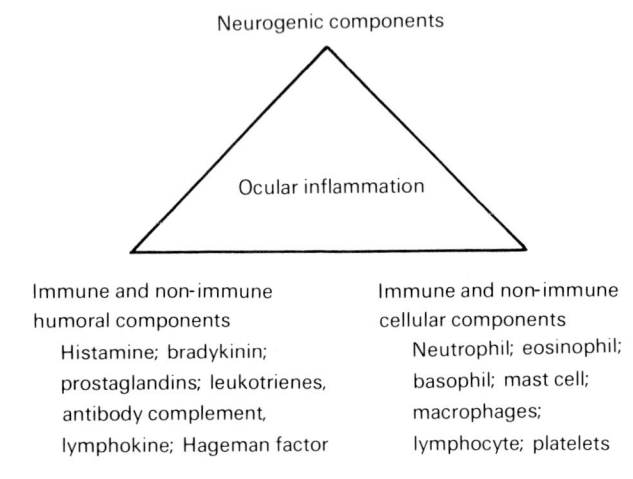

Fig. 9. The three chief components of ocular inflammation.

Responses and Mediators of Ocular Injury

The putative transmitters in the sensory nerve fibres are substance P(SP) and calcitonin-gene related protein (CGRP). Antidromic stimulation of the trigeminal nerve results in the release of SP-like immunoreactivity into the aqueous humour. Thus, stimulation of the sensory fibres of the Vth nerve, local application of nitrogen mustard or formaldehyde, paracentesis of the anterior chamber, or laser burn of the uvea lead immediately to vasodilatation, increased capillary permeability, breakdown of the ciliary epithelial barrier, pupillary constriction and transient rise in intraocular pressure (*Fig.* 10). There is negligible cellular infiltration, however, and the eye recovers from this injury response without developing inflammation.

The vascular and other related changes observed are partly neurogenic in origin; mechanical stimulation of the sensory terminals of the Vth cranial nerve generates antidromic response, and an axon reflex causes vasodilatation. Most of the features of sensory stimulation can be inhibited by removing the Gasserian ganglion in guinea-pigs or by blocking nerve conduction following retrobulbar injection of anaesthetics. A similar neurogenic mechanism accounts for nitrogen mustard and formaldehyde induced inflammation. On the other hand, when aqueous humour is withdrawn from the eye in appreciable quantities, a similar injury response is observed. This response appears to be predominantly dependent on prostaglandins because the intraocular changes and influx of protein into the anterior chamber can be prevented by pretreatment with prostaglandin synthetase inhibitors such as aspirin. Iris lesions, produced by ruby pulse laser, cause transient breakdown of the blood–aqueous barrier with pupillary constriction. The intraocular changes in this case, however, are dependent on both neurogenic influences and locally elaborated biogenic lipids because both local anaesthetic and antiprostaglandin drugs are required to prevent injury response.

Stimulation of the sensory terminals of the Vth nerve or intraocular injection of bradykinin, arachidonic acid or prostaglandins does not lead to cellular infiltration, and therefore inflammation does not develop in spite of increased vascular permeability and vasodilatation. The chemotactic stimulus appears to be provided at least in part by the lipoxygenase pathway of arachidonic acid metabolism resulting in the production of leukotrienes, which is discussed later.

It is known, for example, that the choroidal blood vessels in laboratory animals are innervated by VIP (vasoactive intestinal peptide) containing fibres derived from the VIIth cranial nerve; the stimulation of these fibres by noxious stimuli leads to vasodilatation as a response to injury. Similarly, the anterior uvea is supplied by sensory nerves which, on stimulation cause miosis, vascular changes, aqueous flare and raised intraocular pressure. As SP and VIP containing fibres have also been demonstrated in human ocular tissues, there is reason to believe that neural mechanisms are involved, probably in the early stages of endogenous intraocular inflammation in man.

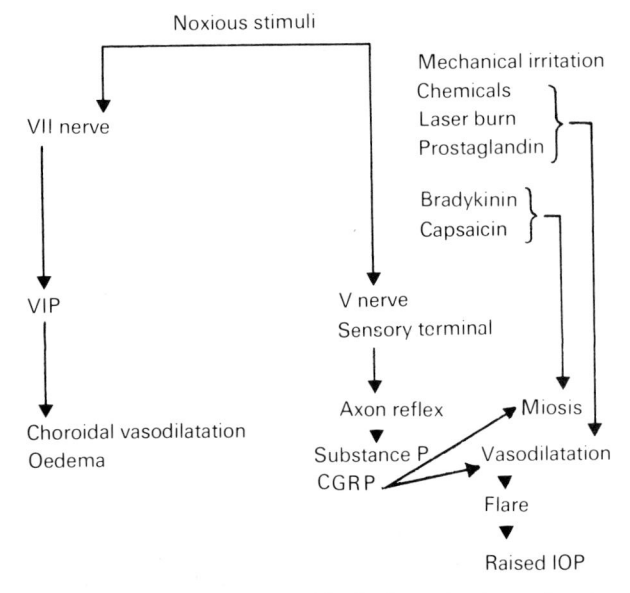

Fig. 10. The role of neuropeptides in the early stages of ocular inflammation. In addition to substance P (SP) and vasoactive interstinal peptide (VIP), calcitonin gene-related protein (CGRP) also seems to be involved in the vascular response of the eye.

Immunogenic and Non-immunogenic Inflammation

Immune and non-immune humoral factors play a significant role in intraocular inflammation and are particularly responsible for prolonged vascular changes, breakdown of the ciliary epithelial barrier and constriction of the pupil. Histamine, kinins and 5-HT at one time or another were thought to be the mediators of inflammation. With the help of the respective antagonist, their relative role in the different type and phase of inflammation has been resolved. It seems that histamine plays a central role in immediate hypersensitivity (type I) reaction but in other types of reaction its role is limited. During inflammation the clotting mechanisms, particularly Hageman factor, and the platelets and the plasmin system are activated, leading to the formation of kinins and release of histamine and serotonin from platelets and probably uveal mast cells (*Fig.* 11) All these substances affect vascular permeability in the eye.

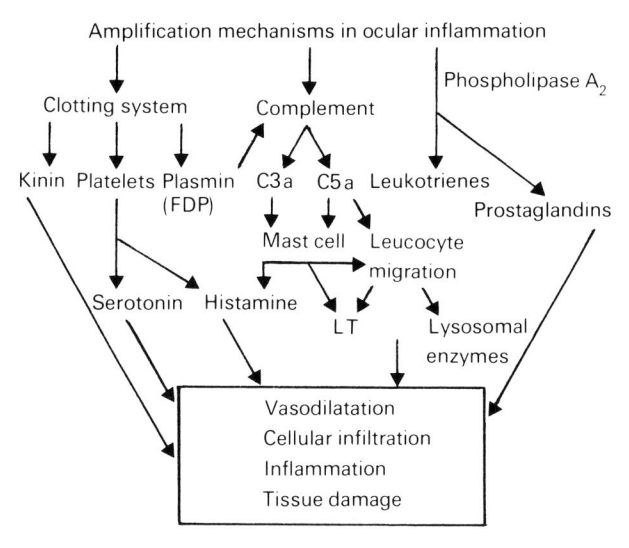

Fig. 11. The complementary roles played by the clotting system, ocular mast cells, complement fragments, lysosomal enzymes, prostaglandins and leukotrienes in the evolution of ocular inflammation.

Antibody-mediated allergic reactions involving IgG and IgM, particularly the type II and type III (i.e. immune-complex mediated) reactions, lead to the activation of the complement system which, apart from releasing cytolytic components, also gives rise to inflammatory fragments which degranulate mast cells, release histamine and are chemotactic for neutrophils. Complement can also be activated in the absence of antibodies, through what is known as the alternative pathway, in which plasmin and fibrinogen degradation products may play a significant role. Inflammatory cells, particularly neutrophils, when activated release various toxic products including oxygen and hydroxyl radicals and hydrogen peroxide which lead to further tissue damage (*Fig.* 12). Since the discovery of inhibitory actions of aspirin-like drugs on prostaglandin synthesis, prostaglandins and related compounds have also been shown to play a role in the inflammatory reactions.

Prostaglandins reproduce signs of inflammation along with other vasoactive substances, such as histamine and bradykinin. For instance, prostaglandins increase vascular permeability to plasma protein, disrupt the blood–aqueous barrier and potentiate oedema formation by histamine and bradykinin.

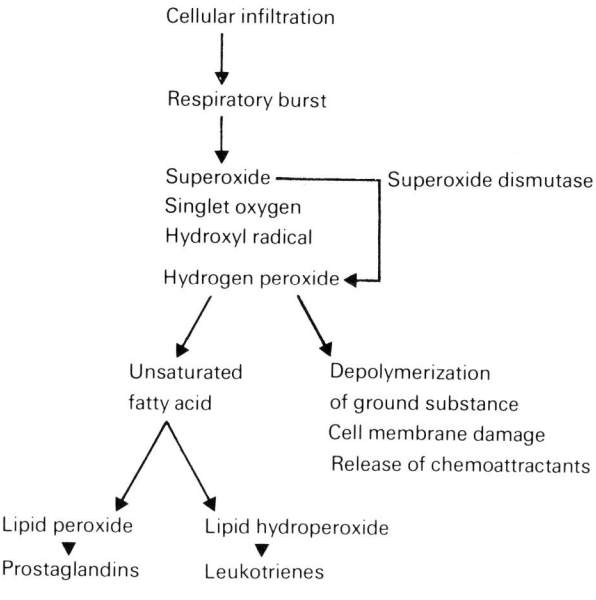

Fig. 12. The role of superoxide and hydroxyl radicals in tissue damage.

They also raise intraocular pressure in rabbits and cats.

In the mid-seventies another pathway of arachidonic acid metabolism was discovered. This pathway of the lipoxygenase system metabolizes arachidonic acid to a group of highly active mono- and dihydroxy products (*Fig.* 13). These products, called leukotrienes, formed by neutrophils, macrophages, lungs, platelets, skin, blood vessels and ocular tissues, have been identified in inflammatory exudates.

Besides mounting immunological responses that have a predominantly beneficial effect, the eye not infrequently shows allergy to a variety of stimuli.

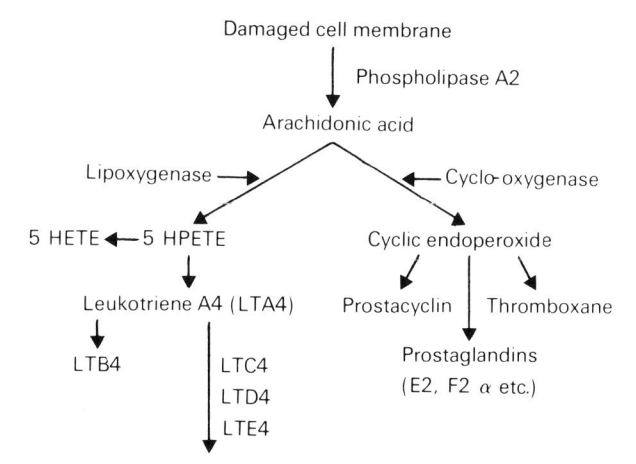

Fig. 13. The metabolic fate of arachidonic acid (AA) released from damaged or activated cell membranes. Steroids induce synthesis of macrocortin which inhibits phospholipase and prevents release of AA. Non-steroidal anti-inflammatory drugs inhibit the cyclo-oxygenase pathway and therefore do not effectively control inflammation. Reliable lipoxygenase inhibitors are currently a focus of attention.

Each of the commonly recognized forms of hypersensitivity has its ocular counterpart and some of the immunological disorders affecting the eye are summarized in *Tables* III and IV. Although these are often attributable to purely immunological mechanisms, these may be modified by local factors such as retention of the antigen within glycosaminoglycan-rich avascular structures and the apparent ease with which antigen–antibody aggregates are deposited in the uvea.

Table III. Allergic and autoimmune disorders of the eye

1. IgE mediated (Type I) hypersensitivity
   Urticarial lid swelling
   Acute allergic conjunctivitis
   Hay fever conjunctivitis
   Chronic allergic conjunctivitis
   Chronic microbial allergic blepharoconjunctivitis
   Vernal keratoconjunctivitis
   Drug induced blepharoconjunctivitis
   Allergic retinitis in animals

2. Ig and complement dependent (Type II) reaction
   Peripheral corneal (including Mooren's) ulcer
   Ocular pemphigus and pemphigoid
   Corneal graft rejection
   Experimental immune retinitis
   Receptor autoimmunity (endocrine exophthalmos, myasthenia gravis)

3. Immune complex induced (Type III) hypersensitivity
   Vernal disease
   Allergic granuloma of conjunctiva
   Corneal immune ring in viral and mycotic keratitis
   Stevens–Johnson syndrome
   Endogenous uveitis
   Lens induced endophthalmitis
   Retinal vasculitis
   Endocrine exophthalmos

4. T-lymphocyte determined (Type IV) allergy
   Phlyctenular conjunctivitis
   Vernal disease
   Herpetic keratitis
   Corneal graft rejection
   Contact lens associated papillary conjunctivitis
   Eczematous keratoconjunctivitis
   Drug induced blepharo conjunctivitis
   Sympathetic ophthalmitis
   Vogt–Koyanagi–Harada syndrome
   Optic neuritis
   Various bacterial, fungal, protozoal and helminthic infections of the eye
   Sjögren's syndrome
   Endocrine exophthalmos

Immunopathology of External Eye Disease

The protection against infections of the conjunctiva and the lid is provided partly by non-specific factors which act independently of the immune system. Fatty acids in tears and sebaceous secretions of the lid are inhibitory to many microorganisms. The mucous secretion from goblet cells protects the conjunctival epithelium against virus penetration. Lysozyme, which is abundantly present in tears, is bacteriolytic in conjunction with complement. During acute inflammation there is egress of phagocytic cells and transudation of bactericidal and antiviral agents, such as C-reactive protein, properdin and interferon.

The aggregates of lymphocytes in the conjunctiva provide specific acquired immunity by elaborating immunoglobulins (IgG, IgA and IgM). The tears also contain immunoglobulins, the predominant being secretory immunoglobulin A (sIgA), which is a special class of immunoglobulin providing a first line of defence against virus infections of mucous surfaces.

Thus, non-specific immunity of ocular tissues depends upon blinking reflex, physical protection afforded by intact conjunctival and corneal epithelium, tears (containing fatty acids from meibomian secretion), lactoferrin, lysozyme, transferrin, interferons, classical and alternative components of the complement systems, phagocytes and natural killer (NK) cells. The specific immunity depends, however, on secretory IgA and IgG in tears and tissues and B- and T-lymphocytes in the subepithelial stroma. Binding of microorganisms to mucosal surfaces depends upon the carbohydrate residues on the surface epithelium which act as receptors. The resistance of the conjunctiva to common cold virus, and of the respiratory epithelium to gonococci, depends partly on these surface glycoproteins.

Microbial Allergic Conjunctivitis (and Blepharitis)

The inflammation of the conjunctiva and the lid is caused by a wide range of infective organisms. The tissue damage in these conditions is due largely to the direct toxic effect of the infection. The inflammatory reaction, however, is accentuated by the host immune response. Antibodies and sensitized T-lymphocytes can damage the host tissue, especially in infections where the organisms are mainly intracellular. Antigen–antibody complexes formed in capillaries and tissue spaces lead to further damage. In such situations the host immune response against the infective organism becomes a hypersensitivity reaction.

Allergic microbial conjunctivitis and blepharitis, however, may develop in the absence of obvious local infection. They are characterized by a sterile conjunctiva or lid, chronic hyperaemia, a little secretion and accentuated subjective symptoms. Chronic microbial allergic blepharo-conjunctivitis is a well-recognized clinical entity. It is associated with mild staphylococcal infection and shows scaling and cuffing of lash bases. A mild mixed papillary and follicular reaction occurs in the conjunctiva and there is often accompanying marginal corneal ulceration. The patients may have high levels of circulating IgE and often

Table IV. Autoimmunity and the eye

	Antigen	Mechanism of tissue damage
1. Isolated eye disturbance		
Mooren's ulcer	Corneal epithelium	Ig and complement dependent cytotoxicity
Lens induced uveitis	Lens crystallins	Immune complex disease
Sympathetic ophthalmitis	Melanocyte	
Vogt–Koyanagi–Harada syndrome	Retinal pigment epithelium	Antibody and T-lymphocyte mediated reactions
	Photoreceptors	
Choroidoretinitis (some cases)	Photoreceptors	Antibody, immune complex and T-lymphocyte dependent reactions
Retinal vasculitis	Photoreceptors	
Optic neuritis	Basic myelin protein	Mainly T-lymphocyte mediated reaction
2. Multisystem disturbance		
Connective tissue diseases with retinal vasculitis, uveitis and scleritis	Cell-nuclei, IgG Tissue breakdown products, e.g. smooth muscle proteins	Mainly immune complex mediated inflammation
Sjögren's syndrome (keratoconjunctivitis sicca)	Secretory duct epithelium Lacrimal glandular tissue	Antibody and T-lymphocyte mediated reaction
Multiple sclerosis with optic neuritis	Basic myelin protein	Antibody and T-lymphocyte mediated reaction
Endocrine exophthalmos	Thyroglobulin Microsome and cell membrane of thyroid cells Extraocular muscle antigen	Antibody, immune complex and T-lymphocyte mediated reaction
Myasthenia gravis	Acetylcholine receptors	Antibody and T-cell mediated reaction

show an immediate type of cutaneous hypersensitivity to staphylococcal extracts.

Allergic conjunctivitis due to hypersensitivity in chronic mycotic and bacterial infections (e.g. tuberculosis), is produced by a cell mediated immune reaction. The inflammation is of gradual onset, much less stormy and runs a non-paroxysmal chronic course. The main histological changes consist of papillary hyperplasia of the epithelium with scattered follicular aggregates of lymphocytes.

Phlyctenulosis is a nodular affection occurring mainly in children and is believed to represent a circumscribed allergic response by the conjunctiva and the cornea to an allergen. In the past a great many sufferers showed a delayed hypersensitivity response to tuberculoprotein. That a cell-mediated allergy to tuberculin may cause phlyctenulosis is supported by the fact that such lesions have been produced in experimental animals and human volunteers by systemic immunization and local instillation of the antigenic protein. A similar lesion, however, can also be produced by local instillation of other antigens such as staphylococcal extracts, horse serum and some protein binding chemicals. Clinically similar lesions have also been observed, though rarely, in protozoal, mycotic and chlamydial infections.

Acute Allergic Conjunctivitis (Type I Hypersensitivity)

Hay Fever Conjunctivitis

This is an IgE-mediated reaction in the eye which develops as part of a generalized atopy. It is characterized by seasonal incidence, moderate redness and itching of the palpebral conjunctiva. The conjunctiva reacts with slight papillary hyperplasia, vasodilatation and infiltration by eosinophils, lymphocytes and other inflammatory cells. The condition usually resolves but may become chronic if there is a constant exposure to allergens.

It is caused by a large number of allergens and the susceptibility to this condition is often hereditary. Most of the allergens are airborne and consist of grass and tree pollens which give rise to other features of hay fever. In western countries hay fever conjunctivitis affects some 3–5 per cent of the population to some degree.

Acute Allergic Conjunctivitis

An acute allergic conjunctivitis not associated with hay fever may develop due to exposure to large doses of allergens including drugs, cosmetics, house dust, animal danders, wool, feathers and certain foods. It is characterized by sudden 'explosive' oedema and hyperaemia of the conjunctiva and of the lids with a very itchy eye. The conjunctiva has a glassy appearance and bulges over the corneal margin. There is rapid complete recovery within 48 h.

Vernal Keratoconjunctivitis

This represents a rather localized manifestation of a predominantly IgE mediated reaction in the conjunctiva. The allergen is still unidentified, although on skin testing the patients show allergy to a variety of extrinsic allergens and in some cases ragweed specific IgE is demonstrable in the serum.

Using sensitive techniques such as radio-allergosorbent test (RAST), increased levels of allergen specific IgE are found in tears and blood of some of the patients, particularly against grass pollens, *Dermatophagoides pteronyssinus* and animal danders. The presence of vasculitis and evidence of delayed hypersensitivity to some common allergens suggest that type III and type IV allergic reactions may also play some role in the pathogenesis of vernal disease. Corneal plaque is an uncommon but serious manifestation of vernal keratopathy; histologically it appears as a stratified amorphous mass consisting of fibrin, cellular debris, IgA, IgG, fibronectin and complement.

Type II Hypersensitivity Reactions

Keratoconjunctivitis may develop in association with diseases of the skin and the mucous membrane.

Pemphigus Vulgaris

Pemphigus vulgaris occurs usually in older people. Bullae appear on apparently normal skin and mucous membranes and heal without scarring. Conjunctival lesions are uncommon; they are intraepithelial, and an antibody to intercellular 'cement' substance is demonstrable in a large percentage of cases. It is believed that these antibodies bind to the junctional zones and produce acantholysis and bullous separation of the epithelium. Antibodies to intercellular cement (ICC) substance have also been demonstrated in dry eye syndrome produced by beta-blockers such as Practolol. Pemphigus vulgaris in the Jewish population is linked to histocompatibility antigens and up to 90 per cent of the patients are positive for HLA-DRW4.

Benign Mucous Membrane Pemphigoid

This disease, on the other hand, is often associated with chronic cicatrizing conjunctivitis. Vesicles, which are subepithelial, are believed to result from the interaction of the basement membrane with specific autoantibodies. Such antibodies have been demonstrated in systemic and ocular pemphigoid, both in tissue sections and in the circulating blood. Apart from this, the subconjunctival stroma always shows the presence of lymphocytes and plasma cells, suggesting a local immune response.

Mooren's Ulcer

Immunopathological studies have shown that immunoglobulin and complement are demonstrable in the involved cornea and the patient's serum contains raised levels of IgA and circulating antibodies to corneal epithelium. In some cases immune complex and cellular immunity to corneal antigen are also demonstrable, suggesting that Mooren's ulcer represents a combination of type II, type III and type IV allergic reactions. In severe cases patients show a reduction in suppressor T-cells in peripheral blood with a high helper/suppressor ratio, suggesting an abnormal homeostasis in this disease.

Type III Allergy (Immune Complex Mediated Conjunctivitis)

Erythema Multiforme (Stevens–Johnson Syndrome)

The lesion consists basically of an immune vasculitis with infiltration by neutrophils, eosinophils and lymphocytes. Some drugs which become attached to a host protein induce antibody responses that give rise to both an IgE mediated reaction as well as an immune complex vasculitis.

Erythema Nodosum

This disease is often associated with immunological diseases, such as sarcoidosis, ulcerative colitis and drug allergy. The lesions consist of subepithelial infiltrations by polymorphs and lymphocytes. It is often possible to demonstrate the presence of immunoglobulins and complement in cutaneous lesions, suggesting that the disease is produced by deposition of circulating immune complexes. It is difficult, however, to rule out the role of cell mediated allergy in these cases. Painful cutaneous nodules, which appear suddenly with fever and multiple joint pains, are reminiscent of experimentally induced immune complex diseases. Ocular lesions include the development of nodules in the conjunctiva, the cornea and the episclera. Sclerokeratitis and anterior uveitis may also develop. The nodules are composed of areas of fibrinoid necrosis and lymphocytic and histiocytic infiltration. The similarity of these nodules to the Aschoff bodies of rheumatic fever is striking.

Serum Sickness

This is a classic example of immune complex disease. Although anterior uveitis is more common in this condition, conjunctivitis is sometimes observed in patients showing allergy to heterologous serum protein.

Type IV Allergy

Contact dermatoconjunctivitis is a well-recognized entity. Locally applied drugs and chemicals can act as active sensitizers. They bind to protein carriers and can convert the body's own proteins into antigens. Although the specificity of the immunological reaction is directed against these small haptens, the local tissues seem to suffer from immunological insults. The allergic response in these situations is mediated by T-lymphocytes and their products (i.e. lymphokines). It is often possible to demonstrate evidence of delayed hypersensitivity by using patch test or *in vitro* techniques such as the lymphocyte transformation test. The early histological changes are characterized by the presence of basophils, mast cells and lymphocytes, but in chronic cases eosinophils appear to dominate the scene. Foreign body associated giant papillary conjunctivitis is found in users of contact lenses. The conjunctival epithelium and the stroma may be infiltrated by mast cells, eosinophils and lymphocytes. IgE levels are raised in tears and in serum of some of the patients, particularly those with a history of atopy, and appear to respond well to sodium cromoglycate.

Immunodeficiency States

The eyelid and the conjunctiva are also involved in certain immunodeficiency states such as Wiskott–Aldrich syndrome and ataxia telangiectasia in which, apart from IgA deficiency, there is also a marked reduction in NK-cell population. Mucocutaneous candidiasis, which is associated with defective MIF production by T-cells, tends to involve the outer eye. Chédiak–Higashi syndrome, with defective phagocyte motility and abnormal melanosomes, is associated with defects in the microtubular system. Its ocular complications are well known.

Immunopathology of the Retina and Optic Nerve

The vertebrate nervous system is derived from a neural tube which arises from infolding of embryonic ectodermal sheets of cells. Adjacent to the neural tube is the neural crest, which gives rise to elements of the autonomic nervous system, Schwann cells and melanocytes. It seems certain that neurones arising from the neural tube are antigenically distinct from neurones arising from the neural crest. Furthermore, antibodies that react with neurones derived from neural tubes do not react with other cell types of the same origin, e.g. astrocyte, oligodendrocytes. Similarly, neurones derived from the neural crest are antigenically distinct from other cells of the same origin, such as melanocytes and Schwann cells. It is conceivable therefore that both the sensory retina and the retinal pigment epithelium, which are derived from neural tube, contain antigens which are not only distinct from neural crest derived cells, but also contain cells such as the photoreceptors, bipolar cells and ganglion cells which are antigenically distinct from Muller cells and astrocytes.

S-100 protein consists of a family of highly acidic proteins that are found mainly in the cytoplasm of glial cells of the retina (as well as the brain), although some may be associated with neuronal membranes and therefore sections of the retina when treated with fluorescein labelled anti-S-100 protein show diffuse fluorescence. Some S-100 proteins are found in Schwann cells, melanocytes and tumours of the melanogenic system and thus act as a marker for the neural crest origin. There is some evidence that S-100 protein is associated with learning and memory, but its precise role in the retina is uncertain.

Myelin basic protein (MBP) is derived from oligodendrocytes, and as far as the eye is concerned it is usually found in the optic nerve. This protein acts as antigen in optic neuritis and other demyelinating diseases and in physiological states acts as a biological glue for holding together lipids and proteins of myelin. Although it has been known for some time that the retina contains both soluble and insoluble (particulate) antigens, and that the former were uveitogenic, the present author, using agar precipitation and passive haemagglutination techniques showed, for the first time, that most of the soluble retinal antigens were located in the photoreceptor outer segments. One of the soluble antigens of rod outer segment (the so-called S-antigen) has been purified; it has a molecular weight of 55 000, avidly produces intraocular inflammation and has similarities with rhodopsin kinase. The photoreceptors contain rhodopsin, which appears to be antigenic and so is the mucopolysaccharide collar which surrounds the visual cells. Reich D'Almeida and Rahi in 1974 first demonstrated the antigenic potential of retinal pigment epithelium and provided evidence of its antigenic specificity. Later it was demonstrated that it also contains cross-reacting cytoskeletal antigens, such as actin.

The advent of monoclonal antibodies has greatly simplified the study of retinal antigens. Barnstable in a review published in 1985 has documented evidence that, using such antibodies, distinct cell specific antigens could be identified in the photoreceptors, the ganglion cells and the astrocytes of the retina.

Retinal Autoimmunity and Inflammatory Eye Disease

Autoimmune phenomena are widespread in human disease. The spectrum of self antigens against which reactive antibodies or sensitized T-cells have been demonstrated is ever increasing. Autoimmunity to retinal antigens in inflammatory eye disease is currently under investigation. Whatever may be the cause of retinal autoimmunity, antiretinal antibodies and sensitized T-cells have been detected in a variety of ocular and non-ocular immune disorders, such as Behçet's disease, SLE and sarcoidosis.

Cell Mediated Immunity to Photoreceptor Antigens

Cell mediated immunity to retinal soluble antigens is well documented in sympathetic ophthalmitis, post-traumatic non-granulomatous uveitis and Vogt–Koyanagi–Harada syndrome. In a recent study a positive lymphoproliferative response to retinal antigens was obtained in 7 of the 31 patients tested. These included patients with pars planitis, ocular sarcoid, choroidoretinitis of unknown origin, ocular toxoplasmosis and chronic uveitis with macular disease. In another study some patients with Behçet's disease, chronic anterior uveitis (with vitriitis and macular cyst), chronic uveitis with acute retinal necrosis and chronic vitriitis with macular oedema also showed evidence of hypersensitivity to retinal S-antigen. Cell mediated immune response to rod outer segment and soluble retinal antigens has been observed, however, in non-inflammatory retinal disease, such as retinitis pigmentosa. Bird shot retinopathy is characterized by choroidoretinitis with cream-coloured lesions throughout the fundus. There is associated vitriitis, retinal vascular leakage and cystoid macular oedema. Although its aetiology is unknown, the disease is strongly associated with HLA-A29 and most of the patients show cell mediated immunity to retinal soluble antigens. A cell mediated immune response has also been noted in patients with retinal detachment.

Photoreceptor Autoantibody and Eye Disease

Antibody to soluble retinal antigens has been demonstrated by enzyme-linked immunosorbent assay (ELISA) in serum samples from patients with several types of uveitis, including toxoplasmosis and sarcoidosis. Raised levels are also found in patients with diabetic retinopathy, particularly after argon laser treatment due to focal disruption of photoreceptors and breakdown of the blood–retinal barrier at the level of retinal pigment epithelium. The cause of retinal autoimmunity in diabetic retinopathy is unclear, but it has been suggested that it is due to disturbed carbohydrate metabolism whereby polyol accumulates in the photoreceptors which leads to its disruption. Retinal antigens thus liberated are probably absorbed directly into the choriocapillaris owing to defective retinal pigment epithelium. Another possibility is that photoreceptor disruption and release of sensitizing antigens may be secondary to osmotic shock. Since some of the diabetic patients develop uveitis following laser therapy it is possible that the intraocular inflammation in these situations has an autoimmune basis.

Optic Neuritis

The optic nerve consists of myelinated nerve fibres. Both human and animal myelin contain strong antigenic basic protein which has been used to produce optic neuritis in experimental animals. The optic nerve lesion may either herald, accompany or follow the brain and spinal cord lesions of multiple sclerosis.

Optic neuritis may sometimes follow exanthemas in childhood and is often a feature of post-vaccinial encephalomyelitis and is regarded as a form of neuro-allergy. Other causes of optic neuritis include Guillain–Barré syndrome, infectious mononucleosis and subacute sclerosing panencephalitis. Multiple sclerosis is associated with lymphocytic and plasma cell infiltration; there is evidence of demyelination and deposition of extracellular and intracellular immunoglobulins. About 90 per cent of the patients show the presence of an oligoclonal band in the CSF, which contains increased numbers of lymphocytes. Oligoclonal IgG in CSF is also present in 30 per cent of patients with optic neuritis. The population of T-lymphocytes is markedly reduced in acute optic neuritis and suppressor cells appear to be defective in multiple sclerosis.

There is a strong association with HLA-DW2 and DR3 in the Caucasian population. In patients of Middle Eastern origin HLA-DR4 is more frequent. About 10 per cent of patients have a family history, and although multiple sclerosis has been described in non-identical twins, the presence of HLA-DW2 does not appear to be essential for the development of the disease. The incidence of multiple sclerosis following optic neuritis is variable (13–73 per cent), but it has been estimated that about 70 per cent of patients who are positive for HLA-DR2 will ultimately develop a generalized disease as compared with only 40 per cent of patients with optic neuritis who do not have this transplantation antigen. It is of interest that patients who develop optic neuritis in winter are more prone to develop this systemic disease.

The retina is involved in 25 per cent of cases and it is associated with sheathing of retinal vessels, capillary leakage and cellular exudates in the vitreous. Women account for three-quarters of patients with optic neuritis. The age of onset is variable, the median age being 29 years. About 57 per cent of cases are unilateral and 19 per cent bilateral; 24 per cent are recurrent. The attack rate tends to be highest from April to July and lowest from August to November. Patients with bilateral optic neuritis or with recurrent disease have a greater risk of developing multiple sclerosis. Many patients have elevated titres of measle antibody in their blood and increased levels of antibody to rubella, parainfluenza and Epstein–Barr virus are found in the CSF from patients with optic neuritis.

An experimental allergic optic neuritis can be produced in guinea-pigs injected with spinal cord emulsion in Freund's complete adjuvant. The animal develops retrobulbar neuritis, with infiltration of the optic nerve, optic chiasma and the brain by mononuclear cells. Focal demyelination of the optic nerve and neuroretinitis may also be seen.

Immunology of Uveitis

The uvea has certain special features which make it a frequent target of immunological reactions. It contains blood vessels, fibroblasts, melanocytes and, in the anterior region, contractile smooth muscle fibres. The connective tissue consists of collagen, elastic and pre-elastic oxytalan fibres and, therefore, the uvea resembles in many ways the joint tissue with which it participates in many disease processes. The uvea can support each of the four classic types of immunological reactions. Uveal inflammation may result directly from bacterial, viral, mycotic, fungal and protozoal infection or may represent a hypersensitivity reaction to microorganismal products. The uveal vessels may act in a manner similar to glomeruli and trap hetero- and auto-immune complexes, leading to an acute or chronic disease which histologically may appear granulomatous or non-granulomatous. Infection, injury and trauma may release and modify tissue specific ocular antigens leading to an autoallergic reaction. It is possible, however, that in certain individuals uveitis represents an immunodeficiency state, particularly involving the suppressor cells. The T-lymphocytes appear numerically or functionally deficient in acute anterior uveitis, heterochromic cyclitis and in uveitis due to leprosy and sarcoidosis.

Acute Anterior Uveitis

Ankylosing spondylitis is a chronic progressive inflammatory arthritis primarily involving the sacroiliac joints and the spine. Ankylosing spondylitis is more common in first degree relatives of patients who have a strikingly high incidence of HLA-B27. About 50 per cent of patients attending the eye clinic for acute anterior uveitis are HLA-B27 positive, and a large proportion of them would have, or would show symptoms suggesting, ankylosing spondylitis. The T-lymphocyte population is normal or reduced in patients with acute anterior uveitis and some patients have functionally deficient suppressor cells.

Chronic Uveitis

This represents a much more heterogeneous group, consisting of at least three subgroups. *Heteroimmune uveitis* results either from chronic infection or is due to allergy to foreign proteins and drugs; the latter may present either as an IgE mediated reaction or an immune complex disease. *Autoimmune uveitis* may follow perforating injury or a possible virus infection and includes sympathetic ophthalmitis and Vogt–Koyanagi–Harada syndrome. *Endogenous uveitis* of unknown aetiology is an undefined group of idiopathic uveitic conditions which possibly represents auto- or heteroimmune complex vasculitis.

Chronic iridocyclitis often occurs in seronegative juvenile rheumatoid arthritis (JRA). About 80 per cent of the patients show the presence of antinuclear antibody in the blood and aqueous humour. The immunoglobulins G, A and M are present in increased amounts in the aqueous humour and the iris is diffusely infiltrated by lymphocytes and plasma cells. Occasionally, antinuclear antibodies are only demonstrable in the intraocular fluids, suggesting their local production and their involvement in intraocular immune complex vasculitis. Antinuclear antibody is of IgG class and shows homogeneous fluorescence implicating DNA protein. Antibodies to double stranded RNA are also present in some patients. Since antinuclear antibodies usually precede uveitis, it is a useful test for identifying patients with JRA who are at risk of developing chronic iridocyclitis. Smooth muscle antibodies are present in a proportion of patients who also show high levels of antibodies to Coxsackie B3 and A9 virus. Isolation of rubella and adenovirus from affected tissues has also been reported.

Behçet's disease is a chronic recurrent inflammatory condition of worldwide distribution. It consists of a triad of recurrent uveitis, and oral and genital ulcers. Autoantibodies to oral mucosa are present in the patient's serum, which also contains high levels of complement, particularly C9. Delayed hypersensitivity to skin antigens and lymphoproliferative response to mucosal antigens are often demonstrable. It is possible that these patients have defective suppressor T-cells. A number of patients show exacerbation of symptoms after ingesting English walnut, which appears to have an initial mitogenic and a subsequent suppressive effect on peripheral blood lymphocytes in tissue culture. An increased incidence of HLA-B5 is found in Japanese and Asian patients and a viral aetiology is suspected on the grounds that as compared with a normal population it is difficult to infect, *in vitro*, lymphocytes from patients with Behçet's disease. Using DNA probes it has been possible to demonstrate herpes associated proteins in the lymphocytes from patients with Behçet's disease. Ocular lesions occur in about 75 per cent of the patients. The majority of the patients with ocular involvement have high levels of circulating immune complexes and respond to immunosuppressive therapy.

Sympathetic Ophthalmitis

This is a bilateral chronic uveitis which develops after perforating injury or surgical trauma. Antibodies to uveal tissue can be demonstrated after perforating injury and in many cases behave as blocking antibodies. Cell mediated immunity plays an important role in the pathogenesis of this disease and lymphocyte transformation and leucocyte migration inhibition tests suggest that the antigen involved may be derived either from the uvea (e.g. melanocytes) or the retina (e.g. photoreceptor cells). Sympathetic ophthalmitis may be associated with lens-induced uveitis, in which case hypersensitivity to lens proteins (i.e. phacoallergy) plays an important pathogenic role. Some patients with sympathetic ophthalmitis have a low T-cell count and others show a transient increase in the number of non-T and non-B-cell populations. The choroid is infiltrated by a large number of helper and suppressor T-cells, the latter being prominent in Dalén–Fuchs nodule. Patients with sympathetic ophthalmitis may show poliosis (of eyelashes), suggesting autoimmunity to antigens associated with melanin producing cells.

Immunopathology of the Lens

The crystalline lens is surrounded by a thick capsule (consisting of type IV collagen) which is lined anteriorly by a single layer of epithelium which multiplies, albeit slowly, throughout the life of the individual and lays down new lens fibres. Most of the soluble antigens (i.e. crystallins) are associated with the lens fibres. Autoantigens are weakly immunogenic in experimental animals and require Freund's complete adjuvant. The myth that lens proteins are sequestered and, therefore, there is no immunological tolerance, requires revision. A generalized inflammation of the uveal tract after liberation of lens protein and subsequent production of chemotactic leukotrienes is a well-known entity. Lens induced intraocular inflammation (e.g. phacoallergic endophthalmitis) usually follows extracapsular lens extraction, discission operations or a perforating injury. As a general rule, the ocular reaction varies directly with the amount of lens material left in the eye. Histologically, there is a zonal reaction in which the lens is infiltrated by neutrophils suggesting an Arthus-type reaction. There is a surrounding mantle of lymphocytes, epithelioid cells and multinucleate giant cells, the neighbouring iris and ciliary body are infiltrated by lymphocytes and plasma cells, and the intraocular tissues contain high levels of prostaglandins. The disease can be produced experimentally by traumatizing the lens in preimmunized animals. The affected lens shows *in vivo* fixation of IgG and complement and the inflammatory reaction can be prevented by pretreatment with agents that either lower the level of complement in blood or the number of circulatory polymorphonuclear leucocytes.

It is possible that lens autoimmunity plays an important role in the development of complicated cataract following intraocular inflammation, such as uveitis and retinitis. An intact lens (maintained in organ culture) when treated with anti-lens or anti-uveal antibody in the presence of complement, shows increased permeability for water and sodium leading to its opacification. It has also been suggested that intraocular inflammatory reactions often activate phospholipases which, in turn, produce cell damage and release lysophosphotidylcholine (LPC) which may act as lens permeability factor; treatment with ganglioside GM1, which reduces the level of LPC, may prevent cataract formation.

There is very little evidence that congenital cataract in man results from immunological disturbance.

LABORATORY INVESTIGATIONS IN OCULAR ALLERGY

For a detailed description of laboratory diagnostic techniques reference should be made to the relevant immunological texts.

1. The diagnosis of *IgE mediated (type I) allergic disorders* depends upon:
    (a) The detection of raised levels of IgE in blood, tears and other body secretions.
    (b) The presence of allergen specific IgE in the blood, tears and body secretions as detected either by the radio-allergosorbent test or by *in vitro* basophil degranulation.
    (c) The demonstration of a positive skin test to a variety of allergen extracts.
2. The diagnosis of *complement dependent (type II) hypersensitivity* reaction is based on:
    (a) The presence of autoantibody to cell surface antigens in blood.
    (b) A positive complement fixation test.
    (c) Increased K-cell activity as demonstrated by the ability of K-lymphocytes to adhere to antibody treated homologous tissue.
    (d) Evidence of lysis in antibody treated tissue culture, a technique used in tumour immunology.
3. A variety of immunological techniques has recently been developed for assessing the *in vivo* formation of immune complexes. The diagnosis of *type III allergy* depends upon:
    (a) A decrease in the blood level of certain components of complement.
    (b) The demonstration of complement breakdown products in the patient's serum, aqueous humour or tears by immunoelectrophoresis.
    (c) The detection of soluble immune complexes in the circulation and the aqueous humour using such techniques as ultracentrifugation, cryoprecipitation, polyethylene glycol (PEG) precipitation, gel filtration, C1q binding assay, inhibition of K-cell activity, and Raji cell assay.
    (d) The demonstration in *in vivo* fixation of antibody and complement in a biopsy of affected tissue by immune-labelling techniques such as immunofluorescence test.
4. The diagnosis of *cell mediated (type IV) hypersensitivity* reaction is achieved in a number of ways:
    (a) The demonstration of a positive intradermal reaction after injection of an appropriate antigen into the skin (i.e. the development of oedema and induration after 24–48 h). This test, however, is difficult to quantitate and has the risk of activating dormant lesions, while concomitant drug therapy (e.g. corticosteroids) often modifies the skin reaction.
    (b) In the lymphocyte transformation test, the degree of sensitization is measured in terms of increased protein and deoxyribonucleic acid synthesis in peripheral blood lymphocytes

when challenged *in vitro* with appropriate antigens.

(c) The leucocyte migration inhibition test is positive if macrophage inhibition factor is produced by the activated lymphocyte. The result is expressed as percentage inhibition after comparison with the size of the 'fan' formed in the absence of antigen.

(d) The degree of cytolysis produced by cytotoxic T-cells is assessed by measuring the release of radioactive chromium from labelled target cells maintained in tissue culture. Alternative techniques include study of deoxyribonucleic acid synthesis in the target cells. An inhibition suggests, however, both cytostasis and cytolysis.

Table V is intended as a general guideline for trainee ophthalmologists and is by no means comprehensive. Relevant immunological investigations and the anticipated findings have been summarized for ready reference. The interpretation of the results may sometimes prove extremely difficult because of wide biological variations and the modifying influences of corticosteroids and non-steroidal anti-inflammatory agents. For antibody measurements clotted blood will be required, but for *in vitro* cellular immune responses blood should be collected in preservative-free heparin and transported to the laboratory immediately; prolonged storage leads to loss of viability and poor yield of lymphocytes. Blood intended for immune complex should be allowed to clot at 37°C to prevent cryoprecipitation of some of the antigen–antibody aggregates. Blood for total and differential T-cell counts should also be collected in heparinized containers and sent to the laboratory immediately. Under no circumstance should it be stored in the refrigerator as it will lead to a false low yield of T-cells, particularly the helper subpopulation (refrigeration associated immunodeficiency – RAIDS!). Since there appears to be a circadian rythm for circulating lymphocytes and blood collected after meals may contain raised levels of immune complexes, it is preferable to collect blood in the morning, or at least at the same time of the day if a meaningful longitudinal study is contemplated.

Table V. Immunological tests in eye disease

Disease category	Ocular manifestations	Immunological tests	Anticipated result
Acute allergy	Vernal conjunctivitis	Skin test using allergen extract	Positive
	Acute drug allergies ? Other forms of allergic keratoconjunctivitis	Radio-immunoassay for total and allergen-specific IgE in tears and blood	Raised (Total IgE >100 i.u./ml) in serum, >10 i.u./ml in tears
		Total and differential T-cell count	Suppressor T-cell may be low
Non-specific acute inflammation	Keratoconjunctivitis Blepharitis Uveitis etc.	Immunoelectrophoresis (of serum, tears, aqueous) for 'acute-phase proteins'	Raised α_1 antitrypsin, C-reactive protein and serum amyloid A (SAA) component
		Quantitative radial immunodiffusion for immunoglobulins and acute phase proteins	Raised
		Tests for circulating immune complex (in diseases of unknown aetiology)	
		(a) Quantitation of complement fraction	Serum C'3 reduced
		(b) Clq and PEG precipitation tests	Precipitable immune complex present
		(c) Cryoglobulins	Single or mixed cryoglobulins present
		Antistreptolysin O titre	Raised in streptococcal infections
		Nitro-blue-tetrazolium (NBT) test for neutrophils	Negative or weakly positive in neutrophil dysfunction
		T-cell	Low in some cases of uveitis
		Helper/suppressor ratio	Altered (normal 1·8)

continued

Table V. Immunological tests in eye disease

Disease category	Ocular manifestations	Immunological tests	Anticipated result
Chronic and recurrent inflammation	Blepharitis Keratoconjunctivitis Mooren's ulcer Herpetic keratitis Uveitis Behçet's syndrome	Quantitative radial immunodiffusion for immunoglobulins	Raised immunoglobulins especially IgG, IgA and IgM
		Antistreptolysin 0 titre	Raised in streptococcal infection
		ELISA or RIA (of serum, aqueous) for Australia antigen	Positive in some cases of uveitis; relevance is unknown at present
		Tests for circulating immune complex	May be positive
		Lymphocyte transformation test (LTT)	'Transformation index' high in delayed tissue allergy, may be low in cases of recurrent infection
		Leucocyte migration inhibition test (MIT)	'Migration index' low in delayed tissue allergy
		Total and differential T-cell count and function	Low T-cell, suppressor cell anomaly, altered H/S ratio
Immune complex disease	Vasculitis of unknown aetiology (involving the uvea, the retina and the outer eye)	Tests for circulating immune complex	
		(a) Quantitation of C'3	Serum C'3 reduced
		(b) C1q precipitation test	Precipitable immune complex may be present in blood
		(c) Polyethylene glycol (PEG) precipitation test	Precipitable immune complex may be present in blood
		(d) Cryoglobulins	Single or mixed cryo-globulins may be present
		Antiphotoreceptor antibody	Positive in retinal disorders
Autoimmune disorders	Ocular manifestation of collagen diseases Endocrine exophthalmos	Quantitation of serum immunoglobulins	Raised IgG and IgM. IgA may be reduced in tears and serum
		Haemagglutination test for thyroid antibodies ELISA test for extraocular muscle antibody	Positive in endocrine exophthalmos
		Immunofluorescence test for antinuclear, anti-nucleolar, anti-mitochondrial and anti-smooth muscle antibodies	Positive in a variety of connective tissue disorders; uveitis, scleritis, KCS and retinopathies
		Tests for rheumatoid factor	Positive in rheumatoid lesions and Sjögren's syndrome
		Immunofluorescence test for antibodies to (i) salivary gland (ii) corneal epithelium (iii) retina	(i) Positive in Sjögren's syndrome (ii) Positive in Mooren's ulcer (iii) Positive in retinal vasculitis, choroidoretinitis etc.
	Sympathetic ophthalmitis Lens induced uveitis Optic neuritis	Haemagglutination test for antibodies against lens, uveal and retinal antigens	Positive in various forms of possible autoimmune uveitis, retinal vasculitis etc.

continued

Table V. Immunological tests in eye disease

Disease category	Ocular manifestations	Immunological tests	Anticipated result
	Other forms of uveitis with unsettled aetiology	Lymphocyte transformation test (LTT): (i) uveo-retinal antigen, (ii) basic myelin protein, (iii) corneal extract Migration inhibition test (MIT)	High 'transformation index' in (i) sympathetic ophthalmitis, Vogt—Koyanagi–Harada syndrome, (ii) optic neuritis, (iii) Mooren's ulcer Low 'migration index' in above mentioned conditions
Immunodeficiency states	Recurrent ocular inflammation in children and persons on immunosuppressive drugs	Quantitation of serum immunoglobulins NBT test for neutrophil function Lymphocyte transformation test (LTT) Migration inhibition test (MIT) Skin tests using purified protein derivative (PPD), candida antigen and dinitrochlorobenzene (DNCB)	Reduced levels of IgG, IgA and IgM Negative or weakly positive in neutrophil dysfunction Low transformation index with PHA, PPD and other recall antigens High 'migration index' Negative or weakly positive
Malignant melanoma	Uveal melanomas, retinoblastomas, conjunctival melanomas etc.	Immunofluorescence test for anti-tumour antibody LTT and MIT	Positive in some cases Positive in some cases

FURTHER READING

Addison D. J. and Rahi A. H. S. Immunoglobulin A deficiency and eye disease. *Trans. Ophthalmol. Soc. UK* 1981; **101**, 8.
Allansmith M. R. *The Eye and Immunology.* St Louis, Mo, Mosby, 1982.
Barnstable C. J. Monoclonal antibodies as molecular probes of the nervous system. In: Springer T. A. (ed.) *Hybridoma Technology in the Biosciences and Medicine.* New York, Plenum Press, 1985; pp. 269–89.
Boke W. and Luntz M. H. *Ocular Immune Responses: Modern Problems in Ophthalmology, Volume 16.* Basle, Karger, 1976.
Buckley R. J. Allergic eye disease: Terminology and classification. In de Laey J. J. (ed.) *Allergic Eye Disease and Sodium Cromoglycate.* Ghent, Belgium, Scientific Society for Medical Information, 1983, pp. 9–15.
Garner A. and Rahi A. H. S. Immunology and the eye. *Practitioner* 1982; **226**, 2035.
Hudson L. and Hay F. C. *Practical Immunology.* Oxford, Blackwell Scientific, 1980.
Murray P. I., Dinning W. J. and Rahi A. H. S. T-lymphocyte subpopulations in uveitis. *Br. J. Ophthalmol.* 1984; **68**, 746.
Murray P. I. and Rahi A. H. S. Pathogenesis of Mooren's ulcer. *Br. J. Ophthalmol.* 1984; **68**, 182.
Roitt I. M. *Essential Immunology.* Oxford, Blackwell Scientific, 1982.
Silverstein A. M. and O'Connor G. R. *Immunology and Immunopathology of the Eye.* New York, Masson, 1979.
Smith R. E. amd Nozik R. M. *Uveitis.* Baltimore, Md, Williams and Wilkins, 1983.
Smolin G. and O'Connor G. R. *Ocular Immunology.* Philadelphia, Lea and Febiger, 1981.
Suran A., Gery I. and Nusenblatt R. B. Immunology of the eye. *Immunology Abstracts* (Suppl.) Washington, 1981.
Theodore F. H., Bloomfield S. E. and Mondino B. J. *Clinical Allergy and Immunology of the Eye.* Baltimore, Md, Williams and Wilkins, 1983.
Rahi A. H. S. Autoimmunity and the retina. I. Antigenic specificity of photoreceptor cells. *Br. J. Ophthalmol.* 1970; **54**, 441–4.
Rahi A. H. S. HLA and eye disease. *Br. J. Ophthalmol.* 1979; **63**, 283.

Rahi A. H. S. Immunological processes and disease. In: Garner A. and Klintworth G. K. (ed.) *Pathobiology of Ocular Disease*. New York, Dekker, 1982.
Rahi A. H. S. and Garner A. *Immunopathology of the Eye*. Oxford, Blackwell Scientific, 1976.
Reich D'Almeida F. and Rahi A. H. S. Antigenic specificity of retinal pigment epithelium and non-immunological involvement in retinal dystrophy. *Nature* 1974; **252,** 307–8.

Immunosuppression

A. M. Denman

An important part of ophthalmological practice concerns the suppression of inflammatory reactions in the sclera, retina and other sites. The most commonly used drugs are usually referred to as 'immunosuppressive' agents, but in reality, most such drugs are still has some validity, it is now clear that immune mechanisms are highly interdependent and that non-specific inflammatory events and immunologically specific events are also inseparable (*Fig.* 1). These principles apply equally to immunopathological

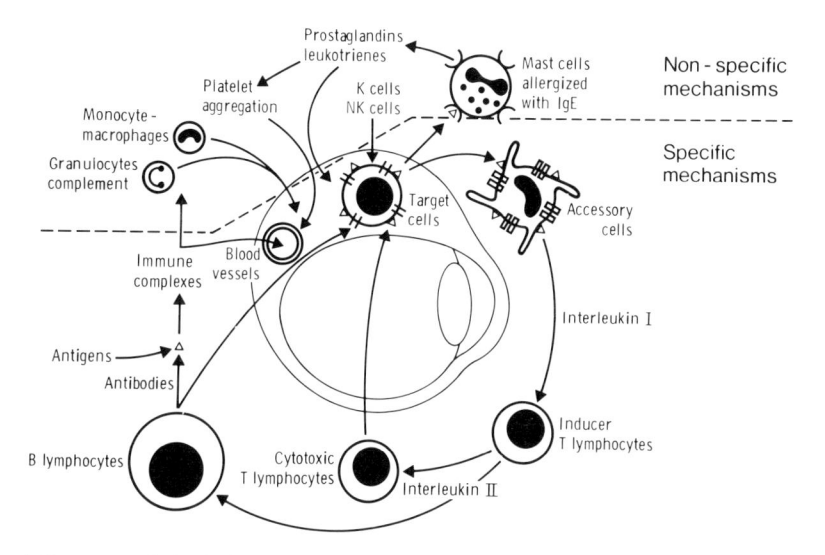

Fig. 1. Immunopathological mechanisms susceptible to immunosuppressive drugs. This schematic outline of the most important pathways is designed to emphasize the following points: the interdependence of cellular and humoral mechanisms; the interdependence of immunologically specific and non-specific mechanisms; the importance of HLA antigens in initiating immune responses. The figure will help clarify the actions of immunosuppressive drugs listed in *Table* I. The hypothetical target cell may exist anywhere in the eye; blood vessels may prove to be the relevant target for immune responses. △, schematic antigens (autoantigens?, blood-borne antigens?); ≣, class I HLA antigens; ≣, class II HLA antigens.

used empirically. This is inescapable given our ignorance of the mechanisms which damage the eye in chronic inflammatory diseases and the multiple effects of the drugs used to treat this inflammation. However, the rational use of immunosuppressive drugs depends upon some insight into the most likely ways in which immune processes damage the eye.

IMMUNOPATHOLOGICAL MECHANISMS AND THE EYE

Several mechanisms inflict immunopathological damage on target organs.[1] While the classic distinction between humoral and cell mediated mechanisms events in the eye with the proviso that relatively little tissue has been available for detailed analysis compared with other diseased organs. In addition, the eye may react peculiarly to immunological stimuli because of local anatomical factors.[2] Of these, the most important are the avascular nature of the cornea and lens and the possibility that the endothelial cell barrier of the retinal vessels limits the entry of lymphocyte populations mediating immune reactions. Furthermore, there is experimental evidence that antigens in the anterior chamber elicit some but not all cell mediated immune responses.[3]

The close association between inflammatory and immunological responses is important in terms of predicting the likely susceptibility of these processes to immunosuppressive drugs. There may be a specifically immunological component in most forms of inflammatory eye disease. Thus in mice, after one eye has been damaged by experimental alkali burning, the process is accelerated when the second eye is subjected to a similar stimulus, suggesting that immunological sensitization contributes to the pathogenesis of the second lesion.[4] There are usually only indirect grounds, such as the nature of the inflammatory infiltrate, for attributing an immunopathological basis to most forms of inflammatory eye disease. In addition, it is vital to distinguish between persistent inflammation, which may respond to immunosuppressive drugs, and terminal, irreversible fibrosis.

As with immunopathological diseases of unknown aetiology at other sites, several immunological hypotheses have been advanced. Each hypothesis suggests a different role for immunosuppressive drugs. The simplest explanation for continued inflammation attributes this response to persistent local antigens. Certainly, there is ample experimental evidence that animals sensitized systemically to a given antigen mount a local reaction if they are subsequently challenged with the same antigen by intraocular injection. The frequent associations between systemic immunopathological disorders and inflammatory eye disease suggest that such mechanisms may operate in human disease. Unfortunately, no exogenous antigen has been identified in most forms of inflammatory eye disease. Nevertheless, the inheritance of certain HLA antigens confers susceptibility to inflammatory uveitis either in isolation or as part of reactive arthritis. Since these clinical conditions are provoked by infectious diseases, notably gut infections, it is logical to conclude that the host response is directed at microbial antigens localized to the eye, or to tissue antigens with which microbial antigens are associated. Persistent local infection induced experimentally displays the immunopathological abnormalities typifying inflammatory eye disease. For example Carreras et al.[5] have shown that the intraocular injection of Sindbis virus in adult mice produces the inflammatory changes characteristic of iridiocyclitis and retinitis in man. Moreover, the histopathological abnormalities in this model result from the immune responses of the host against virus-infected cells.

Anti-viral immune responses inevitably include a phase of ephemeral autoimmunity since viral antigens are recognized in association with histocompatibility antigens. It is attractive therefore to postulate that an initial phase of a specific response to a local infectious agent is perpetuated as an autoimmune response (see review by Denman[6]). Trauma and chemical insults could also initiate persistent autoimmune responses. Sympathetic ophthalmia is the most persuasive example of such a mechanism. In addition, autoimmune reactions to uveal tract antigens have been detected by serological and lymphocyte transformation assays.[7] Autoimmune reactions against the retinal rod antigen termed S-antigen have attracted most attention. However, serological studies in animals in which autoimmune uveitis is induced by immunization with different ocular antigens suggest that autoantibodies may be induced against a wide range of autoantigens.[8] A remarkably sharp distinction between susceptibility to anterior and posterior inflammatory uveitis has also been noted with different HLA antigens,[9] suggesting that topographically distinct target antigens for autoimmune reactions may eventually be discovered. Experimental studies have revealed that virus infections provoke autoimmune reactions against a remarkable range of tissue antigens and hormones.[10] Furthermore these autoantibodies may only be detectable when secreted in isolation by hybridomas produced by fusing autoantibody secreting cells from the affected animals with myeloma cell lines.[11]

Chronic inflammation might also persist when defects in the regulation of immune responses allow the usually ephemeral phase of autoimmune reactivity to continue. Failure of these regulatory mechanisms is usually attributed either to a defect in suppressor T cells or to a failure of anti-idiotype antibody to suppress the proliferation of B cells synthesizing autoantibodies. Indeed, Dumonde et al.[12] have postulated that the circulating immune complexes encountered in patients with inflammatory uveitis may be protective because they consist of anti-retinal antibodies complexed with antibodies reactive with the sequences (idiotypes) that confer immunological specificity on those autoantibodies. Should such theories be confirmed, the differential effects of immunosuppressive drugs on different lymphocyte populations will prove of great practical importance. It would clearly be desirable to avoid agents that inflict further damage on regulatory lymphocytes as the price of suppressing inflammatory reactions.

Inflammatory eye diseases are commonly associated with systemic diseases of unknown aetiology characterized by vasculitis, chronic inflammatory infiltrates in various target organs and polyclonal activation of B-lymphocytes with a variable spectrum of autoantibodies. These features have long prompted speculation that such disorders may be primary lymphoproliferative diseases in which lymphocyte proliferation, although not malignant in conventional terms, is nevertheless autonomous and independent of conventional antigenic stimuli. Indeed intraorbital lesions consisting mainly of proliferating lymphoid cells are encountered in which it may be difficult to distinguish cytologically between a polyclonal lymphoproliferative reaction and a monoclonal disorder characteristic of malignant disease.[13]

Considerations of this kind are important in determining the objectives of immunosuppressive therapy. If the aim of such treatment is to suppress a continuous immune response analogous to that provoked by renal allografts, drug regimes used in transplantation immunology have a logical place in the treatment of ocular inflammation but, equally, such treatment is more likely to be suppressive than curative. In contrast, it would be more rational to use potent cytotoxic drugs in chronic inflammatory eye diseases if these proved to be primary lymphoproliferative disorders.

THE CHOICE OF IMMUNOSUPPRESSIVE DRUGS

Given these uncertainties about the true nature of chronic inflammatory eye diseases, the most rational approach is to interdict such processes at any of the stages indicated in *Fig.* 1 using drugs that carry the least short and long term risks. Any drug with such properties can properly be termed immunosuppressive. The drugs most commonly used in ophthalmological practice are listed in *Table* I. Their properties are described in detail in general texts (*see*, for example, Rees and Lockwood[14]) and only points of ophthalmological relevance are considered here. For simplicity, the combination of specific immunological and non-specific inflammatory reactions are referred to collectively as the 'immune response'.

Non-steroidal Anti-inflammatory Drugs

Many new drugs in this category have become available in recent years, most of which are proprionic acid derivatives, acetic acid derivatives or fenamates. Their most important actions are on arachidonic acid metabolites. There are two principal pathways for arachidonic acid metabolism; metabolites catalysed by cyclo-oxygenase include the platelet aggregating material thromboxane and derivatives that enhance other inflammatory mediators such as histamine; they also augment leukocyte chemotaxis. In contrast, metabolites catalysed by lipoxygenase include prostacyclin, which inhibits platelet aggregation, and other compounds that mediate immediate hypersensitivity reactions. Leucocytes also produce lipoxygenase products with inflammatory properties, termed leukotrienes. These metabolites are generated in response to injury and potentiate inflammatory reactions through the pathways indicated above. In addition, these factors promote platelet aggregation which may in turn lead to thrombosis and occlusion of small blood vessels. The relevance of these pathways to immediate hypersensitivity reactions has been demonstrated in several experimental systems and, to some extent, by direct clinical observation.[15] The short half-life and lability of these mediators makes it difficult to measure their turnover in inflammatory lesions at any site and particularly an inaccessible one such as the eye. Nevertheless, prostaglandin-like activity has been identified in ocular inflammation.[16]

Drugs such as indomethacin and aspirin selectively inhibit cyclo-oxygenase production thereby accounting for their anti-inflammatory activity. Corticosteroids block the metabolism of arachidonic acid at a much earlier stage, inhibiting the formation of both cyclo-oxygenase and lipoxygenase products thus accounting for their ability to depress immediate hypersensitivity reactions so efficiently.

The merits and disadvantages of different non-steroidal anti-inflammatory drugs have been extensively reviewed.[17] Few novel drugs have proved more effective than existing ones judged by their efficacy in common inflammatory disorders such as rheumatoid arthritis and many have been withdrawn because of unacceptable side effects. Relatively few such drugs have been used to treat inflammatory eye disease and there are at present no indications for using drugs other than a small number of proved value. While salicylates and related drugs have no *in vivo* action on the immune system,[18] their anti-inflammatory effects justify their use in some circumstances. Aspirin is still the most commonly prescribed of the salicylic acid derivatives. This drug has been used to treat acute allergic conjunctivitis successfully,[19] but there is little information about its effectiveness in more prolonged inflammatory disorders. In an experimental model of uveitis induced by herpes simplex virus in rabbits, salicylates were ineffective.[20] Clinicians are aware of the most commonly recognized side effects of salicylates, namely gastrointestinal haemorrhage, hepatotoxicity and allergic reactions in susceptible individuals. Less recognized problems are fluid retention and the risk of precipitating pulmonary oedema in patients with pre-existing heart disease.

Proprionic acid derivatives have the lowest incidence of side effects of all non-steroidal anti-inflammatory drugs. While individual authors recommend drugs such as ketoprofen and naproxen in mild inflammatory eye disease, there are no systematic accounts of their value and tolerance in patients with severe or chronic disease.

Of the acetic acid derivatives, indomethacin has been used most widely in inflammatory diseases in general but there are few reports assessing its value in inflammatory eye disease. Inhibition of prostaglandin synthesis by these drugs is readily demonstrable in concentrations which are therapeutically relevant. The drug blocks the conversion of arachidonic acid to inflammatory metabolites catalysed by cyclo-oxygenase. Moreover, it has been shown that indomethacin inhibits prostaglandin synthesis in ocular tissues.[21] Its potential therapeutic usefulness has been demonstrated in a double-blind study in which damage to the iris during the extracapsular extraction of cataracts was significantly reduced by indomethacin drops compared with a placebo preparation.[22] There are uncontrolled reports that indomethacin can be used as an alternative to systemic steroids in patients with polymyalgia rheumatica and its variant, temporal arteritis. Justifiable concern about the visual complications of this disorder almost invariably dictates a prompt recourse to steroids and there has

Table I. Main actions of immunosuppressive agents used in ophthalmological practice

Immunosuppressive agent	Specific									Non-specific					
	Accessory cells	Lymphocytes transformation	T-lymphocytes			B-lymphocytes		Inter-leukins	Prostaglandins		Chemotaxis (granulocytes and monocytes)	NK	Cellular		Monocyte-macrophages
			Inducer	Cytotoxic	Suppressor	1ry antibody response	2ry antibody response		inflammation	immediate hypersensitivity			K		
Non-steroidal anti-inflammatory drugs (e.g. salicylates indomethacin)	Nil	Nil	Nil	Nil	Nil	Nil	Nil	Nil	↓↓↓	Nil	(High dose)	Nil	Nil		Nil
Steroids	Nil	Nil	Nil	?	?	Nil	Conventional: nil autoantibodies ↓ to ↓↓↓ (variable)	↓ to ↓↓↓ e.g. interferon	↓↓↓	↓↓↓	↓	Function ↓ (high dose)	Nil		Enzyme ↓ secretion
Azathioprine	Nil	Nil occas. +	Nil	↓	↓	Nil	Nil	Nil	Nil	Nil	Nil	Production ↓ function ↓	Production ↓ function ↓		Production ↓
Alkylating agents (chlorambucil and cyclophosphamide)	?	Variable may ↓ or +	↓	↓	↓	Nil to ↓	Conventional: nil or ↑ autoantibodies ↓ to ↓↓↓ plasma immunoglobulins ↓	?	Nil	Nil	Nil	Nil	Nil		Nil
Anti-lymphocyte globulin	Nil	Variable may ↓ ↓↓ when combined with other agents	↓	↓	?	May ↓	Nil	?	↓ or nil	↓ or nil	Nil	Nil	Nil		Nil
Cyclosporin	↓ ? ↓	↓↓↓	↓↓↓	Nil	Nil	↓ ?	Nil	Nil	Nil	Nil	Nil	Nil	Nil		Nil

Only clinically important effects are indicated.
Only *in vivo* human data are included; for example, 'lymphocyte transformation' refers to the *in vitro* responses of lymphocytes from patients treated with these agents.
Suppression graded ↓ to ↓↓↓. +, enhancement: Nil, no effect; ?, data unavailable or doubtful.
Doses are within range cited in text.
Key references are given in the text.

been no proper comparative trial of this standard remedy and indomethacin or similar drugs. Some side effects of indomethacin are well recognized, namely headaches, gastrointestinal intolerance and rashes. However dizziness, mild disorientation and difficulty in focusing are often overlooked, particularly in elderly patients.

Corticosteroids (Table I)

The most commonly used glucocorticoids, prednisone and prednisolone, form the mainstay of conventional immunosuppressive treatment in ophthalmological practice. Steroids are given topically, orally and, more recently, as intravenous pulses of methylprednisolone. The vast range of biological effects attributable to steroids makes it difficult to discern which of these are therapeutically relevant. Furthermore, their relative importance is dose-dependent. At low doses, that is less than 7·5 mg of prednisolone or its equivalent daily, the effects on inflammatory mediators are clearly important and steroids represent a more powerful version of the anti-inflammatory drugs already discussed. These considerations apply to the treatment of common ophthalmological disorders using either topical steroids or short courses of systemic treatment. Higher systemic doses of the kind used in the treatment of retinal vascular disease affect lymphocyte function and are more likely to interfere with the execution of specific immune responses. Very high steroid dosage, exceeding 30 mg of prednisolone daily, and pulsed intravenous methylprednisolone, are particularly likely to suppress specific immune responses. However, the literature on this subject is difficult to interpret because investigators have relied on non-specific assays of immune function. These include in vitro lymphocyte transformation by mitogens such as phytohaemagglutinin and in vivo skin reactions or humoral responses to antigens which are irrelevant to controlling the disease in question; indeed, judged by such assays, corticosteroids have little discernible immunosuppressive effect even in doses which allow allografts such as transplanted kidneys to survive. Since the targets for the immune reaction in inflammatory eye disease are unknown, there is no direct means of assaying the relevant immunosuppressive effects of steroids in these disorders. The situation will improve with the current introduction of assays for measuring immunological functions such as antigen presentation and the synthesis of mediators that govern specific immune responses. Since steroids regulate gene expression and thus control the transcription of messenger RNA from DNA and hence protein synthesis, they are likely to influence the rate at which immunological mediators are synthesized. However, systematic studies of this kind have not yet been reported.

The value of topical and systemic corticosteroids is reflected in their routine place in ophthalmological practice. Furthermore, there have been several controlled trials of corticosteroids in the systemic diseases with which inflammatory eye disease is often associated (see review by Rees and Lockwood[14]). Obvious ethical constraints have limited the scope for controlled trials of corticosteroids. However, some systemic studies underscore this clinical impression. For example, Reynard et al.[23] have shown that corticosteroids improve the outlook in sympathetic ophthalmia.

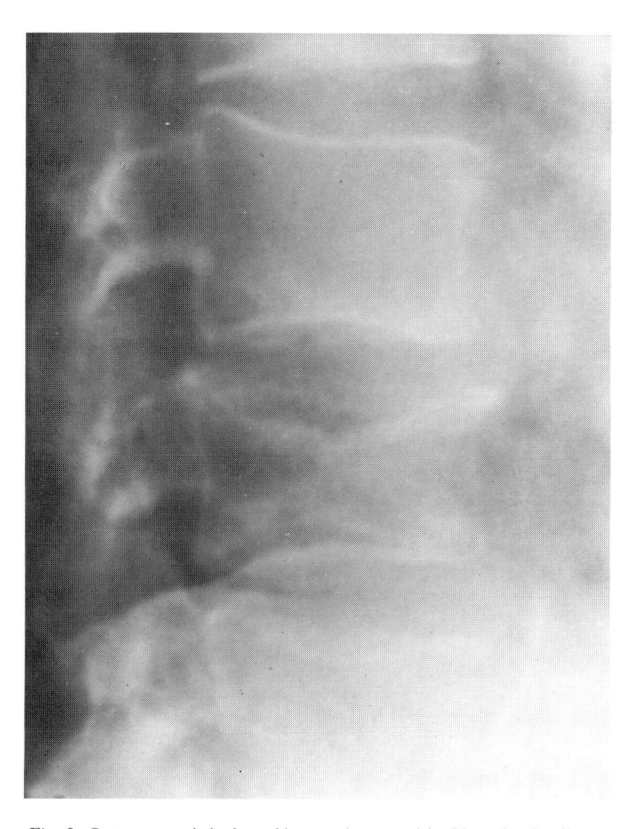

Fig. 2. Osteoporosis induced by corticosteroids. Vertebral collapse in a 70-year-old man with retinal artery occlusion secondary to temporal arteritis treated with high-dose prednisolone for 12 months.

The problems of steroid side effects have received great attention. General awareness of these side effects has greatly reduced their severity but some remain troublesome. Osteoporosis with vertebral collapse is the commonest problem encountered in elderly patients receiving corticosteroids (*Fig.* 2). This is a particular hazard in patients with polymyalgia and temporal arteritis involving the retinal circulation who need such treatment for prolonged periods. Growth retardation is also an important consideration in growing children receiving steroids for the iridocyclitis associated with juvenile chronic arthritis.[24] Avascular necrosis, particularly affecting the femoral and humoral epiphyses, is commonly encountered in young adults and may occur after only a few weeks' treatment. There is also a suspicion that steroids precipitate premature atheromatous degeneration of the coronary arteries and other vessels, particularly in young women. Obesity, largely attributable to increased appetite, is troublesome in all age groups.

The standard means of combating these problems is to maintain patients on the lowest practicable dose. It is important to appreciate that dose reductions may only be feasible in small steps of as little as 0·5 mg of prednisolone daily and at intervals of weeks or even months. It is always preferable and usually practicable to give corticosteroids as a single daily dose in order to preserve the pituitary–adrenal axis as far as possible. Giving prednisone on alternate days only is an accepted means of treatment in many clinical situations but its value in inflammatory eye disease has not been formally proved. Intermittent intravenous injections of methylprednisolone have been advocated as an effective means of giving corticosteroids for chronic immunopathological diseases without incurring the usual side effects. However the place of such treatment has not been established in systemic inflammatory diseases, let alone in inflammatory eye diseases. This procedure is not free from risk and may lead to acute convulsions and cardiovascular collapse. The dangers are reduced by giving the infusion over a period of 4–6 h preceded by a diuretic in patients with known cardiovascular problems. Many simple means of reducing steroid dosage that have proved effective in transplantation practice[25] have not been tested in the management of inflammatory eye disease; for example, the timing of steroid administration in relation to diurnal variations in inflammatory activity may influence the maintenance dose. Patients with systemic connective tissue diseases may have an additional hazard even when receiving topical steroid drops for associated ocular problems since Gaston et al.[26] have shown that such individuals are more susceptible than others to glaucoma induced by corticosteroids.

Cytotoxic Drugs

Azathioprine

Azathioprine is the cytotoxic drug most commonly used to treat non-malignant diseases such as rheumatoid arthritis. Extensive studies in the latter disorder have shown that the drug is well tolerated provided that blood counts are carefully monitored and the dose adjusted accordingly. Azathioprine is a purine analogue which is extensively metabolized first to 6-mercaptopurine and thence to the ribonucleotide thioinosinic acid. The main effects of these active matabolites are to inhibit enzymes involved in DNA synthesis and to substitute for normal bases thereby introducing abnormal base sequences. The main effects of azathioprine on immune function are summarized in *Table* I. Since azathioprine acts as an antiproliferative drug, it inhibits the division not only of progenitor cells of the lymphocyte series but also proliferating cells in the bone-marrow, gastrointestinal tract and other tissues. Nevertheless, since azathioprine is both clinically effective and reasonably safe in many inflammatory diseases its immunosuppressive effects predominate in the relatively low dose range employed in treating such disorders. As in other inflammatory diseases, azathioprine is used in a dose of 2·5–3·0 mg/kg body weight in patients with inflammatory eye diseases. In this dosage, bone-marrow depression is rarely a problem and is almost invariably reversible. Provided the drug is stopped when the granulocyte count falls below $2000/\mu l$ or the platelet count below $100\,000/\mu l$, it is usually safe to resume treatment at a lower dose once the blood count has recovered. However, irreversible bone-marrow suppression may occur, particularly in elderly patients. The most common reason for abandoning treatment is gastrointestinal intolerance, often accompanied by biochemical evidence of hepatoxicity. In addition, a few patients may develop generalized hypersensitivity reactions in the form of fever, malaise and other non-specific symptoms after only a few days' treatment[27,28] and symptoms of this kind must be taken seriously. There are no substantial reports of treating inflammatory uveitis with 6-mercaptopurine.

Alkylating Agents

The alkylating agents chlorambucil and cyclophosphamide have been extensively used in connective tissue diseases and inflammatory uveitis. These agents alkylate the nucleotides in DNA thereby altering their alignment in the DNA strand. In DNA replication preparatory to cell division the alkylated bases mis-pair, thereby producing complementary strands with altered base sequences. These mutations may be lethal or they may persist with a latent propensity for malignant transformation. In addition, the bifunctional alkylating agent cyclophosphamide cross-links the two strands of DNA posing further obstacles to cell division. Mammalian cells contain enzymes for removing the alkylated bases and repairing the resulting gap in the DNA strand. Thus the cumulative effects of treatment with alkylating agents depend partly on the direct effects of the drug and partly on the rate at which the resulting defects are repaired. These effects of cyclophosphamide and hence its immunosuppressive actions are mediated by active metabolites following oxidation by liver microsomes; cyclophosphamide itself has no immunosuppressive effects. Chlorambucil, in contrast, acts directly but less is known about its *in vivo* metabolism in man. The effects of alkylating agents on immune function are listed in *Table* I. Although no controlled studies have been reported in vasculitic diseases in general, impressive results have been obtained with these agents compared with the usually poor response to corticosteroids.[29] Dose schedules have varied greatly; very large single doses of cyclophosphamide of up to 1 g/m² surface area have been given intravenously to patients with severe vasculitic disorders. The doses of alkylating agents used to treat inflammatory uveitis have generally been low, namely 0·05–0·20 mg/kg body weight of chlorambucil and 1·25–2·5 mg/kg body weight of cyclophosphamide.

Like azathioprine, alkylating agents are anti-proliferative and affect precursor cells in the bone-marrow, gastrointestinal tract and gonads as well as lymphocyte precursor cells. Bone-marrow depression may occur and the guidelines for serial blood counts are identical to those indicated for azathioprine; macrocytosis is commonly encountered after prolonged treatment and can be disregarded as it does not presage bone-marrow depression. Some patients develop gastrointestinal intolerance, although in less acute form than that provoked by azathioprine. It can often be overcome by giving these drugs with meals or prescribing standard antispasmodic drugs. Hair loss may occur suddenly and severely, recovering only slowly even after the drug has been withdrawn. Haemorrhagic cystitis is a hazard peculiar to cyclophosphamide but can largely be prevented by the long term, concomitant administration of mesna (Uromitexan) which blocks the urothelial toxicity of the metabolite acrolein.[30]

Infertility is a problem of great concern in patients receiving cytotoxic drugs and particularly alkylating agents. Persistent azospermia is induced by relatively small amounts of cyclophosphamide. In one series it was noted in the majority of patients receiving an average total dose of 168 mg/kg body weight.[31] Similarly cyclophosphamide induced azospermia in the majority of patients treated with this drug for Behçet's syndrome.[32] Side effects are less frequently encountered at the lower end of these dose schedules. However, haemorrhagic cystitis and hair loss may develop acutely even in patients receiving low doses and advanced warning of these possible complications is mandatory.

Opportunistic Infections and Cytotoxic Drugs

There are inadequate data concerning the incidence and severity of opportunistic infections in patients receiving cytotoxic drugs for inflammatory eye disease. Moreover, the situation is complicated by the high percentage of such patients who are receiving concomitant corticosteroids. Most reports of infections consequent upon long term immunosuppressive treatment have concerned transplant recipients or patients with systemic features of the underlying disease, which themselves increase the risk of intercurrent infection; impaired renal function is a good example.[33] There are especial hazards in young children who have not become immune to common virus infections such as measles before treatment is started. Immunization with live viruses should be avoided in immunosuppressed patients unless there is a strong possibility of infection by a virulent virus. Outbreaks of varicella zoster are encountered in patients immunosuppressed for inflammatory uveitis, but they are not of unusual severity and, indeed, it is not clear whether the incidence is increased compared with what would be expected in control individuals of the same age followed over the same number of years. Contrary to conventional belief, it is possible to give immunosuppressive regimes including cytotoxic drugs to patients with severe bacterial infections complicating systemic vasculitic diseases associated with ocular complications. Cytotoxic drugs often restore a normal pattern of lymphocyte proliferation in such individuals, thereby increasing rather than reducing immunological competence.[34] To illustrate the point, 57 patients with Behçet's uveitis have been treated with chlorambucil, azathioprine or ALG (anti-lymphocyte globulin) alone or in combination at this centre since 1970; the majority were also receiving corticosteroids. Only one of these patients has developed a bacterial infection necessitating hospital admission and this patient was found to be suffering from leukaemia.[35] Intercurrent viral infections such as varicella zoster have been of average severity and none has required antiviral chemotherapy.

Cytotoxic Drugs and Malignant Disease

The oncogenic potentiality of cytotoxic drugs is a point of great concern. There is little doubt that alkylating agents are responsible for an increased incidence of leukaemias in children receiving these drugs for juvenile chronic arthritis and other immunological disorders.[36,37] There is some indication that the incidence of lymphomas and other tumours is increased in patients receiving cytotoxic drugs for non-malignant diseases and who are not transplant recipients.[38,39] The exact extent of this problem will not be known until long term surveys currently in progress are completed. Analysis of reported cases emphasizes that the oncogenic risk of chlorambucil is related to the cumulative dose, particularly if this exceeds 4·0 g.[40] The risk of malignancy is related to mutagenic damage exceeding the cell's capacity to repair this damage; sequential counts of sister chromatid exchanges provides a more sensitive measure of this damage than classic cytogenic techniques and confirms that alkylating agents inflict cumulative damage.[35] Moreover, patients with inflammatory uveitis may be particularly susceptible to this damage because of defective repair mechanisms.

Other Immunosuppressive Agents

The non-selective anti-proliferative effects of cytotoxic drugs have prompted a search for more selective immunosuppressive drugs. Anti-lymphocyte globulin, ALG, is relatively selective, predominantly affecting the population of re-circulating T-lymphocytes which initiate both cell mediated and humoral immune responses. However, ALG is cumbersome to administer, requiring prolonged intravenous infusions, and it provokes adverse reactions in 10 per cent of recipients. These take the form of acute anaphylactic or serum sickness reactions and invariably remit without sequelae; nevertheless, their unpredictable appearance necessitates close supervision of patients during infusions. It is likely that anti-sera reactive with specific lymphocyte populations will become available as the result of advances in hybridoma technology for raising monoclonal antibodies. Such anti-sera have already been used to treat some immunopathological diseases.

The fungal metabolite cyclosporin A has a powerful and virtually selective effect on lymphocytes, both T- and B-lymphocytes being affected in man.[41] Its most dramatic effects are on the induction of immune reactions both *in vitro* and *in vivo*.[42] Thus in experimental systems, cyclosporin A suppresses immmunopathological disorders induced by injecting specific tissue antigen; for example, it prevents experimental allergic encephalomyelitis if given at the time of immunization with myelin basic protein. Similarly, cyclosporin A effectively blocks the rejection of experimental allografts including corneal grafts.[43,44] It is not surprising therefore that cyclosporin A also inhibits autoimmune uveitis in rats induced by immunizing with retinal antigen[45] and that immune responses to this antigen are correspondingly inhibited.[46] In clinical practice cyclosporin has been used successfully to limit the appearance of graft-versus-host disease in recipients of bone-marrow grafts and as an adjunct to immunosuppressive regimes in transplant recipients largely because it can be given at the time of grafting.[47]

It suppresses inflammatory uveitis, notably in Behçet's syndrome, through mechanisms which remain unclarified.[48] There are indications that its value will be confirmed in controlled trials.[49] However, it has not been established that remissions induced by cyclosporin A persist once the drug is withdrawn. Whilst most of its side-effects – depression, gingival hyperplasia, hypertrichosis and hepatotoxicity – are reversible, there is less confidence about the nephrotoxicity attributable to this drug.[50] In the majority of patients renal function fully recovers after treatment but chronic toxicity ensues in some patients with auto-immune disease.[51] This must be borne in mind by ophthalmologists contemplating its use and close monitoring of renal function is obligatory. In contrast, earlier concern about its oncogenic potentiality is receding, although one should be wary about this possibility in patients who have already received other immunosuppressive drugs.

OPHTHALMOLOGICAL EXPERIENCE WITH IMMUNOSUPPRESSIVE AGENTS

Cytotoxic drugs have been used to treat individual patients with various forms of inflammatory eye disease which has failed to respond to corticosteroids or has necessitated treatment with unacceptably high maintenance doses of steroids. Patients with some forms of disease, such as the uveitis of Behçet's syndrome, have received cytotoxic drugs as the treatment of first choice. There have been several reports claiming that cytotoxic drugs, and more particularly alkylating agents, produce more impressive responses than are obtained with corticosteroids. Moreover, many authors have described prolonged and even indefinite remissions. For example, cytotoxic drugs have been used to reduce steroid dosage in patients with destructive scleral inflammation[52] and permanent remissions of ocular vasculitic lesions in Wegener's granulomatosis have been reported.[53] Following the first accounts of chlorambucil's value in treating Behçet's uveitis,[54,55] similar results have been recorded by several authors.[56,57] Long term remissions have been described in some patients in whom it has been possible to withdraw all immunosuppressive drugs without subsequent relapse. However, late exacerbations of the disease have also been noted. Steroid-resistant iridocyclitis has also responded to chlorambucil in children with this complication of juvenile chronic arthritis.[58]

Unfortunately the published accounts are of limited value in establishing the true place of cytotoxic drugs in the management of inflammatory eye disease. First, there is a dearth of controlled studies in which the benefits of cytotoxic drugs have been compared with those of conventional steroid treatment. This is understandable given the ethical difficulties in deriving appropriate trials. Secondly, in the majority of these reports, the disease features in treated patients have not been fully described. In comparing the response to cytotoxic drugs with that to other agents, it is essential to take into account potentially responsive features such as inflammatory exudates and irreversible ones, such as vaso-occlusive changes with retinal atrophy. Finally, there have been few attempts to assess the response to immunosuppression quantitatively by allotting scores to each disease feature with appropriate weighting for more important ones, although such methods have been applied in some studies.[12] The ease with which clinical features can be recorded by retinal photography and fluoroscein angiography gives ophthalmologists distinct advantages in this respect. Ideally, sequential assessments should be made by independent observers from whom details of treatment in the controlled trial have been withheld. Sophisticated trials of this kind have been undertaken in diseases with a variable natural history, of which multiple sclerosis is a pertinent example.[59] The place of cytotoxic drugs in the management of inflammatory eye disease will remain undecided until such trials have been undertaken.

The risks of cytotoxic drugs might be more readily acceptable if they cured inflammatory eye disease and did not merely suppress it. This would be plausible if such drugs ablated primed lymphocytes capable of responding to the antigen-provoking disease once the effects of the drug had worn off. Unfortunately, experiments in rabbits locally sensitized to a soluble antigen by the intravitreal injection of bovine gamma globulin suggest that cyclophosphamide for example does not have this effect on 'immunological memory'.[60] The duration of treatment has also been decided pragmatically. As a general rule, cytotoxic drugs should be reduced to the lowest dose needed to maintain clinical remission. It is probably necessary to continue treatment for at least 18 months but there are no accurate data correlating duration of treatment with the subsequent disease course. This is a point of particular concern, given that cumulative dosage is related to oncogenic risks.

No effective remedies are known that influence fibroblastic proliferation. However the anti-proliferative drug fluorouracil suppresses periretinal proliferation in an experimental model of retinal detachment suggesting that the general anti-proliferative effects of cytotoxic drugs may be therapeutically advantageous.[61]

Many immunosuppressive regimes have combined corticosteroids and other agents hoping that these will act synergistically. For example, in a controlled trial of immunosuppressive measures in patients with severe connective tissue diseases a combination of ALG, azathioprine and corticosteroids was more effective than corticosteroids alone.[62] Similarly, ALG has been used as an adjunct in treating inflammatory eye disease (*see* review by Bonnet[56,63]) but controlled trials have not been undertaken to prove the point.

As already stated, there are indications that cyclosporin A is useful in treating some forms of uveitis. However, long term studies of clinical benefit and associated toxicity are still lacking. Analogues of this drug may prove to be equally effective but less nephrotoxic.

LABORATORY MONITORING OF IMMUNOSUPPRESSIVE DRUGS

The only satisfactory means of monitoring treatment with immunosuppressive drugs is to observe their clinical effects and to avoid complications by routine laboratory tests. As will be apparent from *Table* I, the immunosuppressive drugs used in ophthalmological practice do not reproducibly suppress responses such as delayed-skin reactions or humoral antibody responses to standard antigens. Lymphocyte responses *in vitro* to non-specific mitogens such as phytohaemagglutinin have been extensively used for this purpose. However, the technical and biological complexities of lymphocyte transformation tests make this an extremely unsatisfactory means for routinely monitoring immune responses.[64] In Behçet's syndrome, for example, immunosuppressive regimes alter the pattern of proliferative responses to standard mitogens,[65] but the changes represent a return to a more normal pattern of proliferative response rather than 'immunosuppression'. Monoclonal antibodies are widely available which react with different lymphocyte subpopulations. Since studies with these reagents show that the relative numbers of circulating lymphocyte sub-populations are disturbed in inflammatory uveitis,[66] it is possible that assays of this kind will prove a guide to clinical activity and successful treatment. Observations in transplant recipients receiving immunosuppressive drugs suggest that a reduction in the numbers of circulating helper T-lymphocytes detectable by monoclonal antibodies indicates a risk of opportunistic infection by herpes viruses.[67] Thus such assays may help to reduce the complications of immunosuppression. Monoclonal antibodies also identify the effects of immunosuppressive drugs on different lymphocyte populations more precisely than was possible with earlier methods.[68] Correlations between selective effects and clinical response may emerge from further studies of this kind. The assay of mediators secreted by mononuclear cells (interleukins) is also assuming increased importance. Of immediate practical importance, serum immunoglobulin concentrations should be measured at intervals not exceeding 3 months in patients treated with alkylating agents long term because of the risk of hypogammaglobulinaemia.

CONCLUSIONS

Several immunosuppressive agents have been used to treat inflammatory eye disease. Since the pathogenesis of these disorders is unknown, the selection of appropriate drugs is mainly empirical. Thus it is mandatory to use the safest drugs initially, not excluding non-steroidal anti-inflammatory drugs. The undesirable side effects of prolonged steroid treatment, particularly in high doses, are well recognized and it is reasonable to resort to cytotoxic drugs in patients threatened with severe visual impairment. Moreover, there are hints that alkylating agents induce long standing remissions consistent with the idea that these drugs may decisively alter the natural history of these disorders. Unfortunately cytotoxic drugs have long term dangers. There is a dearth of properly controlled trials providing a reliable guide to relatively effective and reasonably safe regimes of treatment with steroids, cytotoxic drugs and combinations of these drugs. Enthusiasm for more selective immunosuppressive agents such as cyclosporin is understandable but premature.

ACKNOWLEDGEMENTS

The author would like to express his thanks to Mr Bill Dinning, to the late Mr Harold Jackson and to Mr Jack Kanski for patiently explaining basic ophthalmological truths to a complete amateur. He would also like to thank Mrs Jenny O'Connor for uncomplaining secretarial assistance.

REFERENCES

1. Roitt I. M. *Essential Immunology*, 4th ed. Oxford, Blackwell Scientific, 1980.
2. Wright P. The eye. In: Lachmann P. J. and Peters D. K. (ed.) *Clinical Aspects of Immunology*, 4th ed. Blackwell Scientific, 1982, pp. 1151–8.
3. Niederkorn J. Y. and Streilein J. W. Alloantigens placed into the anterior chamber of the eye induce specific suppression of delayed-type hypersensitivity but normal cytotoxic T lymphocyte and helper T lymphocyte responses. *J. Immunol.* 1983; **131**, 2670–4.
4. Ben Hanan Y., Landshman N., Avni I. et al. Indication for the role of the immune system in the pathogenesis of corneal alkali burns. *Br. J. Ophthalmol.* 1983; **67**, 635–7.
5. Carreras B., Griffin D. E. and Silverstein A. M. Sindbis-virus-induced ocular immunopathology. *Invest. Ophthalmol. Vis. Sci.* 1982; **22**, 571–8.
6. Denman A. M. Viruses and immunopathology. In: Holborow E. J. and Reeves W. G. (ed.) *Immunology in Medicine*, 2nd ed. London, Academic, 1983, pp. 179–202.
7. Nussenblatt R. B., Gery I., Ballintine E. J. et al. Cellular immune responsiveness of uveitis patients to retinal S-antigen. *Am. J. Ophthalmol.* 1980; **89**, 173.
8. Gregerson D. S. and Abrahams I. W. Immunologic and biochemical properties of several retinal proteins bound by antibodies in sera from animals with experimental autoimmune uveitis and uveitis patients. *J. Immunol.* 1983; **131**, 259–64.
9. Wakefield D., Wright J. and Penny R. HLA antigens in uveitis. *Hum. Immunol.* 1983; **7**, 89–93.
10. Onodera T., Toniolo A., Ray U. R. et al. Virus-induced diabetes mellitus XX polyendocrinopathy and autoimmunity. *J. Exp. Med.* 1981; **153**, 1457–73.
11. Satoh J., Prabhakar B. S., Haspel M. V. et al. Human monoclonal autoantibodies that react with multiple endocrine organs. *N. Engl. J. Med.* 1983; **309**, 217–19.
12. Dumonde D. C., Kasp-Grochowska E., Sanders M. D. et al. Anti-retinal autoimmunity and circulating immune complexes in patients with retinal vasculitis. *Lancet* 1983; **2**, 787–92.
13. Garner A., Rahi A. H. S. and Wright J. E. Lymphoproliferative disorders of the orbit: an immunological approach to diagnosis and pathogenesis. *Br. J. Ophthalmol.* 1983; **67**, 561–9.
14. Rees A. J. and Lockwood C. M. Immunosuppressive drugs in clinical practice. In: Lachmann P. J. and Peters D. K. (ed.) *Clinical Aspects of Immunology*, 4th ed. Oxford, Blackwell Scientific, 1982, pp. 507–64.
15. Lewis R. A. and Austen K. F. Mediation of local homeostasis and inflammation by leukotrienes and other mast cell-dependent compounds. *Nature* 1981; **293**, 103–8.
16. Eakins K. E., Whitelocke R. A. F., Bennett A. et al. Prostaglandin-like activity in ocular inflammation. *Br. Med. J.* 1972; **3**, 452–3.
17. Nuki G. Non-steroidal analgesic and anti-inflammatory agents. *Br. Med. J.* 1983; **287**, 39–43.
18. Higgs G. A., Moncada S. and Vane J. R. The mode of action of anti-inflammatory drugs which prevent the peroxidation of arachidonic acid. In: Huskisson E. C. (ed.) *Anti-Rheumatic Drugs*, Praeger, 1983, pp. 11–35.
19. Abelson M. B., Butrus S. I. and Weston J. H. Aspirin therapy in vernal conjunctivitis. *Am. J. Ophthalmol.* 1983; **95**, 502–5.
20. Dennis R. F. and Oh Jang O. Aspirin, cyclophosphamide and dexamethasone effects on experimental secondary herpes simplex uveitis. *Arch. Ophthalmol.* 1979; **97**, 2170–4.
21. Bhattachewrjee P. and Eakins K. E. Inhibition of the prostaglandin synthetase systems in ocular tissues by indomethacin. *Br. J. Pharmacol.* 1974; **50**, 227–30.
22. Keulen de Vos H. C. J., Van Rij G., Renardel J. C. G. et al. Effect of indomethacin in preventing surgically induced miosis. *Br. J. Ophthalmol.* 1983; **67**, 94–6.
23. Reynard M., Riffenburgh R. S. and Maes E. F. Effect of corticosteroid treatment and enucleation on the visual prognosis of sympathetic ophthalmia. *Am. J. Ophthalmol.* 1983; **96**, 290–4.
24. Ansell B. M. and Bywaters E. G. L. Alternate-day corticosteroid therapy in juvenile chronic polyarthritis. *J. Rheumatol.* 1974; **1**, 176–86.
25. Salaman J. R. Steroids and modern immunosuppression. *Br. Med. J.* 1983; **286**, 1373–4.
26. Gaston H., Absolon M. J., Thurtle O. A. et al. Steroid responsiveness in connective tissue diseases. *Br. J. Ophthalmol.* 1983; **67**, 487–90.
27. King J. O., Laver M. C., Fairley K. F. et al. Sensitivity to azathioprine. *Med. J. Aust.* 1972; **2**, 939–41.
28. Farthing M. J. G., Coxon A. Y. and Sheaff P. C. Polyneuritis associated with azathioprine sensitivity reaction. *Br. Med. J.* 1980; **1**, 367.
29. Scott D. G. I., Bacon P. A., Elliott P. J. et al. Systemic vasculitis in a District General Hospital 1972–1980. Clinical and laboratory features, classification and prognosis of 80 cases. *Q. J. Med.* (New Ser.) 1982; **51**, 292–311.
30. Bryant B. M., Jarman M., Ford H. T. et al. Prevention of isophosphamide-induced urathelial toxicity with 2-mercaptoethane sulphonate sodium (mesna) in patients with advanced carcinoma. *Lancet* 1980; **2**, 657–9.
31. Trompeter R. S., Evans P. R. and Barratt T. M. Gonodal function in males treated with limited cyclophosphamide for steroid sensitive nephrotic syndrome. *Pediatric Res.* 1980; **14**, 1007.
32. Fukutani K., Ishida H., Shinohara M. et al. Suppression of spermatogenesis in patients with Behçet's disease treated with cyclophosphamide and colchicine. *Fertility Sterility* 1981; **36**, 76–80.
33. Cohen J., Pinching A. J., Rees A. J. et al. Infection and immunosuppression. *Q. J. Med.* (New Ser.) 1982; **51**, 1–15.
34. Denman A. M. Immunosuppression and the rheumatic diseases. *Ann. Rheum. Dis.* 1982; **41**, Suppl. 1, pp. 3–8.

35. Palmer R. B., Doré C. J. and Denman A. M. Chlorambucil induced chromosome damage to human lymphocytes is dose-dependent and cumulative. *Lancet* 1984; **1**, 246–9.
36. Buriot D., Prieur A. M., Lebranchu Y. et al. Leucémie aigue chez trois enfants atteints d'arthrite chronique juvénile traités par Chlorambucil. *Arch. Fr. Pediat.* 1979; **36**, 592.
37. Kahn M. F., Arlet J., Bloch-Michel H. et al. Leucémies aigues apres traitement par agents cytotoxiques en rhumatologie. *Nouv. Presse Med.* 1979; **8**, 1393–7.
38. Kinlen L. J., Sheil A. G. R. and Doll R. Collaborative United Kingdom/Australasian study of cancer in patients treated with immunosuppressive drugs. *Br. Med. J.* 1979; **2**, 1461–6.
39. Kinlen L. J., Peto J., Doll R. et al. Cancer in patients treated with immunosuppressive drugs. *Br. Med. J.* 1981; **282**, 474.
40. Palmer R. B. and Denman A. M. Malignancies induced by chlorambucil. *Cancer Treatment Rev.* 1984; **11**, 121–9.
41. Muraguchi A., Butler J. L., Kehrl J. H. et al. Selective suppression of an early step in human B cell activation by cyclosporin A. *J. Exp. Med.* 1983; **158**, 690–702.
42. Glazier A., Tutshka P. J., Farmer E. R. et al. Graft-versus-host disease in cyclosporin A-treated rats after syngeneic and autologous bone marrow reconstitution. *J. Exp. Med.* 1983; **158**, 1–8.
43. Bell T. A. G., Easty D. L. and McCullagh K. G. A placebo-controlled blind trial of cyclosporin-A in prevention of corneal graft rejection in rabbits. *Br. J. Ophthalmol.* 1982; **66**, 303–8.
44. Hunter P. A., Garner A., Wilhelmus K. R. et al. Corneal graft rejection: a new rabbit model and cyclospirin A. *Br. J. Ophthalmol.* 1982; **66**, 292–302.
45. Nussenblatt R. B., Rodrigues M. M., Wacker W. B. et al. Cyclosporin A inhibition of experimental autoimmune uveitis in Lewis rats. *J. Clin. Invest.* 1981; **67**, 1228–31.
46. Nussenblatt R. B., Salinas-Carmona M., Waksman B. H. et al. Cyclosporin A: alterations of the cellular immune response in S-antigen-induced experimental autoimmune uveitis. *Int. Arch. Allergy Appl. Immunol.* 1983; **70**, 289–94.
47. Van Bekkum D. W. and Wagemaker G. Bone marrow transplantation and cyclosporin. *Acuta Sandoz* 4, 1983.
48. Mussenblatt R N. Effectiveness of cyclosporin on sight-threatening endogenous uveitis. In: Schindler R. (ed.), *Cyclosporin in Autoimmune Diseases*. Berlin, Springer-Verlag, 1985, pp. 133–6.
49. Ben Ezra D., Brodsky M., Pe'er J. et al. Cyclosporin (Cy A) versus conventional therapy in Behçet's disease: preliminary observations of a masked study. In: Schindler R. (ed.), *Cyclosporin in Autoimmune Diseases*. Berlin, Springer-Verlag, 1985, pp. 133–6.
50. Myers B. D., Ross J., Newton L. et al. Cyclosporin-associated chronic nephropathy. *N. Engl. J. Med.* 1984, **311**, 699–705.
51. Mihatsh M. J., Thiel G. and Ruffel B. Cyclosporin-associated nephropathy. In: Schindler R. (ed.) *Cyclosporin in Autoimmune Diseases*. Berlin, Springer-Verlag, 1985, pp. 133–6.
52. Watson P. G. The nature and treatment of scleral inflammation. *Trans. Ophthalmol. Soc. UK* 1982; **102**, 257–81.
53. Duncker G., Beigel A. and Lehmann H. Wegenersche Granulomatose: okuläre Manifestationen, Diagnose und Therapie. *Klin. Mbl. Augenheilk.* 1982; **181**, 184–7.
54. Abdalla M. I. and Bahgat N. E. Long-lasting remission of Behçet's disease after chlorambucil therapy. *Br. J. Ophthalmol.* 1973; **57**, 706–11.
55. Dinning W. J. and Perkins E. S. Immunosuppressives in uveitis: a preliminary report of experience with chlorambucil. *Br. J. Ophthalmol.* 1975; **59**, 397–403.
56. Bonnet J. Bilan des immuno-dépresseurs dans le traitement du syndrome de Behçet. *Ann. Ther. et Clin. Ophthalmol.* 1981; **32**, 89–111.
57. Niessen F., Campinchi R. and Bloch-Michel E. Intéret et complications des thérapeutiques immunosuppressives dans les uvéites de la maladie de Behçet ou d'autre origine A propos de 40 cas. *J. Fr. Ophthalmol.* 1982; **5**, 407–416.
58. Kanski J. J. and Ansell B. M. Arthritis and uveitis. In: Wybar K. and Taylor D. (ed.) *Pediatric Ophthalmology*. New York, Marcel Dekker, 1983, pp. 407–12.
59. Mertin J., Rudge P., Kremer M. et al. Double-blind controlled trial of immunosuppression in the treatment of multiple sclerosis: final report. *Lancet* 1982; **2**, 351–4.
60. Hall J. M. and Pribnow J. F. The effect of cyclophosphamide on a secondary ocular immune response in rabbits. *Adv. Exp. Med. Biol.* 1979; **121**, 381–8.
61. Blumenkranz M. S., Ophir A., Claflin A. J. et al. Fluorouracil for the treatment of massive periretinal proliferation. *Am. J. Ophthalmol.* 1982; **94**, 458–67.
62. Hollingworth P., De Vere-Tyndall A., Ansell B. M. et al. Intensive immunosuppression versus prednisolone in the treatment of connective tissue diseases. *Ann. Rheum. Dis.* 1982; **41**, 557–62.
63. Bonnet J. Immunodépresseurs et syndrome de Behçet bilan à long terme. *J. Fr. Ophthalmol.* 1981; **4**, 455–64.
64. Knight S. C. Control of lymphocyte stimulation *in vitro* 'help' and 'suppression' in the light of lymphoid population dynamics. *J. Immunol. Methods* 1982; **50**, 51–63.
65. De Vere-Tyndall A., Knight K., Burman S. et al. Lymphocyte responses in juvenile chronic arthritis and Behçet's disease – cell number requirements and effects of glucocorticosteroid therapy. *Clin. Exp. Immunol.* 1982; **50**, 541–8.
66. Nussenblatt R. B., Salinas-Carmona M., Leake W. et al. T-lymphocyte subsets in uveitis. *Am. J. Ophthalmol.* 1983; **95**, 614–21.
67. Schooley R. T., Hirsch M. S., Colvin R. B. et al. Associations of herpes virus infections with T-lymphocyte-subset alterations, glomerulopathy, and opportunistic infections after renal transplantation. *New Engl. J. Med.* 1983; **308**, 307–13.
68. Bast R. C. jun., Reinherz E. L., Maver C. et al. Contrasting effects of cyclophosphamide and prednisolone on the phenotype of human peripheral blood leukocytes. *Clin. Immunol. Immunopathol.* 1983; **28**, 101–14.

Chapter 21

Systemic Diseases and the Eye

Connective Tissue Disease

J. Williamson

KERATOCONJUNCTIVITIS SICCA

By far the most common eye complication of connective tissue disease is keratoconjunctivitis sicca (KCS).

Definition

KCS is a condition in which there is evidence of inadequate tear film coverage of the conjunctiva and on occasion of the cornea. Under-protection results from reduced or defective tear component production in total or in part. The normal pre-corneal tear film consists of three layers; (a) innermost mucous; (b) middle lacrimal secretion; and (c) outermost oily, probably in the main from Meibomian glands. Defects in any of these may lead to drying of the eye and to a form of KCS.

When considering the significance of dry eyes in connective tissue disease, we must be aware of its incidence and associations in the 'normal' population.

Incidence

The most common form of KCS results from progressive destruction of the lacrimal and accessory lacrimal glands with increasing age.[1,2] The incidence in an otherwise healthy population rises from virtually zero at age 50 to 16 per cent at 80, regardless of the patient's sex.[3]

KCS also occurs unrelated to age in what is now classified as primary Sjögren's syndrome, which includes the well-known sicca syndrome of dry eyes and dry mouth. This is a condition in which the patient does not have evidence of any general systemic disease, but has all the other features associated with the KCS seen in connective tissue diseases. Primary Sjögren's syndrome also encompasses a variety of ocular diseases believed to derive their appearance from fundamental defects in the tear construction. The incidence of primary Sjögren's syndrome in the 'normal' population is unknown.

Secondary Sjögren's syndrome is now the term used to describe keratoconjunctivitis sicca and/or xerostomia found in patients suffering from a connective tissue disease (CTD), usually adult rheumatoid arthritis and more rarely systemic lupus erythematosis, polymyositis, progressive systemic sclerosis or polyarteritis nodosa. According to some authorities, almost three times as many females are affected as males, though opinion on this is divided. KCS occurs in 10–15 per cent of patients suffering from adult rheumatoid arthritis. Its incidence in the other CTDs is so low as to be meaningless in terms of aetiological or prognostic significance.[4,5] Moreover, KCS is also reported in some patients with organ specific auto-immune disease, especially primary biliary cirrhosis and Hashimoto's thyroiditis.

Diagnosis of KCS

There is no single clinical or laboratory test that clinches the diagnosis of KCS. *Table* I shows the range of investigations in current use. These have been arranged in order of the frequency with which they are used.

Questionnaires/Symptoms

The most common symptoms in KCS are grittiness (sometimes described as sandiness in the eyes or scratchiness), tired eyes and itch. Although patients may volunteer dryness as a symptom it is not often directly mentioned, rather 'I can't shed a tear' or 'I feel my eyes are about to water, but they never do'.

Questionnaires are based and weighted on all symptoms and are useful in large surveys, e.g. of a whole population or of all patients attending a centre for rheumatic disease. They should be designed to over-diagnose KCS so that all suspected patients are called for clinical evaluation.

Rose Bengal Dye

One drop of a 1 per cent solution of rose bengal dye instilled into the lower fornix will result in staining of the interpalpebral conjunctiva in 80 per cent of patients suffering from KCS. Only in the minority of patients is the lower third, or even less commonly other parts of the cornea, also stained. Rose bengal is taken up by dead or dying cells and by mucus.

Table I. Diagnostic tests for KCS

	Advantages	Disadvantages
Questionnaires	Non-invasive Over-diagnosis	Ideal questionnaire not yet developed – open to subjective interpretation
Rose bengal dye	Easily interpreted Cheap Simple to use	May cause discomfort
Schirmer tear test	Cheap Simple to use	Unreliable unless a forced test is used Tests reflex lacrimation only
Tear film break up time	Cheap	Difficult to interpret
Impression cytology	Simple to perform	Requires skilled interpretation – open to statistical errors
Conjunctival biopsy	Simple to perform	Requires skilled interpretation. Only performed in research centres
Lacrimal gland biopsy	Extremely accurate	Gland obtainable in only 50% of attempted biopsies. Used in research only
Lysozyme activity	Fairly accurate Easy to perform	Requires enthusiastic bacteriological back up. Time consuming. Rarely performed.

The pattern of staining varies from fine punctate surface conjunctival epithelial to coarse conglomerate, building up to a wedge-shaped area, base towards the limbus (Sjögren's original blunderbuss description). The cornea likewise may demonstrate these patterns and when mucus is attached to the damaged surface cells a filamentous appearance is produced. Plaques of mucus and collections of desquamated epithelial cells in the tear film may be seen in severely affected patients.

Many attempts have been made to grade the severity of the disease according to the extent of staining. However, these have the inherent disadvantage of subjectivity and are only of limited use in therapeutic trials. The biomicroscopic appearances do not always match the patient's symptoms which may indeed be out of all proportion to the severity of the staining. Finally, a rose bengal dye should not be used frequently in patients in whom the diagnosis of KCS has already been made. The discomfort that often follows its use may last for several days and cause great distress.

Schirmer Tear Test

Standardized filter papers (e.g. Contactisol Inc., New York) may be hooked into the lower fornices for 5 min to establish whether enough tear products exist to wet them to a length of 15 mm. This is certainly cheap and simple and estimates the tear flow under minimum stimulation. Some patients are so imperturbable that they appear to produce very few tears during this test, and so there is a tendency for over-diagnosis. If 10 per cent ammonia is inhaled over the 5 min period then a better idea of the ability to produce reflex lacrimation is obtained. This test of course does not measure KCS produced by relative deficiencies in the tear film. Nevertheless, it is extremely useful especially in a busy clinic; wetting below 10 mm is regarded as diagnostic, wetting between 10 and 15 mm as suspicious.

Tear Film Break Up Time (BUT)

Enormous effort and a great deal of time have been spent in measuring the corneal tear film break up time. The inaccuracies of the methods are still so great that we can only generalize about the results. When the eyes are kept open for a unit of time 'dry spots' appear on the cornea due to separation of the surface of the corneal tear film. (It is claimed by some authors that the film separates totally to the corneal epithelium.) The speed with which this occurs is greatly increased in dry eye syndromes.[7,8] However, accurate reproducibility of results is not yet possible. Fluorescein dye is instilled and the break up of the tear film monitored and timed as the dye spreads apart. However, recently it has been shown that the dye itself causes an increased rate of break up. Currently a technique is being developed that uses a grid system projected on to the cornea for direct viewing of the unstained tear film. It will be interesting to see whether this proves more accurate and reproducible.[9]

Impression Cytology

Standardized filter paper plaques pressed on to the conjunctival surface detach surface cells for microscopic examination. In the dry eye flattening and irregularity of surface cells and paucity of goblet cells are diagnostic features. Detailed descriptions of alterations with and between the cells have also been noted and will provide research material for many years.

This again is a simple technique, but there is a caveat. It is in the doubtful cases of KCS that impression cytology should be useful in establishing a diagnosis. However, it is impossible to standardize the pressure applied to the filter piece and the harder the pressure is applied the more likely it is for cells to spread out and for goblet cells to be emptied and thus not counted. Furthermore, the count of cells applies to one plane only; goblet cells lying deeper in the same area than their fellows may be missed. Nevertheless, impression cytology tells us that the conjunctival surface in KCS develops stratification and paucity of goblet cells.[10]

Conjunctival Biopsy

Biopsy of interpalpebral conjunctiva is simple to perform and gives excellent results. Interpretation of the specimen requires skilled histology and may be time consuming. Nonetheless, it can be the only way to determine the difference between true KCS and early Steven–Johnson's syndrome or pemphygoid. Details of the microscopy are set out below.[11]

Lacrimal Gland Biopsy

This is definitely a research technique. The biopsy is obtained under local anaesthesia following an incision of skin and muscle of the upper eyelid through the periorbital membrane close to the superotemporal edge of the bony orbit. Toothed forceps have to be inserted 'blind' into the area of the gland and it is not surprising that in 50 per cent of cases orbital fat is all that is obtained. It is, therefore, unacceptable as a routine diagnostic procedure but the material examined in the one study recorded to date provided a clear picture of progression of KCS in rheumatoid arthritis – secondary Sjögren's syndrome (*see below*)[1]

Lysozyme Activity

In KCS the quantity of lysozyme and lactoferrin enzymatic activity is progressively reduced. Growth of the micrococcus luteus is inhibited by lysozyme and therefore by normal tears. The bacteria flourish in the presence of tears from KCS patients deficient in enzyme activity. It is a pity that this investigation is not more universal; as with the others it has some inherent defects. 'Collected' tears are necessary and the drier the eye the more difficult it is to obtain a representative sample. Paradoxically, profuse tearing may also result in a fluid relatively scarce in enzyme activity.[12–14]

Aetiology

It is not within the remit of this chapter to discuss all possible factors that can result in KCS. To do this we would have to delineate all the theories of causation of connective tissue disease.[4,5]

The influence of histocompatibility antigens and the presence of small molecular weight ribonucleo proteins on the severity of secondary Sjögren's and the sicca syndrome form of primary Sjögren's is interesting. When HLA antigens were first discovered it was not realized that a Pandora's Box had been opened. Opinions of their relative importance change constantly, but at least there is the excitement of a dynamic field of investigation.[15] At the moment, it appears that multiple HLA-D region alloantigens and specifically MT_2 may be the strongest major histocompatibility complex determinant for the sicca syndrome/secondary Sjögren's syndrome. It seems that HLA-DR3 and DR2 mediate the RO/La antibody responses (ribonucleo proteins) characteristic of the more severe forms of the disease. The clinical expression of secondary Sjögren's syndrome and the sicca syndrome appears to result from the complex genetic interplay of the multiple HLA-D region factors.[16] Patients with secondary Sjögren's syndrome are generally 50–60 years old and, like SLE sufferers, show a wider range of autoimmune phenomena than any other disease. In addition to the feature of their CTD, they have a high prevalence of oesophagitis, gastritis, primary biliary cirrhosis and hepatitis. Conversely, patients with primary biliary cirrhosis have higher incidence of KCS than expected and this is reflected in the high incidence of ribonucleo proteins in this group of patients. Moreover, secondary Sjögren's syndrome patients have more than their share of renal tubular defects, Raynaud's phenomenon (20 per cent), purpura, normocytic normochromic anaemia (50 per cent) and arteritis. In brief, secondary Sjögren's syndrome patients tend to have a severe form of rheumatoid arthritis and a multiplicity of complications.[4,5]

Pathology of KCS

Lacrimal Gland – Age Changes

Until recently it was thought that the lacrimal gland underwent a quiet, non-inflammatory involutionary sclerosis with increasing acinar and duct atrophy and replacement with fibrous tissue.[1] It had also been noted that the mucus producing sections of the lacrimal gland stained neutral in youth, stained neutral and acid in middle age, and not only became less evident but stained almost entirely acid in old age.[17] It seemed therefore that the gland not only underwent involution but that the type and form of mucus production was somehow altered with age. However, Damato et al.[2] re-interpreted Williamson's specimens[1] and added considerable fresh material of their own. In a thoughtful study they conclude that bouts of periductal inflammation (*Plate* XVI*a*) occur at all stages in life and result in obliteration of the nutrient blood vessels (*Plate* XVI*b*). This leads to acinar and duct atrophy and on occasion to blockage of the duct, which may develop cystic dilatation (*Plate* XVI*c*). Progressively more of the gland is replaced and atrophies and in due course, if there is sufficient lacrimal fluid depletion, the patient develops age-related KCS. If their interpretation is correct it opens up a whole new field of investigation into the ageing process, at least in tissues of this nature.

Secondary Sjögren's Syndrome and the Sicca Syndrome

The histology in these conditions is well established. Following bouts of severe chronic inflammatory infiltration up to the point of lymphoid follicle formation (*Plate* XVId) the gland is progressively destroyed and replaced with fibrous tissue. It is as though it were an exaggeration and acceleration of the ageing process.[1]

Primary Sjögren's Syndrome other than Sicca Syndrome

Since this 'disorder' contains a variety of conditions all leading from or to an external eye dryness it is to be expected that in many instances the lacrimal gland will be normal. No systematic studies of the lacrimal gland histology have been published to date.

Conjunctival Pathology

Age Changes

The conjunctival epithelium gradually loses its goblet cells and patches of hyperplasia alternate with atrophy.

Secondary Sjögren's Syndrome and Sicca Syndrome

In contrast, the epithelium in these conditions becomes stratified and the surface microplicae depleted and distorted[11] (*Figs.* 1, 2). The superficial layer is mechanically separated, gradually the goblet cells vanish and some show hyaline degeneration (*Plate* XVIe).

Management of KCS

Great efforts are being made to find an ideal replacement for natural tears. Physicists, biochemists and physicians are beavering away measuring surface tension factors, protein content, enzyme activity, stability of artificial tears and so on.[18-20] Since the normal tear film has three layers of different constituents, no one bottle will ever contain a solution capable of replacing the norm.

The present principles of management may be considered under the following headings:

Systemic Therapy

There is no evidence to show that the systemic therapy supplied to secondary Sjögren's syndrome patients consistently improves ocular symptoms and

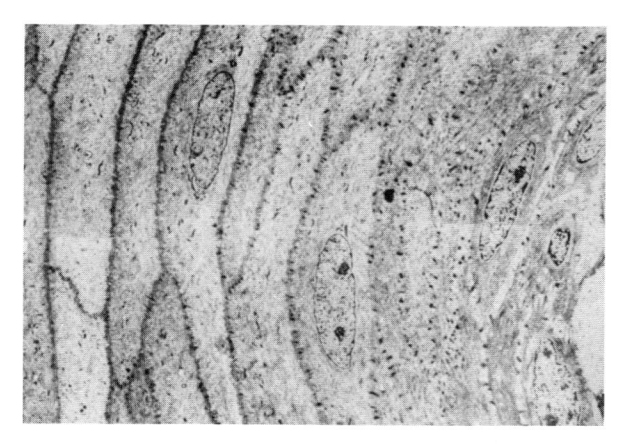

Fig. 1. Electronmicroscopic picture of stratification of the conjunctiva in secondary Sjögren's syndrome.

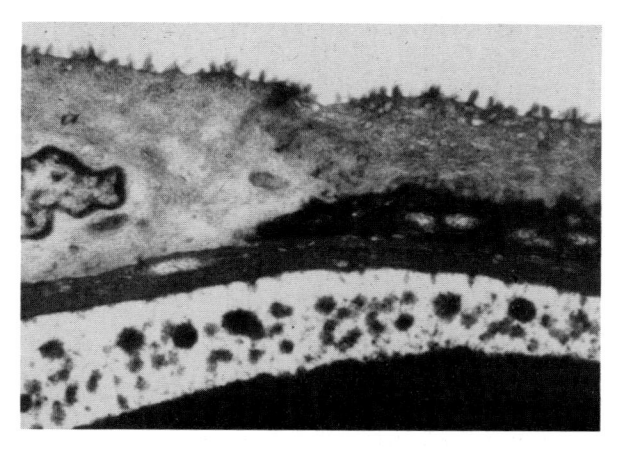

Fig. 2. Electronmicroscopic picture of depleted microplicae on the surface of secondary Sjögren's syndrome. Hyaline degeneration of goblet cell.

signs. In the extremely rare cases in which the patient presents with swollen lacrimal glands, systemic steroids reduce the swelling and produce temporary relief.

Replacement Therapy

The primary reason for the dry eye in secondary Sjögren's syndrome, sicca syndrome, and in the ageing eye is depletion of lacrimal fluid. Most replacement fluids are based on Barrie Jones' Sixth Formula of a dilute alkaline solution of carboxymethyl cellulose, and provided these or similar solutions are instilled regularly and religiously, and especially during spells when the patient is completely asymptomatic, 90 per cent of patients will experience no lasting complications; 50 per cent will require no further treatment. Reservoirs for these artificial tears have been attached to spectacle frames, drip feeding the fluid mechanically or by a pump into the lower fornix. Although they have been around for several years, however, they do not seem to have gained universal approval. Because of hand deformities many severe rheumatoid patients are unable to instil eye drops even when they are packaged in touch-sensitive bottles. Slow release capsules placed in the lower fornix once daily are occasionally useful, although as the capsule finally disintegrates it may cause discomfort and extra artificial tear drops should be inserted at the time (6–8 h after insertion of the capsule). Isosmotic solutions are currently in preparation and are in clinical trials at the time of writing. The results are therefore not to hand, but research experience would suggest that an isosmotic solution should be more suitable as a tear replacement than the existing solutions.

Mucus dispersal

Alteration in the type of 'mucus' and reduction in its total production results from changes in the lacrimal gland and the disappearance of the conjunctival goblet cells (*see above*). In all forms of KCS excess of stringy mucus may collect, causing considerable distress. Five per cent normal acetyl cysteine breaks the sulphylhydryl bonds in the mucoproteins converting tenacious mucus into a harmless soluble solution. Mucus seen in the tear film, as filaments on the cornea or as a ropey mass in the lower fornix, calls for the immediate use of acetyl cysteine drops.

Conservation of Tears

Tear conservation may be achieved by obliteration of both nasolacrimal puncta and ducts, upper and lower. Unless the ducts are also closed the puncta will reopen within 2–3 months. The operation is readily performed under local anaesthesia by passing a diathermy probe along the full length of the canaliculus. The tip of the probe is activated by a current of 50 mA for 5–10 s; when the overlying skin blanches the probe is slowly withdrawn and finally the punctum is sealed. Choice of patients suitable for this procedure can be difficult. The following criteria are helpful:
1. Poor response to replacement therapy for a period of more than one year.
2. Repeated build up of mucus.
3. Recurrent corneal complications – *see below*.
4. Evidence of at least some residual lacrimation using a forced Schirmer tear test.

If these guidelines are followed, 70 per cent of patients so treated benefit over the ensuing 5 years.

Infection

Thirty per cent of secondary Sjögren's syndrome patients who have never been treated for KCS present with a blepharitis, the most common infective form of which is due to *Staphylococcus aureus*. Possible bacterial, viral or fungal infection remain a long term problem in the management of all KCS patients and appropriate steps are required.

Complications

Complications of a worrying nature fortunately only arise in 10 per cent of all secondary Sjögren's syndrome patients, possibly more often in the sicca syndrome, certainly less in the KCS of the aged and variably according to the associated disease in other forms of primary Sjögren's syndrome. Corneal erosions may recur without apparent reason, perhaps associated with excessive drying of patches of the corneal surface. Rarely, they penetrate and are deep enough to perforate. There is no satisfactory management but long term wear contact bandage lenses should be tried while keeping a careful watch for superimposed infection. A corneal graft will only function for 6 months at best when the centre of the graft will perforate, as did the recipient cornea. Occasionally progressive thinning of the cornea starts close to the limbus and encircles the cornea leaving the appearance of the 'contact lens cornea'. It is surprising how may years these patients' eyes continue to function without perforation. If leakage is thought to be eminent a bandage contact lens should be applied.

Symblepharon due to progressive conjunctival and subconjunctival contracture is another rare complication. Care should be taken to distinguish the cause of the 'adhesions' from pemphygoid since in the latter surgical intervention makes matters worse. The symblepharon of secondary Sjögren's syndrome and the sicca syndrome respond well in the early stages to simple incision followed by a month of lubrication with ointment such as Lacrilube or Tanderil.

UVEITIS

Anterior uveitis – inflammation in the iris or ciliary body – is a complication of connective tissue disease in children and young adults. It is not a definitive feature of rheumatoid arthritis except as a complication of scleritis.

Adult Population

Ankylosing Spondylitis, Reiter's Syndrome

Incidence

Between 10 and 15 per cent of patients suffering from ankylosing spondylitis develop anterior uveitis. The longer a patient has had this connective tissue disease, the higher are his chances of acquiring uveitis. The prevalence in Reiter's syndrome is unknown because of the difficulty in standardizing the diagnosis of this syndrome. Strictly applied, the term should be used only in patients who have had urethritis, conjunctivitis and, in the main, an attack of pauci-articular arthritis. Even so, the uveitis of ankylosing spondylitis and Reiter's syndrome is similar in that it is usually benign, responds well to treatment and is unrelated to the degree of activity of the systemic disease. However, onset is variable and the effect on vision is occasionally disastrous.

Aetiology

The presence of HLA-B27 has been shown in some 90 per cent of patients with ankylosing spondylitis and in 75 per cent with Reiter's syndrome. Thirty per cent of the group studied developed anterior uveitis. Moreover, over 50 per cent first degree relatives of the ankylosing spondylitis patients had HLA-B27 antigens. However, in a group of females with uveitis and no connective tissue disease, HLA-B27 was demonstrable in 80 per cent. This may mean that HLA-B27 in young men gives a predilection for ankylosing spondylitis and Reiter's syndrome and a one in three risk of uveitis as a complication. In young women HLA-B27 may predispose to uveitis unaccompanied by a connective tissue disease. In more recent studies the significance of HLA-B27 in ankylosing spondylitis is not quite so strong but still highly relevant.[21]

Ulcerative Colitis

HLA-B27 has been found in 65 per cent of patients suffering from ulcerative colitis, peripheral joint disease or sacro-ileitis but in only 3 per cent of patients without arthropathy. Significantly 10–20 per cent of patients with inflammatory bowel disease and ankylosing spondylitis or peripheral joint disease develop anterior uveitis, compared with less than one per cent of those free of joint problems.

Psoriasis/Psoriatic Arthropathy

When the prevalence of HLA-B27 is shown to be high in a series of patients with psoriasis they either have or are likely to acquire a peripheral arthropathy or spondylitis. In some studies anterior uveitis has been unexpectedly frequent in classic psoriatic arthritis.

Systemic Lupus Erythematosis (SLE)

Anterior uveitis is reported in 0·8 per cent of large series of patients with SLE but there is no method of distinguishing any difference between the SLE sufferers with uveitis from those without this eye complication.

Children

Incidence

If an apparently healthy child develops anterior uveitis the anti-nuclear antibody (ANA) should be determined and a search for juvenile rheumatoid arthritis instigated. Between 2 and 11 per cent of juvenile rheumatoid arthritic children develop anterior uveitis. This may ante-date the arthritis by several years and in such circumstances detection of antinuclear antibodies should alert the physician to the possible development of the arthritis at a later stage.

Aetiology

Antinuclear antibodies are present in 90 per cent of children with chronic polyarthritis and anterior uveitis, but in only 30 per cent of juvenile rheumatoid arthritis patients with no eye disease. In the pathogenesis of juvenile rheumatoid arthritis it would appear that there is a disequilibrium between HLA-DR (especially DR3) on the one hand, and C43Q0 and BPF1 on the other. Subgroups of patients with uveitis cannot be distinguished on this basis from those without eye disease. Thus we still have to depend on the presence of ANA as a marker for uveitis. In the older children with eye disease the prevalence of HLA-B27 is increased.[22]

Management

In general, the ocular prognosis is poorer the younger the age of onset, which is most often, but not exclusively, in girls around 7 years of age. Older children, often boys, develop a milder uveitis but they may continue into young adult life with ileitis and peripheral arthritis. Vigorous management with topical steroids and mydriatics is mandatory and is extremely effective in the older age group. However, recurrences are frequent and in the severe form systemic steroids with all their attendant complications may have to be prescribed. In desperate cases, cyclophosphamide has been successful in stemming the destructive effect of repeated attacks. However, in some children there seems to be no let up in the steady downhill course. Repeated bouts of anterior uveitis in arthritic children cause severe visual loss in 50 per cent, cataract being the most common cause of poor vision. Extraction of the lens opacities by emulsification and suction techniques is less traumatizing than the former ab-externo extracapsular expression, but the results are frequently disappointing. Continued pan-uveitis, vitreous destruction and, on occasion, detachment of the retina follow. Management of secondary glaucoma resulting from blockage of, or damage to, the trabecular meshwork is more often than not unsatisfactory.

Interpalpebral band-shaped keratopathy is a sign of severe visual loss following prolonged recurrent uveitis. Calcium salts are deposited initially in the subepithelium close to the limbus. Eventually they spread throughout the corneal layers and adjacent conjunctiva. Removal of the corneal epithelium and sodium versenate chelation can restore temporary clarity to the cornea when the salts are still superficial. Eventually it is ineffective.

MISCELLANEOUS COMPLICATIONS IN CONNECTIVE TISSUE DISEASE

As expected, since CTD implies involvement of tissues from all embryological origins, it is not surprising to find a bewildering variety of manifestations of connective tissue disease in the eye. Other than those mentioned above, however, these are all quite rare and may be a complication of the spread of the disease rather than a specific pointer to it. *Table* II lists the more common, but still rare, complications.

To date there are only two drugs indisputably proved to cause ocular complications.

Steroid therapy at a level of 15 mg prednisolone per day over 2 years produces posterior subcapsular cataracts in 20 per cent of patients. Children may be more susceptible. Currently these levels are rarely used in connective tissue disease – lower levels carry lower risk, e.g. 5 per cent at 10–15 mg daily over 2 years.

Chloroquine – but not necessarily its derivatives – may cause Bull's eye maculopathy or even a peri-

Table II. Some more common complications of connective tissue disease

CTD	Complications	Comment
Systemic lupus and progressive systemic sclerosis	'Cytoid' bodies	Non specific, but diagnostic
	Unilateral proptosis	Exclude disthyroid disease, tumour, pseudo tumour and intracranial lesions
	Optic neuritis	Responds to systemic steroids
	Retinal arteriolar/venular occlusions	
	Non-specific keratitis	Chronic relatively benign
Progressive systemic sclerosis	Upper lid and fornix shortening	
	Lagophthalmos	
	Atrophy dilator pupillae and iris stroma	Exclude uveitis
Polymyositis, dermatomyositis	Heliotrope discoloration upper lids	
	Extra-ocular myopathy	2 per cent polymyositis
Polyarteritis	Sectional retinal and/or choroidal perivasculitis	<20 per cent untreated cases

IATROGENIC DISEASE

The principles of management of connective tissue disease depend on the employment of first line drugs that reduce pain and inflammation and second line drugs that, hopefully, tackle the fundamental problems causing the disease. Since none is totally effective a wide armoury is employed; from time to time reports of presumed ocular complications appear. Difficulties arise in determining the validity of these side effects, (*a*) due to the multiplicity of factors involved in individual cases – not least of which is the polypharmacy the patient requires, and (*b*) the age group involved, particularly in relation to macular disease. In the latter case most of the patients are in an age group in which macular disease may present spontaneously.

pheral retinopathy and corneal deposits. As in the case of steroids, the doses known to have resulted in maculopathy are infrequently prescribed, 250 mg daily for 7 months (*Plate* XVI*f*).

Individual susceptibility is a major feature in the development of drug complications and as yet there is no way of identifying those at risk.

Steroid cataract is not a worry in its early stages and treatment can be continued. Maculopathy is sight destroying; the chloroquine should be discontinued.

ACKNOWLEDGEMENTS

Colour plates XVI*a*, *b* and *c* are reproduced by kind permission of B. E. Damato et al. and the *British Journal of Ophthalmology*.

REFERENCES

1. Williamson J., Gibson A. A. M., Wilson T. et al. Histology of the lacrimal gland in keratoconjunctivitis sicca. *Br. J. Ophthalmol.* 1973; **57,** 852–8.
2. Damato B. E., Allan D., Murray S. B. et al. Senile atrophy of the human lacrimal gland: the contribution of chronic inflammatory disease. *Br. J. Ophthalmol.* 1984; **68,** 674–85.
3. Whaley K., Williamson J., Wilson T. et al. Sjögren's syndrome and auto-immunity in a geriatric population. *Age Ageing* 1972; **1,** 197–206.
4. Bloch J. H. J., Buchanan W. W., Wohl M. J. et al. Sjögren's syndrome: a clinical, pathological and serological study of 62 cases. *Medicine (Balt.)* 1965; **44,** 187–231.
5. Forestot J. Z., Forestot S. L., Greer R. O. et al. The incidence of Sjögren's sicca complex in a population of patients with keratoconjunctivitis sicca. *Arthritis Rheum.* 1982; **25,** 156–60.

6. Whaley K., Goudie R. B., Williamson J. et al. Liver disease in Sjögren's syndrome and rheumatoid arthritis. *Lancet* 1970; **1,** 861.
7. Norn M. S. Tear secretion in normal eyes estimated by a new method – the lacrimal streak dilution test. *Acta Ophthalmol.* 1965; **43,** 567–73.
8. Stodmeister R., Christ T. and Gaus W. The influence of cut off filter on the tear film break-up time (German). *Klin. Monatsbl. Augenheilkd.* 1984; **184,** 121–4.
9. Bron A. Personal communication, 1984.
10. Nelson J. D., Havener V. R. and Cameron J. D. Cellulose acetate impressions of ocular surface. *Arch. Ophthalmol.* 1983; **101,** 1869–72.
11. Abdel-Khalek L. M. R., Williamson J. and Lee W. R. Morphological changes in the human conjunctival epithelium. 1. In the normal elderly population. *Br. J. Ophthalmol.* 1978; **62,** 792–806.
12. McGill J. I., Liakos G. M., Goulding N. et al. Normal tear protein profiles and age related changes. *Br. J. Ophthalmol.* 1984; **68,** 316–20.
13. Mackie I. A. and Seal D. V. Diagnostic implications of tear protein profiles. *Br. J. Ophthalmol.* 1984; **68,** 321–4.
14. McGill J. I., Liakos G., Seal D. et al. Tear film changes in health and dry eye conditions. *Trans. Ophthalmol. Soc. UK* 1983: **103,** 313–17.
15. Van Rood J. J. Heberden oration: HLA as regulator. *Ann. Rheum. Dis.* 1984; **43,** 665–72.
16. Wilson R. W., Provost T. T., Bias W. B. et al. Sjögren's syndrome: influence of multiple HLA-D region alloantigens on clinical and serological expression. *Arthritis Rheum.* 1984; **27,** 1245–53.
17. Murray S. B., Lee W. R. and Williamson J. Ageing changes in the human lacrimal gland – a histological study. *J. Clin. Exp. Gerontol.* 1981; **3,** 1–27.
18. Coles W. H. and Jaros P. A. Dynamics of ocular surface pH. *Br. J. Ophthalmol.* 1984; **68,** 549–52.
19. Inada K., Baba H. and Okamura R. Studies on human tear proteins; analysis of tears from diseased eyes and detection of secretory sites of tear proteins. *Acta. Soc. Ophthalmol. (Jpn)* 1983; **87,** 1187–91.
20. Marner K. and Prause J. V. A comparative clinical study of tear substitutes in normal subjects and in patients with KCS. *Acta Ophthalmol. (Kbh.)* 1984; **62,** 91–5.
21. Beckingsale A. B., Davies J., Gibson J. M. et al. Klebsiella and acute anterior uveitis. *Br. J. Ophthalmol.* 1984; **68,** 741–5.
22. Arnaiz-Villena A., Comez-Reino J. J., Gamir M. L. et al. DR, C4 and BF allotypes in juvenile rheumatoid arthritis. *Arthritis Rheum.* 1984; **27,** 1281–5.

Carotid Artery Disease and Amaurosis Fugax

R. W. Ross Russell

EMBOLIC AMAUROSIS FUGAX

Uniocular amaurosis fugax is a symptom of transient ocular ischaemia which may affect the retina, the choroid or both. The patient experiences abrupt painless loss of vision lasting a few minutes and recovering rapidly without residual deficit. The loss of vision is often described as a shutter coming downwards or upwards over one eye, and it may sometimes spare the upper or lower half of the visual field.

There are a number of possible causes of reduced ocular perfusion (*see Table* I) but the majority of attacks are due to retinal embolism. The evidence of this may be summarized as follows:

1. The attacks are of very rapid onset consistent with sudden blockage of an artery.
2. The type of visual field loss may suggest occlusion of either the upper or lower retinal artery (upper and lower altitudinal hemianopia).
3. A source of embolism may often be found in the internal carotid artery on the same side.
4. Emboli may sometimes be seen in transit through the circulation during an attack (platelets) or impacted subsequently in the retinal arteries (cholesterol) (*Fig.* 1, Plate XVIIa).
5. Amaurosis fugax is frequently associated with stenosis of the internal carotid artery and the attacks usually cease when occlusion is complete (*Fig.* 2).
6. The attacks may respond to anti-thrombotic treatment.

Emboli may be of varying types. Platelet emboli (*Fig.* 1) resemble white plugs and pass rapidly

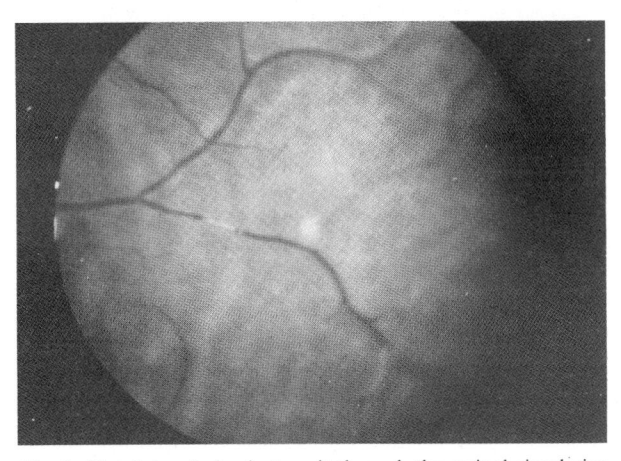

Fig. 1. Platelet embolus in transit through the retinal circulation during an attack of amaurosis fugax.

through the retinal circulation. They are usually derived from mural thrombus in the carotid artery or from an abnormal cardiac valve (e.g. chronic rheumatic mitral stenosis or prolapsing mitral valve). Occasionally spontaneous platelet emboli may occur in blood disorders such as thrombocythaemia.

Table I. Causes of reduced retinal blood flow

	Arterial embolism	Reduced perfusion pressure	Increased venous/intracranial/ intraocular pressure	Increased peripheral resistance
Underlying disorder	Platelet, fibrin, cholesterol emboli carotid atheroma Valvular heart disease	Multiple extracranial occlusion	Retinal vein occlusion Papilloedema Glaucoma	Hypertensive microvascular disease Diabetic microvascular disease Polycythaemia
Retinal appearances	Cloudy swelling, pallor, soft exudates, visible emboli	Dilated retinal veins Peripheral haemorrhages Microaneurysms Ischaemic papillopathy Anterior segment ischaemia	Dilated veins Haemorrhage Microaneurysm Anterior segment ischaemia Disc oedema, atrophy	Artery wall changes Dilated veins, microaneurysms Haemorrhages, neovascularization Soft exudate Hard exudate Disc oedema

Cholesterol emboli are bright yellow flakes which lodge in the retinal arteries for days or weeks. They usually cause temporary or incomplete obstruction because of the flat shape of the crystals. Impaction of a cholesterol embolus causes a white sheathing reaction in the retinal artery walls, which persists

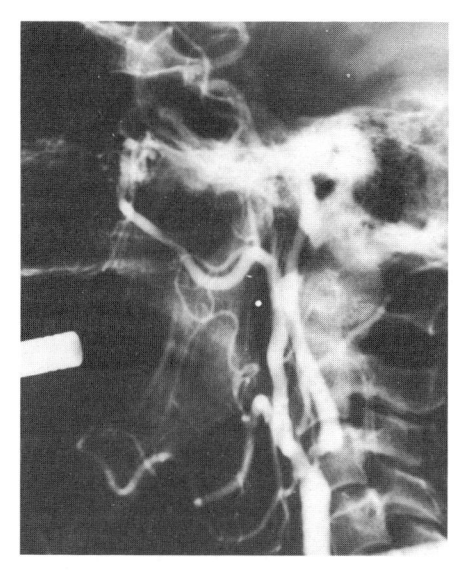

Fig. 2. Angiogram of the carotid arteries from a patient with amaurosis fugax showing severe stenosis of the internal carotid.

after the embolus has disappeared. Calcific emboli (*Plate* XVIIb) derived from scarred and calcified heart valve or mixed thrombus originating in the cavities of the heart tend to cause permanent retinal vascular occlusion rather than amaurosis fugax.

Management of Embolic Amaurosis Fugax

When taking a history from the patient it is important to inquire firstly after a precipitating cause, such as posture, exercise or bright light or following any associated symptom, e.g. ocular pain, chest pain, palpitations. Secondly, discover whether the patient, in addition to amaurosis fugax, has separate transient cerebral ischaemic attacks or symptoms of arterial insufficiency in other sites, such as the heart or legs. On examining the patient the following points are important: the presence of cholesterol emboli or sheathing reaction in the retinal arteries, the pressure on the globe required to empty the central retinal artery, any evidence of retinal venous occlusion or raised ocular tension. General examination should be directed to evidence of valvular heart disease or systemic hypertension, the presence of a carotid artery bruit, or unequal or asynchronous superficial temporal artery pulsations or radial artery pulsations. The following features increase the likelihood of finding a surgically correctable lesion in the internal carotid artery: age over 50 years, hypertension over 110 mmHg diastolic, localized carotid bruit, history of transient ischaemic attacks. If all these features

are absent, carotid angiography is unnecessary. In the detection of carotid stenosis screening tests using Doppler sonography are valuable but the definitive test is carotid angiography, by the intravenous or arterial route. New techniques of digital vascular imaging have greatly improved contrast resolution and have largely replaced other techniques in the detection of extracranial arterial disease.

Treatment

For patients with localized carotid stenosis or atheromatous ulceration at the origin of the internal carotid artery carotid endarterectomy is the most satisfactory treatment provided there are no intercurrent factors which increase the risks of surgery (such as recent myocardial infarction, severe hypertension, advanced age, etc.) and provided expert vascular surgery is available. For all other groups anti-thrombotic treatment with aspirin (300 mg/day) with or without dipyridamole (100 mg t.d.s.) is indicated.

Prognosis

The risk of stroke following amaurosis fugax is approximately 20 per cent in 5 years; the risk of permanent blindness, approximately 10 per cent in 5 years. There is also an increased risk of death and of myocardial infarction. There is some evidence that either endarterectomy or anti-thrombotic treatment may abolish transient attacks and may prevent stroke and prolong survival.

NON-EMBOLIC TYPES OF AMAUROSIS FUGAX

Patients with extensive extracranial arterial disease that affects both right and left carotid arteries or involves the external in addition to the internal carotid circulation may also experience a type of amaurosis fugax (*Fig.* 3).

This is much less common than the embolic variety and is caused by a generalized reduction in ocular blood flow rather than a brief local occlusion. Either one or both eyes may be affected and the following features are characteristic of the syndrome:

1. Longer duration of attack, lasting up to hours in some cases.
2. Less abrupt onset over minutes.
3. Differing symptoms: the loss of vision is described as fragmentation or concentric narrowing of the field of vision, often with a dazzling effect.
4. Transient cerebral hemisphere ischaemia with temporary one-sided weakness or jerking of the limbs may accompany visual loss.
5. The attacks may be related to posture, exercise or exposure to bright light.

The retinal appearances are those of low flow retinopathy – venous dilatation, peripheral blot haemorrhages and microaneurysms. Fluorescein angiography shows leakage from venules in the macular region (*Plate* XVIIc). The central retinal artery pressure is much reduced, the artery collapsing at the slightest pressure on the globe. Sometimes spontaneous pulsation of the artery at the disc may be seen.

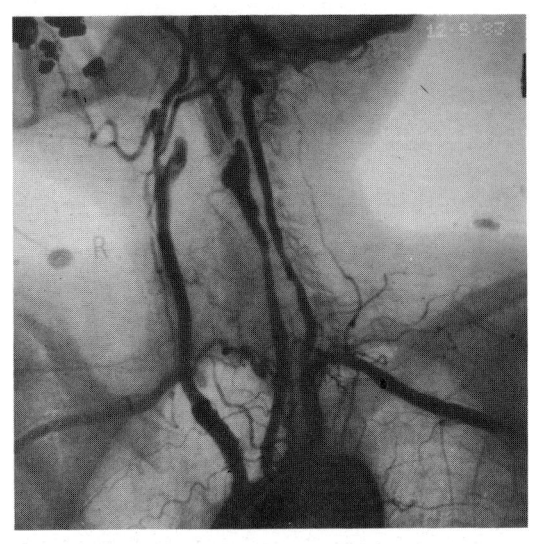

Fig. 3. Angiogram to show extensive bilateral carotid artery disease in a patient with low flow retinopathy on the left side.

The features of the syndrome appear to be caused by generalized ocular oligaemia provoked by a failure of retinal homeostasis.

In these patients the retinal circulation is in a state of critically balanced perfusion maintaining an adequate flow by means of maximal vasodilatation. Any further reduction in systemic blood pressure provoked by postural change or by exercise may be sufficient to cause a fall in blood flow and retinal dysfunction. The symptoms of dazzling and excessive contrast may be caused by a delayed re-synthesis of visual pigment when the metabolic demands of the photoreceptors and pigment epithelium exceed the available blood supply.

In chronic low flow retinopathy loss of sight may occur from permanent occlusion of the retinal arteries. Anastomotic vessels may be seen around the disc. Ischaemic changes also occur in the iris, lens and cornea.

CAROTID ANEURYSMS

Aneurysms of various types may occur on the internal carotid artery at different sites, both extra- and intracranial (*Fig.* 4).
1. At or near the termination of the artery at the base of the brain and within the subarachnoid space (berry aneurysms, occasionally giant aneurysms).
2. In the cavernous sinus (giant saccular aneurysms, occasionally berry aneurysms).
3. In the neck (dissecting aneurysms, rarely saccular aneurysms).

Berry Aneurysms

Intracranial berry aneurysms arise near the termination of the internal carotid artery, on the adjacent

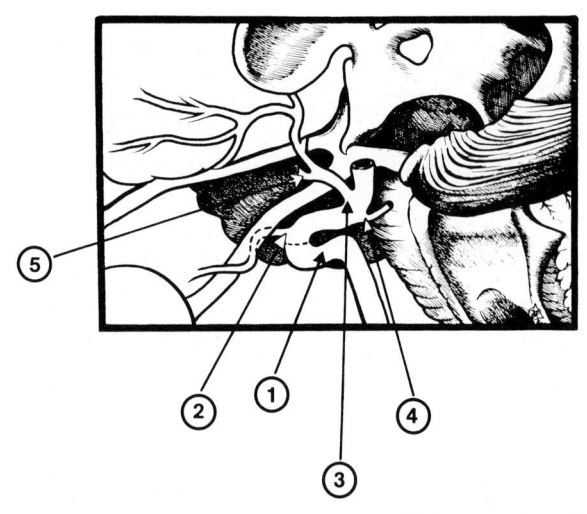

Fig. 4. Distal portion of the internal carotid artery to show the common sites of aneurysm formation: 1, cavernous sinus; 2, ophthalmic artery; 3, terminal carotid; 4, posterior communicating; 5, anterior communicating.

Circle of Willis or on its major branches. These aneurysms may present at any age, most commonly in middle life. The sexes are equally affected. They are sometimes encountered in association with congenital arterial abnormalities (Marfan's syndrome, coarctation of the aorta) or with acquired arterial disease (hypertension, atherosclerosis, fibromuscular hyperplasia). The anterior communicating artery is the most common site.

The usual presentation is with massive subarchnoid haemorrhage causing sudden headache and vomiting with rapidly evolving drowsiness and coma. There is high early mortality (approximately 20 per cent) and about one-third of the survivors have a further bleed within the next 3 weeks. Early clinical features are neck stiffness, cerebral irritation and depressed tendon reflexes with extensor plantar responses. Bilateral papilloedema may develop in a few hours, sometimes with retinal or subhyaloid haemorrhages. The diagnosis is usually confirmed by lumbar puncture or CT scanning and the patient referred to a neurosurgical centre.

Berry Aneurysms of the Posterior Communicating Artery

This common aneurysm may present to ophthalmologists at an early stage before major rupture has occurred. Expansion of the aneurysm or minor leakage may damage the adjacent IIIrd nerve causing an acute painful oculomotor palsy (*Fig.* 5). This occurs over a few hours accompanied by complete ptosis. The pupil on the affected side is large and unreactive. The pain is usually severe and retro-orbital, spreading to the root of the nose; generalized headache and neck stiffness may occur. The corneal reflex is preserved. Although they may not appear seriously ill at this stage, these patients are in grave

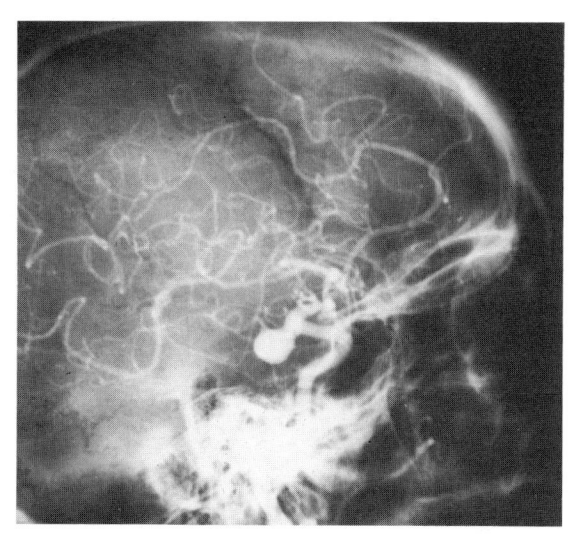

Fig. 5. Aneurysm of the posterior communicating artery from a patient with painful oculomotor palsy and subarachnoid haemorrhage.

danger of major subarachnoid bleeding and they require immediate hospital admission. Once other causes of the IIIrd nerve palsy have been ruled out (e.g. diabetes, cranial arteritis), the diagnosis of an aneurysm is confirmed by angiography. If the patient is fully alert, neurosurgical clipping of the neck of the aneurysm is the treatment of choice, and is carried out within a few days. If the patient is hypertensive, the blood pressure may require to be reduced.

Dissecting Aneurysms

Extracranial carotid aneurysms are usually dissecting in type and affect the internal carotid artery. They may result from indirect trauma such as sudden stretching of the artery and in some cases they may be associated with congenital mesenchymal abnormalities (Marfan's disease, fibromuscular dysplasia, pseudoxanthoma elasticum).

Patients are usually young with no history of degenerative arterial disease. A transverse intimal tear occurs about 1 cm above the origin of the internal carotid artery. A haematoma forms within the wall and the false lumen extends up to the base of the skull.

The clinical symptoms are severe pain in the neck spreading to the retro-orbital region. This is accompanied by oculosympathetic palsy and sometimes by transient or permanent ischaemia of the eye or brain. This is thought to be caused by embolization of thrombus. The diagnosis is made by angiography which shows an attenuated length of internal carotid artery with a normal vessel proximally and distally (string sign) (*Fig. 6*). Treatment is usually conservative since the condition frequently resolves spontaneously.

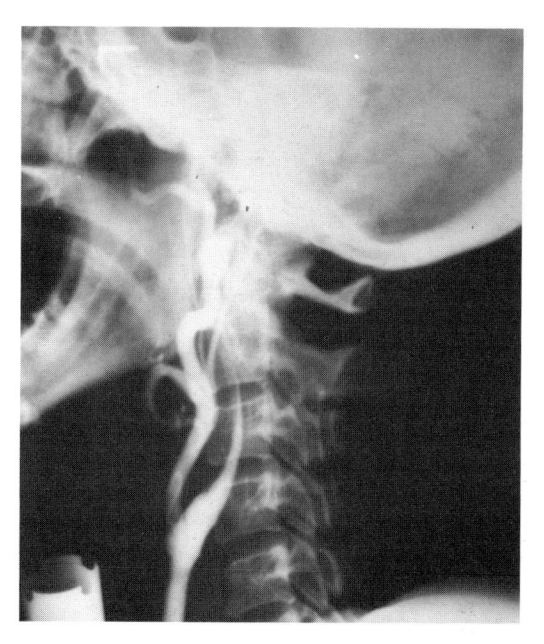

Fig. 6. Carotid dissection. Spontaneous dissection of the internal carotid artery showing the characteristic tapering occlusion of the vessel.

Giant Aneurysms

Although the majority of berry aneurysms tend to rupture when the aneurysm is small, this is not invariable and in some patients the aneurysm may slowly enlarge to compress surrounding structures. When this happens, successive layers of thrombus are formed within the sac thus thickening the wall and lessening the tendency to rupture.

Cavernous Aneurysms

This type of aneurysm is seen almost exclusively in elderly women. It probably begins as a berry aneurysm at the origin of the small hypophyseal branches of the internal carotid artery within the cavernous sinus. Instead of rupturing, these aneurysms slowly expand to fill the cavernous sinus causing pain and affecting the nerves running in the wall of the sinus (*Fig. 7a*). The IIIrd, IVth, Vth and VIth nerves are stretched over the enlarging aneurysm which becomes progressively bigger and may occupy much of the floor of the middle fossa. The aneurysm remains extradural and the danger of subarachnoid haemorrhage is slight (*Figs. 7b,c*).

The clinical presentation is with a VIth nerve palsy which sometimes resolves after a few weeks. This is followed after a variable interval by a combined

IIIrd, IVth and VIth nerve palsy with pain. The pain is trigeminal in distribution, especially affecting the root of the nose. External ophthalmoplegia may be complete, but the pupil is small and unreactive, probably because of additional involvement of sympathetic fibres. The corneal reflex is usually depressed but not lost.

tid angiography is diagnostic. Treatment is usually conservative. If the pain is severe it may be relieved by carotid ligation or by a trapping procedure. This carries some risk of hemiplegia and an external-to-internal carotid bypass is now frequently performed as a preliminary to reduce the risk of cerebral ischaemia.

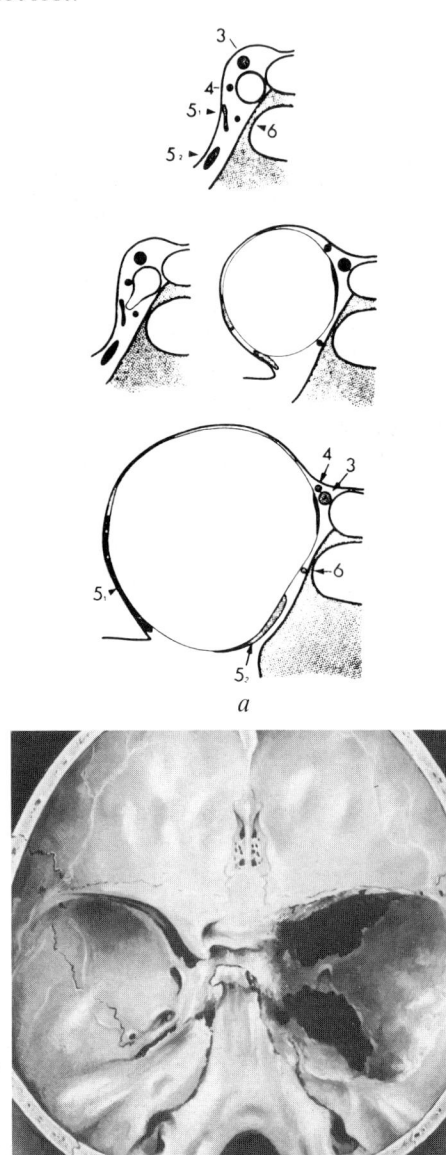

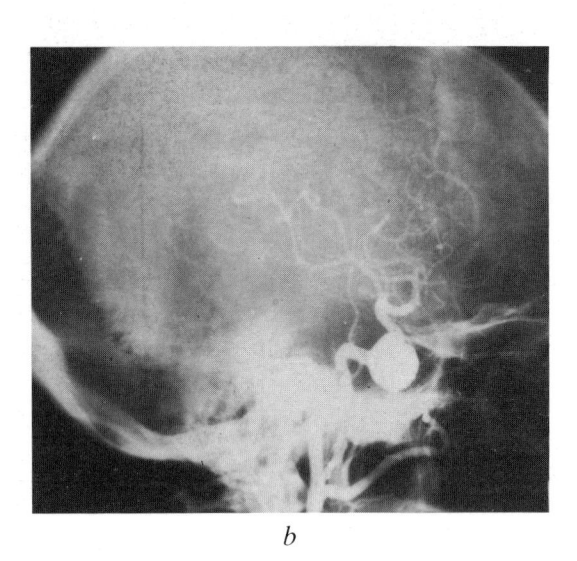

Fig. 7. a, Diagrammatic representation of the growth of a saccular aneurysm of the internal carotid artery in the cavernous sinus, showing the displacement of the IIIrd, IVth, Vth, VIth cranial nerves. (Reproduced from Barr H. W. K. et al. Intracavernous carotid aneurysms. A clinico-pathological report. *Brain* 1971; **94**, 607–724.) *b,* Giant aneurysm of the internal carotid artery in the cavernous sinus in an elderly female with painful cavernous sinus syndrome. *c,* Cavernous aneurysm of the internal carotid artery showing erosion of the floor of the middle fossa and superior orbital fissure.

This condition has a long natural history. The pain may be severe initially but often remits spontaneously. Progressive visual impairment may affect the ipsilateral eye due to optic nerve compression. Slight proptosis may also occur.

The diagnosis of cavernous aneurysm may be suspected on plain X-rays which show erosion of the middle fossa, orbital fissure and clinoid process. There may be calcification in the aneurysm wall. CT scanning shows an enhancing circular lesion and caro-

Supraclinoid Giant Aneurysms

These arise from the termination of the internal carotid artery or at the origin of the ophthalmic artery or (rarely) the posterior communicating artery. The aneurysm enlarges to press on the ipsilateral optic nerve (ophthalmic artery aneurysm) or the lateral side of the chiasma (terminal carotid aneurysm). Pain is usually present at this stage, although it may be intermittent. The visual field defect is usually progressive but may show unexpected fluctuations. Ophthalmic aneurysms produce a central scotoma due to optic nerve compression. Involvement of the temporal field of the contralateral eye may follow after a long interval. This indicates compression of the crossing fibres in the anterior part of the chiasma. Terminal carotid aneurysms characteristically cause hemianopia, unilateral central scotoma with contralateral temporal hemianopia. Frontal lobe signs may be present (seizures, personality change, incontinence).

Diagnosis may be suspected on plain X-ray by local erosion of the pituitary fossa or by calcification in the wall of the aneurysm. CT scanning may show a nasal field loss in the ipsilateral eye progressing to involve central vision and finally causing contralateral temporal field loss as above (*Fig. 8*). Symptoms of hypopituitarism may also occur from erosion of the sella (e.g. amenorrhoea, lassitude, cold intolerance).

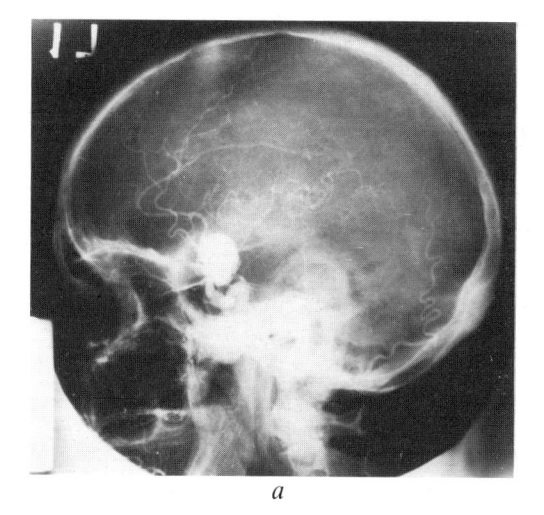

Fig. 8. a, Giant aneurysm of the terminal carotid artery. *b*, Terminal carotid artery giant aneurysm on the left side. The ipsilateral eye shows central and nasal field loss (VA 6/36); the contralateral eye retains good central acuity (VA 6/9) but shows loss of upper temporal field.

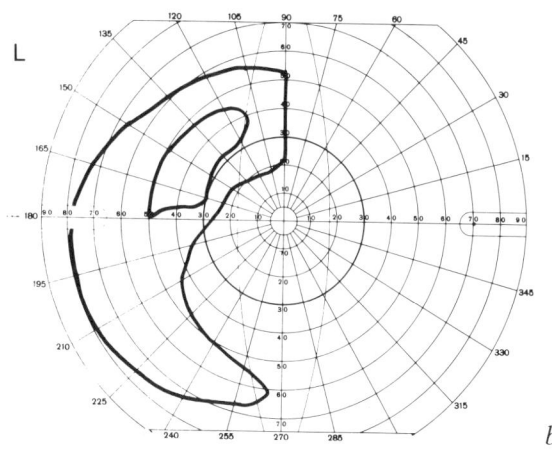

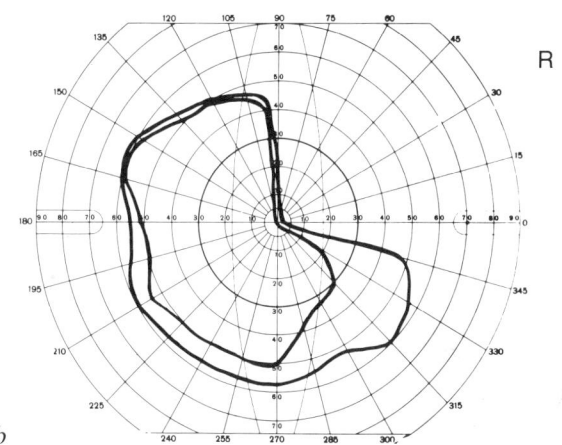

Anterior Communicating Artery Giant Aneurysms

Giant aneurysms in this site may enlarge upwards to compress both frontal lobes. They may also extend downwards impinging on the upper aspect of the chiasma and optic nerves and sometimes bulging between them to produce much distortion, angulation and stretching of the chiasm (*Fig. 9*). The clinical presentation is again of progressive visual loss, usually bilateral, but asymmetrical. A wide variety of different types of field loss have been reported, including bilateral central scotomas, bitemporal

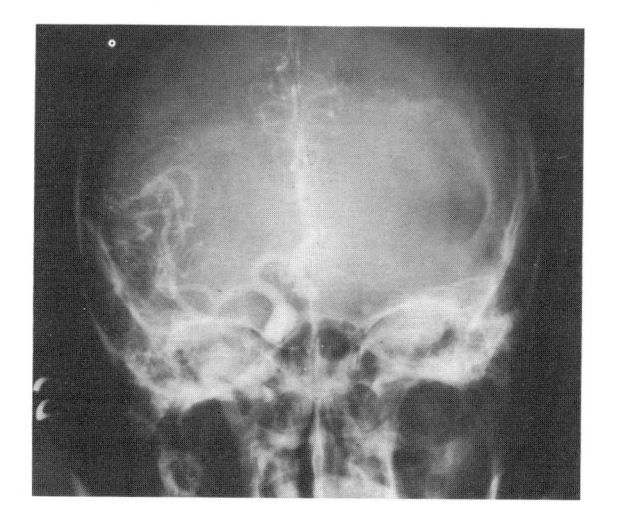

Fig. 9. Anterior communicating artery aneurysm presenting as compression of the optic chiasma.

a circular enhancing lesion. Angiography is usually required for confirmation.

Treatment

Giant aneurysms enlarge very slowly and since radical surgical treatment is always hazardous, some patients are best treated conservatively. Progressive visual loss spreading to involve the second eye is normally an indication for surgical treatment. Carotid ligation in the neck may retard the enlargement of an aneurysm and sometimes causes improvement in vision. It is effective only in aneurysms arising at or near the termination of the carotid. Direct surgical attack is increasingly used even for large aneurysms. After temporary occlusion of the feeding vessels the aneurysm is opened, evacuated and the neck obliterated.

CAROTICOCAVERNOUS FISTULA

Direct communication between the internal carotid artery and the cavernous sinus may develop as a result of rupture of an aneurysm of the artery as it traverses the sinus. At other times the condition may be caused by trauma such as fracture of the base of the skull, or it may occur spontaneously in atherosclerosis or in hereditary mesenchymal dysplasias. Except in the case of trauma or dysplasia the patients are usually elderly females. Shunting of arterial blood through the fistula leads to distension of the cavernous sinus on one or both sides (*Fig.* 10). Depending on the size of the communication a proportion of the carotid blood flow is re-routed directly into the cavernous sinus and the presence of this low-pressure large volume reservoir may also attract blood from other cerebral arteries, causing ocular or cerebral ischaemia. The clinical features consist of a pulsatile tinnitus, sometimes very disturbing to the patient. A loud bruit may be heard on auscultation over one or both eyes. There is usually a cavernous sinus syndrome of which the most constant feature is a VIth nerve palsy followed by a IIIrd, IVth and partial Vth nerve involvement.

The marked elevation of cavernous sinus pressure impedes the venous drainage of the orbit, causing marked conjunctival and scleral hyperaemia with arterialized small venules (*see Fig.* 10). There is also proptosis and chemosis. Vision is usually unaffected but acuity may be impaired by macular oedema.

The retinal veins are markedly dilated and haemorrhages and micro-aneurysms may occur in the periphery. Fluorescein angiography shows markedly retarded flow, venous leakage and microaneurysms.

The natural history is very variable. In some patients the fistula closes spontaneously (or after angiography) and the clinical features rapidly resolve. In other patients the condition may become bilateral and the contralateral eye may be the more severely affected.

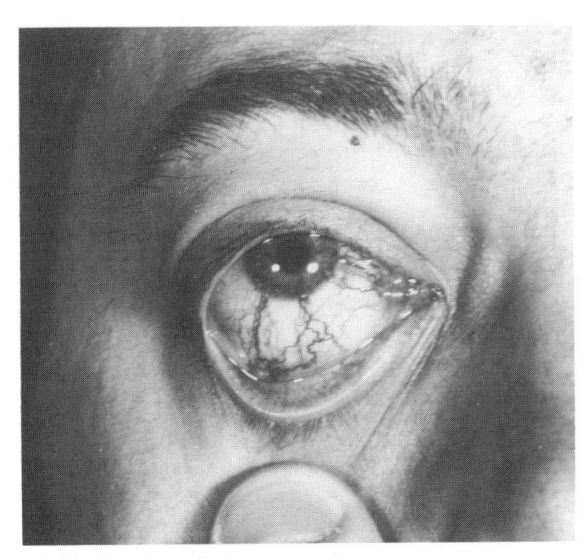

Fig. 10. Caroticocavernous fistula. Marked distension of scleral and conjunctival veins with arterialized blood.

An older form of treatment consisted of carotid ligation; this was sometimes successful but tended to produce cerebral infarction and retinal ischaemia in elderly patients. Trapping of the cavernous portion of the carotid artery or closure of the fistula by muscle embolization proved a more satisfactory technique but still carried some risk of cerebral ischaemia. The most satisfactory method is now closure of the fistula using a small inflatable balloon which leaves the cavernous portion of the carotid artery intact and preserves the cerebral blood supply.

DURAL ARTERIOVENOUS SHUNT

This condition refers to a fistulous communication between a meningeal artery (derived from the external or internal carotid) and the cavernous sinus or adjacent vein (*Fig.* 11). The cause in most cases is

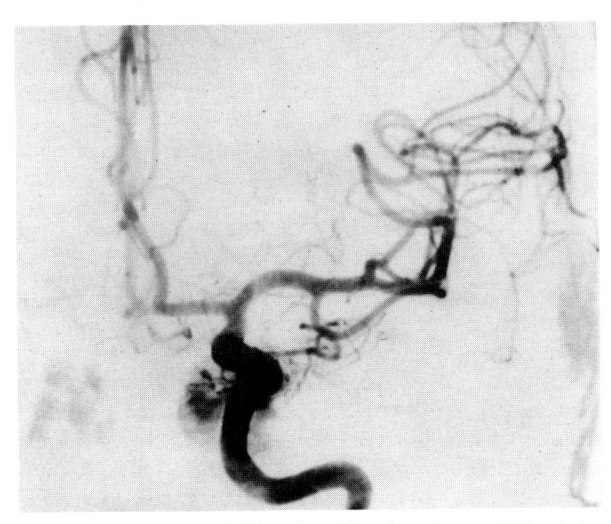

Fig. 11. A dural arteriovenous fistula supplied by small branches from the internal carotid artery and draining into part of the cavernous sinus.

unknown and only a minority of cases follow trauma. In some the condition may be congenital in origin. Dural arteriovenous shunts usually affect middle-aged women and present with unilateral headache or orbital pain, with diplopia due to a VIth nerve palsy and redness of the eye. There may also be unilateral tinnitus or mild proptosis. An orbital bruit is audible in less than half the patients.

Failing vision, severe headache or tinnitus may necessitate treatment by embolization. This gives a satisfactory result provided the shunt is fed by the external carotid vessels. If the fistula persists, the symptoms may return after an interval.

lating cerebral blood flow to the brain stem, usually maintained in a precise relationship to metabolic requirements. Atheroma of the vertebral and basilar arteries may obstruct flow and lower perfusion pressure. This may be compensated for by vasodilatation but the patients become liable to temporary reductions in flow during minor fluctuation in systemic blood pressure or as a result of rotation of the neck, when degenerative discs may further obstruct the vertebral arteries. Arteritis affecting the vertebral arteries may have a similar effect. In the subclavian steal syndrome proximal occlusion of the subclavian artery leads to retrograde flow in the vertebral artery, the

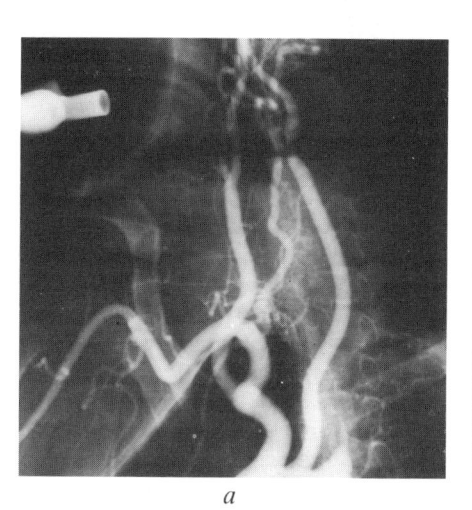

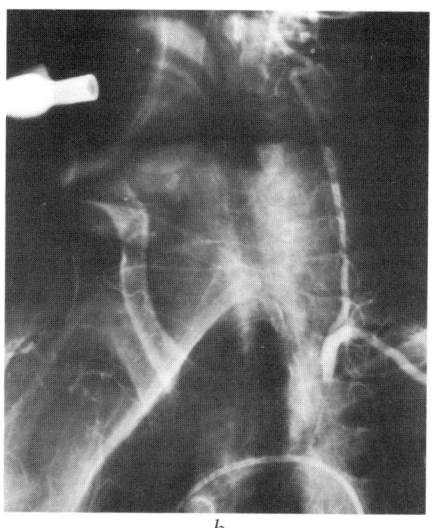

Fig. 12. Subclavian steal syndrome. Note proximal occlusion of left subclavian artery with retrograde filling of left vertebral artery.

BRAIN STEM VASCULAR DISEASE: VERTEBROBASILAR ISCHAEMIA

The features of intermittent ischaemia in the vertebrobasilar territory may include visual and oculomotor disturbances. Loss of vision, patterns or scintillations in one or both half fields are symptoms of ischaemia in the posterior cerebral territories. Diplopia and vertigo signify a disturbance of the vestibular and oculomotor connections within the brain stem, such as the medial longitudinal fasciculus. The resulting disorder of eye movement is more often a type of gaze palsy, such as an internuclear ophthalmoplegia, than a nuclear or infranuclear lesion of a single cranial nerve.

Nystagmus, ataxia, dysarthria and dysmetria of the limbs may be found if the patient is examined during an attack and nystagmus may be accompanied by oscillopsia. Other symptoms of vertebrobasilar ischaemia are limb weakness on one or both sides, tingling around the mouth, transient loss of consciousness or drop attacks (sudden unexpected leg weakness without loss of consciousness).

The cause of vertebrobasilar ischaemia is a temporary breakdown in the homeostatic mechanisms regu-

blood then passing to the arm (*Fig.* 12). Embolism from atheromatous lesions in the basilar artery may cause temporary obstruction in small branches supplying the brain stem, such as the posterior inferior cerebellar artery. This appears to be a less common mechanism than in the carotid territory. Changes in the composition of the blood, such as polycythaemia or dysproteinaemia, tend to raise cerebrovascular resistance and reduce the compensatory reserve of the circulation.

BASILAR ANEURYSM

Aneurysm of the vertebrobasilar circulation may be of two types – small or large. Small berry aneurysms arise on branch arteries, especially the posterior inferior cerebellar artery or posterior cerebral artery. These tend to rupture and present as a subarachnoid haemorrhage. Large aneurysms may be saccular (termination of the basilar) or fusiform (trunk of the basilar) (*Fig.* 13). These do not usually rupture but present as mass lesions or with vertebrobasilar ischaemia. Symptoms are those of multiple cranial nerve palsies combined with long tract signs. Most often

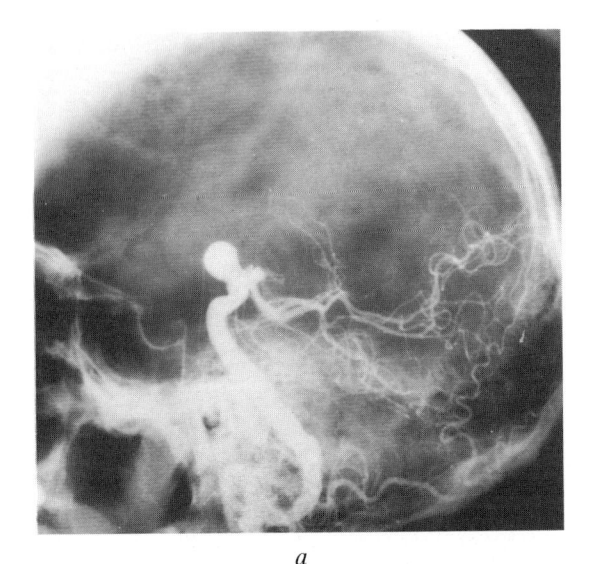

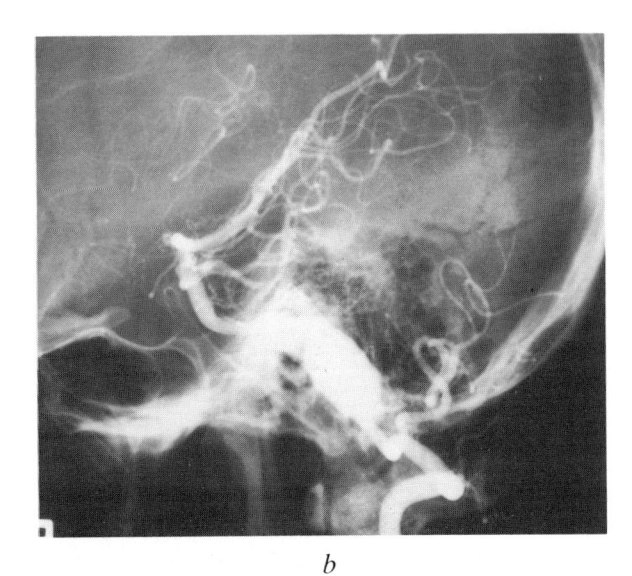

Fig. 13 *a*, Basilar aneurysm in a young male patient presenting with progressive quadriplegia. *b*, Basilar aneurysm. Fusiform enlargement of the lower basilar artery.

there is involvement of the VIIth or VIIIth nerves combined with a pseudobulbar palsy (spastic dysarthria and dysphagia) cerebellar and vestibular symptoms. Sensation is usually normal. Pressure on the diencephalon can cause confusional states, hallucinosis and diabetes insipidus. The symptoms are often intermittent and accompanied by severe occipital headache. The prognosis for giant aneurysms is poor; those having a definable neck can sometimes be operated on directly but fusiform or serpiginous aneurysms arising on the main trunk of the basilar are inoperable.

FURTHER READING

Fisher C. M. Occlusion of the carotid arteries. *Arch. Neurol. Psychiat.* 1954; **72,** 187.
Glaser J. S. *Neuro-ophthalmology.* New York, Harper and Row, 1978.
Gunning A. J., Pickering G. W., Robb Smith A. H. T. et al. Mural thrombosis of the internal carotid artery and subsequent embolism. *Q. J. Med.* 1964; **33,** 155.
Hollenhorst R. W. Carotid and vertebrobasilar arterial stenosis and occlusion: neuro-ophthalmologic considerations. *Trans. Am. Acad. Ophthalmol. Otolaryngol.* 1962; **66,** 166.
McBrien D. J., Bradley R. D., Ashton N. The nature of retinal emboli in stenosis of the internal carotid artery. *Lancet* 1963; **1,** 697.
Meyer J. S. and Denny-Brown D. The cerebral collateral circulation. 1. Factors influencing collateral blood flow. *Neurology (Minn.)* 1957; **7,** 447.
Ross Russell R. W. (ed.) *Vascular Disease of the Central Nervous System.* Edinburgh, Churchill Livingstone, 1983.
Toole J. F. Reversed vertebral artery flow: subclavian steal syndrome. *Lancet* 1964; **1,** 872.

Endocrine disorders

C. S. Cockram and P. H. Sönksen

INTRODUCTION

As the title suggests, this chapter concerns itself with endocrine disorders as they may affect the eye. It is therefore selective in content and does not claim to be a detailed review of endocrinology as a whole. Certain aspects of endocrinology inevitably have greater relevance to the ophthalmologist and these aspects have been given greater consideration. The sections on tumours of the pituitary region and thyroid disorders are given particular prominence. The important topic of diabetic retinopathy is dealt with elsewhere (*see* pp. 238–47) but other aspects of eye disease resulting from diabetes mellitus are discussed.

Endocrine disorders may involve the eye by many different mechanisms. In the case of pituitary tumours, involvement is by direct spread of the primary lesion to involve the neurovisual pathways. In the case of thyroid disorders, involvement either results from the effect of alterations in circulating thyroid hormones, or from a common pathological process (Graves's disease), which produces thyrotoxicosis and exophthalmos. Excess hormone secretion may produce a disorder which in turn, affects the eye. For example, hypertensive retinopathy and diabetic retinopathy may both be encountered in patients with acromegaly, Cushing's syndrome or phaeochromocytoma.

There are rare occasions when endocrine and ophthalmic disorders coexist but where the pathological explanation is less readily understood; for example, the association of testicular atrophy and cataract which may occur in patients with dystrophia myotonica.

DISORDERS OF THE PITUITARY AND HYPOTHALAMUS

General Considerations

The pituitary gland lies within the sella turcica and is anatomically related anteriorly to the sphenoid sinuses, posteriorly to the dorsum sellae, laterally to the cavernous sinuses, carotid siphon and IIIrd, IVth and VIth cranial nerves and superiorly to the diaphragma sellae through which the pituitary stalk passes. The optic nerves, chiasm and tracts lie immediately above the diaphragm sellae and below the relatively unyielding structures of the circle of Willis. Upward extension of pituitary tumours may therefore readily produce compression of the visual pathways or alternatively may compromise their blood supply, thereby producing visual field defects.

The anterior lobe of the pituitary arises from Rathke's pouch and the posterior lobe is comprised of tissue of neural origin (diencephalon). The arterial blood supply is derived from the hypophyseal branches of the internal carotid artery and there is a portal venous system linking the hypothalamus to the anterior pituitary.

The principal hormones secreted by the anterior pituitary are growth hormone (hGH), adrenocorticotrophic hormone (ACTH), thyroid stimulating hormone (TSH), gonadotrophins (luteinizing hormone, LH, and follicle stimulating hormone. FSH), and prolactin (PRL). Secretion is controlled by releasing hormones and inhibitory factors secreted by the hypothalamus into the portal circulation. Most of these releasing hormones and inhibitory factors have now been characterized and their functions ascertained. However, the variety of mechanisms controlling their secretion and release from the hypothalamus are less well understood. Neurotransmitters, particularly noradrenaline, dopamine and serotonin, have important roles and the role of dopamine in inhibiting prolactin secretion is particularly noteworthy as it has a direct therapeutic application with the use of bromocriptine, a dopamine agonist, in the treatment of prolactin secreting pituitary adenomas. Negative feedback inhibition by target hormones is also important and may occur at the pituitary, at the hypothalamus or both. Negative feedback by pituitary hormones upon the hypothalamus may also be important.

The principal hormones secreted by the posterior pituitary are vasopressin (ADH) and oxytocin. These hormones are synthesized in nerve fibres in the hypothalamus and are transferred along these nerve fibres to the posterior pituitary in association with larger molecular weight polypeptides (neurophysins) from whence they are released into the circulation.

The principal disorders of the pituitary and the hypothalamus which have reference to the field of ophthalmology are space-occupying lesions, which may arise from the pituitary itself or from adjacent tissues. A classification is given in *Table* I.

Table I. Space-occupying lesions in the pituitary region

Tumours arising from the pituitary itself

1. Non-secreting — Chromophobe adenoma*
   Sarcoma
2. Hormone secreting — GH secreting
   Prolactin secreting†
   ACTH secreting
   TSH secreting } rare
   Gonadotrophin secreting

Tumours arising from adjacent structures
  Meningioma (mainly sphenoidal ridge)
  Glioma (including optic nerve glioma)
  Craniopharyngioma
  Pineal tumours
  Hypothalamic tumours
  Suprasellar germinomas
  Secondary deposits

Infiltrations and infections
  Sarcoidosis
  Hystiocytosis X
  Syphilis
  Pyogenic abscess

* Many in fact secrete prolactin, some secrete GH, ACTH, or hormone fragments.
† GH and ACTH secreting tumours may also secrete prolactin.

Tumours Arising from the Pituitary Itself

Pituitary tumours are not uncommon, accounting for approximately 10 per cent of primary intracranial tumours. Additionally, small tumours, clinically unapparent during life, are present in 25 per cent of glands examined at post-mortem. The major pathological manifestations result from hormone hypersecretion, destruction of normal tissue or involvement of the pituitary stalk with the production of partial or complete hypopituitarism, and involvement of local structures, particularly the chiasmal region if suprasellar extension occurs. The most convenient classification of these tumours is on the basis of their secretory properties.

Non-secreting Tumours

Chromophobe adenomas are the most common variety of pituitary tumour. They present most frequently between the ages of 30 and 60 and have an equal incidence in both sexes. Although slow growing, they may become very large with considerable invasion of local structures. Very rarely they may metastasize. Although their lack of staining properties indicates a relative absence of stored secretions, they nevertheless commonly secrete prolactin and may occasionally secrete other hormones or hormonal components. Disturbance of vision is the most common presenting feature of these tumours and results from suprasellar extension. Superior bitemporal quadrantinopia is usually the earliest manifestation of visual field loss as the tumours tend to protrude upwards between the arms of the optic nerves producing compression of their inferomedial aspects. This abnormality then progresses to the classic bitemporal hemianopia.

Many patterns of visual field loss can occur, however, depending upon the position of the chiasm and the spread of the tumour, and may ultimately lead to total blindness. Careful visual field examination is therefore mandatory in all cases and should always include the use of a red object which more successfully discriminates minor changes. Repeated visual field examinations should also be an integral part of assessment and follow-up after treatment. Less commonly, diplopia may occur as a result of lateral spread into the cavernous sinus region and involvement of the oculomotor nerves.

Other presenting features include headache (thought to be due to traction on local dural structures), seizures and disturbances of sleep and appetite consequent upon involvement of the hypothalamus. Not uncommonly, delays in growth and sexual development are the reasons for seeking medical advice.

Radiological investigation should include detailed lateral (*Fig.* 1) and anteroposterior coned views of the pituitary fossa and if any abnormality is thought to be present, lateral tomography should be performed. The advent of computerized tomography (CT scanning) has revolutionized radiological assessment (*Fig.* 2). Although requiring a considerable radiation dose, it is a safe, non-invasive technique which is particularly useful for assessing spread beyond the confines of the pituitary fossa and particularly suprasellar and lateral spread. As a result of CT scanning, surgery can be undertaken in many cases without prior resort to the more traumatic air encephalography and arteriography, although in difficult cases this may still be required, particularly if the exact relationship of the tumour to the optic chiasm remains in doubt. Carotid arteriography may also be required if the tumour is very large or if a carotid aneurysm is considered to be a possible alternative diagnosis, although the most recent high resolution CT scanners, as well as digital subtraction angiography, can diagnose carotid aneurysms without recourse to carotid angiography.

Endocrinological assessment is required in all cases. A careful clinical examination should be performed to exclude a hypersecretory syndrome such as Cushing's syndrome or acromegaly and to look for evidence of hypopituitarism (for example hypogonadism, hypoadrenalism, hypothyroidism). It is particularly important to look for the presence of gynaecomastia or galactorrhoea as this may indicate excessive prolactin secretion and may therefore alter

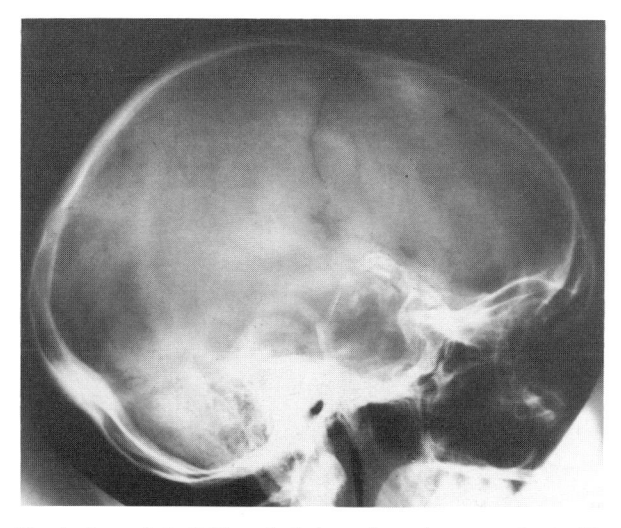

Fig. 1. Lateral skull film of pituitary fossa from a patient with a large craniopharyngioma. Gross expansion of the fossa can be seen and the margins of the tumour are outlined by calcification.

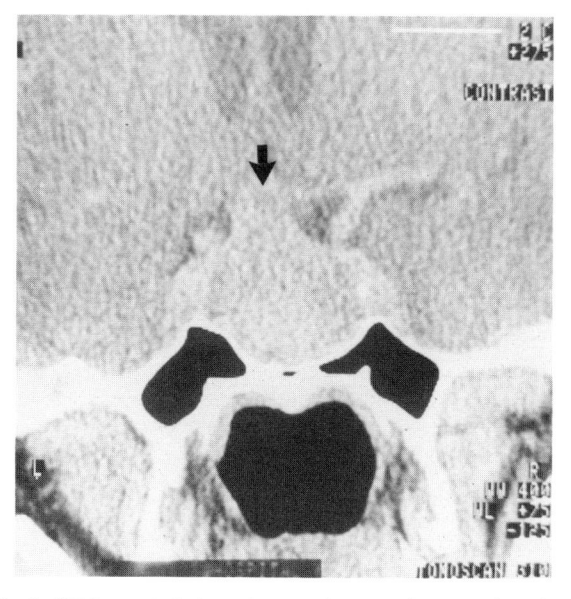

Fig. 2. CT Scan of pituitary fossa region seen in coronal section, from a patient whose visual fields presented bilateral hemianopia to a red object. With contrast enhancement, a large pituitary tumour can be seen extending laterally and superiorly from the fossa. The lateral walls of the fossa have been eroded and the head of the upward extension (arrowed) can be seen lying between the optic tracts.

subsequent management. Galactorrhoea can only be excluded after careful but firm attempts at milk expression. Detailed endocrinological investigation and documentation of pituitary reserve should also be undertaken if time allows; although, if evidence of a hypersecretory syndrome is absent and the need for surgery pressing, then dynamic endocrine testing may be deferred until after surgery, and appropriate hormone cover given during any surgical procedure. It is, however, the view of the authors that the result of a serum prolactin estimation should be obtained in all cases before surgery as it is now clear that even large prolactin-secreting tumours may shrink considerably and quickly in response to bromocriptine with consequent relief of chiasmal compression and improvement in visual fields.

In cases other than prolactinomas, the treatment of choice is usually surgery. Small tumours, confined to the fossa or with limited suprasellar extension, are suitable for trans-sphenoidal hypophysectomy and carry the best prognosis. Significant suprasellar extension requires a transfrontal approach. Very large tumours may not be totally resectable and the surgeon may be forced to confine himself to decompression of the optic pathways. Postoperative radiotherapy has been shown to be effective in reducing recurrence rate with chromophobe adenomas. As already indicated, bromocriptine now has an important role in the management of prolactin secreting adenomas and may obviate the need for palliative surgery in patients with large tumours or any surgery at all in those with smaller tumours. It is usually well tolerated, although constipation can be troublesome and nausea may be dose-limiting.

Sarcomas of the pituitary are fortunately very rare. They are not amenable to surgery, are not radiosensitive and are rapidly fatal. They are only seen in those who have previously received therapeutic radiation to the pituitary region.

Growth Hormone Secreting Tumours

These tumours produce the clinical syndrome of acromegaly in adults, and gigantism in juveniles prior to epiphyseal closure. The clinical features are highly characteristic and the diagnosis can usually be made at the bedside. The diagnosis is usually made incidentally but presenting symptoms are diverse and numerous. Enlargement of the hands and feet, carpal tunnel syndrome, sweating, headache, visual disturbances, catarrh and deepening of the voice are prominent. Physical signs include the characteristic facies with thick, greasy skin, enlargement of the nose and tongue, separation and malocclusion of the teeth, prognathism and broad, spatulate hands and feet. Muscle strength is reduced which belies the rugged physical appearance. Hypertension is commonly present as is diabetes mellitus and insulin resistance. Cardiomyopathy also occurs as do osteoporosis, disorders of calcium metabolism and degenerative joint disease. The morbidity is considerable and an increased mortality rate results from the cardiovascular complications.

The diagnosis is most reliably confirmed by measurement of hGH concentrations during a glucose tolerance test when the normal pattern of suppression is absent and a paradoxical rise may occur. Random or fasting hGH measurements may be misleading, although a low reading (<2 mU/l) excludes the diagnosis. There is little correlation between serum hGH levels (and hence the activity of the disease) and the clinical appearance of the patient.

Additional investigations, as with chromophobe adenomas, should include detailed visual field assessment, pituitary radiology and assessment of the remainder of pituitary function. Growth hormone producing tumours almost inevitably cause enlargement of the pituitary fossa and can occasionally be giant pituitary tumours. When interpreting visual field assessments in these patients, it should be remembered that the considerable enlargement of the eyebrows and supraorbital ridges that can occur may lead to the spurious finding of superior field defects.

Treatment options comprise surgery, radiotherapy and bromocriptine. Trans-sphenoidal hypophysectomy is the most effective treatment in patients with active disease but little or no suprasellar tumour extension. Transfrontal surgery is usually required in patients with visual field defects. Radiotherapy alone produces a significant fall in hGH levels (but the fall is slow over many years) and is helpful in patients for whom surgery is contraindicated. Radiotherapy will also lower hGH levels in those with residual tumour after either transfrontal or trans-sphenoidal surgery. Radiotherapy should be recommended in those in whom hGH levels remain elevated after surgery. Yttrium implantation is also effective but requires considerable expertise and is not widely available.

Bromocriptine reduces hGH levels to normal in a few patients and by a significant amount in others. It may also reduce tumour size but is not as effective as it is with prolactinomas and has not, as yet, established a primary role in the treatment of acromegaly in more than a few patients.

Some degree of hypopituitarism is commonly encountered after both surgery and radiotherapy and careful endocrinological assessment (including dynamic pituitary function tests) and follow-up is therefore required so that hormone replacement can be instituted and supervised as required.

Acromegaly may also come to the attention of ophthalmologists as a result of the presence of retinopathy secondary to diabetes mellitus, hypertension or a combination of both. A proportion of acromegalic patients may develop rapidly progressive proliferative retinopathy. Successful lowering of growth hormone levels with treatment may produce striking regression both of the metabolic abnormality and of the retinopathy. It has been suggested that growth hormone is implicated in the aetiology of diabetic retinopathy and this was the rationale behind the treatment of severe diabetic retinopathy with hypophysectomy, prior to the development of laser photocoagulation.

Prolactin Secreting Tumours

These tumours have been increasingly recognized since prolactin radioimmunoassays have been widely available. They are now known to account for a substantial proportion of chromophobe adenomas. However, it is important to remember that there are numerous other causes of hyperprolactinaemia. Since prolactin secretion from the pituitary is controlled by an inhibitory factor (which is thought to be dopamine) produced by the hypothalamus, raised prolactin concentrations can occur in association with damage to the hypothalamus or pituitary stalk. Tumours, such as chromophobe adenomas and craniopharyngiomas, can therefore produce hyperprolactinaemia by this mechanism and a moderately

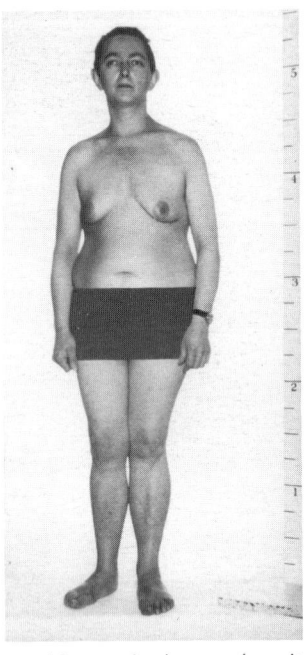

Fig. 3. A patient with a prolactin-secreting pituitary adenoma. Hypopituitarism is combined with pronounced gynaecomastia and galactorrhoea.

raised prolactin concentration does not therefore necessarily imply tumour secretion. Drugs that act as dopamine antagonists can also produce hyperprolactinaemia and a careful drug history must, therefore, be taken. Common examples are phenothiazines, haloperidol and metaclopramide (dopamine receptor blockers), methyldopa and reserpine (which deplete neuronal stores) and monoamine oxidase inhibitors. In general, prolactin levels are greater than 3000 mU/l in patients with true prolactinomas but only rarely exceed 1500 mU/l with other causes.

Hyperprolactinaemia renders the gonads insensitive to the action of gonadotrophins and inhibits the normal patterns of gonadotrophin release (*Fig.* 3). Female patients therefore present with amenorrhoea and infertility in addition to galactorrhoea. Male patients may present with impotence, loss of secondary sexual characteristics, infertility, gynaecomastia and galactorrhoea. Both spermatogenesis and testosterone secretion are reduced. Additionally, of course, other features of hypopituitarism may be present, as may headaches or visual disturbances. Prolactinomas tend to be diagnosed at an earlier stage in woman as a result of the disturbance in menstruation which is usually present.

The primary treatment for prolactinomas is now medical and a course of bromocriptine should always be tried before considering surgery. The response, both in terms of tumour shrinkage and fall in prolactin level, may be immediate and dramatic. Some cases on the other hand respond more slowly and to a larger dose of bromocriptine. In general, but not always, tumour shrinkage and a fall in prolactin levels go hand in hand. Treatment with bromocriptine does not make subsequent surgery more difficult, indeed the converse is usually the case. The long term results of bromocriptine (and it has been in use for nearly 10 years) are all at least as good as surgery and probably substantially better. It removes symptoms, restores hormonal balance and obviates the need for surgery in the majority of cases. When bromocriptine is withdrawn, prolactin levels rise almost immediately in the majority of patients. Treatment is therefore suppressive rather than curative. Medical treatment is the treatment of choice therefore in all except those in whom an adequate trial of treatment has been shown to be ineffective, and those who cannot tolerate the drug. In these patients, surgery is useful in reducing tumour bulk but rarely lowers prolactin levels or restores hormonal balance. Postoperative radiotherapy is nearly always needed to reduce the recurrence rate.

ACTH Secreting Tumours

Basophil adenomas secreting excess ACTH lead to excessive stimulation of the adrenal cortex. Bilateral adrenal hyperplasia results and excessive cortisol production occurs with the production of Cushing's syndrome (*Fig.* 4). In addition, melanophore stimulation leads to increased pigmentation of the skin and this feature aids in the differentiation of pituitary-dependent Cushing's syndrome from adrenal causes such as adrenal adenoma and carcinoma, where such pigmentation is absent. Differentiation has also to be made from ectopic ACTH production by tumours, for example, bronchogenic carcinoma and carcinoid tumours. This may be relatively straightforward if the tumour is clinically apparent and highly malignant but in the case of benign carcinoid tumours may be very difficult and will require detailed endocrinological investigation and discrimination on the basis of ACTH and cortisol responses to dexamethasone suppression and metyrapone stimulation.

Basophil adenomas are frequently small and only a minority of patients present with large space-occupying lesions, suprasellar extension or visual field defects. Presentation, therefore, tends to be with the features of Cushing's syndrome rather than the features of pituitary tumour. Occasionally, however, the converse is true, where Cushing's syndrome may be present in a patient presenting with visual failure due to a large pituitary tumour. In these cases, the histology is that of a chromophobe adenoma and

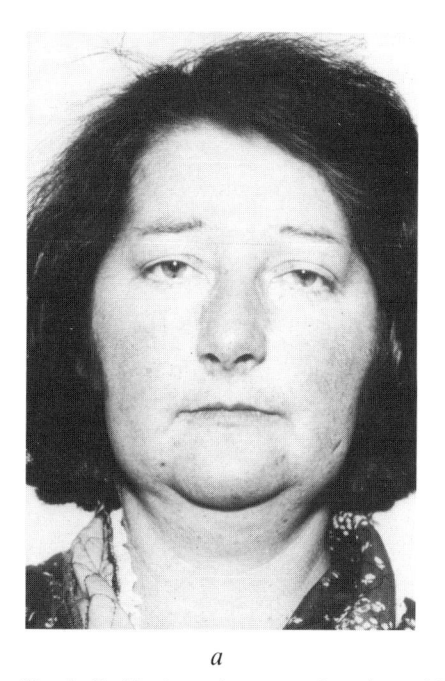

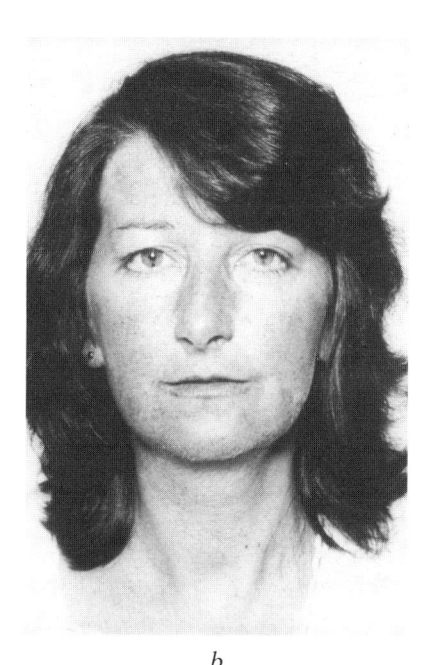

Fig. 4. Cushing's syndrome. *a*, A patient with pituitary-dependent Cushing's syndrome. *b*, The same patient 1 year later, after treatment by bilateral adrenalectomy. This patient subsequently developed Nelson's syndrome (*see* text).

the basophil cells are so few and far between that they may be overlooked. The diagnosis of Cushing's disease in these patients is often also overlooked.

Treatment options are hypophysectomy, bilateral adrenalectomy and radiotherapy. Large tumours are best treated by hypophysectomy. Following bilateral adrenalectomy alone ACTH levels may increase greatly, as may tumour size. This results in the production of Nelson's syndrome (*Fig.* 5), where hyperpigmentation becomes very marked and enlargement

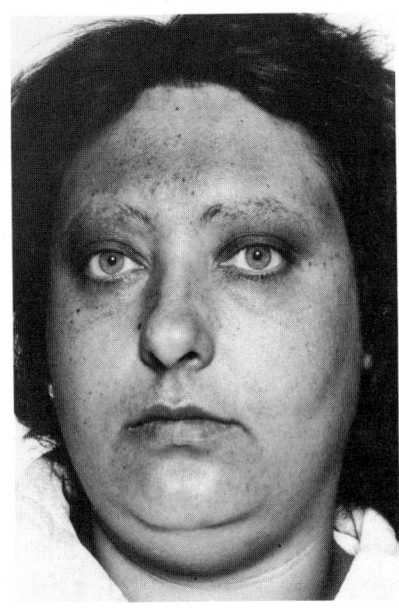

Fig. 5. Nelson's syndrome. Marked facial and periorbital hyperpigmentation can be clearly seen.

of the tumour (due to removal of the restraining influence of excessive cortisol production) may then produce visual field defects. These basophil tumours are commonly invasive locally and difficult to remove. The incidence of Nelson's syndrome may be reduced by combining bilateral adrenalectomy with radiotherapy to the pituitary region.

Following treatment replacement therapy with adrenal corticosteroids is required and panhypopituitarism following hypophysectomy may necessitate additional replacement with thyroxine and sex hormones.

Tumours Arising from Adjacent Structures

Meningiomas and gliomas are not usually the province of the endocrinologist but may become so if they are suspected to be a pituitary tumour, or if hypopituitarism results from involvement of the hypothalamo–pituitary axis.

Craniopharyngioma

These tumours do not arise from the pituitary itself but from remnants of Rathke's pouch tissue. They usually contain cysts and the presence of calcification may lead to the diagnosis being made from plain skull radiographs. They are generally slow growing and are present from birth. They may present at any age but the majority present before the age of 30, and they may become very large. As with chromophobe adenomas they present with headache, visual disturbances due to compression of the chiasmal region and partial or complete hypopituitarism due to destruction of pituitary or hypothalamic tissue or interruption of the pituitary stalk. Occasionally other hypothalamic disturbances may be prominent and include sleep disturbances, hyperphagia, hypodipsia and motor retardation. Hydrocephalus may result from obstruction between the IIIrd and IVth ventricles.

Treatment is fraught with difficulty and the morbidity following treatment remains high. Transfrontal surgery is usually palliative rather than curative as complete removal is technically difficult and recurrences are common. Cysts may be decompressed but reaccumulate if excision of the cyst lining is incomplete. Occasionally aspiration of cysts may be performed by the trans-sphenoidal route. The presence of hydrocephalus may require the insertion of a shunt.

Radiotherapy probably reduces the recurrence rate in cases where radical surgery is not possible.

Pineal Tumours

Pineal tumours are relatively uncommon, but in view of their modes of presentation are of considerable interest both to the ophthalmologist and the endocrinologist.

The pathological classification of tumours in the pineal region is complex and interested readers are advised to consult a more definitive review (*see* Further Reading). Tumours of the pineal organ itself include pineocytoma and pineoblastoma, which arise from the pineocytes, gliomas (astrocytoma and ependymoma) and germ cell tumours (germinoma and teratoma). Tumours of adjacent structures such as meningioma or IIIrd ventricular tumours may present in a similar fashion, as occasionally may non-neoplastic conditions such as pineal cysts and arachnoid cysts.

The neuro-ophthalmic manifestations of these tumours are complex and wide ranging. As a result, visual symptoms are a common presenting complaint and include diplopia, blurred vision and difficulty with reading.

The most common ophthalmic abnormality is paralysis of upward gaze, which is usually supranuclear in origin. Paralysis of downward gaze is rare, and if present, is usually associated with an upward gaze palsy, and implies anterior extension of the tumour. Abnormal or absent pupillary reflexes to both light and convergence are also frequent and are usually associated with paralysis of upward gaze. True light near dissociation of the pupillary reflexes is probably in fact quite rare, both mechanisms usually being affected, although perhaps to differing degrees. Convergence palsies also occur and are the third feature of Parinaud's syndrome.

Other ophthalmic signs which may occur with tumours of the pineal region include lid retraction (of supranuclear origin), skew deviation and pareses of the third and fourth oculomotor nerves (of nuclear origin). Palsies of the VIth nerve may occur if intracranial pressure is raised as a result of aqueduct stenosis. Papilloedema may also be produced by the same mechanism.

Suprasellar germinomas arising from the anterior third ventricle region are histologically identical to pineal germinomas and have been referred to as ectopic pinealomas. They are, however, almost certainly a distinct pathological entity. Because of their suprasellar position they present in a similar way to pituitary tumours with suprasellar extension. Common features therefore include visual field defects, optic atrophy and ophthalmoplegia in addition to hypopituitarism resulting from interruption of the pituitary stalk.

Other neurological manifestations of tumours of the pineal region include headache and epilepsy.

The pineal gland in mammals is a secretory organ, no longer retaining the direct light sensitivity seen in lower vertebrate orders. In mammals it secretes melatonin and other compounds and as a result of sympathetically mediated connections with the eye, its secretory activity is inhibited by light and released from inhibition during darkness. Its secretions are capable of inhibiting gonadal function. It may therefore exert a role in the reproductive cycle in mammals such that during periods of increased light, reproductive function is maximized.

Such a role for the pineal has not been demonstrated in man but one of the principal endocrine disorders associated with pineal tumours is precocious puberty. Isolated gonadotrophin deficiency and hypofunction of both anterior and posterior pituitary also occur and can be explained by involvement of hypothalamus or interruption of the hypothalamo–hypophyseal connections. Precocious puberty may result from loss of a normal inhibitory function of the pineal as a result of tissue destruction, from loss of normal inhibitory functions residing in the hypothalamus or from ectopic production of gonadotrophins or gonadotrophin releasing hormone by the tumour. The assessment of endocrine function in these patients follows the same principles as in patients with pituitary tumours.

Detailed neuroradiological investigation is an essential prerequisite to subsequent neurosurgical management. Skull radiology may reveal abnormal calcification or features of raised intracranial pressure. Computerized tomography with contrast enhancement will usually demonstrate the tumour mass and allow assessment of size and position, and will also demonstrate hydrocephalus, if present. Serial CT scanning is also the ideal procedure for following progress of the tumour and the effect of treatment, and is relatively non-invasive. Arteriography also still has a place but carries greater risks. Ventriculography and air encephalography have largely been replaced by CT scanning.

The management of these tumours requires close liaison with neurosurgeons and radiotherapists. Consideration of the procedures available is beyond the scope of this volume but it should be realized that morbidity and mortality rates are high and direct surgery often impossible. If a benign tumour is thought likely then direct exploration can be considered. In most cases if a diagnosis can be made from the clinical picture together with the CT scan result, then radiotherapy is given without biopsy and surgical intervention is usually confined to those cases in which the presence of hydrocephalus requires an urgent shunting procedure. Radiotherapy, combined if necessary with a shunt, appears to give the best outcome both in terms of complications and survival.

THYROID DISORDERS

Disorders of the thyroid gland provide another area where endocrinologist and ophthalmologist have to work in close cooperation, the major meeting point being in the management of dysthyroid eye disease.

The thyroid gland develops in the embryo as an epithelial downgrowth from the pharyngeal floor, from whence it migrates caudally while its connecting stalk (the thyroglossal duct) elongates. In the adult the gland comprises two lobes joined by a narrow isthmus, affixed closely to the anterior and lateral aspects of the trachea. Two pairs of parathyroid glands are situated on or beneath the posterior surface of the thyroid lobes. The thyroid gland is one of the larger endocrine organs, weighing approximately 20 g, and has a considerable potential for growth. Goitres may become very large. The principal thyroid hormones are thyroxine (T_4) and tri-iodothyronine (T_3), produced by the anterior cells of the thyroid follicle, and calcitonin, which is produced by the parafollicular 'C' cells. The synthesis of adequate quantities of T_4 and T_3 is dependent upon an adequate supply of iodine. The steps involved in synthesis include active uptake and concentration of iodide into the gland, iodination of tyrosyl residues to yield iodotyrosines and coupling of iodotyrosines to form T_4 and T_3. The hormones thus formed are held in peptide linkage within the protein thyroglobulin, which is the major component of follicular colloid. Release of the hormones thus requires prior hydrolysis of thyroglobulin. T_4 and T_3, when released into the circulation, become reversibly protein bound to thyroid hormone binding globulin (TBG). T_3 is the more active hormone and it is now known that a substantial proportion of circulating T_4 is converted to T_3 in the peripheral tissues. Peripheral deiodination of T_4 by an alternative pathway results in the formation of an inert metabolite known as reverse T_3 (rT_3). The balance between these peripheral pathways allows the ratio of T_3 to rT_3 to be varied. This provides a control mechanism for altering energy consumption acutely.

The actions of thyroid hormones are manifest in all tissues. They increase oxygen consumption and thermogenesis and have complex actions on carbohydrate, fat and protein metabolism. They are essential for normal growth. Estimation of basal metabolic rate remains the only satisfactory method of assessing their overall effect.

Regulation of Thyroid Function

Thyroid stimulating hormone (TSH) produced by the anterior pituitary is the major regulator of thyroid function and acts by several mechanisms to increase the synthesis and release of thyroid hormones. TSH release, in turn, is stimulated by thyrotrophin releasing hormone (TRH) from the hypothalamus. TRH is a tripeptide which is commercially available and forms the basis of an important method of assessing thyroid function.

TRH and TSH secretion is in turn controlled by a negative feedback system whereby alterations in circulating concentrations of T_4 and T_3 lead to reciprocal changes in TSH release from the pituitary. In hypothyroid individuals the pituitary responds by increasing the synthesis and release of TSH which in turn stimulates the thyroid. In hyperthyroid subjects the reverse is true.

Thyroid Function Tests

Numerous and diverse methods are available for the assessment of thyroid function and the subject is complex. An understanding of the basis of these tests is essential, however, for those who may be involved in the management of thyroid disorders. Advances in specific radioimmunoassay techniques for T_4 and T_3 have, fortunately, simplified the situation and have led to a move away from the use of procedures using radioactive isotopes. Accurate, sensitive and specific radioimmunoassay for both total T_4 and T_3 is now generally available. However, it must be remembered that since the hormones are largely protein bound in the circulation it is not a measure of the biologically important 'free' hormone and is subject to errors of interpretation if the possibility of changes in binding protein concentration is not appreciated. This problem may be overcome by the use of T_3 uptake tests which allow measurement of unoccupied protein binding sites. A 'free T_4 index' can then be calculated which is a more accurate reflection of free hormone levels. More recent advances in radioimmunoassay techniques have allowed the development of 'free' T_4 and T_3 measurements and they are becoming more generally available. Thyroid binding globulin (TBG) can also be measured directly by either radioimmunoassay or immunoelectrophoresis and this, when available, allows a T_4:TBG ratio to be obtained.

Measurement of serum TSH is particularly important in distinguishing hypothyroidism due to primary thyroid failure (where TSH levels are elevated) from secondary hypothyroidism due to failure of pituitary TSH secretion. Unfortunately, the TSH radioimmunoassay is insufficiently sensitive to detect low levels of TSH and so single TSH values are of no value in the diagnosis of thyrotoxicosis or, for that matter, as a screening test for pituitary function. In these latter circumstances a stimulation test is required, and TRH is the stimulating agent used. An intravenous injection of TRH in normal individuals results in a rise in serum TSH concentration which is evident within a few minutes, peaks at approximately 20 min and then declines to basal levels within 1–2 h. In patients with primary hypothyroidism the basal value will be high (and diagnostic in itself) and the response to TRH exaggerated. In thyrotoxic patients and patients with pituitary failure the response will be subnormal. The TRH test is also of value in the diagnosis of endocrine exophthalmus as the TRH test may be subnormal even in individuals with normal circulating concentrations of thyroid hormones.

As stated earlier, isotopic thyroid uptake tests are now seldom used for diagnostic purposes. Isotopic thyroid scans are, however, of considerable value in the delineation of thyroid anatomy and for ascertaining whether palpable nodules are 'hot' or 'cold'. They are frequently combined with ultrasound of the thyroid which is of particular value in determining whether 'cold' nodules on an isotope scan are cystic or comprised of solid tissue, and therefore possibly malignant.

Measurements of antibodies directed against thyroid tissue or components are of particular value in the diagnosis of thyroid diseases of immunological origin (Hashimoto's thyroiditis and Graves's disease).

Thyrotoxicosis

Thyrotoxicosis or hyperthyroidism results from an excess of circulating thyroid hormones. It is a common disorder, with a greater incidence in females than males. The great majority of cases are due either to Graves's disease, where diffuse thyroid hyperplasia occurs, or to toxic thyroid nodules, which may be single or multiple. Other causes include either deliberate or accidental overdosage with exogenous thyroid hormone and, much more rarely, excess TSH production from pituitary tumours, ectopic TSH production from other tumours (for example choriocarcinoma and hydatidiform mole) and transient thyrotoxicosis in association with thyroiditis.

The clinical features are numerous and affect all

systems. Weight loss is usual, although appetite may be increased. Sweating and heat intolerance are common. Cardiovascular symptoms and signs include palpitation, dyspnoea, angina pectoris, tachycardia, vasodilatation and cardiac failure. Atrial fibrillation may occur and may be the sole overt clinical feature in elderly patients ('masked' thyrotoxicosis). Gastrointestinal abnormalities are common, particularly diarrhoea or steatorrhoea. Neurological abnormalities include agitation, tremor, psychiatric disturbances, muscle weakness and myopathy, periodic paralysis and myasthenic syndrome. The reproductive system is also affected leading to oligomenorrhoea or amenorrhoea in females and gynaecomastia and loss of libido in males. A goitre may be present. The onset is usually gradual but may occasionally present a sudden life threatening acceleration (thyroid storm), which requires emergency treatment. Additional stress, such as surgery or infection, may precipitate thyroid storm.

Ophthalmic Abnormalities in Thyrotoxicosis

Lid retraction and lid lag occur with thyrotoxicosis from any cause. They occur as a result of increased tone in the levator palpebrae superioris muscle. The increased tone is thought to be a direct effect of excess circulating thyroid hormones operating by potentiation of adrenergic synaptic transmission in the sympathetic nerve fibres which partially innervate this muscle.

Diplopia and ophthalmoplegia may occur due to involvement of the extraocular muscles in the more generalized thyrotoxic myopathy although this usually predominantly affects the proximal limb girdle musculature. In Graves's disease, however, involvement of the extraocular muscles is common, the pathological process in this case being a myositis, of similar type to that which may affect skeletal muscles in collagen disorders but selectively involving the extraocular muscles and leading to weakness, limitation of upward gaze and impaired convergence. It has been suggested that these myositic changes occur as a result of damage to the sarcolemma by circulating thyroglobulin–anti-thyroglobulin antibody complexes and it is certainly true that patients with severe ophthalmopathy tend to have high serum levels of anti-thyroglobulin antibodies. The affinity of this immune complex for the sarcolemma is not fully understood but it has been suggested that surface T_3 or T_4 residues may bind with thyroid hormone receptors on the sarcolemma, and that the extraocular muscles may be particularly susceptible as a result of their high level of metabolic activity.

The other striking ophthalmic disorder associated specifically with Graves's disease is exophthalmos (Fig. 6). Marked proptosis may occur with chemosis and ophthalmoplegia. Elevation of retro-orbital pressure may lead to papilloedema and loss of vision. Early symptoms include irritation of the eyes and increased lacrimation. In more severe forms the upper and lower lids may not close, leading to drying and ulceration of the cornea. The degree of exophthalmos may be partially masked by accompanying periorbital oedema and lacrimal gland enlargement. Objective measurements should therefore be made with an exophthalmometer and these measurements allow accurate assessment of progress during follow-up. In extreme cases the consequences may be very severe indeed. Subluxation of the eyeball can occur. Ulceration and infection of the cornea may lead to panophthalmitis and destruction of the eye. Compression of the optic nerve may produce visual field defects. Fortunately such severe consequences are now rarely seen.

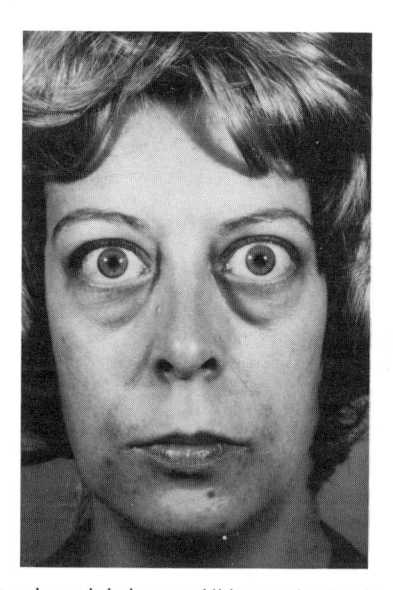

Fig. 6. Bilateral exophthalmos and lid retraction in a female patient with Graves's disease.

Exophthalmos is usually bilateral but often asymmetrical. Accompanying thyrotoxicosis is usually, but not always, evident. Occasionally unilateral exophthalmos may occur in the absence of overt thyrotoxicosis and the cause then has to be differentiated from other causes of raised retro-orbital pressure such as retro-orbital tumours. An intravenous TRH test is most useful in investigating these patients as the TSH response will usually be found to be reduced to the thyrotoxic range even when other thyroid function tests are normal. The 'flat' TSH response to TRH suggests latent thyrotoxicosis, which is not apparent from the conventional thyroid function tests. It may well be that the more sophisticated 'free' T_3 and T_4 assays are abnormal when total T_4 and total T_3 are normal.

Graves's disease is an autoimmune disorder in which hyperthyroidism results from the stimulating effect of thyroid stimulating immunoglobulins acting via TSH receptors. These immunoglobulins include long acting thyroid stimulator (LATS), which appears not to be the aetiological factor in man, and

LATS-protector or human-specific thyroid stimulating antibody (HSTS), which probably is the important immunoglobulin responsible for thyroid hyperactivity. A group of closely allied immunoglobulins appears also to be present and react with TSH-sensitive receptors in other tissues. One group of immunoglobulins (ophthalmopathic immunoglobulins) may be responsible for the proliferation of retro-orbital adipose tissue and connective tissues seen in exophthalmos. A separate group may be responsible for the other specific features of Graves's disease, pretibial myxoedema and thyroid acropachy. It is well established that adipose cells in certain sites including retro-orbital fat have TSH receptors and stimulation of these receptors by an immunoglobulin that mimics TSH could explain both the observed pathological changes of proliferation and the associated inflammatory infiltrate.

Treatment of Thyrotoxicosis

Excessive secretion of thyroid hormone can be reversed by the use of anti-thyroid drugs, by radioactive iodine (^{131}I) or by thyroidectomy. In general it is worth trying a full course of up to 24 months of anti-thyroid drugs first, but if subsequent relapse occurs then radioactive iodine or surgery is required. Surgery is preferable if a large goitre is present, if there is compression of local structures, or in patients who find tablet treatment difficult. Radioiodine is the treatment of choice in 'toxic nodules' where the cure rate is high and post-treatment hypothyroidism uncommon. Surgery is generally preferred for patients of reproductive age because of the theoretical risks of genetic damage or malignancy associated with radioactive iodine. Both radioactive iodine therapy and surgery carry a risk of rendering the patient hypothyroid, and in the case of radioactive iodine the risk is substantial and may be delayed for many years.

Treatment of Ophthalmopathy

Re-establishment of the euthyroid state corrects those ophthalmic abnormalities which are directly due to the excessive action of thyroid hormones. However, those features of Graves's disease, particularly exophthalmos, which are not due to the effect of T_4 and T_3 are uninfluenced by anti-thyroid treatment and may indeed be worsened if a hypothyroid state is induced.

The assessment of therapeutic measures is also made difficult by the unpredictable natural history of the condition, which is characterized by remissions and exacerbations, and eventually regresses spontaneously.

If the disorder is mild, symptomatic measures only are required. Dark glasses provide protection and aid photophobia and light sensitivity. Methyl cellulose drops aid xerophthalmia due to incomplete apposition of the eyelids and benefit may also be gained at night if the patient sleeps with the head of the bed elevated.

If the condition is more severe, large doses of systemic steroids may produce improvement or at least halt progression. As an alternative to systemic corticosteroids, external radiotherapy has been employed but is seldom helpful. Corneal ulceration and infection should be treated appropriately and tarsorrhaphy performed. Further progression despite these measures, particularly if vision is threatened by corneal or retinal changes, warrants surgical decompression of the orbit.

Hypothyroidism

The clinical picture of thyroid hormone deficiency is that of insidious slowing of all body functions. The clinical picture, once recognized, appears obvious but the insidious onset and non-specific nature of the symptoms mean that the diagnosis is easily missed. Since the morbidity of the disorder is high and treatment with thyroxine highly effective, a missed diagnosis is a tragedy for the patient. Although hypothyroidism is unlikely to present to an ophthalmologist, it is nevertheless important that he, as all clinicians, should be alert to the disorder. Common symptoms include fatigue, lethargy, mental and physical slowness, deepening of the voice and puffiness around the eyes (*Fig.* 7). As with thyrotoxicosis all systems may be affected and other manifestations include constipation, menorrhagia, dry skin and alopecia, psychiatric disturbances, anaemia, ischaemic cardiac pain, cardiac failure and neurological manifestations (peripheral neuropathy and cerebellar dysfunction). Myxoedema coma is the most serious complication and carries a high mortality rate, despite treatment. Examination reveals a dry skin, coarse brittle hair, puffiness of the eyes and face and evidence of the disorders listed above. Particularly useful physical signs include bradycardia, difficulty with palpation and auscultation of the heart (due to pericardial effusion) and slow-relaxing reflexes. A goitre may also be present.

The more common causes of primary hypothyroidism are Hashimoto's thyroiditis or iatrogenic hypothyroidism. Hashimoto's thyroiditis is an autoimmune disorder in which anti-thyroid antibodies can be detected and the gland is destroyed by inflammation and fibrosis. As with Graves's disease, it is more common in women. Iatrogenic hypothyroidism may follow treatment with anti-thyroid drugs (when a goitre may be present due to compensatory TSH stimulation), surgery, or most commonly radioactive iodine treatment. Iodine deficiency can rarely also produce goitrous hypothyroidism. Cretinism in children may result from thyroid agenesis when thyroid tissues will not be palpable, or from hereditary enzyme defects in hormone synthesis, when a goitre will be present, again due to high TSH drive (dyshormonogenetic goitre). Neonatal screening with measurement of TSH is now routine in the United Kingdom.

Treatment in all cases involves appropriate replacement with thyroxine or tri-iodothyronine. The adequacy of replacement is best assessed by measurement of TSH levels to ensure that they are adequately suppressed.

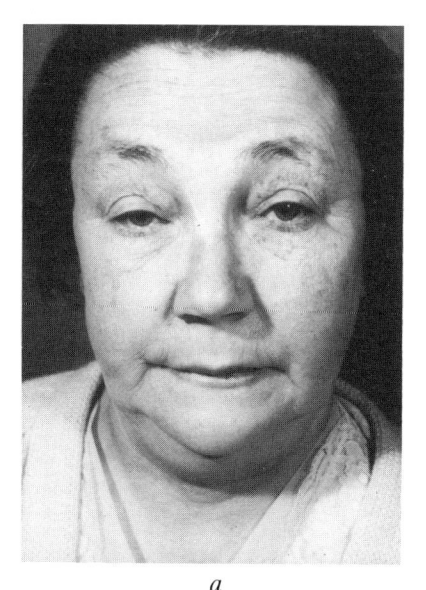

crine neoplasia. Associated disorders then include a high frequency of phaeochromocytoma, multiple neuroma, hyperparathyroidism and a Marfanoid habitus. Each of these associated disorders has implications for the ophthalmologist.

Phaeochromocytoma will be discussed later. Neuromas may be present in the eyelids. Corneal calcification may occur with hyperparathyroidism and

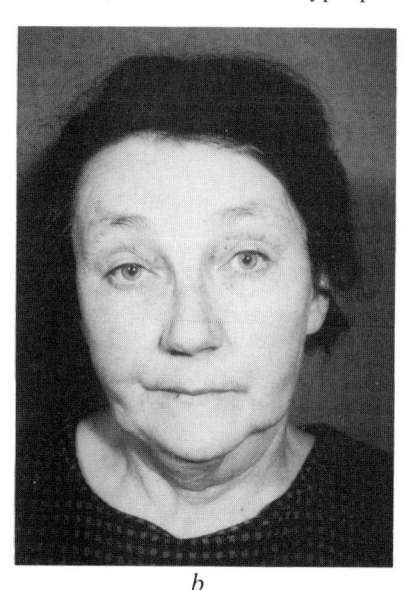

Fig. 7. a, A patient with the classic facies of myxoedema. *b*, The same patient after 4 months' treatment with thyroxine.

Although ocular involvement in the disorder is rare, the ophthalmologist may become involved in a number of ways. A patient with puffy eyes may be referred. Patients with secondary hypothyroidism due to pituitary failure may have ocular complications from an associated pituitary tumour. Patients with autoimmune hypothyroidism may have associated B_{12} deficiency due to pernicious anaemia and may therefore have optic neuritis, or may have diabetes mellitus with the presence of diabetic retinopathy.

Thyroid Cancer

Malignant disease of the thyroid is of several types. Carcinomas may arise from the follicular epithelium (papillary carcinoma, follicular carcinoma, anaplastic carcinoma) or from the parafollicular C-cells (medullary carcinoma). More rarely, the thyroid may be the seat of a primary lymphoma or of metastatic spread from carcinoma, lymphoma or sarcoma arising elsewhere.

Ophthalmological consequences of thyroid malignancy are unusual. Local spread, particularly with anaplastic carcinoma, may involve the carotid sheath and predispose to the development of Horner's syndrome, or transient ischaemic attacks.

A familial form of medullary thyroid carcinoma may occur as part of a syndrome of multiple endo-

subluxation of the ocular lens is a complication of Marfan's syndrome.

Malignant thyroid disease usually presents as nodular enlargement of the thyroid which can be shown to be 'cold' on an isotope scan and solid rather than cystic on ultrasound. Thyroid function tests are usually normal. Medullary carcinomas secrete calcitonin and assay of calcitonin levels in the blood provides a tumour marker.

ADRENAL DISORDERS

The Adrenal Cortex

The adrenal cortex secretes steroid hormones. The most important of these are cortisol and aldosterone. Others include corticosterone, androgens (testosterone and andostenedione) and oestrogens. Cortisol has an important role in the control of carbohydrate metabolism and gluconeogenesis. It also has some mineralocorticoid action and is important in the maintenance of blood pressure. Cortisol deficiency also leads to an inability to excrete a water load. Aldosterone is the major mineralocorticoid hormone in man. It influences sodium and potassium transport across cell membranes and this effect is most noticeable in the kidney where sodium retention is promoted and potassium excretion into the urine enhanced. Aldosterone secretion is controlled primarily by the renin-angiotensin system and remains unimpaired after hypophysectomy. It is the absence of aldosterone that makes primary adrenal failure much more lethal than adrenal failure secondary to hypopituitarism, since it adds sodium depletion, potassium retention, loss of ECF volume and circulatory collapse to the effects of cortisol deficiency.

Cushing's Syndrome

Cushing's syndrome results from increased circulating levels of cortisol. This may be due to therapeutic administration of exogenous cortisol or to increased secretion of endogenous cortisol. Endogenous cortisol secretion may be increased due to the presence of an adrenal adenoma or carcinoma, or due to bilateral adrenal hyperplasia consequent upon excessive stimulation by ACTH. Excessive ACTH production most commonly arises from a pituitary basophil adenoma (Cushing's disease), or as a result of ectopic ACTH production by benign or malignant tumours elsewhere (for example, carcinoid tumours and bronchogenic carcinoma). Adrenal androgen secretion may also be increased, particularly in the case of adrenal carcinoma.

The clinical features of Cushing's syndrome include truncal obesity with a buffalo hump and moon-faced appearance, acne, striae, hypertension, peripheral oedema, menstrual abnormalities, excessive bruising, atrophy of the skin, muscle weakness and wasting, psychiatric and sleep disturbances and osteoporosis. Hirsutism may be prominent if adrenal androgen production is increased. Skin pigmentation may be noticed in patients with excessive ACTH production, and is then an important clue to the diagnosis, as a pituitary tumour or source of ectopic ACTH production becomes the likely cause.

The diagnosis can be confirmed by measurement of plasma cortisol and ACTH levels, cortisol secretion rate and 24 hour urinary excretion of cortisol metabolites (oxogenic steroids).

The simplest and most effective screening investigation is an overnight dexamethasone suppression test. The patient is instructed to take 1 mg (or 1·5 mg in those whose weight exceeds 100 kg) of dexamethasone on retiring to bed and a single cortisol estimation is performed at 9.00 am the following morning. This cortisol value should then be suppressed to low levels (less than 50 nmol/l). If suppression does not occur and it is confirmed that the patient took the dexamethasone, then further investigation is essential. Additional investigations are as stated above, together with high and low dose dexamethasone suppression tests and a metyrapone test (which is particularly useful in distinguishing pituitary dependent Cushing's syndrome from ectopic ACTH production). If the diagnosis is confirmed, then appropriate imaging techniques of either the pituitary region or the adrenal glands are required for anatomical confirmation.

Cushing's syndrome, although rare, is a serious disorder with high morbidity and mortality. The treatment of pituitary dependent disease has already been discussed. Adrenal adenomas and carcinomas are resected as far as possible. Small tumours are usually benign but local recurrences often occur, sometimes many years later. Malignant tumours can only be diagnosed with certainty when distant metastases are present. These respond poorly to radiotherapy; palliative chemotherapy may then be tried with metyrapone which controls cortisol overproduction or with the adrenal cytotoxic agent o,p^1–DDD. The latter drug, however, is toxic and has numerous side effects. In the case of ectopic ACTH production treatment of the local lesion, if possible, produces resolution. Otherwise adrenal blockade with metyrapone may be helpful in relieving symptoms and controlling the associated hypokalaemia.

Ophthalmological complications of the disease can occur. Chemosis is a constant feature. Opportunistic infections of the eye may occur (for example herpes virus and cytomegalovirus infections). Hypertension may lead to retinopathy and this may be aggravated by polycythaemia. Diabetes mellitus may be present and also associated with retinopathy. Occasionally, giant ACTH secreting pituitary tumours may produce visual field defects. Adrenal carcinomas may rarely metastasize to the brain as may tumours associated with ectopic ACTH production, and such metastases may involve the neurovisual pathways or occipital cortex. Cataract formation and raised intraocular pressure have been recorded in association with long term use of exogenous steroids.

Conn's Syndrome

Primary hyperaldosteronism is due to autonomous hypersecretion of aldosterone by the adrenal cortex (Conn's syndrome). Hyperaldosteronism may also occur secondary to hypersecretion of renin. In true Conn's syndrome, renin levels will be suppressed. The syndrome presents with hypertension and hypokalaemia, and hypertensive retinopathy may be present. The presence of hypokalaemia allows the condition to be distinguished from essential hypertension.

Addison's Disease

This condition is due to destruction or atrophy of the adrenal cortex with consequent failure of secretion of cortisol and aldosterone. The most common cause is autoimmune destruction of the cortex. Tuberculosis of the adrenal is now less common than it was in Addison's era. Other causes include metastatic carcinoma and amyloidosis, and iatrogenic Addison's disease following bilateral adrenalectomy.

Lack of aldosterone produces sodium depletion and a fall in ECF volume, blood pressure and glomerular filtration rate. Cortisol lack accentuates these changes and also predisposes to hypoglycaemia. A fall in circulating cortisol levels activates the feedback loop and leads to increased ACTH secretion by the pituitary. Pigmentation of the skin results. The circulatory changes induced by a fall in circulating aldosterone levels lead to increased renin secretion by the juxtaglomerular apparatus in the kidney.

Adrenal failure secondary to pituitary disease produces a rather different picture because aldosterone secretion will be preserved and ACTH levels will be low so that pigmentation changes do not occur. Hypoglycaemia becomes a more prominent feature and dilutional hyponatraemia may occur as a result of the inability to excrete a water load induced by the cortisol deficiency. True 'Addisonian crises' do not occur.

Common symptoms of Addison's disease include tiredness, malaise, anorexia, nausea, weight loss, pigmentation and fainting attacks. Useful physical signs include the presence of abnormal pigmentation and postural hypotension. Occasionally Addison's disease may be an incidental finding and the presence of associated conditions may alert one to the diagnosis. Autoimmune adrenal destruction is commonly associated with other autoimmune disorders, notably diabetes mellitus, Hashimoto's thyroiditis, vitiligo, pernicious anaemia, primary gonadal failure, primary hypoparathyroidism and chronic mucocutaneous candidiasis. Ophthalmic manifestations may therefore include diabetic retinopathy, optic atrophy and abnormal retinal pigmentation. Clearly also the presence of tuberculous destruction of the adrenals may be suspected from the presence of tuberculosis elsewhere and the optic fundi should always be inspected for the presence of choroidal lesions.

The presence of vomiting or of abnormal urea and electrolytes (classically a raised plasma urea and potassium and reduced plasma sodium) indicate that treatment is required urgently and definitive investigation should wait. Blood may, however, be collected for ACTH, cortisol and adrenal antibody estimations prior to commencement of treatment. If time is available, definitive investigation may be completed first. It must be stressed that if the adrenocortical failure is incomplete, cortisol values may be maintained in the normal range by high ACTH drive, and normal cortisol values do not therefore exclude the diagnosis. The definitive diagnosis can usually be made using a short ACTH (Synacthen) stimulation test, although in cases of doubt a prolonged depot ACTH stimulation test is required. It should also be remembered that if the aldosterone deficiency is more severe than the cortisol deficiency, the patient may be very ill and yet retain some basal cortisol levels but no response to ACTH. In these patients the findings of low circulating aldosterone levels and elevated renin levels may be diagnostic.

Acute cortisol and aldosterone deficiency may produce an Addisonian crisis before the diagnosis is made. In these severely shocked, ill patients intravenous fluid replacement and intravenous cortisol administration is urgent. Maintenance therapy is then required with glucocorticoid (cortisone acetate, hydrocortisone or dexamethasone) and mineralocorticoid (fludrocortisone). In practice, Addisonian crises most commonly occur in patients in whom the diagnosis is already known and result either from poor compliance to therapy or from failure to increase the steroid dose in the face of intercurrent illness, particularly if vomiting is a feature.

Adrenal Medulla and Phaeochromocytoma

The adrenal medulla secretes catecholamines. It is, however, a relatively minor source of catecholamines and there are no known diseases associated with adrenal medullary insufficiency. Catecholamine secreting tumours of the adrenal medulla (phaeochromocytoma), although rare, are, however, of a degree of importance which far outweighs their prevalence. They constitute a treatable cause of paroxysmal or persistent hypertension which if untreated will eventually prove fatal. Their presence may herald other occult, potentially fatal but treatable diseases and there is often a marked familial incidence. The clinical manifestations of phaeochromocytoma are protean and may be confused with acute anxiety, thyrotoxicosis, diabetes mellitus, Cushing's syndrome, carcinoid syndrome and acute surgical abdominal emergencies.

Pathology

Ninety per cent of phaeochromocytomas occur in the adrenal medulla while the remainder occur in ectopic sites, usually within the abdomen but sometimes within the neck or thorax. Bilateral medullary tumours are present in approximately 10 per cent of cases. The tumours are malignant in approximately 10 per cent of cases. The tumours secrete excessive amounts of catecholamines, particularly adrenaline and noradrenaline. Malignant tumours may also secrete dopamine. When only noradrenaline is secreted in excess it is said that the tumour is more likely to be in a non-adrenal site. They may arise from any chromaffin tissue and tumours arising from the orbital paraganglia have been recorded as producing proptosis.

Associated Disorders

Certain disorders are frequently associated with phaeochromocytoma and some of these have implications for the ophthalmologist. Autosomal dominant inheritance (with variable penetrance) occurs with each. Neurofibromatosis or von Recklinghausen's disease, is the most common association. About 5 per cent of patients with phaeochromocytoma have neurofibromatosis and about 10 per cent of patients with neurofibromatosis will develop phaeochromocytoma.

The incidence of meningioma and glioma is also increased and glioma of the optic nerve and chiasm may occur in childhood and should always be considered in the differential diagnosis of unilateral blindness, proptosis or extraocular muscle paralysis in childhood, especially if there is other evidence of von Recklinghausen's disease. Patients with von Hippel–Lindau's disease also have a high incidence of phaeochromocytomas. This disease is characterized by vascular abnormalities of the retina, capillary angiomas, which are usually multiple and cause progressive loss of vision, cerebellar haemangioblastomas, occasionally cystic haemangioblastomas elsewhere and polycythaemia. Sturge–Weber syndrome and tuberous sclerosis may also co-exist with neurofibromatosis and further ophthalmological associations will therefore include those associated with these conditions, for example, retinal fibromas, optic atrophy, cataract and involvement of the neurovisual pathways due to destruction of the cerebral tissue within the parietal and occipital lobes.

Multiple endocrine neoplasia type II describes the association between phaeochromocytomas, medullary carcinoma of the thyroid and hyperparathyroidism. Some of these patients may also have a Marfanoid habitus and mucosal neuromas (which may be present in the conjunctivae). These patients tend to present at a later age than those with simple familial phaeochromocytoma and very frequently have bilateral disease.

Clinical Features

Symptoms are most marked with paroxysmally functioning tumours. Hypertension may be paroxysmal, labile or sustained. The most common symptoms are headache which is throbbing in nature, excessive sweating and palpitation. Weight loss is also commonly reported. Other features include chest pain (which resembles angina), abdominal pain, breathlessness, nausea, vomiting and anxiety. Syncopal attacks and visual disturbances may also occur. Features of associated disorders may be present. Diabetes mellitus may occur. Hypertensive retinopathy may be present, particularly in patients with sustained hypertension, as may retinopathic features attributable to diabetes and polycythaemia. Paroxysmal attacks can be triggered by a number of events such as exercise, postural changes, pressure upon the abdomen, surgery, Valsalva's manoeuvre and pain.

Diagnosis

The diagnosis is based upon the finding of elevated levels of catecholamine metabolites in the urine. The test usually employed is estimation of the metabolite vanillylmandelic acid (VMA) in 24 hour urine collections, preferably collected during and after an attack. Certain interfering substances (dietary and medicinal) such as bananas, ice cream, chocolate, methyldopa, phenothiazines and monoamine oxidase inhibitors, should be withheld as they may produce false positive results. The diagnosis can be further confirmed by estimation of plasma adrenaline and noradrenaline concentrations using enzyme assay. There is no longer a case for provocation tests using histamine or tyramine as these are unreliable and potentially dangerous. The intravenous injection of 5 mg of phentolamine may be helpful in the management of severe hypertensive episodes but a considerable fall in diastolic pressure occurs with most forms of hypertension and is not (as previously thought) pathognomonic of phaeochromocytoma. If the diagnosis is confirmed then the tumour has to be located by appropriate radiological procedures. Nephrotomography, CT scanning and angiography are the investigations of choice and it must always be remembered that the tumours may be multiple or in an ectopic position. Selective venous sampling of plasma catecholamines also has a place, but the results may be difficult to interpret.

Treatment

The treatment of choice is surgical excision after preparation of the patient with alpha- and beta-adrenergic blockade. Such preparation is essential both to minimize the risk of a hypertensive crisis and to reduce the risk of postoperative hypovolaemic shock which may follow the release of long standing vasoconstriction. The anaesthetic management of these patients requires considerable skill and experience.

Following surgery urinary catecholamine metabolite secretion should be checked annually in order to detect recurrence. This is particularly important in patients with a positive family history.

DISORDERS OF THE PARATHYROID GLANDS

Hyperparathyroidism

Primary hyperparathyroidism may be due to an adenoma, multiple adenomas, carcinoma or hyperplasia of the parathyroid gland. The excessive parathyroid hormone production results in hypercalcaemia. Secondary hyperparathyroidism is said to be present when parathyroid hormone production is increased as a compensatory response to hypocalcaemia due to, for example, osteomalacia or chronic renal disease. The calcium concentration is therefore normal or low in secondary hyperparathyroidism. The development of hypercalcaemia in patients with secondary hyperparathyroidism indicates progression to tertiary hyperparathyroidism. In this situation, adenoma formation develops from a background of secondary parathyroid hyperplasia.

The more common presenting features of primary and tertiary hyperparathyroidism include renal stones, bone pain due to osteitis fibrosa, peptic ulceration, symptoms of hypercalcaemia and psychiatric disorders. Routine biochemical screening in asymptomatic patients is, however, the most common reason for the diagnosis being made. Hereditary hyperparathyroidism may occur on its own or as part of a syndrome of multiple endocrine neoplasia, either in association with prolactin secreting pituitary tumours and tumours of the pancreatic islets (gastrin producing tumours, Zollinger–Ellison syndrome), or in association with phaeochromocytoma and medullary carcinoma of the thyroid. Physical signs are few. Parathyroid nodules are rarely palpable.

Hypertension and proximal myopathy may be present. Corneal calcification or band keratopathy may be clinically recognizable or recognizable on slit lamp examination. Calcium phosphate crystals may rarely be deposited in the conjunctiva. Difficulty in focusing of the eyes also occurs.

Diagnosis depends upon finding the appropriate biochemical abnormalities (hypercalcaemia, hypophosphataemia and elevation of alkaline phosphatase). Additional confirmatory investigations include measurement of renal phosphate threshold, radioimmunoassay of parathyroid hormone and appropriate radiology, particularly of the hands to demonstrate abnormalities of bone. Thallium scans with subtraction of the thyroid image may be helpful in localizing tumours.

The major differential diagnosis is from other causes of hypercalcaemia, notably malignant tumours involving bone, vitamin D intoxication, milk-alkali syndrome and sarcoidosis. The diagnosis of sarcoidosis is particularly likely to involve the ophthalmologist as there may be numerous ophthalmic abnormalities, notably uveitis, retinal vasculitis or cranial nerve involvement secondary to granulomatous basilar meningitis.

The treatment of choice for primary and tertiary hyperparathyroidism is surgical removal of any abnormal tissue.

Hypoparathyroidism

This condition is much less common than hyperparathyroidism and produces a metabolic abnormality characterized by hypocalcaemia and consequent neuromuscular symptoms. It most commonly follows removal of the parathyroids or damage to the glands or their vascular supply as a result of surgery for thyroid disorders, hyperparathyroidism or radical neck dissection. It may be either transient or permanent.

Idiopathic hypoparathyroidism is rare. It may occur in isolation, in association with thymic agenesis and aortic arch anomalies (Di George syndrome), or in association with multiple failure of adrenal, thyroid and ovarian function, pernicious anaemia and diabetes mellitus.

The clinical features of hypoparathyroidism include tetany, epilepsy, psychological disturbances, intracranial calcification (particularly of the basal ganglia) and soft tissue calcification. A surgical scar may be present in the neck. Ophthalmological abnormalities include cataract and, less commonly, papilloedema due to raised intracranial pressure as well as ophthalmic manifestations of associated conditions such as diabetes mellitus, pernicious anaemia and Addison's disease. Early calcium deposits in the lens may be detected with the slit lamp. Later changes include nuclear degeneration, vacuolation, fissuring and diffuse opacities.

The major aim of treatment is to maintain normocalcaemia by use of vitamin D and calcium supplements. Other causes of hypocalcaemia have to be considered in the differential diagnosis, notably dietary deficiency, or malabsorption of vitamin D, or vitamin D resistance consequent upon renal disease.

Pseudohypoparathyroidism is a rare genetic disorder in which hypocalcaemia occurs in association with characteristic skeletal and other abnormalities including short stature and mental retardation. Ocular problems can occasionally occur, notably strabismus, soft tissue calcification and, again, cataract. This condition is characterized by tissue resistance to the action of parathyroid hormone.

Pseudo-pseudohypoparathyroidism is a term used to describe cases which have many of the physical features of pseudohypoparathyroidism but no detectable abnormality of calcium metabolism.

DISORDERS OF THE ENDOCRINE PANCREAS

Endocrine cells of the pancreas reside largely within the Islets of Langerhans which are ovoid clusters of cells lying between the pancreatic acini. Some endocrine cells also exist outside the islets. The principal hormones normally secreted by the pancreatic islets are insulin, glucagon, somatostatin and pancreatic polypeptide. Two important groups of disorders of pancreatic endocrine function need to be considered. First, deficiency states, of which the only important example is diabetes mellitus due to impaired or absent insulin secretion. Secondly, hormone secreting tumours of the pancreas, of which the most important are tumours secreting insulin (insulinomas) and tumours secreting gastrin. A variety of hormones can, however, be produced by tumours of the pancreatic islets and further examples include glucagonomas, somatostatinomas, ACTH producing tumours and tumours secreting serotonin with the production of carcinoid syndrome. Some tumours may secrete several hormones.

Diabetes Mellitus

A detailed discussion of this subject is beyond the scope of this chapter. The important topic of diabetic retinopathy is dealt with in Chapter 8 (pp. 238–47). There are, however, numerous and diverse ophthalmic manifestations of diabetes mellitus in addition to retinopathy and these will be briefly discussed.

Aetiological Associations

In a small proportion of cases, diabetes mellitus occurs either in association with other disorders, or as a result of another disorder, and in some of these cases additional ophthalmic problems may arise.

A rare inherited form of diabetes mellitus occurs in association with diabetes insipidus, optic atrophy and nerve deafness (DIDMOAD syndrome). Diabetes mellitus may be part of the autoimmune syndrome associated with multiple endocrine organ failure. Several very rare syndromes also link diabetes mellitus with retinitis pigmentosa. Patients with dystrophia myotonica have an increased incidence of diabetes mellitus. Progeria may link diabetes mellitus with the premature formation of cataracts.

Diabetes occurs as a secondary phenomenon in patients with tumours that secrete hormones that have opposing actions to insulin, notably in Cushing's syndrome, acromegaly and phaeochromocytoma. The potential ophthalmic manifestations of these disorders have been discussed above.

Complications

Acute alterations in visual acuity are common symptoms of hyperglycaemia and are thought to result from osmotic changes within the lens. Patients not infrequently attend their optician as a result of this and they should be advised not to change their glasses at this time as the changes gradually reverse when their diabetes is controlled.

Chronic ophthalmic complications include cataract, oculomotor nerve palsies, neuropathy of the optic nerve, autonomic neuropathy, which may affect pupillary function, an increased incidence of cerebrovascular disease and manifestations of hyperlipidaemia.

Cataract formation is a common diabetic complication. In adult patients nuclear opacities are most common and are similar in appearance to senile cataracts. In juvenile diabetics 'snowflake' cataracts may occur. Multiple small cortical opacities occur deep to the lens capsule and may progress very rapidly indeed. These cataracts are associated with the accumulation of sorbitol within the lens. Osmotic changes then occur and produce disorganization of lens fibres. A similar aetiological explanation has been invoked in the case of cataract associated with galactosaemia, when high levels of galactose within the lens lead to increased production of dulcitol and similar osmotic changes.

Progression of these cataracts can be halted or even reversed at the early stages by good control of blood glucose concentration as this minimizes glucose metabolism via the sorbitol pathway. Aldose reductase inhibitors have been shown to be effective in animals with experimentally induced cataracts and may prove to have a place in the treatment of diabetic patients with cataract.

Oculomotor nerve palsies in diabetic subjects are usually a result of mononeuritis multiplex secondary to disease of the vasa nervorum. They are usually abrupt in onset and the prognosis is generally good.

The existence of optic neuropathy in diabetic patients has been the subject of considerable controversy. It has recently been shown, however, that a substantial proportion of diabetics who have reasonably normal retinal function have abnormal visual evoked potentials with considerable prolongation of latency. This suggests that the optic nerve is not uncommonly involved in the neuropathy of diabetes.

Abnormalities of the pupil are also common in diabetic patients, an abnormally small pupil being a salient finding. Smith and Smith showed in 1983 that the small pupil in diabetes is supersensitive to phenylephrine and this is evidence in favour of a neuropathic rather than a myopathic aetiology. The small pupil is commonly associated with evidence of autonomic neuropathy elsewhere. The abnormality of sympathetic innervation of the pupillary muscle may explain the clinical observation that the small diabetic pupil is difficult to dilate, anticholinergic mydriatics alone being insufficient when sympathetic tone is reduced. Smith and Smith have shown that the addition of a directly acting sympathomimetic will improve the mydriasis.

The major complication of the treatment of diabetes is hypoglycaemia. The protean clinical manifestations of hypoglycaemia result from a combination of neuroglycopenia and compensatory stimulation of the autonomic nervous system. Visual symptoms, particularly blurred vision and diplopia, are common. It has been the authors' experience that visual symptoms with hypoglycaemic attacks are more frequent in patients with retinopathy and especially maculopathy. A recent study in the authors' department into the effects of hypoglycaemia upon vision has shown some changes in refraction, deterioration of colour discrimination and prolongation of the latency of the visual evoked response in the absence of changes in visual acuity. It is clear that, if visual evoked responses are measured in diabetic patients, then care should be taken to ensure that the patient is not hypoglycaemic at the time as the result may otherwise be misleading.

Pancreatic hormone secreting tumours

Insulinoma

These tumours may be benign or malignant. Patients classically present with manifestations of hypoglycaemia, which are particularly likely to occur when the patient is fasted or taking vigorous exercise and which respond to the ingestion of food or glucose. In view of the many manifestations of hypoglycaemia the symptomatology can be very diverse indeed and many alternative diagnoses may be entertained, particularly epilepsy and psychiatric disorders. Visual disturbances occur in approximately 30 per cent of patients. Weight gain is usual. Diagnosis depends upon documentation of hypoglycaemia, documentation of inappropriately elevated circulating insulin concentrations and identification of the pancreatic tumour. Identification of the tumour may, however, be difficult, even with the most sophisticated imaging techniques.

For benign tumours, surgical resection should be performed where possible. In patients for whom surgery is deemed inappropriate, treatment with diazoxide may be of considerable benefit. Treatment of malignant insulinomas is difficult and the results very poor despite the trial of a number of chemotherapeutic agents.

Gastrinoma

Gastrin producing tumours are responsible for the Zollinger–Ellison syndrome which is characterized by intractable multiple peptic ulceration and gastric hyperacidity. Hormone secreting pancreatic tumours may be part of a multiple endocrine neoplasia syndrome and this is particularly true in the case of gastrinoma, where there is a strong association with hyperparathyroidism and pituitary tumours (usually prolactinomas) and a positive family history (multiple endocrine neoplasia, type I).

Other Tumours

Tumours secreting other hormones such as vasoactive intestinal polypeptide, pancreatic polypeptide and glucagon are all known to occur but are rather unlikely to enter the province of the ophthalmologist. Somatostatin secreting tumours are exceptionally rare and as yet the related clinical syndrome cannot be fully defined. Associations are, however, known to include hypochlorhydria and malabsorption and B_{12} deficiency must therefore be a theoretical possibility. Islet cell tumours may also be a source of ectopic ACTH secretion, may secrete serotonin, thereby producing carcinoid syndrome, and may secrete a mixture of hormones (for example gastrin, insulin and serotonin).

GONADAL DISORDERS

Primary disorders of the testis and ovary are relatively unlikely to involve the ophthalmologist and will therefore only receive brief discussion. However, hypogonadism secondary to pituitary or hypothalamic disease is often associated with ocular disturbances.

Primary Gonadal Failure

Among the numerous causes of primary testicular or ovarian failure is autoimmune destruction. Antibodies against ovarian or testicular tissue may then be demonstrable in the serum, and the disease is commonly associated with autoimmune destruction of other endocrine organs. This syndrome of multiple endocrine organ failure has been discussed before and includes diabetes mellitus, Addison's disease, hypothyroidism (Hashimoto's thyroiditis) and hypoparathyroidism.

Hypogonadism may also occur in association with other systemic diseases with ocular manifestations such as thyrotoxicosis, inflammatory bowel disease and rheumatoid arthritis. Leprosy, and occasionally other granulomatous diseases, may produce testicular damage.

Dystrophia myotonica in the male is associated with testicular atrophy, in addition to cataracts and its other manifestations. Gonadal dysgenesis in the female (Turner's syndrome) may be associated with ptosis, and carries an increased risk of hypertension (both as a result of coarctation of the aorta and 'essential' hypertension). Hypertensive retinopathy may therefore be present.

Secondary Gonadal Failure

Secondary gonadal failure occurs when gonadotrophin release is impaired. It may result from a wide variety of hypothalamic and pituitary disorders. If the disorder is present before puberty then it will present with delayed puberty and persistent sexual infantilism. If it develops in the adult, it will present with the features of adult hypogonadism, notably loss of secondary sexual characteristics and infertility or secondary amenorrhoea. If only gonadatrophins are deficient prior to puberty, then height will usually be normal or increased. If other pituitary hormones are also deficient then a variety of other abnormalities may be present. Growth hormone deficiency in particular will result in the additional feature of short stature. The most common cause of secondary gonadal failure (hypogonadotrophic hypogonadism) tumours of the pituitary region. Gonadal failure is commonly the earliest manifestation of generalized hypopituitarism secondary to tumours, adrenal and thyroid function failing at a later stage. It has then to be differentiated from isolated gonadotrophin deficiency occurring in the absence of detectable structural disease.

Tumours of the pituitary region may impair gonadotrophin release either by direct destruction of the pituitary or hypothalamic tissue or by interruption of the pituitary stalk and interruption of the portal circulation by which gonadotrophin releasing hormone reaches the pituitary. It should be remembered that prolactin secreting tumours are particularly likely to produce hypogonadism as a result of the additional effect of elevated prolactin levels upon both pituitary gonadotrophin release and directly upon the gonad itself. The presentation, diagnosis and management of these tumours has already been discussed.

Secondary gonadal failure can be distinguished from primary gonadal failure by measurement of gonadotrophin (FSH and LH) concentrations both basally and following the intravenous injection of gonadotrophin releasing hormone (LHRH). In primary failure gonadotrophin levels will be high as a result of reduced negative feedback by gonadal sex steroids, as seen in post-menopausal females. If the pituitary is destroyed, then LH and FSH levels will be low and will not rise following administration of LHRH. In patients with hypothalamic disease basal LH and FSH levels will again be low but there will usually be a response to LHRH, and this response may be delayed and sometimes exaggerated.

Isolated gonadotrophin deficiency may occur sporadically or as a familial disorder. These patients present with delayed puberty and have eunuchoid features. Rarely the deficiency is of LH alone, FSH secretion being preserved, and this produces the condition known as 'fertile eunuch' in which spermatogenesis occurs although fertility is, in fact, rare. Isolated gonadotrophin deficiency also occurs in association with growth hormone deficiency when short stature is superimposed and this contrasts with the situation arising with gonadotrophin deficiency alone, where the patients are of normal height or even tall, due to the lack of gonadal sex steroid influence on skeletal maturation.

A number of different syndromes are also identifiable in which isolated gonadotrophin deficiency occurs in association with a number of other abnormalities: Kallman's syndrome, which occurs in males, probably by X-linked recessive inheritance, is a combination of hypogonadotrophic hypogonadism due to hypothalamic dysgenesis; anosmia, due to agenesis of the olfactory bulb; colour blindness and nerve deafness. The Prader–Willi syndrome and Laurence–Moon–Biedl syndrome provide further examples of hypogonadotrophic hypogonadism secondary to hypothalamic dysfunction. Prader–Willi syndrome is also associated with mental retardation, short stature and obesity. The Laurence–Moon–Biedl syndrome also displays obesity (a common accompaniment of all hypothalamic disorders) and important ocular abnormalities, notably retinitis pigmentosa and nystagmus. A superficially similar, but probably separate, entity is the Alström syndrome in which are found, obesity, childhood blindness due to retinal degeneration, aminoaciduria and nephrogenic diabetes insipidus, primary hypogonadism, hypotriglyceridaemia, hyperuricaemia and acanthosis nigricans. The Biemond syndrome is another very similar syndrome but can be distinguished by the presence of iris coloboma.

Precocious Puberty

True precocious puberty, due to inappropriate secretion of gonadotrophins, may result from premature activation of the hypothalamo–pituitary axis or may occur with certain disorders involving the hypothalamus such as encephalitis, and with pineal tumours (*see above*). Very rarely other tumours may be associated with ectopic secretion of gonadotrophins (for example malignant melanoma and ovarian chorioepithelioma). These patients require full investigation and differentiation must be made from other causes of precocious puberty (precocious 'pseudopuberty') where gonadotrophins are not detectable. These disorders include testicular tumours in the male; ovarian tumours in the female and adrenal tumours or congenital adrenal hyperplasia in both sexes.

MISCELLANEOUS DISORDERS

Before concluding this chapter, mention should be made of a number of disorders, not previously discussed, in which ophthalmic manifestations may occur.

Hyperlipidaemias

A detailed discussion of the classification of hypercholesterolaemia and hypertriglyceridaemia is beyond the scope of this chapter. It should be remembered, however, that important physical signs may be elicited on examination of the eye, notably xanthomas, xanthelasma, arcus senilis and lipaemia retinalis. The presence of these signs should alert the clinician to a diagnosis which may not otherwise be apparent and which carries an increased risk of the development of atherosclerosis.

Inborn Errors of Metabolism

Some of these conditions have already been mentioned. Other examples may also have ophthalmological implications.

Galactosaemia

In this condition galactose accumulates in the blood as a result of deficiency of the enzyme galactose-1-phosphate uridyl transferase. In addition to other abnormalities, cataracts may develop within a few weeks of birth, or occasionally may be present at birth. They can be prevented by removal of lactose from the diet.

Hypoliproteinaemias

These exceptionally rare conditions may be associated with corneal infiltration by lipid or cholesterol esters. Abetalipoproteinaemia is additionally associated with nystagmus, visual impairment with scotomas and pigmentary retinal degeneration in addition to other progressive neurological deficits.

Alcaptonuria and Ochronosis

This is a disorder of the metabolism of the amino acid tyrosine. Homogentisic acid accumulates as a result of the deficiency of the enzyme homogentisic acid oxidase and spills over in the urine (alcaptonuria). Ochronosis results from deposition of an oxidized brown–black pigment of homogentistic acid in connective tissue. This pigment may be deposited in the cornea and sclera of the eye.

Homocystinuria

This is a disorder of the metabolism of the amino acid methionine which leads to accumulation of homocysteine. Homocysteine is oxidized to homocystine and excreted in the urine. Excess homocysteine interferes with the structure of collagen and elastin and impairs its function. Damage to elastin in the ocular lens creates marked instability which is manifest as iridodonesis and subsequent downward dislocation. Pupillary entrapment may occur with glaucoma, optic atrophy and subsequent blindness.

Lens dislocation is also seen with Marfan's syndrome, although upward rather than downward dislocation is usual. The causal defect is unknown.

Paget's Disease of Bone

Paget's disease is characterized by localized areas of bone remodelling, resulting from increased osteoclastic and osteoblastic activity. It is a quite common disorder of unknown aetiology. The clinical features include skeletal deformity, bone pain and symptoms related to compression of neural structures. Compression of cranial nerves may occur and if the optic nerve or oculomotor nerves are affected the condition may present to the ophthalmologist. The most effective form of treatment is calcitonin administration. However, this is rather more effective at producing pain control than in reversing skeletal deformity. Treatment with mithramycin (a cytotoxic drug) and disphosphanates ('bone crystal poisons') can also be used.

Congenital Rubella

The syndrome of congenital rubella may include hypothalamic dysfunction as part of a generalized microcephaly or subsequent progressive subacute panencephalitis presenting in later life. Ocular manifestations are also common and include corneal opacities, cataracts, chorioretinitis and microphthalmia. Among the many other described abnormalities a higher instance of diabetes mellitus in later life is said to occur.

ACKNOWLEDGEMENTS

Thanks are due to Mr P. Riley of the Department of Medicine and to the Photographic Department of St Thomas's Hospital, London, for assistance in the preparation of the illustrations and to Lisbeth Lawrence for invaluable secretarial assistance.

FURTHER READING

Donald R. A. (ed.) *Endocrine Disorders: a Guide to Diagnosis.* New York, Marcel Decker, 1984.
Gray C. H. and James V. H. T. (ed.) *Hormones in Blood*, vol. 4, 3rd ed. London, Academic Press, 1983.
Irvine W. J. (ed.) Autoimmunity in endocrine disease. *Clin. Endocrinol. Metabol.* 1975; **4**, no. 2.
Marble A., White P., Bradley R. F. et al. *Joslin's Diabetes Mellitus*, 11th ed. Philadelphia, Lea and Febiger, 1971.
Puvanendren K., Devathesen G. and Wong P. K. Visual evoked responses in diabetes. *J. Neurol. Neurosurg. Psychiat.* **46**, 643–7.
Scanlon M. F. (ed.) Neuroendocrinology. *Clin. Endocrinol. Metabol.* 1983; **12**, no. 3.
Schmidek H. H. (ed.) *Pineal Tumours.* New York, Masson, 1977.
Smith S. A. and Smith S. E. Evidence for neuropathic aetiology in the small pupil of diabetes mellitus. *Br. J. Ophthalmol.* 1983; **67**, 89–93.
Smith S. E., Smith S. A., Brown P. M. et al. Pupillary signs in diabetic autonomic neuropathy. *Br. Med. J.* 1978; **2**, 924–7.
Volpé R. (ed.) Thyrotoxicosis. *Clin. Endocrinol. Metabol.* 1978; **7**, no. 1.
Williams R. H. (ed.) *Textbook of Endocrinology*, 6th ed. Philadelphia, Saunders, 1981.

Haematological Diseases

P. I. Condon and G. R. Serjeant

INTRODUCTION

Involvement of the eye in blood disorders may be classified according to the affected blood constituent
1. Red cell disorders
   (a) Decreased haemoglobin level (anaemias) classified by the morphological appearance of the red cells into microcytic, normocytic and macrocytic forms.
   (b) Increased haemoglobin level (erythraemias), including polycythaemia rubra vera and the secondary polycythaemias.
   (c) Qualitatively abnormal red cells, as in sickle cell disease.
2. White cell disorders
   (a) Decreased numbers of white cells (leucopenia).
   (b) Increased numbers of white cells (leukaemia) classified according to the types of white cell affected into myelocytic, lymphocytic and monocytic varieties.
3. Platelet disorders
   (a) Decreased number of platelets as in thrombocytopenic purpura
   (b) Increased numbers of platelets in thrombocythaemia.
4. Coagulation disorders.
5. Dysproteinaemia
   Conditions associated with large amounts of abnormal plasma proteins produced by plasma cells (multiple myeloma) or other cells (macroglobulinaemia).

ANAEMIAS

All anaemias are characterized by a reduction in haemoglobin level, and a variety of compensatory mechanisms occur to reduce the resulting tissue hypoxia. In the vascular system there is a reduction in peripheral vascular resistance and an increase in cardiac output so that the blood is circulated more rapidly. At the cellular level there is an increased tissue extraction of oxygen leading to an increased arteriovenous oxygen difference and this is aided by an increase in erythrocyte 2,3 DPG which shifts the oxygen dissociation curve to the right, allowing release of greater amounts of oxygen.

The retinal vasculature contains no sympathetic or parasympathetic nerve fibres, local conditions acting directly on the retinal arterial wall muscle to adjust local blood flow (autoregulation). In response to the anoxia in anaemia there is an increase in blood flow and also an increased permeability. The resulting retinal changes are generally similar regardless of the aetiology of the anaemia and the most common findings are retinal haemorrhages,[1] appearance of which depends upon their site and level within the retina.

Preretinal and sub-hyaloid haemorrhages originate directly from the retinal vessels and spread in front of the retina in the space between the posterior vitreous face and the retina. Sub-hyaloid haemorrhages may be large but are generally shallow with a circular outline and often a fluid level. Occasionally large preretinal haemorrhages may rupture the posterior vitreous face leading to vitreous haemorrhage and sudden decrease in visual acuity. Flame shaped haemorrhages resulting from blood tracking in the superficial nerve fibre layer are common. Intraretinal haemorrhages have a rounded appearance with dark periphery and pale centre (Roth's spots) and result from blood tracking anteroposteriorly along the vertical elements of the retina. Deep subretinal haemorrhages originate in the choriocapillaris and appear as dark slate grey, circumscribed areas with vague margins.

Retinal haemorrhages in anaemia are often striking since they occur against the background of a pale fundus. The pathological mechanism leading to retinal haemorrhage in anaemia is poorly understood but is presumed to result from anoxic damage of the retinal vessel wall, with a possible contribution from the hyperdynamic circulation common in anaemia.

Other ocular changes include loss of the granular texture of the retina due to mild retinal oedema, and dilatation of the retinal arterioles and venules. Soft cotton-wool exudates, which are signs of focal capillary shutdown, with formation of minute superficial retinal infarcts occur only in severe anaemia. Hard exudates, sometimes taking the form of a 'macular star', can occur with resolving retinal oedema or cotton-wool spots. Non-rhegmatogeneous retinal detachment may rarely occur in severe congestive cardiac failure.

Microcytic Anaemia

A microcytic hypochromic anaemia characterizes iron deficiency which results most frequently from inadequate intake of dietary iron, failure of intestinal iron absorption or chronic blood loss. This anaemia develops slowly, low haemoglobin levels are surprisingly well tolerated and retinal changes are rare.

Acute hypotension from haemorrhage may result in an ischaemic optic neuropathy.[2] Blood vessels supplying the optic nerve do not autoregulate and sudden sustained hypotension may cause infarction of the nerve fibres in the optic nerve. As a result there may be deterioration of the visual acuity, dilatation and unresponsiveness of the pupil in the affected eye, scattered retinal haemorrhages, cotton-wool exudates and swelling of the optic disc. The late appearance is of optic atrophy with a pigmentary retinal disturbance. Symptoms are generally delayed for 3–16 days after the haemorrhage, and blindness, often with other focal neurological signs, may occur.

Treatment of sudden severe blood loss requires correction of the underlying condition, transfusion and general supportive therapy. Treatment of chronic blood loss or malabsorption requires correction of the underlying pathology and oral or parenteral iron. Treatment of dietary deficiency requires only oral or parenteral iron.

Normocytic Anaemias

Normocytic anaemias may result from deficient production or excessive destruction of red cells.

Deficient production may be caused by congenital abnormalities in the process of haemoglobin synthesis, by toxic chemicals interfering with haemoglobin synthesis or damaging red cell precursors, by marrow hypoplasia associated with chronic infection and renal failure and by crowding out of the red cell precursors by malignant disease or myelofibrosis.

Haemolytic anaemias may be congenitally determined (hereditary spherocytosis, paroxysmal nocturnal haemoglobinuria, haemoglobinopathies), the result of infection (malaria), the result of chemical poisons (phenylhydrazine) or brought about by red cell antibodies (Rhesus incompatibility).

None of these conditions, other than sickle cell disease, has specific ocular or retinal findings other than those occurring in anaemias generally.

Macrocytic (Megaloblastic) Anaemias

Megaloblastic change in the bone-marrow may occur from either deficiency of vitamin B_{12} or of folic acid.

Deficiency of vitamin B_{12} is recognized to occur from a dietary deficiency in strict vegetarians, from fish tapeworm infestation, which competes for supplies of vitamin B_{12}, from malabsorption secondary to disease or surgical resection of the ileum, and from the deficiency of intrinsic factor necessary for its absorption. The latter condition, called pernicious anaemia, is probably the most common cause and may occur in adults from gastric atrophy and lack of synthesis of intrinsic factor or in children when antibodies to intrinsic factor are usually responsible. The conditions may be diagnosed by the finding of macrocytic anaemia in the peripheral blood, a megaloblastic bone-marrow and a low level of serum vitamin B_{12}. If the underlying pathology cannot be corrected, both forms respond to the parenteral administration of B_{12}.

Symptoms include those of the underlying condition and those of anaemia. Subacute combined degeneration of the spinal cord and optic neuropathy[3] may both complicate this condition and may be precipitated by the administration of folic acid. Treatment should be confined to the hydroxycobalamin form of vitamin B_{12} since the cyanocobalamin form may cause deterioration.

Folic acid deficiency may result from dietary deficiency but is more frequently the sequel of malabsorption associated with coeliac disease, tropical sprue, steatorrhoea and extensive gastric surgery.

No specific ocular changes are recognized in folate deficiency.

Polycythaemia

Polycythaemia is characterized by red cell counts exceeding $6 \times 10^{12}/l$. Polycythaemia rubra vera is a neoplastic condition of the red cell precursors and is frequently associated with marked increases in platelet counts. Secondary polycythaemia results from increased erythropoietic drive secondary to tissue anoxia. This may occur in cyanotic congenital heart disease, pulmonary disease and in certain haemoglobinopathies characterized by an increased oxygen affinity.

Clinically, polycythaemia is characterized by headache, lassitude, dyspnoea, a florid dusky-red appearance of the skin and hepato-splenomegaly. The course is determined by the underlying cause. Death is usually due to cerebral haemorrhage or thrombosis.

Visual symptoms are frequent, even in the absence of retinal changes, and have been attributed to angiospasm, thrombosis or haemorrhage in the regions of the optic nerve, visual pathways and cerebral cortex. Amaurosis fugax, secondary to vertebrobasilar artery insufficiency, is common, but permanent scotomas and visual loss can also occur.

This condition is one of the causes of a hyperviscosity retinopathy,[4] which may also occur in leukaemia, the hypereosinophilic syndrome and dysproteinaemias. Symptoms include dizziness, vertigo, paraesthesiae, headaches and seizures. Ocular manifestations include large dilated retinal veins, disc oedema, retinal haemorrhages and microaneurysms, areas of capillary non-perfusion and peripheral neovascularization. Occasionally subretinal and choroidal exudation may cause non-rhegmatogenous retinal detachment at the posterior pole. In addition to these features of hyperviscosity, platelet emboli may be observed causing interruption of the red blood columns in the retinal vessels. The possibility that multiple platelet emboli contribute to these symptoms in the eye and central nervous system was suggested by the increase in platelet adhesiveness and a 50 per cent reduction in blood platelet count during symptomatic attacks.[5] Thrombosis of the central retinal veins or their branches in one or both eyes may also occur and be followed by central retinal artery occlusion.

The treatment of polycythaemia rubra vera is beyond the scope of the present chapter but includes repeated venesection, administration of radioactive ^{32}P, irradiation of the skeleton and spleen and the use of cytotoxic agents.

Sickle Cell Disease

Sickle cell disease includes a group of conditions characterized by pathology attributable to the presence of the sickle cell gene. This abnormal gene has a single point mutation in the DNA structure which determines an abnormal beta polypeptide chain. Normal adult haemoglobin (HbA) is composed of two pairs of polypeptide chains, each chain folded around a haem molecule. In HbA, these polypeptide chains are designated alpha and beta chains and the structure of HbA may be written $alpha_2 beta_2$. The beta chain is 146 amino acids long and the sixth amino acid from the amino terminus, which in normal people is glutamic acid, has been replaced by valine as a result of the DNA mutation in the sickle cell gene. This substitution changes the character of the molecule so that when deoxygenated, molecules of sickle haemoglobin (HbS) polymerize into long chains which distort the red cell membrane. The resulting sickled cells have a high internal viscosity and a stiff membrane, both factors causing these cells to become lodged in capillaries leading to their destruction (haemolysis) and causing ischaemia or death of tissue supplied by those capillaries.

There are four principal genotypes of sickle cell disease. Homozygous sickle cell (SS) disease results from the inheritance of the sickle cell gene from both parents. Sickle cell–haemoglobin C (SC) disease results from the inheritance of the sickle cell gene from one parent and the gene for another abnormal haemoglobin (HbC) from the other. Two conditions result from the interaction of HbS and the beta thalassaemia gene. In the $beta^0$ thalassaemia gene there is complete suppression of beta chain synthesis and sickle cell–$beta^0$ thalassaemia is a severe condition similar to SS disease. In the $beta^+$ thalassaemia gene there is only a partial suppression of beta chain synthesis and sickle cell–$beta^+$ thalassaemia is a mild condition similar to SC disease. Of these four principal genotypes, two are clinically mild (SC and S $beta^+$ thalassaemia) and two are generally severe (SS and S $beta^0$ thalassaemia). The sickle cell trait is the heterozygous form of HbS, is a benign carrier state and should never be classified as a form of sickle cell disease. Differentiation of these conditions is relatively simple with haemoglobin electrophoresis (*Fig.* 1).

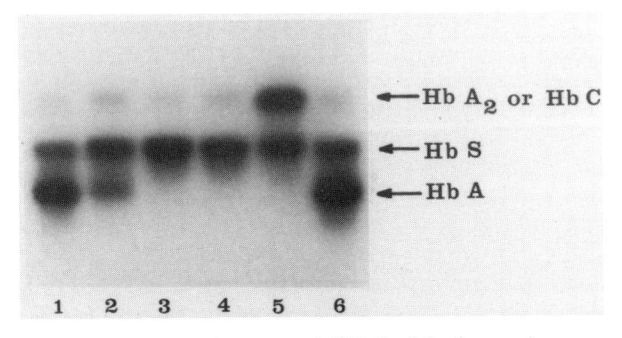

Fig. 1. Electrophoretic patterns (pH 8·4) of the four major genotypes of sickle cell disease. 1,6. Sickle cell trait controls. 2, Sickle cell–$beta^+$ thalassaemia. 3, Homozygous sickle cell disease. 4, Sickle cell–$beta^0$ thalassaemia. 5, Sickle cell–haemoglobin C disease.

The pathophysiology of sickle cell disease results partly from anaemia and partly from the tendency to small vessel obstruction. Although haemoglobin levels in SS disease are generally in the range 6–9 g/dl, symptoms of anaemia are unusual because HbS behaves as a low affinity haemoglobin within the red cell and unloads oxygen much more readily in the periphery than HbA. The ocular findings in SS disease differ from those seen in anaemia of other conditions and generally result from small vessel obstruction.

Conjunctival Vessel Changes

Examination of the conjunctival vessels by slit lamp or by direct ophthalmoscope reveals multiple short dark truncated vessel segments apparently unconnected to the rest of the conjunctival vessel network (*Fig.* 2). These abnormal vessel segments are transient obstructions of capillaries believed to be caused

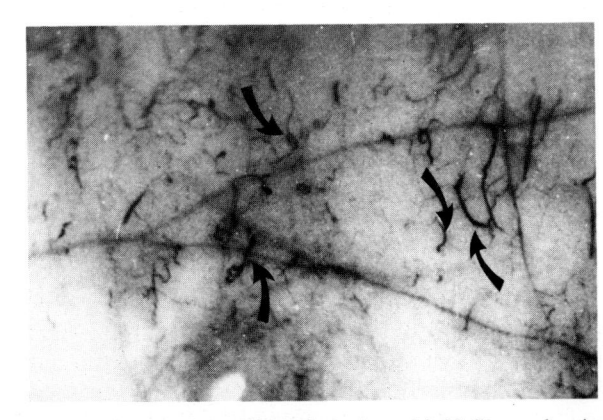

Fig. 2. Conjunctival vasculature in patient with SS disease showing anomalies of conjunctival vessels (arrows).

by sickled cells on the following evidence. Vessel anomalies are more common in patients with high counts of irreversibly sickled cells,[6,7] are uncommon in patients with high levels of fetal haemoglobin which are known to inhibit sickling, and disappear following transfusion. These changes are most marked in SS disease and S beta[0] thalassaemia and less frequent in SC disease and in S beta[+] thalassaemia. The pattern of obstructions constantly changes and although clinically unimportant, they may present a useful diagnostic sign at the bedside.

Anterior Segment Ischaemia

Obstruction of the long posterior ciliary and anterior ciliary arteries with the development of anterior segment ischaemia may occur spontaneously or following surgery that may interfere mechanically with these vessels. Such procedures include scleral buckling, detachment of the extraocular muscles, or diathermy or cryopexy in the region of the long posterior ciliary arteries. This complication has been reported to occur as frequently as in 71 per cent of patients with SC disease[8] and preoperative exchange transfusion has been recommended to reduce the frequency of this complication.

Glaucoma secondary to obstruction of the anterior chamber outflow tract can occur in sickle cell disease and in the sickle cell trait following relatively minor traumatic hyphaemas. Even modestly raised intraocular pressure may be associated with unexpectedly frequent visual loss from central retinal artery occlusion in these patients.[9] Hyphaema in sickle cell disease or the sickle cell trait should therefore be considered an emergency requiring early surgical intervention with mechanical decompression and anterior chamber washout.

Choroidal Abnormalities

Wedge shaped choroidal infarcts have been described, as well as pathological evidence compatible with choroidal ischaemia.[10] Another form of probable choroidal vessel occlusion resulting in sectoral choroidal retinal degeneration, pigmentary disturbance and visual field defect has also been reported.[11]

POSTERIOR POLE

Occlusion of the capillary vessel network around the macula leads to avascular zones which, if extensive, may result in reduced visual acuity.[12] Microaneurysmal dilatation of capillaries may occur on the disc or around the posterior pole[13,14] but is not associated with recognized functional impairment. Major retinal vessel obstruction is rare but central retinal artery occlusion[15] and branch arteriolar occlusions[13] have been described.

Angioid streaks, resulting from defects in Bruch's membrane, are an acquired abnormality common in older patients with SS disease.[16] Although generally benign, streaks occasionally spread out to involve the macula with the development of disciform degeneration and sometimes vitreous haemorrhage. The aetiology of angioid streaks in SS disease is not well understood but there is no evidence that affected patients have a generalized elastic tissue degeneration similar to that occurring in pseudoxanthoma elasticum.[17]

Non-proliferative Peripheral Retinal Changes

The most striking feature of ocular involvement in sickle cell disease is the development of arteriolar occlusion and capillary loss at the periphery (*Fig.* 3).

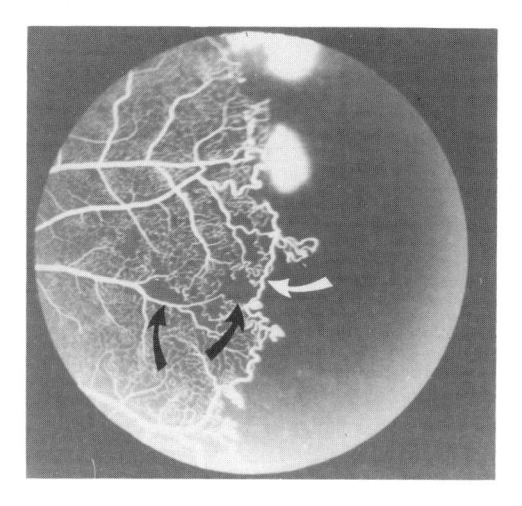

Fig. 3. Fluorescein angiogram of left temporal retina in a 31-year-old patient with SS disease showing areas of capillary loss (black arrow), abnormal arteriovenous connections (white arrow) and small proliferative lesions.

With advancing age there is a general progression of occlusion and ischaemia, although extensive remodelling of the peripheral vasculature may occur.[18] This process is apparent even in young children in whom vaso-occlusion is significantly more frequent in SS than in SC disease.[19]

Associated with this vaso-occlusive process is a variety of retinal signs usually deriving from haemorrhage, the size and site of which determine their appearance. Preretinal haemorrhages are circumscribed generally by red lesions lying between the sensory retina and the internal limiting membrane. Intraretinal haemorrhage may resolve leaving schisis cavities and iridescent spots. Haemorrhage close to the subretinal space may cause a pigmentary reaction known as the 'black sunburst' sign.[20]

Eventually avascular and vascular areas of the retinal periphery become clearly defined and abnormal arteriovenous communications develop at the border. It is from these abnormal vessels that the lesions of proliferative sickle retinopathy (PSR) develop (*Fig.* 4).

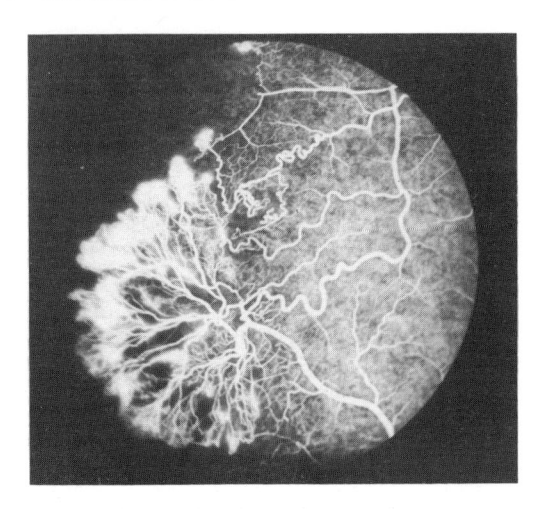

Fig. 4. Fluorescein angiogram of right temporal retina in a 26-year-old patient with SC disease showing moderate sized proliferative lesion supplied by a tortuous artery.

Proliferative Sickle Retinopathy

AETIOLOGY

Genotype: Comparison of the prevalence of PSR in the different genotypes of sickle cell disease (*Table I*) indicates this complication to be most frequent in SC disease, followed by sickle cell–beta+ thalassaemia, SS disease and sickle cell–beta⁰ thalassaemia.

Table I. Sample prevalence of PSR in different genotypes of sickle cell disease

Genotype	Average age of patients examined (yr)	No. examined	Patients with PSR No.	%
Sickle cell–haemoglobin C (SC) disease	25·5	282	101	36
Sickle cell–beta+ thalassaemia	28·8	50	9	18
Homozygous sickle cell (SS) disease	30·2	306	36	12
Sickle cell–beta⁰ thalassaemia	21·3	23	2	9

The actual prevalences quoted are subject to selection biases and vary with the age structure of the population, but the relative prevalences are probably correct.

Age: Since the lesions of PSR are cumulative, being always recognizable even if avascular, the prevalence of PSR rises with age. Comparisons of SS and SC disease indicate that the prevalence of PSR rises at an earlier age and to a higher level in SC disease than in SS disease.[21]

Haematological Factors: Analysis of haematological factors in patients with and without PSR has given information on haematological indices which may contribute to its development. A high haemoglobin level was significantly related to PSR in SS disease in males but not in females.[22] In SC disease, initial investigation suggested a highly significant relationship of PSR with high haemoglobin levels but further analysis indicated this to be entirely accounted for by a steep age-related increase in haemoglobin at between 15 and 30 years. Within each age group, PSR did not occur more frequently in patients with high haemoglobin levels. The data therefore from SS and SC disease differ in the apparent role of total haemoglobin level.

Fetal haemoglobin (HbF), which persists in SS disease and in some patients with SC disease, inhibits sickling, and high levels tend to be associated with decreased intravascular sickling. It was of interest therefore that low levels of HbF were significantly associated with PSR in males with SS disease and in both sexes with SC disease.[22,23]

NATURAL HISTORY OF PROLIFERATIVE RETINOPATHY

Early longitudinal observations of sickle cell eye disease[24] suggested a rapidly progressive course culminating in vitreous haemorrhage or retinal detachment. However, the rapid progression that was apparent in some patients[25] conflicted with the relative infrequency of severe visual dysfunction or blindness in the population as a whole. This apparent inconsistency may be reconciled by the tendency of proliferative lesions to undergo obstruction of their own blood supply leading to autoinfarction.

Autoinfarction or spontaneous regression of proliferative lesions[25–27] results from a variety of mechanisms, the most common of which is a progressive centripetal retraction of vascular arcades. Although representing progression in pathological terms, since more vascular bed has been occluded, this process brings about a clinical 'regression' since proliferative lesions are rendered ischaemic and less likely to bleed. Another mechanism is vitreo-retinal traction which compromises flow in the feeder vessels and may even cause avulsion of PSR lesions leaving a fibrotic PSR lesion floating in the vitreous. In other patients, haemorrhage into a PSR lesion appears to initiate regression.

A recent longitudinal study of 313 patients with different genotypes of sickle cell disease observed over periods of 1–8 years[25] revealed that autoinfarction of PSR lesions had occurred in 19 out of 29 (66 per cent) eyes in SS disease and in 41 out of 75 (55 per cent) eyes in SC disease. However, despite this tendency to spontaneous regression and cure, sickle cell eye disease cannot be considered entirely benign. In the patient group mentioned above, 14 of 119 (12 per cent) eyes affected by PSR became blind (visual acuity 6/60), and this occurred in four eyes during the 8-year study period.

TREATMENT

Feeder Vessel Occlusion: The anatomy of PSR lesions with discrete feeding arteries and draining veins renders them amenable to closure by photocoagulation of the arterial supply.

The most widely used method has been photocoagulation with either the xenon arc or the argon laser. Uncontrolled observations indicated that both the xenon arc[28-30] and the argon laser[31] were capable of occluding feeding arterioles and rendering PSR lesions avascular although complications of therapy included choroidal neovascularization,[32-34] retinal tears,[35] acute choroidal ischaemia[36] and vitreous haemorrhage.[37]

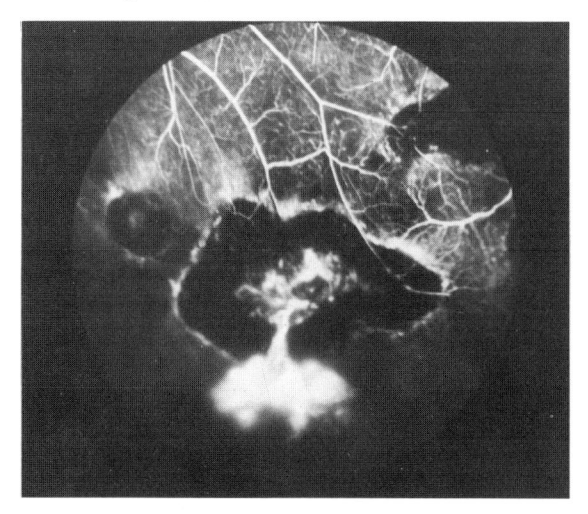

Fig. 5. Fluorescein angiogram of right inferonasal region showing old xenon arc burn area with choroidal vessel in centre.

The preliminary results of the first controlled trial using either xenon arc or the argon laser[38] indicated that the risk of vitreous haemorrhage was significantly reduced in the treated eyes. However, after 4 years' follow-up, choroidal neovascularization (*Fig.* 5) had developed in 80 per cent of eyes treated with the xenon arc and in 20 per cent of eyes treated with the argon laser. The natural history of this complication is not known, although in the majority of cases it was of the flat chorioretinal type, which is believed to be benign.[33,34]

Choroidal neovascularization commonly follows the feeder vessel technique because the energy needed to occlude large vessels, frequently with increased flows at a peripheral location, causes extensive damage to Bruch's membrane,[39] through which choroidal vessels invade. The frequency of this complication has led to alternative approaches to therapy sparing the feeder vessels.

Scatter Technique: By analogy with the diabetic retinopathy study, scatter photocoagulation has been proposed as a means of destroying ischaemic retina believed to be responsible for proliferative retinopathy. Two procedures have been proposed in the therapy of PSR – sectoral[40] and circumferential[41] retinal ablation. Both methods have been followed by striking regression of PSR, most marked in the small flat lesions. Neither has been subject to controlled assessment and a trial of sectoral retinal ablation is currently under way.

Current Status of Therapy: Rendering PSR lesions avascular significantly reduces the risk of vitreous haemorrhage. Small lesions appear to respond well to both feeder vessel and scatter techniques but their clinical significance is unclear and some may autoinfarct spontaneously. The prognosis with large elevated lesions is poor, the response to scatter therapy doubtful and feeder vessel techniques inappropriate unless the feeder vessels are in the plane of the retina. Such lesions would require indirect therapy such as cryotherapy or diathermy. Large lesions could be prevented by prospective examination of all patients and therapy of early small lesions. However, a greater understanding of the factors determining autoinfarction might enable therapy to be confined to those cases in which the PSR lesions are unlikely to occlude spontaneously.

Leukaemias: Leukaemia is a serious neoplastic disease resulting from the uncontrolled proliferation of white cells. It is usually characterized by large numbers of immature or abnormal leucocytes in the peripheral blood. The leukaemias are classified according to the type of white cell affected. The most common types are myeloid, lymphoid and monocytic varieties. The clinical course of leukaemia may be acute or chronic and is characterized by relapse and remissions. Approximately two-thirds of leukaemias are of the chronic myeloid or chronic lymphatic type, and one-third of the acute type tend to be lymphoblastic in children and myeloblastic in adults.

Acute leukaemias usually present with infection, haemorrhage or the sequelae of anaemia. In children, there may be ulcerative stomatitis, excessive bleeding after dental extraction or tonsillectomy, resistant respiratory infections and increased fatigue due to anaemia. Splenomegaly is common in the myeloid type and generalized lymphadenopathy in the lymphatic type. Diagnosis is based on examination of the peripheral blood, which may contain very high numbers of white cells, and confirmed by bone-marrow examination.

The pathophysiology of leukaemias is extremely complex, bone-marrow infiltration by abnormal white cells crowding out red cell and platelet precursors with resulting anaemia and thrombocytopenia. The white cells are functionally abnormal, giving rise to frequent infections, and leukaemic cells may directly infiltrate other tissue. These processes may be further influenced by therapy of leukaemia, which includes radiation, cytotoxic drugs and corticosteroids.

Estimates of ocular involvement in the leukaemias range from 50 to 70 per cent and appear to complicate acute leukaemias approximately four times more commonly than the chronic forms. There is some evidence that the prevalence of ocular involvement has fallen in the past 20 years, perhaps attributable to the success of modern anti-leukaemic therapy. The spectrum of ocular changes has been well described in two comprehensive reviews.[42,43]

In the anterior segment, sterile ring ulcers and pannus may affect the cornea. Blood flow in the conjunctival capillaries may manifest sludging or trucking of the red cell column, presumably related to hyperviscosity. Scleral infiltration by leukaemic cells is common and iris involvement may take the form of iritis, hypopyon and leukaemic nodules extending to the pupil margin or diffuse infiltrates causing a colour change.[44] Glaucoma may complicate these anterior segment changes.

Choroidal involvement has been reported in over half the cases, the greatest significance of this observation being that the choroid may act as a sanctuary for leukaemic cells allowing them to persist when radiation or cytotoxic therapy may destroy cells elsewhere. Leukaemic infiltration of the choroid may also be reflected in a shallow serous retinal detachment at the posterior pole characterized by multiple leaking points in the retinal pigment epithelium apparent on fluorescein angiography.

Retinal involvement has been reported in 30 per cent of all leukaemias but is most common in the acute type. It is caused by a combination of pathological processes, including the associated anaemia, infiltration of the retina by large numbers of immature white cells and by the hyperviscosity syndrome. Preretinal haemorrhages occasionally rupture into the vitreous and subretinal haemorrhage may produce a non-rhegmatogenous retinal detachment. Characteristic of leukaemia is a flame shaped haemorrhage with a pale centre (boat shaped haemorrhage) probably due to haemorrhage around a leukaemic nodule. Perivascular infiltration of the retinal vessels by white cells resembles sheathing and is probably an exaggerated form of the periaxial leucocyte streaming normally present in the retinal circulation.

Leukaemic infiltration of the optic nerve may cause papilloedema and usually signifies involvement of the central nervous system. The papilloedema may result from either raised intracranial pressure secondary to involvement of the central nervous system or from direct invasion of the optic nerve itself. Patients complain of nausea, vomiting, lethargy and seizures, and blurred vision, diplopia and signs of papilloedema are common.

Involvement of the orbit may take the form of leukaemic infiltration of the extraocular muscles or orbital fat and the bones composing the orbital margins are particularly prone to tumour involvement. Lymphoblastomas may occur in acute leukaemia and greenish tumour masses of leukaemic cells (chloromas) may complicate chronic myeloid leukaemia. Symptoms include painful lid oedema, bulbar chemosis and proptosis.

Treatment

The treatment of leukaemia is beyond the scope of this text except for the measures relevant to the eye. The observation that the eye, especially the choroid but also the retina, acts as a sanctuary for leukaemic cells has led to the use of prophylactic irradiation of the eye (100 rad daily spread over 5–6 days), the low dose being spread over several days to reduce the chance of radiation induced lens damage. Decreased vision from leukaemic infiltration of the optic nerve is an ophthalmic emergency requiring larger doses of up to 2000 rad.

Measures used in the therapy of leukaemia, which include cytotoxic therapy, steroids, radiation and bone-marrow transplantation, may themselves give rise to ocular complications. Immune suppression may allow opportunistic infection by a variety of viruses, bacteria, fungi and protozoa. Cytomegalovirus may cause retinal necrosis and haemorrhage occasionally leading to visual loss from exudative retinal detachment. Occasionally chorioretinal biopsy in a blind eye may be needed to differentiate this infection from a relapse of the leukaemic process. Herpes simplex, herpes zoster, measles and mumps viruses can occur and fungal lesions such as candida, aspergillus and other organisms may cause uveitis and retinitis.

The cytotoxic drugs vincristine and vinblastine may cause oculomotor palsies, corneal hypothesia and optic atrophy. Busulphan may cause posterior subcapsular cataracts and cytosine arabinoside may be toxic to the corneal epithelium. Radiation may cause necrosis of the optic nerve.

Bone-marrow transplantation may be complicated by graft versus host disease, ocular manifestations of which may include pseudomembranous conjunctivitis, ectropion of the eyelids, uveitis and dry eyes from a Sjögren's disease-like syndrome.

HYPEREOSINOPHILIC SYNDROME

The hypereosinophilic syndrome is a condition of unknown aetiology, probably allied to the leukaemias. It is characterized by high blood eosinophil counts and eosinophilic infiltration of the bone-marrow, heart, lungs and central nervous system.

Ocular manifestations[45] result from thromboemboli of the choroid and retina and there may be features of a hyperviscosity retinopathy.

THROMBOCYTOPENIA

Thrombocytopenic purpura may be primary (idiopathic) or secondary to antimitotic agents affecting platelet production. In both, platelets fall below $90 \times 10^9/l$, and a haemorrhagic tendency may be manifest as widespread purpura or haemorrhage from the gastrointestinal or genitourinary tracts. Diagnosis depends upon the low blood platelet count and typical bone-marrow findings. In the absence of a generalized purpuric rash, purpura may be provoked by the Hess' test employing a sphygmomanometer. Treatment of acute haemorrhage requires fresh blood or platelet concentrates and splenectomy may be valuable in the management of idiopathic thrombocytopenic purpura.

Ocular findings occur in about 50 per cent of patients with both primary and secondary forms of thrombocytopenia,[46] and consist principally of retinal haemorrhages, oedema and soft cotton-wool spots similar to the findings in general anaemias. The haemorrhagic tendency may also lead to recurrent hyphaemas which may provoke iritis, choroidal haematomas, subconjunctival haemorrhages, purpura involving the lids and haematridosis (blood-stained tears).

Thrombotic thrombocytopenic purpura is an uncommon condition of unknown aetiology characterized by haemolytic anaemia, thrombocytopenia and multiple vessel occlusions which may cause neurological manifestations and renal disease. It is a cause of disseminated intravascular coagulation (DIC) in which release of thromboplastin from either platelets or damaged endothelial cell walls, activates coagulation. When such intravascular coagulation exceeds the capacity for fibrinolysis, multiple and widespread vaso-occlusions may occur. The condition is recognized in obstetric complications, drug sensitivities, septicaemias, sickle cell disease and extensive tissue damage in burns. Diagnosis is based on evidence of increased consumption of coagulation factors, decreased platelet counts and increased fibrin degradation products.

The frequency of ocular involvement in DIC is unknown and manifestations include the sequel to both thrombosis and haemorrhage. The haemorrhagic tendency may be manifested in hyphaema, subconjunctival, retinal, intravitreal and sometimes subarachnoid haemorrhage.[47] Visual acuity may deteriorate because of occlusion of the submacular choriocapillaris with damage to the overlying retinal pigment epithelium and serous retinal detachment.[48]

COAGULATION DISORDERS
Decreased Coagulability

Deficiency of factors involved in the coagulation process may be either congenitally determined (haemophilia, Christmas disease) or acquired (haemorrhagic disease of the newborn). The resulting pathology common to these conditions is haemorrhage, often precipitated by minor trauma. The eyes may be affected by haemorrhage and tortuosity and dilatation of retinal vessels, and retinal vasculitis associated with gross optic disc swelling has been described.

Increased Coagulability

Increased intravascular coagulation occurs in the syndrome of disseminated intravascular coagulation (DIC), which has been previously described (see p. 226).

DYSPROTEINAEMIAS

Uncontrolled and usually malignant proliferation of lymphocytes or plasma cells may synthesize large amounts of monoclonal plasma proteins. This occurs in Waldenström's macroglobulinaemia, lymphomas, multiple myeloma and benign monoclonal gammopathy. The pathology in these conditions results partly from the invasive nature of the underlying cellular proliferation and also from the effects of the large amount of specific plasma protein synthesized by the abnormal cells. This is usually a gamma globulin and the condition is known as a monoclonal gammopathy. This protein may be deposited in tissues throughout the body, as in secondary amyloidosis, but may also have circulatory effects due to a hyperviscosity syndrome.

Waldenström's Macroglobulinaemia

This condition results from a malignant proliferation of IgM secreting B-lymphocytes. The high levels of IgM result in a hyperviscosity syndrome in about one-third of cases, and cryoglobulins may cause Raynaud's phenomenon and peripheral vessel disease. IgM coats the red cells, white cells and platelets and a bleeding diathesis is common. Males are most commonly affected, initial symptoms including fatigue, weakness and epistaxis and later symptoms including congestive cardiac failure, recurrent infections and renal failure. Diagnosis is based on findings in the peripheral blood and bone-marrow and the demonstration of a monoclonal gammopathy by plasma protein electrophoresis. Treatment is based on chemotherapy for the underlying condition and plasmaphoresis for removing the abnormal plasma protein.

The ocular manifestations in this condition[49] are principally those of a hyperviscosity retinopathy and of a haemorrhagic diathesis.

Multiple Myeloma

This condition is much more common than Waldenström's macroglobulinaemia and arises from neoplasia of plasma cells. The paraprotein synthesized depends upon the affected plasma cell line, but two-thirds secrete IgG and approximately one-third IgA.

Symptoms of the condition result partly from a hyperviscosity syndrome but mainly from the invasion of the bone-marrow by deposits of myeloma cells.

Local deposits of neoplastic cells may occur in the conjunctiva, uvea and scleral tissues and less commonly in the orbit. Fine crystals in the stroma of the cornea and cysts in the pars plana also occur. Intracranial extension of the disease may cause papilloedema, ocular nerve palsies and involvement of the ocular pathways.

REFERENCES

1. Holt J. M. and Gordon-Smith E. C. Retinal abnormalities in diseases of the blood. *Br. J. Ophthalmol.* 1969; **53**, 145–60.
2. Drance S. M., Morgan R. W. and Sweeney V. P. Shock induced optic neuropathy: a cause of nonprogressive glaucoma. *N. Engl J. Med.* 1973; **288**, 392–5.
3. Stambolian D. and Behrens M. Optic neuropathy associated with vitamin B_{12} deficiency. *Am. J. Ophthalmol.* 1977; **83**, 465–8.
4. Carr R. E. and Henkind P. Retinal findings associated with serum hyperviscosity. *Am. J. Ophthalmol.* 1963; **56**, 23–31.
5. Kuriyama M., Ishii N., Umazaki H. et al. Polycythaemia vera and transient monocular blindness. *Eur. Neurol.* 1977; **16**, 127–35.
6. Serjeant G. R., Serjeant B. E. and Condon P. I. The conjunctival sign in sickle cell anemia. *JAMA* 1972; **219**, 1428–31.
7. Nagpal K. C., Asdourian G. K., Goldbaum M. H. et al. The conjunctival sickling sign, hemoglobin S and irreversibly sickled erythrocytes. *Arch. Ophthalmol.* 1977; **95**, 808–11.
8. Ryan S. J. and Goldberg M. F. Anterior segment ischemia following scleral buckling in sickle cell hemoglobinopathy. *Am. J. Ophthalmol.* 1971; **72**, 35–50.
9. Goldberg M. F. The diagnosis and treatment of secondary glaucoma after hyphema in sickle cell patients. *Am. J. Ophthalmol.* 1979; **87**, 43–9.
10. Dizon R. V., Jampol L. M., Goldberg M. F. et al. Choroidal occlusive disease in sickle cell hemoglobinopathies. *Surv. Ophthalmol.* 1979; **23**, 297–306.
11. Condon P. I., Serjeant G. R. and Ikeda H. Unusual chorioretinal degeneration in sickle cell disease. *Br. J. Ophthalmol.* 1973; **57**, 81–8.
12. Asdourian G. K., Nagpal K. C., Busse B. et al. Macular and perimacular vascular remodelling in sickling haemoglobinopathies. *Br. J. Ophthalmol.* 1976; **60**, 431–53.
13. Condon P. I. and Serjeant G. R. Ocular findings in homozygous sickle cell anemia in Jamaica. *Am. J. Ophthalmol.* 1972; **73**, 533–43.
14. Goldbaum M. H., Jampol L. M. and Goldberg M. F. The disc sign in sickling hemoglobinopathies. *Arch. Ophthalmol.* 1978; **96**, 1597–600.
15. Jampol L. M., Condon P., Dizon-Moore R. et al. Salmon-patch hemorrhages after central retinal artery occlusion in sickle cell disease. *Arch. Ophthalmol.* 1981; **99**, 237–40.
16. Condon P. I. and Serjeant G. R. Ocular findings in elderly cases of homozygous sickle-cell disease in Jamaica. *Br. J. Ophthalmol.* 1976; **60**, 361–4.
17. Hamilton A. M., Pope F. M., Condon P. I. et al. Angioid streaks in Jamaican patients with homozygous sickle cell disease. *Br. J. Ophthalmol.* 1981; **65**, 341–7.
18. Galinos S. O., Asdourian G. K., Woolf M. B. et al. Spontaneous remodelling of the peripheral retinal vasculature in sickling disorders. *Am. J. Ophthalmol.* 1975; **79**, 853–70.
19. Talbot J. F., Bird A. C., Serjeant G. R. et al. Sickle cell retinopathy in young children in Jamaica. *Br. J. Ophthalmol.* 1982; **66**, 149–54.
20. Welch R. B. and Goldberg M. F. Sickle-cell hemoglobin and its relation to fundus abnormality. *Arch. Ophthalmol.* 1966; **75**, 353–62.
21. Condon P. I., Hayes R. J. and Serjeant G. R. Retinal and choroidal neovascularization in sickle cell disease. *Trans. Ophthalmol. Soc. UK* 1980; **100**, 434–9.
22. Hayes R. J., Condon P. I. and Serjeant G. R. Haematological factors associated with proliferative retinopathy in homozygous sickle cell disease. *Br. J. Ophthalmol.* 1981; **65**, 29–35.
23. Hayes R. J., Condon P. I. and Serjeant G. R. Haematological factors associated with proliferative retinopathy in sickle cell-haemoglobin C disease. *Br. J. Ophthalmol.* 1981; **65**, 712–17.
24. Goldberg M. F. Natural history of untreated proliferative sickle retinopathy. *Arch. Ophthalmol.* 1971; **85**, 428–37.
25. Condon P. I. and Serjeant G. R. Behaviour of untreated proliferative sickle retinopathy. *Br. J. Ophthalmol.* 1980; **64**, 404–11.
26. Condon P. I. and Serjeant G. R. Ocular findings in hemoglobin SC disease in Jamaica. *Am. J. Ophthalmol.* 1972; **74**, 921–31.
27. Nagpal K. C., Patrianakos D., Asdourian G. K. et al. Spontaneous regression (autoinfarction) of proliferative sickle retinopathy. *Am. J. Ophthalmol.* 1975; **80**, 855–92.
28. Goldberg M. F. Treatment of proliferative sickle retinopathy. *Am. Acad. Ophthalmol. Otol.* 1971; **75**, 532–56.
29. Condon P. I. and Serjeant G. R. Photocoagulation and diathermy in the treatment of proliferative sickle retinopathy. *Br. J. Ophthalmol.* 1974; **58**, 650–62.

30. Condon P. I. and Serjeant G. R. Photocoagulation in proliferative sickle retinopathy: results of a 5-year study. *Br. J. Ophthalmol.* 1980; **64**, 832–40.
31. Goldberg M. F. and Acacio I. Argon laser photocoagulation of proliferative sickle retinopathy. *Arch. Ophthalmol.* 1973; **90**, 35–44.
32. Galinos S. O., Asdourian G. K., Woolf M. B. et al. Choroido-vitreal neovascularization after argon laser photocoagulation. *Arch. Ophthalmol.* 1975; **93**, 524–30.
33. Dizon-Moore R. V., Jampol L. M. and Goldberg M. F. Chorioretinal and choriovitreal neovascularization. *Arch. Ophthalmol.* 1981; **99**, 842–9.
34. Condon P. I., Jampol L. M., Ford S. M. et al. Choroidal neovascularization induced by photocoagulation in sickle cell disease. *Br. J. Ophthalmol.* 1981; **65**, 192–7.
35. Jampol L. M. and Goldberg M. F. Retinal breaks after photocoagulation of proliferative sickle cell retinopathy. *Arch. Ophthalmol.* 1980; **98**, 676–9.
36. Goldbaum M. H., Galinos S. O., Apple D. et al. Acute choroidal ischemia as a complication of photocoagulation. *Arch. Ophthalmol.* 1976; **94**, 1025–35.
37. Goldbaum M. H., Goldberg M. F., Nagpal K. et al. Proliferative sickle retinopathy. In: L'Esperance (ed.) *Current Diagnosis and Management of Chorio-Retinal Diseases.* St Louis, Mo, Mosby, 1977, Ch. 7, pp. 132–45.
38. Jampol L. M., Condon P., Farber M. et al. A randomised clinical trial of feeder vessel photocoagulation of proliferative sickle cell retinopathy. *Ophthalmology* 1983; **90**, 540–5.
39. Wallow I. H. L. and Davis M. D. Clinicopathologic correlation of xenon arc and argon laser photocoagulation. *Arch. Ophthalmol.* 1979; **97**, 2308–14.
40. Rednam K. R. V., Jampol L. M. and Goldberg M. F. Scatter retinal photocoagulation for proliferative sickle cell retinopathy. *Am. J. Ophthalmol.* 1982; **93**, 594–9.
41. Cruess A. F., Stephens R. F., Magargal L. E. et al. Peripheral circumferential retinal scatter photocoagulation for treatment of proliferative sickle retinopathy. *Ophthalmology* 1983; **90**, 272–8.
42. Allen R. A. and Straatsma B. R. Ocular involvement in leukemia and allied disorders. *Arch. Ophthalmol.* 1961; **66**, 490–508.
43. Kincaid M. C. and Green W. R. Ocular and orbital involvement in leukaemia. *Surv. Ophthalmol.* 1983; **27**, 211–32.
44. Fonken H. A. and Ellis P. P. Leukaemic infiltrates in the iris. Successful treatment of secondary glaucoma with X-irridiation. *Arch. Ophthalmol.* 1966; **76**, 32–6.
45. Chaine G., Davies J., Kohner E. M. et al. Ophthalmic abnormalities in the hypereosinophilic syndrome. *Am. Acad. Ophthalmol.* 1982; **89**, 1348–56.
46. Rubenstein R. A., Yanoff M. and Albert D. M. Thrombocytopenia, anemia and retinal hemorrhage. *Am. J. Ophthalmol.* 1968; **65**, 435–9.
47. Azar P., Smith R. S. and Greenberg M. H. Ocular findings in disseminated intravascular coagulation *Am. J. Ophthalmol.* 1974; **78**, 493–6.
48. Cogan D. J. Fibrin clots in the choriocapillaris and serous detachment of the retina. *Ophthalmologica* 1976; **172**, 298–307.
49. Ackerman A. L. The ocular manifestations of Waldenström's macroglobinemia and its treatment. *Arch. Ophthalmol.* 1962; **67**, 701–7.

Chapter 22

The Management of Visual Disability

Janet H. Silver

It is only in this century that visually handicapped people have been encouraged to use residual vision and to employ optical and other appliances to maximize it. Although most of the principles have been understood for centuries, within the past 25 years aids have become less expensive and more acceptable in weight and performance. These developments have coincided with changes in attitude both by patients and clinicians and a wide variety of aids is now available.

Much benefit can be derived from very simple strategies such as the exploitation of contrast. Steak will be difficult to see on a brown plate, boiled fish disappears on white, reverse them and add a green vegetable and a common problem is resolved. If one or two such examples are brought to the patient's notice the principles are generally adopted and applied. The simplest way of gaining magnification is simply to move closer to the object (*Fig.* 1). Patients frequently believe that it is possible to

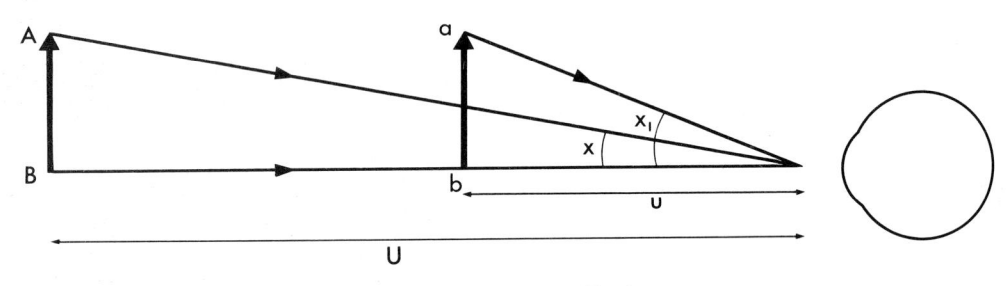

Fig. 1. Simple geometric magnification.

AB = ab = height of object
U = distance of AB from the eye (m)
u = distance of ab from the eye (m)
X = angle projected by AB
X′ = angle projected by ab

$$\frac{X'}{X} = \frac{U}{u}$$

An ophthalmic service must include the supply of equipment that will allow the visually handicapped to function to the limit of their capability. The prescription of low vision aids enables many employed people with an acquired visual disability to keep their job and maintain their skills, allows many visually handicapped children to remain in open education,[1] and can maintain the independence of old people.

In countries where statistics on visual disability are available, the age distribution is remarkably similar. Less than 5 per cent of all recognized visual disability occurs in children under 16 years of age and more than 70 per cent occurs in the retired age group.[2] In the United Kingdom less than one in 3000 children under the age of 16 years is known to have a visual disability, but one in 30 of those over the age of 75 years is registered as 'blind' or 'partially sighted'.[3]

damage the remaining vision by watching too much television, or sitting close to the screen. There is also an unspoken belief that the residual vision can in some way be used up and should, therefore, be conserved. Alternatively, it is believed that using already damaged eyes will further exacerbate the disease process. Until these superstitions are dispersed, true cooperation cannot be gained.

THE APPLIANCES

Effective prescribing for the low vision patient depends upon the availability of a comprehensive range of aids which should include a fitting set such as the ones devised by William Feinbloom or Charles Keeler. Every practitioner develops preferences for certain aids but these should never be allowed to become exclusive. Alternatives of every type of aid should be available.

Every type of aid has both advantages and disadvantages, and ultimately the function of the practitioner is to prescribe for the individual patient the aid that confers the greatest advantages combined with the minimum disadvantages. For near vision there are many alternatives:

Hand and Stand Magnifiers (Fig. 2)

The simple magnifier is probably the most widely used and best accepted aid.[4] Hand and stand magnifiers are available in a wide variety of power and quality. They are made of glass or plastic material and classified by focal length in inches or centimetres, by the diameter of the lens, or most usefully in dioptres. It is unfortunate that no agreed method of classifying them has been adopted.

The optics of such lenses is a complex subject. Even if the effective dioptric power is quoted this may be the back vertex power, the front vertex power or the equivalent power. In low powered lenses the difference between front vertex power, back vertex power and equivalent power is negligible, but in high powered or combinations of lenses the differences may be significant.[5]

Magnification is normally considered to be equivalent power (in dioptres) divided by four, although hand lenses are usually held well within the focal length and resultant magnification may in practice be considerably less.

Hand and stand magnifiers meet different needs. For both types integral illumination may be an advantage and both have a relatively small field unless the patient can be persuaded to use the appliance close to the eye. Stand magnifiers are often bulky but they have applications in industry if low power is adequate, and may allow the user to carry out a task requiring both hands. They have particular advantages when there are additional handicaps, a need for extra light or when a large field is essential and low power acceptable.

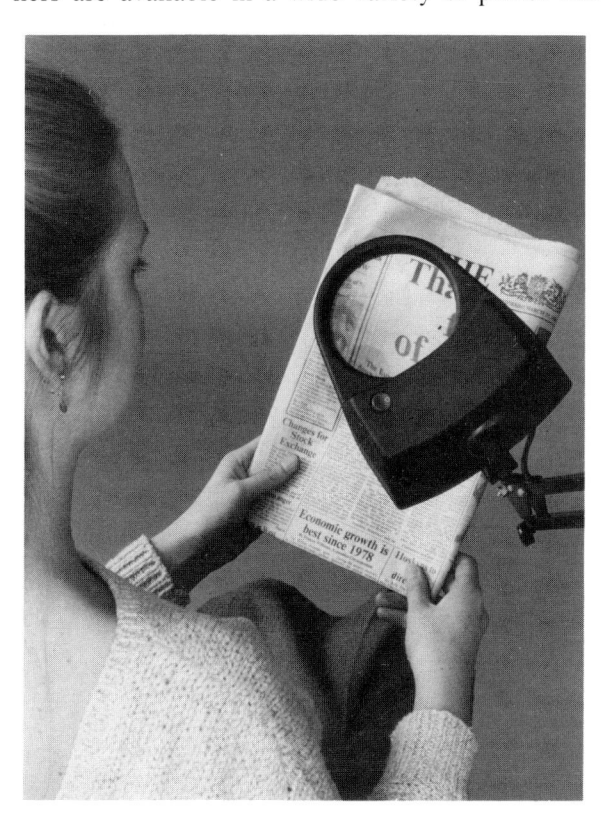

Fig. 2 Stand magnifier with illumination. Power +3·00 dioptres. (1001 Lamp Company.)

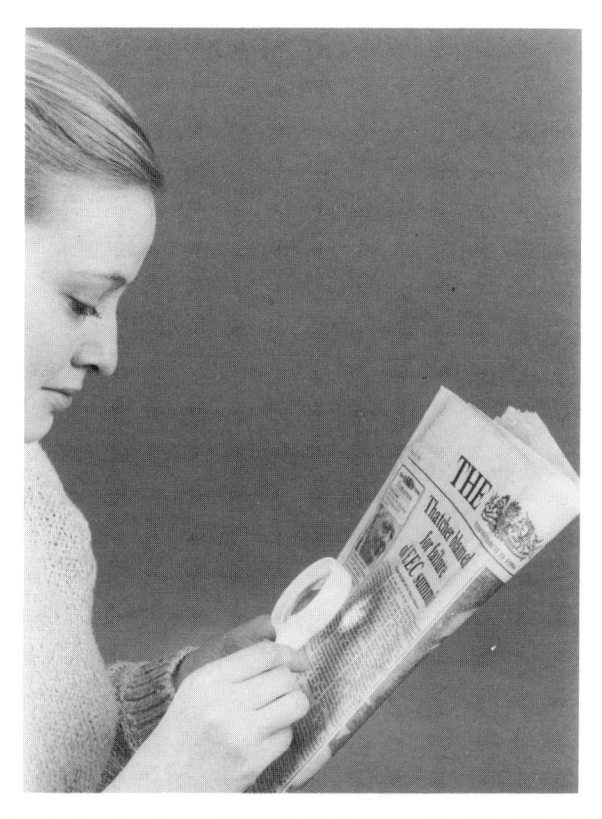

Fig. 3. Hand held magnifier. +20·00 dioptres. (Combined Optical Industries Ltd.)

Even where other aids are used, a hand lens is a great advantage in a pocket or handbag (*Fig.* 3). A busy low vision clinic will hold at least 50 alternative hand and stand magnifiers, each of which will have significantly different characteristics. Theoretically magnifiers should be used with a distance vision correction. In practice, the patient will often prefer to wear a normal reading correction, selecting the material with spectacles, then reading the small print with a magnifier (*Fig.* 4).

Spectacle Magnifiers (Fig. 5)

High powered convex lenses may be mounted in spectacle frames (*Fig.* 6), attached to them with clips,

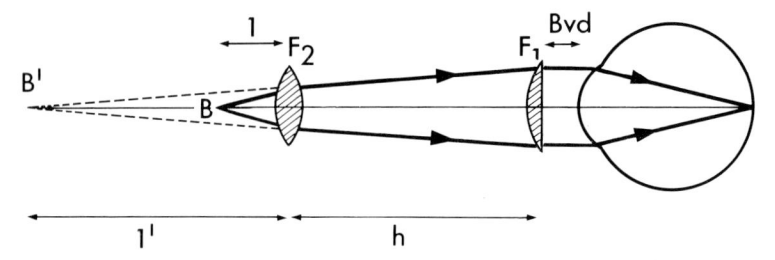

Fig. 4. Optics of presbyopic correction lens plus simple magnifier.

B   = Object
F1 = Presbyopic correction lens
F2 = Magnifier (focal length f′)
BVD = Back vertex distance (mm)
l   = Object distance (m)
l′ = Image distance (m)
h   = Spectacle lens to magnifier distance (m)

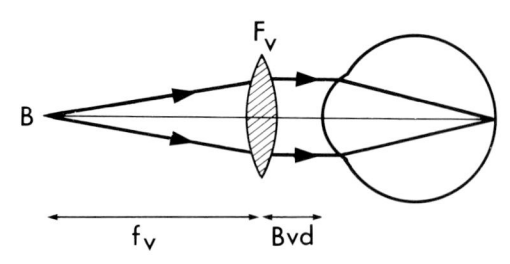

$$\frac{1}{l'} = \frac{1}{l'} + \frac{1}{f}$$

Fig. 5. Spectacle magnifier.

B   = Object
Fv = Spectacle Magnifier (Power in Dioptres)
BVD = Back vertex distance
fv   = Work distance = 1/FV (Metres)

or simply used as watchmaker's loupes. (*Fig.* 7). Such lenses, which may be spherical or aspheric, are usually described by magnification powers. Certain spectacle magnifiers have been produced with surfaces designed to reduce aberrations. These are usually described as hyperoculars.[6] The formula for simple magnifiers can be applied in reverse, thus a 4× spectacle magnifier will have the power of 16 dioptres. However, it is generally accepted that the main function of the lens is to focus the image at the retina; most of the magnification is due to the proximity of the object (*Fig.* 3).[7]

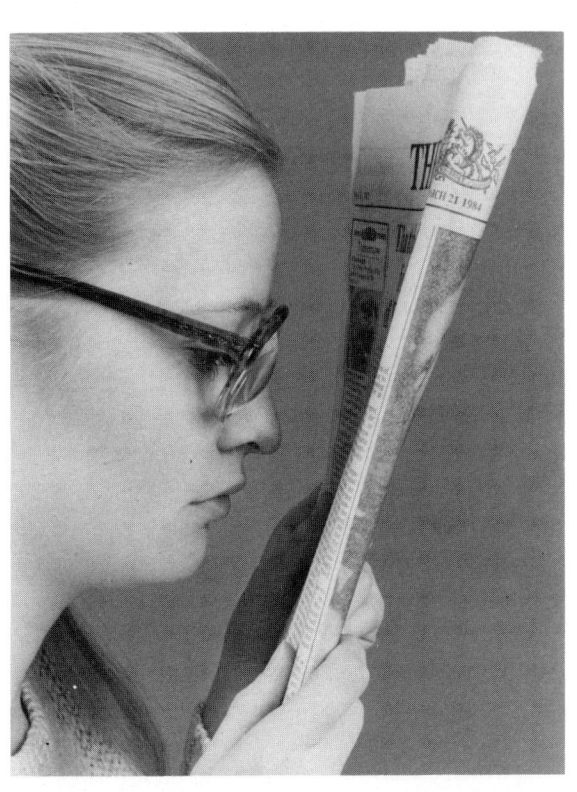

Fig. 6. 15× Peak Light Lupe. (Carton Industries.)

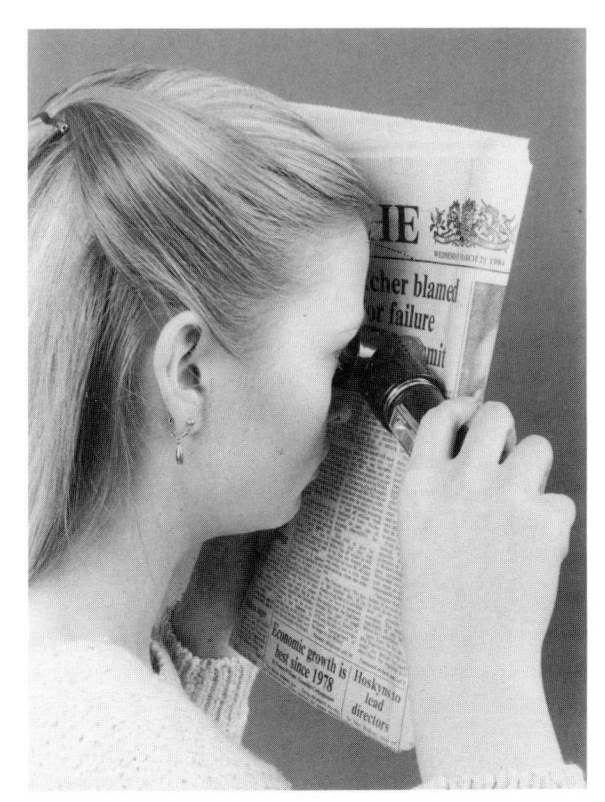

Fig. 7. +16·00 dioptre Full Field Spectacle Magnifier used monocularly. (Combined Optical Industries.)

It must be remembered that magnification and working distance will be modified by the patient's own refractive error. If a 5× spectacle magnifier is used by an aphake where 12 dioptres is used to correct the aphakic hypermetropia, only 8 dioptres will remain for the near vision correction. This will give 2× magnification and a working distance of 12 cm. Conversely, if a similar lens is put before a 12 dioptre myopic eye the total positive power would be 32 dioptres, the working distance 3 cm and the actual magnification 8×. Spectacle magnifiers are excellent cosmetically and have a relatively good field. Several manufacturers produce them in bifocal form, which is frequently an advantage. Disadvantages are the short working distance in higher powers and the inevitable decision to abandon binocular vision where more than about 2× magnification is indicated. Spectacle magnifiers are usually single lenses, although sometimes two or more lenses in combination are used. Powers available at the time of writing are up to 20× or thereabouts, and again integral illumination is available for some high powered aids.

Clearly if high reading additions are to be given binocularly problems will arise with convergence. In practice, patients can rarely cope with more than 10 or 12 dioptres addition and then base-in prisms are needed to relieve the convergence. Fonda[8] suggests that it is appropriate to incorporate one prism dioptre in each eye for each dioptre of addition and as convergence reduces interpupillary distance, spectacles with small eye sizes are essential. Inevitably chromatic aberration is increased and a heavy thick lens is created.

Telescopes

For a larger working distance, that is from 25 cm to infinity, telescopic systems are needed (*Fig.* 8). The major disadvantages of telescopes are that they reduce field, are very heavy, have a bizarre appearance, disrupt normal spatial relationships and are relatively expensive.

Small low powered telescopes can be mounted on spectacle frames – several different types are available (*Fig.* 9). Simple binocular 'sports spectacles' are mass produced with adjustable interpupillary distances and are often focusable, with one of the elements being movable to allow for the correction of spherical refractive errors up to perhaps plus or minus 6 dioptres, and magnification of up to 3×.

Several manufacturers produce monocular or binocular telescopes which incorporate a correction for ametropia. These can sometimes be mounted high on a carrier spectacle lens to allow normal vision below; the head is dropped slightly to allow vision 'along the tubes', these are called 'bioptic telescopes'. Magnification is again no more than 3×. They have obvious applications in the classroom. Certain States in America allow visually disabled people to drive using such appliances. Similar telescopes are placed

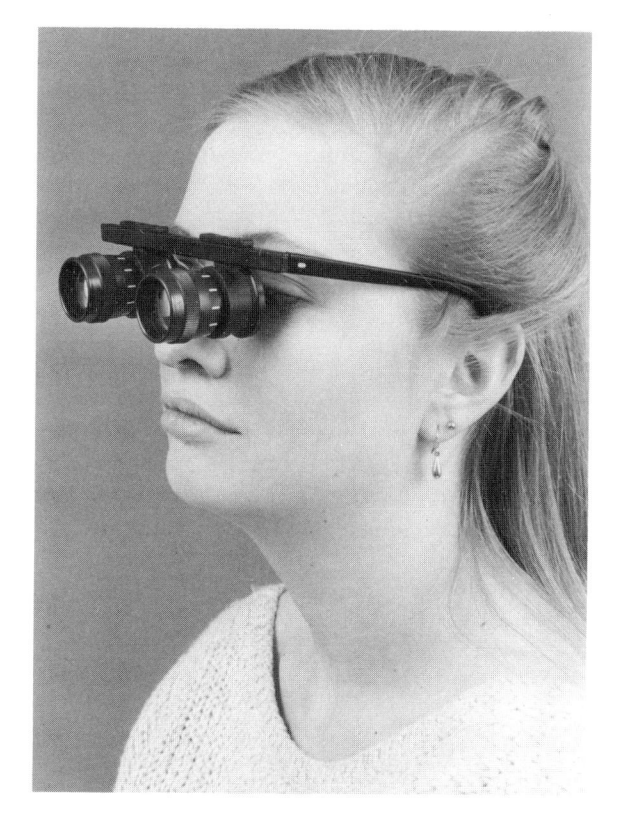

Fig. 8. 5× Binocular Near vision Telescope incorporating correction of refractive error. (Keeler Instruments)

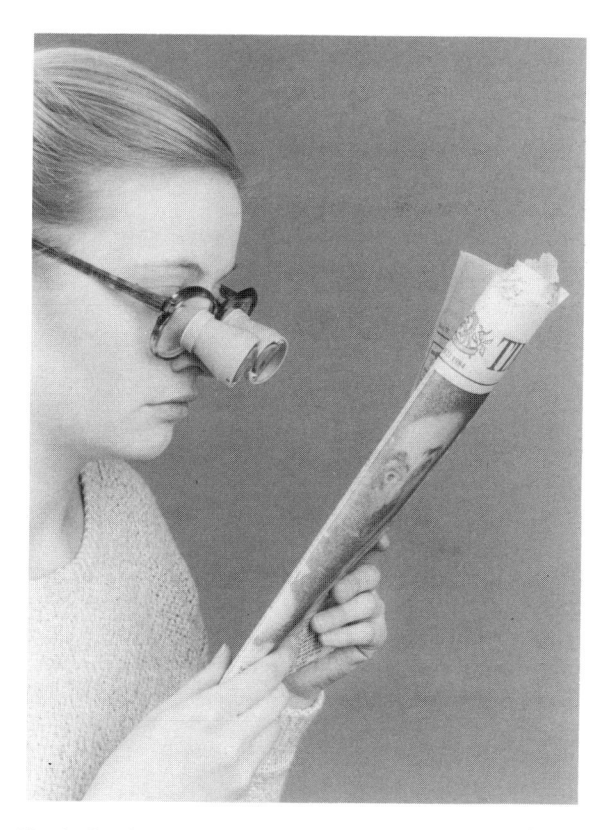

Fig. 9. 3× Spectacle Mounted focusable Telescopes. (Eschenbach.)

centrally on the carrier lens and also have convex 'cap' lenses of varying power over the objective. These effectively reduce the working distance but produce a very flexible device (*Fig.* 4).

Most face mounted telescopes use a straightforward Galilean principle (*Fig.* 10) (*Fig.* 5). These lenses are relatively lightweight. For practical purposes few face mounted aids are made at more than 3× magnification for distance use, although up to

scope. A high power negative contact lens forms the eyepiece and a high plus lens the objective. Superficially the system is most attractive, but the maximum practical back vertex distance, which acts as the space between the elements, is rarely more than 15 mm, and much more than 20 is unlikely to be tolerated; therefore the maximum effective magnification will be considerably less than 2×. Very few of these telescopes are actually in use.[11]

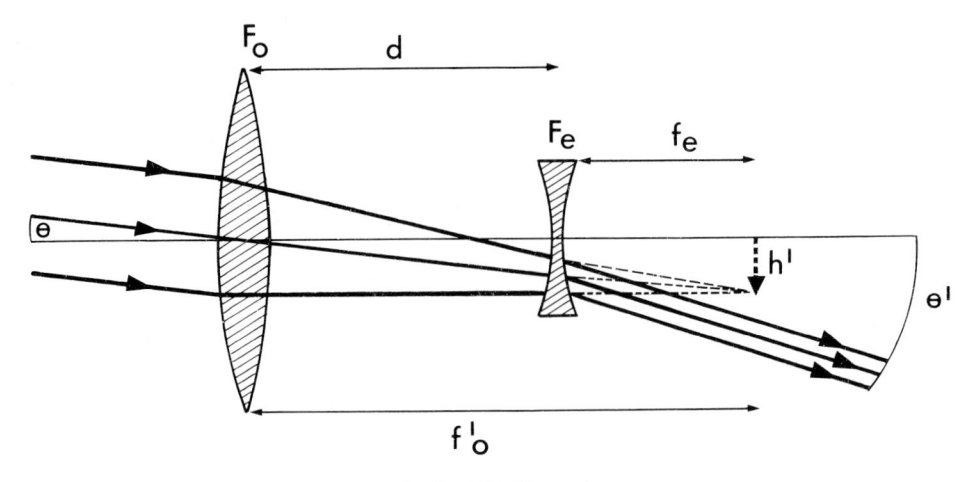

Fig. 10. Simple afocal Galilean telescope.

F_o = Objective lens (Power in Dioptres)
F_e = Eye Piece lens (Power in Dioptres)
F'_o = Focal length of objective ($1/F_o$ metres)
f_e = Focal length of Eye Piece ($1/F_e$ metres)
h' = Height of image
θ = Incident Angle
θ' = Emergent Angle
d = Separation of elements ($f_o' - f_e$)

$$\text{Magnification (M)} = \frac{F_e}{F_o}$$

about 12× monocularly and 8× binocularly are available for near. Near vision telescopes are the only optical appliance that can allow manipulative skills such as writing or sewing to be sustained. The same disadvantages apply to near as distance vision telescopes, but because they are often used for longer periods, to neglect refractive errors may result in discomfort.

Small hand held monocular or binocular telescopes can also be used for a wide range of purposes. For most patients the maximum is around 8×. A few telescopes will clip on to or suspend from spectacles, thus producing the best of both worlds, but they are monocular and only up to 4×. Hand held telescopes are frequently Galilean but may also be astronomical, when an inverting prism is used to create an erect image. Several manufacturers now produce roof prism telescopes using a Pechan Schmidt prism to present a compact system with a bright image[9,10] (*Fig.* 11).

Mention must be made of the contact lens tele-

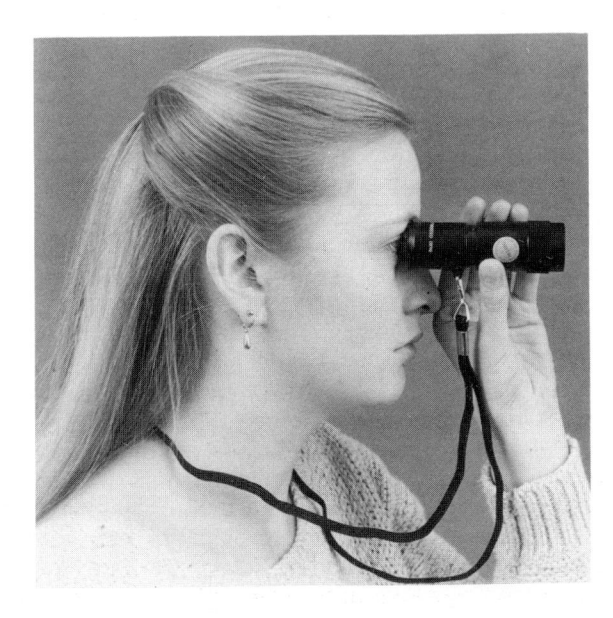

Fig. 11. 8× Roof Prism Monocular Telescope. (Greenkat.)

Other Aids

Various devices have been suggested for improving the field for patients limited to a small central area or with hemianopia. These are either variants on a reversed Galilean telescope (with the disadvantages of such systems) or use mirrors or prisms to allow a lateral view. Although these devices are effective in the laboratory, in normal use, patients prefer to scan.

Electronic Aids

In the past decade electronic aids utilizing closed circuit television (CCTV) techniques have become widely used as low vision aids. They can produce far higher levels of magnification than have previously been available (up to 50× on most machines), allow image reversal, that is white print on a black background, and a normal reading position with the distance from the screen selected by the subject. Pictures from two cameras can be combined onto a split screen to permit copying. Such aids are enormously flexible, particularly when a zoom lens is incorporated providing a wide range of magnification by a simple adjustment. Disadvantages are the cost, currently at least £1000, and its bulk – CCTV is transportable rather than portable. Recently a new device has been introduced. A hand held multiple photoreceptor is moved across the line of print. The image is orange on very dark red, and the fidelity of the image is limited by the number of receptors. But the machine is about briefcase size and allows up to 64×.

Several electronic reading machines are now compatible with computer systems, and new developments are being announced constantly in this rapidly developing area.

Image intensifiers originally developed for military use have been suggested as an aid for those with night blindness. They are still relatively expensive, and not very easy to use. Under most circumstances it is easier and more effective simply to increase the light.

Illumination

The subject of the hardware cannot be left without mention of illumination. Every practitioner needs to be familiar with the principles and be equipped with flexible lighting in order to be able to demonstrate ideal conditions for the individual patient. Certain diagnostic groups, notably the macular diseases, benefit from very high levels of illumination.[12] Most patients with corneal or vitreous disorders need very high contrast levels if they are to read ink print. A normal tungsten bulb produces an unacceptable level of heat at high wattage, but this can be significantly reduced by using a focused luminaire which at 60 W will give 3000 lux at 30 cm from source compared with 500 for a standard tungsten bulb.[13] The luminaries need to be carefully sited to avoid glare.

Patients with early opacities of the media frequently complain about 'glare'. The real problem is light scatter due to oblique light and a tinted lens does very little if anything to alleviate this, but may reduce contrast to below safety level under some circumstances. A shady hat will often provide protection from oblique light. The only exception to the no-tints rule is the group where cone function is severely reduced. This group frequently derive benefit from very dark tinted lenses with perhaps 2 per cent transmission. This can be achieved by coating a solid tint. The lenses must be mounted in a frame that affords protection from stray light from the sides and above.

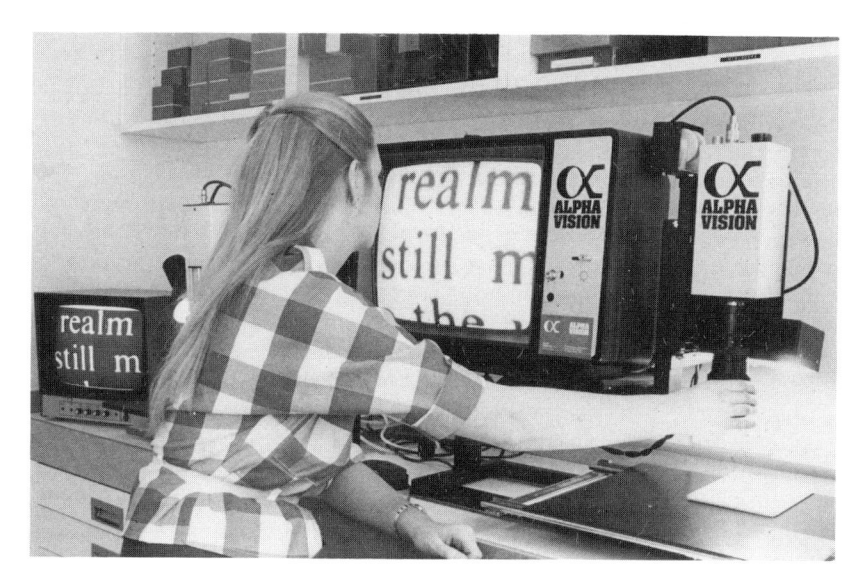

Fig. 12. Closed Circuit Television. (Focus and Alphamed.)

THE LOW VISION ASSESSMENT

The patient who wishes to perform tasks that cannot be managed with a normal spectacle correction should be seen in the low vision clinic. A complete ophthalmological report should be available at the first attendance. This information gives the low vision practitioner some insight into how patients perceive their environment and a prognosis for preservation of vision, both long and short term, is valuable.

The most important part of the procedure is the full elucidation of the patient's visual needs. They must be described as accurately and as specifically as possible and put in order of priority. It is common to find patients with unrealistic expectations of what can be achieved with optical appliances. On the other hand, particularly among the elderly, expectations may be very low. Patients should be encouraged to bring examples of 'problem materials' with them to the clinic, along with any aids prescribed, purchased or improvised. It is important to create a sympathetic environment as, without fear of disapproval or ridicule, patients will disclose their own unconventional solutions. These may include wearing two or more pairs of glasses, or convex lenses 'borrowed' from other devices. This provides invaluable information about the motivation and adaptability of the patient. Most patients request help with reading, but for one person it will be checking the occasional telephone number; for another reading notes at meetings and large numbers of letters; for a third, checking printers' proofs for publication.

It is of benefit if some priority order is established, with the most important tasks taking precedence. Best vision should be established for each eye and near vision acuity recorded with a +4·00 addition. This makes a useful starting point as it repesents not only unit magnification but also the limit to which reading material is normally held. In most disorders one eye has rather better vision than the other and the appropriate magnification level should be established for each eye in turn, starting with the better eye. Plus lenses can be added in 2·00 dioptre steps, with the print moved closer at each step. A normal trial case will give up to 5× magnification with a working distance of 5 cm. This process will allow the patient to become accustomed to holding things closer in several steps rather than one jump. If more than 5× magnification is indicated it is necessary to use hyperoculars or magnifiers (see Table I). The main magnification effect is due to the increased angle projected at the retina by the print, the main function of the lens is simply to bring this larger retinal image into focus.[7] The second eye should be assessed in the same way.

The choice of appropriate aids is, of course, governed by the tasks.

Most patients attend the clinic with an escort and it is of benefit to involve this person towards the end of the assessment, both to confirm that the desired level has indeed been reached and to reinforce the message of illumination and range.

Few patients can absorb too many changes into their way of life at one time, therefore it is wise to supply the aid that appears to meet the first priority need and allow that aid to be absorbed into the patient's lifestyle, introducing other appliances to meet other needs as indicated.

The importance of follow-up cannot be overstressed. Even the most experienced practitioner may not prescribe the ideal appliance at the first visit. Indeed many patients reject the 'ideal' appliance, particularly if it is conspicuous or demands major behaviour modifications. Such a rejection is probably multi-factorial, but changes in attitudes and skill will have taken place by the first follow-up visit and a better alternative may then be accepted.

Many patients are seen with progressive disease or active disease that will ultimately stabilize. Such patients are given either a series of simple magnifiers until stability is reached or aids such as the Stigmat telescope which, by the addition of alternative caps, can be modified in the light of changed circumstances.

A reasonable follow-up regime is to see the patient

Table I. Summary of aids

Type	Magnification	Main advantages	Main disadvantages
Hand magnifiers	to 15×	Well accepted, cheap, immediately available	Hands occupied Small field in high power
Stand magnifiers	to 8×	Alleviate problems caused by other disabilities – leave hands free (low powers)	Bulk
Spec. magnifiers	to 12× (20× with illumination)	Good appearance Good field	Short working distance ∴ problems with illumination Monocular only over 2×
Spec. telescopes	to 8× (binoc) to 10× (monoc)	Increased working distance Binocular vision possible	Appearances, reduced field, weight, disruption of spatial relationships
CCTV	to 80×	Reversed image Adjustable magnification Enhanced contrast	Expensive, fixed

3 months after any aid is supplied and, once the aids are stabilized, at yearly intervals.

Training

Certain authorities, mainly in Sweden and the United States, claim that both the number of people able to use aids successfully and the reading speed obtained, can be improved if the patient is trained to find the most useful area of retina, and hold the print in the best position.[14,15] So far no report of a controlled trial of these rather time-consuming techniques has appeared in the literature. In their absence, the clinician should give advice on eccentric fixation to patients with a central scotoma who have not learned to do so spontaneously.

More recently impressive results have been claimed by a method of using prisms to shift the image.[16] The technique is based on insecure theory and cannot be advocated.

Eccentric fixation may be easier to learn if one line of print is isolated by a device such as the Prentice Typoscope,[17] this is simply a piece of black card with a slit which can be placed over the paper.

The practitioner needs a good working relationship with others involved in rehabilitation – social workers, mobility teachers, educationalists, technical officers etc. – and close interaction with the ophthalmologist responsible overall. An arrangement where information can be given informally (and fast) by telephone can be greatly to the advantage of all concerned.

There are, of course, methods of obtaining information that do not involve the use of sight at all. These include tape-recording and tactile systems. But more and more the trend is towards methods that do not impose a delay, i.e. microprocessors interpreting optical information and giving an audible or tactile output. These are still at a relatively early stage of development and, inevitably, expensive.

DELIVERY OF SERVICE

Internationally, there are several ways in which aids are provided. Clinics may be associated with medical and surgical units, medical or optometry schools, the rehabilitation services or special schools.

In the United Kingdom through the National Health Service low vision aids are prescribed at the request of an ophthalmologist. Treatment is completely free and all aids are given to patients 'on loan'. Patients may also seek help from optometrists or opticians privately. The ethical practitioner will see patients only with a referral or at least the acquiescence of the ophthalmologist concerned.

Under the Manpower Services 'Aids to Employment' scheme, any aid or modification to the environment that can be considered essential can be supplied on loan at the work place. By this means several hundred persons have been supplied with electronic reading aids. These are prescribed through low vision clinics at centres able to perform a full assessment.

REFERENCES

1. Parlett M., Jamieson M. and Pocklington K. *Towards Integration.* Slough, National Foundation for Education Research, 1976. pp. 40.
2. Sorsby A. *The Incidence and Causes of Blindness in England and Wales, 1963–1968.* London, DHSS (Reports on Health and Medical Subjects), 1972, No. 128.
3. Silver J. H. and Jackson J. Visual disability series: Part 1. *Ophthalmic Optician*, 18 December 1982, pp. 841–2.
4. Sloan L. L. *Reading Aids for the Partially Sighted.* Baltimore, Md, Williams and Wilkins, 1977, ch. 2, 4.
5. Bennett A. G. Review of ophthalmic standards. Part 11: Hand and Stand Magnifiers. *Manufacturing Optics International* 1977; **30,** 67–73.
6. Bennett A. G. Igard hyperoculars, their origin and development. *Ophthalmic Optician* 27 December 1975, pp. 1151–4.
7. Bennett A. G. Spectacle magnification and loupe magnification. *The Optician* 1982; **183,** 16–18, 36.
8. Fonda G. E. Binocular reading additions for low vision. *Arch Ophthalmol.* 1978; **83,** 294–9.
9. Bailey I. L. Principles of near vision telescopes. *Optometric Monthly* 1981; **72,** 32–4.
10. Daniels E. J. and Gottlob H. New low vision aids based on the Kepler telescope (Zeiss prism magnifying spectacles and prism magnifiers). *Neuesoptiker Journal* 1978.
11. Silver J. H. and Woodward E. G. Driving with a visual disability – a case report. *Ophthalmic Optician* 28 October 1978, pp. 794–5.
12. Sloan L. L., Habel A. and Feiock K. High illumination as an auxilliary reading aid in diseases of the macula. *Am. J. Ophthalmol.* 1971; **76,** 745.
13. Gill J. M. and Silver J. H. Illumination from domestic lamps. *Ophthalmic Optician* 24 April 1982, **22,** 28.
14. Backman O. and Inde K. *Low Vision Training.* Malmo, LiberHermods, 1979.
15. Groodrich G. L. and Quillman R. D. Training eccentric viewing. *J. Impairment Blindness* 1977; **71,** 377–81.
16. Romayanda M., Wong S. W., Elzeneny I. H. et al. Prismatic scanning with low vision. *Ophthalmology* 1982; **89,** 937–45.
17. Mehr E. B. and Freid A. N. *Low Vision Care.* Chicago, Professional Press, 1975, p. 125.

FURTHER READING

Bennett A. G. *Ophthalmic Lenses*. London, Hatton Press, 1968.
Faye E. (ed.) *Clinical Low Vision*. Boston, Mass., Little Brown, 1976.
Fonda G. *Management of Low Vision*. New York, Thieme-Stratton, 1981.
International Guide to Aids and Appliances for Blind and Visually Impaired Persons, 2nd ed. New York, American Foundation for the Blind, 1977.
Mehr E. B. and Freid A. N. *Low Vision Care*. Chicago, Professional Press, 1975.
Silver J. H. The place of optimum low vision aids in the management of visual handicap. MPhil Thesis, Department of Ophthalmic Optics and Visual Science, City University, London, August 1976.
Silver J. H. and Jackson A. J. The visual disability series. *Ophthalmic Optician*. Pt 1: Introduction and epidemiology. 18 December 1982, pp. 841–2; Pt 2: Hand magnifiers. 15 January 1983, pp. 29–35; Pt 3: Stand magnifiers. 12 February 1983, pp. 85–97; Pt 4: Spectacle and head-borne magnifiers. 26 March 1983, pp. 214–23; Pt 5: Magnification of non-telescopic low vision aids used for near vision. 7 May 1983, pp. 313–17; Pt 6: Telescopic systems (1). 16 July 1983, pp. 489–96; Pt 7: Telescopic systems for near vision (2). 24 September 1983, pp. 597–607; Pt 8: Setting up the clinic. 5 November 1983, pp. 699–706; Pt 9: Patient management. 17 December 1983, pp. 804–13.

Chapter 23

The Epidemiology of Blindness

T. R. Cullinan

DEFINITIONS OF BLINDNESS

There are at least 65 different definitions of 'blindness' in use around the world,[1] based either on levels of measured distance visual acuity or on estimates of functional ability – or, occasionally, on both. Each definition reflects a society's cultural attitude to the social and financial needs of a group of people it is prepared to identify, and its willingness to relieve them of certain responsibilities. Unfortunately, demographic, social and economic changes have tended to overtake definitions that once may have been both sensitive and specific so that they neither identify all those who may need help nor provide what is most needed to those that do. This is especially so in industrialized countries where definitions designed to bring educational and employment help to younger people are hardly adequate for the growing numbers 'blinded' in later life. Different definitions, and outdated ones, also make it very difficult to compare data between countries.

In the United Kingdom a Register of Blind Persons was first established in 1919, although many local voluntary Blind Societies kept their own registers before then. The Blind Persons Act of 1920 defined blindness for the purposes of registration as 'so blind as to be unable to perform any work for which eyesight is essential' – a neat tautology. This definition was subsequently written into the National Assistance Act 1948, and remains the basis for registration to this day. Two objections to this essentially functional definition are immediately obvious – it is 'any work' that is the basic criterion and specifically not work for which an individual is trained or best suited, and the majority of 'blind' people are now well past their working years. The definition has much of the old Poor Law about it.

Guidelines issued with the statutory definitions suggest that distance acuity of less than 3/60 (corrected) with full visual field, achievable in the better eye or, where present, both eyes, should qualify a person for registration as blind.

If the visual field is 'considerably' contracted, then 3/60 vision, but not better, qualifies. The 1948 National Assistance Act also made provision for a Partial Sight Register which became established in 1951; partial sight has never been statutorily defined, but guidelines from the Ministry of Health at the time suggested that visual acuity no better than 6/60 with full field, or better if there is marked field loss, should be used as a general guide. Such looseness of definition, both for 'blind' and 'partial sight' allows individual ophthalmologists some latitude in interpreting the Acts in the light of individual patients' needs and, judging by the range of acuities represented in registration data, this undoubtedly occurs.

The only other countries to include a functional element in defining blindness are some of the developing nations, such as Zambia and Ghana, with younger populations and, perhaps, fewer resources to measure visual acuity. Functional definitions in these countries are invariably related to mobility rather than near vision tasks; Zambia, for instance, defines a blind person as one who is unable 'to move about in unfamiliar surroundings unaided, such aid including the blind man's stick'.[2]

Outside the United Kingdom, no European countries include any functional aspects in their statutory definitions, relying solely on some 'cut-off' point of measured visual acuity. This is usually 3/60 or less, thus including as blind those who would be considered partially sighted in the UK. However, the United States, Canada and the USSR use a more liberal definition of 6/60 or less to define 'legal' blindness;[3] the higher 'cut-off' point certainly makes it possible to include more people with needs, but no easier to define what these needs are, especially with ageing populations whose difficulties may be as much with near vision as distant. A considerable literature has grown up around this point.[4–7]

Registration as 'blind' or 'partially sighted' in the UK is always by way of an assessment from a specialist ophthalmologist who completes a BD8 form (BP1 in Scotland). Social service departments, medical services or voluntary bodies may refer people for assessment. The fiscal benefits of blind registration presently include a special pension to those over 40 years of age, an added income tax allowance and extra supplementary benefits for those who need them. Talking books are provided nationally and sent by free post, but other social and adult educational benefits depend to an extent on local authority resources, as well as on voluntary bodies, local and national. They may include the help of social workers with special training, financial help towards rehabilitation, guide dog or long cane training, education in Braille or the Moon alphabet, access to clubs and societies, free or reduced bus fares, talking newspapers, the provision of aids such as closed circuit television for work, and several other possibilities. Registration is also usually needed for children to gain access to special education. Somewhat surprisingly, reduced television licence fees are available to those registered as blind as well as a reduction in rates for council house tenants. There is, at the time of going to press, a move to review and simplify the whole process of registration. Although some of the above services may be available to those registered as partially sighted, depending in large part on which area of the country they live, and on how liberally local voluntary societies for the 'blind' interpret their remit, no monetary allowances are made.

In 1972 a World Health Organisation Study Group,[8] proposed a definition of Visual Impairment (*Fig.* 1) to embrace most national definitions of 'blindness' based on measurement of visual acuity. It suggested that all those with no more than 1/60 visual acuity in the better eye (WHO categories 3, 4 and 5) should be regarded as 'blind' for the purposes of international comparison, though category 3 should also include those with adequate acuity, but a field of no more than 10° round central fixation and category 4 those with a field of 5° or less. (In fact, grossly contracted fields account for no more than 8 per cent of those registered as blind in most Western countries). Despite the obvious advantages of common definitions, most countries that do analyse their statistics continue to do so according to their own criteria and there are only a few examples of analyses that fit the WHO suggestions.[7]

BLINDNESS STATISTICS – ENGLAND AND WALES

Fairly detailed analyses of blind registration data have been made for England and Wales covering the years from 1948–68[9,10] and for England alone from 1969 to 1976.[11] There are also summary figures for England, and its regions, for the year ending 1980.[12] Similar estimates and analyses are available for the USA,[3] Canada,[13] New Zealand[14] and several other industrialized countries.

Comparing data between countries is not always easy. Not only are different population bases involved, but different age groups and even disease definitions are often used in presentation. Changes and trends must also be seen against considerable demographic shifts in the population which, in Western countries at least, are far greater determinants of 'blindness' than changes in the incidence of specific diseases or in therapeutic intervention.

Fig. 2 shows bi-annual new additions to the blind

CATEGORY	MAXIMUM LESS THAN	MINIMUM EQUAL TO OR BETTER THAN
1	6/18 3/10 20/70	6/60 1/10 (0·1) 20/200
2	6/60 1/10 (0·1) 20/200	3/60 1/20 (0·05) 20/400
3	3/60 1/20 20/400	(Finger counting at 1 metre) 1/60 1/30 (0·02) 5/300 (20/1200)
4	(Finger counting at 1 metre) 1/60 1/50 5/300	Light perception
5	No light perception	
6	Undetermined or unspecified	

Fig. 1. WHO categories of visual impairment and blindness. (Visual acuity both eyes best possible correction.)

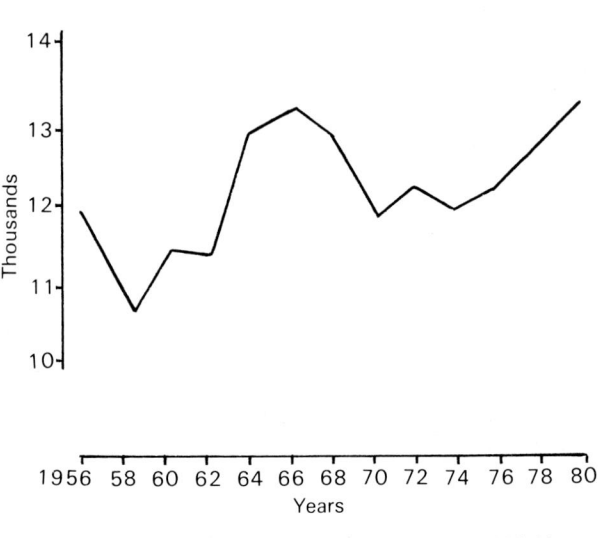

Fig. 2. New blind registrations in England and Wales, 1956–80.

register in England and Wales between 1956 and 1980. (Age adjusted figures have been estimated for Wales in the latter years.) Each year about 50 per cent of men becoming registered were aged 75 years or more; for women, the percentage rose from 63 per cent in 1956 to 65 per cent in 1976, the last year for which analyses by sex were made. In 1980 12 614 people were newly registered as blind in England.

*Fig.*3 analyses age groups for the newly registered from 1970 to 1980; the recent rise in elderly people becoming registered has not been accompanied by changes at any other age.

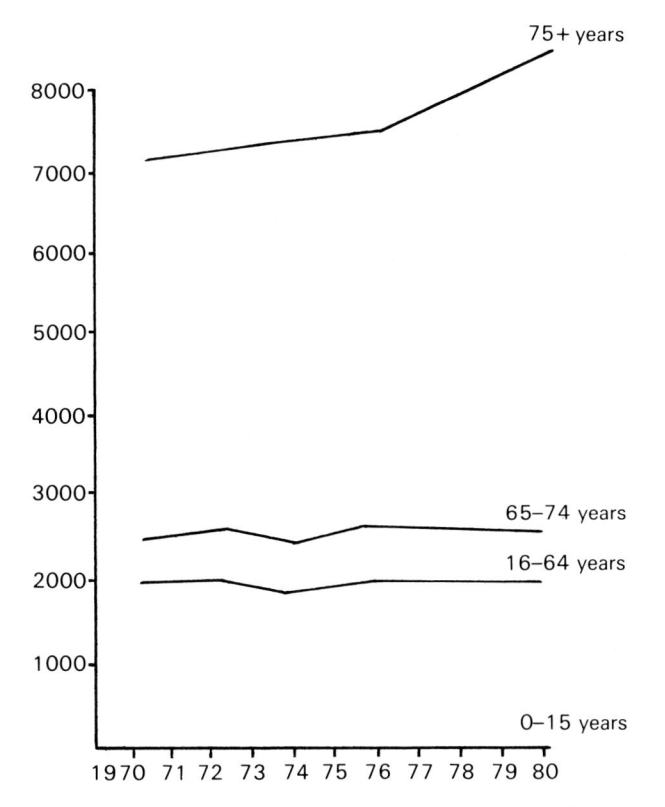

Fig. 3. New blind registrations by age group in England and Wales, 1970–80.

In 1980 there were 107 765 people on the Blind Register in England – adding estimated numbers for Wales to allow comparison with previous years brings the total for the two countries to about 115 000 (*Fig.* 4). This is a rise of about 20 per cent since 1958 (*Table* I), almost entirely caused by an increasing number of elderly people over the age of 74 years on the Register, and especially elderly women. The percentage in this group rose from 45 per cent in 1958 to 57 per cent in 1976. The reasons are not only more elderly people seeking registration, but also the increasing longevity of those already registered, although at least half of the total number of registered blind people have some other significant handicap.[7]

Until retirement years there are always more men on the Blind Register than women (*Table* I). This is not a demographic effect and since there is little evidence of sex bias in any of the major blinding diseases of young adult life, with the possible exception of diabetic retinopathy, it probably reflects the fiscal and retraining benefits of registration, which may appear greater for men than women.

During the years 1958–76 (*Table* I) there were no significant changes in the number of children registered as blind (1200–1300 boys aged 0–15 and 1000 girls). The all age prevalence of registered blindness in 1980 was 2·3 per 1000 in England and Wales, having risen slightly with the age of the population from 2·1 per 1000 in 1956. The age/specific preva-

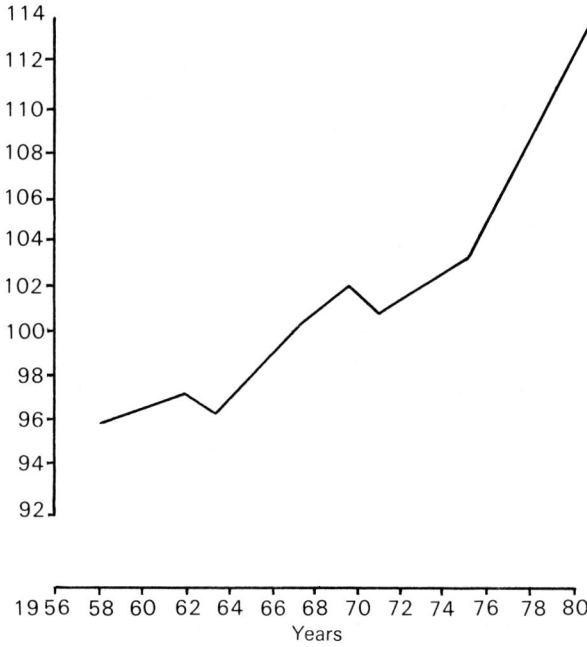

Fig. 4. Total registered blind in England and Wales, 1956–80.

Table I. Adults (16 years +) on the Blind Register in England and Wales in selected years

Age groups		1958 (10³)	1962 (10³)	1966 (10³)	1970 (10³)	1976 (10³)
16–49	M	7·7	7·2	6·8	6·7	6·4
	F	5·6	5·2	4·9	4·8	4·8
50–59	M	5·2	5·2	5·1	4·8	4·6
	F	5·0	4·8	4·6	4·1	3·9
60–69	M	7·5	7·2	7·3	7·6	7·5
	F	9·4	9·0	9·1	9·8	9·1
69–74	M	4·7	5·3	6·2	4·9	5·1
	F	5·5	6·8	7·3	6·1	7·2
75+	M	14·0	14·0	13·9	14·4	16·2
	F	29·3	31·1	35·1	36·1	40·5
Total M		39·1	38·9	39·3	38·4	39·8
Total F		54·8	56·7	61·0	61·0	65·5
Total registered adults (10³)		93·9	95·8	100·3	99·4	105·3

lence rates are illustrated in *Table* II; they have remained substantially unchanged for the past 20 years. Finally, it can be calculated that by 1992 the numbers on the Blind Register will have risen to over 130 000, purely as a result of demographic changes in the population of England and Wales.

Table II. Age specific prevalence rates among the registered blind in England and Wales, 1980

Age group	Prevalence (/1000)
0–4	0·09
5–15	0·23
16–64	0·85
65–74	4·48
75+	23·24

PARTIAL SIGHT AND VISUAL DISABILITY

No analyses of partial sight registration have been made for the years before 1970, but since then trends in new registrations have been very similar to those for blindness, with the same increases of elderly people (*Fig.* 5). There are many parts of the country where registration as partially sighted brings few

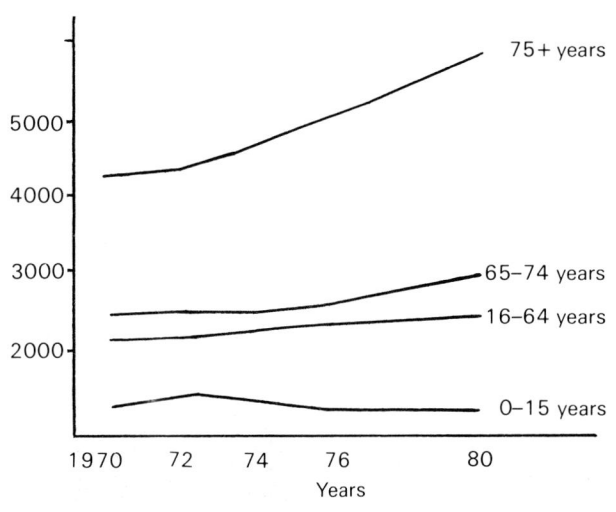

Fig. 5. Partial sight register, new registrations in England and Wales, 1970–80.

benefits to an elderly person, except access to 'talking books', and it must in part be seen as a 'holding operation' before a decision is made about blind registration; nevertheless, it has been estimated[15] that the 'Partial Sight' Register underestimates by at least 50 per cent the number of people in the community who might qualify, while the Blind Register may underestimate by 20 per cent.[16] Inevitably, most of those not registered will be in the older age groups. In 1980 there were 51 420 people on the Partial Sight Register – almost half as many as on the Blind Register.

No routine data are collected in England and Wales, or in any other country, that fit the more recent WHO criteria for Visual Disability (Impairment). However, a national random household survey of some 18 000 households in 1977 (England and Wales)[7] established the approximate population prevalence of visual disability according to these criteria (less than 6/18 vision in the better eye) and ascribed, as far as possible, the causes of reduced vision. The estimated prevalence of visual disability in the population is 5·2 per 1000 home based adults, two and a half times the number of people registered as blind. Again, over half are aged 75 years or more and three-quarters are in their retirement years. Two somewhat surprising findings from this survey were that nearly half of visually disabled people had, apparently, never had a specialist eye assessment and over half were able to see slightly or markedly better when acuity was measured at a hospital clinic than when measured at home. This was subsequently shown to be almost entirely due to poor home lighting.[17]

STATISTICS FROM OTHER COUNTRIES

Prevalence figures for England and Wales accord fairly well with those from other countries with similar populations, such as Canada,[13] United States,[3] and New Zealand.[14] Most, however, share the same difficulties in relying upon incomplete registration data, although an attempt was made in the United States to overcome some of these by setting up a Model Reporting Area (MRA) of 16 states who agreed to abide by common criteria and do their utmost to ensure both accurate and complete registration. Reports from MRA[3] between 1962 and 1964 suggested an overall prevalence of registered blindness of about 150 per 100 000 total population.

The population at the time was a little younger than that of England and Wales and the definition of blindness (less than 6/60 in the better eye) somewhat more liberal; nevertheless, the prevalence of blindness still seems low in comparison, and may have represented under-registration by socially disadvantaged groups.[3] The MRA was abandoned in 1970, due to lack of funds.

A summary of world statistics, as far as they were known, was made by WHO in 1966[1] and later unpublished reports have added to the data. Some 60 countries have made estimates, though many of them are based only on limited surveys in regions showing particular needs. Nevertheless, the differences in prevalence of 'blindness' (however variously defined) between 'developed' countries with populations suffering largely from the degenerative diseases of old age and the younger populations of less developed countries exposed to infections and nutritional deficiencies stand out starkly.

Kenya, for instance, estimates a prevalence of blindness (less than 3/60) as high as 10 per 1000 (1960), and Zambia 22 per 1000 (1978). India, Sudan and Egypt with prevalence figures for their rural population of 35, 45 and 48 per 1000 respectively have all produced figures of less than half these for their urban dwellers, while the highest prevalence appears in rural Tunisia in which some villages reach 70 per 1000 total population blind. But, even among the 'developed' countries with supposedly similar populations and social conditions some differences seem remarkable. The Netherlands, for instance, estimate a prevalence of 0·55 per 1000 (1959) while Iceland records six times that at 3·0 per 1000 (1954). Many of these data clearly need updating using modern techniques of study design and analysis so that accurate comparisons can be made and the reasons for apparent differences sought.

CONDITIONS LEADING TO BLINDNESS IN 'WESTERN' POPULATIONS

In all age groups after childhood, registrable blindness is usually the end result of a progressive disease.

Similar proportions at different ages apply to the 7000 or so newly registered as partially sighted each year; and to those becoming registered as blind in other countries with populations and social conditions similar to those in the UK.[2,13,14] However, national data can mask considerable regional and racial differences within a country. For instance, the rate of blind registration for glaucoma in the USA is almost four times higher among non-whites than whites.[18]

Many attempts to survey populations for the prevalence of diseases eventually leading to blindness

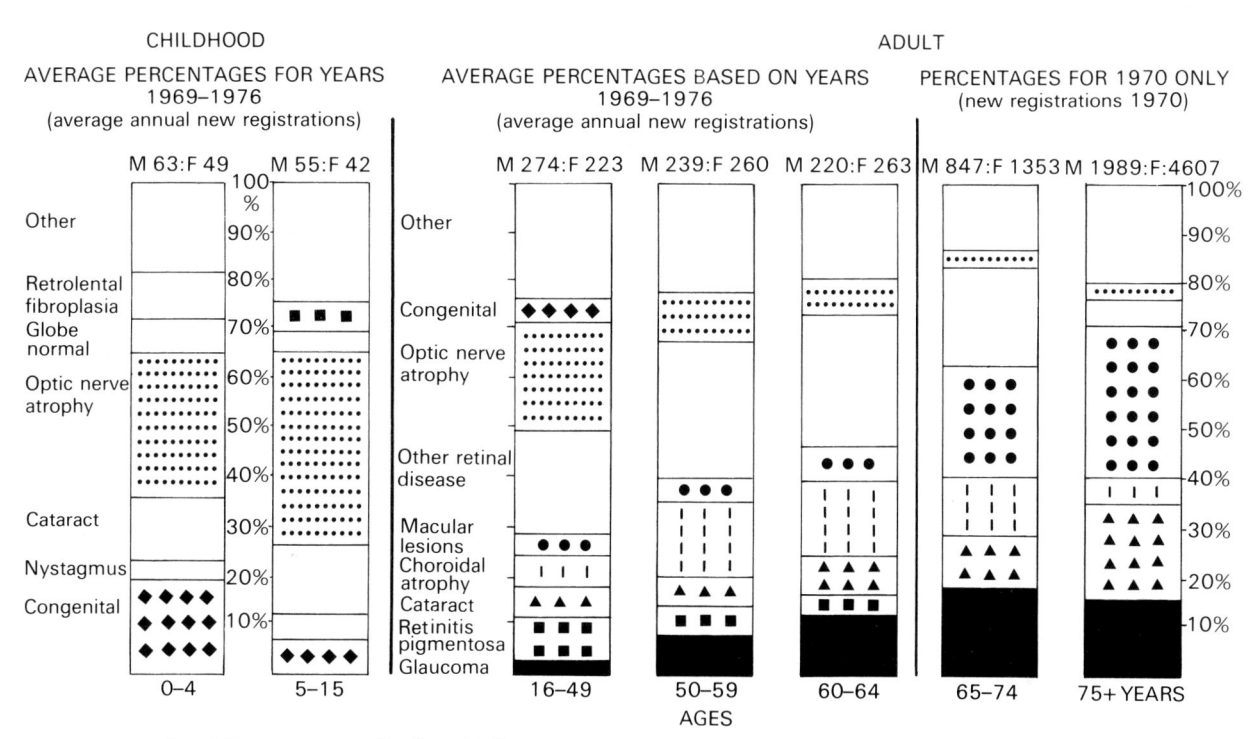

Fig. 6. Percentage contribution of different diseases at blind registration in England. M, male; F, female.

Since progress towards blindness depends on many factors other than age, and age-at-onset of disease, the analysis of registration data to esimate the incidence or prevalence of any major sight threatening disease is hazardous. The best that can be done is to list the diseases leading to new registration at different age groups and then look elsewhere for estimates of population occurrence.

Fig. 6 summarizes the latest available data for England. Averages have been taken for the years 1969–76 for children and younger adults; for the elderly 1970 alone is used. The proportional importance of retinal lesions in middle age stands out; most analyses do not categorize those that are diabetic in origin, but it is undoubtedly the majority. Macular changes assume more importance than cataracts only after the age of 65 years. New registrations for retinitis pigmentosa (about 100 in each of the years from 1969 to 1976) cover a wide range of some 60 years.

have been reported,[7] but they have usually been limited to selected age groups or clinic attenders, or have used arbitrary 'cut-off' points of visual acuity. Undoubtedly the most comprehensive is the Framingham Eye Study;[19] it is nearer to a true population study than any previously achieved, but is still limited in age range (52–85 years) and dependent on a somewhat distorted final sample. The following summaries of incidence and prevalence data are based on Framingham, but include other data where they are relevant.

SENILE MACULAR DEGENERATION

Ferris[20] deduces from the Framingham study a population prevalence of senile macular degeneration in men rising from 1·6 per cent at ages 52–64 years to 24·4 per cent at 75–85, and in women from 2·0 per cent to 30·1 per cent. Moderate or severe macular changes were defined as 'obvious or severe macular pigmentary disturbance; or 10 or more small macular drusen or large macular drusen or serous, haemorrhagic or proliferative elevation of the pigment or neurosensory epithelium; or peri-macular circinate exudate (in people without diabetes)'.[21] Senile macular degeneration was considered to be present when any of the above was accompanied by vision of 6/9 or less. This excludes the mere appearance of a few small drusen which were seen in 25 per cent of all eyes examined. Of those eyes considered to have definite macular disease 80 per cent showed either drusen alone or 'dry' atrophic changes in the pigment epithelium; 20 per cent were of the 'wet', exudative type with sub-retinal fluid. But definitive examination was performed only where acuity was 6/9 or less so that other pathology (such as early lens changes) made accurate classification of the macula more likely.[20]

Ferris quotes other evidence from the National Health and Nutrition Survey in the USA (1971–2) suggesting a prevalence of drusen of between 7 and 10 per cent in approximately the same age groups as Framingham, but this was based on the unvalidated observations of many individual ophthalmologists. Other recent estimates[7] suggest that 18 per cent of visually disabled adults (WHO definition), who make up about 1 in 200 of the adult population of England and Wales, have their visual disability ascribed to macular degeneration.

Estimates of annual incidence have been calculated from the Framingham study.[21] For macular changes not associated with sight loss (excluding less than 10 small drusen) the annual incidence rises from 3 per cent at age 55 to nearly 6 per cent at 75; for macular degeneration associated with sight loss, from 0·5 to 6·5 per cent. Finally, Hyman and colleagues[22] have shown in a case control study a positive association between senile macular degeneration and a maternal family history, exposure to chemicals at work and smoking (men only), a history of cardiovascular disease, blue or medium pigment iris colour, decreased hand/grip and hyperopia. They point to the need for further studies to confirm and explore these associations.

SENILE CATARACTS

Similar estimates have been made, from the Framingham study, of the population incidence and prevalence of senile cataracts.[23] Cataracts were defined as 'lens opacities (excluding early cortical changes) [which] could not be ascribed to congenital, secondary or other specific causes and were accompanied by visual acuity of 6/9 or worse'. Once again, defining a pathological entity in terms both of clinical appearance and an arbitrary level of functional impairment has its semantic limitations, but there is every reason in epidemiological studies to distinguish between senile cataracts and the lens changes normally associated with ageing.

Leske and Sperduto[23] calculate prevalence figures for men, ranging from 4·3 per cent at ages 52–64 to 40·9 per cent at ages 75–85; and for women, 4·7 per cent and 48·9 per cent. For senile lens changes alone, without sight loss, the corresponding figures for men are 38 per cent and 88 per cent, and for women 45 per cent and 93 per cent. Using the same data, Podgor and colleagues have calculated age/specific annual incidence rates varying from 1·2 per cent at age 55 to 15·3 per cent at 75 years.[21] The equivalent figures for the annual incidence of senile lens changes are 10 per cent and 37 per cent.

An annual incidence of more than 1 per cent at the age of 55, rising to 15 per cent at 75, puts cataracts far ahead of any other degenerative disease of later life and it is no surprise to find them the most commonly ascribed cause of visual disability, short of blindness, in population surveys.[7,19] In parts of England and Wales the annual extraction rate is almost 1 per cent in that part of the population aged 70 years or more.[24]

Although in 'western' countries the great majority of cataracts are not associated with any known cataractogenic factors, apart from age, the much higher prevalence of cataract in countries with high annual exposure to ultraviolet radiation is becoming increasingly well documented. A report from the Royal Australian College of Ophthalmologists (1980)[25] found an age-adjusted prevalence of cataract, aphakia or subluxation of 73 per thousand among rural non-Aborigines. High figures occurred in all age groups, but particularly in those aged 50–59 where the rate in Aborigines and non-Aborigines was as high as 11 per cent. There was a positive correlation among both Aborigines and non-Aborigines between levels of climatic ultraviolet radiation and cataract occurrence.[26] There have been similar reports from the Punjab[27] and Nepal.[28] However, as Hollows points out,[26] there is scant evidence of the effect of other possible factors such as genetic or family history or nutritional disadvantage in such studies.

Statistically, and apart from well-recorded occupational risks in vibration and intense ultraviolet light, the strongest risk factors associated with senile cataract in western populations seem to be diabetes, hypertension, heart disease, high blood urea, use of diuretics, eye ointments (especially miotics and steroids), eye injury and, for women, abstinence from or excessive intake of, alcohol.[29] Most of these associations remain statistical and their interactions have yet to be adequately explored. Although the association between diabetes and senile cataract has been questioned, Hiller and colleagues[30] have used data from the 1971–2 National Health and Nutrition Examination Survey in the USA to deduce a relative risk associated with diabetes of 1·9. Increased risk was also shown for poor education (1·5), race black/white (1·3), rural living (1·4) and high exposure to ultraviolet light (1·6). These relative risks compare with a relative risk of 13·3 associated with being over 70 years of age. Similarly, the Poole Diabetic Eye Survey found a prevalence of cataract in insulin-treated diabetic patients of 60 per cent in the 71–80 years age group and 40 per cent in the non-insulin-treated group.[31] At these ages this prevalence for insulin-dependent diabetics is considerably higher than in the general population at Framingham, though not so for non-insulin diabetics. Both groups showed considerably higher prevalences than in Framingham at younger ages, but numbers were small. Lastly, the evidence linking exposure to supposed radiation from visual display units (VDUs) and cataracts is at present no more than conjectural.[32]

DIABETIC RETINOPATHY

Rand[33] has summarized and collated the numerous attempts that have been made over the years to estimate the incidence and prevalence of visible retinopathy among diabetic patients, and hence figures for the general population. He deduces an *incidence* of 25 per cent to 53 per cent in the 5–7 years following the diagnosis of insulin dependent diabetes, assuming that, after 15 years of diabetes, almost all diabetic patients have some evidence of retinopathy. The WHO Multinational Study[34] quotes somewhat lower figures than these with 6 year incidences ranging from 4·5 per cent for men in West Germany to over 30 per cent in Japan. The percentage prevalence of visible retinopathy after 14–20 years' duration of diabetes ranged from 56 per cent among men in the UK to 78 per cent in Bulgaria. In most of the 14 countries reporting, diabetic retinopathy was more prevalent among men than women at each duration period (0–6 years, 7–13 years, 14–20 years); in the UK, however, this only applied to the shortest period (21·3 per cent men, 18·6 per cent women). Corresponding figures for 7–13 were 34·4 per cent and 40·0 per cent, and for 14–20 years 56·1 per cent and 75·0 per cent. In the Framingham study 2 per cent of the population aged 52–64 were diagnosed as having diabetic retinopathy, 3 per cent at 65–74 and 7·0 per cent at 75–85. Only in the eldest age group did prevalence among women exceed that among men.[19] But these were small numbers of actual diabetic sufferers and retinopathy was not related to type of diabetes, time since diagnosis or control. Other studies in the UK, however, have found an excess of men with severe retinopahy in insulin dependent diabetes of long standing:[35] most, however, were not population based.

Age at onset must be a compounding factor in and between different study populations, but its precise relationship to disease duration or control has yet to be clarified. For these and other reasons comparative data from cross-sectional studies are bound to be hazardous and it is probable that only population based prospective studies will settle the points; several such studies are now under way.

GLAUCOMA

Problems of definition make population studies of the prevalence of chronic open angle glaucoma very difficult. If the classic triad of field defects, disc cupping and persistently raised intraocular pressure is used, the all age prevalence of open angle glaucoma in western countries is probably between 0·3 and 0·4 per cent, rising to 1 per cent around the age of 70 and 3 per cent over the age of 75.[18] But if disc cupping and field defects alone are used, the prevalence in middle age (approximately 40–70 years) is between 0·5 per cent[36] and 0·9 per cent[37]. Leske[18] calculates that one-third to one-half of people with glaucoma type field loss have 'normal' intraocular pressures (21 mmHg) at diagnosis. No adequate estimates of age specific annual incidence are available except among very selected cohorts; the problems of definition are compounded by the size and duration of longitudinal studies needed to derive statistically sound results.

Many attempts to find systemic, behavioural and genetic risk factors for chronic open angle glaucoma have been made, with varying degrees of success. Age is by far the strongest predictor and is independent of other factors.[18] Prevalence is probably higher among black people than white, but this may be an indirect association with systemic blood pressure and a greater tendency among coloured people to raised intraocular tension. Too few good studies on mixed race populations have been made to confirm or refute this. Several hypotheses have been advanced for the apparent association between systemic hypertension and glaucoma[38] and vascular hypothesis for field loss remains epidemiologically attractive, but it is far from proved.

However, the evidence for genetic associations, though not their precise mechanism, is accepted. There is a reported risk in first degree relatives of glaucoma sufferers ranging from 4 to 16 per cent.[18] There is also a supposed association with diabetes, though this was not found in the Framingham study nor in Bengtsson's study in Dalby.[39] It may have been that both studies were too small because a strong association between diabetes and high intraocular pressure (21 mmHg) was found in Framingham.[37] There is controversy over associations with cardiovascular disease, alcohol intake and short stature; each has been found to be statistically correlated with glaucoma in some studies, but not confirmed in others.

REFERENCES
1. WHO Blindness (Information collected from various sources). Epidemiology Vital Statistics Report 19, 1966, pp. 437–511.
2. Goldstein H. *Demography and Causes of Blindness*. New York, American Foundation for the Blind, 1968.
3. Goldstein H. Incidence, prevalence and causes of blindness. Statistics for the United States and selected countries in Asia and Europe. *Publ. Health Rev.* 1974, **3**, pp. 5–37.
4. Fitzgerald R. G. Reactions to blindness; an exploratory study of adults with recent loss of sight. *Arch. of Gen. Psychiat.* 1970, p. 22.
5. Gray P. G. and Todd J. *Mobility and Reading Habits of the Blind*. Government Social Survey, London, HMSO, 1965.
6. Kemp N. J. Social psychological aspects of blindness. *Curr. Psychol. Rev.* 1981, **1**, 69–89.
7. Cullinan T. R. The epidemiology of visual disability. Studies of visually disabled people in the community. University of Kent, Canterbury, HSRU Report No. 28, 1977.
8. WHO *The Prevention of Blindness*. (Report of a WHO Study Group) Geneva, WHO, Technical Report Series, No. 518, 1973.
9. Sorsby A. The Incidence and Causes of Blindness in England and Wales. 1948–1962. (Reports on Public Health and Medical Subjects No. 114.) London, HMSO, 1966.
10. Sorsby A. The Incidence and Causes of Blindness in England and Wales. 1963–1968. (Reports of Public Health and Medical Subjects No. 128.) London, HMSO, 1972.
11. DHSS Blindness and Partial Sight in England. 1969–1976. (Reports on Public Health and Medical Subjects No. 129.) London, HMSO, 1979.
12. DHSS Registered Blind and Partially Sighted Persons: year ending 31 March 1980. England. London, DHSS A/F80/7.
13. MacDonald A. E. Causes of blindness in Canada. An analyses of 24 605 cases registered with Canadian National Institute for the Blind. *Canad. Med. Assoc. J.* 1965 **92**, 264–79.
14. Sturman D. A statistical approach to eye problems in New Zealand. *Trans. Ophthalmol. Soc. NZ* 1969; **1**, 74–84.
15. Page J. Definition of blindness and partial sight. In: *Technological Prosthetics for the Partially Sighted*. International Institute for Applied Systems Analysis, Schloss Laxenburg Austria, 1974.
16. Graham P. A., Wallace J., Welsby E. Evaluation of postal detection of registrable blindness. *Br. J. Prev. Soc. Med.* 1968 **22**, 238.
17. Cullinan T. R., Gould E. S., Silver J. H. et al. Visual disability and home lighting. *Lancet.* 1979; **1**, 642–4.
18. Leske, C. M. The epidemiology of open-angle glaucoma: a review. *Am. J. Epidemiol.* 1983; **118**, 166–91.
19. Ederer F. *The Framingham Eye Study. Blindness (1977–1978)*. Washington, DC, American Association of Workers for the Blind, 1977/8.
20. Ferris F. Senile macular degeneration: review of epidemiological features. *Am. J. Epidemiol.* 1983, **118**, 132–51.
21. Podgor M. J., Leske C. and Ederer F. Incidence estimates for lens changes, macular changes, open-angle glaucoma and diabetic retinopathy. *Am. J. Epidemiol.* 1983; **118**, 206–12.
22. Hyman L. G., Lilienfeld A. M., Ferris F. L. et al. Senile macular degeneration: a case-control study. *Am. J. Epidemiol.* 1983; **118**, 213–27.
23. Leske M. and Sperduto R. D. The epidemiology of senile cataracts: a review. *Am. J. Epidemiol.* 1983; **118**, 152–65.
24. Brennan M. and Knox E. The incidence of cataract and its clinical presentation. *Community Health* 1975; **7**, 13.
25. National Trachoma and Eye Health Programme (1980) Royal Australian College of Ophthalmologists, Sydney.
26. Hollows F. and Moran D. (1981) Cataract – the ultraviolet risk factor. *Lancet* 1981 **2**, 1249–50.
27. Chatterjee J. Cataract in the Punjab. In: *Symposium on the Human Lens in Relation to Cataract*. Amsterdam, Associated Scientific Publishers, Ciba Foundation Symposium 19 (new series) 1973, pp. 265–79.
28. Brilliant L., Grasset N., Pokhrel R. P. et al. Associations among cataract prevalence, sunlight hours and altitude in the Himalayas. Paper presented at Symposium on Eye Disease Epidemiology. National Eye Institute, Bethesda, Md, June 1982.
29. Clayton R. M., Cuthbert J., Duffy J. et al. Some risk factors associated with cataract in S.E. Scotland: a pilot study. *Trans. Ophthalmol. Soc. UK*. 1982; **102**, Part 3, pp. 331–6.
30. Hiller R, Sperduto R. and Ederer F. Epidemiologic Associations with Cataract in the 1971–1972 national health and nutrition examination. *Am. J. Epidemiol.* 1983; **118**, 239–49.
31. Houston A. C. (1982) Preliminary communications.
32. Cakir A., Hart D. and Stewart T. *The V.D.T. Manual*. Inca-Fiej Research Association, Washingtonplatz, 1, D – Darmstadt, Federal Republic of Germany.
33. Rand L. I. Recent advances in diabetic retinopathy. *Am. J. Med.* 1981 **70**, 595–602.
34. Jarrett R. J. and Keen H. The WHO Multinational Study of Vascular Disease in Diabetes: 3. Microvascular Disease. *Diabetes Care* 1979; **2**, 196–201.
35. Bodansky J. H., Cudworth A. G., Drury P. L. et al. Risk factors associated with severe proliferative retinopathy in insulin-dependent diabetes mellitus. *Diabetes Care Bull.* 1982; pp. 97–100.
36. Hollows F. C. and Graham P. A. Intraocular pressure, glaucoma and glaucoma suspects in a defined population. *Br. J. Ophthalmol.* 1966; **50**, 570–86.
37. Leske M. C. and Podgor M. J. Intraocular pressure cardiovascular risk variables and visual field defects. *Am. J. Epidemiol.* 1983; **118**, 280–7.
38. Maunenee A. E. The pathogenesis of visual field loss in glaucoma. In: Brocklehurst R. J. (ed.) *Controversy in Ophthalmology*. Philadelphia, Saunders, 1977; pp. 300–11.
39. Bengtsson B. Aspects of the epidemiology of chronic glaucoma. *Acta Ophthalmol. (Suppl.)* 1981; **146**, 4–26.

Index

A-pattern squint, 415–16
A-scan ultrasonography, 81–82
Abducens
   neurones, 426
   palsy, 437–41
Abduction nystagmus, 434
Abetalipoproteinaemia, 473, 550
Abiotrophies, optic, 325–8
Abrasion, corneal, 138
Abscess, lacrimal sac, 400
Accommodation in infants, 452
Accommodative esotropia, 416–17
Acetazolamide, 53–54
Acetic acid derivatives, 507
Acetylcholine, 47–48
   activity in retina, 40
Acetylcysteine drops for keratitis, 114
Achromatopsia see Cone dystrophy
Acid burns, 375
   corneal, 138
Acne rosacea in staphylococcal
      blepharitis, 110
Acromegaly, 535–6
ACTH-secreting tumours, 537–8
ACTH secretion, 544, 545
Actinomycosis, canalicular, 119, 408
Acycloguanosine, 56
Acyclovir, 56
   for herpes zoster uveitis, 172
Addison's disease, 544–5
Adenine arabinoside, 56
Adenocarcinoma, eyelid, 390
Adenoma
   renal, 544
   basophil, 537
   chromophobe, 534
   pituitary, 346
Adenosine utilization in cornea, 26
Adenovirus infections, 115
   causing membranous conjunctivitis,
      125
   to cornea, 138–9
Adjuvants, 484
Adnexa involvement in sarcoidosis, 178
Adrenal gland
   disorders, 543–6
      adrenal cortex, 543–5
      medulla, 545
Adrenaline, 50–51
   for glaucoma, (Table VII) 311
Adrenergic drugs, 50–51
   for glaucoma, 33
Adrenergic neurone-blocking drugs, 52
   alpha, 51
   beta, 51–52
Adverse reactions from drugs, 58–60
Ageing effects
   on anterior chamber, 316
   in cataract, 30
   in conjunctiva, 519
   on ERG, 99

Ageing effects (cont.)
   lacrimal secretion and, 392, 518–19
   in Leber's disease, 327
   ptosis and, 383, 384
   on retina, 42
   in sickle cell disease, 556
   on VEG, 103
   vitreous humour and, 33
Agnosia, visual, 350
Aicardi's syndrome in infants, 461
Aids
   for blindness, 571–2
   for visual disability, 562–9
AIDS, uveitis and, 181–2
Air tamponade, intravitreal, 253–4
Albinism, 456, (Table III) 457, 458,
      473–4, 478
Albuminoids, 28
Alcaptonuria, 551
Alcohol-tobacco amblyopia, 328–9
Alcuronium, 53
Aldose reductase
   diabetic retinopathy and, 42
   inhibitors for cataract therapy, 30, 31
   for diabetes, 548
Aldosterone
   deficiency, 544–5
   secretion, 543–4
Alexia without agraphia, 349–50
Alkali burns, 375
   corneal, 138
Alkylating agents, 510–11
   main actions, (Table I) 508
Allen Braley Thorpe lens, 64–65
Allergy, 487
   autoimmune disorders of eye and,
      (Table III) 494
   conjunctivitis, 119–22, 125, 494–5
      acute, 495–6
   drug, 59
   episcleritis and, 150
   laboratory tests for, 500–3
   mechanisms involved in, 493
   staphylococcal, 111
   type I, 487–8, (Table III) 494, 495–6,
      500
   type II, 488, (Table III) 494, 496, 500
   type III, 488–9, (Table III) 494, 496–7,
      500
   type IV, 489–90, (Table III) 494, 497,
      500–1
Alpha beta agonists for glaucoma, (Table
      VII) 311
Alport's syndrome in infants, 462
Alström syndrome, 550
Amacrine
   cells in retina, 14, 18–20
   neurochemistry, 40–42
Amaurosis
   fugax, carotid artery disease and,
      524–43

Amaurosis, fugax (cont.)
   aneurysms, 526–30
   basilar aneurysms, 531–2
   brain stem vascular disease, 531
   caroticocavernous fistula, 530
   dural arteriovenous shunt, 530–1
   embolic, 524–5
   non-embolic, 525–6
   Leber's, 200, 203, 456–7, 462
   differential diagnosis, 481
Amblyopia, 412–14
   of disuse, VEP in, 103, (Fig. 7) 104
   in handicapped children, 455
   hysterical, VEP in, 104
   neurophysiology of, 412–13
   test, 322
   tobacco-alcohol, 328
   toxic, 60
Amethocaine hydrochloride, 52
Amino acids
   in aqueous humour, 32
   in retina, 41
γ-Aminobutyric acid see GABA
Aminocaproic acid for haemorrhage,
      363
Aminoglycosides, 55
Amniotocoele, 398
Amoebic keratitis, 140
Amoxycillin, 55
cAMP
   in aqueous humour, 32
   fluid transport in retina and, 36
Amphotericin B, 57
Ampicillin, 55
Amsler grid test, 322
Amyloidosis, vitreous, 264
Anaemia, eye and, 552–8
   macrocytic, 553
   microcytic, 553
   normocytic, 553
   polycythaemia, 553–4
   sickle cell disease, 554–8
Anaesthetics
   general, 53
   for lacrimal surgery, 400–1
   local, 52–53
Anaphylaxis following fluorescein
      angiography, 75
Anergy, 487
Aneuploidy, 467
Aneurysm
   basilar, 531
   carotid, 536–40
      berry, 526–7
      dissecting, 527
      giant, 527–30
   intracranial, 347
   ophthalmic artery, 91
   posterior communicating arterial,
      440–1

579

Angiography
  for chiasmatic investigation, 350
  fluorescein *see* Fluorescein angiography
  orbital, 89–90
Angioid streaks, 233, (Fig. 9) 234
  in sickle cell disease, 555
Angle
  abnormalities, 67–68
  closed, 67, 68
  fine capillaries, 68
  inflammatory changes, 68
  neovascularization, 67–68
  trauma effects on, 68
  widths in anterior chamber, 66–67
  see also under Glaucoma
Aniridia, 162
  congenital, 468
  sporadic, 468
Anisometropia in infants, 463–4
Ankylosing spondylitis, uveitis and, 169, 499, 520–1
Antazoline, 57
Anterior chamber
  angle irritation following lens implant, 299–300
  measurement by gonioscopy, 64–69
  cleavage syndrome, classification of, (Table V) 135
  collapse during lens implant, 299
  haemorrhage during lens implant, 299
  lenses, 293–4, 295–6
  reformation following penetrating injury, 370
  shallowing, 315–16, 317
Anterior segment
  injury, 362–4
    reconstruction following, 371
  ischaemia in sickle cell disease, 555
Antibiotics, 54–56
  for bacterial keratitis, 140
  for endophthalmitis, 290, 370
  polyene, 56–57
  for staphylococcal hypersensitivity, 111
  for trachoma, 118
Antibodies
  -mediated allergy, 488, 493
  in pemphigoid, 126
  in tears, 107
Anticholinesterase drops, 48–49
Anticholinergic drugs, 49–50
Antifibrinolysis for haemorrhage, 363
Antifungal agents, 56–57
  for mycotic keratitis, 140
Antigens, 484
  mechanism of action, 486
  photoreceptor, 498
  sequestered in vitreous, depot effect of, 491
  tissue specific, 491
  see also S antigen
Antiglaucoma agents, (Table VII) 311
Antihistamines, 57
  for vernal disease, 121
Anti-inflammatory drugs, 57–59
  for scleritis, 160
  non-steroidal, 507–9
Antilymphocyte globulin, 511–12, 513
  main action, (Table I) 508
Antimetabolic drugs for corneal herpes simplex, 139
Antimicrobial agents, 54–56
Antithyroid therapy, 542

Antiviral
  agents, 56
  immune responses, 506
Aphakia
  lens implants for, 292–303
  retinal detachment and, 248
APMPPE *see* Pigment epitheliopathy, acute posterior multifocal placoid
Aponeurosis, 383
  surgery for, 383–4
Apoplexy, pituitary, 346
Applanation, 62
Aqueous humour, 32–33
  abnormal sugar levels in, 277
  accumulation in retro-iridic region, 319
    in retrolentricular space, (Fig. 13) 313
  appearance in uveitis, 165
  -blood barrier, 490–1
  composition, 32
  function, 32
  glaucoma and, 32–33
  pathway through trabecular meshwork, 306
  production, 32
  secondary, 32
Arachidonic acid metabolic pathways, 493, 507
Arachnoiditis, chiasmatic, 348
Arcus
  juvenalis, 137
  senilis, 142
Arden Index, 101
Arnold-Chiari syndrone, nystagmus and, 465
Areolar dystrophy, central, 212–13
Argon laser, 238
Argyrosis corneae, 136
Arterial aneurysms, posterior communicating, 440–1
Arteriolar lesions in diabetic retinopathy, 239–40
Arteriography, carotid orbital, 89–90
Arteriovenous malformation, 91
Arteritis, ischaemic optic neuropathy and, 335–6
Artery *see under* Carotid; Ophthalmic; Retinal
Arthritis
  in Behçet's disease, 177
  juvenile chronic *see* Still's disease
  juvenile rheumatoid, iridocyclitis in, 499
  rheumatoid *see* Rheumatoid arthritis
Arthropathy, psoriatic, uveitis and, 521
Arthrophthalmopathy, hereditary progressive, 470
Artificial tears, 123
Ascension phenomenon, 261
Ascorbate
  in aqueous humour, 32
  for corneal breakdown prevention, 376
  in vitreous humour, 33, 34
Ascorbic acid, lens metabolism and, 29
Aspartate, retinal, 41
Aspergillus endophthalmitis, 195
Asteroid hyalosis, 262
Astigmatism, 129
  in infants, 464
Ataxia telangiectasia, 497
Atenolol, 52
Atheroma, vertebrobasilar, 531
Atopy, 488
ATP utilization in retina, 37

ATPase, corneal fluid transport and, 27
Atrophy, optic, 325–8
Atropine, 49–50
  for uveitis, 167
Autoantibody, photoreceptor, 498
Autofluorescence, 77
Autoimmune disorders diagnosis, (Table V) 502–3
Autoimmunity, 490, 506
  retinal, 497–8
Autonomic drugs, 47–53
Autonomic system, stimulation effects on, (Table I) 47
Autosomal dominant inheritance, 469–470
  cataract, 478
  optic atrophy, 480
  retinitis pigmentosa, 472
Autosomal recessive inheritance, 470–1
  cataract, 478
  ocular albinism, 474
  optic atrophy, 482–1
  retinitis pigmentosa, 472
Avascular necrosis, corticosteroid-induced, 509
Axenfeld's syndrome, 67, (Table V) 135
Axial opacities removal, 273
Azathioprine, 510
  main actions, (Table I) 508
  for uveitis, 168
Azlocillin, 55

B lymphocytes *see under* Lymphocytes
Bacterial
  culture for conjunctival disorders, 108–9
  endophthalmitis, 290
  infiltration to cornea, 140
  sensitivity of antibiotics, (Table III) 55
'Bag of worms', 460
Band keratopathy, 142
Barkan's membrane, 67
Barrie Jones' sixth formula, 519
Basal gel fibrosis, 266
Basilar aneurysm, 531–2
Basophil adenomas, 537
Bassen-Kornzweig syndrome, 473
Batten-Mayou syndrome, 473
Batten's disease
  infantile, 460
  juvenile, 473
Bathorhodopsin, 5
Behçet's disease
  cytotoxic therapy, 511
  immunology, 499
  retinal lesions in, 188–9
  uveitis and, 177–8
Behr's syndrome, 325, 481
Berry aneurysms, 526–7
Best's disease
  clinical aspects, 209–10
  pathogenesis, 210
Betamethasone sodium phosphate, (Table VI) 58
Betaxolol for glaucoma, (Table VII) 311
Bielschowsky head tilt test, (Fig. 6) 418, 437
Biemond syndrome, 550
Bietti's crystalline dystrophy, 202
Bimedial rectus recessions, 247
Binkhorst
  clip, 293

Binkhorst *(cont.)*
  lens, (Fig. 2) 294
Binocular vision
  functioning, 425
  single, in infants, 452–3
Biochemistry of eye, 24–45
Biometry before lens implants, 295
Biomicroscopy, slit lamp, 71
Biopsy
  conjunctival, 518
  lacrimal gland, 518
Bipolar cells of retina, 13, 16–18
Bird shot retinochoroidopathy, 178, 179, 187, 498
Bjerrum screen test, 349
'Black cornea', 137
Black sunburst sign, 555
Bleb, filtering, 288
Blepharitis, 389
  dry eye and, 124
  microbial allergic, 494–5
  seborrhoeic, 109
  Sjögren's syndrome and, 520
  staphylococcal, 110
  tear film instability and, 113
  trigeminal irritation and, 392
Blepharoptosis, 383
Blind spot in chiasmatic disease, 346
Blindness
  conditions leading to, 575
  definitions, 571–2
  diabetic retinopathy and, 577
  epidemiology, 571–8
  glaucoma and, 577
  in infants
    causes, (Table III) 457
    effect on general development, 454
    examination, 455–6
    facial signs, 451
  partial *see* Visual acuity loss;
    disorders; field loss; loss
    registration, 572
  senile cataracts and, 576–7
  senile macular degeneration and, 575–6
  stationary night, 214
  statistics, 572–4
  trachoma and, 117–18
Blinking test, 451
Blood
  -aqueous barrier breakdown, 32
  coagulation disorders, 559
  deposition in cornea, 137
  filling Schlemm's canal, 66
  flow, measurement by fluorescein angiography, 79
  for immunological study, 501
  -ocular barriers, 490–1
  -retina barrier failure, 223, 224
'Blue stone', 137
Blue-dot cataract, 278
Blunt injuries, 362–8
Bobbing, ocular, 446
Bone
  defects in infants, 462
  disease, Paget's, 551
  -marrow transplant in leukaemia, 558
  spicular pigmentation in syphilis, 194, (Fig. 16) 195
Bourneville's disease *see* Tuberous sclerosis
Bowel disease, uveitis and, 182–3
Bowen's disease, 352–3

Bowman's layer, 24, 130
Brain stem
  organization of eye movements
    horizontal, 426
    vertical, 426–7
  vascular disease, 531
Bridle suture, 283
Bromocriptine therapy
  for growth hormone-secreting tumours, 536
  for pituitary tumours, 535
  for prolactinoma, 537
Brow *see* Eyebrow
Brown's syndrome, 420–1
  acquired, 422–3
Bruch's membrane
  abnormalities, 227–9
    causing angioid streaks, 233
  breaks, myopia and, 234
Brushfield's spots, 467
BSS Plus solution, 26
Bucket handle tear, 259
Buckles, scleral, 251
Bulbar tumours, 354–60
Bullae, epithelial, 136
Bull's eye dystrophies, 212
Buphthalmos, 133, 314
Bupivacaine hydrochloride, 53
Burns
  chemical, 138, 375–6
  conjunctivitis and, 125
  eyelid, 390
Burst cells, 425, 427
Busacca nodules, 164, 166, 178
Butterfly-shaped dystrophy, 210–11
Bypass surgery, lacrimal, 406–8

C-scan ultrasonography, 82–83
Café-au-lait spots, 476
Calcific emboli, 525
Calcification, orbital, 87
Calcium
  deposits in cornea, 136, 142
  metabolism defect, cataract and, 281
  phototransduction and, 39
  release from rods, 8
  voltage-gated mechanism in rods, 11
Camera adaptation for angiography, 74
Canaliculi, lacrimal, 392–3
  agenesis, 398
  lacerations, 409
  obstructions, 397, 404–8
Canaliculitis, 408
Canaliculodacryocystorhinostomy, 405–6, 409
Candida retinitis, 194–5
Canine dysplasia, 43
Canthal sling, 383
Capillary lesions in diabetic retinopathy, 238–9
Capsular
  opacifications, posterior, 289
  polishing, posterior, 285
  rupture, 284, 285–6
    posterior, during lens implant, 299
  thickening, following lens implant, 301–2
Capsulectomy
  anterior, 285, 287
  posterior, 287
Carbachol, 48
Carbenicillin, 55

Carbon dioxide, corneal, 131–2
Carbonic anhydrase
  corneal fluid transport and, 27
  inhibitors, 53–54
    for glaucoma, 33
Carcinoma
  basal cell eyelid, 389
  lacrimal passages, 400
  squamous cell eyelid, 389
  thyroid, 543
Carcinomatosis, optic nerve involvement by, 339
Caroticocavernous fistula, 530
Carotid arteriography, orbital, 89–90
Carotid artery disease, amaurosis fugax and, 524–32
Caruncle excision, 407
Cataract
  aetiology in first year of life, (Table II) 479
  anterior polar, 278
  in blunt trauma, 364, (Fig. 1a) 365
  classification, 276–7
  complicated, 280–1
  congenital 478–80
    complete, 278
  coronary, 278
  cortical, 279
  development, 30–31, 278
  diabetes and, 548
  in Fuch's heterochromic cyclitis, 171
  genetically determined, 478–80
  hypermature, 280
  incipient, 279–80
  irradiation, 277
  juvenile complete, 278
  lamellar, 278
  lens implants for, 292–303
  maturation, 280
  miotic, 49
  Morgagnian, 280
  non-hereditary, 480
  nuclear, 278–9
  posterior polar, 278
  punctate, 278
  senile, 277, 278–80, 576–7
  steroid-induced, 168
  surgery for
    extracapsular, 284–6
    general principles, 282–3
    intracapsular, 283–4
    lensectomy, 286–7
    phacoemulsification, 286
    postoperative complications, 287–90
  symptoms and signs, 281
  systemic disease and, 277–8, 281
  traumatic, 277
  ultrasonography, (Fig. 26) 82, 83
  uveitis and, 166
Catecholamine
  activity in retina, 40
  secretion, 545
Catford drum test, 452
Cat's eye appearance following lens implant, 301
Cavernous sinus syndrome, 530
Cell-mediated
  allergy, 489–90
  immunity to photoreceptor antigens, 498
Cellular infiltration, conjunctival, 108
Cellulitis, orbital, 95
Cephalosporins, 55

Cerebellar
  influence on eye movement, 428
  lesions, acute nystagmus and, 464–5
    causing downbeat nystagmus, 445
Cerebello-pontine angle disease, nystagmus of, 445
Cerebral
  artery occlusion causing optic lesions, 349
  blindness in infants, (Table III) 467, 468
  tumours causing optic radiation lesions, 349
Ceroid-lipofuscinosis, neuronal, 473
Chalcosis, 137
Chamber see Anterior;Posterior
Chandler's manoeuvre, 67, 313
CHARGE associations with coloboma, 462
Chediak-Higashi syndrome, 497
  retinal effects in, 42
Chemical
  abrasion, corneal, 138
  burns, 375–6
    conjunctivitis and, 125
Cherry red spot
  myoclonus syndrome, 445
  in Tay–Sach's disease, 460
Chiasma
  anatomy, 346
  arachnoiditis, 348
  compression, disc cupping in, (Table IV) 308
  diseases, 346–51
  gliomas, 338, 462, (Figs 18–19) 463
  investigations, 350–1
Chlamydial
  conjunctivitis, 117–18
  isolation from conjunctiva, 109
  zoonosis, 119
Chlorambucil, 510–11
Chloramphenicol, 56
Chloroma, 558
Chlorophyll, Refsum's syndrome and, 208
Chloroquine
  retinal effects of, 59
    EOG in, 101
  side effects, 522
Chlortetracycline, 56
Cholesterol emboli, 525
Cholinergic drugs, 47–49
Cholinesterase inhibitors
  irreversible, 49
  reversible, 48–49
Chondroitin sulphate, 25
Choriocapillaris atrophy, 212–13
Chorioretinal see Retinochoroid
Choroid
  abnormalities in fundus flavimaculatus, 211–12
    in leukaemia, 558
    in retinitis pigmentosa, 207
    in sarcoidosis, 179
    in sickle cell disease, 555
  central areolar dystrophy, 212–13
  detachment ultrasonography, (Fig. 3f, g) 83, 84–85
  disturbances causing fluorescence leakage, 77
  fluid accumulation, 224, 226–9
  folds in papilloedema, 342
  gyrate atrophy, 471

Choroid (cont.)
  haemangioma, 236, 355
  haemorrhage following SRF drainage, 253
  infiltrate in sympathetic ophthalmitis, 180
  knuckle transillumination, (Fig. 3) 253
  local vasculopathy, 226
  melanocytoma, 355–7
  melanoma, 237
  naevi, 236, 355
  neovascularization, 227–9, 557
  osteoma, ultrasonography of, (Fig. 4f) 84, 85
  phase in normal angiogram, 75
  tears, 234
    from blunt injury, 367
  tumours, 355–7
  ultrasonography, 84–85
  vascular disease, 226–9
  vasculature, 223
  venous obstruction, 227
Choroideraemia, 207–8, 478
  ERG in, 99
Choroiditis
  geographic see Choroiditis, serpiginous
  Jensen's juxtapapillary, 173
  serpiginous, 186–7, 190
  uveitis and, 163
Choroidoretinitis see Retinochoroiditis
Chromophobe adenomas, 534
Chromosome
  11p13 deletion, 468
  13q14 deletion, 469
  aberrations, 467–9
    in infants, 462
  Lyon hypothesis, 477–8
Cicatricial
  ectropion, 383
  entropion, 380–1
Cicatrizing conjunctivitis, 125
Ciliary
  band appearance, 66
  body
    and aqueous humour production, 32
    coloboma, 162
    tumours, 355
Cilio-lenticular block, 313
Cilium in photoreceptor cells, 36
Ciné-fluorescein angiography, 79
Citric acid for collagen repair, 376
Climatic droplet keratopathy, 142
Clindamycin, 56
  for toxoplasmosis, 173, 192
Clobetasone butyrate, 58
  for uveitis, 168
Clotrimazole, 57
Cloxacillin, 55
Coagulation disorders, 559
'Cobblestone' papillae, 124
Cocaine, 51
  hydrochloride, 52–53
Cochet and Bonnet instrument, 148
Cogan lid twitch, 441
Cogan's syndrome, 141, 143
Cold opposite warm same (COWS), 435, 443
Colitis, ulcerative, uveitis in, 521
Collagen
  corneal, 129, 130, 141, 152
    disease and, 27
    transparency and, 27
  repair, 376

Collagen (cont.)
  scleral, 152
  stromal, 25
  vitreous humour, 33
    fibrosis and, 265–6
'Collar stud' appearance, 356
Coloboma
  associations, 462
  ciliary body, 162
  eyelid, repair of, 390
  field defects in, (Table V) 308
  in infant, 456
  optic disc, 234
    cupping in, (Table IV) 308, (Fig. 10) 310
  optic nerve head, 323
Colour
  intensity test, 321–2
  opponency, 15, 17–18
  vision
    defects, 212
      from optic nerve disorders, 321
    in infants, 453
Commotio retinae, 365–6
Complement-mediated allergy, 488, 493
Computerized tomographic scanning
  for chiasmal lesions, 350, 351
  for chromophobe adenoma, 534
  of foreign bodies, 373
  for pineal tumours, 539
  orbital, 88–89
Cones
  bipolar cells, 17–18
  coupling, 12
  defects, 213–14
  dystrophies, 209–13
    in infants, (Table III) 457, 458
  light adaptation by, 9
  metabolic function disorders, 199
  pathways, 19–20
  pedicle, 14–15
  photoresponses from, 2
  pigments, 6–7
  retinitis pigmentosa effects on, 203, 206
  spectral sensitivity, 15
  structure, 4, 34
  visual cycle, 7
Congenital
  abnormalities
    corneal, 133–5
    lacrimal drainage, 396–9
    optic disc, 234
    uveal tract, 162
    vascular, causing fluid accumulation, 235
  aniridia, 467
  cataract, 478–80
    complete, 278
  disc dysplasias, 323–4
  ectropion, 382
  entropion, 380
  esotropia, 414–15
  glaucoma, 314
  nystagmus, 444
  optic nerve pits, 234–5
  ptosis, 383
  rubella, 461–2, 551
  syphilis, ocular effects of, 174–5
  toxoplasmosis, 459–461
  venous malformation, 92
Conjugate ocular movements, 425–6
  supranuclear and vestibular influences on, 427

Conjunctival
  age effects, 519
  allergic reaction, 59
  biopsy, 518
  copper deposition, 137
  disorders, diagnostic aids in, 108–9
  epithelial ingrowth, 289
  examination for assessment of tear
    drainage, 394
  hyperaemia in uveitis, 164
  inflammatory response patterns, 108
  inserts, 123
  lymphocytes, 491, 494
  melanoma, 353
  plexus, superficial, 147–8
  response to staphylococcal
    hypersensitivity, 111
  scarring, 107
  stratification in Sjögren's syndrome,
    (Fig. 1) 519
  vessel changes in sickle cell disease,
    554–5
Conjunctivitis
  acute allergic, 119–20, 125, 495–6
  atopic, 120
  chlamydial, 117–18
  chronic atopic, 120
  cicatrizing, 125
  epidemic haemorrhagic, 116–17
  Epstein–Barr virus causing, 117
  eye medication causing, 119
  follicular, 114–24
    acute, 114–18
  herpes simplex, 115
  herpes zoster, 117
  immune complex-mediated, 496–7
  inclusion, 139–40
  ligneous, 114
  membranous, 125
  microbial allergic, 494–5
  in molluscum contagiosum, 117
  neonatal inclusion, 118–19
  papillary, 119–24
    contact lens-induced, 124–5
  phlyctenular, 110–11
  vernal, 120–2
  see also Keratoconjunctivitis
Conjunctivodacryocystorhinostomy, 406
Connective tissue disease, 516–23
  scleritis in, 158
Conn's syndrome, 544
Contact lenses
  corneal metabolism and, 132–3
  for hypermetropia, 292–3
  -induced papillary conjunctivitis, 124–5
  in infants, 464
  for keratoconus, 145
  painted scleral, 133
  soft, for drug delivery, 47
  telescope, 566
  use in fundus examination, 70–71
    in gonioscopy, 64
    in specular microscopy, 62
Contrast medium for CT scanning, 89
Contusion
  following blunt injury, 362–8
  following penetrating injury, 368
Convergence
  in infants, 452
  movement testing, 428
  retraction nystagmus, 444–5, 465
  spasm, 444
Convulsions in infants, 459–61

Copper
  deposition in cornea, 137
  foreign bodies, 373
  levels in lens, 278
Corneal
  abrasion and erosion, 138
    causing uveitis, 163
  acclimatization following ptosis
    surgery, 386
  angiography, 79
  avascularity, 490
  cellular infiltration, 138–41
  changes in episcleritis, 150
    in herpes simplex conjunctivitis, 115
    in scleritis, 148, 153–4
    in vernal disease, 121
  congenital abnormalities
    size, 133–4
    transparency, 134–5
  contusion injury, 362
  decompensation following lens
    implant, 299
  defects, posterior, 134
  degeneration
    age-related, 141–2
    pathological, 142
  deposition, 136–8
    from drug effects, 59
  dermoid, 135
  disease, biochemistry of, 27
  drying, 136
  dystrophy, 27, 142–3, (Table VI) 144–5
  ectasia, 143–6
  epithelium, 24, 130
    abrasion, 138
    breakdown and repair, 376
    oedema, 362
  erosions in sicca syndrome, 520
  grafts, 490
  lesions in phlyctenular conjunctivitis,
    110
  marginal guttering, 153–4
  metabolism, 25–27
  microvillae, 112
  normal
    Bowman's layer, 130
    components, (Table II) 130
    Descemet's membrane, 130
    dimensions, 129
    endothelium, 130–1
    epithelium, 130
    histology, 129
    hydration, 131
    limbal vessels, 133
    metabolism, 131
      contact lens and, 132–3
      oxygen and carbon dioxide, 131–2
    power, 129
    shape, 129
    thickness, 129–131
    transparency, 131
  oedema, 135–6
    following blunt injury, 362
    following cataract surgery, 288, 289
    formation, 131
    prolonged contact lens wear and, 133
    thickness in, 136
  opacity, 134, 135–41
  rupture, 133
  scarring, 141
  sensitivity in scleritis, 148
  specular microscopy, 61–63
  structure and function, 24–25

Corneal (cont.)
  thinning, 154
    in sicca syndrome, 520
  transport and transparency, 27
  ulcer, 134
  vascularization, 141
  verticillata, 138
  wound
    healing, 27
    penetrating, 368
Corneo-retinal potential, 97
  in EOG, 101
Coronary cataract, 278
Cortical
  cataract, 279
  cells, 412
  clean-up in extracapsular surgery, 285
  in phacoemulsification, 286
Corticosteroids see Steroids
Cortisol
  deficiency, 544–5
  secretion, 543
Cosmetic shell, 133
Cotton-wool spots, 239
  in AIDS, 181–2
  in anaemia, 552
Craniofacial abnormalities, lacrimal
  passages and, 399
Craniopharyngioma, 346–7, 538
  in infants, 462
  investigation of, 350, (Fig. 1) 535
Cretinism, hypothyroidism and, 542–3
Crocodile tears, 392
Crohn's disease, uveitis and, 182
Cryosurgery
  for abnormal eyelashes, 382
  for bleb, 288
  for cataract surgery, 283–4
  for eyelid tumours, 389
  for penetrating injury prophylaxis, 370
  for retinal detachment, 250–1
    prophylaxis, 256
  for retinoblastoma, 359
Cryptococcal retinochoroiditis, 196
Crystallins, 28
Cultures in conjunctival disease, 108
Cushing's syndrome, 537–8, 544
Cyanide toxicity in Leber's disease, 328
Cyclic nucleotides
  corneal wound healing and, 27
  in retina, 38–39
Cyclitic membrane formation, 266
Cyclitis
  chronic see Uveitis, intermediate
  heterochromic, 68
  Fuch's, 171
Cyclodialysis
  following lens implant, 300
  traumatic, 68
Cyclo-oxygenase production, 507
Cyclopentolate, 50
Cyclophosphamide, 510–11
  for scleritis, 160–1
Cycloplegia, drug-induced, 59, 414
Cyclosporin A, 512
  for Behçet's disease, 177
  main actions, (Table I) 508
  for uveitis, 168–9
Cyst
  ciliary body, 355
  craniopharyngeal, 538
  Meibomian, 389
  of Moll, 389

Cyst *(cont.)*
  orbital, CT scan of, 89, 93
    ultrasonography, (Fig. 5e) 85, 87
  of Zeis, 389
Cystathionine synthase deficiency, 475
Cysticercosis, retinal, 191
Cystinosis in infants, 462
Cystitome, irrigating, 285
Cystoid macular oedema, 289–90
Cytology
  of conjunctival scrapings, (Table I) 109
  impression, 517–18
Cytomegalovirus
  retinal involvement, 193–4
  in AIDS, 182
Cytotoxic drugs, 510–11
  for leukaemia, 558
  malignant disease and, 511
  opportunistic infections and, 51
  side effects, 511
  for uveitis, 168

Dacryoadenitis from mumps virus, 139
Dacryocystitis
  acquired, 399–400
  acute, 398, 400
    intermittent, 400
  chronic, 398
  in congenital nasolacrimal duct obstruction, 397
  secondary, 400
Dacryocystography, 395–6
Dacryocystorhinostomy, 397
  closure, 403
  complications, 404
  failed, reoperation for, 404
  history, 401
  incision, 401–3
  preparation of mucosal flaps, 403
Dacroliths, 400
Dalen-Fuch's nodules, 180, 374
Daranide for glaucoma, (Table VII) 311
Daraprim for toxoplasmosis, 192
Dark adaptation, 9–10
  effects on ERG, 99
  in fleck retina of Kandori, 215
  in fundus albipunctatus, 215
  in Oguchi's disease, 214
de Morsier syndrome, 323, 462
Deafness, blindness and, 455
Dellen, 150
Demecarium, 49
Demyelinative disease, primary, 331
Dermatitis, contact, 59
Dermatoconjunctivitis, contact, 125, 497
Dermatomyositis, eye signs in, (Table II) 522
Dermoid cyst
  corneal, 135
  CT scan, 89, 93
Descemetocele, 130
  in marginal guttering, 154
Descemet's membrane, 24, 130
  dystrophy, 143
  rupture, 136
  tears, 133, 134
Deuteranomaly, 213
Deuteranopia, 213
Development in children
  abnormalities, 463
  handicaps and, 454–5
  milestones, 453–4

Development in children *(cont.)*
  visual, 449–53
    defects and, 454
Devic's disease, 331
Dexamethasone, (Table VI) 58
  suppression test, 544
Di George syndrome, 547
Diabetes
  cataract and, 277, 281, 576
  glaucoma and, 577
  ischaemic optic neuropathy in, 336–7
  juvenile, recessive optic atrophy and, 325–6
  maculopathy, 244–7
  mellitus, eye and, 547–8
  optic atrophy and, 481, 548
  retinopathy, 42, 238–43
    ERG in, 99–100
    retinal autoimmunity in, 498
    statistics, 577
  vitreous humour and, 33
    detachment, 272
Diamox for glaucoma, (Table VII) 311, 317
Dichlorphenamide, 54
DIDMOAD syndrome, 481, 548
Digitalis side effects, 60
Dihydroxypropoxymethyl for cytomegalovirus infection, 182, 194
Diplopia, 436
  in chiasmal disease, 346
  developmental palsy and, 418–19
  differentiation of concomitant and incomitant strabismus causing, 437
  examination of, 436–7
  intermittent, 436
  in thyrotoxicosis, 541
Disc shedding in photoreceptor cells, 35–36
  see also Optic disc
Disodium cromoglycate
  for contact lens-induced papillary conjunctivitis, 124
  for vernal disease, 121–2
Disseminated intravascular coagulopathy, eye signs in, (Fig. 1) 226, 559
Distichiasis, 382
Doll's head movements, 428, (Fig. 3c) 430
Dopamine activity in retina, 40
Dorsal midbrain syndrome, 431
Down's syndrome, 467
Doxycycline, 56
Drugs
  absorption, 46
  adverse reaction, 58–60
  antifungal, 56–57
  anti-inflammatory, 57–59
  antimicrobial, 54–56
  antiviral, 56
  autonomic, 47–53
  causing corneal abrasion, 138
  causing hyperprolactinaemia, 536
  causing optic neuropathy, 329
  compliance, 46
  deposition in cornea, 138
  disposal, 46
  follicular changes following, 119
  hypotensive, 53–54
  ocular side effects, 522
  topical, causing inflammation, 127–8

Drugs *(cont.)*
  toxicity, ERG in, 100
  vehicles, 46–47
  see also Immunosuppressive drugs; Steroids
Drusen
  optic disc, 235
  optic nerve head, 323–4
  prevalence, 576
Dry eye syndrome, 122–4, 516–20
Duane's retraction syndrome, 419–20, 438
Dural
  arteriovenous shunt, 530–31
  fistula, orbital hypoxia and, 443
DUSN *see* Neuroretinitis, diffuse unilateral subacute
Dysplasia, developmental, 323–4
Dysproteinaemia, 559–60
Dysthroid eye disease, 421
  exophthalmos, 90–91
  ophthalmoplegia and, 442
Dystrophia myotonia in males, 549
Dystrophy
  corneal, 142–3, (Table VI) 144–5
    biochemical defects and, 27
  endothelial, 134–5
  receptor *see under* Photoreceptor
  tapetoretinal, 471
  vitreoretinal, 471
  vortex, 138
Dwarf eye, 133
Dye tests for lacrimal drainage patency, 395

Eales's disease, 175, 176–7, 190
Early receptor potentials, 23
  in retinitis pigmentosa, 205
Eccentric fixation, 569
Econazole, 57
Ecothiopate iodide, 49
Ectasia, corneal, 134, 143–6
Ectopia lentis, 475
  causes, (Table I) 476
  in homocystinuria, 475
Ectropion, 382–3, 394
  cicatricial, 383
  congenital, 382
  involutional, 382–3
  mechanical, 383
  paralytic, 383
Eczema, atopic, eye symptoms in, 120
Edrophonium, 49
Eisner indentation funnel, 72
Elastosis, senile, 148
Electrode
  effects on ERG, 98–99
  for VEP, 102
Electrodiagnosis, 97–106
Electrolysis for abnormal eyelashes, 382
Electronic aids for visual disability, 567
Electro-oculogram, 22, 101
  in retinitis pigmentosa, 205
Electrophoresis, haemoglobin, (Fig. 1) 554
Electroretinogram, 1–3, 20–23, 97–101
  effect of disease on response, 99–101
  factors influencing response, 98–99
  in infants, 451
  nature of response, 97–98
  recording method, 97

Electroretinogram *(cont.)*
  in retinitis pigmentosa, 205
Embolic amaurosis fugax, 524–5
Embryology, nasolacrimal drainage system, 396
Embryotoxon, posterior, (Table V) 135
Empty sella syndrome, 348
Emulsification, nuclear, 286
Encephalopathy, Leigh's subacute necrotizing, 462
Encephalotrigeminal angiomatosis *see* Sturge–Weber syndrome
Endocrine
  diseases, eye and, 533–51
  pancreas disorders, eye and, 547–9
  studies of optic chiasma, 350
Endophthalmitis
  aspergillus, 195
  following cataract surgery, 290
  following lens implant, 300
  prevention, 370
Endoscopy of lacrimal drainage system, 396
Endothelial
  cell shape, 63
  dystrophy, late hereditary *see* Fuch's dystrophy
  examination by Vogt's method, 61
Endothelium, corneal, 24, 130–1
  oedema, 135–6
Enkephalins, retinal, 41
Enophthalmos following enucleation, 390
Entropion, 379–82
  cicatricial, 380
  congenital, 380
  in erythema multiforme, 127
  eyelid problems following, 390
  following enucleation, 390
  involutional, 380
  trichiasis, 382
  upper lid, 381–2
Enucleation
  for malignant melanoma, 357
  for retinoblastoma, 359–60
  for scleritis, 155, 156
  for sympathetic ophthalmitis, 375
Enzyme deficiency, inherited, 471
Eosinophils, allergic reaction and, (Fig. 5) 487
  levels, raised, 558
Epiblepharon, 380
Epibulbar tumours, 352–4
Epicanthic fold, 380
  squint and, 413
Epidemic
  haemorrhagic conjunctivitis, 116–17
  keratoconjunctivitis, 116
Epidermoid tumour, orbital, 93
Epileptic fits in infants, 459–61
Epiloia *see* Tuberous sclerosis
Epimacular membranes, 268
Epipapillary gliosis, 260
Epiphora, 391
  control, 407
Epiretinal membranes
  fibrocellular, 268
  fibrovascular, 268–9
Episclera, 149
  examination, 150
  vessels, deep, 148
    superficial, 148
Episcleritis, 149–51
  aetiology, 150

Episcleritis *(cont.)*
  corneal changes, 150
  differentiation, 147–8
  diffuse, 150
  nomenclature, 148–9
  treatment, 150–1, 160
Epithelial basement membrane dystrophy, 143
Epithelium *see under* Conjunctiva; Cornea;Pigment
Epstein–Barr virus, conjunctivitis from, 117
Erosion, corneal, 138
Erythema
  multiforme, 127, 496
  nodosum, 496
Erythrocyte sedimentation rate in arteritis, 335–6
Erythromycin, 56
Eserine, 48–49
  for glaucoma, 317
Esotropia
  A- and V-pattern, 415–16
  abduction and, 414
  accommodative, 416–17
  congenital, 414–15
ESP technique, 62
Esterase D gene, 469
Ethambutol
  causing optic neuropathy, 329
  side effects, 60
Ethchlorvynol causing optic neuropathy, 329
Examination of eye, 61–63
Excretory mechanism, 392–3
Exophthalmos
  dysthroid, 90–91
  endocrine, diagnosis of, 540
  in thyrotoxicosis, 541
  unilateral, 91–95
Exotropia, 415
  A- and V-pattern, 415–16
Expressivity, hereditary, 475–6
Expulsive haemorrhage, 284
Extracapsular extraction, 284–6
Extraretinal neovascularization, 268
Exudates, hard
  in anaemia, 552
  in diabetic retinopathy, 238–9
  in papilloedema, 342
Exudative maculopathy, 244–5
Eye medications *see* Drugs, topical
Eyebrow suspension procedure, 385–6
Eyelashes, abnormal, 382
Eyelids
  allergic reaction in, 59
  anatomy, 379
  epicanthic folds, 380, 413
  examination for assessment of tear drainage, 394
  eye protection by, 107
  function requirements, 107
  lag in thyrotoxicosis, 541
  lesions, 389–90
  lowering, 386
  malposition, 379–88
  margin disorders, 109–11
  problems following enucleation, 390
  repair, 390
  retraction, 386–8
    in thyrotoxicosis, 541
  shortening, 107
  tumours, 389–90

Fabry's disease, corneal deposition in, 138
Facial signs in blindness, 451
Faden operation, bilateral, 417
Familial dysautonomia, 122
Fasanella Servat operation, 384
Fatty acids in photoreceptors, 35
Fazadinium, 53
Fibrocellular epiretinal membranes, 268
Fibrovascular epiretinal membranes, 268–9
Filamentary keratitis, 113
Filters for fluorescein angiography, 74
Fistulizing surgery failure, 313
Fixation in infants, 453
  test for, 450
Fleck retina of Kandori, 215
Fleischer's ring, 137
Floaters
  in bird shot retinochoroidopathy, 187
  in uveitis, 165, 166, 176
Florid retinopathy, diabetic, 243
Flubiprofen for episcleritis, 151
Flucloxacillin, 55
Flucytosine, 57
Fluid, ocular, 31–34
  accumulation at macula, diseases associated with, 226–36
  pathophysiology of, 223–5
  requirements in gonioscopy, 65
  transport, corneal, 27
  in lens, 29
  in retina, 36
Fluorescein angiography, 74–80
  abnormal, 77–79
  centroserous, 231
  instruments, 74
  in macular elevation, 225
  normal, 75–77
  in optic nerve pits, 235
  in papilloedema, 342
  in pigment epithelial detachment, 230–1
  principles, 74
  in retinitis pigmentosa, 201
  side effects, 75
  technique, 74–75
Fluorescein test
  for dry eye, 123
  for precorneal film, 113
Fluorescence
  leakage, active, 77–78
  reversed, 77
  transmitted, 77
Fluorometholone, 58
  for uveitis, 168
Folate deficiency, optic neuropathy and, 329
Folic acid deficiency, 553
Folinic acid for toxoplasmosis, 192
Follicular
  conjunctival hypertrophy, 119
  conjunctivitis, 113–24
    acute, 114–18
'Following' test, 450
Forced
  choice preferential looking test, 452
  duction test, 436
Foreign bodies
  in angle, 68
  corneal, 136–7
  differential diagnosis, 150
  eyelid, 390

Foreign bodies (cont.)
  intraocular, 372–4
  lacrimal passages, 400
  in vitreous, 34
Foster Kennedy syndrome, 341
Fourth nerve palsy, 439
  developmental, 420
  traumatic bilateral, 423
Foveal
  cones see Cones
  electroretinogram, 21
Framycetin, 55
Frontal
  eye fields, 427
  gaze palsy, 430
FSH levels, 550
FTA-ABS test, 175
Fuch's
  dystrophy, 131, 143, 298
    corneal biochemical defects and, 27
  heterochromic cyclitis, 171
Fundus
  albipunctatus disease, 10, 215
  biomicroscopy of macular elevation, 225
  changes in histoplasmosis, 182
    in lipoproteinaemia, 208
    in posterior scleritis, 155
    in retinitis pigmentosa, 199–202
  examination, 70–73
  flavimaculatus, 211–12
  fluorescence, 77
  'ketchup' appearance, 460
  lesions in serpiginous choroiditis, 186
  pepper and salt, 174
  reflectometry for investigating visual pigments, 4
Fungal
  infections
    canaliculus, 408
    corneal, 140
    endophthalmitis, 290
    retinal, 194–6
  sensitivity of antibiotics, (Table V) 57

GABA activity in retina, 40
Galactokinase deficiency, cataract and, 480
Galactorrhoea, 534–5
Galactosaemia, 550
  cataract and, 277, 281, 480
Ganglion cells in retina, 13–14, 18–20
Gangliosidoses, infantile, 460–1
Ganzfield illumination, 23
Gas tamponade, intravitreal, 254
Gastrinoma, 549
Gaze
  deviation ultrasonography, 82–85
  evoked nystagmus, 446
  palsy, 430–1
    in pineal tumours, 538–9
Gelatine occlusion in dry eye, 123
Gels, intraocular, 34
Genetic effects
  glaucoma and, 577
  heterogeneity, 472–5
  retinitis pigmentosa and, 199–200
  retinoblastoma and, 357–8, 469
  uveitis and, 163, 169
Geniculate body lesions, 348
Genotypes in sickle cell disease, 556
Gentamicin, 55

Geographic choroiditis see Serpiginous choroiditis
Germ cell tumours, pineal, 538
Germinoma, suprasella, 539
Ghost vessesl, 141
Giardiasis, uveitis and, 183
Gigantism, 535
Girard phacoemulsifier, 286
Glass wool opacities, 264
Glaucoma, 304–20
  atropine-induced, 49–50
  in buphthalmos, 133
  chronic simple, (Table III) 307
    inheritance, 481
  classification, 304–5
  congenital, 314
  drug therapy for, 47, (Table VII) 311
  epidemiology, 305
  IOP and, 32–33
  juvenile, 314
  low tension, 314
  malignant, 312–13
  neuroma and, 477
  phacolytic, 181
  pigmentary, 68
  primary, (Table I) 304, 306–19
    closed angle, 68, (Table I) 304, 314–19
      acute, 315–16
      chronic, 318–19, 314–15
      mixed, 319
      pathogenesis, 314–15
      subacute, 318
      treatment, 319
    combined mechanism (Table I) 304
    congenital, 67
    narrow angle, 319
    open angle, (Table I) 304, 306–19
      pathogenesis, 306–7
      symptoms and signs, 307–8
      treatment, 308–14
  scleritis and, 154–5
  secondary, (Table II) 305, 319–20
    closed angle with pupil block, (Table II) 305
    without pupil block, (Table II) 305
    control, 372
    due to trauma, 68
    hyphaemia and, 363, 364
  in sickle cell disease, 555
  statistics, 577
  steroid-induced, 59, 122, 154–5, 167–8
  therapy for, 33
  uveitis and, 166–7
  VEP in, 104
Glaukumflecken, 317
Glioblastoma, optic, 338
Glioma
  chiasmatic, 462, (Figs 18–19) 463
  optic nerve, 337–8, 347–8
    investigations, 350
  phaeochromocytoma and, 546
  pineal, 538
Globe perforation causing sympathetic ophthalmitis, 179
Glucagon secreting tumour, 549
Glucocorticoids in aqueous humour, 33
Glucose
  in aqueous humour, 32
  metabolism, corneal, 131, 25–26
    lens, 29
    retinal, 37
  in vitreous humour, 33

Glutamate, retinal, 41
Glutathione
  -bicarbonate Ringer's, 26
  lens metabolism and, 29
  utilization in cornea, 26
Glycerol, 54
Glycine, retinal, 41
Glycoproteins in tear film, 113
Glycosaminoglycans, corneal, 25
cGMP
  phototransduction and, 39–40
  release from rods, 8–9
  retinal, 38–39
Goblet cells, conjunctival, 112
Goldmann lens, 64–65, 70, 71
Gonadal disorders, eye and, 549–50
Gonadotropin release, 549–50
Goniolenses, 64–65
Gonioscopy, 64–69
  indentation, 315
Gonococcal infection causing ophthalmia neonatorum, 118
Gout
  episcleritis and, 150
  therapy, 160
G-protein, 8
Gradenigo's syndrome, 438
Granuloma
  orbital, CT scan of, 89
  in sarcoidosis, 178, 179
  scleral, 155, 156–7, 161
  in sympathetic ophthalmitis, 179
  in toxocariasis, 174, 191
Granulomatous uveitis, 164, 165, 166
Graves's disease, 540–2
  ophthalmoplegia in, 442
  optic neuropathy in, 337
Growth
  hormone secreting tumours, 535–6
  retardation, corticosteroid-induced, 509
Guanethidine, 52
  for glaucoma, (Table VII) 311, 312
Guillain-Barré syndrome, 441
Gyrate atrophy, 43, 208–9, 471
  ERG in, 99

Haab's striae, 133, 134
Haemangioma
  choroidal, 236, 355
  eyelid, 389
  orbital, 91
    capillary, 91
    cavernous, (Fig. 5a) 85, 88, 91
Haematological diseases, eye and, 552–61
Haemorrhage
  anterior chamber, during lens implant, 299
  from blunt injury, 362–3
  choroidal, 253
  in diabetic retinopathy, 239
  expulsive, 284
  intraretinal, 552, 555
  during lacrimal surgery, 401, 404
  papilloedema and, 342
  from pituitary tumours, 346
  preretinal, 552, 555, 558
  retinal, 253, 552
  sub-hyaloid, 552
  subretinal, 253, 552
  vitreous, 34, 264–5, 369

Haemorrhagic cystitis, cytotoxic drug-induced, 511
Hair loss, cytotoxic drug-induced, 511
Hallucinations, visual, 350
Haloes, testing for, 318
Halothane, 53
Hamartoma, pigment epithelium, 236–7
Handicapped children, visual defects in, 454
Haptens, 484
Harada's disease, 227
Hashimoto's thyroiditis, 542
Hay fever conjunctivitis, 119–20, 495–6
Head
 injury, causing chiasmatic damage, 348
 postures, abnormal/compensatory, 417–18
  in strabismus, 437
 shake, nystagmus and, 465
 tilt tests, (Fig. 6) 418, 437
Heerfordt's syndrome, lacrimal infiltration in, 178
'Helper' protein, 8
Hemianopia
 homonymous, VEP in, 103–4
  from optic radiation lesions, 349
  from optic tract lesions, 348
Hepatic disease in infants, 462
Hepatitis, non-infective, 141
Hepatolenticular degeneration, 137
Hereditary diseases, 467–82
 progressive arthropathy, 470
 retinoblastoma, 357–8
Heredofamilial optic atrophies, 325–8
Herpes simplex
 canaliculitis, 408
 conjunctivitis, 115
 corneal, 139
 keratitis, 134
  uveitis and, 172
 retinitis, 194
Herpes virus associated with acute retinal necrosis, 188
Herpes zoster ophthalmicus
 conjunctivitis, 117
 corneal, 139, 154
 optic neuritis, 332
 retinitis, 194
 scleritis, 159
 uveitis, 171–2
Hess screen, 424
Hessburg lens, (Fig. 1) 294
Heterochromia, 171
 cyclitis, 68
Heterogeneity, 472–5
Hexokinase
 lens metabolism and, 29
 utilization in retina, 37
High-water mark, 249
Histiocytosis X in infants, 463
Histology
 corneal, 129
 in scleritis, 156–8
Histoplasmosis
 chorioretinitis, presumed, 233
 ocular, 182
History taking in paediatric ophthalmology, 449
HLA A29, 187
 B5, 177, 499
 B27, 169–70, 521
 D, 518

HLA (cont.)
 DR, 498
 DR5, 170
 DW2, 498
HMP shunt in lens, 29
Hogan's syndrome, 120
Homatropine hydrobromide, 50
Homocystine in lens, 278
Homocystinuria, 475, 551
Horizontal
 cells in retina, 13–16
 eye movements, 426
Hormones
 adrenal, 543–4
 pancreatic, 547
 pituitary, 533
 thyroid gland, 539–40
HTLV-III virus, 181
Hudson-Stähli line, 137
Humeral protection of eye, 107–8
Hyaloid membrane, detached posterior, 267–8
Hyaloideo-retinal degeneration, Wagner's, 470
Hyaluronic acid, 25
 in vitreous humour, 33, 34
Hydrocephalus, nystagmus and, 465
Hydrocortisone acetate, (Table VI) 58
Hydrogel lenses properties, 132
Hydrops cornea, 136
Hydroxyquinolines causing optic neuropathy, 329
5-Hydroxytryptamine see Serotonin
Hyoscine hydrobromide, 50
Hyperaemia
 conjunctival, 108
 in uveitis, 164
Hyperaldosteronism, 544
Hypercalcaemia
 corneal effects in, 142
 in hyperparathyroidism, 546–7
Hypereosinophilic syndrome, 558
Hyperergy, 487
Hyperfluorescence, 77–79
Hyperlipidaemia, eye and, 550
Hypermetropia
 correction choices for, 292
 exotropia and, 415
 in infants, 452, 463
Hyperornithinaemia, 471
 gyrate atrophy and, 209
Hyperparathyroidism, 546–7
Hyperprolactinaemia, 536
Hypersensitivity see Allergy
Hypertension, ocular, 309–10
 risk factors, (Table VI) 311
 see also Intraocular pressure, raised
Hyperthyroidism see Thyrotoxicosis
Hyphaema
 from blunt injury, 362–4
 following cataract surgery, 288
 iris, 354
 in sickle cell disease, 555
Hypocalcaemia
 cataract and, 31
 hypoparathyroidism and, 547
Hypofluorescence, 79
Hypoglycaemia
 epilepsy and, 461
 vision and, 548
Hypoglycaemic agents for glaucoma, 317
Hypogonadism, eye and, 549–50

Hypolipoproteinaemias, 550
Hypoparathyroidism, 547
Hypopyon
 in Behçet's disease, 189
 in uveitis, 165, 177
Hypotensive agents, ocular, 53–54
Hypothalamic disorders
 in infants, 463
 eye and, 533–9
Hypothyroidism, 542–3
 diagnosis, 540
Hypotony
 acute ocular, 229
 chronic ocular, 229
Hypoxia causes, 131, 135

Idoxuridine, 56
IgA, 484–5
 antibody in dermatitis herpetiformis, 127
 disease, linear, 127
 in tears, 107–8
IgD, 485
IgE, 485
 -mediated allergy, 487–8
 in tears, 107
IgG, 484
 in tears, 107
IgM, 485
 in tears, 107
Illumination for visual disability, 567
Imidazole antifungals, 57
Immune
 complex diseases
  allergy, 488–9
  Behçet's, 177–8
  conjunctivitis, 496–7
  diagnosis, (Table V) 502
  scleritis, 157–8
  uveitis, 163
 mechanisms
  basic, 483–6
  pathological, 487–90
 response
  regulation, 486
  in scleritis, 157, 159–60
  in sympathetic ophthalmitis, 374–5
  in toxoplasmosis, 173
 rings
  in cornea, 137
  in scleritis, 154
Immunodeficiency states
 AIDS in, 181
 conjunctivitis in, 497
 cytomegalovirus retinitis in, 193
 diagnosis, (Table V) 503
Immunogen, 484
Immunogenic inflammation, 492–4
Immunoglobulins, 484–5
 in aqueous humour, 32, 490
 in lymphocytes, 484
 proliferation, 559–60
 production, 486
 properties, (Table I) 485
 in tear film, 31–32, 107–8
 in thyrotoxicosis, 541–2
Immunological
 disorders of eye, 490–500
  laboratory tests for, 500–3
 tolerance, 490
Immunology, 483–515
 dysthyroid ophthalmoplegia, 442

Immunopathological mechanisms in eye, 505–7
  external, disease and, 494–7
  lens, 500
  retina and optic nerve, 497–8
  uveitis, 499–500
Immunosuppression, 505–15
  in leukaemia, 558
  in scleritis, 160
Immunosuppressive agents
  choice of, 507–12
  experiments with, 512–13
  immunopathological mechanisms susceptible to, (Fig. 7) 505
  laboratory monitoring of, 513
  main actions, (Table I) 508
  for systemic ophthalmitis, 375
Implants
  for cataract, 295–303
  -induced papillary conjunctivitis, 124
  for lacrimal bypass surgery, 406–8
  silastic sponge, 251
Incision
  for cataract, 282, 284–7
  for dacryocystorhinostomy, 401–3
Indomethacin, 57, 507–9
Infantile recessive atrophy, 325
  see also Paediatric
Infections
  adenovirus, 115
  cytotoxic drugs and, 511
  eyelid, 389
  following lacrimal surgery, 404
  following lens implant, 300
  orbital acute, 95
    chronic, 95
  picornavirus, 116–17
  silastic sponge, 251
  Sjögren's syndrome and, 520
  see also Endophthalmitis;Ophthalmitis
Infertility, cytotoxic drug-induced, 511
Inflammation
  in acute closed glaucoma, 316, 317–18
  in allergy, 487, 489
  chronic cicatrization and, 127–8
  in conjunctivitis, 494–5
  diagnosis, (Table V) 501–2
  in episcleritis, 150
  eyelid, 389
  mechanisms of, 108, 491–4
  optic nerve, 332–3
  orbital, 95
  persistent, 506
  in scleritis, 157, 159
  in sympathetic ophthalmitis, 374, 375
  in toxocariasis infestation, 174
  in uveitis, 163, 164–5
Inflammatory
  cell infiltration to cornea, 138–41
  diseases, retinal, causing fluid accumulation, 233
  invasions into vitreous, 265
  reaction, conjunctival, 108
    causing ocular palsy, 419
    control following penetrating injury, 371
    immunology of, 505–7
Infranuclear disorders, 436–7
Inheritance
  Mendelian, 469–81
  multifactorial, 481–2
Injury *see* Perforating injury;Trauma

Ink blot
  haemorrhage in diabetic retinopathy, 239
  pattern on fluorescein angiography, 231
Inositol
  in aqueous humour, 32
  triphosphate release in rods, 9
Insulin
  in aqueous humour, 32
  secretion deficiency, 547
Insulinomas, 548–9
Interferon in tear film, 32
Interleukins, 486
Internuclear
  disorders, 433–5
  neurones, abducens, 426
  ophthalmoplegia, 433–4
Interplexiform cell of retina, 20
Intracapsular extraction, 283–4
Intracranial
  aneurysms, 347
  tumours, epilepsy and, 461
Intraocular
  damage following penetrating injury, 369, 370
  diagnosis by ultrasonography, 83–85
  foreign bodies, 372–4
  gels, 34
  lens implantation, 292–303
  opacities, clearance of, 371
  pressure, collapse in hypotony, 229
    fall, following acetazolamide, 54
    in general anaesthesia, 53
    following pilocarpine, 48
    glaucoma and, 32–33
    low, restoration of, 254
    raised, in angle closure, 316
      following cataract surgery, 289
      in hyphaema, 288, 363
      from laser iridotomy, 318
      lowering, 309–14, 317–19
      pathogenesis of, 306
      from steroids, 151
      symptoms of, 307
      visual field loss and, 310–14
  tumours, ultrasonography of, 85
Intraorbital space-occupying lesions, 91–95
Intraretinal
  cyst formation, 249
  fluid accumulation, 224–5
  haemorrhage, 552, 555
  neovascularization, 239
Intubation
  of canaliculus, 405
  of nasolacrimal duct, 398
Iodine, radioactive, for thyrotoxicosis, 542
Ions transport
  in aqueous humours, 27, 32
  corneal, 27
  in lens, 29
  in pigment epithelium, 36
  in vitreous humour, 33
Iridectomy
  accidental, 287
  in closed angle glaucoma, 316
  peripheral, 283
  prophylactic, 317
  in uveitis, 166
Iridocyclitis
  chronic, 499

Iridocyclitis *(cont.)*
  uveitis and, 163, 170
Iridodonesis, 475
Iridogoniodysgenesis, (Table V) 135
Iridotomy laser, 318
Iridotrabecular
  adhesions, 67
  neovascularization, 67–68
Iris
  angiography, 79
  atrophy in uveitis, 166
  bombé, 66, 315
    in uveitis, 166
  changes in Fuch's heterochromic cyclitis, 171
  in herpes zoster uveitis, 172
  coloboma, 162
  disorder following lens implant, 300
  freezing, 284
  naevus, 354
  nodules, 164, 166, 178
    in trisomy 21, 467
  plateau, 67, 318–19
  processes, 66
  prolapse following cataract surgery, 288
  rubeosis, 67–68
  -supported lenses, 294, 296
  surgery following penetrating injury, 370
  thickening, 316
  tumours, 68, 354
Iritis
  in Behçet's disease, 189
  uveitis and, 163
Iron
  -deficiency anaemia, 553
  deposition in cornea, 136–7
  foreign body, 372–3
Irradiation cataract, 277
  see also Radiotherapy
Irrigating solutions, corneal, 26–27
Irvine-Gass syndrome, 289–90
Ischaemia choroidal, 226–9
Ischaemic
  maculopathy, 247
  optic neuropathy, clinical characteristics of, (Table IV) 330, 334–7
    disc cupping in, (Table IV) 308, (Fig. 8) 310

Jamaican optic neuropathy, 329
Jensen's juxta-papillary choroiditis, 172–3
Juvenile
  complete cataract, 278
  glaucoma, 314

K cells, 484
  -dependent allergy, 488
Kallman's syndrome, 550
Kandori, fleck retina of, 215
Kelman
  multiflex lens, (Fig. 1) 294
  phacoemulsifier, 286
Keratan sulphate, 25
Keratic precipitates, 164, 165, 171, 178
Keratinization of tear film, 32

Keratitis
  adenoviral, 138–9
  amoebic, 140
  bacterial, 140
  filamentary, 113–14
  fungal, 140
  herpes simplex, 139, 172
    zoster, 139
  interstitial, 140–1
  nummular, 154
  paramyxoviral, 139
  phlyctenular, 110
  sclerosing, 154
  superficial punctate, 116
    Thygeson's, 141
  vernal, 122
Keratoacanthoma, 389
Keratoconjunctivitis
  epidemic, 116
  from mechanical injury, 138
  sicca, 113, 122–4, 516
    aetiology, 516–18
    definition, 516
    diagnosis, 516–18
    incidence, 516
    management, 519–20
    pathology, 518–19
  vernal, 120–2, 496
Keratoconus, 143–5
  biochemical defects and, 27
  posterior, 134
  in trisomy 21, 467
Keratocytes, corneal, 130
Keratoglobus, 133
Keratomalacia, corneal, 142
  biochemical defects and, 27
Keratopathy
  band, 142
  climatic droplet, 142
  interpalpebral band-shaped, 521
  striate, following cataract surgery, 288
Keratoplasty, penetrating, for chemical burns, 376
Keratosis, eyelid, 389
Ketamine, 53
'Ketchup'-like fundus, 460
Ketoconazole, 57
Kinase enzyme, phosphorylation of rhodopsin by, 6
Klebsiella pneumonia, uveitis and, 170
Koeppe
  lens, 64
  nodules, 164, 166, 178
Koerber-Salus-Elschnig syndrome, 431
Krill's disease, pigment epithelium involvement in, 183
Krypton lasers, 238
Kuhnt-Zymanowski procedure, (Fig. 6c) 382
Kveim test, 179

Lachesine chloride, 50
Lacquer cracks, 234
Lacrimal
  drainage system, 392–3, 396–409
    congenital abnormalities, 396–8
    determination of anatomical state of, 395
    disease, acquired, 399–400
    fistula, 399
    insufficiency, 396

Lacrimal *(cont.)*
    obstruction, 395–6, 401–4
    surgery
      anaesthesia for, 400–1
      indications for, 400
      reparative, 409
    tests for patency, 394–5
    trauma, 408–9
  gland, 391
    age changes, 518–19
    biopsy, 518
    cyst ultrasonograph, (Fig. 5e) 85
    disorders, 122
    innervation, 391–2
    involvement in sarcoidosis, 178
    tear production by, 112
    tumours, 94–95
  pump, 393–4
  sac, 393
    lacerations, 409
    swelling, 398
  see also Tears
Lacrimation *see* Tears
Lactate
  in aqueous humour, 32
  utilization in retina, 37
Lactic acid accumulation in cornea, 131
Lactoferrin enzyme activity, 518
Lamellae, 47
  cataract, 278
Lancaster red-green test, 436
Laser
  iridotomy, 318, 320
  photocoagulation *see* Photocoagulation
  therapy for capsular thickening, 302
  types, 238
Lattice
  degeneration of retina, 256
  theory of Maurice, 131
Laurence-Moon-Biedl syndrome, 209, 462, 550
Leber's
  amaurosis, 200, 203, 327–8
    differential diagnosis, 481
    in infants, 456–7, 462
  optic atrophy, 481
Lees screen, 424
Leigh's subacute necrotizing encephalopathy, 462
Leiske lens, (Fig. 1) 294
Lens
  anatomy, 275–6
  antigens, 491
  avascularity, 490
  capsule, 28
    pseudo-exfoliation of, 68
    rupture, 284
  changes in uveitis, 166
  condensing, 71
  delivery, 283
  developmental defects, 276–81
  displacement
    from blunt trauma, 364, (Fig. 2) 365
    causes, (Table I) 476
    following lens implant, 300–1
    in homocystinuria, 475
    in Marfan's syndrome, 475
    posterior, 287
    ultrasonograph, (Fig. 2c) 82, 83
  embryology, 275
  excision, 287
  extraction in uveitis, 166
  immunopathology, 500

Lens, implants *(cont.)*
    anterior chamber, 293–4
    biometry, 295
    for blunt trauma, 364
    complications, 298–302
    history and development, 293–5
    indications, 298
    insertion, 295–6
    intraocular lens material and sterilization, 302
    iris-supported, 294
      insertion, 296
    posterior chamber, 294–5
      insertion, 206–7
    secondary, 297–8
    surgical considerations, 295–7
    triple procedure, 298
  -induced uveitis, 181
  metabolism, 29
  opacities
    from blunt trauma, 364
    from steroids, 58–59
    subcapsular lamellar cortical, 317
    in trisomy, 21, 467
  pathology, 275–81
  perforation causing uveitis, 180
  physiology, 27–81
  pre-set, 71
  residual material following cataract surgery, 289
  rupture, ultrasonograph, (Fig. 2d) 82, 83
  shape, 276
  structure and composition, 28
  transparency, 29
  ultrasonography, 83
  see also Cataract; Contact lenses
Lensectomy, 286–7
  following intraocular damage, 370
  in uveitis, 166
Leucocoria, 174
Leucocytes in aqueous humour, 165
Leukaemia, 557–8
  optic effects in, 339
Leukotrienes, 487, 493
Leukovorin for toxoplasmosis, 192
Levamisole for uveitis, 168
Levator muscle
  function assessment, 384
  resection, 385
LH release, 550
Lids *see* Eyelids
Light
  absorption by rhodopsin, 3–5
  adaptation, 9–10
  effects on photoreceptor cell renewal, 35
  incident, percentage reflected equation, (Footnote) 61
  refraction by lens, 275–6
  retinal response to, 1–23
  sensitivity in optic nerve disorders, 322
  stimulus effect on ERG, 98
    for VEP, 102
Ligneous conjunctivitis, 114
Lignocaine hydrochloride, 53
Limbal
  anatomy, 282
  paracentesis for hyphaema, 363
  vessels, 133
Limbitis, scleritis and, 154
Lipidosis
  infantile, 460

Lipidosis *(cont.)*
  ophthalmoplegic, 431–2
Lipids, 484
  abnormalities, 113
  deposition, corneal, 137
  diseases, corneal, 134
  peroxidation, cataract formation and, 30
  in photoreceptors, 35
  in tear film, 31, 107
Lipofuscin granule formation, 37
Lipoproteinaemia, A-beta, 208
Lissamine green stains for dry eye, 123
Long-acting thyroid stimulator (LATS), 541–2
Lowe's oculocerebrorenal syndrome, 480
  in infants, 463
Lung involvement in sarcoidosis, 178
Lycopodium disc, 318
Lyell's syndrome, 127
Lymphatic vessel absence in ocular tissue, 490
Lymphoblastoma in leukaemia, 558
Lymphocytes
  accumulation in conjunctiva, 491, 494
  activation, 486
    B, 484
    K, 484
    natural killer, 484
    null, 484
    T, 483–4
  effects of immunosuppressants on, 506
  hypersensitivity, 489–90
  infiltration in sympathetic ophthalmitis, 374, 375
  proliferation, 559–60
  transformation tests, 513
Lymphoid
  cells, conjunctival, 127
  system, 483–4
Lymphoma
  eyelid, 390
  orbital, 94
  subconjunctival, 352–3
  ultrasonograph, (Fig. 5b) 85, 86
Lyon hypothesis, 477–8
Lysosomes, pigment epithelium, 37
Lysozyme
  activity in keratoconjunctivitis sicca, 518
  in tear film, 32

McCannel suture, 300, (Fig. 5) 301
Macro square wave job, 432
Macroaneurysm, 235
Macrodacryocystography, 396
Macroglobulinaemia, Waldenström's, 559
Maculae occludentes, 131
Macular
  degeneration, disciform, (Figs 3–4) 228
    EOG in, 101
    senile, 575–6
  deposit in Best's disease, 209–10
  detachment, with abnormal retinal deposits, 236
    coloboma and, 234
    in congenital vascular abnormality, 235, (Fig. 11) 236
    from fluid accumulation, 224
    from optic nerve pits, 235
    from perforating injury, 237

Macular, detachment *(cont.)*
    rhegmatogenous, 236
    serous, 227
    traction and, 237
    from tumours, 237
  disease, associated with retinal elevation, 223–7
  examination, 225
  exudates, hard, 244–5
  fluid accumulation, diseases associated with, 226–36
    pathophysiology, 223–5
  functional anatomy, 223
  holes, 236
  ischaemia, 237
  oedema, 246
    cystoid, 289–90
    in posterior scleritis, 155
    in uveitis, 167
    intermediate, 176
  photostress test, 322
  scar from toxoplasmosis, (Fig. 10) 459
  sparing, 349
  star, 552
  tears from blunt injury, 366–7
  terminology, 223
Maculopathies, 235
  definition, 240
  diabetic, 244–7
Magnifiers
  hand or stand, 563
  spectacle, 563–5
Main Intrinsic Protein, 28
Maltese Cross lens, (Fig. 2) 294
Mannitol, 53, 54
Marcus Gunn
  pupil, 333
  test, 322
Marfan's syndrome, 474–5
  expressivity, 476
  in infants, 462
Masking, fluorescent, 79
Measles
  corneal effects of, 139
  retinal effects of, 193
Medial longitudinal fasciculus disorders, 433–4
Megalocornea, 133
Megalopapilla, disc cupping in, (Table IV) 308
Meibomian
  cyst, 389
  glands, 379
    disorders, 110
    response to staphylococcal hypersensitivity, 111
Meibomianitis, 389
Melanin
  deposition in cornea, 137
  migration in retinitis pigmentosa, 206
Melanocyte
  changes in heterochromia, 171
  distribution, 162
Melanocytoma, choroidal, 355–7
Melanoma
  choroidal, 237
  malignant, choroidal, 355–7
    ciliary body, 35
    conjunctival diffuse, 353–4
    diagnosis, (Table V) 503
    eyelid, 389
    iris, 354
    ultrasonograph, (Fig. 4a-c) 84, 85

Melanosis
  benign scleral, 148
  precancerous, 353–4
Melanosomes, 36
  giant, in X-linked ocular albinism, 474
Melatonin, disc shedding and, 36
Membrane formation
  cyclitic, 266
  'ochre', 265
  retinal detachment and, 249–50, 255
  see also Epiretinal, Hyaloid membranes
Membranous conjunctivitis, 125
Mendelian inheritance, 469–81
Meningioma
  chiasmatic, 346
  optic nerve, 339–40
    ultrasonograph, (Figs 5f, g) 85
  orbital, CT scan, (Fig. 1) 87
  primary intraorbital, 92
  secondary, 93
Meningitis, optic neuritis and, 332
Mercury deposition in cornea, 137
Mesenchymal dysgenesis of anterior segment classification, (Table V) 135
Metabolic disorders in infants, 462
Metabolism, inborn errors of, 550–1
Metallic foreign bodies, 372
  removal, 373–4
Metapyrone test, 544
Metarhodopsin, 5–6, 38–39
Metastases
  choroidal tumour from, 357
  optic nerve, 339
  orbital, 94
Methacholine, 48
Methicillin, 54
Methyl cellulose inserts, 124
Methylprednisolone, (Table VI) 58, 509, 510
  for scleritis, 160
Miconazole, 57
Microaneurysms in diabetic retinopathy, 238
Microangiopathy, pre-morbid peripapillary telangiectatic, 328
Microbial
  allergic conjunctivitis, 494–5
  foreign bodies, 373
Microcornea, 133
Microphthalmos, 133
Microscopy, specular, 61–63
Microspectrophotometry, for investigating visual pigments, 4
Microsurgery for penetrating wounds, 369–70
Microvillae, corneal, 112
Mikulicz's syndrome, lacrimal infiltration in, 178
Milestones of development in children, 453–4
Millard-Grubler syndrome, 438
Miller-Fisher syndrome, 441
Minocycline, 56
Miosis
  following physostigmine, 48
  following pilocarpine, 48
Miotics for glaucoma, 33
Mizuo phenomenon, inverse, 202
Mizuo-Nakamura phenomenon, 214
Moebius syndrome, 438
Molluscum contagiosum, 117

Mongolism *see* Trisomy 21
Monoamines, retinal, 40
Monochromatism, 213–14
Monoclonal
　antibody tests, 513
　gammopathy, 559
Mooren's ulcer, 142, 496
Morgagnian cataract, 280
Morning glory syndrome, 234
Mosaicism, 477–8
Motility of eyes in infants, 452
　disorders, 464–5
Motor neurones, abducens, 426
Mouse dysplasia, 43
Mucin
　deficiency, 136
　in tear film, 31
Mucocele
　dacryocystitis and, 399
　sinus, optic neuritis and, 332
Mucocutaneous candidiasis, 497
Mucolipidosis, 134
　in infants, 462
Mucopolysaccharidoses, 134
　in infants, 462
Mucosal flaps in dacryocystorhinostomy, 403
Mucous
　membrane pemphigoid, 126–7
　plaques, superficial, 114
Mucus
　dispersal, 420
　production deficiency, 113–14
　in tear film, 107, 112–13
Mueller cells, 20
　effects of retinitis pigmentosa on, 207
Mulberry tumours, 460
Multifactorial inheritance, 481–2
Multiple
　evanescent white dot syndrome, 188
　myeloma, 559–60
　sclerosis, optic neuritis and, 331–2, 498
　uveitis and, 182
Mumps, corneal effects of, 139
Muscles in eyelids, 379
'Mutton fat' keratic precipitates, 164, 165
Myasthenic ptosis, 383
Mydriasis
　following adrenaline, 40
　following atropine, 49
　in pupil block, 319–20
Mydriatics for uveitis, 167
Myelin-basic protein, 497
Myeloma, multiple, 559–60
Myoclonus, ocular, 465
Myogenic ptosis, 383
Myokymia, superior oblique, 446
Myopia
　disc cupping in, (Fig. 11) 310
　ERG in, 99
　field defects in, (Table V) 308
　in gyrate atrophy, 209
　in infants, 463
　　handicapped, 454
　retinal elevations of, 234, 248
Myositis in thyrotoxicosis, 541
Myxoedema, 542–3

Naevi
　choroidal, 236, 355
　eyelid, 389
　iris, 354

Naevi *(cont.)*
　malignant change in, 353
Naevoxanthoendothelioma, 354
Nalidixic acid side effects, 60
Nanophthalmos, 133
Nasal examination for lacrimal drainage, 396
Nasolacrimal duct, 393
　obstruction, 398
　　congenital, 397
Natamycin, 57
Natural killer cells, 484
Nelson's syndrome, 538
Nematode, intraocular, associated with DUSN, 189
Neomycin, 55
Neonatal inclusion conjunctivitis, 118–19
Neoplasia *see* Tumour
Neostigmine, 49
Neovascularization
　angle, 67–68
　choroidal, 227–9, 557
　corneal, 141
　extraretinal, 268
　intraretinal, 239
　optic, 498
　　disc, 241–3
　preretinal, 241
　subretinal, 367
Nephroblastoma, aniridia and, 162
Nervous system, lacrimal system and, 391
Neurilemma, orbital, CT scan of, 88
Neuritides, optic, 329–34
Neuritis, chronic optic, 333–4
Neuroblastoma in infants, 462–3
Neurofibroma, eyelid, 390
Neurofibromatosis, 476–7
　glioma and, 338
　in infants, 460
　orbital, 93
　phaeochromocytoma and, 545–6
Neurogenic
　mechanism of ocular inflammation, 492
　ptosis, 383
Neurolipidoses, infantile, 460, 462
Neurological disease, uveitis and, 182
Neuroma in neurofibromatosis, 477
Neuromyelitis optica, 331
Neuronal ceroid-lipofuscinosis, 473
Neurones
　immunology of, 497
　inner retina, 36
　see also Motor neurone
Neuropathy
　hypertrophic interstitial peripheral, 208
　optic, nutritional and toxic, 328–9
　　diabetic, 548
Neuropeptides
　activity in retina, 41–42
　role in ocular inflammation, (Fig. 10) 492
Neuroretinitis, diffuse unilateral subacute(DUSN), 189
Neuroretinopathy, acute macular, 189
Neurotensin, retinal, 41
Neurotransmitters, retinal, 40–42
Neutral density filter test, 322
Niemann Pick type C disease, 460
Night blindness, stationary, 214
Nocardia chorioretinitis, 195–6
Non-accidental injury, 461

Nuclear magnetic resonance, orbital, 87
Nucleus
　cataract, 278
　delivery, 285
　emulsification, 286
Null cells, 484
Nutrient
　transport in retina, 36
　uptake by cornea, 25
Nyctalopia, 187
Nystagmus
　abduction, 434
　cerebello-pontine angle disease and, 445
　charting features of, (Fig. 20) 464
　classification, 443
　congenital, 444
　　esotropia and, 414
　　idiopathic, 464
　convergence retraction, 444–5, 465
　dissociated, 444
　in dormant optic atrophy, 326, 327
　downbeat, 445, 465
　gaze-evoked, 446
　in glioma, 338
　head shake and, 465
　induction in child with squint, 414
　non-localizing, 446
　optokinetic, 428, (Fig. 7) 434
　　in infants, 451–2
　　in occipital lesions, 349
　　in optic radiation lesions, 348
　periodic alternating, 445, 465
　physiological, 443–4
　rebound, 446
　secondary, 464–5
　see-saw, 444
　upbeat, 445, 465
　vertical, 465
　vestibular, 445
　voluntary, 444
Nystatin, 56

Objective lenses, accessory, 61
Oc. Tanderil for episcleritis, 151
Occipital lobe lesions, 349
Occlusion therapy, 413, 414
Ochre membrane formation, 265
Ochronosis, 551
Ocular
　albinism, 473, 474, 478
　bobbing, 446
　flutter, 432, 465
　inserts, 46–47
　motor function disorders in optic radiation lesions, 348
　nerve palsies, 437–41
　pathways, 426–8
　system, 425–48
　　anatomical and physiological substrates, 425–8
　　disorders, 430–42
　　examination, 428–30
　muscle palsy, 418–24
　　acquired, 423–4
　myasthenia, 441
　myoclonus, 465
Oculocerebrorenal syndrome, 480
Oculocutaneous
　albinism, 473–4
　disorders, 125–6
Oculogenital chlamydial disease, 118

Oculomotor apraxia, 465
Oculopalatal myoclonus, 445
Ocusert-pilo, 47
Oedema
  conjunctival, 108
  corneal, 131, 135–6
  macular, 246
  retinal, in diabetic retinopathy, 238
    in retinitis pigmentosa, 202
Oguchi's disease, 214–15
Ointments, 46
One and a half syndrome, 434–5
Opacities
  axial, removal of, 273
  obscuring view of detached retina, 255
Ophthalmia
  neonatorum, 118–19
    bacterial, 134
  sympathetic, 233
Ophthalmic artery aneurysm, 91
Ophthalmitis sympathetic, 179–81, 374, 499–500
Ophthalmopathy in thyrotoxicosis, 541–2
Ophthalmoplegia
  chronic progressive external, 441–2
  dysthyroid disease and, 442
  in giant aneurysm, 528
  internuclear, 433–4
  in thyrotoxicosis, 541
Ophthalmoplegic lipidosis, 431–2, 460
Ophthalmoscopy
  direct, 70–71
  indirect, 70, 72
  of macular elevation, 225
Opsin structure, 4
Opsoclonus, 433, 465
Optic
  atrophy, 480–1
    heredofamilial
      dominant, 326–7
      indeterminate, 327–8
      recessive, 325–6
    in infants, (Table III) 457, 458
    Leber's, 481
  cup in papilloedema, 342
  disc
    checking appearance following surgery for glaucoma, 314
    congenital abnormalities, 234
    crescent, 323
    cupping, 306–7
      differential diagnosis of, 307–8
      in glaucoma, (Figs 5–7) 309
    degenerative changes, 235
    elevation, 323–4
    fluorescence, 77
    hypoplasia, 323
    in infants, 456–8
    neovascularization, 241–3
    oedema, 332, 340–3
      differential diagnosis of, 343
      in closed angle glaucoma, 317
      in uveitis, 179
      with tumour, 338–9
    pit, congenital, disc cupping in, (Table IV) 308, (Fig. 9) 310
    pseudopapilloedema, 323–4
  nerve
    diseases, 321–45
      symptoms and signs, 321–3
    glioma, 347–8
    immunopathology, 497–8
    incision, 342–3

Optic, nerve (cont.)
  injury, contusional, 367–8
  leukaemic infiltration, 558
  meningioma, ultrasonograph, (Fig. 5f, g) 85, 86)
  pits, 234–5
  tumours, 337–40
    CT scans, 88
  vascular disorders, 334–7
  neuritis, 329–34, 498
    chronic, 333–4
  neuropathy
    diabetes and, 548
    nutritional and toxic, 328–9
  papilloedema, clinical characteristics, (Table IV) 330
  radiation lesions, 348–9
  tract lesions, 348
Optokinetic
  drum, 443–4
  nystagmus, 428, (Fig. 7) 434
    in infants, 451–2
Orbicularis muscle, 379
  anatomy, (Fig. 3) 393
Orbital
  calcification, 87
  changes in leukaemia, 558
  diagnosis by ultrasonography, 86
  erosion, 87
  floor fractures, squint and, 421–2
  phlebography, 90
  pseudotumours, optic neuritis and, 332
  radiography, 87–96
  size changes, 87
  tumours
    in neurofibromatosis, 477
    radiography of, 87, 92–95
  varices, 92
Organophosphorus compounds, 49
Ornithine
  aminotransferase, deficiency, 43
  raised, 471
Orthoptics, 424
Oscillations
  abnormal ocular, 428–33
  resembling nystagmus, 446
  see also Nystagmus
Oscillatory potential, 98
Oscillopsia, 434
Osmotic agents, 54
Osteoporosis
  in infants, 462
  corticosteroid-induced, 509
Osteotomy in dacryocystorhinostomy, 403
Ovarian failure, 549–50
Ox-eye, 133
Oxidation, retinal, 42
Oxybuprocaine hydrochloride, 52
Oxygen
  in aqueous humour, 32
  corneal, 25, 131–2
Oxyphenbutazone, 57
Oxytetracycline, 56

Pachometer, 129, 136
Paediatric ophthalmology, 449–66
Paget's disease of bone, 551
Pain
  in optic nerve disorders, 321
  in scleritis, 147, 151, 155
  in uveitis, 164

Palsy
  abducens, 437–41
  abnormal head position in, 418
  gaze, frontal, 430
    in pineal tumours, 538–9
    pontine, 430–1
  monocular elevator, (Fig. 14) 443
  nerve
    in giant aneurysms, 527–8
    ocular motor
      adult, mechanical restriction of ocular rotations in, 421–4
      investigations of, 441
      management of, 441
      multiple, 441
      seventh, 388
    ocular muscle, 418–23
      acquired, 423–4
      developments, 419–21
    progressive supranuclear, 431, (Fig. 6) 433
Pancreatic disorders, endocrine, eye and, 547–9
Pancuronium, 53
Panencephalitis, subacute sclerosing, in measles, 193
Panfunduscope, 70, 71, 72
Panretinal photocoagulation, 243
Panuveitis, 164, 179
  in VKH syndrome, 183
Papillae, conjunctival, 119–20
Papillary
  conjunctivitis, 119–24
    contact lens-induced, 124–5
  retinal vasculitis, 333
  vascular anomalies, 235
Papillitis, optic, 330, 332–3
Papilloedema, optic, 340–3
  clinical characteristics, (Table IV) 330
Papilloma, eyelid, 389
Papillopathy, ischaemic, 335
Parafovea, effects of retinitis pigmentosa on, 206
Paralytic ectropion, 383
Paramedian pontine reticular formation, 426
Paramyxovirus infiltration to cornea, 139
Parasitic infestations of retina, 190–2
  see also Toxocariasis
Parasympatholytic drugs, 49–50
Parathyroid gland disorders, eye and, 546–7
Parinaud's syndrome, 431, 539
Pars plana electromagnet extraction, 373
Pars planitis see Uveitis, intermediate
Patau's syndrome see Trisomy 13
Paton's lines, 342
Pattern
  bombing, 243
  ERG, 23
Pause cell, 426
Pectinate tissue, 66
Pellucid margin degeneration, 146
Pemphigoid, benign mucous membrane, 496
Pemphigus vulgaris, 496
Penetrance, hereditary, 475–6
Penetrating injuries, 368–72
Penicillins, 54–55
Perceptual abilities in infant, 453
Perforating injury, macular disease and, 237
Periphlebitis, retinal, 182

Periretinal
　fibrosis, 255
　proliferation, massive, 271
Peter's anomaly, (Table V) 135
Phacoemulsification, 286
Phacolytic glaucoma, 181
Phacomatosis, 360
Phacouveitis see Uveitis, lens-induced
Phaeochromocytoma, 545–6
Phagocytosis by PE cells, 36
Phakoma
　in Sturge-Weber syndrome, 460
　in tuberous sclerosis, (Figs 11–12) 459
Phakomatoses, 476–7
Pharyngoconjunctival fever, 115–16, 139
Phenocopy, 478–81
Phenothiazine
　pigmentation, 59
　retinal effects of, 59
Phentolamine in phaeochromocytoma, 546
Phenylbutazone, 57
Phenylephrine, 51
Phlebography, orbital, 90
Phleboliths, orbital, 88
Phlyctenular conjunctivitis, 110–12
Phlyctenulosis, 495
Phosphodiesterase
　activation in rods, 8
　activity in retina, 38–39, 40
Phosphofructokinase utilization in retina, 37
Phospholine, 49
　for esotropia, 417
Photo refraction, 452
Photocoagulation
　for centroserous chorioretinopathy, 232
　for choroidal neovascularization, 229
　for diabetic maculopathy, 244–7
　for macular vascular abnormalities, 235
　for pigment epithelium detachment, 231
　for proliferative sickle retinopathy, 557
　for retinal detachment prophylaxis, 256
　for retinal neovascularization, 241–3
Photo-oxidation, cataract formation from, 30
Photoreceptor, 1–23
　adaptation, 9–10
　antigens, 498
　autoantibody, 498
　coupling between, 11–12
　dystrophies, 199–222
　　as part of multisystem disease, 209
　　central, 209–13
　　congenital, 213–15
　　peripheral, 199–208
　　with known metabolic defect, 208–9
　electrical signals from, 1–3
　hand-held multiple, 567
　investigating techniques, 4
　macular, 223
　renewal, 35–36
　structure, 3–4, 34
　synaptic transmission, 10–11
Photo-slit lamps, 61
Photostress test, macular, 322
Phototransduction, 39–40
Phthisical eye, (Fig. 4h) 84
Phycomycetes, retinal, 195
Physostigmine, 48–49

Phytanic acid levels in Refsum's disease, 208
Picornavirus infections, 115–16
Pigments, visual
　investigation techniques of, 4
　iron-containing, 137
　spectra, 7
　structure, 304
　see also Cone pigments; Rhodopsin
Pigment epitheliitis, acute retinal, 189
Pigment epitheliopathy, 183
　acute posterior multifocal placoid (APMPPE), 189–90, 226
　serous bullous retinal detachment with, 226–7
Pigment epithelium
　breakdown, 77, (Fig. 2) 78
　changes in bull's eye dystrophies, 212
　in butterfly-shaped dystrophy, 210–11
　in centroserous retinopathy, 231
　in choroideraemia, 207
　in fundus albipunctatus, 215
　in fundus flavimaculatus, 211
　in gyrate atrophy, 209
　in retinitis pigmentosa, (Fig. 1) 200, 206
　-choroid, 36
　　metabolism and function, 36–37
　detachment, 224, 230–1
　　with angioid streaks, 233
　　with bullous retinal detachment, 232–3
　hamartoma, 236–7
　response to light, 22
　-retina unit, 34–37
　retinoid movement and, 38
Pigmentary glaucoma, 68
Pigmentation
　phenothiazine, 59
　racial difference in, 66
　scleral, 148
Pigmented malignant epibulbar tumours, 353–4
Pilocarpine, 48, (Table VII) 311, 312
　for glaucoma, 317, 318
Pindolol, 52
Pineal gland
　role, 539
　tumours, 431, 538–9
Pingueculae, 150
Piperacillin, 55
Pituitary gland, 533
　adenoma, 346
　apoplexy, 346
　disorders, eye and, 533–9
　hormone secretion, 533
　tumour, 534–8
　　adjacent, 538–9
　　CT scan of, (Fig. 2) 350
　　gonadotrophin release and, 549
Placoid lesions in APMPPE, 189–90
Plaque, corneal, 137
Plasma cell proliferation, 559–60
Plateau iris, 318–19
Platelet abnormalities, 558–9
　polycythaemia and, 554
Pneumo-encephalography for chiasmatic lesion investigation, 350
Poliosis in VKH syndrome, 183
Polyarteritis, eye signs in, (Table II) 522
Polycythaemia, 553–4
Polymethylmethacrylate lenses, 302

Polymorphs, chemical burns and, 376
Polymyositis, eye signs in, (Table II) 522
Polymyxin B, 56
Polyphloretin, 57
Polyploidy, 467
Polypropylene lens loops, 302
Pontine gaze
　centre, 426
　palsy, 430–1
Port wine stain, 460
Position of eyes in infants, 452
Posterior
　chamber lens, 294–5, 296–7
　corneal rings, 62
　polymorphous dystrophy of Schlichting, 143
　segment injury, 364–8
　reconstruction, 371
　synechiae formation in uveitis, 165–6
Potassium, Mueller cell sensitivity to, 20–21
Practolol syndrome, 59
Prader-Willi syndrome, 550
Precorneal film disorders, 112–13
Prednisolone, 509, 510
　semilog dilution of, (Table II) 111
　sodium phosphate, (Table VI) 58
Pregnancy, retinopathy in, 243
Preproliferative retinopathy, 241
Preretinal
　haemorrhage, 552, 555, 558
　neovascularization, 241
Presbyopia, 276
Prism cover test, 424
Prismatic scanning, 569
Prochlorperazine phenothiazine side effects, 60
Pro-drugs, 46
Prolactin secreting tumours, 536–7
　hypogonadism and, 549
Proliferative retinopathy, 240–3
Proprionic acid derivatives, 507
Proptosis in posterior scleritis, 155
Prostaglandins
　in aqueous humour, 32
　-induced inflammation, 493
　inhibitors, non-steroidal, 57
　for uveitis, 168
Prosthesis see Contact lens; Implants
Prostigmin, 49
Protanomaly, 213
Protanopia, 213
Protection of eye, physical, 107
Proteins
　in aqueous humour, 32, 165
　disorders, corneal, 134
　in lens, 28
　myelin-basic, 497
　in photoreceptors, 35
　in pigment epithelium, 38
　in retina, 38
　ribonucleo, 518
　S-100, 497
　in tear film, 31
　in vitreous humour, 33
Proteoglycan, corneal, 24–25, 130
Protozoal infiltration to cornea, 140
Proxymetacaine hydrochloride, 52
Pseudo-dendrites, 139
Pseudo-exfoliation of lens capsule, 68
Pseudofluorescence, 78
Pseudo-Foster Kennedy syndrome, 335
Pseudohypoparathyroidism, 547

Pseudointernuclear ophthalmoplegia, 435
Pseudoisochromatic test, 322
Pseudoneuritis, 323
Pseudopapilloedema, optic disc, 323–4
Pseudopemphigoid, 127–8
Pseudophakodonosis, 293
Pseudopodia lentis, 264
Pseudo-pseudohypoparathyroidism, 547
Pseudoptosis, 383–4
Pseudopuberty, precocious, 550
Pseudoretinitis pigmentosa in syphilis, 194
Pseudotumour
 cerebri, 342
 orbital, 95, 442–3
  CT scan, 89
  optic neuritis and, 332
  ultrasonograph, (Fig. 5c) 85, 86
Pseudoxanthoma elasticum, 233
Psoriasis, uveitis in, 521
Psychic weeping, 392
Pterional meningioma, (Fig. 7) 93
Ptosis
 assessment, 384
 causes, 383–4
 in chronic progressive external ophthalmoplegia, 441–2
 following enucleation, 390
 management, 384
 surgery, 384–6
  complications of, 386
Puberty, precocious, 539, 550
Pullman disease, 181
Pulse-echo techniques, 81–83
Puncta, 393, 394
 agenesis, 398
 lesions, 409
 occlusion in dry eye, 123
 supernumerary, 398–9
Punctate cataract, 278
Pupil
 accommodation problems after drugs, 59
 block, 315, 316
  acute aphakic, 319–20
  following cataract surgery, 288
 defect, afferent, following injury, 369
  following lens implant, 300
 Marcus Gunn, 333
 mobility loss following lens implant, 293
 reaction in infants, 449–50
 semi-dilated oval, 316
 small, diabetes and, 548
 during lens implant, 299
Purkinje shift, 9
Pursuit movements, 427
 disorders of, 433, (Fig. 7) 434
 testing for, 428
Pyridoxine see Vitamin B6
Pyrimethamine, 56
Pyrimidine antifungal, 57

Quinine side effects, 60

Race
 Behçet's disease and, 177, 189
 glaucoma and, 577
 malignant melanoma and, 355
 uveitis and, 163

Race (cont.)
 VKH syndrome and, 183
Radiation causing corneal abrasion, 138
Radiography
 for chiasmatic investigation, 350
 orbital, 87–96
 tests for lacrimal drainage patency, 395
Radionucleotide tests for lacrimal drainage patency, 395
Radiotherapy
 for eyelid carcinoma, 389
 for growth-hormone secreting tumours, 535
 for leukaemia, 558
 for malignant melanoma, 357
 for retinoblastoma, 359
RCS rat, 43
Reaching for objects test, 450–1
Receptors see Photoreceptors
Reconstruction following penetrating injury, 370–1
Red blood cell disorders, 552–7
Red eye
 differential diagnosis of, (Table XIII) 317
 in episcleritis, 150
 in uveitis, 164, 166
Reflectometry, fundus, for investigating visual pigments, 4
Refraction
 errors in infants, 463–4
 tests in infants, 452
Refsum's syndrome, 208, 473
Reis-Buckler's ring-shaped dystrophy, 27
Reiter's disease, uveitis and, 169, 520–1
Relief mode, 62
Renal disorders in infants, 462
Reticulogeniculate pathway abnormalities in albinos, 474
Reticulum cell sarcoma, optic nerve involvement by, 339
Retina, 186–98
 arterial occlusion, ERG in, 100
  phase in normal angiogram, 76–77
 arteriovenous phase in normal angiogram, 77
 atrophy in retinitis pigmentosa, 202
 blood flow, reduced, (Table I) 524, 526
 breaks see Retinal tears
 changes in abetalipoproteinaemia, 473
  in amaurosis fugax, 525–6
  in anaemia, 552
  in leukaemia, 558
  in sickle cell disease, non-proliferative, 555
   proliferative, 556–7
  in uveitis, 167
 coloboma, 162
 damage from blunt injury, 365–7
  from foreign bodies, 372
  identification following penetrating injury, 371–2
 degeneration, lattice, 256
  snail track, 256
 deposits, abnormal, macular detachment and, 236
 detachment, from blunt injury, 366–7
  bullous, with pigment epithelial detachment, 232–3
  centroserous, 231–2
  from cataract surgery, 290
  coloboma and, 234
  differential diagnosis of, 356

Retina, detachment (cont.)
 ERG in, 100
 from fluid accumulation, 224
 macular disease associated with, 223–37
 malignant melanoma and, 356
 membrane formation and, 249–50
 from necrosis, 188
 pathogenesis, 248–9
 in posterior scleritis, 155
 preoperative management and assessment, 250
 presentation, 250
 prophylaxis, 255–6
 repair following preretinal injury, 372
 rhegmatogenous, 248, 270
  and traction, 270–1
 serous bullous, 226–7
 subretinal fluid accumulation and, 249
 surgery, choice of operation in, 250–3
  complications of, 253–5
  postoperative management, 255
 traction, 270
 types, (Fig. 7) 271
 ultrasonograph, (Fig. 2h) 82, (Fig. 3) 83, 84
 dialysis following lensectomy, 287
 drug effects on, 59
 electrical signals from photoreceptors in, 103
  recording, 97–101
 fluorescence leakage, 78, (Fig. 4) 79
 function, 38–40
 ganglion cells, 412
 gyrate atrophy, 471
 haemorrhage, 253
  in anaemia, 552
 holes, 248–9, 255, 270
  prophylaxis for, 255–6
  scleral buckling for, 251
 immunopathology, 497–8
 infectious diseases, 190–6
 infiltration in Behçet's disease, 177
 inflammatory diseases, 186–98
  causing fluid accumulation, 233
 inner, neurones, 36
 lesions in infant, 456
 metabolism, 37, 38
 necrosis syndrome, acute(ARN), 187–8
 neurochemistry, 40–42
 occlusion from phycomycetes, 195
 oedema in diabetic retinopathy, 238
  in retinitis pigmentosa, 202
 papillary vasculitis, 333
 parallel functional pathways in, 12–16
 pathology, 42–43
 peripheral vaso-occlusion see Eales's disease
 periphlebitis, 182
 pigment epithelium see Pigment epithelium
 placoid lesions in APMPPE, 189–90
 processing in, 18–20
 receptor dystrophies, 199–222
 'S' antigen, 163, 180–1, 187, 374–5, 497
 structure, 5, 34–36
 tears from blunt injury, 366–7
  mobilization, 273
  tractional, 270

Retina, tears (cont.)
  traumatic, 269
  trophic, 270
  tumours, 236–7, 357–60
  ultrasonography, 84
  vascular supply, 491
  vasculitis, 176–7
    in sarcoidosis, 179
  venous occlusion, ERG in, 100
    phase in normal angiogram, 77
    pulsation, papilloedema and, 342
  vessel changes in sickle cell disease, 555
Retinitis
  candida, 194–5
  cytomegalovirus, 193–4
    in AIDS, 182
  herpes simplex, 194
  herpes zoster, 194
  measles, 193
  necrotizing, 187–8
  pigmentosa, 42–43, 472–3, 478
    electrophysiology, 205
    EOG in, 99
    ERG in, 99
    histopathology, 206–7
    inheritance, 199–200
    ophthalmoscopic appearance, 200–2
    pattern of visual loss in, 203
    rhodopsin metabolism, 203–4
  punctata albescens, 202
    ERG in, 99
  sclopetaria, 367
  toxocara/toxoplasmosis, 191–2, 233, (Fig. 8) 234
  see also Retinochoroiditis
Retinoblastoma, 357–60
  autosomal dominant, 468–9
  penetrance, 475–6
  retinal detachment and, 237
  somatic mutation, 468
  ultrasonograph, (Fig. 4e) 84, 85
Retinochoroid
  coloboma, 162
  rupture, 367
Retinochoroiditis
  cryptococcal, 196
  herpes simplex, 172
  histoplasmosis, presumed, 233
  nocardia, 195–6
  toxoplasmosis and, 172–3
Retinochoroidopathy
  bird shot, 179, 187
  centroserous, 231–2
  vitiliginous see under Birdshot
Retinoid movement, 38
Retinol formation, 6
Retinoma, 468–9
Retinopathy
  in AIDS, 181–2
  bird shot, 498
  cataract and, 480
  central serous, 77, (Fig. 3) 78
  chloroquine, EOG in, 101
  diabetic, 42, 238–43
    autoimmunity and, 498
    ERP in, 99–100
    florid, 243
    in pregnancy, 243
    statistics, 577
  hyperviscosity, 553
  peripheral vascular see Eales's disease
  proliferative, 240–3

Retinopathy (cont.)
  sickle, aetiology of, 556
    natural history of, 556–7
    treatment, 557
  rubella, 233
  salt and pepper, 192, (Fig. 11) 193
  vascular, 238–57
  see also Neuroretinopathy; Retinochoroidopathy
Retinoschisis, X-linked, 471–2
Retractors, 386
  recession, 387
Retrobulbar neuritis, 339
  VEP in, 103
Retrohyaloid haemorrhage, ultrasonograph, (Fig. 2f) 92
Retrolental fibroplasia, 42
Retro-orbital
  calcification, 87–88
  pseudotumours, 95
Retzlaff regression formula, 295
Rhabdomyosarcoma, orbital, 93–94
Rheumatoid
  arthritis
    juvenile, uveitis and, 521
    scleritis and, 158
    scleromalacia perforans and, 153
  disease, dry eye and, 122
Rhinostomy, 403, 405
Rhodopsin
  bleaching, 5–6, 7–8, 38
  light absorption by, 3–5
  metabolism, retinitis pigmentosa and, 203–4
  photolysis, 38–39
  regeneration, 6, 10
  structure, 4–5, 34
Riboflavin deficiency, cataract and, 31
Ribonucleo proteins, 518
Ridley's lenses, 293
Rieger's anomaly, 67, (Table V) 135
Riley-Day alacrimia, 122
Ritten-type TEN, 127
Rodenstock panfunduscope, 70, 71, 72
Rods
  biochemistry of transduction in, 7–9
  coupling, 12
  defects, 214–15
  light/dark adaptation, 9–10, 16
  metabolic function disorders, 199
  pathways, 19–20
  photoresponses from, 103
  pigment see Rhodopsin
  retinitis pigmentosa effects on, 203, 204, 206
  structure, 3–4, 34
  synaptic transmission and voltage-dependent mechanisms in, 11
Rolling ball test, 450
Rose bengal dye test, 516–17
  for dry eye, 123–4
Roth's spots, 552
Rubella
  cataract and, 480
  congenital, 461–2, 551
  retinal involvement, 192
  retinopathy, 233

'S' antigen, retinal, 42, 163, 180–1, 187, 374–5, 497
S–100 protein, 497

Saccadic
  eye movements, disorders, 430–3
    failure to sustain, 441
    horizontal, in infants, 452
    supranuclear influence on, 427
    testing for, 428, (Fig. 2) 429
  pulse, 425
  step, 425
Saccadomania, 433
Salbutamol, (Table VII) 311
Salicylates, 507
Salmon patch, 141
Salt and pepper pattern
  in retina in syphilis, 194, (Fig. 16) 195
  retinopathy, 192, (Fig. 11) 193
Salts in tear film, 31
Salzmann's nodular degeneration, 142
Sandhoff's disease, 461
Sarcoidosis
  hyperparathyroidism and, 547
  uveitis and, 178–9
Sarcoma reticulum cell, pigment epithelium detachment and, 237
Scarring
  corneal, 141
  following lacrimal surgery, 404
Scheie operation, 312
Schirmer tear test, 517
  for dry eye, 123
Schlemm's canal, 66
  aqueous pathway to, 306
Schwalbe's line appearnce, 66
Sclera, 24
  avascular areas, 153
  buckling, 250, 251
  explants, 370
  glow, (Fig. 2b) 78, 79
  graft for eyelid retraction, 387
  hyaline plaque, 148
  indentation, 71–72
  lysis, 153
  spur appearance, 66
  thinning, 148
  translucency, 148
  vessels, 147–8
  wounds, 368
Scleritis, 147–61
  anterior diffuse, 151–2
  corneal changes, 153–4
  histology, 156
  investigations, 159
  necrotizing, 152–3
  nodular, 152
  nomenclature, 148–9
  pathogenesis, 157–9
  posterior, 155–6, 229–30
  symptoms, 147–8
  treatment, 159–61
Sclerocornea, 134
Sclerokeratitis, acute necrotizing, 154
Scleromalacia perforans, 153, 157, 161
Sclerostomy for glaucoma, 312
Scotoma
  in acute macular neuroretinopathy, 189
  bilateral central, causes of, (Table III) 328
  in dominant optic atrophy, 326
  in macular oedema, 155
  tests for, 322
Seborrhoeic
  blepharitis, 109–10
  keratosis, 389
Secretory apparatus, 391–2

See-saw nystagmus, 444
Sella syndrome, empty, 348
Senile
    cataract, 277, 278–80, 576–7
    elastosis, 148
    keratoses, 389
    macular degeneration, 575–6
    ptosis, involutional, 383, 384
Senior's syndrome, 462
Septo-optic dysplasia, 323, 462
Septum pellucidum absence, 462
Serotonin activity in retina, 40
Serpiginous choroiditis, 186–7, 190
Serum sickness, 496–7
    uveitis and, 163
Setting sun syndrome, (Fig. 6) 301
Sex effects
    on diabetic retinopathy, 577
    on ERG, 99
    on Leber's disease, 327
    on uveitis, 163
    on VEP, 103
Shipyard eye, 115
Shock phacoemulsifier, 286
Sickle cell disease, 544–7
    anterior segment ischaemia, 555
    conjunctival vessel changes, 544–5
    choroidal abnormalities, 555
    non-proliferative peripheral retinal changes, 555
    proliferative sickle retinopathy, 556–7
Siderosis, 137
    bulbi, ERG in, 100
    from foreign bodies, 372–3
Siedel test, 288
Silicone
    oil tamponade, intravitreal, 254
    rubber lenses, properties of, 132
Silver deposition in cornea, 136
Sinskey-type lens, (Fig. 4) 297
Sinusitis, optic neuritis and, 332
Sixth (VIth) nerve palsy
    bilateral weakness, 439
    in children, 439
        handicapped, 455
    development, 420
    fascicular lesions, 438–9
    in giant aneurysm, 527–8
    nuclear, 438
Sjögren's syndrome, 516–20
Skew deviation, 439
    coefficient of, 63
Skin
    disease, eye involvement in, 125–8
    involvement, in Behçet's disease, 177
    in sarcoidosis, 178
Slit lamp biomicroscopy, 71
'Smoke stack' pattern on fluorescein angiography, 231
Snail track degeneration, 248, 256
'Snow balls', 265
    in retina, 182
    in vitreous gel, 176
'Snowbank' overlying inferior pars plana, 176
Sodium cromoglycate, 57–58
Sodium hydroxide, lenses packed in, 302
Solutions, aqueous, 46
Somatostatin secreting tumours, 549
Sorbitol pathway in lens, 29
Spasmus nutans, 444
Spectacles
    for hypermetropia, 292

Spectacles (cont.)
    magnifiers for, 563–5
    for squint, 414
    telescopes for, 565–6
    tinted, 567
Spectrophotometry for investigating visual pigments, 4
Specular microscopy, 61–63
    analyses, 62–63
    clinical, 61
    large field, 61–62
    non-contact, 61
Speilmeyer-Vogt syndrome, 473
Spinning for visual testing in children, 452
Spiramycin for toxoplasmosis, 192
Sponge anterior vitrectomy, 284
Square wave jerks, 432
Squint
    detection, 412–18
    in handicapped child, 454, 455
    management in infants, 413–14
    from ocular motor lesions, 525–48
    ocular muscle palsy and, 418–23
    tests in infants, 451
Staphylococcal
    blepharitis, 110
    hypersensitivity, 111
Staphylococcus epidermidis causing endophthalmitis, 290
Starch endophthalmitis, 290
Stargardt's disease, 211
Steele-Richardson-Olzewski syndrome, 431
Stereo-illusion tests, 322
Steroids, 58–59, 509–10
    absorption, 46
    in aqueous humour, 32
    for arteritis, 336
    cataract formation from, 31
    for corneal burns, 376
    for episcleritis, 151
    for fungal keratitis, 140
    for glaucoma, 33, 317, 319
    for herpes simplex keratitis, 139
    for keratoconjunctivitis, 116
    main actions, (Table I) 508
    for optic neuritis, 333
    for scleritis, 160
    side effects, 60, 509–10, 522
    for sympathetic ophthalmitis, 375
    for thyrotoxicosis, 542
    topical, 111
    for uveitis, 167–8
    for vernal disease, 122
Stevens–Johnson syndrome, 59, 127, 496
Stickler's syndrome, 262, 470
Still's disease, uveitis and, 165, 170–1
Stones in canaliculus, 408
Strabismus, 412–24
    differentiation of concomitant and incomitant, 437
    fixus, 421
    head posture with, 437
    primary and secondary deviations in, 437
Streptothrix, 119
    of canaliculus, 408
String of pearls, 262
Stroma, 130
    corneal, 24–25
    dystrophy, 143
    oedema, 136

Sturge–Weber syndrome, 477
    in infants, 460
    phaeochromocytoma and, 546
Stycar mounted ball test, 450
Subclavian steal syndrome, 531
Sub-hyaloid haemorrhage, 552
Subretinal
    fluid accumulation, 249
        drainage, 252–3
            complications, 253–5
    haemorrhage, 253, 552, 555
    neovascularization, 367
    pigment epithelial space, 224
    space, 224
Substance P, retinal, 41
Sugar
    cataract, 30
    levels in aqueous, abnormal, 277
Sulphacetamide, 54
Sulphadiazine for toxoplasmosis, 173
Sulphahexafluoride tamponade, 254
Sulphonamides, 54
Sulphur for toxoplasmosis, 192
Superior
    collicular influence on eye movement, 427
    oblique tendon sheath syndrome, 429
    rectus suture, 284
Supraclinoid giant aneurysms, 528–9
Supranuclear
    influence in conjugate eye movements, 427
    palsy, gaze, 430
        progressive, 431, (Fig. 6) 433
Suprasellar
    extension, 535
    germinoma, 539
    glioma, 462, (Fig. 18) 463
Suspensions, aqueous, 46
Sutures
    for cataract, 282–3
    corneal shape following, 129
    for dacrocystorhinostomy, 403
    for ectropion, 380–1
    for eyelid retraction, 388–9
    -induced papillary conjunctivitis, 124–5
    for lens implant, 300, (Fig. 5) 301
        iris-supported, 296
    for penetrating wounds, 369
    for ptosis, 384–5
Suxamethonium, 53
Swinging flashlight test, 322, 450
Sylvian aqueduct syndrome, 431, (Fig. 5) 432
Symblepharon in sicca syndrome, 520
Sympathetic
    ophthalmia, 233
    ophthalmitis, 374–5, 499–500
Sympatholytic drugs, 51
Synechiae
    anterior, 317–18
    peripheral, 67, 68
Syphilis
    retinal involvement in, 194, (Fig. 16) 195
    uveitis and, 174–5
Syringeing
    lacrimal, 395, 401
    nasolacrimal duct, 397
Systemic
    disease, eye and, 516–61
    lupus erythematosus, uveitis and, 521
    sclerosis, eye signs in, (Table II) 522

Systemic *(cont.)*
    sclerosis, progressive, eye signs in, (Table II) 522
    vasculopathy, eye signs in, 266

Tactile systems, 569
Taenia solium infestation, 191
Tape recording systems, 569
Tapetal reflexes, 202
Tapetoretinal dystrophy, 471
Tarsal manoeuvres for entropion, 380–1
Tarsorrhaphy
    central, 388
    lateral, 387–8
    medial, 383
Tarsotomy, 386–7
Taste tests for lacrimal drainage patency, 394
Taurine activity in retina, 41
Tay–Sach's disease, infantile, 460–1
TBG assay, 540
Tear film, 31–32, 112
    break up time, 517
    composition, 31, 112–13
    corneal transparency and, 136
    disruption in staphylococcal blepharitis, 110
    dysfunction, 32
    function, 31–32
    stability, 113
Tears
    artificial, 123, 519–20
    conservation, 520
    constituents, 107
    crocodile, 392
    drainage, 392–4, 409
    functions, 107
    gas transmission by, 130
    immunity and, 494
    production, 112
        deficiency, 122–4
        stimulation, 123
    secretion following drug administration, 46
        surgery to limit, 392
    secretory apparatus, 391–2
    surfeit, 391, 394
    volume, 391
    see also Lacrimal
Telescopes, 565–6
Television, closed-circuit, 567
Tenotomy, 386–7
Terrien's marginal degeneration, 142
Testicular failure, 549–50
Tetracyclines, 56
    side effects, 60
Thalassaemia, 554–8
Thiabendazole, 57
Thiamine deficiency, optic neuropathy and, 328
Thiopentone, 53
Thioridazine side effects, 59
Third (IIIrd) nerve
    lesions
        from arterial aneurysms, 440–1
        fascicular, 440
        nuclear, 440
    palsy, 439–40
        in children, 440
        developmental, 420
Thrombocytopenia, 558–9

Thrombotic thrombocytopenia purpura, 559
Thygeson's superficial punctate keratitis, 141
Thymoxamine, 51
Thymus-derived lymphocytes *see* Lymphocytes, T
Thyroid gland
    carcinoma, 543
    disorders, eye and, 539–43
        cataract, 281
        ophthalmoplegia, 442
    function regulation, 540
        tests, 540
    hormones, 539–40
    ophthalmopathy, 419
    scans, 540
Thyroidectomy, 542
Thyrotoxicosis, 540–2
    diagnosis, 540
    eye signs, 541–2
    treatment, 542
Thyroxine, 539
Ticarcillin, 55
Tight junctions, 130
    focal, 131
Timolol, 52
    for glaucoma, (Table VII) 311, 312
Tissue characterization by ultrasonography, 83
Tobacco-alcohol amblyopia, 328–9
Tobramycin, 55
Tolazine, 51
Tolerogen, 484
Tonic
    cells, 426
    deviation of eyes, 452
Toxic epidermal necrolysis, 127
Toxocariasis
    retinal, 190–1, 233
    uveitis and, 173–4
Toxoplasmosis
    congenital, 459, 461
    retinal, 191–2, 233, (Fig. 8) 234
    uveitis and, 172–3
TPHA test, 175
Trabecular meshwork
    appearance, 66
    aqueous pathway through, 306
    damage from hyphaemia, 364
Trabeculectomy, postoperative complications, (Table VIII) 313
Trachoma, 117–18, 408
    corneal effects, 139
    resembling inclusion conjunctivitis, 118
Traction macular detachments, 237
Tranexamic acid for haemorrhage, 363
Transducin, 8, 39
Transgel fibrosis, 266–7
Transhydrogenation in lens, 29
Transudate, conjunctival, 108
Trantas' dots, 121
Trauma to eye, 362–78
    angle effects of, 68
    blunt, 363–8
    Brown's syndrome and, 422–3
    causing cataract, 277
    causing chronic ocular hypotony, 229
    causing fluid accumulation at outer retina, 233–4
    causing ocular palsy, 419, 423

Trauma to eye *(cont.)*
    causing ptosis, 383
    causing scleritis, 158–9
    causing sympathetic ophthalmitis, 179–80
    causing varices, 92
    causing vertical movement disorders, 431
    chiasmatic, 348
    corneal, 138, 362
    ERG in, 100
    eyelid, 390
    lacrimal passages, 408–9
    penetrating, 368–72
    see also Perforating injury
Treponaema, 174
TRH
    assay, 540
    secretion, 540
Triamcinolone, 58
TRIC *see* Conjunctivitis, inclusion
Trichiasis, 382
Triethylene melanine for retinoblastoma, 360
Trifluorothymidine, 56
Trigeminal nerve irritation, 392
Tri-iodothyronine, 539
Trisomy
    13, 467
    21, 467–8
Tritan dyschromotopsia, 326
Tritanomaly, 213
Tritanopia, 213
Trochlear nerve palsy, 439
Tropicamide, 50
TSH
    assay, 540
    secretion, 540
Tuberculosis
    miliary infantile, 462
    uveitis and, 175
Tuberous sclerosis, 477
    in infants, 459–60
    phaeochromocytoma and, 546
Tubocurarine, 53
Tumours, 352–61
    adrenal, 544, 545–6
    bulbar, 354–60
    causing macular elevation, 236–7
    cytotoxic therapy-induced, 511
    epibulbar, 352–4
    eyelid, 389–90
    gonioscopy in, 68
    in infants, 462–3
    intraocular, ultrasonography of, 85
    investigations, 350–1
    in neurofibromatosis, 477
    nystagmus and, 445
    optic nerve, 337–40
    pancreatic hormone-secreting, 548–9
    pituitary, 534–8
    punctum, 409
    radiography of, 87–90, 92–95
    retinal, 357–60
    in Sturge–Weber syndrome, 477
    thyroid, 543
    in tuberous sclerosis, 477
    uveal, 354–7
Turner's syndrome, 293
Tyrosinase
    -negative OCA, 473
    -positive OCA, 474
    test for albinism, 473

Uhthoff's symptom, 331
Ulceration
  in Behçet's disease, 177
  corneal, 134
  Mooren's, 142, 496
Ulcerative colitis, uveitis in, 521
Ultrasonography, 81–86
  for macular elevation, 225
  thyroid, 540
'Umbrella' pattern on fluorescein angiography, 231
Unconsciousness, vestibulo-ocular reflex in, 435
Urea, 54
Usher's syndrome, 209
UV radiation, cataract and, 576
Uveal tract, 162–85
  congenital anomalies, 162
  effusion syndrome, 227
  pigment epitheliopathies, 183
  prolapsed tissue replacement, 370
  tumours, 354–7
  uveitis, 162–83
Uveitis, 162–83
  angle inflammation in, 68
  anterior
    acute, 164–5, 169–70, 499
    chronic, 164, 165, 170–1, 499
      extracapsular surgery contraindicated in, 285
    episcleritis with, 150
  causes, 163
  chronic, following lens implant, 300
  classification, 163–4
  clinical presentation, 164–6
  cytotoxic therapy for, 511
  immunology and, 499–500, 506
    acute anterior, 499
    chronic, 499
  intermediate, 164, 175–6
  lens-induced, 180, 181
  pan-, 165, 169
  phacoallergic see U. lens-induced
  posterior, 164, 166
  scleritis with, 148, 154
  systemic disease and, 520–2
  treatment, 167
  types, 169–83
  visual loss, 166–7
Uveoretinal autoimmune disease, 42
Uveo-scleral outflow, 306
  impairment of, 229–30

V-pattern squint, 415–16
Vanillylmandelic acid test, 546
Varices, orbital, 92
Vascular
  abnormalities
    cerebral, 350–1
    congenital, causing fluid accumulation, 235
    optic nerve, 334–7
    orbital, 91–92
    papillary, 235
  filling defects, 79
  occlusion, retinal, ERG in, 100
  pattern in scleritis, 147–8, 153
  retinopathies, 238–57
  supply to lens, imperfect regression of primitive, 278
    to uveal tract, 162
Vascularization, corneal, 141

Vasculitis
  choroidal, 226–9
  retinal, 176–7
    in sarcoidosis, 179
  in scleritis, 157, 159
Vasoactive intestinal polypeptide
  retinal, 41
  -secreting tumour, 549
Vaso-occlusion, peripheral retinal see Eales's disease
VDRL test, 175
Venous
  changes in retinopathy, 240
  malformation, congenital, 92
  obstruction, choroidal, 227
Vergence movement testing, 428
Vermis influence on eye movement, 428
Vernal
  disease, 120–2, 137
  keratoconjunctivitis, 496
  plaques, 114
Vertebrobasilar ischaemia, 531
Vertical
  deviation and head tilt test, 437
  eye movements, 426–7
    disorders, 431–3
Vestibular
  eye movement disorders, 435
  influence on conjugate eye movements, 427
  nystagmus, 445
Vestibulo-ocular reflex, 427–8
  testing for, 428–9
  in unconscious patient, 435
Vidarabine, 56
Virus infection
  conjunctival, 115–18, 125
  corneal, 138–9
  immune response to, 486
  isolation, 10
  retinal, 192–4
Visceral larva migrans, 174
Viscodelamination, 268
Visual
  acuity, definition for blindness, 571
    development in infants, 453
    following penetrating trauma, 368
    following sympathetic ophthalmitis, 180
  loss, in cataract, 281
    in centroserous chorioretinopathy, 231, 232
    definition for partial blindness, 571, 572
    in diabetes mellitus, 548
    in posterior scleritis, 155
    in retinal detachment, 250
    in uveitis, 165
    recovery following retinal detachment surgery, 255
  testing, 322, 568–9
  adaptation, 3
  agnosia, 350
  aids, 562–9
  assessment in infants, 449–52
  cortex lesions, 349
  cycle, 38
  defects, effects on general infant development, 454
    in glaucoma, 307
    management of, 562–9
    nystagmus and, 464
  deprivation effects, 412

Visual (cont.)
  development in infants, 452–4
    delayed, (Table III) 457, 458–9
  field
    defects, in chiasmatic disease, 346
      in dominant optic atrophy, 326–7
      glaucomatous, differential diagnosis of, (Table V) 308
      in glioma, 338
      in growth hormone-secreting tumours, 535
      in occipital lesions, 349
      from optic radiation, 348
      in pituitary adenoma, (Fig. 1) 347
    definition for blindness, 571
    loss, in chromophobe adenomas, 534
      definition for partial blindness, 571, 572
      elevated IOP and, 309–14
      in low tension glaucoma, 314
      in meningioma, 347
      in papilloedema, 341
    testing in infants, 451
      handicapped, 454
  function disorders, higher, 349–50
    tests, 225
  hallucinations, 350
  loss in amaurosis figax, 524
    in APMPPE, 189–90
    in Behçet's diease, 177, 189
    in birdshot chorioretinopathy, 187
    following blunt injury, 368
    in disc drusen, 324
    in histoplasmosis, 182
    in ischaemic optic papillopathy, 336
    in Leber's disease, 328
    in macular elevation, 225
    in MEWDS, 188
    in optic neuritis, 330
    in papillitis, 333
    in Refsum's syndrome, 208
    in retinitis pigmentosa, 203, (Fig. 5) 204–5
    in sarcoidosis, 179
    in scleritis, 152
    in serpiginous choroiditis, 186
    statistics of, 574
    in toxoplasmosis, 173
    in uveitis, 166–7
    see also Blindness
  pathways disorders, 321–51
  pigment see Pigment
  symptoms in optic neuritis, 331
Visually
  directed reaching, 450–1
  evoked cortical responses in infants, 451
  evoked potential, 97, 101–4
    factors influencing, 103–4
    normal, 102–3
    recording equipment for, 102
Vitamin
  A, corneal disease and, 27
    deficiency, dark adaptation in, 10
      lipoproteinaemia in, 208
      tear film and, 32
    in pigment epithelium cell, 37
    supply to cornea, 25
    therapy, for abetalipoproteinaemia, 473
    side effects, 60
  B deficiency, optic neuropathy and, 328–9

Vitamin *(cont.)*
  B₆ therapy for gyrate atrophy, 209
    for homocystinuria, 475
  B₁₂ deficiency, 553
  D therapy for hypoparathyroidism, 547
  deficiency, optic neuropathy and, 328–9
  E
    deficiency
      cataract and, 31
      corneal effects of, 142
      lipoproteinaemia and, 208
      retinal effects of, 42
    in photoreceptors, 35
Vitiliginous chorioretinopathy *see* Bird shot chorioretinopathy
Vitiligo in VKH syndrome, 183
Vitrectomy, 273
  anterior, 287
    automated, 284
    sponge, 284
  criteria, 290
  for endophthalmitis, 290
  for foreign body removal, 374
  prophylactic, 274
  for retinal detachment, 255
  technique, 258–9
  for toxocariasis, 174
  for uveitis, 166
Vitreolenticular attachment, 259
Vitreopapillary adhesion, 260
Vitreo-retinal
  adhesions, acquired, 260
    developmental post-basal, 260
  disease, 237
  dystrophy, 471
  juncture, post-basal, 260
  sequelae of penetrating trauma, (Fig. 6) 368, (Fig. 8) 369
  traction, 269
    prevention or relief, 273, 371
Vitreo-retinopathy, proliferative, 249, 271
Vitreous, 33–34
  adhesions, 259–60
  amyloidosis, 264
  aspiration in endophthalmitis, 290
  base, 259–60
    evulsion, 366
  cellular infiltration in uveitis, 165, 166
  collapse in membrane formation, 249
  composition and structure, 33
  degeneration, 261–2

Vitreous *(cont.)*
  depot effects of antigens sequestered in, 491
  detachment, 248, 262–4
    non-rhegmatogenous, 264
    rhegmatogenous posterior, 263–4
    ultrasonograph, (Figs 2c, e, g) 82, 83–84
  disorders, 258–74
  displacement and incarceration, 260–1
  fibrosis, 265–7
  fluorophotometry, 79–80
    of macular elevation, 225
  function, 33
  haemorrhage, 264–5
    following penetrating injury, 369
    in retinal detachment, 250
  infiltration in uveitis, 176
  injections, 259
    for retinal detachment surgery, 253–5
  invasions, 264–9
  leak during secondary lens implantation, 298
    during cataract surgery, 284
  pathology, 33–34, 258
  removal for sampling, 274
  retraction, 264, 267
  structure, 258
  surgery, 273
  touch syndrome, 289
  traction, 249
  ultrasonography, 83–84
  wick syndrome, 289
Vitritis, 265
Vogt–Koyanagi–Harada syndrome, 183
Vogt's
  limbus girdle, 141
  method of endothelial examination, 61
Voltage-dependent mechanisms in photoreceptors, 10–11, 12
Von Hippel–Lindau syndrome, 477
  phaeochromocytoma and, 546
Von Recklinghausen's disease *see* Neurofibromatosis
Vortex dystrophy, 138
Vossius' ring, 277

Wand diplopia test, 436
Wagner's hyaloideo-retinal degeneration, 470
Waldenström's macroglobulinaemia, 559

Watery eye, 391
Wernicke's hemianopic pupillary reaction, 348
Wessely ring, 137
Wetting agents for drugs, 46
Whipple's disease, uveitis and, 182–3
White
  cell disorders, 557–8
  dot syndrome, multiple evanescent, 188
  streaks, retinal, 239, (Fig. 4) 240
Whitnall's ligament maintenance, 385
Wilm's tumour
  aniridia and, 162
  in infants, 463
Wilson's disease, 137, 278
  in infants, 462
'Window' defect, 77, (Fig. 2) 78
Windscreen wiper syndrome, 301
Wipe-out syndrome, unilateral, 189
Wiskott-Aldrich syndrome, 497
Wolfram's syndrome, 481
Word blindness, acquired, 349–50
Wound
  appearance following penetrating injury, 368
  leak following cataract surgery, 288

X-linked inheritance, 471–2
  choroideraemia, 478
  isolated cataracts, 480
  ocular albinism, 474, 478
  retinitis pigmentosa, 472–3, 478
Xanthelasma, 389
Xanthoma, eye lesions and, 354
Xerosis, corneal, 142

YAG laser, 238

Z-myotomy, 387
Zeiss
  four-mirror lens, 65
  gonioscopy lens, 315
Zellweger's syndrome in infants, 462
Zollinger-Ellison syndrome, 549
Zonulae occludentes, 130
Zonular rupture during anterior capsulotomy, 285
Zonulysis, 283
Zoonoses, chlamydial, 119